Fungal Infections
in the
Immunocompromised
Patient

INFECTIOUS DISEASE AND THERAPY

Series Editor

Burke A. Cunha

Winthrop-University Hospital
Mineola, and
State University of New York School of Medicine
Stony Brook, New York

Fungal Infections in the Immunocompromised Patient

edited by

John R. Wingard
University of Florida College of Medicine
Gainesville, Florida, U.S.A.

Elias J. Anaissie
The University of Arkansas for Medical Sciences
Little Rock, Arkansas, U.S.A.

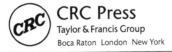

CRC Press
Taylor & Francis Group
Boca Raton London New York

CRC Press is an imprint of the
Taylor & Francis Group, an **informa** business
A TAYLOR & FRANCIS BOOK

CRC Press
Taylor & Francis Group
6000 Broken Sound Parkway NW, Suite 300
Boca Raton, FL 33487-2742

First issued in paperback 2019

© 2005 by Taylor & Francis Group, LLC
CRC Press is an imprint of Taylor & Francis Group, an Informa business

No claim to original U.S. Government works

ISBN-13: 978-0-8247-5428-0 (hbk)
ISBN-13: 978-0-367-39236-9 (pbk)

Library of Congress Cataloging-in-Publication Data

Catalog record is available from the Library of Congress

Visit the Taylor & Francis Web site at
http://www.taylorandfrancis.com

and the CRC Press Web site at
http://www.crcpress.com

Preface

Opportunistic infections have always been accompaniments of medical conditions that compromise host defenses. Because of the severe morbidity and mortality that result from such infectious complications, these pose substantial challenges for the clinician who cares for such individuals. With medical progress, the number of immunocompromised patients is steadily climbing. Moreover the types of host defense compromises are changing. As transplant practices evolve, as critical care procedures advance, and as HIV management strategies change, the spectrum of opportunistic pathogens shifts.

Initially, bacterial infections were most problematic. As strategies to control bacterial infections improved, the herpesviruses came to increasing attention of clinicians. Herpes simplex and varicella zoster virus cause considerable morbidity and occasional mortality. Cytomegalovirus (CMV) became recognized as a major killer of transplant recipients, but morbidity declined due to advances in rapid diagnostics and the introduction of effective antiviral agents such as acyclovir and ganciclovir.

Today, the invasive fungal pathogens have seized center stage from the above historically important opportunistic pathogens. During the 1980s the rate of nosocomial invasive fungal disease in U.S. hospitals doubled with no sign of slowing during the 1990s. *Candida* has become the fourth leading bloodstream isolate in U.S. hospitals, surpassing many historically important bacterial pathogens. Estimates are that the United States spends approximately one billion dollars annually for *Candida* infections, and more than $650 million annually for *Aspergillus* disease. However, accurate diagnostics and effective therapies have lagged for this emerging group of opportunists. As survival from bacteria and the herpesviruses has improved, more immunocompromised patients are now living to develop infection from fungi.

Candida is the most common genus of fungal pathogens. *C. albicans* long was recognized as a cause of mucosal disease of the mouth, esophagus, and vagina in patients with T-cell deficiency, as seen in patients with HIV infection, those treated with corticosteroids or other potent immunosuppressive drugs, and patients with lymphoreticular neoplasms. Fungemia is especially problematic in cancer patients with chemotherapy-induced myelosuppression, blood and marrow transplant recipients, and patients in critical care units on multiple antibiotics with venous, bladder, or endotracheal catheters. With the increasing use of potent immunosuppressive purine analogues, such as fludarabine, pentostatin, and cladribine, and anti-T and anti-B cell antibodies (e.g., rituximab, alemtuzumab, and anti-thymocyte globulin) in the management of hematolymphoreticular malignancies, increasing emphasis on chemotherapy dose intensity in oncologic practice, and the growth in critical care, the number of patients at risk for fungal diseases is growing.

In recent years, the non-albicans *Candida* species have become increasingly recognized as fungal pathogens in immunocompromised patients. In cancer patients, *C. tropicalis and C. glabrata* are especially problematic. In critical care patients, the rates of *C. glabrata* infections are climbing. A variety of risk factors for different *Candida* species has been identified.

Aspergillus species have been the chief non-*Candida* fungal opportunistic pathogens. The major portals of entry for these airborne organisms are the nasal passages, sinuses, and respiratory tract, in contrast to the gastrointestinal tract for *Candida* organisms. In bone marrow transplant recipients and in patients with acute leukemia, the mortality is in excess of 75%.

Mold pathogens other than *Aspergillus* are increasing. The agents of mucormycosis are quite difficult to culture and the syndromes caused by these infections are indistinguishable from those caused by *Aspergillus* species; response to therapy is poor. *Fusarium*, a soil fungus, has been historically impervious to most therapeutics. *Scedosporium*, another emerging pathogen, is being increasingly reported in blood and marrow transplant recipients.

Difficulty in accurate diagnosis has been a tremendous impediment hindering therapeutic advances. Noninvasive techniques have been limited for most opportunistic fungal pathogens. Blood culture techniques have improved for detection of *Candida*, but still are not foolproof. *Aspergillus* is poorly diagnosed by bronchoscopy, and reliable diagnosis requires a thoracotomy, an invasive procedure which is quite dangerous in many of the patients that are suspected to be infected. There is an urgent need for noninvasive, rapid, accurate diagnostics. Antigen detection assays have been helpful aids to diagnosis for only a few fungal pathogens, such as *Cryptococcus* and *Histoplasma*. Recent studies suggest that antigen detection assays (such as galactomannan and glucan) and PCR methods for detecting fungal antigens may finally yield promising tools for a broader array of fungal pathogens and these will be discussed in the book.

Antifungal therapy had been quite limited in the past. The gold standard of therapy has been amphotericin B, a polyene antifungal agent with considerable toxicity. This concern was somewhat eased by the development of lipid formulations of amphotericin B, permitting delivery of high doses of amphotericin B with substantially less toxicity. The introduction of antifungal azoles offered considerable promise, but because of limited spectrum of activity and poor or erratic bioavailability, little progress was realized until fluconazole was introduced a decade ago. With excellent bioavailability, little toxicity, and both oral and intravenous formulations, fluconazole was quickly embraced by clinicians treating immunocompromised patients with suspected or proven *Candida* infection. The only blemish of fluconazole is a limited spectrum of activity: excellent activity against many yeast pathogens, but none against mold pathogens. Selection of fluconazole resistant yeasts was also a concern, especially in patients with advanced HIV disease failing anti-retroviral therapy.

New antifungal agents have been introduced into the clinical arena and more are arriving. Caspofungin, a member of a unique class of agents, the echinocandins, was licensed several years ago. This class of agents acts on the fungal cell wall, interfering with the biosynthesis of beta glucan, the main constituent of the fungal cell wall, whereas both polyenes and azoles act on a constituent of the fungal cell membrane, namely ergosterol. With excellent activity against the two most frequent invasive fungal pathogens, *Candida* and *Aspergillus*, and an outstanding safety profile, caspofungin has rapidly become widely used. Anidulafungin and micafungin are also on the horizon. New extended spectrum azoles have been introduced and others are in development. One, voriconazole, has been shown to be more effective than amphotericin B as first-line therapy of invasive aspergillosis, in a randomized trial. The drug is now available worldwide. New oral and intravenous formulations of itraconazole were approved to expand that agent's utility in clinical practice. Other broad spectrum azoles, such as posaconazole, are in clinical trials.

Even with effective and safe therapeutics, treatment is frequently started late during the course of infection, when the burden of organisms is high and the likelihood of therapeutic success low. This accounts for much of the extraordinarily high mortality. Accordingly, considerable attention has been paid to different antifungal strategies. Prophylaxis and empiric therapy have been evaluated in groups of immunocompromised patients at high risk for fungal infection. Today, there are good evidence-based data to support use of a broad array of antifungal agents and strategies for different patient settings.

Considerable progress has been achieved during the past decade. The cumulative mortality from *Candida* infections is finally beginning to recede. However, the collective mortality from aspergillosis continues to climb. Moreover, infection rates from fungi also are increasing. More work is needed. Yet, with new diagnostics and the expanding array of antifungals, the future looks bright.

The goal of this book is to provide an up-to-date overview of the fungal syndromes in immunocompromised patients, describe the shifts in fungal pathogens and the reasons behind them, indicate the setting in which they cause illness and the risk factors for infection, cover the pros and cons of current and emerging diagnostic measures, and discuss treatment modalities and strategies. The book is divided into five sections to cover the above topics, with individual chapters devoted to specific syndromes, infections, and settings.

This book is targeted to the clinician caring for immunocompromised patients at risk for invasive fungal infections. This includes transplant clinicians, critical care specialists, oncologists, stem cell transplant specialists, and infectious disease physicians. Both academic physicians and practitioners will find this book informative. Clinical microbiologists, mycologists, and individuals with research interests in developing new antimicrobial agents will also find very useful information related to their respective fields.

An international group of expert clinicians who have defined many of the pertinent issues in fungal epidemiologic studies and clinical trials have contributed to this effort. The authors review the published data, offer critical insights as to the interpretation of the literature, and provide timely summaries of the current state of knowledge. We are truly grateful for their hard work in making this project happen.

John R. Wingard
Elias J. Anaissie

Contents

Contributors

Elias J. Anaissie   The University of Arkansas for Medical Sciences, Myeloma and Transplantation Research Center, Little Rock, Arkansas, U.S.A.

Gregory M. Anstead   Department of Medicine, South Texas Veterans Healthcare System, San Antonio, Texas, U.S.A.

Anucha Apisarnthanarak   Division of Infectious Diseases, Washington University School of Medicine, St. Louis, Missouri, U.S.A.

Lindsey R. Baden   Division of Infectious Disease, Brigham and Women's Hospital and Dana-Farber Cancer Institute, Harvard Medical School; The Center for Experimental Pharmacology and Therapeutics, Harvard-MIT Division of Health Sciences and Technology, Boston, Massachusetts, U.S.A.

M. A. Boogaerts   Department of Hematology, University Hospital Gasthuisberg, Leuven, Belgium

E. J. Bow   Sections of Infectious Diseases and Hematology/Oncology, Department of Internal Medicine, University of Manitoba, Department of Medical Oncology and Hematology, Infection Control Services, Cancer Care Manitoba, and Health Sciences Center, Winnipeg, Manitoba, Canada

Robert W. Bradsher   Division of Infectious Diseases, University of Arkansas for Medical Sciences and Central Arkansas Veterans Health Care System, Little Rock, Arkansas, U.S.A.

Stephen J. Chanock   Section of Genomic Variation, Pediatric Oncology Branch, National Cancer Institute, National Institutes of Health, Bethesda, Maryland, U.S.A.

Ben E. de Pauw   Department of Blood Transfusion and Transplant Immunology and Mycology Research Center Nijmegen, University Medical Center, St. Radboud, Nijmegen, The Netherlands

Daniel J. Diekema   Department of Pathology and Department of Medicine, University of Iowa College of Medicine, Iowa City, Iowa, U.S.A.

María Cecilia Dignani   Head Infectious Diseases FUNDALEU (Foundation for the Fight Against Leukemia), Uriburu, Buenos Aires, Argentina

John Dotis   Third Department of Pediatrics, Hippokration Hospital, Thessaloniki, Greece

Rhonda V. Fleming   Division of Infectious Diseases, Texas Tech University Health Sciences Center, El Paso, Texas, U.S.A.

Charles B. Foster   Division of Pediatric Infectious Diseases, Johns Hopkins Hospital, Baltimore, Maryland, U.S.A.

John R. Graybill   Department of Medicine, Division of Infectious Diseases, University of Texas Health Science Center, San Antonio, Texas, U.S.A.

Monica Grazziutti   University of Arkansas for Medical Sciences, Little Rock, Arkansas, U.S.A.

Reginald Greene   Massachusetts General Hospital, Boston, Massachusetts, U.S.A.

Andreas H. Groll   Infectious Disease Research Program, Center for Bone Marrow Transplantation, Department of Pediatric Hematology/Oncology, University Children's Hospital, Münster, Germany

Paul O. Gubbins   Department of Pharmacy Practice, College of Pharmacy, University of Arkansas for Medical Sciences, Little Rock, Arkansas, U.S.A.

John Hiemenz   Sections of Hematology, Oncology and Infectious Diseases, Medical College of Georgia, Augusta, Georgia, U.S.A.

Helen L. Leather   BMT/Leukemia, Shands at the University of Florida, Gainesville, Florida, U.S.A.

Juergen Loeffler   Medizinische Klinik, Labor Prof. Dr. Einsele In der Hals- Nasen- Ohren- Klinik, Tübingen, Germany

José L. López-Ribot   Department of Medicine/Division of Infectious Diseases, The University of Texas, Health Science Center at San Antonio, San Antonio, Texas, U.S.A.

J. A. Maertens   Department of Hematology, University Hospital Gasthuisberg, Leuven, Belgium

Kieren A. Marr   Program in Infectious Diseases, Fred Hutchinson Cancer Research Center, and Department of Medicine, University of Washington, Seattle, Washington, U.S.A.

Francisco M. Marty   Division of Infectious Disease, Brigham and Women's Hospital and Dana-Farber Cancer Institute, Harvard Medical School; The Center for Experimental Pharmacology and Therapeutics, Harvard-MIT Division of Health Sciences and Technology, Boston, Massachusetts, U.S.A.

Jacques F. G. M. Meis Department of Medical Microbiology and Infectious Diseases, and Mycology Research Center Nijmegen, Canisius-Wilhelmina Hospital, Nijmegen, The Netherlands

Thomas F. Patterson Department of Medicine/Division of Infectious Diseases, The University of Texas, Health Science Center at San Antonio, San Antonio, Texas, U.S.A.

Michael A. Pfaller Department of Pathology and Department of Epidemiology, University of Iowa College of Medicine and College of Public Health, Iowa City, Iowa, U.S.A.

William G. Powderly Division of Infectious Diseases, Washington University School of Medicine, St. Louis, Missouri, U.S.A.

Sandra S. Richter Department of Pathology, University of Iowa College of Medicine, Iowa City, Iowa, U.S.A.

Emmanuel Roilides Third Department of Pediatrics, Hippokration Hospital, Thessaloniki, Greece

Robert H. Rubin Division of Infectious Disease, Brigham and Women's Hospital; Health Sciences and Technology, Harvard Medical School; The Center for Experimental Pharmacology and Therapeutics, Harvard-MIT Division of Health Sciences and Technology, Boston, Massachusetts, U.S.A.

Joseph S. Solomkin Department of Surgery, University of Cincinnati College of Medicine, Cincinnati, Ohio, U.S.A.

William J. Steinbach Division of Pediatric Infectious Diseases, Duke University Medical Center, Durham, North Carolina, U.S.A.

David A. Stevens Department of Medicine, Santa Clara Valley Medical Center, Stanford University Medical School, San Jose, California, U.S.A.

K. Theunissen Department of Hematology, University Hospital Gasthuisberg, Leuven, Belgium

Thomas J. Walsh National Institutes of Health, National Cancer Institute/ Pediatric Oncology Branch, Bethesda, Maryland, U.S.A.

John R. Wingard Department of Medicine, University of Florida College of Medicine, Gainesville, Florida, U.S.A.

1

Overview of Host Defenses: Innate and Acquired Immunity

Monica Grazziutti and Elias J. Anaissie
University of Arkansas for Medical Sciences, Little Rock, Arkansas, U.S.A.

John R. Wingard
Department of Medicine, University of Florida College of Medicine, Gainesville, Florida, U.S.A.

I. INTRODUCTION

Invasive fungal infections remain a serious challenge to clinicians caring for immunocompromised patients. The proportion of vulnerable patients is increasing, paralleling the increased use of immunosuppressive therapies and the more effective supportive care in high-risk populations.

Fungi responsible for these infections can be separated in two groups: the pathogenic and the opportunistic. The true pathogenic fungi cause self-limited disease in normal hosts but may cause devastating infections in compromised patients. Examples of such pathogens include *Cryptococcus neoformans* and the endemic fungi *Histoplasma capsulatum*, *Coccidioides immitis*, *Paracoccidioides brasiliensis*, and *Blastomyces dermatitidis*. These infections may remain in a latent state only to recrudesce when the patient is immunosuppressed. Opportunistic fungi rarely cause serious disease in normal hosts but are responsible for life-threatening infection in the setting of weakened host defenses. These fungi include *Candida* spp. and *Aspergillus* spp. and less commonly *Zygomycete* spp., *Trichosporon* spp., *Fusarium* spp., and *Pseudoallescheria boydii* among others.

Innate and acquired immunities work together as part of an integrated host immune response to prevent fungal infections (Fig. 1).

II. INNATE IMMUNITY

Innate immunity, also called natural or native immunity, consists of cellular and biochemical defense mechanisms that are in place before the exposure to the offending pathogen and, thus, can rapidly respond to prevent infection. This response remains unchanged upon reexposure to the pathogen.

The principal components of the innate immunity include physical barriers, soluble components and cell membrane receptors, the complement system, and the phagocytes.

A. Physical Barriers

Intact epithelium, fatty acids, mucus, and cilia act as physical barriers to invading pathogens. In the airways, the mechanism of cough helps to eliminate potential pathogens.

B. Soluble Components

Antimicrobial peptides (lysozymes, lactoferrin, secretory leukoprotease inhibitors, and defensins) are present in mucosal secretions. In the respiratory tract, these substances inhibit the entry of fungi through the epithelial barriers by disrupting crucial microbial structures, sequestering essential nutrients, interfering with microbial metabolism, and inhibiting microbial replication. Defensins are peptides produced by epithelial cells and phagocytes (neutrophil azurophilic granules) and possess broad antimicrobial activity, including fungi. Defensins also act as chemotactic factors for mononuclear cells (a-defensins) and T-cells (b-defensins) and stimulate the release of interleukin-8 (IL-8), a potent neutrophil chemotactic agent from epithelial cells

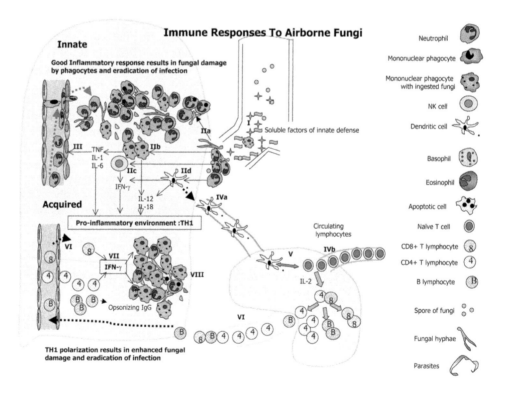

Figure 1 (*Caption on Facing Page*)

Various antimicrobial substances attack particular microbial targets and co-operate to enhance antimicrobial defenses (1) (Table 1).

C. Recognition of the Pathogen Through Pattern-Recognition Receptors

If microbes penetrate the epithelial barrier, defense mechanisms act to distinguish self from the potentially harmful pathogens through "pattern-recognition receptors" (PRRs) that are soluble molecules or present on cellular membranes.

1. Cellular Membrane PRRs

The PRRs that are present on the cellular membrane are the toll-like receptors (TLRs), mannose, and Fc receptors (Fig. 2).

TLRs are a family of membrane proteins present in phagocytes and epithelial cells that recognize microbial sugars. The interaction of TLRs with the pathogen-associated molecular patterns (PAMPs) activates host immune cells leading to the production of microbicidal peptides and proteins, cytokines, induction of respiratory

---

Figure 1 (*Facing Page*) Immune response to airborne fungi. Protective immunity against airborne fungi developed in two stages shown in sequence: Immediate by innate immunity (*upper part*) and delayed by acquired immunity (*lower part*). Immediate: (I) Three lines of defense against airborne fungi: epithelial barrier, soluble factors (antimicrobial and opsonizing molecules), and phagocytes. (II) If the spores invade the epithelium, the epithelial cells respond with chemokines production that activate immune cells: (a) Neutrophils attack intracellular and extracellular fungi; (b) macrophages attack intracellular fungi and produce proinflammatory cytokines such as IL-1, TNF, and IL-6; (c) NK cells secrete IFN-γ; and (d) DCs phagocytose the fungi and process and present fungal antigens to naive or memory T-cells. They also secrete IL-12, IL-18, and IFN-γ. A proinflammatory environment is thus created. (III) Proinflammatory cytokines upregulate the expression of adherence molecules in the recruitment of neutrophils and monocytes to the site of infection. Delayed (IV) (a) DCs process the antigens and migrate to the lymph nodes. (b) naive and memory T-cells also migrate from the circulation to lymph nodes. (V) DCs present the fungal antigen to naive and memory lymphocytes. T lymphocytes are specifically activated, which secrete IL-2 and promote the proliferation of B cell, CD4+, and CD8+ T-cells. (VI) Specific B and T-cells migrate through lymphatic vessels, thoracic duct, and general circulation and leave the circulation driven by chemoattractant released at the site of infection. (VII) In a proinflammatory environment, specific T lymphocytes polarize to type 1 and secrete IFN-γ. IFN-γ stimulates neutrophils and macrophages for a more effective killing of the pathogen. B cells produce (IgG), which opsonizes the pathogen for better phagocytosis. (VIII) Effective killing and clearance of the pathogen. Resolution of the infection. In contrast, a deleterious immune response to airborne fungal pathogens may develop in immunocompromised hosts. Immediate: Damaged epithelium, decreased number or function of phagocytes, or decrease in the concentration of antimicrobial and opsonizing molecules allow fungi to invade the host, reach the parenchyma and proliferate. Decreased number and function of phagocytes result in fungal proliferation and infection. Poor recruitment of inflammatory cells deprives the host from a strong phagocytic defense. A proinflammatory environment is not present. Delayed: Suppressed DC function results in inadequate antigen presentation to T-cells and little T-cell proliferation. The specific T-cells that migrate to the site of infection reach an environment devoid of proinflammatory cytokines. Without the proinflammatory cytokines (IL-12 and IFN-γ), the polarization of lymphocytes is to type 2 with production of IL-4 and IL-5 by T-cells and IgE from B cells. This type of response results in proliferation of fungi and progressive infection.

Table 1 Soluble Factors of the Innate Immunity

Polypeptide	Source	Probable mechanism of action	Known fungal target
Defensins	Neutrophils (azurophilic granules), epithelial cells	Disruption of microbial membrane, chemotaxis, complement modulation	*Candida* spp. (126–128), *Histoplasma capsulatum*, *Cryptococcus neoformans* (129,130)
Lysozyme	Neutrophils (azurophilic and specific granules), monocytes, macrophages, epithelial cells	Cleavage of glycosidic links in fungal membrane	*Candida* spp. (131)
Lactoferrin	Neutrophils (specific granules)	Iron sequestration	*Candida* spp.
Histatins	Salivary glands	Binding to metals (Zn and Cu)	*Candida* spp. *Aspergillus* spp. *C. neoformans, Saccharomyces cerevisiae* (132)
Antileukoproteases	Respiratory and genital epithelial cells	Protease inhibition	*Candida* spp. *Aspergillus* spp. (133)
Peroxydases	Neutrophils, monocytes, eosinophils, epthelial cells	Generation of microbicidal hypohalites from hydrogen	*Aspergillus* spp. *Candida* spp. (29,134)

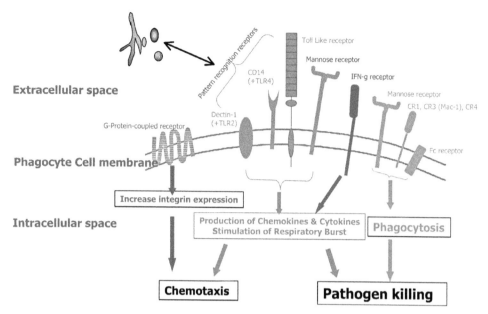

Figure 2 Role of phagocyte membrane receptors in immune defenses against fungi. G-protein-coupled receptor: Allows leukocytes to respond to chemoattractants (chemokines, chemotactic splits of complement and *N*-formylmethionyl-derived molecules) and migrate toward fungi. Pattern-recognition receptors (PRRs): Dectin-1, CD14, Toll-like receptors and mannose receptors. PRRs recognize fungal components known as pathogen-associated molecular patterns (PAMPs) that include zymosan, mannan, and mannoproteins. PRRs trigger phagocyte functions such as phagocytosis, respiratory burst, degranulation, and cytokine and chemokine production. IFN-γ receptor: Mediates the phagocyte response to IFN-γ. Mannose receptor: Recognizes mannan and induces phagocytosis. CR recognizes the complement fraction bound to fungi resulting in phagocytosis. Fc receptors recognize immunoglobulin-bound fungi and stimulate phagocytosis.

burst, and phagocyte degranulation. Fungal PAMPs on the fungal cell wall include polysaccharides as α- and β-glucans, galactomannans, chitin, and zymosan (2).

TLR4 and TLR2 receptors interact with CD14 and Dectin-1 receptor, respectively (3). Dectin-1 mediates the biological effects of fungal-derived β-glucans and zymosan and acts with TLR2 receptor to produce tumor necrosis factor (TNF) in response to fungi (4).

Our understanding of the role of TLRs in immunity against fungi is rapidly evolving. Most studies suggest that TLR2 and TLR4 are involved in the production of proinflammatory cytokines in response to *Aspergillus fumigatus* conidia and hyphae (2,5,6). In one study, however, TLR2 binding to hyphae from *A. fumigatus* resulted in an anti-inflammatory cytokine response (7). Studies with *C. neoformans* and *Candida albicans* further support the proinflammatory cytokine response induced by TLR2 and TLR4 (7,8).

Mannose receptors present on phagocytic membranes bind to fucose and mannose (absent in mammalian cells but abundant in fungi) and trigger phagocytosis.

Chemokines bind to G-protein-coupled receptors and stimulate chemotaxis.

2. Soluble PRRs

Soluble PRRs are present in body fluids and on mucosal surfaces and include two collectins: mannose-binding lectins (MBLs) and surfactant protein-A (SP) and SP-D;

ficolins, and pentraxin. These soluble PRRs recognize unique sugar patterns on microbes and act as opsonins presenting the microbe to the phagocyte directly or through complement activation (9–12) (Table 2).

D. Complement System

The complement system consists of plasma proteins normally present in an inactive state; when activated, the complement system plays a key role in opsonization, chemotaxis, and killing of microbes (Fig. 3). The proteins of the complement system are activated along an enzymatic cascade of sequential proteolysis resulting in bioactive molecules that facilitate opsonization, osmotic lysis of targeted cells, and recruitment of phagocytic cells. There are three major pathways of complement activation: the classical pathway in which activation results from binding of complement split Clq to IgG or IgM bound to an antigen; the alternative pathway, which is activated without the need for such antibodies, and the lectin pathway, which is activated by a plasma lectin that binds to mannose residues on microbes. The common event in complement activation is the cleavage of the complement protein C3, leading to C3b and C3a. C3b binds to the microbial surface and participates in the activation of C5, splitting it into C5b and C5a. C5b is followed by deposition of C6, C7, and C8, and the assembling the membrane attack complex (MAC) with a polymer of C9 inserted in the cell membrane of the microbe leading to microbial lysis. The opsonization of pathogens is mediated by C3b or C4b, which promotes phagocytosis by the cell bearing the appropriate receptors.

C3a, C4a, and C5a stimulate inflammation through chemotaxis and activating neutrophils and mast cells. MAC formation has not been found to play an important role against fungi as the fungal wall may block the formation of this complex, but another mechanism of complement system plays a role in host defense against certain fungi. Fungi are potent activators of the alternative and lectin pathway.

The phagocytic cell membrane has complement receptors (CRs) of four different types. Type 1 receptor, CR1 promotes phagocytosis of C3b- and C4b-coated particles and acts synergistically with the Fc γ receptor. Type 2 receptor, CR2 stimulates humoral immune response. Type 3 receptor, CR3 also called Mac-1, is an integrin composed of two chains (CDllb, CD18), is expressed on phagocytes and natural killer (NK) cells and promotes phagocytosis of C3-coated pathogens. CR3 also interacts with intercellular adhesion molecule (ICAM)-1 from endothelial cells during the recruitment of leukocytes. Type 4 receptor, CR4 (CD11c, CD18), is similar to CR3 and has similar functions but is more abundant on dendritic cells (DCs).

C3 acts as a major opsonin for *C. neoformans* in the *C. neoformans* naive host, whereas C5a seems to play a protective role against infections caused by *C. albicans, A. fumigatus, C. neoformans,* and *Saccharomyces cerevisiae* but not against dimorphic fungi (*H. capsulatum, C. immitis,* or *P. brasiliensis*) (13–15).

E. Phagocytes

The effector cells of the innate immunity are neutrophils, circulating monocytes, and tissue-based macrophages. As described earlier, these cells express surface receptors: mannose receptors, Dectin-1 receptors and TLRs that recognize pathogens, chemokine receptors and CRs for migration to the site of infection, cytokine receptors to respond to cytokines, mannose, and CRs and Fc receptors to increase phagocytosis (Fig. 2). Neutrophils and monocytes are recruited from the blood to sites of infection

Table 2 Pattern Recognition Receptors and Their Fungal Interaction

	Origin	Mechanism of Action	Fungal pathogen	Biological correlates
MBL (collectin)	Hepatocytes	Binding to MASP and activation of the complement system to increase phagocytosis	Acapsular *C. neoformans Candida* spp. *Aspergillus* spp. *Pneumocystis carinii*	Decreased MBL levels is associated with decreased opsonization; increased infections in patients receiving chemotherapy (135) and those with cystic fibrosis; recurrent vulvovaginal candidiasis (26); chronic necrotizing pulmonary aspergillosis (28)
SP-A and SP-D (collectin)	SP-A: alveolar type II cells, other respiratory cells, synovial cells SP-D: alveolar type II cells, gastrointestinal epithelium	Opsonization. Stimulation of chemotaxis, phagocytosis, production of proinflammatory cytokines, and fungal killing by phagocytes. Inhibition of IgE-mediated response to fungi	*Pneumocystis carinii,* acapsular *C. neoformans, A. fumigatus* (increase phagocytosis), *Candida albicans* (SP-A: anti-inflammatory effect on pulmonary alveolar macrophages) (136)	Decreased in patients with cystic fibrosis, adult respiratory distress syndrome, smokers, asthma, and conditions associated with increased risk for pneumonia. Increased in patients with interstitial lung diseases (137).
Ficolins	L ficolins: liver, H ficolins: liver and alveolar type II cells and bronchial epithelial cells, M ficolins: monocytes	Binding to MASP and activation of the complement system to increase phagocytosis	Bind to acapsular *C. neoformans*	None documented
Long Pentraxin 3	Macrophages and DCs	Binding to C1q to increase phagocytosis	*Aspergillus fumigatus, A. flavus, A. niger*	Pentraxin deficient (−/−) mice have increased mortality when challenged with *Aspergillus* spores. Administration of Pentraxin 3 to these animals increases survival

Abbreviations: MASP, Mannose-binding protein-associated serine protease; MBL, mannose-binding lectin; SP-A, surfactant protein-A; SP-D, surfactant protein-D.

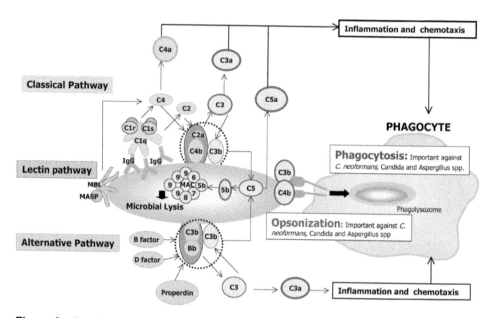

Figure 3 Complement system. Three pathways of complement activation lead to opsonization, chemotaxis, and the formation of the membrane attack complex (MAC). Classical pathway: Several molecules of IgG (or one molecule of IgM) bound to the fungal surface and bind to Clq, Clr, and Cls. Activated C1 leads to cleavage of C4 and C2 in C4a and C4b, C2a, and C2b. C4b and C2a have the function of C3 convertase. C3 convertase cleaves C3, leading further to C3a and C3b. Lectin pathway: Mannan-binding lectin (MBL) with a similar structure to Clq binds to the surface of fungi and to the MBL-associated serum proteases (MASP) and can cleave C4 or C2 in a fashion similar to that of the classical pathway. Alternative pathway: Antibodies are not required in this pathway. C3 cleaves spontaneously, binds to Factor B, and is cleaved by Factor D resulting in C3bBb, which has the function of a C3 convertase, analogous to the C4bC2a complex of the classical pathway (shown in gray as egg-shaped drawings). Properdin stabilizes the C3-convertase cleaves. The addition of C3b to the C3 convertases from classical or alternative pathway leads to C5 convertase that cleave C5 into C5a and C5b. C5b initiates the formation of the MAC that will cause lysis of the organism, although the importance for fungi is not clear. C3a and C5a are chemotactic molecules that favor inflammation. C3b and C4b are opsonins that will favor phagocytosis.

by binding to adhesion molecules on the endothelial cells and by chemoattractants produced in response to infection (Fig. 4).

There are three families of adhesion molecules: selectins, integrins, and immunoglobulin (Ig) superfamily adhesion molecules. Selectins are found on all type of leukocytes. Selectins participate in the process of leukocyte rolling along vascular endothelium, whereas integrins and the Ig superfamily adhesion molecules are important for stopping leukocyte rolling and mediating leukocyte aggregation and trans-endothelial migration. The integrins include the very-late antigen (VLA) molecules, leukocyte function-associated antigen (LFA)-1, and Mac-1. The Ig superfamily adhesion molecules include the ICAMs, vascular adhesion molecules (VCAM), LFA-2 and LFA-3, and platelet endothelial cell adhesion molecule (PECAM)-l.

Resident tissue macrophages that recognize microbes secrete cytokines such as TNF, IL-1, and chemokines. TNF and IL-1 act on the endothelial cells of postcapillary venules adjacent to the infection and induce the expression of selectins by

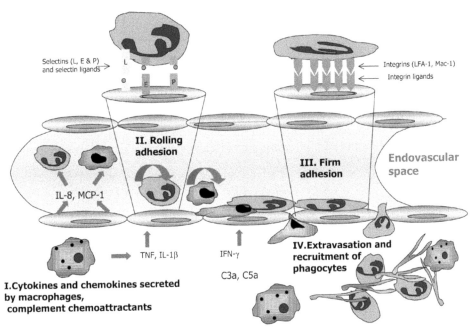

Figure 4 Recruitment and migration of inflammatory cells to site of fungal infection. (I) Secretion of cytokines: Macrophages secrete cytokines, IL-1, and TNF, which increase the expression of selectins on endothelial cells (E and P) and leukocytes (L) and the expression of the corresponding ligand on the opposite cell. Endothelial cells secrete chemokines as IL-8, which attract neutrophils and monocyte chemotactic protein (MCP)-1 to attract monocytes. (II) Rolling adhesion: The light attachment of leukocytes to endothelial cells is disrupted by the forces of the circulating blood resulting in a rolling motion for leukocytes. (III) Firm adhesion: Chemokines (IL-8 and MCP-1) and IFN-γ increase the expression of integrins on leukocytes (LFA-1, Mac-1) and their corresponding ligands on endothelial cells resulting in a change in the shape of leukocytes and their firm adhesion to the vascular wall. (IV) Extravasation and recruitment of phagocytes: Platelet-endothelial cell adhesion molecules (PECAMs) are upregulated on leukocytes and endothelial cells. PECAMs guide the extravasation of the leukocytes to the site of infection with further recruitment in the presence of C5a (chemoattractant to neutrophils) and C3a (chemoattractant to macrophages).

endothelial cells. Lymphocytes, monocytes, and neutrophils express ligands that bind to the endothelial selectins and cause leukocytes to roll along the endothelial surface.

TNF and IL-1 also induce endothelial expression of ligands for integrins, mainly VCAM-1, the ligand for the VLA-4 integrin, and ICAM-1, the ligand for the LFA-1 and Mac-1 integrin. Leukocytes express the integrin in low-affinity fashion. Chemokines and IFN-γ produced at the site of the infection are released into the bloodstream, bind to endothelial cells, and stimulate leukocytes to enhance the expression of leukocyte integrins. The binding of leukocyte integrins and endothelial cell ligands results in a firm binding of leukocytes to the endothelial interface. The leukocytes are attracted by PECAM-1 molecules, which are abundant in the interendothelial junction and migrate through the interendothelial spaces to the site of infection.

1. Neutrophils

Neutrophils are the most abundant phagocytic cells and the earliest to be recruited to the infectious foci. They contain azurophilic and specific granules in their cytoplasm (Fig. 5). The azurophilic granules are similar to lysosomes filled with myeloperoxidase, a variety of proteolytic enzymes, including acid hydrolase, glucoronidase, mannosidase, arylsulfatase, cathepsin, elastase, lysozyme, collagenase, elastase, protease, and antimicrobial peptides such as defensins and bactericidal permeability-increasing protein. The specific granules contain lactoferrin, lysozymes, monocyte chemotactic factor, C3 and C5 cleaving proteases, membrane-bound components of

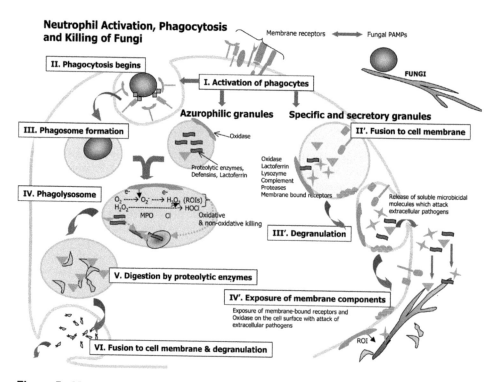

Figure 5 Neutrophil activation: phagocytosis and killing. (I) Membrane receptors recognize the presence of the pathogen and activate the neutrophil. (II) Phagocytosis begins. (III) The phagocytosed particles form a phagosome, which attracts the azurophilic granules. (IV) A phagolysosome is formed from the fusion of the phagosome with azurophilic granules. The organism is attacked within the phagolysosome by oxidative and nonoxidative mechanisms. Oxidative-dependent mechanisms consist of the respiratory burst performed by the oxidase complex, resulting in toxic reactive oxygen intermediates (ROIs). Hydrogen peroxide (H_2O_2) is a substrate for myeloperoxidase (MPO) with formation of hydrochlorus acid (HOC1), a very potent antimicrobial compound. Defensins and proteolytic enzymes attack the pathogen in an oxygen-independent manner. (V) The pathogen is digested in the phagolysosome by proteolytic enzymes. (VI) The phagolysosome degranulates its content, mainly to the extracellular space, but can also form a vacuole in the phagocyte. (II') Upon cell activation, the specific granules migrate toward the cell membrane and fuse with it. (III') The specific granules degranulate to the extracellular space delivering microbicidal molecules to extracellular fungi. (IV') Exposure of membrane-bound receptors (complement, immunoglobulin, chemokine receptors) and the oxidase complex delivers ROIs to the extracellular fungi.

NADPH oxidase system, cytochrome-b_{558} and membrane-bound receptors, CR3, CR4, and the chemotactic receptor for C5a.

After the phagocytes recognize the pathogen, they ingest it through phagocytosis. In this process, they form vesicles called phagosomes, the contents of which bind to lysosomes forming the phagolysosomes in which pathogens can be killed. In the phagolysosomes, the molecular O_2 is converted to reactive oxygen intermediates (ROIs) by the oxidase system in a process called respiratory burst. The ROIs are highly reactive oxidizing agents that destroy pathogens. Superoxide is one of the ROIs that can be converted to hydrogen peroxide and used by myeloperoxidase to produce more microbicidal products. Neutrophils also have nonoxidative killing mechanisms mediated by enzymes and defensins contained in their granules.

Azurophilic granules fuse with the phagosome and deliver high concentration of lytic proteins to the microbes while specific granules fuse preferentially with the plasma membrane releasing their contents in the extracellular space. This brings to the cell surface various functionally important membrane structures such as integrins, receptors for chemokines and opsonins, and the oxidase system.

Neutrophils play a major role in the defense against *Candida* spp. and *Aspergillus* spp. The normal number of circulating neutrophils is between 1500 and 2000 cells/mm^3, and when the number drops below 100 cells/mL, the risk for fungal infections increases. There are several categories of impairments of neutrophils.

a.   **Neutropenia.** Patients can have a deficient number of neutrophils as a consequence of myelosuppressive antineoplastic chemotherapy, induction of autoantibodies, or genetic disorders. The hereditary forms of neutropenia can be severe such as Kostmann's syndrome, which is a rare autosomal recessive disorder with granulocyte-maturation arrest and early death, or benign such as cyclic or familial neutropenia. Patients with invasive fungal infections remain a major complication among neutropenic cancer patients and stem cell transplant recipients. The most common pathogens of fungal infections are *Aspergillus* spp. and *Candida* spp., mucormycosis and the emerging fungal pathogens *Fusarium* spp., *Scedosporium* spp., and *Trichosporon* spp. The likelihood of fungal infection not only correlates with the depth and duration of the neutropenia, but also with the presence of neutrophil dysfunction resulting from suppression of acquired immunity by drugs (glucocorticoids) or the presence of graft versus host disease. The severity of fungal infections in profoundly neutropenic patients with hematological malignancies is reflected by the poor survival rate, unless marrow recovery is complete (16,17)

Hematopoietic growth factors, granulocyte colony-stimulating factor (G-CSF), and granulocyte–macrophage colony-stimulating factor (GM-CSF) stimulate proliferation, maturation, and activation of phagocytes (Table 3). These cytokines are administered as prophylaxis to shorten the duration of neutropenia and as preemptive therapy at the onset of febrile neutropenia (18–21). Another strategy is the use of granulocyte transfusions from G-CSF and corticosteroid-stimulated donors. This approach has been used for treatment and for prophylaxis with variable results. Success appears to correlate with the higher numbers of granulocytes transfused and the host-performance status (22,23).

b.   **Functional Defects of Neutrophils.** *Chronic granulomatous disease (CGD):* It is a hereditary disease, which can be autosomal or crosslinked, resulting from a defect in the cytochrome-b_{558} with failure to generate a respiratory burst in response to pathogens. CGD patients suffer from infections caused by catalase positive microorganisms, such as *Staphylococcus aureus, Pseudomonas* spp., *Salmonella* spp.,

Table 3 Cytokines and Fungal Immunity: Protective and Deleterious Effects

Cytokine	Source	Functional effect	Effect on fungi
Cytokines with a protective effect on fungal immunity			
Tumor necrosis factor (TNF)	Monocytes and macrophages	Stimulates and recruits neutrophils, monocytes, and lymphocytes. Increases expression of adhesion molecules and chemokine secretion. Stimulates IL-1 secretion by macrophages. Increases killing activity of phagocytes in large amounts, produces systemic effects: fever, increases liver production of acute phase reactants: C reactive protein, fibrinogen, and serum amyloid A protein (↑ESR). High levels produce hypotension and shock, reduces synthesis of lipoprotein lipase and causes cachexia, it is more typically produced in a type 1 response but can be present in a type 2 response (138).	Critical for protecting mice against infection by *Aspergillus* spp. (139), *Cryptococcus neoformans* (99,100) *H. capsulatum* (140). Increases the fungicidal activity of neutrophils against hyphae and phagocytic activity of macrophages against conidia *of Aspergillus* spp. (100,141) Use of anti-TNF in humans has been complicated with aspergillosis and histoplasmosis (114,115,142).
Interferon-γ (IFN-γ)	NK cells in (innate immunity) T lymphocytes (in adaptive immunity)	Activates killing mechanisms of phagocytes, promotes T_H1 polarization of the immune response and inhibits T_H2 differentiation, stimulates production of IgG involved in opsonization for phagocytosis.	Enhances neutrophil and monocyte fungicidal effect against yeasts and molds (143–146). Increases in vitro neutrophil fungal damage against *Aspergillus* hyphae in CGD patients (147). Exhibits synergistic effect with Amphotericin B against cryptococcosis in SCID mice (148). Critical in protection against invasive aspergillosis (139) and histoplasmosis (111,140,149) in mice but not against candidiasis (150).
Granulocyte-colony stimulating factor (G-CSF)	Lymphocytes and bone marrow stromal cells, monocytes, fibroblasts, endothelial cells	Regulates proliferation, survival, and differentiation of neutrophil precursors, increases the phagocytic function and oxidative burst, induces CD34+ cell mobilization, increases the ratio of DC2/	Increases neutrophil antifungal activity against *A. fumigatus*, *Candida albicans*, *Rhizopus arrhizus*, *Fusarium solani* (143,145,146,153,154). Improves antifungal damage by phagocytes of HIV+ patients against *A. fumigatus* (33,155). Increases in vitro

Cytokine	Cellular source	Function	Role in antifungal host defense
Granulocyte–macrophage colony-stimulating factor (GM-CSF)	Monocytes, macrophages, endothelial cells, fibroblasts	DC1, and polarizes to a T_H2 response during mobilization and when used to accelerate engraftment after bone marrow transplant (151,152). Promotes differentiation of multipotential hematopoietic progenitor cells, activates neutrophils, eosinophils, monocytes, and macrophages. Improves phagocytosis, oxidative metabolism, release of chemotactic factors, and antigen presentation. Can be produced in the context of a T_H1 or T_H2 response. Inhibits IL-12 production by mouse DCs (157). Induces T_H2 differentiation (158).	phagocytic fungal damage against *Candida* spp., *A. fumigatus, and R. arrhizus* after in vivo administration (153). Reverses the corticosteroid-mediated detrimental effect on antifungal activity of neutrophils (35). Improves the outcome of mice with acute disseminated candidiasis but not those with subacute or chronic candidiasis (156). Activates monocytes and macrophages antifungal activity against *C. albicans, Fusarium solani, A. fumigatus* (145), *H. capsulatum,* and *C. neoformans.* Prevents the deleterious effect of corticosteroids on monocyte-mediated antifungal activity and cytokine production (39,159).
Interleukin (IL)-1	Macrophages, neutrophils, epithelial and endothelial cells	Stimulates acute phase plasma proteins, induces central fever and cachexia	It is part of the proinflammatory response against *Aspergillus* spp. *Candida* spp., and *C. neoformans* (160–163).
IL-2	T lymphocytes	Promotes T- and B-cell proliferation.	IL-2-activated NK cells inhibit *C. albicans* yeast growth in vitro (164).
IL-6	Monocytes, macrophages, T lymphocytes, endothelial cells, fibroblasts	Stimulates the acute phase response (innate immunity). Promotes B-cell proliferation (adaptive immunity).	Enhances resistance to invasive aspergillosis and candidiasis in mice (165,166).
IL-12	Monocytes, macrophages and DCs	Induces T_H1 immune response, stimulates production of IFN-γ from T and NK cells. Increases the cytolytic activity of CD8+ and NK cells.	Critical in protecting against infection by most fungi including *Aspergillus* spp. *Candida* spp. *C. Neoformans* (61,106,167) and *H. capsulatum* (110). Enhances oxidative anti fungal activity of human mononuclear phagocytes against *A. fumigatus* (168).

(Continued)

Table 3 Cytokines and Fungal Immunity: Protective and Deleterious Effects (*Continued*)

Cytokine	Source	Functional effect	Effect on fungi
IL-15	Bone marrow stroma cells, gut and skin epithelia, macrophages	Stimulates production of IL-8 from neutrophils and monocytes and macrophages. Stimulates production of IFN-γ from NK cells, favors T$_H$1 polarization.	Increases the oxidative antifungal activity of neutrophils against *A. fumigatus* and induces IL-8 release in vitro after exposure to *A. fumigatus* and *A. flavus* (169). Increases oxidative antifungal activity of monocytes against *C. albicans* (170). Critical for cytotoxic T lymphocyte activity against *C. neoformans* (105).
IL-18	Monocytes, macrophages, DCs, and fibroblasts	Synergizes IL-12 by stimulating IFN-γ production by T-cells mediating a T$_H$1 response. IL–18 + IL–10 in the absence of IFN-γ stimulate secretion of IL–13, which is a type 2 cytokine	Improves the antifungal activity of murine peritoneal exudates against *C. neoformans* (171). Critical for an effective clearance of *A. fumigatus* conidia in the context of allergic fungal airway disease in a murine model (172). Protects mice against disseminated candidiasis through endogenous IFN-γ (173).
IL-8 and CXCL chemokines	Monocytes, macrophages, endothelial cells, epithelial cells, T-cells	Recruits neutrophils	Important in chemotaxis against aspergillosis (174)
CCL chemokines	Monocytes, macrophages, endothelial cells, epithelial cells, T-cells	Chemoattractant to monocytes, chemoattractant and activator to eosinophils and basophils	Monocyte chemotactic protein-1 (MCP-1) is necessary for clearance of *C. neoformans* and *Aspergillus* from murine lungs (46,102,103) MIP-1 α is necessary for the development of a T$_H$1 response to *C. neoformans*
Cytokines with deleterious effect on fungal immunity			
IL-4	T lymphocytes, mast cells and basophils	Promotes B- and T-cell proliferation and production of IgGl and IgE. Inhibits macrophage activation, antagonizes T$_H$1 development	Plays a role in the pathogenesis of allergic aspergillosis (175). IL-4-deficient mice are more resistant to invasive aspergillosis and cryptococcosis than wild-type mice (78,176). Impairs pulmonary clearance of *H. capsulatum* in mice (177).

	Source	Function	Role in aspergillosis
IL-5	T lymphocytes and mast cells	Promotes production of IgM, IgA, and IgE, eosinophil expansion, and activation	Favors allergic bronchopulmonary aspergillosis (175,178,179)
IL-10	Monocytes, macrophages, CD4+ T-cells, B cells, keratinocytes	Anti-inflammatory effect, inhibits proinflammatory cytokine secretion. Decreases phagocytosis, oxidative burst, intracellular killing and antigen presentation to T-cell, decreases inflammation in a T_H2 context, upregulates perforin expression and the Fas/Fas ligand system by cytotoxic T lymphocytes	Decreases antifungal activity of monocytes against *Aspergillus* hyphae in vitro (180). Detrimental in invasive aspergillosis in a murine model (80). Beneficial effect in mice with allergic pulmonary aspergillosis (82). Increased levels in non-neutropenic patients with invasive aspergillosis correlates with poor outcome (79).
IL-25	Lymphocytes	Induces airway hyper-reactivity, induces type 2 cytokine response, activates eosinophils	Produced in response to *Aspergillus* spp. in the airway of animals. May mediate allergic diseases related to *Aspergillus* spp. (181).

Aspergillus spp., and *Candida* spp. (24). Antibiotics and IFN-γ prevent serious infections in these patients (25). Neutrophils of CGD patients improve their antiaspergillar activity when the patient is treated with IFN-γ (9).

Leukocyte adhesion deficiency (LAD): It is an autosomal recessive disorder in which the number of neutrophils may be increased; neutrophils, however, are unable to migrate to the site of infection. LAD-1 is associated with a defect in integrins, which affects the neutrophil's ability to adhere firmly to the endovascular endothelium, and LAD-2 is related to a defect in selectins, which affects the neutrophil's capacity to roll over the endothelium. These disorders cause early death as a result of life-threatening infections, mostly bacterial.

Chediak–Higashi syndrome (CHS): It is an autosomal recessive disorder affecting neutrophils and other cells. The lysosomes are giant and dysmorphic. In these patients, leukocyte counts are decreased and neutrophils have poor chemotactic response and delayed degranulation of phagolysosomes resulting in deficient and delayed microbial killing and severe infections.

Job's syndrome: This syndrome is characterized by defective neutrophil chemotactic response, recurrent cutaneous bacterial infections, and mucocutaneous candidiasis.

Abnormal phagocytosis because of decreased MBL: Patients with low levels of MBL are at increased risk for infections particularly after cytotoxic chemotherapy. Low levels of MBL have been associated with recurrent vulvovaginal candidiasis, and polymorphism of the MBL gene was described in patients with chronic necrotizing pulmonary aspergillosis (26–28).

Myeloperoxidase deficiency: Neutrophils with MPO deficiency have delayed microbial killing, though without an apparent increase in incidence of infections in humans. Myeloperoxidase deficiency produces a delay in the clearance of *A. fumigatus* and decreased cytotoxicity to *C. albicans, C. tropicalis,* and *Trichosporon asahii* in experimental murine infections (29).

Specific granule deficiency: A rare congenital disease characterized by dysfunction of the neutrophils resulting in recurrent severe bacterial infections, but uncommon fungal infections, starting from early infancy. The disease is characterized by abnormal migration and decreased killing activity of neutrophils lacking defensins, lactoferrin, BPI, and collagenase. Eosinophils, monocyte, and macrophages are also affected.

    c. Functional Defects of Neutrophils in Systemic Conditions. Several examples of this are notable:

1. Diabetes mellitus: Neutrophils in diabetic patients have decreased chemotaxis, phagocytic capacity, and killing capacity, especially during hyperglycemia (30,31).
2. AIDS: Neutrophils from patients with advanced AIDS have decreased migration, phagocytosis, and killing when stimulated by encapsulated *C. neoformans* in vitro (32). Neutrophils from HIV-infected patients with low CD4+ lymphocyte counts also have decreased antifungal activity against *A. fumigatus* in vitro that can be partially corrected with G-CSF pretreatment (33).
3. *Glucocorticoid therapy*: Glucocorticoids affect multiple neutrophil functions: suppress migration, phagocytosis, oxidative burst and free radical generation, degranulation, nitric oxide release, and cytokine production, although neutrophil survival is increased (decrease apoptosis). In vitro, *A. fumigatus* is stimulated in the presence of pharmacological doses of

hydrocortisone (34). IFN-γ and G-CSF prevent the suppression of *A. fumigatus* hyphal damage by neutrophils induced by glucocorticoids (35).

2. Mononuclear Phagocytes

Resident tissue macrophages encounter the pathogen upon initial infection, and their central role is to inhibit it and kill it. Monocytes are also recruited from the circulation to the site of infection attracted by chemokines. Alveolar and interstitial macrophages from the lungs play a very important role against fungi because most fungal infections are acquired through the airborne route.

Mononuclear phagocytes kill pathogens by oxygen-dependent and oxygen-independent mechanisms, as described with neutrophils. In the oxidative antimicrobial killing, oxygen is converted into ROIs by the oxidase system. In addition to ROIs, macrophages produce nitric oxide (NO), which can combine with hydrogen peroxide or superoxide and generate more potent antimicrobial molecules.

Macrophages produce cytokines including TNF, IL-β, IL-6, IL-12 and chemokines such as MCP-1 and possess the machinery required for antigen presentation.

Macrophages live longer than neutrophils and persist longer in the site of the infection. G-CSF, GM-CSF, M-CSF, and IFN-γ enhance the antifungal activity of phagocytes by augmenting oxidative and nonoxidative mechanisms to damage the membrane and cell wall of fungi (Table 3).

Of note, antifungal agents affecting the integrity of the fungal cell membrane and wall have a synergistic and/or additive effect with phagocytes against fungi with increased fungal damage in vitro (36) and in animal models of murine aspergillosis (37).

Macrophages are the main effector cells against *H. capsulatum, C. neoformans,* and *Penicillium marneffei* yeast cells but they require cytokine activation to destroy these fungi.

Glucocorticoids induce reversible monocytopenia and impair the maturation, chemotaxis, migration, and phagocytosis and cytokine production by monocytes. The killing effect of alveolar macrophages against *A. fumigatus* conidia is mediated through ROIs. This effect is reduced by corticosteroids and may be responsible of the increased susceptibility to invasive infections (38). GM-CSF prevents in vitro the inhibitory effect of glucocorticoids on cytokine production by alveolar macrophages challenged with *Aspergillus* conidia (39) (Table 3).

In contrast to the damaging effect of phagocytes on fungal cells, fungi have their own protective mechanisms against phagocytes. Spores of *Aspergillus* spp. inhibit phagocytosis in vitro (40,41), and toxins such as gliotoxin and proteases produced by *Aspergillus* spp. and other pathogenic fungi inhibit neutrophil activation, respiratory burst, and chemotaxis (41–43). Unidentified products from *A. fumigatus* also inhibit the effect of macrophages on conidial germination and hyphal damage by neutrophils (44).

3. NK Cells

NK cells are lymphocytes that can secrete IFN-γ, recognize cells lacking the major histocompatibility complex (MHC) class I molecule with resulting NK-cell activation and killing of these cells. NK cells are especially important for defense against viruses, but can also kill cells infected with other intracellular pathogens.

NK cells are activated by cytokines, mainly IL-15 and IL-12 and high levels of IL-2. Through the secretion of IFN-γ, NK cells activate macrophages and favor polarization of T-cells to type 1 response. NK cells kill target cells (infected cells, tumor cells), by creating pores in the cellular membranes with perforins, and inducing apoptosis of target cell through granzymes. Apoptosis can also result from a Fas–Fas ligand activation. NK cells play a role against *C. neoformans* and *A. fumigatus* through secretion of IFN-γ (45,46).

4. Platelets

Platelets aggregate and are able to damage non-albicans *Candida* spp. and *A. fumigatus* (47,48) in in vitro assays. Whether this is clinically important is unclear.

III. ACQUIRED IMMUNITY

Adaptive, acquired, or specific immunity, like innate immunity, is stimulated by exposure to infectious agents. However, adaptive immunity is characterized by its extraordinary capacity to distinguish among different, even closely related agents, and its ability to generate an enhanced immune response through the production of memory cells after exposure to a particular agent. The main characteristics of acquired immunity are its specificity and its memory allowing response to a previously known antigen.

There are two types of acquired immunity: humoral and cell-mediated.

A. Humoral Immunity

Humoral immunity is mediated by antibodies secreted by B lymphocytes and can be transferred by serum from an immunized individual to a nonimmunized one. Antibodies bind to the antigens of extracellular microbes and function to neutralize and eliminate these microbes. The elimination of different types of microbes requires several effector mechanisms, which are mediated by distinct classes, or isotypes of antibodies. B lymphocytes populate peripheral lymphoid tissues, which are the sites of interaction with foreign antigens. Antigen binds to the membrane IgM and IgD on naive cells and activates these cells. B cells proliferate in response to the antigen, resulting in clonal expansion of antigen-specific cells and differentiation into effector cells that actively secrete antibodies and into memory cells. The B cell internalizes the antigen and processes it. If the antigen is a protein, the antibody response requires CD4+ helper T lymphocytes that recognize the antigen and play an essential role in further activation of B cells (Fig. 8B). Polysaccharides and lipid antigens activate B cells through a T-independent pathway.

The IgM and IgD are two chains, and Igα and Igβ are the receptors for the antigen. They form the B-cell receptor complex (similar to T-cell receptor (TCR) with CD3 and ζ in T-cells). Once the antigen is recognized, the complex starts the first signal of activation and the second signal is provided by complement: C3b bound on the surface of the microbe is degraded to C3d, and this binds to CR2 (type 2 CR), CD19, and CD81. These three receptors represent the coreceptor complex, and when the microbe is bound to the BCR and the complement is bound to this coreceptor complex, the B-cell activation begins. Activated B cells upregulate the expression of class II MHC, costimulatory molecules, and chemokine and cytokine receptors. They process the antigen into peptides that bind to the MHC class II molecule. The complex of class II MHC and peptide migrates toward CD4 lymphocytes and results in stimulation of B-cell clonal expansion, isotype switching, and differentiation in memory B cells (Fig. 8B). When the memory cells are exposed to the antigen again, the secondary response develops faster and produces larger amounts of antibodies.

Humoral immunity plays a limited role in host defense against fungi. B-cell depleted mice are susceptible to systemic but not to mucosal candidiasis (49).

Vaccination of mice with a liposome-mannan vaccine elicits monoclonal antibodies that are protective against disseminated and vaginal candidiasis. The passive administration of these antibodies is also protective against these infections. Protection is elicited by binding of these antibodies to complement (activating the classical pathway) with opsonization of the yeast cell for faster and more effective phagocytosis (50–52). Mycograb, a human monoclonal antibody against *Candida* heat shock protein (Hsp) 90, is present in patients with disseminated candidiasis, and its presence correlates with recovery from infection. This antibody is protective against murine disseminated candidiasis and acts synergistically with amphotericin B against *albicans* and *non-albicans Candida* spp. This action may be mediated by decreasing the adherence of circulating yeast cells to tissues (53,54). MAb C7, a monoclonal antibody against a protein epitope from a mannoprotein, has three mechanisms of protection against candidiasis: decreasing the adherence of *Candida* to epithelial cells, inhibiting germination, and damaging the yeast by direct candidacidal effect. This antibody is also fungicidal against *C. neoformans*, *A. fumigatus*, and *Scedosporium prolificans*, mimicking the activities of a killer toxin (52). An anti-idiotipic antibody to antibodies recognizing killer toxin and mimicking natural antikiller toxin receptor is protective against experimental candidiasis, cryptococcosis, aspergillosis, and pneumocystosis (55).

Antibodies against *C. neoformans* can be protective, nonprotective, or deleterious, depending on dose, antibody isotype, inoculum size, and availability of T-cells and mediators of cell immunity (56). Vaccines with polysaccharide conjugate and peptide vaccines that elicit antibodies to the capsule are protective against experimental Cryptococcosis. In addition, monoclonal antibodies against glucuronoxylomannan (GXM), a capsule component, protect against *C. neoformans*, probably by facilitation of cellular response (57,58).

Humoral immunity does not appear to play an important role in the defense against infections by other fungi such as *Aspergillus* spp. *H. capsulatum*, or *Coccidioides immitis*, despite the role that antibodies against these pathogens play in diagnosis.

B. Cell-mediated Immunity

Cell-mediated immunity is the most important mechanism of acquired immunity against fungal pathogens. In cell-mediated immunity, T lymphocytes recognize the antigen and act to destroy the micro-organism and/or infected cell. Its mode of action relies to a great degree on stimulating phagocytic immune response.

The principal cells of the cell-mediated immune system are the antigen-presenting cells (APCs) and lymphocytes. The most highly specialized APCs are DCs, although monocytes, macrophages, and B lymphocytes may also act as APCs. DCs are the best at stimulating naive T-cells while DCs, macrophages, and B cells can stimulate specific T-cells previously primed for the same antigen.

The adaptive immune response starts when the antigen is presented to the T-cell, and the T-cell recognizes it. The T-cell responds with proliferation leading to clonal expansion and activation. The activated T-cells stimulate the response, which will eliminate the pathogen through stimulation of phagocytic cells. Once the elimination of the pathogen is achieved, the homeostasis is reached by a decrease of the immune response. Most of the immune cells die because of the lack of antigen stimulation, but some cells are preserved as memory cells that will respond faster than naive cells during a second encounter with the same pathogen (Fig 6).

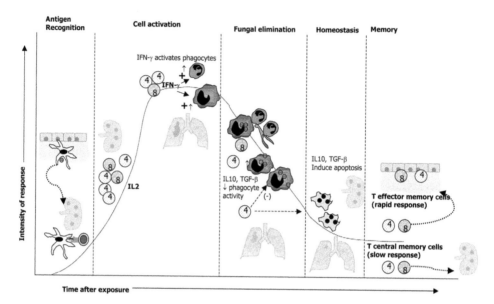

Figure 6 Evolution of the adaptive immune response to fungi. After the antigen is recognized, T-cells proliferate and get activated and then stimulate phagocytes to effectively eliminate the pathogen. With successful elimination of the pathogen, the immunity declines by cell apoptosis, but memory cells survive to rapidly respond upon encounter of the same antigen. Antigen recognition: DCs phagocytose the pathogen, migrate to lymph nodes where they process the pathogen, and present it to T-cells. Cell activation: Antigen-specific T lymphocytes are activated, secrete IL2, and proliferate into CD4+ and CD8+ lymphocytes. These cells migrate to sites of infection and stimulate phagocytes through IFN-γ production to control the infection. Fungal elimination: Primed phagocytes attack the pathogen and control the infection. With resolution of the infection, anti-inflammatory cytokines act locally to reduce inflammatory damage to organs. Homeostasis: Apoptosis of immune cells throughout the immune system and at sites of infection returns the immune system to homeostasis. Only memory cells survive. Memory: Memory cells survive to respond upon encountering the same antigen. Response is rapid through T effector memory cells and slower through T central memory cells.

1. Antigen Recognition

To present the antigen to T-cells, the APCs, mainly immature DCs, have to uptake and process the antigen. Immature DCs are located in the skin and mucosa (gastrointestinal, respiratory tract, genitourinary tract) where they capture microbial protein antigens, process them, and transport them to the draining lymph nodes where they present them to T-cells. During this process, DCs become mature (Fig. 1–IV).

The process is different according to the source of the antigen, which can be extra- or intracellular (Fig. 7):

    a. Extracellular antigens are attracted by the APCs through receptors such as mannose, Fc, complement, and TLR. The APCs endocytose the antigen to process it into peptides (antigen processing) and present the peptides bound to MHC to T-cells (antigen presentation) to initiate a T-cell response to the given antigen (priming).
        DCs and macrophages also can phagocytose the pathogen; the phagosome then fusing with the lysosome to form a phagolysosome.

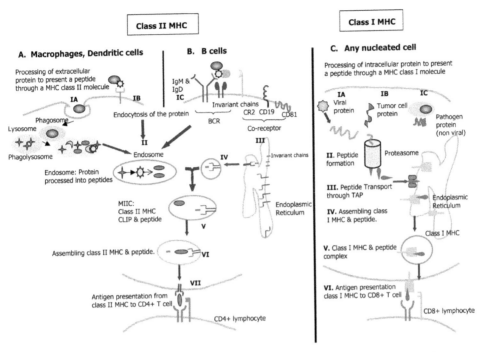

Figure 7 Antigen uptake and processing. A and B: Class II MHC. (I) (A) DCs and macrophages phagocytose the fungal element, and the phagosomes fuse with the lysosomes forming phagolysosomes. The fungi are destroyed with formation of proteic antigens. (B) Proteins from the fungi can be endocytosed from the extracellular space. (C) The antigen binds to IgM or IgD and opsonizing complement and its receptor on the surface of a B cell. The antigen is internalized by endocytosis. (II) The endocytosed proteins are in the endosome where the proteolytic enzymes will degrade it into peptides that will assemble with the MHC class II molecule. (III) MHC class II molecules are synthesized in the endoplasmic reticulum where they bind to the invariant chain. The invariant chain stabilizes the MHC class II molecule and prevents the union of the MHC class II molecules with peptides in the endoplasmic reticulum by occupying the pocket that will bind the foreign peptide. (IV) The invariant chain guides the movement of the MHC class II toward the endosome. (V) The fusion of the endosome and the vesicle containing the class II MHC molecule results in the formation of a new vesicle called MIIC. (VI) In the MIIC, the invariant chain is released from the MHC class II molecule by a class II-like molecule called HLA-DM and the peptides replace the invariant chain and form the complex to be presented to a T lymphocyte. (VII) The MHC class II molecule presents the antigen in the cell surface to the CD4+ T-cell. C: Class I MHC. (I) The source of peptides presented by class I molecules is proteins originated in the cytosol. These proteins may result from: (A) the product of virus; (B) a mutated protein produced by a tumor cell; or (C) a protein produced by a nonviral intracellular pathogen. (II) Cytosolic proteins are processed by the proteasome resulting in peptides. (III) Peptides are transported into the endoplasmic reticulum by a TAP. (IV) Inside the endoplasmic reticulum, the peptide binds the MHC class I molecule. (V) The class I–MHC peptide complex moves to the Golgi complex and is transported to the cell surface by exocytic vesicles. (IV) Once on the cell surface, the antigen is presented to a CD8+ cell.

The pathogen is destroyed and results in formation of proteic antigens and peptides. In B cells, protein antigens bind to BCR and coreceptor on the cell surface, which induce endocytosis of the antigen. Endocytosed proteins in the DC, macrophage, or B cell reside in the endosome where proteolytic enzymes degrade them into peptides that will be assembled with the MHC class II molecule. MHC class II molecules are synthesized in the endoplasmic reticulum where they bind to an invariant chain. The invariant chain stabilizes the MHC class II molecule and guides its movement toward the endosome. The endosome and the vesicle containing the MHC class II molecule fuse together, and the new vesicle is called MIIC. In the MIIC, the invariant chain is released from the MHC class II molecule and the peptides replace the invariant chain to form the complex to be presented on the APC cell surface to the CD4+ T-cell.

b. Intracellular antigens are those produced by virally infected cells, mutated proteins produced by tumor cell, or less frequently, produced by an intracellular pathogen other than virus (Fig. 7C). The proteins from the cytosol are processed by the proteasome resulting in peptides. These peptides are transported into the endoplasmic reticulum by a transporter associated with antigen presentation (TAP). In the endoplasmic reticulum, the peptide binds the MHC class I molecule. The complex MHC class I–peptide moves toward the Golgi complex and is transported to the cell surface by exocytic vesicles. Once on the surface, the antigen is presented to a CD8$^+$ cell. Any nucleated cell having the MHC class I molecule can present intracellular antigens to CD8$^+$ cells.

During antigen processing, DCs lose their adhesion molecules to epithelial cells and express a chemokine receptor called CCR7 (receptor for CC chemokine) that is specific for lymph node chemokines. These chemokines attract DCs bearing CCR7 receptor to the lymph node. Because naive T-cells also express CCR7, they are also attracted to the lymph node where they will encounter the DCs with resulting antigen presentation to naive T-cells.

In order to respond, the T-cell has to recognize the MHC molecule, and the peptide from the MHC–peptide complex. Naive T-cells will accept any peptide, but memory specific T-cells will only respond to the same antigen recognized during prior contact. This gives T-cells a dual MHC and antigen specificity.

The activation of T-cells requires two signals: the antigen itself triggers the first signal and a second signal is induced by microbial products or cytokines produced in response to a microbial product. The requirement for a second signal triggered by microbes or cytokines ensures that immune responses are triggered only when needed and not against harmless substances, including self-antigens (Fig. 8).

The T-cells are first attracted by adhesion receptors and their ligands. Once in contact, the T-cells recognize the MHC–peptide complex in the APC through the TCR. The presence of the CD4+ and CD8+ molecules on the surface of T-cells is indispensable for the lymphocyte to respond, initiate the first-signal transduction event leading to cell maturation and promotion of adhesion of the TCR to the MHC–peptide complex. Once the peptide is recognized, CD3 and ζ can lead to functional activation of the T-cell. CD2 binds to LFA-3 and is important for both adhesion and activation.

The second signal is provided by the costimulatory APC molecules B7-1 (CD80) and B7-2 (CD86). These molecules bind to CD28 on the lymphocyte surface, which results in an antiapoptotic signal to cells, proliferation and production of cytokines, and growth factors. The expression of B7 is upregulated by microbial substances such as endotoxins, and by cytokines produced by the innate immune reaction to an antigen. Activated T-cells also express CD40 ligand, a molecule that

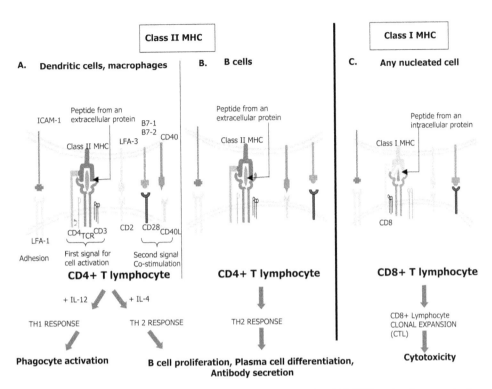

Figure 8 Antigen presentation A and B: Class II MHC. Class II MHC molecule presents the bound peptide to CD4+ lymphocyte by binding to the T-cell receptor (TCR). CD4 molecule is the coreceptor that binds to an invariable region of the MHC molecule and participates in signal transduction. CD3 and ζ are invariable proteins and, together with TCR and CD4, form the TCR complex, which send the first signal for activation of the cell. CD28 in the T-cell binds to B7.1 (CD80) or B7.2 (CD86) which provides the second signal for activation. They are costimulatory molecules. LFA-1 binds to ICAM-1 and CD2 binds to LFA-3. These are adhesion molecules that facilitate antigen presentation. CD2 is also a signal transducer molecule. CD40 ligand is expressed in T lymphocytes and bind to CD40 is expressed in the antigen-presenting cell (APC). When CD40 is expressed in B cells stimulates T helper, which will activate B cell for production. Once the CD4+ lymphocyte is activated, it triggers a T_H1 or T_H2 response. In contrast, when a B cell acts as the APC, the activated CD4+ cell triggers a T_H2 response. C: Class I MHC. Class I MHC molecule presents the peptide to a CD8+ lymphocyte. The coreceptor in the lymphocyte is the CD8 molecule; otherwise, the TCR complex and the costimulatory molecules are the same as the molecules involved in class II MHC presentation. The result is the stimulation for proliferation, cytokine production, and differentiation in cytotoxic T lymphocytes (CTL).

binds CD40 expressed on APC and also upregulates B7. After lymphocyte activation, another receptor, the CTLA-4 (CD 152) is expressed on T-cells and binds to B7 receptors to deactivate the lymphocyte and terminate the TCR. CTLA-4 plays an important role in self-tolerance

2. Cell Activation

After the first encounter with the antigen, naive T-cells get activated and respond with proliferation, differentiation, and synthesis of new proteins (Fig. IV). Proliferation, mediated by IL-2 in an autocrine pathway, results in expansion of the T-cell pool and differentiation into memory and effector T-cells. Each antigen originates a clone of cells that will only recognize that given antigen presented by the MHC molecule. Upon subsequent exposures to this antigen, the specific pre-existing clone will be activated.

Effector T-cells migrate to the site where the antigen is located (Fig. VI). This migration is not antigen specific, but once in the inflamed tissue, only lymphocytes specific for the attracting antigen will stay, whereas the other lymphocytes may return to circulation. At this stage, CD4+ lymphocytes are called T helper precursor. When they get to the site of inflammation, they become effector CD4+ cells and can produce two subsets of cytokines, T helper 1 (T_H1) or T helper 2 (T_H2) also called type 1 and type 2 immunity because the response involves not only T helper lymphocytes, but also other cells. The polarization to T_H1 or T_H2 is determined by the type of antigen and APCs, by the presence of hormones, and most importantly by the cytokine environment (Fig. 9). The presence of IL-12 produced by monocytes and DCs at the site of the infection will polarize toward a T_H1 response whereas during the lack of IL-12, the presence of IL-4 will induce a T_H2 response. When the APC is a B cell, T_H2 ensues, but a T_H1 response occurs when the APC is a macrophage. DCs can induce a T_H1 or T_H2 response.

The type of antigen also influences the response with bacteria and fungi stimulating T_H1 and helminths stimulating T_H2. A T_H2 response also occurs in the presence of a high antigen burden (including fungi and bacteria). Thus, reducing the fungal burden by antifungal agents favors T_H1 polarization, while the administration of glucocorticoids or anti-IL-2 agents (cyclosporine, tacrolimus) favors type 2 immunity, even when responding to antigens that normally would elicit type 1 immune response. Estrogens decrease the activation of macrophages by increasing the production of hepatic inhibitory substance Apo-I. On the other hand, testosterone decreases the production of the inhibitory Apo-I, favoring T-cell–macrophage contact and the subsequent macrophage activation (59), although the role of hormones in cell-mediated immunity is still not well understood (60). Pregnancy is associated with abrogation of cell-mediated immunity and a T_H2 immune response. Fungal dissemination during pregnancy has been described with *H. capsulatum* and *C. immitis* (61,62). Acute stress favor type 1 response while chronic stress favors type 2 response (63).

The hallmark of type 1 response is the production of IFN-γ, which is the most potent stimulus for the macrophage's ability to kill intracellular pathogens including fungi. Activated macrophages increase inflammation through secretion of TNF, IL-1, chemokines, prostaglandins, leukotriens, and platelet-activating factors. Finally, macrophages remove dead tissue and facilitate damage repair.

Type 2 response is characterized by the production of IL-4, IL-5, IL-9, and IL-13. Effector cells are B lymphocytes and plasma cells with production of IgE antibodies that opsonize helminths. IL-5 activates eosinophils that bind to the opsonized helminths and destroy them. The relative proportions of T_H1/T_H2 subsets induced during an immune response are major determinants of the protective functions and pathologic consequences of the response to a pathogen. Once a type of response is established, T_H1 favors its own expansion by an autocrine mechanism with T_H1 response expanded by IFN-γ and IL-2 while T_H2 response is perpetuated by IL-4.

Lymphocytes that are not completely polarized are called T_H0 and they can simultaneously produce IFN-γ and IL-10.

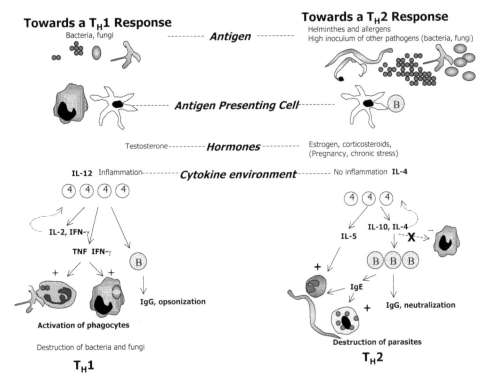

Figure 9 Polarization of T helper Cells. Polarization of T helpers depends on the type of antigen: typically, bacteria and fungi elicit T_H1 and helminths elicit T_H2 response. High inoculum of bacteria and fungi can also elicit T_H2 response. APC: Macrophages drive the response to type 1 and B cells elicit type 2 while DCs can induce both types of response. The environment of the infection site influences in the development of the response: IL-12 produced by macrophages and DCs induce a T_H1 response. T_H1 lymphocytes produce IL-2 and IFN-γ, which will favor their own expansion and will stimulate phagocytes to kill the pathogens. It also induces B cells to produce opsonizing IgG, which will also improve phagocytosis. In the absence of IL-12 production, minimal amount of IL-4 produced by lymphocytes trigger a T_H2 response. T_H2 lymphocytes produce more IL-4, continue their own expansion, and stimulate proliferation and differentiation of B cells and secretion of neutralizing IgG and IgE. IL-4 and IL-10 decrease the phagocytic and killing activities of macrophages. IL-5 stimulates eosinophils. T_H2 is important for the elimination of helminths and ectoparasites. The production of antihelminth-specific antibodies results in opsonization of helminths by these antibodies. Both eosinophils and basophils degranulate after binding to IgE-bound helminth. TNF can be part of the cytokine response in both, T_H1 and T_H2. T_H2 is the default response in the absence of IL-12. Hormones such as corticosteroids, estrogens, progesterone, and adrenaline favor a T_H2 response as a result of their inhibition of the inflammatory response.

A positive correlation has been found between the occurrence of T_H1 cell responses and resistance to experimental infections by various fungi including *C. immitis, P. brasiliensis, H. capsulatum, B. dermatitidis, C. neoformans, A. fumigatus,* and *C. albicans* (64). A type 2 response is associated with fungal proliferation and invasive infection or an allergic reaction (65–68).

The effector CD8+ subset differentiates into Cytolytic T lymphocytes (CTLs) with the ability to kill infected cells (mainly virally infected cells) and tumor cells bearing a specific MHC–antigen complex.

The principal mechanism of CTL killing is through the delivery of granules containing perforins and granzymes. Perforins form aqueous channels in the membrane of the target cell through which granzymes penetrate into the cell and activate caspases, which in turn lead to apoptosis. Caspase activation with cell death can also result from the binding of Fas ligand to T-cells. The role of cytotoxicity in fungal infections is not clear. CD8+ T-cells also produce IFN-γ.

3. Homeostasis

After the elimination of the pathogen, the immune system returns to its basal resting state, in large part because of the apoptosis of antigen-stimulated lymphocytes. The survival of these lymphocytes depends on antigens and antigen-induced growth factors. The elimination of the antigen by the immune response deprives these lymphocytes of their essential survival stimuli leading to their death.

The immune response can be suppressed by T regulatory cells (Tr, CD4+ CD25+) through direct contact with APCs and/or naive T-cells and through secretion of IL-10 and transforming growth factor β (TGF-β), which inhibit T_H1. The role of regulatory cells is to prevent an exaggerated T-cell-mediated response that may result in severe tissue damage. Tr cells may prevent complete eradication of the infection thus allowing the induction of long-term immunity, a mechanism described with candidiasis (69). Tr lymphocytes are also considered tolerance inducers.

4. Memory

Memory T-cells are a population of antigen-specific T lymphocytes that survive for long periods of time even after elimination of the antigen and get rapidly activated when encountering the same antigen.

Memory T-cells accumulate through life and account for about 50% of the adult T-cells. Memory T-cells present in peripheral tissues exhibit a rapid response to encounter with the antigen and are called T effector memory (TEM) while the slower responding T central memory (TCM) are present predominantly in lymphoid organs. TCM is CCR7-high memory and TEM is CCR7-low memory (70,71).

a. Compromised Cell-Mediated Immunity and Fungal Infections. Patients with altered cell immunity include those with AIDS, the recipients of stem cell and organ transplantation, and patients receiving corticosteroids and other immunosuppressive drugs (OKT3, azathioprine, methotrexate, mycophenolate mofetil, tacrolimus, cyclosporine, rapamycin/sirolimus), anti-TNF and anti-IL-2 antibodies.

Patients with altered cell-mediated immunity are susceptible to infections caused by various fungi including *H. capsulatum*, *C. neoformans*, *Pneumocystis carinii*, and *P. marneffei* and dermatophytes including *Aspergillus* spp. and *Candida* spp.

IV. HOST DEFENSES AGAINST THE MOST COMMON FUNGI IN IMMUNOCOMPROMISED HOSTS

A summary of the host defenses against the most common fungal pathogens affecting immunocompromised hosts is shown in Table 4.

Table 4 Host Defenses Against the Most Common Fungi in the Immunosuppressed Host

	Molds	Candida spp.	Cryptococcus neoformans	Dimorphic fungi
Soluble factors	Airway opsonizing and microbicidal substances improve phagocytosis	Lysozyme and Histatin 5 has anticandidal activity (182,183)	Airway opsonizing and microbicidal substances improve phagocytosis	Defensins are fungistatic against Histoplasma capsulatum (130)
Complement	Opsonization, chemotaxis and phagocytosis (13)	C5-deficient mice with disseminated candidiasis have a worse outcome (15)	Opsonization, chemotaxis, and phagocytosis (13)	Histoplasma capsulatum can activate the alternative pathway, although importance for host defense is unknown.
Neutrophils	Hyphal destruction by oxidative and nonoxidative mechanisms. Function and number are critical in host defense (16,73) White blood cell transfusion useful for neutropenic patients with mold infections (22,23).	Critical role. Candida hyphae damaged by oxidative and nonoxidative mechanisms (184) The anticandidal activity is increased by IFN- γ and G-CSF (145,154) Neutropenia is the main risk factor for disseminated candidiasis, CDG patients (defective neutrophils) develop invasive candidiasis	Limited role. Neutropenic mice survive longer than controls (98)	Neutrophils can destroy H. capsulatum through the contents of azurophilic granules (130).
Macrophages	Conidial phagocytosis and destruction, secretion of inflammatory cytokines and chemokines (74,75)	Phagocytes are the effector cells but need T-cell augmentation. Macrophages are indispensable for antifungal killing (185).	Fungal phagocytosis and destruction, secretion of inflammatory cytokines and chemokines. However, yeasts can multiply in the macrophage and kill in the absence of macrophage activation by cytokines (101).	Histoplasma capsulatum: Fungal phagocytosis and destruction, secretion of inflammatory cytokines and chemokines (109), but the fungus can multiply in the macrophage and kill in the absence of macrophage activation by cytokines (186). Penicillium marneffei: Fungal phagocytosis and destruction, secretion of inflammatory cytokines and chemokines (120)
NK cells	Production of IFN-γ favoring a type 1 response. Increased mortality of NK cell-depleted (neutropenic) mice (46)	Production of IFN-γ after exposure to Candida spp. yeasts (164)	Production of IFN-γ favoring a type 1 response (45)	Production of IFN-γ favoring a type 1 response (113). May have cytotoxic activity because perforin-deficient mice have increased mortality (112)

(Continued)

Table 4 Host Defenses Against the Most Common Fungi in the Immunosuppressed Host (*Continued*)

	Molds	*Candida* spp.	*Cryptococcus neoformans*	Dimorphic fungi
DCs	Phagocytosis of fungi (conidia and hyphae), migration to lymph nodes, antigen presentation to T-cells, production of IL-12 and induction of a type 1 response (76)	T_H1 response after stimulation with yeasts, germ-tube forms and hyphae of *Candida albicans* (187). In another study, exposure to conidia results in T_H1 response whereas exposure to hyphae leads to T_H2 response (188)	Phagocytosis of fungi, migration to lymph nodes, antigen presentation to T-cells, production of IL-12, and induction of a type 1 response (189). The fungal capsule interferes with phagocytosis, but anticapsular antibodies improve phagocytosis through Fc receptors (190)	*Histoplasma capsulatum:* Phagocytosis of yeast form, migration to lymph nodes, antigen presentation to T-cells, production of IL-12, and induction of a type 1 response. *Coccidioides immitis:* DC pulsed by a *Coccidioides* lysate mature and induce a specific T_H1 response in vitro (191).
CD4+ cells	Production of IFN-γ and polarization towards a T_H1 protective response.	Critical role in oropharyngeal candidiasis as observed in AIDS (192,193). Local CD4+ lymphocytes may play a role in experimental vaginal candidiasis (194,195)	Production of IFN-γ and polarization toward a T_H1 protective response. Critical role in protection against disseminated and meningeal cryptococcosis (107,196–198)	*Histoplasma capsulatum:* Production of IFN-γ and polarization towards a T_H1 protective response. Critical role in protection in primary infection (111,118). CD4+ cells from spleen of immunized mice transfer protection to animals (199,200). *Penicillium marneffei:* Critical role for host defense (120). *Coccidioides immitis:* low CD4+ lymphocytes correlates with active disease (201,202).
CD8+ cells	Role unknown	Decrease tissue damage in experimental candidiasis (203). Probable protective role of local CD8 cells in experimental vaginal candidiasis (204).	May play a complementary cytotoxic role in the presence of CD4+ cells (104,105).	*Histoplasma capsulatum:* In secondary infection, either CD4 or CD8 is necessary for survival (111). CD8+ may have cytotoxic role (112). Depletion of CD4 and CD8 in mice worsens experimental infections (CD4 depletion alone is worse than CD8 depletion) (205)
Type 1 response	Type 1 cells and cytokines (Table 3) critical for protection in animal models of infection (75,77) IFN-γ as adjuvant	Critical role for protection in animals (87). Failure to develop type 1 response may be the cause of CDC after recovery from	Type 1 cells and cytokines (Table 3) critical for protection in animal models (107). IFN-γ adjuvant therapy is under evaluation in	*Histoplasma capsulatum:* Type 1 cells and cytokines (Table 3) critical for protection in animal models (113). *Paracoccidioides brasiliensis:* Type 1

	therapy for invasive infections in non-neutropenic patients	neutropenia. CMC is associated with the inability to generate a T_H1 response against Candida spp. (91)	humans	response is associated with asymptomatic infection in humans (resistance) (206,207). *Coccidioides immitis*: critical to control the infection (208).
				Histoplasma capsulatum: Type 2 cells and cytokines (Table 3) deleterious in animal models (177). *Paracoccidioides brasiliensis*: Type 2 response is associated with symptomatic infection in humans (206).
Type 2 response	Type 2 cells and cytokines (Table 3) deleterious in animal models of infection. Plays a role in allergic complications, asthma, and allergic broncho-pulmonary aspergillosis (179,209).	Deleterious in animal models of candidiasis (87). Pseudohyphae generate type 2 response (210).	Not protective. IL-4-deficient mice develop weak delayed-type hypersensitivity after challenge with *C. neoformans* (176).	*Histoplasma capsulatum*: A monoclonal antibody against a yeast surface protein increases phagocytosis and intracellular killing by macrophages and prolongs animal survival (116)
Antibodies	Not protective	Protective role in experimental vulvovaginal, disseminated and systemic candidiasis(211,50,51,53,54)	Promote phagocytosis IgG1 > IgG2a = IgG2b > IgG3 (56)	
Vaccines	Partial protection shown in experimental aspergillosis with vaccines based on DCs, recombinant *Aspergillus* antigen, and *Aspergillus* filtrate (83,85,86)	Partial protection against experimental disseminated candidiasis in immunosuppressed mice using a *Candida* membrane antigen (212–214) or Dc-based vaccine (215)	Partial protection in experimental cryptococcosis with various vaccines: culture filtrates (107), recombinant proteins (108), capsular polysaccharide mimotope (57) and APC- based (pulsed with a capsular glucuronoxylmanarman) (198).	*Histoplasma capsulatum*: Partial protection in experimental histoplasmosis with various vaccines: recombinant protein H (117) and Hsp 60 (118). *Coccidioides immitis*: Partial protection in experimental coccidioidomicosis with various vaccines (216–220).

A. Molds

Most of the information related to immunity against molds is based on work on *Aspergillus* spp.

After inhalation in the respiratory tract of a healthy individual, conidia are efficiently eliminated by the innate mucosal local defense. Alveolar macrophages selectively kill conidia (38,72), get activated in response to fungi, and release pro-inflammatory cytokines and chemokines that will result in a second wave of phagocyte recruitment and fungal phagocytosis. Conidia that escape the first line of cellular defense may germinate and grow as hyphae. Protection against hyphae is mediated by neutrophils (73), which is illustrated by the strong clinical association of severe neutropenia and defect of the oxidative killing of neutrophil with invasive aspergillosis (16,24). NK cells may also play a role as depletion of NK cells in neutropenic mice with invasive aspergillosis results in increased fungal burden and mortality (46,74,75).

APCs, mainly DCs, activate B and T-cells resulting in humoral and cellular response. DCs transport the antigen to the draining lymph nodes and present the antigen to T-cells. T-cells will result activated, will proliferate, and migrate to the infected tissue, where they will be polarized to a T_H1 or T_H2 response (76). The presence of IL-18 upregulates the IL-12 receptor on T-cells driving the response to a protective T_H1 type, with production of IFN-γ, which recruits and stimulates the phagocytic and fungicidal activity of neutrophils and macrophages (75,77). Patients who cannot develop a $T_H I$ response are vulnerable to invasive aspergillosis.

Type 2 response is associated with increased susceptibility to invasive aspergillosis in animal models (65,78). Higher serum levels of IL-10 were found in patients with progressive invasive aspergillosis, where as patients with good response to treatment have lower or undetectable levels (79). However, IL-10 is necessary to limit tissue damage and to the development of regulatory CD4+CD25+ T-cells that may lead to long-lasting memory lymphocytes and antifungal immunity (80,81).

Atopic patients initiate a type 2 response characterized by IL-4 and IL-5 cytokine production. IL-4 leads to production by B cells of IgE antibodies against *Aspergillus* antigens, followed by increased sensitization of mast cells. IL-5 recruits eosinophils from the bone marrow to the airways. These patients develop *Aspergillus-associated* asthma or the more complicated manifestation, allergic bronchopulmonary aspergillosis (ABPA). The continuous presence of the fungus on the epithelial surface will result in abundant liberation of antigens eliciting strong antibody production. IL-10 reduces the inflammation seen in animal models of ABPA (82). Studies in animals suggest that it could be possible to drive the immune defense to a beneficial T_H1 type even in immunosuppressed animals by using adoptive transfer of antigen specific CD4+ T-cells producing IFN-γ and IL-2 or by conidial RNA-transfected DCs. Vaccination with *Aspergillus* filtrates or a recombinant antigen with cytosine phosphate guanosine oligodeoxynucleotides as adjuvant promotes a dominant T_H1 response with protective effect in experimental aspergillosis (83–86).

B. Yeasts

1. *Candida spp.*

Candida spp. colonize the gastrointestinal and genital tract of the normal host. The innate and adaptive immunities regulate candidal resistance to prevent progression from simple mucosal colonization to symptomatic infection. Phagocytic cells are the effector cells (neutrophils and mononuclear phagocytes), but intact T-cells are critical for an effective antifungal activity of phagocytes. T_H1 is considered the protective mechanism of defense, and IFN-γ the key cytokine in resistance to *Candida* spp. (87).

IL-10 and the development of regulatory Tr cells are necessary for long-lasting protection. These cells dampen the type 1-mediated antifungal resistance, avoiding inflammatory pathology at the expense of fungal persistence as a commensal. Thus, preventing reactivation rather than complete sterilization of ubiquitous fungal pathogens may represent the ultimate expectation of vaccine-based strategies (69).

The most important manifestations of candidiasis include the following:

- Acute disseminated candidiasis: Neutropenia, neutrophil dysfunction and breakage of the mucosal barrier are the main risk factors for disseminated infections (88). At least two routes of entry are thought to predispose to invasive disease in immunocompromised hosts: translocation from the gastrointestinal tract and infection via intravascular catheters (89).
- Chronic disseminated candidiasis (CDC): develops after marrow recovery following myelosuppressive therapy. Myeloid cells expressing CDllb can inhibit T-cells. These cells are abundant at sites of intensive hematopoiesis and in tumor-bearing hosts. Inhibition of lymphocytes by these cells may be responsible for the failure to develop a type 1 response to overcome the infection. The inhibitory effect of suppressor granulocytes appears to be mediated by CD80/CD28. CD80 is upregulated in neutrophils after exposure to hyphae from *Candida*. It was demonstrated that mice with overwhelming *Candida* infection have an expanded population of granulocytes expressing CDllb and CD80, which suggests that these neutrophils act as myeloid suppressor cells, skewing the adaptive immunity to a type 2, non protective response (90).
- Mucosal candidiasis: defense against this infection relies on cell-mediated immunity. As a consequence, mucosal candidiasis is common in patients with AIDS. Of interest, patients with deficit in IFN-γ or IL-12 receptor are not susceptible to this infection.
- Chronic mucocutaneous candidiasis (CMC): is a chronic, debilitating disease secondary to a failure to develop T_H1 response to *Candida,* leading to persistence of fungi in the skin, nails, and mucosa (91). In CMC patients, the innate immunity and antibody response are normal but a defect in the cell-mediated immunity with a switch to a T_H2 type of cytokine response against *Candida* antigens is present (91–93).
- Vulvovaginal candidiasis develop in immunocompetent women, which can be acute, chronic, or recurrent, sometimes very difficult to treat. Local response is more important than the systemic immune response in the defense of this form of infection.

2. *Cryptococcus neoformans*

Cryptococcosis is a rare disease in individuals with normal host defenses, despite the presence of relatively common asymptomatic infection (94). Cell-mediated immunity is critical in protecting against cryptococcal infections because deficit in T-cells is the most common risk factor associated with cryptococcosis (95–97).

Cryptococcus neoformans is acquired via the respiratory tract and the normal host develops immunity against it during self-limited, asymptomatic infection.

Alveolar macrophages are the first cells to encounter cryptococcal yeasts and are able to kill the fungi. TNF and chemokines are essential for the recruitment of inflammatory cells and CD4+ T lymphocytes. NK cells are important in the development of a T_H1 response (45). Neutrophils can efficiently ingest and kill *C. neoformans* in vitro, but their role in the clinical setting is not important (98). DCs process and present the antigen to T-cells and generate the protective T_H1 response. IFN-γ stimulates macrophages to finally eliminate the fungi. Failure to produce TNF or IL-12 is associated with increased levels of IL-4 and IL-5, pulmonary eosinophilia, and persistence of fungi (99–103). CD8+ cells can be cytotoxic against *C. neoformans*, but the clinical significance of this response is not clear. CD8+ cells are dependent on CD4+ signals (104,105).

The capsule and melanin of *C. neoformans* downregulate the immune response, and encapsulated *C. neoformans* are more protected from phagocytosis than nonencapsulated variants. Monoclonal antibodies against GXM can reduce fungal burden in infected mice. The antibodies can enhance host defense against *C. neoformans* by promoting more effective cellular immunity. However, studies in animal models have shown that the effect depends on dose, type of antibody, and inoculum size (56). Passive antibody-mediated protection against *C. neoformans* requires both type 1 and type 2-associated cytokines (106).

Animal studies using vaccines with different antigens from *C. neoformans* confer protection to animals by inducing T_H1 response (107,108).

C. Dimorphic Fungi

Sporothrix schencki and agents of chromomycosis have worldwide distribution, but diseases are common only in tropical and subtropical areas and are secondary to traumatic inoculation with subcutaneous and osteoarticular involvement. More invasive and disseminated infections occur in patients with AIDS or those receiving immunosuppressive therapy.

Histoplasma capsulatum, B. dermatitidis, C. immitis, and *P. brasiliensis* cause endemic infections, which can be life-threatening in patients with defects in cellular-mediated immunity. Acquisition of infection is through inhalation of airborne fungi, although *P. brasiliensis* is usually acquired through cutaneous inoculation.

1. Histoplasma Capsulatum

Normal host may develop self-limited respiratory or systemic symptoms of histoplasmosis but immunocompromised host, such as patients with AIDS or patients receiving immunosuppressive therapy for cancer, transplantation, and autoimmune diseases can develop disseminated infections.

Histoplasma capsulatum is a facultative intracellular parasite that lives in macrophages. Macrophages are the principal effector cells in host resistance. The yeast can replicate inside the macrophage and inhibit the fusion of lysosomes with phagosomes until host resistance develops with the subsequent activation of macrophages to destroy the yeast and eradicate the infection (109). TNF, IL-12, GM-CSF, and induction of CD4+ T-cell type 1 response are critical for the successful killing of the intracellular yeast during primary infection. In secondary infection, CD4+ or CD8+ cells are necessary for survival, and TNF becomes the key regulator of host resistance (110–113). The development of disseminated histoplasmosis among recipients of TNF antibodies highlights the importance of TNF in the protection against this infection (114,115). Antibodies to the cell wall of *H. capsulatum* can also have a role. They opsonize the yeast and increase macrophage phagocytosis and killing and are associated with increased IL-4, IL-6, and IFN-γ in murine lungs (116).

Protective vaccines have been developed that induce type 1 cytokine response in experimental pulmonary histoplasmosis (117). Recombinant Hsp60 from *H. capsulatum* also confers protection to mice mediated by CD4+ cells and production of IFN-γ and IL-12 (118).

2. Penicillium Marneffei

Penicillium marneffei is another dimorphic fungi that can cause disseminated infections in immunocompromised patients, specially in AIDS patients in southeast Asia (119). This observation suggests that cell-mediated immunity is the main host defense against these fungi.

Penicillium marneffei conidia reach the lungs and are ingested by macrophages, where they multiply as yeast.

Macrophages can kill the yeast by release of nitric oxide, but macrophage activation by T-cell derived cytokines, mainly IFN-γ, is critical for this activity (120).

D. Dermatophytosis and Other Cutaneous Fungal Infections

The normal skin is not suitable for the development of fungi, because of the presence of bacteria and keratin. Keratinocytes are the most common cells in the epidermis, not only form a physical barrier to micro-organisms, but also mediate immune reactions. They secrete cytokines that regulate the immune response including basic fibroblast growth factor, platelet-derived growth factors, transforming growth factor β, and TNF, IL-1, IL-3, IL-6, IL-7, IL-8, GM-CSF, G-CSF, and M-CSF. Keratinocytes express constitutively MHC class I and express MHC class II molecules when exposed to IFN-γ produced by infiltrating lymphocytes.

Local cutaneous conditions (warmth, moisture, and occlusion) are important factors in the development of dermatophytosis. Underlying diseases such as diabetes, or immunosuppressive therapy, and peripheral vascular diseases are associated with chronic infections. If the fungi progress beyond the stratum corneum of the skin, neutrophils and macrophages will be recruited to the infection site and initiate the inflammatory response (121). Endothelial cells participate in wound healing, angiogenesis, production of clotting factors, and secretion of cytokines and chemokines to recruit the immune cells. DCs are distributed in the dermis and epidermis while T-cells are mainly beneath the dermal–epidermal junction. DCs migrate with the antigen to lymph nodes where they initiate activation and clonal expansion of T-cells that migrate back to the dermis and epidermis by homing to cytokine-activated microvascular endothelial cells in the area. At the infection site, the T-cells can be restimulated to continue clonal expansion and generation of more effector T-cells to eliminate the micro-organisms. When the infection is cleared, some of memory T-cells may stay locally. Antibodies against fungal agents of the skin are present in the circulation in higher levels in patients who have cutaneous fungal infection.

Dermatophytes and *Candida* spp. hydrolyze keratin and facilitate the development of fungal infection in the stratum corneum where the cells of the immune system are barely present. The dermatophytes generally cause infections confined to the skin, but *C. albicans*, *Malassezia furfur* (the causative agent of tinea versicolor or pityriasis), *Trichosporon beigelii* (the causative agent of White piedra), and

T. pullulans are able to disseminate in patients with defective immunity (122). Most patients with chronic dermatophytosis are relatively intact immunologically. It is possible that an IgE response in some patients with chronic dermatophytes may inhibit the development of protective cell-mediated immune response (123).

The CD4+ lymphocytes and activated lymphocytes from peripheral blood of patients with dermatophytosis are significantly lower than in healthy individuals suggesting a role for cell-mediated immunity (124). Adequate cell-mediated immune response to *Malassezia* antigens has been demonstrated in noninfected human subjects, whereas patients with tinea versicolor (*Malassezia* infection) appear to have deficient cell-mediated immune response to the same antigen. Dermatophytosis, pityriasis, and mucocutaneous candidiasis are common in AIDS patients, which also suggests the importance of cell-mediated immunity against these fungal infections (125).

V. CONCLUSION

Susceptibility for invasive fungal infection is a function of both the virulence capacity of the fungal organism and the integrity of host defenses. Impairment of normal host defenses can occur by disease or by treatment of a disease that results in unintended compromise of one or more of the elements of innate or acquired immunity. After exposure to a potential fungal pathogen, the likelihood that invasive infection will occur which results in illness depends on the type of host defense compromised, the degree and duration of compromise, and the importance of the compromised host defense element for control of the given potential pathogen. Advances in understanding of host innate and adaptive immunities have led to new insights into the risks for infection and new strategies to improve control of infection.

REFERENCES

1. Ganz T. Antimicrobial proteins andpeptides in host defense. Semin Respir Infect 2001; 16(1):4–10.
2. Meier A, et al. Toll-like receptor (TLR) 2 and TLR4 are essential for Aspergillus-induced activation of murine macrophages. Cell Microbiol 2003; 5(8):561–570.
3. Brown GD, Gordon S. Immune recognition. A new receptor for beta-glucans. Nature 2001; 413(6851):36–37.
4. Brown GD, et al. Dectin-1 mediates the biological effects of beta-glucans. J Exp Med 2003; 197(9):1119–1124.
5. Wang JE, et al. Involvement of CD14 and toll-like receptors in activation of human monocytes by *Aspergilhts fumigatus* hyphae. Infect Immun 2001; 69(4):2402–2406.
6. Braedel S, et al. *Aspergillus fumigatus* antigens activate innate immune cells via toll-like receptors 2 and 4. Br J Haematol 2004; 125(3):392–399.
7. Netea MG, et al. The role of toll-like receptor (TLR) 2 and TLR4 in the host defense against disseminated candidiasis. J Infect Dis 2002; 185(10):1483–1489.
8. Shoham S, et al. Toll-like receptor 4 mediates intracellular signaling without TNF-alpha release in response to *Cryptococcus neoformans* polysaccharide capsule. J Immunol 2001; 166(7):4620–4626.
9. Ahlin A, Elinder G, Palmblad J. Dose-dependent enhancements by interferon-gamma on functional responses of neutrophils from chronic granulomatous disease patients. Blood 1997; 89(9):3396–3401.

10. Lu J, et al. Collectins and ficolins: sugar pattern recognition molecules of the mammalian innate immune system. Biochim Biophys Acta 2002; 1572(2–3):387–400.

11. Garlanda C, et al. Non-redundant role of the long pentraxin PTX3 in anti-fungal innate immune response. Nature 2002; 420(6912):182–186.

12. Neth O, et al. Mannose-binding lectin binds to a range of clinically relevant microorganisms and promotes complement deposition. Infect Immun 2000; 68(2):688–693.

13. Kozel TR. Activation of the complement system by pathogenic fungi. Clin Microbiol Rev 1996; 9(1):34–46.

14. Clemons KV, Stevens DA. Overview of host defense mechanisms in systemic mycoses the basis for immunotherapy. Semin Respir Infect 2001; 16(1):60–66.

15. Ashman RB, et al. Role of complement C5 and T lymphocytes in pathogenesis of disseminated and mucosal candidiasis in susceptible DBA/2 mice. Microb Pathog 2003; 34(2):103–113.

16. Chang HY, et al. Causes of death in adults with acute leukemia. Medicine (Baltimore), 1976; 55(3):259–268.

17. Warnock DW. Fungal infections in neutropenia: current problems and chemotherapeutic control. J Antimicrob Chemother 1998; 41(suppl D):95–105.

18. Roilides E, et al. Immunomodulation of invasive fungal infections. Infect Dis Clin North Am 2003; 17(1):193–219.

19. Hubel K, Dale DC, Liles WC. Therapeutic use of cytokines to modulate phagocyte function for the treatment of infectious diseases: current status of granulocyte colony-stimulating factor, Granulocyte–macrophage colony–stimulating factor, macrophage colony-stimulating factor, interferon-gamma. J Infect Dis 2002; 185(10):1490–1501.

20. Dale D. Current management of chemotherapy-induced neutropenia: the role of colony- stimulating factors. Semin Oncol 2003; 30(4 suppl 13):3–9.

21. Dale DC. Colony-stimulating factors for the management of neutropenia in cancer patients. Drugs 2002; 62(suppl 1):1–15.

22. Dignani MC, et al. Treatment of neutropenia-related fungal infections with granulocyte colony-stimulating factor-elicited white blood cell transfusions: a pilot study. Leukemia 1997; 11(10):1621–1630.

23. Jendiroba DB, Freireich EJ. Granulocyte transfusions: from neutrophil replacement to immunereconstitution. Blood Rev 2000; 14:219–227.

24. Liese J, et al. Long-term follow-up and outcome of 39 patients with chronic granulomatous disease. J Pediatr 2000;137(5):687–693.

25. The International Chronic Granulomatous Disease Cooperative Study Group. A controlled trial of interferon gamma to prevent infection in chronic granulomatous disease. N Engl J Med 1991; 324(8):509–516.

26. Babula O, et al. Relation between recurrent vulvovaginal candidiasis, vaginal concentrations of mannose-binding lectin, and a mannose-binding lectin gene polymorphism in Latvian women. Clin Infect Dis 2003; 37(5):733–737.

27. Eisen DP, Minchinton RM. Impact of mannose-binding lectin on susceptibility to infectious diseases. Clin Infect Dis 2003; 37(11):1496–1505.

28. Crosdale DJ, et al. Mannose-binding lectin gene polymorphisms as a susceptibility factor for chronic necrotizing pulmonary aspergillosis. J Infect Dis 2001; 184(5):653–656.

29. Aratani Y, et al. Differential host susceptibility to pulmonary infections with bacteria and fungi in mice deficient in myeloperoxidase. J Infect Dis 2000; 182(4):1276–1279.

30. Geerlings SE, Hoepelman AI. Immune dysfunction in patients with diabetes mellitus (DM). FEMS Immunol Med Microbiol 1999; 26:259–265.

31. Lionakis MS, Kontoyiannis DP. Glucocorticoids and invasive fungal infections. Lancet 2003; 362(9398):1828–1838.

32. Monari C, et al. Neutrophils from patients with advanced human immunodeficiency virus infection have impaired complement receptor function and preserved Fc gamma receptor function. J Infect Dis 1999; 180(5):1542–1549.

33. Roilides E, et al. Impairment of neutrophil antifungal activity against hyphae of *Aspergillus fumigatus* in children infected with human immunodeficiency virus. J Infect Dis 1993; 167(4):905–911.
34. Ng TT, Robson GD, Denning DW. Hydrocortisone-enhanced growth of *Aspergillus* spp.: implications for pathogenesis. Microbiology 1994; 140(Pt 9):2475–2479.
35. Roilides E, et al. Prevention of corticosteroid-induced suppression of human polymorphonuclear leukocyte-induced damage of *Aspergillus fumigatus* hyphae by granulocyte colony-stimulating factor and gamma interferon. Infect Immun 1993; 61(11):4870–4877.
36. Vora S, et al. Activity of voriconazole, a new triazole, combined with neutrophils or monocytes against *Candida albicans*: effect of granulocyte colony-stimulating factor and granulocyte–macrophage colony-stimulating factor. Antimicrob Agents Chemother 1998; 42(4):907–910.
37. Sionov E, Segal E. G-CSF in combination with polyenes or polyene-intralipid admixtures in treatment of murine aspergillosis. ISHAM, San Antonio, Tx, 2003.
38. Philippe B, et al. Killing of *Aspergillus fumigatus* by alveolar macrophages is mediated by reactive oxidant intermediates. Infect Immun 2003; 71(6):3034–3042.
39. Brummer E, Maqbool A, Stevens DA. In vivo GM-CSFprevents dexamethasone suppression of killing of *Aspergillus fumigatus* conidia by bronchoalveolar macrophages. J Leukoc Biol 2001; 70(6):868–872.
40. Hobson RP. The effects of diffusates from the spores of *Aspergillus fumigatus* and *A. terreus* on human neutrophils, *Naegleria gruberi* and *Acanthamoeba castellanii*. Med Mycol 2000; 38(2):133–141.
41. Yoshida LS, Abe S, Tsunawaki S. Fungal gliotoxin targets the onset of superoxide-generating NADPH oxidase of human neutrophils. Biochem Biophys Res Commun 2000; 268(3):716–723.
42. Hasegawa Y, et al. The effect of an *Aspergillus fumigatus* derived elastolytic proteinase on human neutrophils. Nippon Ishinkin Gakkai Zasshi 1999; 40(4):235–238.
43. Tsunawaki S, et al. Fungal metabolite gliotoxin inhibits assembly of the human respiratory burst NADPH oxidase. Infect Immun 2004; 72(6):3373–3382.
44. Murayama T, et al. Effects of *Aspergillus fumigatus* culture filtrate on antifungal activity of human phagocytes in vitro. Thorax 1998; 53(11):975–978.
45. Kawakami K, et al. NK cells eliminate *Cryptococcus neoformans* by potentiating the fungicidal activity of macrophages rather than by directly killing them upon stimulation with IL-12 andIL-18. Microbiol Immunol 2000; 44(12):1043–1050.
46. Morrison BE, et al. Chemokine-mediated recruitment of NK cells is a critical host defense mechanism in invasive aspergillosis. J Clin Invest 2003; 112(12):1862–1870.
47. Willcox MD, et al. Interactions between *Candida* species and platelets. J Med Microbiol 1998; 47(2):103–110.
48. Christin L, et al. Human platelets damage *Aspergillus fumigatus* hyphae and may supplement killing by neutrophils. Infect Immun 1998; 66(3):1181–1189.
49. Wagner RD, et al. B cell knockout mice are resistant to mucosal and systemic candidiasis of endogenous origin but susceptible to experimental systemic candidiasis. J Infect Dis 1996; 174(3):589–597.
50. Han Y, Riesselman MH, Cutler JE. Protection against candidiasis by an immunoglobulin G3 (IgG3) monoclonal antibody specific for the same mannotriose as an IgM protective antibody. Infect Immun 2000; 68(3):1649–1654.
51. Han Y, et al. Complement is essential for protection by an IgM and an IgG3 monoclonal antibody against experimental, hematogenously disseminated candidiasis. J Immunol 2001; 167(3):1550–1557.
52. Moragues MD, et al. A monoclonal antibody directed against a *Candida albicans* cell wall mannoprotein exerts three anti-*C. albicans* activities. Infect Immun 2003; 71(9):5273–5279.

53. Matthews R, Hodgetts S, Burnie J. Preliminary assessment of a human recombinant antibody fragment to hsp9O in murine invasive candidiasis. J Infect Dis 1995; 171(6): 1668–1671.

54. Matthews RC, et al. Preclinical assessment of the efficacy of mycograb, a human recombinant antibody against fungal HSP90. Antimicrob Agents Chemother 2003; 47(7): 2208–2216.

55. Polonelli L, et al. Therapeutic activity of an engineered synthetic killer antiidiotypic antibody fragment against experimental mucosal and systemic candidiasis. Infect Immun 2003; 71(11):6205–6212.

56. Taborda CP, et al. More is not necessarily better: prozone-like effects in passive immunization with IgG. J Immunol 2003; 170(7):3621–3630.

57. Fleuridor R, Lees A, Pirofski L. A cryptococcal capsularpolysaccharide mimotope prolongs the survival of mice with *Cryptococcus neoformans* infection. J Immunol 2001; 166(2):1087–1096.

58. Casadevall A, Feldmesser M, Pirofski LA. Induced humoral immunity and vaccination against major human fungal pathogens. Curr Opin Microbiol 2002; 5(4):386–391.

59. Burger D, Dayer JM. Cytokines, acute-phase proteins, and hormones: IL-1 and TNF-alpha production in contact-mediated activation of monocytes by T lymphocytes. Ann NY Acad Sci 2002; 966:464–473.

60. Cutolo M, et al. Androgens and estrogens modulate the immune and inflammatory responses in rheumatoid arthritis. Ann NY Acad Sci 2002; 966:131–142.

61. Powell BL, et al. Relationship of progesterone- and estradiol-binding proteins in *Coccidioides immitis* to coccidioidal dissemination in pregnancy. Infect Immun 1983; 40(2):478–485.

62. Whitt SP, et al. Histoplasmosis in pregnancy: case series and report of transplacental transmission. Arch Intern Med 2004; 164(4):454–458.

63. Dhabhar FS. Stress-induced augmentation of immune function—the role of stress hormones, leukocyte trafficking, and cytokines. Brain Behav Immun 2002; 16(6):785–798.

64. Romani L. The T-cell response against fungal infections. Curr Opin Immunol 1997; 9(4):484–490.

65. Cenci E, et al. Th1 and Th2 cytokines in mice with invasive aspergillosis. Infect Immun 1997; 65(2):564–570.

66. Magee DM, Cox RA. Interleukin-12 regulation of host defenses against *Coccidioides immitis*. Infect Immun 1996; 64(9):3609–3613.

67. Decken K, et al. Interleukin-12 is essential for a protective Th1 response in mice infected with *Cryptococcus neoformans*. Infect Immun 1998; 66(10):4994–5000.

68. Mencacci A, et al. Low-dose streptozotocin-induced diabetes in mice. II. Susceptibility to *Candida albicans* infection correlates with the induction of a biased Th2-like antifungal response. Cell Immunol 1993; 150(1):36–44.

69. Montagnoli C, et al. B7/CD28-dependent CD4+ CD25+ regulatory T-cells are essential components of the memory-protective immunity to *Candida albicans*. J Immunol 2002; 169(11):6298–6308.

70. Langenkamp A, et al. Kinetics and expression patterns of chemokine receptors in human CD4+ T lymphocytes primed by myeloid or plasmacytoid dendritic cells. Eur J Immunol 2003; 33(2):474–482.

71. Esser MT, et al. Memory T-cells and vaccines. Vaccine 2003; 21(5–6):419–430.

72. Ibrahim-Granet O, et al. Phagocytosis and intracellular fate of *Aspergillus fumigatus* conidia in alveolar macrophages. Infect Immun 2003; 71(2):891–903.

73. Schaffner A, Douglas H, Braude A. Selective protection against conidia by mononuclear and against mycelia by polymorphonuclear phagocytes in resistance to *Aspergillus*. Observations on these two lines of defense in vivo and in vitro with human and mouse phagocytes. J Clin Invest 1982; 69(3):617–631.

74. Schelenz S, Smith DA, Bancroft GJ. Cytokine and chemokine responses following pulmonary challenge with *Aspergillus fumigatus*: obligatory role of TNF-alpha and GM-CSF in neutrophil recruitment. Med Mycol 1999; 37(3):183–194.

75. Brieland JK, et al. Cytokine networking in lungs of immunocompetent mice in response to inhaled *Aspergillus fumigatus*. Infect Immun 2001; 69(3):1554–1560.

76. Bozza S, et al. Dendritic cells transport conidia and hyphae of *Aspergillus fumigatus* from the airways to the draining lymph nodes and initiate disparate Th responses to the fungus. J Immunol 2002; 168(3):1362–1371.

77. Cenci E, et al. Cytokine- and T helper-dependent lung mucosal immunity in mice with invasive pulmonary aspergillosis. J Infect Dis 1998; 178(6):1750–1760.

78. Cenci E, et al. Interleukin-4 causes susceptibility to invasive pulmonary aspergillosis through suppression of protective type I responses. J Infect Dis 1999; 180(6):1957–1968.

79. Roilides E, et al. Elevated serum concentrations of interleukin-10 in nonneutropenic patients with invasive aspergillosis. J Infect Dis 2001; 183(3):518–520.

80. Clemons KV, et al. Role of IL-10 in invasive aspergillosis: increased resistance of IL-10 gene knockout mice to lethal systemic aspergillosis. Clin Exp Immunol 2000; 122(2): 186-191.

81. Montagnoli C, et al. A role for antibodies in the generation of memory antifungal immunity. Eur J Immunol 2003; 33(5):1193–1204.

82. Grunig G, et al. Interlenkin-10 is a natural suppressor of cytokine production and inflammation in a murine model of allergic bronchopulmonary aspergillosis. J Exp Med 1997; 185(6):1089–1099.

83. Ito JI, Lyons JM. Vaccination of corticosteroid immunosuppressed mice against invasive pulmonary aspergillosis. J Infect Dis 2002; 186(6):869–871.

84. Cenci E, et al. T-cell vaccination in mice with invasive pulmonary aspergillosis. J Immunol 2000; 165(1):381–388.

85. Bozza S, et al. A dendritic cell vaccine against invasive aspergillosis in allogeneic hematopoietic transplantation. Blood 2003; 102(10):3807–3814.

86. Bozza S, et al. Vaccination of mice against invasive aspergillosis with recombinant *Aspergillus* proteins and CpG oligodeoxynucleotides as adjuvants. Microb Infect 2002; 4(13):1281–1290.

87. Romani L, et al. Gamma interferon modifies CD4$^+$ subset expression in murine candidiasis. Infect Immun 1992; 60(11):4950–4952.

88. Maertens J, Vrebos M, Boogaerts M. Assessing risk factors for systemic fungal infections. Eur J Cancer Care (Engl) 2001; 10(1):56–62.

89. Nucci M, Anaissie E. Revisiting the source of candidemia: skin or gut? Clin Infect Dis 2001; 33(12):1959–1967.

90. Mencacci A, et al. CD80+ Gr-I+ myeloid cells inhibit development of antifungal Th1 immunity in mice with candidiasis. J Immunol 2002; 169(6):3180–3190.

91. Lilic D, et al. Deregulated production of protective cytokines in response to *Candida albicans* infection in patients with chronic mucocutaneous candidiasis. Infect Immun 2003; 71(10):5690–5699.

92. Zuccarello D, et al. Familial chronic nail candidiasis with ICAM-1 deficiency: a new form of chronic mucocutaneous candidiasis. J Med Genet 2002; 39(9):671–675.

93. Kalfa VC, Roberts RL, Stiehm ER. The syndrome of chronic mucocutaneous candidiasis with selective antibody deficiency. Ann Allergy Asthma Immunol 2003; 90(2): 259–264.

94. Chen LC, et al. Antibody response to *Cryptococcus neoformans* proteins in rodents and humans. Infect Immun 1999; 67(5):2218–2224.

95. Chuck SL, Sande MA. Infections with *Cryptococcus neoformans* in the acquired immunodeficiency syndrome. N Engl J Med 1989; 321(12):794–799.

96. Mitchell TG, Perfect JR. Cryptococcosis in the era of AIDS—100 years after the discovery of *Cryptococcus neoformans*. Clin Microbiol Rev 1995; 8(4):515–548.

97. Cheung MC, Rachlis AR, Shumak SL. A cryptic cause of cryptococcal meningitis. CMAJ 2003; 168(4):451–452.
98. Mednick AJ, et al. Neutropenia alters lung cytokine production in mice and reduces their susceptibility to pulmonary cryptococcosis. Eur J Immunol 2003; 33(6):1744–1753.
99. Bauman SK, Huffnagle GB, Murphy JW. Effects of tumor necrosis factor alpha on dendritic cell accumulation in lymph nodes draining the immunization site and the impact on the anticryptococcal cell-mediated immune response. Infect Immun 2003; 71(1):68–74.
100. Huffhagle GB, et al. Afferent phase production of TNF-alpha is required for the development of protective Tcell immunity to *Cryptococcus neoformans*. J Immunol 1996; 157(10):4529–4536.
101. Huffiagle GB. Role of cytokines in T-cell immunity to a pulmonary *Cryptococcus neoformans* infection. Biol Signals 1996; 5(4):215–222.
102. Huffnagle GB, et al. The role of monocyte chemotactic protein-1 (MCP-1) in the recruitment of monocytes and CD4+ Tcells during a pulmonary *Cryptococcus neoformans* infection. J Immunol 1995; 155(10):4790–4797.
103. Traynor TR, et al. CCR2 expression determines T1 versus T2 polarization during pulmonary *Cryptococcus neoformans* infection. J Immunol 2000; 164(4):2021–2027.
104. Syme RM, et al. Both CD4+ and CD8+ human lymphocytes are activated and proliferate in response to *Cryptococcus neoformans*. Immunology 1997; 92(2):194–200.
105. Ma LL, et al. CDS T-cell-mediated killing of *Cryptococcus neoformans* requires granulysin and is dependent on CD4 T-cells and IL-15. J Immunol 2002; 169(10):5787–5795.
106. Beenhouwer DO, et al. Both Thl and Th2 cytokines affect the ability of monoclonal antibodies to protect mice against *Cryptococcus neoformans*. Infect Immun 2001; 69(10):6445–6455.
107. Murphy JW, et al. Antigen-induced protective and nonprotective cell-mediated immune components against *Cryptococcus neoformans*. Infect Immun 1998; 66(6):2632–2639.
108. Biondo C, et al. Identification and cloning of a cryptococcal deacetylase that produces protective immune responses. Infect Immun 2002; 70(5):2383–2391.
109. Newman SL. Cell-mediated immunity to *Histoplasma capsulatum*. Semin Respir Infect 2001; 16(2):102–108.
110. Deepe GS Jr, Gibbons R, Woodward E. Neutralization of endogenous granulocyte–macrophage colony-stimulating factor subverts the protective immune response to *Histoplasma capsulatum*. J Immunol 1999; 163(9):4985–4893.
111. Allendorfer R, Brunner GD, Deepe GS Jr. Complex requirements for nascent and memory immunity in pulmonary histoplasmosis. J Immunol 1999; 162(12):7389–7396.
112. Zhou P, et al. Perform is required for primary immunity to *Histoplasma capsulatum*. J Immunol 2001; 166(3):1968–1974.
113. Cain JA, Deepe GS Jr. Evolution of the primary immune response to *Histoplasma capsulatum* in murine lung. Infect Immun 1998; 66(4):1473–1481.
114. Wood KL, et al. Histoplasmosis after treatment with anti-tumor necrosis factor-alpha therapy. Am J Respir Crit Care Med 2003; 167(9):1279–1282.
115. Lee JH, et al. Life-threatening histoplasmosis complicating immunotherapy with tumor necrosis factor alpha antagonists infliximab and etanercept. Arthritis Rheum 2002; 46(10):2565–2570.
116. Nosanchuk JD, et al. Antibodies to a cell surface histone-like protein protect against *Histoplasma capsulatum*. J Clin Invest 2003; 112(8):1164–1175.
117. Deepe GS Jr, Gibbons R. Protective efficacy of H antigen from *Histoplasma capsulatum* in a murine model of pulmonary histoplasmosis. Infect immun 2001; 69(5):3128–3134.
118. Deepe GS Jr, Gibbons RS. Cellular and molecular regulation of vaccination with heat shock protein 60 from *Histoplasma capsulatum*. Infect Immun 2002; 70(7):3759–3767.
119. Supparatpinyo K, et al. Disseminated *Penicillium marneffei* infection in southeast Asia. Lancet 1994; 344(8915):110–113.

120. Sisto F, et al. Differential cytokine pattern in the spleens and livers of BALB/c mice infected with *Penicillium marneffei*: protective role of gamma interferon. Infect Immun 2003; 71(1):465–473.

121. Calderon RA, Hay RJ. Fungicidal activity of human neutrophils and monocytes on dermatophyte fungi, *Trichophyton quinckeanum* and *Trichophyton rubrum*. Immunology 1987; 61(3):289–295.

122. Wagner DK, Sohnle PG. Cutaneous defenses against dermatophytes and yeasts. Clin Microbiol Rev 1995; 8(3):317–335.

123. Leibovici V, et al. Imbalance of immune responses in patients with chronic and widespread fungal skin infection. Clin Exp Dermatol 1995; 20(5):390–394.

124. Maleszka R, Adamski Z, Dworacki G. Evaluation of lymphocytes subpopulations and natural killer cells in peripheral blood of patients treated for dermatophyte onychomycosis. Mycoses 2001; 44(11–12):487–492.

125. Odom RB. Common superficial fungal infections in immunosuppressed patients. J Am Acad Dermatol 1994; 31(3 Pt 2):S56–S59.

126. Hoover DM, et al. Antimicrobial characterization of human beta-defensin 3 derivatives. Antimicrob Agents Chemother 2003; 47(9):2804–2809.

127. Thevissen K, et al. Defensins from insects and plants interact with fungal glucosylceramides. J Biol Chem 2004; 279(6):3900–3905.

128. Yoshio H, et al. Antimicrobial polypeptides of human vernix caseosa and amniotic fluid: implications for newborn innate defense. Pediatr Res 2003; 53(2):211–216.

129. Mambula SS, et al. Human neutrophil-mediated nonoxidative antifungal activity against *Cryptococcus neoformans*. Infect Immun 2000; 68(11):6257–6264.

130. Newman SL, et al. Identification of constituents of human neutrophil azurophil granules that mediate fungistasis against *Histoplasma capsulatum*. Infect Immun 2000; 68(10):5668–5672.

131. Samaranayake YH, et al. Antifungal effects of lysozyme and lactoferrin against genetically similar, sequential *Candida albicans* isolates from a human immunodeficiency virus-infected southern Chinese cohort. J Clin Microbiol 2001; 39(9):3296–3302.

132. Lupetti A, et al. Antimicrobial peptides: therapeutic potential for the treatment of *Candida* infections. Expert Opin Investig Drugs 2002; 11(2):309–318.

133. Tomee JF, et al. Antileukoprotease: an endogenous protein in the innate mucosal defense against fungi. J Infect Dis 1997; 176(3):740–747.

134. Aratani Y, et al. Relative contributions of myeloperoxidase and NADPH-oxidase to the early host defense against pulmonary infections with *Candida albicans* and *Aspergillus fumigatus*. Med Mycol 2002; 40(6):557–563.

135. Peterslund NA, et al. Association between deficiency of mannose-binding lectin and severe infections after chemotherapy. Lancet 2001; 358(9282):637–638.

136. Rosseau S, et al. Surfactant protein A down-regulates proinflammatory cytokine production evoked by *Candida albicans* in human alveolar macrophages and monocytes. J Immunol 1999; 163(8):4495–4502.

137. Holmskov U, Steffen T, Jensenius JC. Collectins and ficolins: humoral lectins of the innate immune defense. Annl Rev Immunol 2003; 21:547–578.

138. Lappin MB, Campbell JD. The Th1–Th2 classification of cellular immune responses: concepts, current thinking and applications in haematological malignancy. Blood Rev 2000; 14(4):228–239.

139. Nagai H, et al. Interferon-gamma and tumor necrosis factor-alpha protect mice from invasive aspergillosis. J Infect Dis 1995; 172(6):1554–1560.

140. Deepe GS Jr, Gibbons RS. Protective and memory immunity to *Histoplasma capsulatum* in the absence of IL-10. J Immunol 2003; 171(10):5353–5362.

141. Roilides E, et al. Tumor necrosis factor alpha enhances antifungal activities of polymorphonuclear and mononuclear phagocytes against *Aspergillus fumigatus*. Infect Immun 1998; 66(12):5999–6003.

142. Warris A, Bjorneklett A, Gaustad P. Invasive pulmonary aspergillosis associated with infliximab therapy. N Engl J Med 2001; 344(14):1099–1100.

143. Roilides E, et al. Enhancement of oxidative response and damage caused by human neutrophils to *Aspergillus fumigatus* hyphae by granulocyte colony-stimulating factor and gamma interferon. Infect Immun 1993; 61(4):1185–1193.

144. Roilides E, et al. Antifungal activity of elutriated human monocytes against *Aspergillus fumigatus* hyphae: enhancement by granulocyte–macrophage colony-stimulating factor and interferon-gamma. J Infect Dis 1994; 170(4):894–899.

145. Gaviria JM, et al. Modulation of neutrophil-mediated activity against the pseudohyphal form of *Candida albicans* by granulocyte colony-stimulating factor (G-CSF) administered in vivo. J Infect Dis 1999; 179(5):1301–1304.

146. Liles WC. Immunomodulatory approaches to augment phagocyte-mediated host defense for treatment of infectious diseases. Semin Respir Infect 2001; 16(1):11–17.

147. Rex JH, et al. In vivo interferon-gamma therapy augments the in vitro ability of chronic granulomatous disease neutrophils to damage *Aspergillus* hyphae. J Infect Dis 1991; 163(4):849–852.

148. Clemons KV, Lutz JE, Stevens DA. Efficacy of recombinant gamma interferon for treatment of systemic cryptococcosis in SCID mice. Antimicrob Agents Chemother 2001; 45(3):686–689.

149. Zhou P, Seder RA. CD40 ligand is not essential for induction of type 1 cytokine responses or protective immunity after primary or secondary infection with histoplasma capsulatum. J Exp Med 1998; 187(8):1315–1324.

150. Qian Q, Cutler JE. Gamma interferon is not essential in host defense against disseminated candidiasis in mice. Infect Immun 1997; 65(5):1748–1753.

151. Arpinati M, et al. Granulocyte-colony stimulating factor mobilizes T helper 2-inducing dendritic cells. Blood 2000; 95(8):2484–2490.

152. Volpi I, et al. Postgrafting administration of granulocyte colony-stimulating factor impairs functional immune recovery in recipients of human leukocyte antigen haplotype-mismatched hematopoietic transplants. Blood 2001; 97(8):2514–2521.

153. Liles WC, et al. Granulocyte colony-stimulating factor administered in vivo augments neutrophil-mediated activity against opportunistic fungal pathogens. J Infect Dis 1997; 175(4):1012–1015.

154. Gaviria JM, et al. Comparison of interferon-gamma, granulocyte colony-stimulating factor, and granulocyte–macrophage colony-stimulating factor for priming leukocyte-mediated hyphal damage of opportunistic fungal pathogens. J Infect Dis 1999; 179(4):1038–1041.

155. Roilides E, et al. Defective antifungal activity of monocyte-derived macrophages from human immunodeficiency virus-infected children against *Aspergillus fumigatus*. J Infect Dis 1993; 168(6):1562–1565.

156. Kullberg BJ, et al. Modulation of neutrophilfunction in host defense against disseminated *Candida albicans* infection in mice. FEMS Immunol Med Microbiol 1999; 26(3–4):299–307.

157. Tada Y, et al. Granulocyte/macrophage colony-stimulating factor inhibits IL-12 production of mouse Langerhans cells. J Immunol 2000; 164(10):5113–5119.

158. Ritz SA, et al. Granulocyte–macrophage colony-stimulating factor-driven respiratory mucosal sensitization induces Th2 differentiation and function independently of interleukin-4. Am J Respir Cell Mol Biol 2002; 27(4):428–435.

159. Brummer E, Kamberi M, Stevens DA. Regulation by granulocyte–macrophage colony-stimulating factor and/or steroids given in vivo of proinflammatory cytokine and chemokine production by bronchoalveolar macrophages in response to *Aspergillus* conidia. J Infect Dis 2003; 187(4):705–709.

160. Kamberi M, Brummer E, Stevens DA. Regulation of bronchoalveolar macrophage proinflammatory cytokine production by dexamethasone and granulocyte–macrophage

colony-stimulating factor after stimulation by *Aspergillus* conidia or lipopolysaccharide. Cytokine 2002; 19(1):14–20.

161. Netea MG, et al. The role of endogenous interleukin (IL)-18, IL-12, IL-1beta, and tumor necrosis factor-alpha in the production of interferon-gamma induced by *Candida albicans* in human whole-blood cultures. J Infect Dis 2002; 185(7):963–970.

162. Steele C, Fidel PL Jr. Cytokine and chemokine production by human oral and vaginal epithelial cells in response to *Candida albicans*. Infect Immun 2002; 70(2):577–583.

163. Retini C, et al. Capsular polysaccharide of *Cryptococcus neoformans* induces proinflammatory cytokine release by human neutrophils. Infect Immun 1996; 64(8):2897–2903.

164. Mathews HL, Witek-Janusek L. Antifungal activity of interleukin-2-activated natural killer (NK1.1+) lymphocytes against *Candida albicans*. J Med Microbiol 1998; 47(11): 1007–1014.

165. Cenci E, et al. Impaired antifungal effector activity but not inflammatory cell recruitment in interleukin-6-deficient mice with invasive pulmonary aspergillosis. J Infect Dis 2001; 184(5):610–617.

166. van Enckevort FH, et al. Increased susceptibility to systemic candidiasis in interleukin-6 deficient mice. Med Mycol 1999; 37(6):419–426.

167. Pietrella D, et al. Interleukin-12 counterbalances the deleterious effect of human immunodeficiency virus type 1 envelope glycoprotein gp120 on the immune response to *Cryptococcus neoformans*. J Infect Dis 2001; 183(1):51–58.

168. Roilides E, et al. Interleukin-12 enhances antifungal activity of human mononuclear phagocytes against *Aspergillus fumigatus*: implications for a gamma interferon-independent pathway. Infect Immun 1999; 67(6):3047–3050.

169. Winn RM, et al. Selective effects of interleukin (IL)-15 on antifungal activity and IL-8 release by polymorphonuclear leukocytes in response to hyphae of *Aspergillus* species. J Infect Dis 2003; 188(4):585–590.

170. Vazquez N, et al. Interleukin-15 augments superoxide production and microbicidal activity of human monocytes against *Candida albicans*. Infect Immun 1998; 66(1): 145–150.

171. Zhang T, et al. Interleukin-12 (IL-12) and IL-18 synergisticatty induce the fungicidal activity of murine peritoneal exudate cells against *Cryptococcus neoformans* through production of gamma interferon by natural killer cells. Infect Immun 1997; 65(9): 3594–3599.

172. Blease K, Kunkel SL, Hogaboam CM. IL-18 modulates chronic fungal asthma in a murine model; putative involvement of Toll-like receptor-2. Inflamm Res 2001; 50(11):552–560.

173. Stuyt RJ, et al. Role of interleukin-18 in host defense against disseminated *Candida albicans* infection. Infect Immun 2002; 70(6):3284–3286.

174. Mehrad B, et al. CXC chemokine receptor-2 ligands are necessary components of neutrophil-mediated host defense in invasive pulmonary aspergillosis. J Immunol 1999; 163(11):6086–6094.

175. Chu HW, et al. Immunohistochemical detection of GM-CSF, IL-4 and IL-5 in a murine model of allergic bronchopulmonary aspergillosis. Clin Exp Allergy 1996; 26(4): 461–468.

176. Blackstock R, Murphy JW. Role of interleukin-4 in resistance to *Cryptococcus neoformans* infection. Am J Respir Cell Mol Biol 2004; 30(1):109–117.

177. Gildea LA, et al. Overexpression of interleukin-4 in lungs of mice impairs elimination of *Histoplasma capsulatum*. Infect Immun 2003; 71(7):3787–3793.

178. Murali PS, et al. *Aspergillus fumigatus* antigen induced eosinophilia in mice is abrogated by anti-IL-5 antibody. J Leukoc Biol 1993; 53(3):264–267.

179. Kurup VP, et al. Anti-interleukin (IL)-4 and -IL-5 antibodies downregulate IgE and eosinophilia in mice exposed to *Aspergillus* antigens. Allergy 1997; 52(12):1215–1221.

180. Roilides E, et al. IL-I0 exerts suppressive and enhancing effects on antifungal activity of mononuclear phagocytes against *Aspergillus fumigatus*. J Immunol 1997; 158(1): 322–329.

181. Hurst SD, et al. New IL-17 family members promote Th1 or Th2 responses in the lung: in vivo function of the novel cytokine IL-25. J Immunol 2002; 169(1):443–453.

182. Anil S, Samaranayake LP. Impact of lysozyme and lactoferrin on oral *Candida* isolates exposed to polyene antimycotics and fluconazole. Oral Dis 2002; 8(4):199–206.

183. Baev D, et al. Killing of *Candida albicans* by human salivary histatin 5 is modulated, but not determined, by the potassium channel TOK1. Infect Immun 2003; 71(6):3251–3260.

184. Christin L, et al. Mechanisms and target sites of damage in killing of *Candida albicans* hyphae by human polymorphonuclear neutrophils. J Infect Dis 1997; 176(6):1567–1578.

185. Romani L. Innate and adaptive immunity in *Candida albicans* infections and saprophytism. J Leukoc Biol 2000; 68(2):175–179.

186. Porta A, Maresca B. Host response and *Histoplasma capsulatum*/macrophage molecular interactions. Med Mycol 2000; 38(6):399–406.

187. Romagnoli G, et al. The interaction of human dendritic cells with yeast and germ-tube forms of *Candida albicans* leads to efficient fungal processing, dendritic cell maturation, and acquisition of a Th1 response-promoting function. J Leukoc Biol 2004; 75(1): 117–126.

188. d'Ostiani CF, et al. Dendritic cells discriminate between yeasts and hyphae of the fungus *Candida albicans*. Implications for initiation of T helper cell immunity in vitro and in vivo. J Exp Med 2000; 191(10):1661–1674.

189. Syme RM, et al. Primary dendritic cells phagocytose *Cryptococcus neoformans* via mannose receptors and Fc gamma receptor II for presentation to T lymphocytes. Infect Immun 2002; 70(11):5972–5981.

190. Vecchiarelli A, et al. The polysaccharide capsule of *Cryptococcus neoformans* interferes with human dendritic cell maturation and activation. J Leukoc Biol 2003; 74(3):370–378.

191. Richards JO, et al. Dendritic cells pulsed with *Coccidioides immitis* lysate induce antigen-specific naive T-cell activation. J Infect Dis 2001; 184(9):1220–1224.

192. Farah CS, et al. Primary role for CD4(+) T lymphocytes in recovery from oropharyngeal candidiasis. Infect Immun 2002; 70(2):724–731.

193. Farah CS, et al. T-cells augment monocyte and neutrophil function in host resistance against oropharyngeal candidiasis. Infect Immun 2001; 69(10):6110–6118.

194. Santoni G, et al. Immune cell-mediated protection against vaginal candidiasis: evidence for a major role of vaginal CD4(+) T-cells and possible participation of other local lymphocyte effectors. Infect Immun 2002; 70(9):4791–4797.

195. de Bernardis F, et al. Local anticandidal immune responses in a rat model of vaginal infection by and protection against *Candida albicans*. Infect Immun 2000; 68(6): 3297–3304.

196. Buchanan KL, Doyle HA. Requirement for CD4(+) T lymphocytes in host resistance against *Cryptococcus neoformans* in the central nervous system of immunized mice. Infect Immun 2000; 68(2):456–462.

197. Aguirre K, Miller S. MHC class II-positive perivascular microglial cells mediate resistance to *Cryptococcus neoformans* brain infection. Glia 2002; 39(2):184–188.

198. Blackstock R. Roles for CD40, B7 and major histocompatibility complex in induction of enhanced immunity by cryptococcal polysaccharide-pulsed antigen-presenting cells. Immunology 2003; 108(2):158–166.

199. Allendoerfer R, et al. Transfer of protective immunity in murine histoplasmosis by a CD4+ T-cell clone. Infect Immun 1993; 61(2):714–718.

200. Deepe GS Jr. Protective immunity in murine histoplasmosis: functional comparison of adoptively transferred T-cell clones and splenic T-cells. Infect Immun 1988; 56(9): 2350–2355.

201. Ampel NM. Delayed-type hypersensitivity in vitro T-cell responsiveness, and risk of active coccidioidomycosis among HIV-infected patients living in the coccidioidal endemic area. Med Mycol 1999; 37(4):245–250.

202. Ampel NM, Dols CL, Galgiani JN. Coccidioidomycosis during human immunodeficiency virus infection: results of a prospective study in a coccidioidal endemic area. Am J Med 1993; 94(3):235–240.

203. Ashman RB, Fulurija A, Papadimitriou JM. Both CD4+ and CD8+ lymphocytes reduce the severity of tissue lesions in murine systemic candidiasis, and CD4+ cells also demonstrate strain-specific immunopathological effects. Microbiology 1999; 145(Pt 7): 1631–1640.

204. Ghaleb M, Hamad M, Abu-Elteen KH. Vaginal T lymphocyte population kinetics during experimental vaginal candidosis: evidence for a possible role of CD8+ T-cells in protection against vaginal candidosis. Clin Exp Immunol 2003; 131(1):26–33.

205. Schnizlein-Bick C, et al. Effects of CD4 and CDS Tlymphocyte depletion on the course of histoplasmosis following pulmonary challenge. Med Mycol 2003; 41(3):189–197.

206. Oliveira SJ, et al. Cytokines and lymphocyte proliferation in juvenile and adult forms of paracoccidioidomycosis: comparison with infected and non-infected controls. Microb Infect 2002; 4(2):139–144.

207. Kashino SS, et al. Resistance to *Paracoccidioides brasiliensis* infection is linked to a preferential Th1 immune response, whereas susceptibility is associated with absence of IFN-gamma production. J Interferon Cytokine Res 2000; 20(1):89–97.

208. Ampel NM. Measurement of cellular immunity in human coccidioidomycosis. Mycopathologia 2003; 156(4):247–262.

209. Skov M, Poulsen LK, Koch C. Increased antigen-specific Th-2 response in allergic bronchopidmonary aspergillosis (ABPA) in patients with cystic fibros is. Pediatr Pulmonol 1999; 27(2):74–79.

210. Spellberg B, et al. Parenchymal organ, and not splenic, immunity correlates with host survival during disseminated candidiasis. Infect Immun 2003; 71(10):5756–5764.

211. Magliani W, et al. New immunotherapeutic strategies to control vaginal candidiasis. Trends Mol Med 2002; 8(3):121–126.

212. Tansho S, et al. Protection of mice from lethal endogenous *Candida albicans* infection by immunization with *Candida* membrane antigen. Microbiol Immunol 2002; 46(5): 307–311.

213. Mizutani S, et al. Immunization with the *Candida albicans* membrane fraction and in combination with fluconazole protects against systemic fungal infections. Antimicrob Agents Chemother 2000; 44(2):243–247.

214. Mizutani S, et al. CD4(+)-T-cell-mediated resistance to systemic murine candidiasis induced by a membrane fraction of *Candida albicans*. Antimicrob Agents Chemother 2000; 44(10):2653–2658.

215. Bacci A, et al. Dendritic cells pulsed with fungal RNA induce protective immunity to *Candida albicans* in hematopoietic transplantation. J Immunol 2002; 168(6):2904–2913.

216. Abuodeh RO, et al. Resistance to *Coccidioides immitis* in mice after immunization with recombinant protein or a DNA vaccine of a proline-rich antigen. Infect Immun 1999; 67(6):2935–2940.

217. Shubitz L, et al. Protection of mice against *Coccidioides immitis* intranasal infection by vaccination with recombinant antigen 2/PRA. Infect Immun 2002; 70(6):3287–3289.

218. Pappagianis D. Seeking a vaccine against *Coccidioides immitis* and serologic studies: expectations and realities. Fungal Genet Biol 2001; 32(1):1–9.

219. Jiang C, et al. Role of signal sequence in vaccine-induced protection against experimental coccidioidomycosis. Infect Immun 2002; 70(7):3539–3545.

220. Li K, et al. Recombinant urease and urease DNA of *Coccidioides immitis* elicit an immunoprotective response against coccidioidomycosis in mice. Infect Immun 2001; 69(5):2878–2887.

2

Impact of Invasive Fungal Infection on Patients Undergoing Solid Organ Transplantation

Francisco M. Marty and Lindsey R. Baden
Division of Infectious Disease, Brigham and Women's Hospital and Dana-Farber Cancer Institute, Harvard Medical School; The Center for Experimental Pharmacology and Therapeutics, Harvard-MIT Division of Health Sciences and Technology, Boston, Massachusetts, U.S.A.

Robert H. Rubin
Division of Infectious Disease, Brigham and Women's Hospital; Health Sciences and Technology, Harvard Medical School; The Center for Experimental Pharmacology and Therapeutics, Harvard-MIT Division of Health Sciences and Technology, Boston, Massachusetts, U.S.A.

I. INTRODUCTION

Solid organ transplantation has made remarkable progress over the past three decades, evolving from a fascinating experiment in human immunobiology into the most effective means of rehabilitating patients with end-stage organ dysfunction of a variety of types. Today, at the best transplant centers, more than 90% long-term patient and allograft survival are being achieved following kidney, heart, and liver transplantation, with about 75% of lung-transplant recipients achieving these positive results. Because of these successes, the transplant community has been encouraged to "extend the envelope," by bringing new forms of transplantation to the care of affected individuals. For example, in a number of transplant centers, bowel transplantation and transplantation of needed organs into patients with AIDS are now being explored in a responsible fashion (1–3).

The success that has occurred in organ transplantation has been achieved because of the progress in a number of areas in which multidisciplinary skills have been joined for the benefit of the patient (1):

1. *Technical success* in the conduct of the transplant operation itself, and the perioperative management of the endotracheal tube, vascular access catheters, and the variety of surgical drains that are required.
2. The appropriate use of *tissue typing* and sensitive *cross-matching* techniques to optimize the match of donor and recipient pretransplant and to

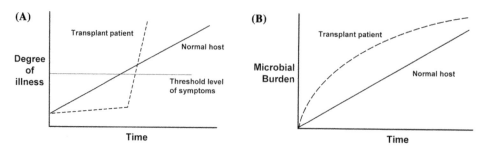

Figure 1 The effects of an impaired inflammatory response on infection in the solid organ-transplant recipient. (**A**) Effects on symptoms and there can be a delay in recognizing disease because of attenuation of symptoms until late in the course. (**B**) Effects on microbial burden and on transmissibility.

permit early recognition and treatment of *post-transplant humoral responses* that can threaten the allograft.

3. Careful *evaluation* of *donor* and *recipient* (in particular, eradicating all *treatable infection* prior to transplant) as well as meticulous care in the procurement and preservation of the donor organ.

4. Recognition of the clinical consequences of *the impaired inflammatory response* that exists in the transplant patient. This renders infection more occult and subtle, which often delays its recognition and compromises subsequent therapeutic efforts. Microbial load is often increased because of delay in diagnosis (as well as the amplification effect of immunosuppressive therapy), again making therapy more difficult (as well as more prolonged), and antimicrobial resistance more common. To prevent these events, early intervention is necessary and should trigger a more aggressive strategy in the use of high-resolution imaging studies and in the use of tissue sampling to effect early diagnosis and therapy (Fig. 1).

5. Precise, *individualized management* of the *immunosuppressive regimen*, on the one hand, effectively preventing or treating allograft rejection, and, on the other, minimizing the severe depression of a broad range of host defenses against infection that can be the consequence of overly aggressive immunosuppressive therapy.

6. *Prevention* of infection in the transplant patient rather than treatment of established disease is the goal. A time-honored example is the use of trimethoprim–sulfamethoxazole prophylaxis for the prevention of human pneumocystosis and other infections.

7. The integration of the prior two principles in clinical practice leads to a dynamic concept that we call the *therapeutic prescription*. The therapeutic prescription has two components: an immunosuppressive program to prevent and treat rejection, and an antimicrobial program to make it safe. Just as changes in the immunosuppressive program may be needed to deal with particular problems with the allograft, the ability to make changes in the antimicrobial program that are linked to the nature of the immunosuppression required is essential. The pre-emptive administration of ganciclovir to renal- or liver- transplant recipients who receive antilymphocyte antibody therapy to treat rejection is a well-studied example of this concept (4,5).

II.   INVASIVE FUNGAL INFECTION IN SOLID ORGAN-TRANSPLANT PATIENTS

The range of organisms capable of causing significant infection in the organ-transplant recipient is quite broad, and these lend themselves to a simple classification system: true pathogens, sometime pathogens, and nonpathogens. True pathogens are the classic plagues of humankind (influenza, bubonic plague, smallpox, and others) that produce toxins and cross-tissue planes, and are able to evade the protection provided by innate immunity. Specific immunity or effective antimicrobial therapy are essential for their control. Sometime pathogens are those organisms that normally reside on mucocutaneous surfaces without clinical impact; injury to these surfaces provides access for these organisms to sites vulnerable to invasive infection (e.g., peritonitis after colonic perforation). Nonpathogens are those saprophytes that are ubiquitous in the environment and are kept in check by innate immune mechanisms and only cause disease in the significantly immunocompromised species (e.g., *Aspergillus species*, *Pneumocystis jiroveci*, zygomycetes, and a variety of other microbial species). The term opportunistic infection is applied to an invasive infection caused by a nonpathogen or to an infection caused by an organism that causes a trivial infection in the normal host but life threatening infection in the immunocompromised individual (e.g., candidal vaginitis vs. disseminated candidiasis). Transplant patients are subject to all three classes of infection, with amplification of a particular clinical syndrome being created by the immunosuppressed state (1,4).

In general, the fungal infections that occur in the transplant patient are caused by sometime and nonpathogenic organisms and can usefully be divided into three general categories:

1.   *The endemic, geographically restricted, systemic mycoses* (caused by *Blastomyces dermatitidis*, *Coccidioides immitis*, *Histoplasma capsulatum*, and others). These organisms share a number of characteristics in common: they are dimorphic in their growth pattern, with the mycelial or mold form present in the soil of endemic areas; in this state, they produce spores, which are infectious for humans. The spores or conidia are aerosolized when the soil is disturbed, making possible the inhalation of these infectious agents and their deposition in the lower respiratory tract. Conversion of the conidia to the invasive yeast form then occurs, with these events initiating the infective process (6,7).

Innate immunity—as mediated by neutrophils, monocytes, and alveolar macrophages—can kill the conidia and block the conversion to the yeast form if the infecting inoculum is relatively small, but is overwhelmed by large inocula, such that invasive primary infection of the lung develops. In the transplant patient, there is abundant evidence of pulmonary disease as a consequence of these events with subsequent hematogenous dissemination. Over time, other forms of clinical infection may develop: reactivation of quiescent infection (again with the possibility of bloodstream seeding), which is not only more common among the immunocompromised, but also has a greater clinical impact than in the general population and *reinfection*. Reinfection is perhaps the most interesting form of these infections: there is a prior minimally symptomatic infection that confers immunity on the individual. With the initiation of antirejection therapy post-transplant, the immunity is attenuated and re-exposure then leads to reinfection and the events that normally follow primary exposure (1,7).

2.   *Opportunistic Fungal Infection.* The most common causes of invasive fungal infection in the transplant recipient are the commensal organisms present on the mucocutaneous surfaces of the body (*Candida* species) and the saprophytic organisms

that are ubiquitous in the environment (e.g., *Aspergillus*, *Cryptococcus*, and the zygo-mycetes). *Candida* species are present as part of the normal gastrointestinal flora in the vagina and on diseased skin. Overgrowth of these organisms is a critical first step in the pathogenesis of candidal infection. Factors that contribute to such overgrowth include decline in immune surveillance because of immunosuppression or neutrope-nia, diabetes mellitus, and other endocrinopathies, and the elimination of competing flora, especially anaerobes, by use of broad-spectrum antibiotics. Mucocutaneous candidal overgrowth can result in clinical entities such as oropharyngeal thrush, candidal esophagitis, vaginitis, intertrigo, paronychia, and onychomycosis (1,8).

Of greater clinical significance is mucocutaneous overgrowth associated with penetration of these surfaces. In transplant patients, this is usually because of tech-nical factors: for example, contaminated vascular access lines or complicated liver-transplant operations in which *Candida* species from the gastrointestinal tract are spilled into devitalized tissue, hematomas, or ascites. If bloodstream invasion occurs, dissemination with the potential for metastatic infection occurs in more than half of transplant patients (1,8–10).

Invasive aspergillosis is the most fearsome of the opportunistic fungal infections occurring in transplant patients. It is acquired through inhalation of an aerosol laden with this mold, with the primary portal of entry being the lungs, sinuses, or damaged skin, although surgical site infections are encountered occasionally because of airborne or surgical supplies' contamination. Exposure to this organism can occur in the hospital or in the community and is particularly associated with construction activities (1,9,10).

Cryptococcal infection and Mucorales infection also have pulmonary (and sinusal in the case of the Mucorales) portals of entry, with the potential for hemato-genous spread and metastatic infection [e.g., the central nervous system (CNS) with *C. neoformans*] or contiguous spread (the Mucorales can cause bloodstream dissemi-nation, but contiguous spread is more characteristic) (1,9,10).

3. *New and Emerging Fungi.* The nature of the fungal species causing invasive infection in the transplant patient is undergoing significant change. Although fluconazole-susceptible *Candida albicans*, *Aspergillus fumigatus*, and *Cryptococcus neoformans* remain the most common causes of invasive fungal infection in solid organ-transplant recipients, 2–10% of invasive fungal infections today are caused by such organisms as fluconazole-resistant *Candida* (both *albicans* and non-*albicans* strains), *Scedosporium*, *Trichosporon*, *Fusarium*, and other heretofore unusual organ-isms. The selective pressures of antifungal prevention strategies, the increased potency of modern immunosuppressive programs, and increased exposures (both in the hospital and in the community) undoubtedly have contributed to the growing importance of this category of infection. What is particularly important is that many of these organisms are poorly responsive to amphotericin B, requiring voriconazole or some other innovative therapy. This group of infections is almost assuredly going to continue to grow in importance over the next few years and will demand not only new therapies, but also new diagnostic approaches (1,11).

III. RISK OF INVASIVE FUNGAL INFECTION IN THE SOLID ORGAN-TRANSPLANT RECIPIENT

The risk of invasive fungal infection in the solid organ transplant patient is largely determined by the interaction of three factors: *technical-anatomic factors, environ-mental exposures, and the net state of immunosuppression.*

A. Technical-Anatomic Factors in the Pathogenesis of Fungal Infection in the Solid Organ-Transplant Patient

The technical-anatomic factors that constitute a risk of infection are those that lead to devitalized tissue, fluid collections, and an ongoing need for invasive devices for vascular access, drainage catheters, and other foreign bodies that abridge or otherwise attenuate the primary mucocutaneous barriers to microbial invasion. *Candida* species are among the most common microbial pathogens that serve as secondary invaders of these technical mishaps. Indeed, the reports of >40% incidence of fungal infection in the early days of liver transplantation were largely because of these technical-anatomic considerations. Factors associated with a particularly high risk of post-transplant candidal infection include hyperglycemia, undrained fluid collections, need for re-exploration, hepatic artery thrombosis, the use of a choledochojejunostomy biliary anastomosis, and a large blood-replacement requirement. Some centers recommend fluconazole prophylaxis for all liver-transplant recipients; we have restricted the use of fluconazole to those patients with one or more risk factors. Although no antimicrobial agent takes the place of technically perfect surgery, the use of fluconazole will improve outcomes further, such that the incidence of this type of fungal infection is now <2% in many centers (1,9,10,12–14).

The technical demands of liver transplantation easily explain the relatively high incidence of these infections, as they do for lung and pancreatic transplantation. In the case of diabetes, the organism burden is far higher on the skin and gastrointestinal mucosa of the individual, significantly adding to the risk of invasive fungal infections. As a general rule, the incidence of such events is determined by the complexity of the surgery involved—being most common following liver, lung, and pancreas transplants, somewhat less common following heart transplantation, and, least often, in association with the renal allograft (1,10).

Two uncommon problems with candidal infection in transplant patients may be encountered: infection and obstruction at the ureteropelvic junction in renal-transplant recipients (observed particularly in those with a neurogenic bladder), which results in obstructive uropathy, ascending pyelonephritis, and the possibility of bloodstream infection. A similar process occurs occasionally in the bile duct of liver-transplant recipients. Because of the difficulty in treating these entities once they are fully developed, we advocate pre-emptive antifungal therapy for those patients with microbiologic evidence of candidal colonization at either of these two sites (1).

If the patient is free of technical-anatomic abnormalities, the risk of infection, particularly opportunistic infection, is largely determined by the semi-quantitative relationship that exists between the environmental exposures and the net state of immunosuppression: if the epidemiologic exposure to a microbial agent is intense enough, even nonimmunosuppressed individuals can develop significant infection; conversely, if the net state of immunosuppression is great enough, then minimal exposure to non-invasive, commensal organisms can result in life-threatening infection (1,4,10).

B. Environmental Exposures of Importance in the Pathogenesis of Fungal Infection in the Solid Organ-Transplant Recipient

The inhalation of fungal conidia is usually the first step in establishing invasive pulmonary infection in the transplant patient. Whereas the endemic mycoses and cryptococcal infection are almost always acquired in the community, *Aspergillus* and *Scedosporium* species may be acquired either in the community or nosocomially (1).

The epidemiology of cryptococcal infection in transplant patients is very different from that of *Aspergillus* and other invasive molds. Asymptomatic primary infection of the lungs with *C. neoformans* is common in the general population, with latent infection controlled by a granulomatous response in a manner analogous to tuberculosis. Immunocompromise, as seen in transplant patients, those with AIDS, and patients with lymphoma under treatment, will result in reactivation of the infection in the lungs and systemic spread, particularly to CNS, skin, skeletal system, and prostate. It is believed that inhalation of infectious propagules of the organism from aerosols created from contaminated soil (particularly that enriched with pigeon and other avian excreta) is the source of the infection, but this concept has yet to be validated.

Acute, progressive primary disease in immunosuppressed patients exposed to a high density of organisms may occur but has not been documented (15–17). One exception is the report of vascular access-associated bloodstream infection (with hematogenous seeding of the lung) caused by *C. neoformans* that was found to spread from a pigeon roost located adjacent to the air intake for an unfiltered air conditioner (18).

In the community, acquisition of infection caused by the endemic mycoses, *Aspergillus*, and the other invasive molds is related to activities in which infectious aerosols are created. The most common scenario is exposure to construction activities in which older structures are being rehabilitated or the soil is being disturbed. The inhalation of these infectious agents then can lead directly to invasive infection or to colonization of the respiratory tract, with the degree of immunocompromise determinmg if invasive disease develops. There are two other situations that should be avoided by transplant patients because of the risk of invasive mold infection: marijuana use and gardening. Marijuana is commonly contaminated with *Aspergillus* species, and the smoking of contaminated marijuana can lead to invasive pulmonary infection; gardening in which the soil is being disturbed can likewise lead to invasive opportunistic infection because of the presence of a variety of *Aspergillus* species (as well as other organisms such as *Nocardia asteroides*). We have cared for a successful renal transplant patient (normal renal function, minimal maintenance immunosuppression, and 4 years post-transplant) who presented with disseminated infection due to *Aspergillus fumigatus*, *A. niger*, *A. flavus*, and *Nocardia asteroides*. All four agents were present on admission. This illness began ~1 week after a spending weekend tending to the patient's rose bushes where considerable digging in the soil was involved. Samples of the soil from the patient's rose garden yielded all of these organisms and other species of mold. Although the patient survived this infection with aggressive and extended therapy, considerable morbidity was encountered in what must be regarded as a preventable infection (1).

Nosocomial acquisition of the invasive molds, particularly *A. fumigatus* and *A. flavus*, and also including emerging agents such as *Scedosporium*, remains a significant problem for the transplant recipient, and is usually associated with hospital construction (1,19).

Water-borne aspergillosis associated with contaminated hospital water tanks or locally in patient room showers has been documented. Patients are exposed either by ingestion of conidia or by aerosolization of water droplets (20,21). The operative principle is that the transplant recipient, like other immunosuppressed hosts, is an epidemiologic "sentinel chicken" (1) within the hospital environment—any excess traffic in microbes will be seen first in this patient population, and constant surveillance is essential to prevent catastrophic outbreaks of life-threatening infection.

C. Net State of Immunosuppression in the Organ-Transplant Recipient

The net state of immunosuppression is a complex function determined by the interaction of a number of factors: the driving force is the dose, duration, and temporal sequence in which immunosuppressive drugs are being deployed; the presence of immunodeficiencies unrelated to therapy (e.g., those associated with the underlying disease, as well as newly acquired deficiencies like the acquired hypoglobulinemic state that has been linked to intensive therapy with tacrolimus and mycophenolate); compromise of mucocutaneous surfaces such that the barrier function is incomplete; degree of neutropenia; metabolic disorders (protein-calorie malnutrition, and perhaps diabetes and uremia); the two extremes in age; infection with one of the immunomodulating viruses [cytomegalovirus (CMV), Epstein–Barr virus (EBV), the hepatitis viruses, and the human immunodeficiency virus]; and, perhaps, race.

Modern immunosuppressive therapy is based on two general principles: multiple drugs that act by different mechanisms should be deployed in combination in order to achieve adequate control of the rejection process and to decrease toxicity and complicating infection. Of all the drugs that are employed, prednisone is thought to be associated with the greatest number of side effects (Table 1), and most regimens devised in the past two decades have been, in large part, designed to be steroid sparing. The most profound effect of currently used regimens is to block the microbe-specific cytotoxic T-cell response, thus putting the patient at special risk for such pathogens as certain classes of viruses, particularly the herpes group viruses, bacteria such as mycobacteria, *Nocardia*, and *Listeria*, and the fungi. Although the specific effects of different immunosuppressive agents in transplant recipients have been reviewed in some detail, as have the nature of the net state of immunosuppression, a few general points bear emphasis:

a. Although corticosteroids at high doses (e.g., pulse doses of >500mg intravenously to treat rejection) are immunosuppressive, the majority of their effects are

Table 1 Effects of Corticosteroids on Inflammation and Immune Function[a]

Anti-inflammatory effects
Inhibition of proinflammatory cytokine production
Increase in the circulating level of polymorphonuclear leukocytes (PMNs), but decrease in the
  accumulation of PMNs at site of tissue injury
Decrease the number of circulating lymphocytes and increase the ratio of B to T cells and
  CD8 to CD4 cells
Decrease the number of circulating monocytes, eosinophils, and basophils
Inhibit all arachidonic acid metabolites, as well as platelet-activating factor (inflammatory
  mediators)
Decrease vascular permeability
  Inhibit the inducible form of nitric-acid synthase
  Inhibit the mediators of vasodilatation
Immunosuppressive effects
Inhibit T-cell activation and proliferation
  Block clonal expansion in response to antigenic stimulation
  Block IL-2 release, resulting in impaired cell-mediated immunity
Inhibit activation of immature B cells; little effect on recall

---

[a]Adapted from Ref. 1.

anti-inflammatory. The result, particularly with fungal infections, is not only to increase the incidence of opportunistic infections, but also to attenuate signs and symptoms, making clinical recognition of invasive disease difficult, increasing the organism burden, and mandating prolonged therapeutic courses (Fig. 1).

b. The immunomodulating viruses, most notably CMV, contribute significantly to the net state of immunosuppression, with 90% of opportunistic infections occurring in patients with active infection with one or more of these viruses. Indeed, occurrence of invasive fungal infection in a patient without viral replication is a clue to the presence of an unsuspected environmental exposure (1,4,10).

c. In addition to the direct immunosuppressive effects of the agents used, their particular effects on the reactivation of such viruses as CMV also help to determine the net state of immunosuppression. Agents like anti-lymphocyte antibodies (e.g., OKT3 and antithymocyte globulin) have a powerful effect in causing reactivation of latent virus. The cytotoxic agents azathioprine, mycophenolate, and cyclophosphamide have a moderate effect in this regard. In contrast, the calcineurin inhibitors (tacrolimus and cyclosporine), sirolimus, and prednisone have no ability to reactivate virus. However, once replicating virus is present, these agents, particularly the calcineurin inhibitors, have profound effects in increasing the risk of invasive fungal infections and of amplifying the infection if present. Candidemia and invasive aspergillosis are both significantly increased in patients with active CMV, and it is likely that other invasive fungal infections are as well (1,4,10).

d. Metabolic factors contribute to the net state of immunosuppression as well. In particular, protein-calorie malnutrition is important, with hyperglycemia and uremia likely to have an effect as well. If one segregates transplant patients on the basis of a serum albumin of greater than or less than 2.5 g/dL, there is a 10-fold difference in the incidence of opportunistic infection, including invasive fungal infection in those with lower albumin levels (1,4,10).

e. Genetically determined aspects of both innate and specific immunities probably control susceptibility to opportunistic infection. Racial background may be a surrogate marker for susceptibility. For example, when compared with Caucasians and Asians, African-Americans have a significantly lower incidence of cadaveric renal allograft survival; they also have a lower incidence of invasive infection. As all these groups receive essentially the same immunosuppressive program, these observations suggest that the net state of immunosuppression produced in African-Americans by standard anti-rejection programs is less than in other population groups. Therefore, unless other factors intervene, it would be expected that the incidence of invasive fungal infection in African-Americans subjected to standard immunosuppressive protocols is less than among other ethnic groups and that more intensive anti-rejection strategies would be safe in these individuals, perhaps improving the rate of allograft survival, emphasizing the importance of a judicious therapeutic prescription (22).

IV. TEMPORAL ASPECTS OF FUNGAL INFECTION IN THE SOLID ORGAN-TRANSPLANT RECIPIENT

There is an expected timetable of infection following organ transplantation. It is useful to divide the post-transplant course into three time periods: the first-month post-transplant, the period 1–6 months post-transplant; and the late period, >6 months post-transplant (Fig. 2). This timetable can be useful in three ways: in constructing a differential diagnosis in a patient who presents with a clinical infectious disease

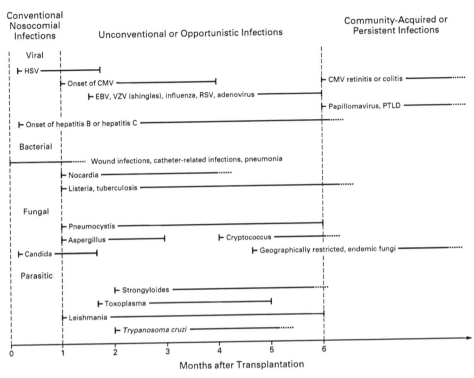

Figure 2 Timetable of infection following solid organ transplantation. Exceptions to the usual sequence of infections after transplantation suggest the presence of unusual epidemiologic exposure or excessive immunosuppression. HSV denotes herpes simplex virus, CMV cytomegalo virus, EBV Epstein–Barr virus, VZV varicella–zoster virus, RSV respiratory syncytial virus, and PTLD post-transplantation lymphoproliferative disease. "0" indicates the time of transplantation. Solid lines indicate the most common period for the onset of infection; dotted lines and arrows indicate periods of continued risk at reduced levels. (*Source:* Reproduced from Ref. 10 with permission.)

syndrome; as a tool of infection control, as exceptions to the timetable are usually because of, heretofore, unrecognized environmental exposures; and as the cornerstone for prescribing cost-effective, focused preventative antimicrobial strategies (1,4,10).

A. Fungal Infection in the First Month Post-transplant

In the first month post-transplant, there are essentially three types of infection observed: active infection that was present pre-transplant and is now clinically apparent post-transplant; active infection that was conveyed through a contaminated allograft; and perioperative infection of the surgical wound, lungs, urinary tract, vascular access devices, and surgical drains (which account for >95% of infections in this time period). In terms of infection that was present prior to transplant, a significant minority of patients coming to lung, liver, or cardiac transplant (rarely, kidney recipients) have been recipients of immunosuppressive therapy in an attempt to control their underlying disease. As a result, these patients can present with invasive candidal, cryptococcal, *Aspergillus* infection, or other fungal infection early in the post-transplant period due to previously unrecognized disease. A cardinal rule of transplantation is that pre-existing infection should be eradicated prior to transplant. A corollary of this rule is that any patient who comes to transplant significantly immunosuppressed merits an evaluation for active infection, especially fungal infection. This evaluation includes blood cultures, cryptococcal antigen measurement, and a chest computed tomography (1,4,10).

Both histoplasmosis (23) and cryptococcosis (24) have rarely been transmitted via an allograft, representing dormant or active infection of the allograft acquired via the hematogenous route. Candidal contamination of the allograft as a consequence of terminal care of a cadaveric donor, the acquisition and transport of the allograft, and the handling of the organ is an uncommon cause of infection. Such contamination threatens the vascular suture line, with potentially grave consequences such as the formation and rupture of arterial pseudoaneurysms (1,4,10,25).

As noted, transplant patients are susceptible to the same infections that complicate comparable surgical procedures in nonimmunosuppressed individuals, although the consequences are usually greater in transplant patients. The occurrence of such infections is directly related to the skill with which the operation is performed, and how invasive care devices (endotracheal tubes, drains, and vascular access devices) are managed. *Candida* species infecting fluid collections, devitalized tissue or drainage catheters, and vascular access devices are the usual clinical problems caused by fungi in this time period. Antifungal prophylaxis with drugs such as fluconazole or an amphotericin B preparation can limit the impact of such infections, but nothing is as important as impeccable surgical and perioperative technical management. Antifungal prophylaxis is particularly useful in liver-transplant patients with one or more of the following risk factors: patients requiring re-exploration diabetes, a history of recent broad spectrum antibacterial therapy, and those with a choledochojejunostomy biliary anastomosis (1,4,10,12–14).

Notable by their absence during this time period are infections caused by opportunistic fungi such as *Aspergillus*, *Cryptococcus*, *Scedosporium*, etc., despite the fact that this is the time period when the highest daily doses of immunosuppression are prescribed. There are two important implications of these findings: if infection caused by one of these opportunistic fungi occurs in the first month, this is *prima facie* evidence of an unexpected environmental exposure that needs correction; it also emphasizes that the prime determinant of the net state of immuno suppression is sustained immunosuppression ("the area under the curve"), rather than the daily dose (1,4,10).

B. Fungal Infection 1 to 6 Months Post-transplant

Residual effects of infection acquired earlier may still be important at this time point. However, there are two types of clinical infections that are of particular relevance in this period. The major cause of infectious disease morbidity and mortality is the immunomodulating viruses, particularly CMV, EBV, and *human herpesvirus 6* (HHV-6), which not only directly cause infectious disease syndromes, but also contribute significantly to the net state of immunosuppression. The combination of these effects and what is now sustained immunosuppression makes possible an array of opportunistic infections, including fungi such as *Aspergillus* species, *Scedosporium*, and *Candida* species, even in the absence of a particularly intense epidemiologic exposure. Prevention of fungal infection during this time period is accomplished by CMV prevention, provision of uncontaminated air (within the hospital, HEPA-filtered), and avoidance of construction sites both inside and outside the hospital. Systemic antifungal therapy plays little role unless colonization is demonstrated, at which point pre-emptive therapy should be considered (1,4,9,10).

C. Fungal Infection More than 6 Months Post-transplant

The great majority of transplant patients in this time period are at relatively low risk of invasive fungal infection, unless an intense environmental exposure occurs. These are patients who have had a good outcome from transplantation: good allograft function, minimal maintenance immunosuppression (particularly, a prednisone dose of ≤10 mg/day), and no ongoing viral infection. Their biggest risk is from community-acquired viral infections such as influenza. Fungal infections seen in these patients are primarily mucocutaneous and can be effectively treated with topical or systemic therapy. The most common invasive fungal infection observed during this time period is that caused by *C. neoformans*, usually presenting as asymptomatic nodules on incidental chest imaging.

Approximately 10% of patients maintained on immunosuppression with a functioning allograft are at high risk for opportunistic infections of all types, but particularly fungal ones. These are patients who have had a relatively poor outcome from transplantation: borderline allograft function, too much acute and/or chronic immunosuppression and often, chronic viral infection. These "chronic n'er do wells" are at high risk for such fungal infections such as those caused by *C. neoformans*, *Aspergillus* species, the newly emerging fungi, and—if the epidemiologic history is appropriate—disseminated infection due to *Histoplasma capsulatum or Coccidioides immitis*. Prevention in these patients requires decreased immunosuppressive therapy, close supervision for possible environmental exposures, treatment of viral infection, and consideration of prophylactic azole administration (although guidelines for this last have not been established) (1,4,10,25).

V. FUNGAL INFECTIONS OF IMPORTANCE IN THE ORGAN-TRANSPLANT RECIPIENT

A. Candidiasis

Candida species are the most common causes of fungal infection in the organ-transplant recipient, causing a broad range of syndromes that range from the trivial to the life threatening. These organisms are part of the normal oral flora. Other sites of colonization are the skin, gastrointestinal tract, and the female genital tract. Candidal colonization is constantly being abetted by the ingestion of food and by exposure to the hospital environment. Of particular importance, the nosocomial spread of *Candida* species has been traced to the contaminated hands of hospital personnel. This mode of transmission has been particularly important in the acquisition of azole-resistant species (8–10,12–14,26).

Oropharyngeal candidiasis can take a variety of forms:

a. An acute exudative, pseudomembranous candidiasis.
b. Chronic atrophic stomatitis.
c. Chronic hyperplasic candidiasis (*Candida* leukoplakia).
d. Acute atrophic stomatitis.

Candida infection of the *esophagus* is not an uncommon finding in these immunocompromised individuals, often linked with oropharyngeal infection. Diagnosis is made by endoscopic evaluation, including biopsy. A rigorous approach to diagnosis is necessary as similar x-ray findings and even endoscopic appearance can be produced by herpetic, CMV, radiation, and reflux esophagitis. It is important to recognize that candidal esophagitis requires systemic antifungal therapy (oral or IV fluconazole being the drug of choice), with topical therapy being ineffective (1,8,12,26).

Urinary tract candidiasis is not uncommon in transplant patients, being made possible by instrumentation of the urinary tract (particularly an indwelling bladder catheter), diabetes, vulvovaginal infection, and the presence of a neurogenic bladder. Although hematogenous renal infection is well recognized as a consequence of bloodstream infection with *Candida*, the great majority of cases of urinary tract infection occur via the ascending route. A particularly virulent form of candiduria occurs when obstruction due to a fungal ball occurs at the ureterovesical junction, with resulting pyelonephritis and bloodstream invasion; papillary necrosis and/or renal cortical abscess can occur in the most severe of these cases. To prevent fungal balls from occurring, we advocate pre-emptive therapy of asymptomatic candiduria after removal of a bladder catheter and control of metabolic derangements. This is in direct contrast to the approach in nonimmunocompromised patients, where watchful waiting is advocated after catheter removal (1,27,28).

Candidemia and disseminated candidal infection occur most commonly because of infection of vascular access catheters, although intestinal translocation in critically ill patients can also occur. The importance of the vascular access device in the pathogenesis of this process is underlined by the observation that the response to systemic therapy is greatly improved in those patients whose catheters are removed promptly as therapy is initiated. In this setting, the maintenance of a bladder catheter and/or the insertion of a three-way bladder catheter to deliver antifungal washes are to be avoided. Once bloodstream infection occurs, metastatic infection can develop anywhere, producing renal infection, hepatosplenic disease, and eye disease (candidal endophthalmitis). It should be emphasized that metastatic infection to the skin can be the first sign of invasive candidal infection in as many as 20% of patients with disseminated disease (26,29,30).

Candidal pneumonia via the tracheobronchial route is vanishingly rare, whereas pulmonary invasion due to bloodstream infection is well recognized. This statement remains true even when the sputum has easily demonstrable candidal forms on microscopic exam and culture and even when blood cultures are positive. In this latter instance, the sequence of events is sputum to skin (with a marked increase in the skin microbial burden) to vascular access site, with this being the portal of entry to the bloodstream. The one situation in which *Candida* species in the sputum should be treated vigorously is the lung-transplant patient with a relatively fresh bronchial suture line. This site has a borderline blood supply, and the combination of organisms at the site and poor perfusion are synergistic in causing breakdown of the bronchial anastomosis. Hence, the principle that *Candida* in the sputum should be treated pre-emptively or to protect the suture line in this patient group (1,26,31).

Uncommon forms of invasive candidal infection. As previously noted, metastatic seeding of distant organs is not uncommon in transplant patients with candidemia. Hence, entities such as endocarditis, meningitis, osteomyelitis, septic arthritis, and other forms of focal infection result. Diagnosis of these entities requires the combination of state-of-the-art imaging techniques, surgical biopsy, and serial cultures. In addition, surgical debridement or excision, in combination with appropriate antifungal therapy, can be particularly useful in the management of candidal endocarditis, osteomyelitis, and other focal lesions (1).

B. Aspergillosis

Aspergillus species are ubiquitous saprophytes in our environment, growing as a mold that produces the infective form, conidia, which is inhaled into the respiratory tract to initiate disease. Once inhaled, these conidia can produce a variety of clinical syndromes that are grouped into four categories of disease (32,33):

a. *Hypersensitivity syndromes.* Asthma, extrinsic allergic alveolitis, and allergic bronchopulmonary aspergillosis (ABPA) are all possible hypersensitivity responses to the inhalation of this organism. In addition, allergic sinusitis can occur, typically in individuals with other evidence of an allergic diathesis—allergic rhinitis, asthma, nasal polyps—in response to chronic colonization with *Aspergillus* species. ABPA is of particular importance, with a clinical syndrome of transient pulmonary infiltrates, asthma, sputum that contains brown particles, eosinophilia, and the presence of immunologic reactivity to *Aspergillus* antigens (as demonstrated by skin testing, the presence of precipitating antibodies, and *Aspergillus* specific IgE). If left untreated, central bronchiectasis and/or pulmonary fibrosis will develop. At present, the therapy of choice is the combination of corticosteroids and an anti-*Aspergillus* drug (e.g., itraconazole or voriconazole) (33–35).

b. *Colonization syndromes.* The best example of this manifestation of *Aspergillus* colonization is the formation of an "aspergilloma" or "*fungal ball*" at the site of such pre-existing lung cavities as those produced by tuberculosis, bronchiectasis, bullous emphysema, or sarcoidosis (Fig. 3). Indeed, sustained colonization of the lung usually connotes a significant abnormality of the tracheobronchial tree. One variant of tracheobronchial disease caused by *Aspergillus* species is obstructing bronchial aspergillosis in which exuberant colonization by these organisms obstruct the airway, with resultant atelectasis, and the production of a pseudomembranous tracheobronchitis. In transplantation, this is a particular problem among lung allograft recipients, particularly those patients with bronchial anastomotic problems or those who may need a bronchial stent because of breakdown of the anastomosis

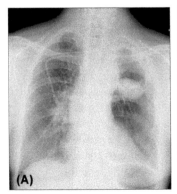
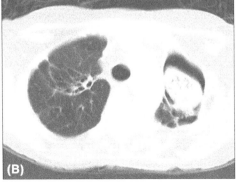

Figure 3 An aspergilloma in a bronchiectatic cavity in a patient with known history of sarcoidosis. (**A**) Conventional chest radiograph (posteroanterior view). (**B**) Computerized tomography scan of the chest of the same patient.

(32,36,37). Aspergillomas consist of a meshwork of fungal hyphae held together by reactive debris (fibrin and inflammatory cells). Clinical symptoms resulting from the presence of an aspergilloma have usually been considered irritative: cough, sputum production, and hemoptysis. Erosion of an aspergilloma into an adjacent large blood vessel can be life threatening. However, increasingly, local invasion has been noted pathologically, and, in select patients, anti-*Aspergillus* therapy can effect clinical improvement and avoidance of surgery in those whose overall lung function is poor.

c. *Semi-invasive aspergillosis*. This is a relatively recently recognized entity characterized by slowly progressive necrosis of the involved lung in individuals not classically considered immunosuppressed, but who have underlying conditions such as diabetes, liver disease, or recent influenza. It has been suggested that a deficiency in mannose-binding protein may be the underlying defect responsible for this condition. Surgical excision under coverage of antifungal therapy appears to be the therapy of choice for this entity, as—unlike invasive aspergillosis in the truly immunosuppressed host—progression of this process is by contiguous spread, not by hematogenous dissemination (32,38,39).

d. *Invasive aspergillosis*. This is the important form of aspergillosis for solid-organ transplant recipients. The great majority of cases involve the lung, with invasive sinusitis being the second most common portal of entry. Damaged skin is also susceptible to invasion by this organism. Studies of hematopoietic stem-cell transplant (HSCT) patients have shown that deficiencies of important host defenses put patients at high risk of invasive disease: a severe deficit in the number and function of polymorphonuclear leukocytes, and significant impairment in cell-mediated immunity. In the solid organ-transplant patient, the latter is the primary deficit that leads to this infection, particularly when infection with one of the immunomodulating viruses, especially CMV, is also present. Acquisition of this infection can occur either in the community or in the hospital and is associated with activities such as construction, the creation of a warm and wet environment (as with a leaking pipe in the ceiling), and even gardening. Two epidemiologic patterns have been identified within the hospital: domiciliary and nondomiciliary. In the domiciliary form, the infection is acquired by the inhalation of conidia laden air in the room or on the ward where the patient is housed. This usually results in the clustering of cases in time and space, and the hazard is relatively easily identified. Nondomiciliary exposures occur as patients travel through the hospital for essential procedures. Thus, outbreaks or single cases have been documented as resulting from exposures in a contaminated operating suite, the radiology suite, or while awaiting bronchoscopy or endomyocardial biopsy in an anteroom. Because of the nature of these exposures and the lack of clustering of cases, nondomiciliary hazards are often difficult to detect, with the best clue being the occurrence of this opportunistic infection at a time when the net state of immunosuppression is not great enough for such infection to occur without a particularly intense exposure (19,32,40).

This division of disease caused by *Aspergillus* species is a clinically useful concept provided that the clinician recognizes that "cross-over" syndromes occur. Thus, invasive disease can occur as a result of steroid use to control allergic manifestations. A cavity caused by necrotizing infection can subsequently develop an aspergilloma. Increasingly, the possibility that some patients with what was regarded as "non-invasive" disease may benefit from antifungal therapy, particularly in conjunction with surgical manipulations, is being recognized. The advent of less-toxic therapies (e.g., voriconazole and caspofungin) has made this management decision considerably easier.

1.   Clinical Aspects of Invasive Aspergillosis *in Solid Organ-Transplant Recipients*

The genus *Aspergillus* encompasses close to 200 different species, with only a few of these being of significance in man. *Aspergillus fumigatus* is responsible for about 90% of the cases of *invasive* disease, with a variety of virulent factors being defined to account for this remarkable pathogenicity. *Aspergillus flavus* accounts for the majority of the remaining cases, particularly those involving the paranasal sinuses. Other species, such as *A. terreus, A. nidulans,* and *A. niger* occasionally produce disease, with there being some evidence that these unusual infections are increasing, particularly among lung-transplant recipients. This is an important trend to follow, as these uncommon species have a greater tendency to be drug resistant; for example, *A. terreus* is amphotericin resistant (32,40–42).

The key characteristic of invasive aspergillosis, whatever the portal of entry, is its angioinvasive behavior. This means that the three cardinal features of invasive aspergillosis are hemorrhage, infarction, and metastases. Of particular importance is the occurrence of metastatic infection, for example, to the brain. As many as half of patients with invasive aspergillosis have evidence of dissemination when initially diagnosed, which greatly decreases their chances for survival. For example, in our experience with renal, cardiac, and hepatic transplant patients, >65% of patients with a single pulmonary lesion were cured with amphotericin B therapy, whereas those with disseminated disease had a survival rate of <25%, and those with CNS disease had a survival rate that approached "zero" (1,32,40,43).

The clinical presentation of invasive aspergillosis is non-specific: fever, hemoptysis, pleurisy, cough, headache, etc. Depending on how suppressed the inflammatory response is, invasive disease can even be relatively asymptomatic. Hence, the need for early diagnosis is great, and a variety of approaches to accomplish this are becoming available:

a.   *Radiology.* Organ-transplant patients with nodules, an infarct pattern, or focal infiltrates with or without cavitation on high-resolution CT scan of the chest should be suspected as harboring invasive *Aspergillus* infection. Conventional chest radiography is not sensitive enough, as the impaired inflammatory response of these patients attenuates the findings on conventional radiographs, and a CT scan should be ordered when the clinician is evaluating respiratory symptoms, unexplained fever, symptoms of sinusitis, or other subtle signs of possible infection. In the even more susceptible HSCT patient, protocol CT scans in the absence of symptoms have been suggested (44,45); such a recommendation does not appear to be warranted with the organ-transplant patient. In HSCT patients, a halo sign (Fig. 4) has been correlated with a high probability of the presence of invasive pulmonary aspergillosis. This halo effect (a ground-glass abnormality thought to be a result of local invasion and hemorrhage that surrounds a focal lesion) is far less common in organ-transplant patients; further, it is non-specific, as we have observed halo signs in HSCT patients with such other processes as nocardiosis, recurrent esophageal cancer, and fungal infections caused by *Scedosporium* and *Fusarium* species. Air-crescent lesions (45) are late manifestations of angioinvasive infection and do not fulfill the need for early diagnosis (1,43,45,46).

b.   *Conventional mycology.* Although the isolation of *Aspergillus* species from respiratory secretions has long been a marker for the presence of significant disease

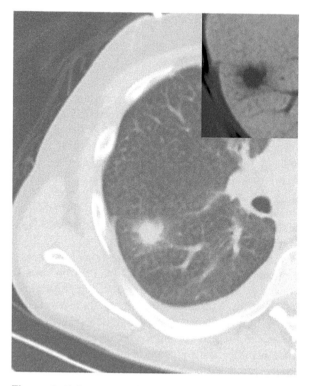

Figure 4 Pulmonary nodule with a halo sign in a hematopoietic stem-cell transplant patient. Subsequent video-assisted thoracic surgical (VATS) resection demonstrated invasive pulmonary aspergillosis. Inset shows the negative image to illustrate the subtlety of the halo sign.

of the tracheobronchial tree (e.g., bronchiectasis and chronic bronchitis), it has not been a major part of the diagnostic approach in transplant patients. Recent observations have suggested that the isolation of these organisms from sputum is a useful part of the diagnostic approach. Thus, high-risk HSCT patients studied in Seattle who are colonized with *Aspergillus* species have a >60% risk of having or developing invasive disease; in liver-, heart-, and kidney-transplant patients, the risk is >50%, and pre-emptive antifungal therapy is advocated. In lung-transplant patients, the positive predictive value is somewhat less (presumably because of the presence of tracheobronchial disease), but pre-emptive approaches are still recommended. The bigger problem is that the sensitivity of this approach is only about 30%. In this circumstance, tissue sampling (for culture and pathology) is needed to make the appropriate diagnosis at this point in time (Fig. 5) (1,32,46,47).

c. *Non-cultural diagnostics.* A significant effort has been expended to develop serologic techniques for the diagnosis of invasive aspergillosis. These have been largely abandoned because of two factors: circulating antibody to this ubiquitous organism is not uncommon in the general population, making interpretation of these results difficult; conversely, in immunocompromised patients such as these, an antibody response may be either delayed or blunted. Two other approaches, however, appear promising: a double sandwich ELISA assay (Platelia® Aspergillus, Bio-Rad Laboratories, Redmond, Washington, U.S.A.) that detects *Aspergillus* cell-wall galactomannan when done serially on a biweekly schedule in HSCT patients has had a negative and positive predictive values around 90%. Thus, this assay could

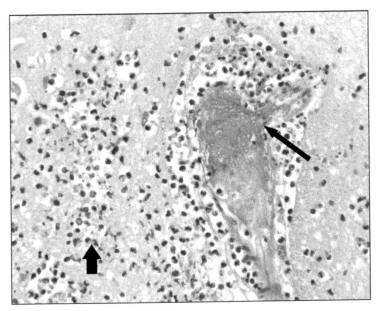

Figure 5 Brain biopsy from a transplant patient with disseminated aspergillosis. The classic behaviors of metastatic infection, angioinvasion (*thin arrow*), and tissue infarction (*thick arrow*) are illustrated. (*Source*: Photomicrograph courtesy of Danny Milner, MD, Department of Pathology, Brigham & Women's Hospital; Hematoxylin & Eosin, 100×.)

allow for a pre-emptive antifungal strategy (32,48,49). Alternatively, molecular amplification techniques to detect fungal nucleic acids appear to be comparably useful. Both these approaches will permit prospective surveillance, provide an estimate of microbial load, and insight into the response to therapy ("proof of cure") (50).

Details of drug therapy will be discussed subsequently. The points to be emphasized, however, are clear-cut: there are a variety of drugs available for the treatment of invasive aspergillosis at present, with voriconazole offering the best results as a single agent (51); combination therapy with multiple drugs, particularly in the treatment of CNS or disseminated infection, is being actively pursued and should be studied systematically. Surgical extirpation, together with antifungal therapy, is appropriate in the presence of a single lesion and no metastatic disease elsewhere. The key is to recognize that invasive aspergillosis is a medical emergency requiring the immediate initiation of therapy (1,32,46).

C. Cryptococcosis

The precise source of human cryptococcal infection in the United States remains unclear, but it is thought to stem from the inhalation of infectious propagules derived from sites contaminated with pigeon excreta. There are three potential outcomes from this inhalation: clearance of infection, development of latent infection, and acute infection with or without hematogenous dissemination. The first two of these are the usual outcome of this initial encounter with *C. neoformans*. Latent *C. neoformans* capable of being reactivated to cause clinical disease, especially after the onset of immunocompromise, is not uncommon in the general population. The pathologic response to cryptococcal invasion is quite variable: from no response (in those patients most immunocompromised) to a strong granulomatous response, which is the cornerstone of the individual's ability to control this infection. The activated macrophage is the most prominent cell type in this attempt to limit the extent of cryptococcal infection. The capsular polysaccharide of *C. neoformans* serves to impede phagocytosis and is thought to be an important virulence factor (17).

Clinical disease caused by *C. neoformans* in the organ-transplant recipient usually occurs more than 6 months post-transplant. The major exception to this general pattern is the group of patients who come to transplant with a history of immunosuppression for their underlying disease or a previous failed transplant. It is our practice to evaluate such individuals for the possibility of cryptococcal (and such other opportunistic infections as pneumocystosis) prior to the performance of a new transplant (1).

The most common presentation of cryptococcosis post-transplant is that of an asymptomatic chest nodule discovered by chance on a chest x-ray. Diagnosis usually requires a biopsy, as antigen testing in this circumstance is often negative; in addition, evaluation of the transplant patient for other sites of cryptococcal disease (CNS, skin, prostate, and skeletal system) is recommended. For those patients with cryptococcal nodules with no evidence of other sites of infection, fluconazole therapy is prescribed for 2–4 weeks after diagnosis to protect against the development of metastatic infection, which is not uncommon after such surgical manipulation. Those with other sites of infection are treated for systemic cryptococcosis as outlined in what follows. The transplant patient presenting with an asymptomatic nodule is often a patient whose net state of immunosuppression is not very great (the patient with a good outcome from transplantation who is receiving only maintenance immunosuppression); in contrast, the patient with disseminated infection is usually the patient with a poor outcome from transplantation, whose net state of immunosuppression is greater than it should be (the previously described "chronic n'er do well") (1,17,46).

Cryptococcal pneumonia, ranging from asymptomatic to that causing significant respiratory compromise, can also occur. Pulmonary disease in general, whether true pneumonia or just a nodule, may present with a negative serum cryptococcal antigen test, thus mandating more invasive tests (bronchoscopy and/or biopsy) for diagnosis. Patients with cryptococcal pneumonia also merit evaluation for other sites of infection. The evaluation should include brain CT, lumbar puncture, bone scan, urine culture and prostate exam, and a careful examination of the skin for evidence of cryptococcal lesions. In 20% of patients with cryptococcosis, skin findings (nodules, papules, ulcerations, etc.) are the first signs of cryptococcosis. Synchronous dual infection is not uncommon in this setting: such combinations including tuberculosis, nocardiosis, and aspergillosis with cryptococcal disease (17).

The key issue with cryptococcal infection is whether or not hematogenous dissemination occurs, and if so, is the CNS involved? Cryptococcal CNS infection is properly termed a meningoencephalitis, although the meningitis component is usually the most evident. The pathologic changes are those of a granulomatous process, both in the meninges and in the brain itself (with cerebral mass lesions occasionally being found on brain imaging). The most common presentation of CNS cryptococcosis in the transplant patient is a febrile headache of gradual onset, often over several weeks. However, other symptoms such as change in the level of consciousness, difficulty concentrating, and memory loss may be present. Less than half of the patients with cryptococcal meningitis will exhibit signs of meningeal inflammation on physical exam. A variety of ocular findings may be present in these patients, most commonly cranial nerve palsies (e.g., of the sixth cranial nerve), but also papilledema, endophthalmitis, and visual loss because of increased intracranial pressure (17).

Virtually, any bodily site can be infected by *C. neoformans*, with two of these warranting special mention here: the bones and joints and the prostate gland. Cryptococcal osteomyelitis may be present as an isolated site of infection; alternatively, it is present as part of disseminated infection involving multiple sites. The prostate gland can serve as a protected site of cryptococcal infection that is relatively resistant to antifungal therapy. Although best demonstrated among AIDS patients, active cryptococcal infection of the prostate has been demonstrated in transplant patients post-therapy. Because of this, more intensive therapy is advocated in men with evidence of prostatic infection at the time of presentation (17).

Of all the fungal infections that can occur in transplant patients, the diagnosis of cryptococcal disease is perhaps the easiest to accomplish, provided the possibility of this infection is considered. Blood cultures, particularly when the lysis centrifugation method is used, have a sensitivity around 70%. The classical cerebrospinal fluid (CSF) formula for cryptococcal meningitis is a lymphocytic pleocytosis, low sugar, and elevated protein, with increased intracranial pressure. The India ink test on CSF is positive in ~50% of transplant patients with CNS disease and is a measure of the organism burden present. The ability to measure cryptococcal capsular polysaccharide, both in serum and in CSF, has become the cornerstone of the diagnosis of cryptococcal disease and should be employed in the evaluation of any transplant patients with unexplained febrile illnesses, as well as in patients with the focal findings described. The titer of antigen present on diagnosis is a good estimate of the organism burden and prognosis, although serial measurements to monitor therapy have had mixed results (17).

D. Zygomycosis (Mucormycosis)

These two terms, usually used interchangeably, describe a group of invasive fungal infections characterized by rapid progression, tissue necrosis, angioinvasion, and the need for aggressive surgery in addition to antifungal therapy. These infections are caused by fungi of the class Zygomycetes, which is currently subdivided into three orders: the Mucorales, the Mortierellales, and the Entomophthorales (52). The Mucorales and Mortierellales are responsible virtually for all the diseases that occur in organ-transplant patients, with a rapid course that constitutes a medical emergency; the Entomophthorales are usually found in tropical areas and cause a slowly progressive disease involving the skin and/or sinuses of relatively normal individuals. We will restrict our attention to the Mucorales, which are ubiquitous in the environment (easily isolated from the soil) and are present in particularly high numbers in decaying organic materials such as fruit and bread. Most cases of infection with these organisms are a result of inhalation of spore-laden air, although direct inoculation of damaged skin is also possible (53).

Risk factors that predispose to infection with the Mucorales include three major categories of abnormality: *immunosuppression*, caused by both neutropenia and post-transplant immunosuppressive therapy, especially corticosteroids; *metabolic derangement* such as diabetic ketoacidosis, chronic metabolic acidosis, deferoxamine therapy, and protein-calorie malnutrition; and *skin and soft-tissue injury*: burn wounds, skin macerated by compression dressings laden with spores, and traumatic or surgical injury. There appear to be two important stages in the evolution of these infections where host defenses are of critical importance: suppression of spore germination and the killing of hyphal elements. Hence, neutrophil number and function, as well as macrophage/monocyte number and function, are critical variables in dealing with these organisms, with the effects of both immunosuppression and metabolic derangement likely to be exerted through their impact on neutrophil and macrophage function (53).

The association between zygomycosis (especially the rhinocerebral form) and diabetic ketoacidosis has long been recognized. In addition, chronic acidosis itself can predispose to zygomycosis. For example, we have observed necrotizing pneumonia caused by these organisms in a nondiabetic man with a failing renal transplant, whose renal failure rendered him chronically acidotic. Similarly, rhinocerebral disease has been observed in patients with combined renal/pancreas transplants in which the exocrine secretions of the pancreatic allograft have been excreted through a bladder anastomosis, resulting in a bicarbonate leak, which is not compensated if kidney function deteriorates. This results in a euglycemic, formerly diabetic individual with chronic acidosis, and an increased risk of life-threatening Mucorales infection. Finally, deferoxamine therapy for iron overload, particularly if immunosuppression is also present, has emerged as a major risk factor for this infection. Iron is a critical growth factor for these (and other) organisms, and this iron chelator provides the organism with access to large amounts of the metal, thus promoting infection (1,53,54).

The clinical syndromes produced by the Mucorales are characterized by the following features: it is angioinvasive, causing necrosis and infarction, as well as hemorrhage; it is rapidly progressive and is relatively resistant to available antifungal agents. The most common syndromes are rhinocerebral, pulmonary, skin and soft tissue, and disseminated. When compared with *Aspergillus* infection, another angioinvasive fungus, the Mucorales, cause less disseminated disease and much more rapid spread into contiguous structures (1,53).

Rhinocerebral zygomycosis involves sequentially the nose, sinuses, eyes, and brain. Presenting symptoms include nasal congestion, epistaxis, sinus tenderness, retroorbital headache, and local swelling. As the process progresses, swelling of involved tissues becomes more noticeable and ocular symptoms (blurred vision, diplopic, proptosis, and blindness) become evident, with loss of cutaneous sensation at involved sites being caused by infarction of nerves. On physical examination, a black eschar in the nasal cavity or hard palate is characteristic. As the infection invades the cranial vault, cavernous sinus thrombosis, carotid thrombosis, and focal brain disease result. This is a medical emergency requiring urgent surgical excision (1,53).

Only slightly less dramatic is the rapidly progressive, necrotizing pneumonia that the Mucorales can cause. Not only the lungs are involved, but also contiguous spread across fascial planes to involve the great vessels, the pericardium, the chest wall, and the diaphragm is not uncommon. Again, rapid recognition and aggressive surgery are the only hope for an increasingly desperate situation (1,53).

The normal skin is remarkably resistant to invasion by the Mucorales, but skin damaged by a variety of means, including the placement of vascular access devices, becomes quite vulnerable. A particular problem in the past was the placement of pressure dressings tapes, which not only damaged the skin, but also were often laden with fungal spores, an ideal situation for producing necrotizing skin infection. Hematogenous seeding of the skin is also possible, but is relatively less common, presumably because of the rapid progression of the primary site of infection (1).

The diagnosis of zygomycosis requires pathologic assessment and/or culture. Early biopsies of sites of necrotizing infection are of critical importance. One of our rules of thumb in the evaluation of immunocomprornised hosts is that no necrotic lesion should be left without biopsy, as it may be the earliest clinical manifestation of these or other angioinvasive molds.

High-dose amphotericin B should be used as adjunctive therapy to surgical debridement in the management of this infection. Voriconazole and the echinocandins are unfortunately not active against the Mucorales, but there are promising in vitro data and initial clinical experience with the use of posaconazole in treating this infection, although it is not yet approved for this indication.

E. New and Emerging Fungi

With the licensure of a number of broad-spectrum antifungal agents (e.g., the new azoles and echinocandins) and their rapid deployment, it is not surprising that new fungal species are coming to attention. In general, these fungi are most apt to occur in HSCT and oncology patients, where they now account for ≥5% of the invasive fungal infections. For the most part, these have not been important pathogens as yet in solid organ-transplant patients, with the notable exception of lung allograft recipients. Such angioinvasive molds as *Scedosporium* and *Fusarium* have been noted to produce clinical syndromes akin to those produced by *Aspergillus* species: colonization being associated with increased risk of invasion; infarction, hemorrhage, and metastatic infection being the norm; and amphotericin B— as well as other drugs— resistance being common. These infections appear to be increasing in number. When infection with one of these agents is documented, every effort should be made to speciate the isolate and to test for drug susceptibility, as the incidence of primary resistance is higher with these organisms than with the usual fungal pathogens (11).

Agents of phaeohyphomycosis (the black or pigmented fungi in tissue sections) are occasionally found as causes of infections in organ-transplant recipients. These are usually cutaneous and subcutaneous infections, although they can rarely cause more invasive disease. Acquisition is usually through skin trauma or contamination of wounds. Treatment of localized disease with excision and ablation is usually preferred. Amphotericin B, itraconazole, voriconazole, and terbinafine have been used successfully for the treatment of both localized and systemic infections (55).

VI. PRINCIPLES OF ANTIFUNGAL THERAPY IN SOLID ORGAN-TRANSPLANT RECIPIENTS

A. Modes of Therapy

There are four different modes in which antimicrobial therapy may be deployed in the management of the infectious disease problems of the transplant recipient (1,4):

1. A *therapeutic* mode, in which antimicrobial agents are prescribed to control and, hopefully, cure clinical and microbiologically identified disease. Early diagnosis and initiation of therapy is the key to the successful therapeutic use of antimicrobial agents. This truism applies particularly to fungal infections.
2. An *empiric* mode, in which a pre-determined antimicrobial prescription is administered without knowledge of the specific etiologic agent or agents causing a certain syndrome. It is based on knowledge of prior epidemiology for such a syndrome and the risk of a bad outcome in a specific population. The empiric use of antibiotics in patients with fever and neutropenia

or in patients with community-acquired pneumonia is now a standardized avenue of such empiric therapy.

3. A *prophylactic* mode, in which *everyone* in a cohort receives an antimicrobial program before an event to prevent important infection. Antifungal prophylaxis has a particular role to play in the management of liver-transplant recipients who receive routine fluconazole prophylaxis to prevent perioperative *Candida* infections and lung-transplant recipients who are treated with amphotericin B nebulizations to prevent pulmonary infections, especially anastomotic site infections caused by *Candida* or *Aspergillus*.

4. A *pre-emptive* mode, in which a subgroup of patients is identified as being at particularly high risk of invasive infection on the basis of a laboratory marker and/or a clinical or epidemiologic characteristic. For example, colonization of the respiratory tract of a heart- or liver-transplant patient with *Aspergillus* species is correlated with a >50% risk of invasive aspergillosis. If a surgical procedure (e.g., an excisional biopsy of a nodule in the lung) reveals the presence of an endemic fungus, there is a 10% risk that hematogenous spread of the organism to the CNS bone, or eyes occurred because of surgical manipulation of infected tissue. In both instances, pre-emptive therapy with the appropriate azole agent (e.g., fluconazole) can eliminate these problems.

It is likely that as new diagnostic tests such as polymerase chain reaction (PCR) and fungal antigen detection become available, pre-emptive therapy will become even more important in the management of these patients.

B. Drug Interactions

Antimicrobial therapy in the organ-transplant patient is associated with frequent drug interactions, particularly with the mainstays of modern immunosuppression: tacrolimus and cyclosporine. There are essentially three classes of interactions that are observed, two of which are related to effects on the hepatic cytochrome P450 enzyme isoforms that catalyze the metabolism of the two calcineurin inhibitors (1,4):

1. *Upregulation* of cytochrome P450 isoforms, resulting in low blood levels, inadequate levels of immunosuppression, and a high probability of allograft rejection. Although currently available antifungal agents do not have this effect, it should be remembered that antimicrobial drugs such as rifampin, isoniazid, and nafcillin do (and it is not unlikely that other drugs may have this effect as well).

2. *Downregulation* of cytochrome P450 isoforms, resulting in high blood levels, renal toxicity, the possibility of over immunosuppression, and an increase in the risk of opportunistic infection. The azoles have a significant effect of this type, with ketoconazole being greater than itraconazole or voriconazole, and all these greater than fluconazole. All azoles have the same effect but of differing magnitude. A potentially dangerous interaction is that of sirolimus and voriconazole because the introduction of voriconazole inhibits the CYP-2C19 causing a steep increase in sirolimus levels.

3. The third mechanism has to do with the causation of *significant renal injury* by the administration of an antifungal agent (usually an amphotericin B preparation) in patients with appropriate therapeutic (not toxic) blood levels of tacrolimus or cyclosporine. There are at least two forms of this interaction: (a) single doses as small as 10 mg of conventional amphotericin B (deoxycholate) have induced acute, oliguric renal failure in transplant patients, probably because of polymorphisms in

the Toll-like receptors that bind amphotericin B and make this patients uniquely susceptible to amphotericin B toxicity and (b) renal function will deteriorate much earlier in the course of amphotericin therapy (e.g., after as little as 200 mg of amphotericin B as opposed to a similar effect only after more than 500 mg of cumulative amphotericin B dose) when therapeutic levels of a calcineurin inhibitor are present, in a principle that we have called *synergistic nephrotoxicity* (1).

The end result is that the nature of the antimicrobial agents employed will be somewhat different. It is imperative that evaluation for direct and indirect drug interactions in organ-transplant recipients be part of the clinical assessment of any confirmed or suspected fungal infection and that treatment is tailored to minimize drug toxicities. Furthermore, transplant patients should acquire the habit of consulting with their treating teams concerning *any* new medication they are prescribed. This includes over-the-counter and herbal medications. We have witnessed patients who have lost their allografts or developed new infections when this basic practice was overlooked. The assessment of acute and cumulative toxicity of amphotericin B should be part of the ongoing care of these patients, and the use of lipid formulations of amphotericin B, azoles, or echinocandins should be reevaluated if any significant toxicity develops.

These considerations on the nature, dynamics, and treatment of invasive fungal infections have also led us to view antifungal therapy as having several stages: (a) *induction* therapy, in which the most potent regimen available is administered to gain control of the disease process as quickly as possible; toxicity and cost issues are of relatively minor consequence until the patient stabilizes; (b) *consolidation* therapy, in which cure of the patient is sought over a prolonged period of, when feasible, oral therapy; at this stage, toxicity and cost are major considerations; (c) *maintenance* therapy (also conceived as secondary prophylaxis), in which the fungal process has been brought into remission, but, because of the need for continuing immunosuppression, relapse is possible and needs to be prevented. Again, the use of non-toxic, relatively inexpensive oral therapy is emphasized. This approach, borrowed from oncology, is illustrated in Table 2 for the different forms of fungal infection seen in solid organ-transplant patients.

The remaining therapeutic general principle that merits attention is how to determine the duration of therapy in the individual patient, an area in which there is relatively little data. Indeed, as stated by the esteemed Professor Louis Weinstein, "there are only two things we don't know in infectious disease: how much to treat with and how long to treat for." This observation is particularly applicable to antifungal therapy for transplant patients, as changes in the immunosuppressive regimen can have profound effects on the antifungal program. The approach we advocate does not utilize fixed courses of therapy for a particular infection; rather, our plan is to treat until all signs and symptoms referable to the fungal infection are eliminated, and then add an additional buffer or consolidation period. The duration of the buffer period will depend on the seriousness of the condition, the rapidity of response, the net state of immunosuppression (if it can be improved), the consequences of relapse, and the toxicities of the therapy. For example, CNS infection merits consideration of long-term maintenance therapy, as well as a prolonged buffer period. In sum, the complexity of antifungal therapy for this population of patients requires not a standard regimen for all, but rather individualized therapy that encompasses all parts of the clinical situation and the therapeutic milieu in which the therapy is being deployed.

Table 2 Treatment of Systemic Mycoses in Solid Organ-Transplant Patients

Infection	Induction therapy	Consolidation therapy	Maintenance therapy	Additional interventions
Aspergillosis	Voriconazole or amphotericin B, or caspofungin[a]	Voriconazole or caspofungin	Voriconazole	Consider excision and ablation of singleton lesions
Blastomycosis	Amphotericin B	Itraconazole	Itraconazole	
Candidemia (and/or deep tissue infection)	Amphotericin B, or caspofungin, or fluconazole[b]	Fluconazole, or caspofungin, or amphotericin B	Only if vascular anastomosis at risk or prosthetic devices cannot be removed	Remove contaminated indwelling devices
Coccidioidomycosis	Amphotericin B	Fluconazole Itraconazole	Fluconazole Itraconazole	Consider secondary prophylaxis in seropositive patients undergoing solid organ transplantation
Cryptococcosis	Amphotericin B and flucytosine[c]	Fluconazole	Fluconazole	Management of intracranial pressure critical with CNS involvement
Fusariosis	Voriconazole or amphotericin B	Voriconazole or amphotericin B	Voriconazole	
Histoplasmosis	Amphotericin B[d]	Itraconazole	Itraconazole[e]	
Paracoccidioidomycosis	Amphotericin B	Itraconazole or TMP-SMX	TMP-SMX or Itraconazole	
Penicilliosis	Amphotericin B	Itraconazole	Itraconazole	
Phaeohyphomycosis	Local excision and itraconazole, or voriconazole, or terbinafine	Itraconazole, or voriconazole, or terbinafine	Only if disseminated disease suspected	

Scedosporonosis			
S. apiospermum,	Voriconazole	Voriconazole	Voriconazole
S. prolificans	Voriconazole and terbinafine	Voriconazole and terbinafine	Unknown
Trichosporonosis	Fluconazole or voriconazole, and amphotericin B	Fluconazole or voriconazole	Fluconazole or voriconazole
Zygomycosis	Amphotericin B (>1.25 mg/kg/day or lipid formulation equivalent)	Amphotericin B	Excision and ablation is the cornerstone of therapy. Consider expanded access posaconazole

[a] The benefit of combination therapy is currently under investigation.

[b] Antifungal susceptibility testing and final species identification results should guide final therapy. Empiric therapy should be based on local epidemiology, bearing in mind that some *Candida* species are likely fluconazole resistant (*C. krusei*), amphotericin B resistant (*C. lusitaniae*), or caspofungin resistant (*C. guillermondii*) and some strains of *C. parapsilosis*.

[c] Avoid flucytosine use if there is renal dysfunction unless drug level determinations are readily available in "real clinical time."

[d] We prefer use of a lipid formulation of amphotericin B in this situation, given preferential targeting of the reticuloendothelial system.

[e] Consider fluconazole for CNS histoplasmosis or if no other alternatives are feasible.

Abbreviations: TMP-SMX, trimethoprim–sulfamethoxazole.

C. Antifungal Agents

After decades in which amphotericin B deoxycholate was the only form of systemic antifungal therapy available, there has been a much-needed expansion in drugs approved for the treatment of invasive fungal infection. This welcome occurrence is tempered by the fact that the information base on which therapeutic decisions are made is presently incomplete; so the recommendations made in Table 2 should be regarded as subject to change, as more information is garnered and even more useful drugs become available. The following observations, however, are important adjuncts to Table 2.

1. Amphotericin B is well known for two major toxicities: acute infusion toxicity ("cytokine storm"), particularly with the first few doses, with fever, chills, hypotension being the rule, and dose-related nephrotoxicity. The lipid formulations of amphotericin B significantly attenuate the first of these and decrease, but do not eliminate, the incidence and severity of the renal injury. As far as efficacy is concerned, available information suggests that all of the amphotericin B preparations have comparable efficacy.

2. The advent of azole antifungal therapy has been a major advance. Fluconazole, as a treatment of many yeast infections, both candidal and cryptococcal, is well tolerated, pharmacologically ideal, and only limited by two factors: its antifungal spectrum does not encompass the molds; resistance is beginning to be an issue and the possibility of resistance needs to be assessed as part of the therapeutic decision making. Itraconazole is a broad-spectrum drug, including *Aspergillus* species, but its use has been hampered by pharmacokinetic issues: unreliable absorption orally (the new oral suspension formulation and the availability of an IV form help greatly in this area); poor penetration into respiratory secretions, the urinary tract, the CNS, and the eye; and the limited information available on efficacy in serious human disease. Voriconazole is a broad-spectrum drug, shown to be superior to amphotericin B in the treatment of invasive aspergillosis, as well as to several of the new and emerging fungi (e.g., *Scedosporium apiospermum*, but not *S. prolificans*), and although transient visual symptoms and liver dysfunction can occur, the drug is generally well tolerated.

3. The advent of caspofungin provides a new approach for the treatment of both *Candida* and *Aspergillus* infection. Its mechanism of action by glucan synthetase inhibition resulting in impairment of fungal cell-wall synthesis is of interest not only used alone, but also raises the possibility of synergistic multidrug regimens for greater efficacy (indeed, it has been suggested that echinocandins could be the "penicillins of antifungal therapy," the cell-wall effects potentiating the entry of the other antifungal agents). Until more data become available, our policy is to consider multidrug therapy in the face of disseminated disease, particularly that which is involving the CNS and to participate in trials of systematic evaluations of antifungal combinations.

4. Antifungal susceptibility testing of most pathogenic yeasts has now been standardized (56). Although the correlation between in vitro resistance and clinical failure is not precise, routine susceptibility testing of all invasive yeast isolates will provide useful information both to refine the management of an individual patient and to provide epidemiologic information to guide future empiric therapy. We hope that this valuable information will be incorporated into routine clinical practice.

5. In addition to the choice of an appropriate antifungal agent, optimal management of these patients includes several other considerations: (a) decrease the net state of immunosuppression, primarily by decreasing the doses of the immunosuppressive

drugs being administered; (b) augment host defenses whenever possible, such as reversing neutropenia—whether disease or drug related—by use of colony stimulating factor or neutrophil transfusions in the case of HSCT recipients; (c) always consider the possibility of surgical resection of the site of infection: *excision* and cursive to first *ablation* rather and incision and drainage of infected tissues; (d) diagnosis and control of CMV and other immunornodulating viruses; (e) optimize other aspects of the patient's care: for example, the prompt removal of vascular access devices in patients with candidemia.

VII. SUMMARY AND CONCLUSIONS

Fungal infections remain a significant problem among solid organ-transplant recipients, with the incidence of such infections being determined by the interactions of three factors: technical-anatomic abnormalities, environmental exposures, and the net state of immunosuppression. Prevention of infection remains the goal, failing which early recognition and prompt therapy remain major factors determining outcome. Early diagnosis remains challenging because of the impaired inflammatory response present in transplant patients. This renders signs and symptoms of fungal infection, as well as radiological findings in this patient population subtler, and necessitates closer follow-up and an aggressive diagnostic approach that usually includes invasive procedures and tissue sampling. Recent advances have made the possibility of detecting fungal infection earlier by means of antigen-detection approaches (e.g., the sandwich EIA assay for galactomannan) or the detection of circulating fungal DNA by PCR quite possible. These approaches, if effective, will not only permit early diagnosis, but also make possible a more targeted pre-emptive therapy and an assessment of the response to therapy ("proof of cure"), and help in establishing optimal durations of therapy. Therapy of fungal infection, both preventative and treatment related, is currently in a state of flux, at least in part because of the advent of new therapies. It is clear that voriconazole and caspofungin are significant additions to our therapeutic armamentarium, but optimal use and the utility of combination therapy remain to be determined. Drug interactions with the calcineurin inhibitors, sirolimus, and other medications remain important issues. In sum, much has been accomplished in this field, but much remains to be done.

REFERENCES

1. Rubin RH. Infection in the organ transplant recipient. In: Rubin RH, Young LS, eds. Clinical Approach to Infection in the Compromised Host. New York: Kluwer Academic/Plenum Publishers, 2002:573–679.
2. Calabrese LH, Albrecht M, Young J, McCarthy P, Haug M, Jarcho J, Zackin R. Successful cardiac transplantation in an HIV-1-infected patient with advanced disease. N Engl J Med 2003; 348:2323–2328.
3. Roland ME, Stock PG. Review of solid-organ transplantation in HIV-infected patients. Transplantation 2003; 75:425–429.
4. Rubin RH, Dconen T, Gummert JF, Morris RE. The therapeutic prescription for the organ transplant recipient: the linkage of immunosuppression and antimicrobial strategies. Transpl Infect Dis 1999; 1:29–39.
5. Turgeon N, Fishman JA, Basgoz N, Tolkoff-Rubin NE, Doran M, Cosimi AB, Rubin RH. Effect of oral acyclovir or ganciclovir therapy after preemptive intravenous ganciclovir

therapy to prevent cytomegalovirus disease in cytomegalovirus seropositive renal and liver transplant recipients receiving antilymphocyte antibody therapy. Transplantation 1998; 66:1780–1786.

6. Cano MV, Hajjeh RA. The epidemiology of histoplasmosis: a review. Semin Respir Infect 2001; 16:109–118.
7. Wheat LJ, Kauffman CA. Histoplasmosis. Infect Dis Clin North Am 2003; 17:1–19, vii.
8. Vazquez JA, Sobel JD. Mucosal candidiasis. Infect Dis Clin North Am 2002; 16:793–820, v.
9. Singh N. Fungal infections in the recipients of solid organ transplantation. Infect Dis Clin North Am 2003; 17:113–134, viii.
10. Fishman JA, Rubin RH. Infection in organ-transplant recipients. N Engl J Med 1998; 338:1741–1751.
11. Fleming RV, Walsh TJ, Anaissie EJ. Emerging and less common fungal pathogens. Infect Dis Clin North Am 2002; 16:915–933, vi–vii.
12. Paya CV. Fungal infections in solid-organ transplantation. Clin Infect Dis 1993; 16: 677–688.
13. Hadley S, Karchmer AW. Fungal infections in solid organ transplant recipients. Infect Dis Clin North Am 1995; 9:1045–1074.
14. Hibberd PL, Rubin RH. Clinical aspects of fungal infection in organ transplant recipients. Clin Infect Dis 1994; 19(suppl 1):S33–S40.
15. Garcia-Hermoso D, Janbon G, Dromer F. Epidemiological evidence for dormant *Cryptococcus neoformans* infection. J Clin Microbiol 1999; 37:3204–3209.
16. Husain A, Wagener MM, Singh N. *Cryptococcus neoformans* infection in organ transplant recipients: variables influencing clinical characteristics and outcome. Emerg Infect Dis 2001; 7:375–381.
17. Perfect JR, Casadevall A. Cryptococcosis. Infect Dis Clin North Am 2002; 16:837–874, v–vi.
18. Ramsey PG, Rubin RH, Tolkoff-Rubin NE, Cosimi AB, Russell PS, Greene R. The renal transplant patient with fever and pulmonary infiltrates: etiology, clinical manifestations, and management. Medicine (Baltimore) 1980; 59:206–222.
19. Hopkins CC, Weber DJ, Rubin RH. Invasive *Aspergillus* infection: possible non-ward common source within the hospital environment. J Hosp Infect 1989; 13:19–25.
20. Anaissie EJ, Penzak SR, Dignani MC. The hospital water supply as a source of nosocomial infections: a plea for action. Arch Intern Med 2002; 162:1483–1492.
21. Anaissie EJ, McGinnis MR, Pfaller MA. Clinical Mycology. 1st ed. New York: Churchill Livingstone, 2003.
22. Meier-Kriesche HU, Ojo A, Magee JC, Cibrik DM, Hanson JA, Leichtman AB, Kaplan B. African-American renal transplant recipients experience decreased risk of death due to infection: possible implications for immunosuppressive strategies. Transplantation 2000; 70:375–379.
23. Limaye AP, Connolly PA, Sagar M, Fritsche TR, Cookson BT, Wheat LJ, Stamm WE. Transmission of *Histoplasma capsulatum* by organ transplantation. N Engl J Med 2000; 343:1163–1166.
24. Ooi BS, Chen BT, Lim CH, Khoo OT, Chan DT. Survival of a patient transplanted with a kidney infected with *Cryptococcus neoformans*. Transplantation 1971; 11:428–429.
25. Gottesdiener KM. Transplanted infections: donor-to-host transmission with the allograft. Ann Intern Med 1939; 110:1001–1016.
26. Ostrosky-Zeichner L, Rex JH, Bennett J, Kullberg BJ. Deeply invasive candidiasis. Infect Dis Clin North Am 2002; 16:821–835.
27. Rex JH, Walsh TJ, Sobel JD, Filler SG, Pappas PG, Dismukes WE, Edwards JE. Practice guidelines for the treatment of candidiasis. Infectious Diseases Society of America. Clin Infect Dis 2000; 30:662–678.
28. Kauffman CA, Vazquez JA, Sobel JD, Gallis HA, McKinsey DS, Karchmer AW, Sugar AM, Sharkey PK, Wise GJ, Mangi R, Mosher A, Lee JY, Dismukes WE. Prospective multicenter surveillance study of funguria in hospitalized patients. The National Institute

for Allergy and Infectious Diseases (NIAID) Mycoses Study Group. Clin Infect Dis 2000; 30:14–18.

29. Rex JH, Bennett JE, Sugar AM, et al. The NIAID Mycoses Study Group, the Candidemia Study Group: intravascular catheter exchanges and the duration of candidemia. Clin Infect Dis 1995; 21:994–996.

30. Wenzel RP. Nosocomial candidemia: risk factors and attributable mortality. Clin Infect Dis 1995; 20:1531–1534.

31. Masur H, Rosen PP, Armstrong D. Pulmonary disease caused by *Candida* species. Am J Med 1977; 63:914–925.

32. Marr KA, Patterson T, Denning D. Aspergillosis. Pathogenesis, clinical manifestations, and therapy. Infect Dis Clin North Am 2002; 16:875–894, vi.

33. Stevens DA, Kan VL, Judson MA, Morrison VA, Dummer S, Denning DW, Bennett JE, Walsh TJ, Patterson TF, Pankey GA. Practice guidelines for diseases caused by *Aspergillus*. Infectious Diseases Society of America. Clin Infect Dis 2000; 30:696–709.

34. Stevens DA, Schwartz HJ, Lee JY, Moskovitz BL, Jerome DC, Catanzaro A, Bamberger DM, Weinmann AJ, Tuazon CU, Judson MA, Platts-Mills TA, DeGraff AC Jr. A randomized trial of itraconazole in allergic bronchopulmonary aspergillosis. N Engl J Med 2000; 342:756–762.

35. Wark P, Gibson P, Wilson A. Azoles for allergic bronchopulmonary aspergillosis associated with asthma. Cochrane Database Syst Rev 2003; 3:CD001108.

36. Kramer MR, Denning DW, Marshall SE, Ross DJ, Berry G, Lewiston NJ, Stevens DA, Theodore J. Ulcerative tracheobronchitis after lung transplantation. A new form of invasive aspergillosis. Am Rev Respir Dis 1991; 144:552–556.

37. Mehrad B, Paciocco G, Martinez FJ, Ojo TC, Iannettoni MD, Lynch JP III. Spectrum of *Aspergillus* infection in lung transplant recipients: case series and review of the literature. Chest 2001; 119:169–175.

38. Denning DW. Chronic forms of pulmonary aspergillosis. Clin Microbiol Infect 2001; 7(suppl 2):25–31.

39. Gefter WB. The spectrum of pulmonary aspergillosis. J Thorac Imaging 1992; 7:56–74.

40. Marr KA, Carter RA, Crippa F, Wald A, Corey L. Epidemiology and outcome of mould infections in hematopoietic stem cell transplant recipients. Clin Infect Dis 2002; 34: 909–917.

41. Moore CB, Sayers N, Mosquera J, Slaven J, Denning DW. Antifungal drug resistance in *Aspergillus*. J Infect 2000; 41:203–220.

42. Sutton DA, Sanche SE, Revankar SG, Fothergill AW, Rinaldi MG. In vitro amphotericin B resistance in clinical isolates of *Aspergillus terreus*, with a head-to-head comparison to voriconazole. J Clin Microbiol 1999; 37:2343–2345.

43. Patterson TF, Kirkpatrick WR, White M, Hiemenz JW, Wingard JR, Dupont B, Rinaldi MG, Stevens DA, Graybill JR. Invasive aspergillosis. Disease spectrum, treatment practices, and outcomes. I3 *Aspergillus* Study Group. Medicine (Baltimore) 2000; 79:250–260.

44. Caillot D, Casasnovas O, Bernard A, Couaillier JF, Durand C, Cuisenier B, Solary E, Piard F, Petrella T, Bonnin A, Couillault G, Dumas M, Guy H. Improved management of invasive pulmonary aspergillosis in neutropenic patients using early thoracic computed tomographic scan and surgery. J Clin Oncol 1997; 15:139–147.

45. Caillot D, Couaillier JF, Bernard A, Casasnovas O, Denning DW, Mannone L, Lopez J, Couillault G, Piard F, Vagner O, Guy H. Increasing volume and changing characteristics of invasive pulmonary aspergillosis on sequential thoracic computed tomography scans in patients with neutropenia. J Clin Oncol 2001; 19:253–259.

46. Rubin RH, Greene R. Clinical approach to the compromised host with fever and pulmonary infiltrates. In: Rubin RH, Young LS, eds. Clinical Approach to Infection in the Compromised Host. New York: Kluwer Academic/Plenum Press, 2002:111–162.

47. Horvath JA, Dummer S. The use of respiratory-tract cultures in the diagnosis of invasive pulmonary aspergillosis. Am J Med 1996; 100:171–178.

48. Maertens J, Verhaegen J, Demuynck H, Brock P, Verhoef G, Vandenberghe P, Van Eldere J, Verbist L, Boogaerts M. Autopsy-controlled prospective evaluation of serial screening for circulating galactomannan by a sandwich enzyme-linked immunosorbent assay for hematological patients at risk for invasive aspergillosis. J Clin Microbiol 1999; 37:3223–3228.
49. Maertens J, Verhaegen J, Lagrou K, Van Eldere J, Boogaerts M. Screening for circulating galactomannan as a noninvasive diagnostic tool for invasive aspergillosis in prolonged neutropenic patients and stem cell transplantation recipients: a prospective validation. Blood 2001; 97:1604–1610.
50. Einsele H, Hebart H, Roller G, Loffler J, Rothenhofer I, Muller CA, Bowden RA, van Burik J, Engelhard D, Kanz L, Schumacher U. Detection and identification of fungal pathogens in blood by using molecular probes. J Clin Microbiol 1997; 35:1353–1360.
51. Herbrecht R, Denning DW, Patterson TF, Bennett JE, Greene RE, Oestmann JW, Kem WV, Marr KA, Ribaud P, Lortholary O, Sylvester R, Rubin RH, Wingard JR, Stark P, Durand C, Caillot D, Thiel E, Chandrasekar PH, Hodges MR, Schlamm HT, Troke PF, de Pauw B. Voriconazole versus amphotericin B for primary therapy of invasive aspergillosis. N Engl J Med 2002; 347:408–415.
52. de Hoog GS, Guarro J, Gene J, Figueras MJ. Atlas of Clinical Fungi. 2nd ed. Utrecht, The Netherlands: Centraalbureau voor Schimmelcultures, 2000.
53. Gonzalez CE, Rinaldi MG, Sugar AM. Zygomycosis. Infect Dis Clin North Am 2002; 16:895–914, vi.
54. Boelaert JR, de Locht M, Van Cutsem J, Kerrels V, Cantinieaux B, Verdonck A, Van Landuyt HW, Schneider YJ. Mucormycosis during deferoxamine therapy is a siderophore-mediated infection. In vitro and in vivo animal studies. J Clin Invest 1993; 91:1979–1986.
55. Husain S, Alexander BD, Munoz P, Avery RK, Houston S, Pruett T, Jacobs R, Dominguez EA, Tollemar JG, Baumgarten K, Yu CM, Wagener MM, Linden P, Kusne S, Singh N. Opportunistic mycelial fungal infections in organ transplant recipients: emerging importance of non-*Aspergillus* mycelial fungi. Clin Infect Dis 2003; 37: 221–229.
56. NCCLS. Reference Method for Broth Dilution Antifungal Susceptibility Testing of Yeasts; Approved Standard. 2nd ed. NCCLS document M27-A2. Wayne, Pennsylvania: NCCLS, 2002.

3

Fungal Infections in Blood and Marrow Transplant Recipients

Kieren A. Marr
Program in Infectious Diseases, Fred Hutchinson Cancer Research Center, and Department of Medicine, University of Washington, Seattle, Washington, U.S.A.

I. INTRODUCTION

Patients who undergo blood or marrow transplantation (BMT) are at risk for death because of relapse of the underlying condition (e.g., malignancy), as well as complications that arise from the transplant itself. Common causes of transplant-related mortality include opportunistic infections and organ toxicities resultant from receipt of cytotoxic conditioning or other immunosuppressive therapies. Over the last few decades, multiple changes in transplantation practices have occurred, including changes in stem cell sources, conditioning regimens, and supportive care strategies used. These changes have impacted the relative proportion of relapse-related vs. transplant-related mortality, and have led to a changing spectrum of opportunistic pathogens.

During the last two decades, fungi have become important pathogens in BMT patients, and the fungi of importance have changed as well, with yeasts giving way to molds as the most common fungi causing death after BMT. Infections thus remain a dominant cause of non-relapse related deaths after BMT, even late after receipt of stem cells (1,2). To optimize outcomes after BMT, efforts continue to focus on developing effective strategies to prevent and treat infections. This chapter focuses on the epidemiology of fungal infections in BMT patients. The incidence of, risks for, and outcomes of the most common fungal infections are discussed.

II. FUNGAL INFECTIONS: OVERALL INCIDENCE AND RISKS

For fungal infections to develop after BMT, microbial exposure is required, but exposure alone will not result in infection without the presence of other factors to impair host defenses. Immunologic defects that pose risks for fungal infections in BMT recipients include severe neutropenia, and defects in cell-mediated immunity, which typically last for a longer duration, especially in people who require therapy for graft vs. host disease (GVHD) or receive T-cell depleted stem cell products. Thus, multiple host factors, transplantation variables, and microbial factors impact overall risks for infection (Fig. 1).

The magnitude of risks is not constant, but it expands and contracts during the course of BMT. Early post-transplant infection risks are largely influenced by severe neutropenia. A second high-risk period occurs later after transplantation with the onset of GVHD. In fact, severe acute GVHD may currently be the most important risk for invasive fungal infections (IFI), especially for those caused by molds. In one study, 50% of allogeneic BMT patients who developed severe (grades III–IV) acute GVHD developed an IFI, compared to 8% of patients who had minimal GVHD (3). Similarly, 57% of patients with clinically extensive chronic GVHD developed IFI, compared to 5% of those with limited chronic GVHD. Type of therapy for GVHD may also impact overall risks; this same study noted that 77% of patients who received high-dose steroids (methylprednisolone 0.25–1 g/day for 5 days) developed IFI, compared with 5% of patients who received lower doses (<2 mg/kg/day) of prednisone for GVHD therapy (3). Multiple studies have now shown that steroid containing regimens used to prevent and treat GVHD are associated with particularly high risks for infection and infection-related death (4–6). Unfortunately, transplanters are often forced to negotiate between the effects of GVHD and the overwhelming immunosuppression that may be required to suppress it.

Other transplantation variables, such as stem cell source and type of conditioning therapy, alter risk periods by impacting the duration and magnitude of immune reconstitution and other complications (e.g., gastrointestinal mucositis, GVHD). For instance, people who receive transplantation after non-myeloablative condi-

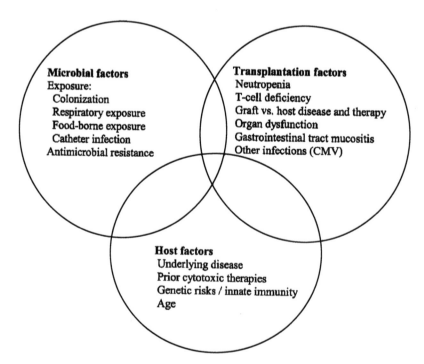

Figure 1 Multiple factors that impact risks for fungal infections after BMT. Overall risks for infection are influenced by microbial, host, and transplantation variables. The magnitude of each variable may expand and contract during the course of BMT, creating time periods that correspond to low and high risks for infection.

tioning therapy, which relies on graft versus host effects to elicit an adequate anti-tumor response, appear to develop infections later, during the period of GVHD (7–9). On the other hand, people who undergo transplantation using cord-blood as a stem cell source appear to have higher risks early after BMT, prior to stem cell engraftment (1,10,11). Typical risk periods for the most common fungal infections that occur after BMT, and corresponding host factors, are outlined in Figure 2. This time course provides a helpful guideline for understanding typical risk periods, which can be utilized to develop appropriate preventative strategies. However, it is important to appreciate that these generalizations do not account for important individual variables that may impact the risk for infection, such as severity of underlying disease and prior cytotoxic therapies, stem cell dose, and genetic differences in immunity. Incidence of, and specific risks, for the most common fungal infections are discussed in more detail in the following sections.

A. *Candida* Species

1. *Manifestations, Incidence of Infection, and Risks*

Candida species cause both mucosal infections and invasive diseases, such as candidemia and hepatosplenic candidiasis. More information on the pathogenesis of disease, clinical presentation, and diagnosis and management of candidal infections

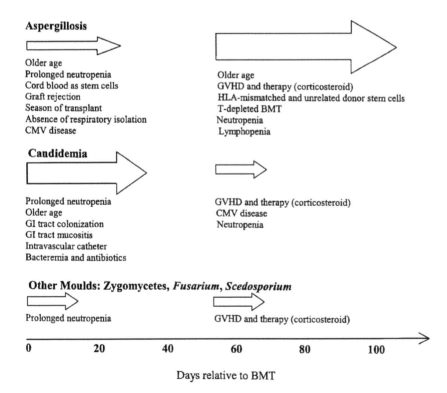

Figure 2 Risk periods for specific fungal infections, according to risk factors and time relative to receipt of stem cells (day 0). Size of arrows represents relative risk of infection during early and late time periods. Variables listed are those that have been identified with multivariable modeling (1,64–68).

is presented in Chapter 10. This section focuses on the epidemiology of mucosal and invasive candidiasis in BMT recipients.

Oral complications are important in BMT recipients, often causing pain and debilitation, with decreased oral intake potentially leading to systemic complications. Although *Candida* species are known to be a common cause of oral mucositis, few studies have specifically examined the incidence of, or risk factors for mucosal disease in BMT recipients. This may in part be due to diagnostic uncertainties attributable to the fact that *Candida* species are common colonizing organisms, and ulcerative mucositis and plaque-like lesions are caused by multiple factors, such as cytotoxic therapy, Herpes viruses, and GVHD. Older studies performed prior to the use of prophylactic azole antifungals in BMT recipients noted that the majority of patients have oral colonization with *Candida* species during the early post-transplant period, corresponding with mucositis associated with cytotoxic and/or radiation conditioning therapy (12,13), however, the causative role of *Candida* is not clear. Infections may progress to involve the esophagus in BMT patients, however, the incidence of esophageal candidiasis in the BMT setting is not well described. A review of esophageal infections that occurred in patients who underwent BMT without prophylactic antimicrobials in the early 1980s noted that the prevalence of esophageal infection is high, however, causative organisms (viral vs. fungal) could not be identified based on symptoms, oropharyngeal culture, or X-ray (14). Also, the concept of diagnostic parsimony does not hold for mucosal infections with *Candida* species, as in several studies, yeasts were found to cause esophageal infection with cooperation of an underlying Herpes virus (HSV or CMV) and/or GVHD (14,15).

Data on clinical significance of mucosal disease may be more reliable from the prospective studies performed to evaluate the efficacy of fluconazole for prophylactic therapy. In the placebo-controlled trials of the early 1990s, the incidence of "superficial" candidal infections ranged from 10% to 30% (16,17). In these studies, fluconazole administration decreased the incidence of both symptomatic mucosal candidiasis and gastrointestinal tract colonization.

Subsequent to the use of prophylactic therapy in allogeneic BMT patients, the morbidity of mucosal candidiasis declined dramatically. In part, this is related to the fact that azole-susceptible *C. albicans* more frequently cause oropharyngeal candidiasis than azole-resistant non-*albicans Candida* species (18,19). However, it is noteworthy that fluconazole-resistant *C. albicans* has not appeared as a common cause of mucosal candidiasis in BMT patients, as it did in the AIDS population (20). This is somewhat surprising since azole-resistant *C. albicans* species have been documented to colonize the GI tract and cause invasive disease in BMT patients receiving fluconazole prophylaxis (20–22). These differences may be due to multiple factors, including the relative durations of impairment in cell-mediated immunity, mucosal factors that impact microbial colonization, or to the use of topical or empiric antifungals in BMT patients.

The epidemiology of invasive candidiasis is better documented in this patient population. Several large studies have examined the clinical significance of, and risk factors for invasive candidal infections, both before and after the use of azoles for prophylactic therapy. In one institution, prior to the use of azoles for prophylaxis, the 1-year cumulative incidence of candidemia and/or deep tissue infection following allogeneic or autologous BMT was 12.5% (23). Investigators from another institution reported that the incidence of candidemia and/or deep tissue infection increased between the years 1980 and 1986, ranging from 11.4% to 40% (24). Outcomes of candidemia during this time period were poor; attributable mortality in these studies ranged from 32–37% (23,24).

Risks for candidemia that have been identified using multivariable modeling include the factors that increase exposure to the organism (e.g., GI tract colonization, presence of IV catheters) and factors that increase susceptibility of the host (e.g., prolonged neutropenia (Fig. 2) (23–25). Although the majority of candidemias occur during the early post-transplant period, patients who have severe GVHD have continued risks for candidemia, largely because of continued portals of entry via GI tract mucositis and indwelling catheters. Other factors that have been identified as risks for candidemia include bacteremia, CMV disease, and receipt of antibiotics (23–27). Whether these factors truly increase the risk for infection by altering microflora in the gut (28–30), or by modulating immune responses to fungi (31,32), or whether these events serve as markers of increased susceptibility is not clear.

2. Microbial Epidemiology

A change in the microbial epidemiology of candidiasis has been well described in large studies performed by networks of hospitals located throughout the world; nearly all studies performed in the latter 1990s noted a relative increase in non-*albicans Candida* species as pathogens, however, *C. albicans* has remained an important cause of invasive disease (33–35). In BMT patients, the use of azole antifungals has been a factor contributing to the change in epidemiology; prophylaxis has decreased the incidence of both candidemia and hepatosplenic candidiasis in BMT recipients, and changed the spectrum of *Candida* species that cause disease (25,36). In one institution, the use of prophylactic fluconazole was associated with a decreased incidence of candidemia (11–5%) and hepatosplenic candidiasis (9–3%) (25,36). The *Candida* species that cause disease have changed, with fewer infections by species that are typically azole-susceptible, and more caused by azole-resistant organisms (25,36,37). In the 1980s and early 1990s, *C. albicans* and *C. tropicalis* were the most frequent causes of invasive infection, with risks largely related to GI tract colonization (23,24,37,38). One surveillance study reported that *C. albicans* and *C. tropicalis* were the most frequent colonizing organisms, detected in 43% and 10.8% of BMT patients in the 1980s (38). Fluconazole administration appears to decrease colonization with *C. albicans* and encourage colonization with azole-resistant non-*albicans Candida* species, especially *C. glabrata* and *C. krusei*, resulting in increased risks for invasive disease with the potentially resistant organisms (25,39–41).

Case reports and series of infections caused by non-*albicans Candida* species emphasize that the mode of acquisition and risks for infection are species-dependent. Detailed cases of infection with *C. krusei, C. parapsilosis, C. dubliniensis, C. lusitaniae, C. lipolytica,* and *C. guilliermondii* have been presented in the literature (25,42–52). Candidemia is most common in patients with heavy GI tract colonization, and animal studies have shown that *C. albicans* and *C. tropicalis* are particularly adept at invading GI mucosa (3,25). Several other *Candida* species, including *C. parapsilosis, C. lusitaniae,* and *C. lipolytica* may more frequently be acquired through an exogenous route, potentially through IV catheters or infusates (25,37,49,51). Hence, risks for infection in particular patient populations impact microbial epidemiology to a large degree. More information on the pathogenesis of candidal infections is found in Chapter 10.

B. *Aspergillus* Species

1. Manifestations, Incidence of Infection, and Risks

During the 1990s, invasive infections caused by molds became more common in BMT patients. Currently, *Aspergillus* species are a frequent cause of invasive fungal infections, and in some centers, aspergillosis has become the most common cause of infection-related death (53). Disease caused by these organisms usually involves the respiratory tract, as organisms are usually acquired through aerosolization. Sinusitis and invasive pulmonary infection are the most common manifestations, however, complications can develop from local invasion into the orbit and brain, as well as hematogenous dissemination (Fig. 3). *Aspergillus* species can also cause locally invasive gastrointestinal disease in BMT patients (Fig. 3) (54), as well as a primary cutaneous infection involving areas of skin breakdown (55). More information on clinical manifestations and pathogenesis of *Aspergillus* infections is found in Chapter 10. The following discussion is focused on the risks for, and epidemiology of pulmonary aspergillosis in BMT recipients.

Aspergillus species were recognized as an important cause of pneumonia and death in BMT patients in the late 1970s and 1980s (56,57). During this period of time, the nosocomial nature of these infections became apparent; in one hospital, *Aspergillus* species were recognized as the single most common agent of nosocomial pneumonia, causing 36% of episodes (58,59). Infection typically occurred early after BMT; in a large review of patients who received BMT in one institution between 1974 and 1989, 58% of infections (including aspergillosis) occurred prior to neutrophil engraftment (60). Risks identified during this early period include prolonged neutropenia and graft rejection, especially in combination with nosocomial exposure to the organism (61).

During the 1980s aspergillosis was also recognized as a common cause of infection late after BMT (4,62,63). In a survey of European BMT centers, aspergillosis was identified as one of the most common infections that occurred greater than 3 months after BMT, along with CMV disease, *Pneumocystis carinii* pneumonia, and invasive infection with *Pseudomonas* species (63). A review of infections that occurred in 549 patients who received BMT in one transplant center during the 1980s showed that the majority of *Aspergillus* infections in allogeneic BMT patients occurred post-engraftment, especially in association with corticosteroid receipt for GVHD (4).

The results of most recent studies emphasize that aspergillosis now occurs more frequently late after allogeneic BMT, creating two peaks of infection, or a 'bimodal' incidence (1,64–68). In cohorts of patients who underwent transplantation during the latter 1990s, the median day of diagnosis ranged from day 92 to day 136 after receipt of stem cells (1,65–69). In these series, only 10–14% of *Aspergillus* infections occurred during neutropenia (65,68,70). The reason that aspergillosis occurs more frequently as a late complication of allogeneic BMT is not well understood. Potential explanations include reporting bias, increased diagnostic certainty, changes in GVHD therapies, increased environmental exposure, and shifts in microbial resistance patterns (1,36,71).

Factors that are important in conferring risks for aspergillosis during the early or late time periods after BMT are different; in general, early aspergillosis is associated with delayed neutrophil engraftment and late aspergillosis is associated with factors that impair cell-mediated immunity (Fig. 2) (1). Host and transplant variables that extend the duration of neutropenia and factors that lead to increased

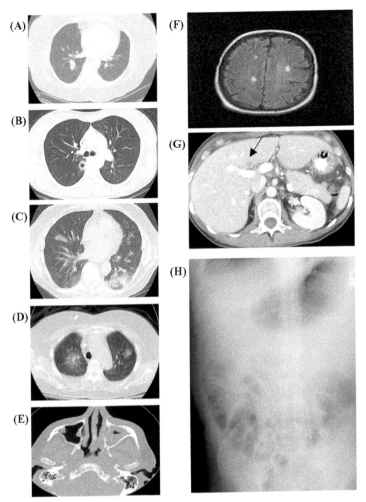

Figure 3 Radiographic images of diseases caused by *Aspergillus* species. Panels A–D demonstrate multiple presentations of pulmonary aspergillosis. This infection can present as isolated nodular lesions (**A**), cavitated lesions (**B**), pleural-based infiltrates (**C**), and scattered ground-glass appearing infiltrates (**D**). *Aspergillus* species may cause sinus opacification (**E**) with thickening of membranes and potentially bone destruction. Disease can disseminate to sites distant from lungs, including brain (**F**), liver (**G**, arrow), and other organs. *Aspergillus* species can also involve the GI tract. The patient in panel H presented with abdominal distress and ileus, which were found to be caused by *Aspergillus* gastritis and enterocolitis.

exposure to the organism increase the risk for early infection. Hence, stem cell sources and graft rejection are important factors associated with early disease (1,64); in one study, receipt of bone marrow or cord blood instead of peripheral blood as a stem cell source was associated with increased risks for early aspergillosis (1). Likewise, cohort studies have noted that patients who receive CD34-selected stem cells for either autologous or allogeneic transplantation may have relatively higher risks for infections early after BMT (72–74). Factors associated with an increased risk for post-transplant exposure to the organism, such as hospital construction and transplantation in the absence of protective isolation have also been identified as important variables in risk factor models focusing on the early time period (64). In one study, season of BMT was associated with increased risks during the early period; whether this is associated with increased environmental or hospital exposure is unknown (64).

Host factors that increase the likelihood of GVHD, such as receipt of stem cells from an unrelated or HLA-mismatched donor, increase the likelihood of aspergillosis later after BMT (1,65). Multivariable modeling noted a trend to increased risks for aspergillosis in patients who received peripheral blood instead of bone marrow as a stem cell source (1), possibly related to increased severity of GVHD (75,76). Type of therapy for GVHD is important; the highest risks for infection have been noted in people with severe GVHD (acute grades 3–4 and chronic clinically extensive disease) that is treated with high doses of corticosteroids (1,4,66,67). The relative magnitude of risks in people who undergo BMT using T-cell depleted stem cell products is unclear, as few comparative studies have been performed. However, the results of cohort studies suggest that T-cell depletion increases relative risks for aspergillosis late after BMT (77,78). The finding that T cells may be important in conferring risks for aspergillosis is not entirely surprising; multiple animal studies and a small clinical study showed that CD4+ T cells are important determinants for both infection risk and outcome (79–82). Precisely how these cells function to impact *Aspergillus* host defenses is not well understood.

The results of multiple studies have also demonstrated increased risks for aspergillosis in patients who have bacterial (27) and viral (1,32) infections after BMT. An association between CMV disease and aspergillosis has been particularly well described and noted in other immunosuppressed patients (e.g., solid organ transplant) (1,32,83). Other recent studies also found that certain respiratory viruses (Parainfluenza 3 and respiratory syncytial virus) are associated with increased risks for aspergillosis in multivariable models (1). It has been proposed that some viruses may impact risks by having a direct impact on fungal host defenses (32,84–88). However, other studies have noted that CMV disease and receipt of corticosteroids are statistically linked, raising the possibility that the infection serves as a marker of generalized impaired immunity, rather than a risk in itself (66).

Underlying diseases impact risk for aspergillosis both early and late after BMT. These factors may be important for a number of reasons, including age of the host, receipt of prior cytotoxic therapies, and type of BMT typically used to treat the underlying condition. In multiple studies, the underlying diseases of aplastic anemia and acute leukemias not in remission were associated with increased risks for post-transplant aspergillosis, especially early post-transplantation (1,64). Also, patients who have myelodysplastic syndromes have been noted to have increased risks for aspergillosis, both early and late after BMT (1,65). Underlying diseases may impact risks by specific impairments in host defenses, impacting prior cytotoxic therapies, or impacting the frequency (or severity) of GVHD or organ dysfunction.

Finally, different types of conditioning therapy impact risks for aspergillosis during the early and late time periods. Recent attention has been focused on the sustained risks for aspergillosis after non-myeloablative transplantation, despite decreased cytotoxic therapy and neutropenia in these patients. In studies performed to date, risks for late aspergillosis appear to be roughly equivalent in patients who underwent BMT after non-myeloablative and myeloablative conditioning therapy, although the rate of infection is likely to be dependent on specific treatment regimens (8,9,78). Not surprisingly, specific risks during the late time period include severe GVHD and CMV disease (9).

2. Microbial Epidemiology

The vast majority (>90%) of aspergillosis cases are caused by *A. fumigatus* (53,89). This is most likely reflective of an increased virulence of this organism, as relative exposure does not appear to be increased compared to other molds (90). Other *Aspergillus* species, notably, *A. terreus*, *A. niger*, and *A. flavus*, also cause diseases, possibly with increasing frequency in most recent years (53,91). These organisms cause disease that is limited to the sinuses more frequently than *A. fumigatus*, although all species appear to be able to cause invasive and disseminated disease in particularly immunosuppressed hosts. It is becoming increasingly apparent that different transplant centers may have unique patterns in microbial epidemiology, potentially because of a geographic impact on environmental mold quantity and differences in factors that impact nosocomial exposure. For instance, one center reported an outbreak of *A. terreus* infections associated with contamination of potted plants in their hospital (91). As the reported frequency of infection is influenced by both the patient populations at risk for disease and reporting bias, it is unclear how much variation in *Aspergillus* species exists between centers. Surveillance studies currently underway to track infections in transplant centers may allow us to assess better regional differences in the epidemiology of molds.

The source of exposure to *Aspergillus* species has recently come into question. For many years, these organisms were thought to be acquired by inhalation of aerosols produced in or around areas of construction. In one study, the presence of hospital construction increased rates *of Aspergillus* recovery in BMT patients (92). Regression modeling and molecular typing studies have also documented a relationship between aspergillosis in hospitalized patients and air contamination with *Aspergillus* spores (93–95). However, other studies have not been able to establish correlations with infections and results of air sampling (92,96–98). Potential explanations include the insensitivity of air sampling for *A. fumigatus* (99,100), biodiversity of isolates (96), identification of pseudo-epidemics' that result from contamination of culture media in the microbiology laboratory (101), as well as the possibility that *Aspergillus* species may be acquired through alternative sources (102,103). One suggestion is that *Aspergillus* species may be acquired from hospital water supplies. In several studies, molds were isolated in up to 70% of water sources (71,103–108). However, the frequency of recovery of molds from water supplies also appears to be variable; it is likely that mold contamination is impacted both by geography and the mechanism by which hospitals acquire, and deliver water to patient's rooms (106,108). Finally, it is possible that water-borne and food-borne *Aspergillus* species may also allow for acquisition through the gastrointestinal tract, although the relative frequency of "primary gastrointestinal aspergillosis" is not well described (102).

Hence, microbial epidemiology and clinical syndromes observed in different patient populations are likely to be impacted by air and water distribution practices in both the hospital and the environment. Multiple mechanisms of acquisition, including aerosolization of air and water, and ingestion may contribute to high risks for disease post-transplantation.

C. Other Fungi

Other molds and yeasts cause invasive diseases in BMT recipients. Other molds that are most frequent include the Zygomycetes, *Fusarium* spp., and *Scedosporium* spp. One BMT center reported that infections caused by Zygomycetes and *Fusarium* have increased in frequency during the latter 1990s (53). Although *Scedosporium* spp. did not appear to be increasing in frequency in this center located in Seattle, Washington, centers located in different geographic regions report increasing invasive infections with these molds. The epidemiology of these infections is discussed in more detail in the following sections.

1. Infections Caused by Zygomycetes

The class Zygomycetes is split into two orders: *Mucorales* and *Entomophthorales*. Although invasive infections with organisms in the *Entomophthorales* order occur (109–113), the vast majority of infections in humans are caused by the *Mucorales*. *Mucorales* is split into six families: *Mucoraceae, Cunninghamellacaea, Thamnidiaceae, Syncephalastraceae,* and *Mortierellaceae* (114). The most common causes of invasive infections in humans are caused by *Rhizopus* spp., *Mucor* spp., *Absidia* spp., and *Rhizomucor* spp., members of the family *Mucoraceae* (53,114,115), although increasing reports of infections caused by *Cunninghamella* spp. have appeared in the literature (116–119).

The majority of invasive infections caused by Zygomycetes originate in the sinopulmonary tract, and can invade through local tissues or by hematogenous dissemination (53,115). In our experience, pulmonary lesions caused by these organisms tend to be large and bulky, and local invasion through the chest wall can occur (Fig. 4). Some Zygomycetes infections may also be acquired through the GI tract, causing local colonic invasion and dissemination to the liver (109–111,115). It is likely that a certain number of these infections are acquired by contaminated food products. In one report, hepatic abscesses caused by Zygomycetes in a BMT patient was traced to ingestion of contaminated herbal medicines (120).

The incidence of Zygomycetes infections in BMT centers is not well defined. In retrospective studies performed in cancer centers, the incidence of invasive disease ranged from <1% to 2.5% (53,60,115), however, two recent studies reported that the frequency of disease increased in the latter 1990s (53,115). Severe neutropenia and corticosteroid therapy are important risks (53,114,115). Given the association

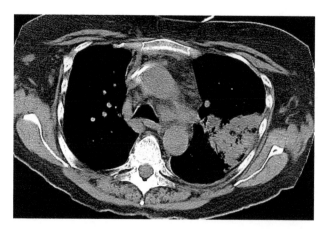

Figure 4 Radiographic manifestation of pulmonary zygomycosis in a BMT patient. Pulmonary zygomycosis can appear as nodular lesions, infiltrates, or large, necrotic masses. In the patient shown in the figure, disease progressed directly through the chest wall before successful therapy was achieved by a combination of systemic and locally applied antifungals and surgical debridement.

with GVHD and corticosteroid use, these infections may occur very late after BMT
(53). There is some evidence that the median duration of survival after Zygomycetes
infections is longer than infection with other molds (*Aspergillus* spp., *Fusarium* spp.,
and *Scedosporium* spp.); however, survival 1 year after infection appears equivalent
and poor (20%) (53). Many of these patients die despite successful antifungal therapy
with other complications of severe GVHD.

2. Infections Caused by Fusarium *species*

Fusarium species, common plant pathogens, also cause disease in immunocompromised patients. The majority of invasive infections are caused by *F. solani*, although
infections with *F. moniliforme* and *F. oxysporum* occur as well (121,122). These
organisms cause both cutaneous infections, such as onychomycosis and wound infections, as well as invasive infections, which can originate in the sinopulmonary tract,
gastrointestinal tract, IV catheter, or through skin breakdown (114,122).

The incidence of invasive *Fusarium* infections is variable among centers worldwide. A large cancer center in Texas reported that the frequency of infection
increased over the years spanning 1970–1995, although with approximately four
cases per year, the annual incidence is low, when compared to aspergillosis (123).
In contrast, European centers report few infections with these organisms (123).

Explanations for geographic clustering remain elusive. Because *Fusarium* spp.
can be isolated from water supplies, it was suggested that these infections may be
primarily nosocomial, with acquisition related to shower exposure (121). However,
another study failed to find an association between water culture of *Fusarium* spp.
and infection; instead, the organisms were more frequently recovered from environmental air (124). These investigators noted that recovery increased in rainy weather,
which corresponded with the seasonal distribution of infection (122,124). As with
other fungi, it is most likely that these organisms can be acquired through multiple
sources.

Few risk factor analyses for fusariosis in BMT recipients have been performed,
however, nearly all reports have linked infection with severe neutropenia after
conditioning therapy (53,122). Prolonged neutropenia and an underlying disease
of multiple myeloma have been identified as risks for fusariosis (53). Outcomes with
these infections have been poor during the amphotericin B era, with few patients
(≤30%) responding to therapy (53,122). Factors that improve prognosis include
neutrophil recovery, limited GVHD, and local disease (53,122). More discussion
on antifungal therapy of these infections is provided in Chapter 10.

3. Infections Caused by Scedosporium *Species*

Scedosporium prolificans and *S. apiospermum* (the sexual anamorph of
Pseudallescheria boydii) both cause disease in BMT patients. *Scedosporium apiospermum* is a well-known agent of mycetomas. In immunosuppressed patients, this
organism generally causes a spectrum of disease that is similar to those caused by
Aspergillus species, including sinusitis, inflammatory pneumonitis, cutaneous infections, and invasive pulmonary infection (125,126). *Scedosporium prolificans*,
although reported as a cause of invasive disease less frequently than *S. apiospermum*,
has become an important pathogen in certain parts of the world, especially Spain,
Australia, and parts of the United States (127,128). Variability in epidemiology is
likely to be related to the observation that this fungus proliferates best in a Mediter-
ranean climate (129), although nosocomial sources are also possible. In one recent

report, an outbreak of *S. prolificans* infections was found to be associated with contamination of the ambient air in hospital rooms (130).

Both *S. prolificans* and *S. apiospermum* infections are associated with a very poor prognosis in BMT patients (<20% survival). *Scedosporium prolificans* appears particularly resistant to current therapies, owing possibly to antifungal drug resistance and potentially, an increase in virulence of the organism (53,129–131). Correction of underlying neutropenia, the primary risk factor, is critical (127). More information on treatment of these infections is provided in Chapter 10.

*4. Infections Caused by non-*Candida *Yeasts and Endemic Fungi*

Patients who undergo BMT are at risk for infections with organisms that can be considered less pathogenic, "normal" flora, such as *Trichosporon* species, *Blastoschizomyces capitatus*, *Rhodotorula* spp., *Cryptococcus laurentii*, and *Malassezia furfur*, and infection in this setting is most likely to occur through IV catheters (132–137). Other relatively more pathogenic organisms that occur frequently among other immunosuppressed patients (e.g., AIDS) also occur infrequently in BMT patients. *Cryptococcus neoformans* can cause meningitis in this setting (138), however, these infections are notably rare. Agents of endemic mycoses, such as *Coccidioides immitis*, *Penicillium marneffei*, and *Histoplasma capsulatum*, also cause disease infrequently, even within endemic regions. Among 137 patients who received allogeneic BMT within a hyperendemic region for histoplasmosis, none of the patients developed invasive disease (139). Whether the infrequency of infection is associated with degree or duration of impairment in cell-mediated immunity, use of antifungals or some other factor in BMT patients is not known.

III. CONCLUSION

The pathogens of importance in BMT patients have evolved over the last 30 years, with emphasis shifted from gram-negative bacteria and gram-positive bacteria to Herpes viruses and fungi. Although early infections caused by Herpes simplex virus, CMV, and *C. albicans* have decreased, the late risk period has become more prominent. Recent studies showed that CMV still causes a great deal of morbidity and mortality after BMT. However, compared to in the 1980s (140), molds now are frequent pathogens during GVHD (1). These changes in epidemiology result from multiple variables, such as supportive care strategies that prevent early infection, changes in the population of patients who undergo transplantation, and changes in methods to perform the transplant itself. It is likely that new conditioning regimens, immunosuppressive drugs, and stem cell sources will continue to impact the epidemiology of infection in upcoming years. Although host variables are critically important, microbial virulence factors and microbial ecology play a role in defining the pathogens of importance. The combinatorial impact of all of these factors has led to the emergence of non-*albicans* Candida species, *Aspergillus* species, and other molds as important causes of death after BMT. Given the poor outcomes of treating documented infections, current efforts are focused on developing effective strategies to prevent these infections, particularly aspergillosis, during GVHD. We can thus expect to see more changes in epidemiology in the future, however, given the ubiquitous nature of these organisms, fungi are likely to continue to play a prominent role in transplantation-related mortality for years to come.

REFERENCES

1. Marr KA, Carter RA, Boeckh M, Martin P, Corey L. Invasive aspergillosis in allogeneic stem cell transplant recipients: changes in epidemiology and risk factors. Blood 2002; 100:4358–4366.
2. Ochs L, Shu X, Miller J, Wagner J, Filipovich A, Miller W, Weisdorf D. Late infections after allogeneic bone marrow transplantation: comparison of incidence in related and unrelated donor transplant recipients. Blood 1995; 86:3979–3986.
3. Hovi L, Saarinen-Pihkala UM, Vettenranta K, Saxen H. Invasive fungal infections in pediatric bone marrow transplant recipients: single center experience of 10 years. Bone Marrow Transpl 2000; 26:999–1004.
4. Wingard JR, Beals SU, Santos GW, Merz WG, Saral R. Aspergillus infections in bone marrow transplant recipients. Bone Marrow Transpl 1987; 2:175–181.
5. Ribaud P, Chastang C, Latge J, Baffroy-Lafitte L, Parquet N, ADevergie, Esperou H, Selimi F, Rocha V, Derouin F, Socie G, Gluckman E. Survival and prognostic factors of invasive aspergillosis after allogeneic bone marrow transplantation. Clin Infect Dis 1999; 28:322–330.
6. Sayer HG, Longton G, Bowden R, Pepe M, Storb R. Increased risk of infection in marrow transplant patients receiving methylprednisolone for graft-versus-host disease prevention. Blood 1994; 84:1328–1332.
7. Junghanss C, Marr K, Carter R, Sandmaier B, Maris M, Maloney D, et al. Incidence of bacterial and fungal infections after nonmyeloablative compared to myeloablative allogeneic stem cell transplantation (HSCT). Biol Blood Marr Transpl 2002; 8:512–520.
8. Hagen EA, Stern H, Porter D, Duffy K, Foley K, Luger S, Schuster SJ, Stadtmauer EA, Schuster MG. High rate of invasive fungal infections following nonmyeloablative allogeneic transplantation. Clin Infect Dis 2003; 36:9–15.
9. Fukuda T, Boeckh M, Carter RA, Sandmaier BM, Maris MB, Maloney DG, Martin PJ, Storb RF, Marr KA. Invasive fungal infections in recipients of allogeneic hematopoietic stem cell transplantation after nonmyeloablative conditioning: risks and outcomes. Blood 2003; 102:827–833.
10. Benjamin DK Jr, Miller WC, Bayliff S, Martel L, Alexander KA, Martin PL. Infections diagnosed in the first year after pediatric stem cell transplantation. Pediatr Infect Dis J 2002; 21:227–234.
11. Saavedra S, Sanz GF, Jarque I, Moscardo F, Jimenez C, Lorenzo I, Martin G, Martinez J, De La Rubia J, Andreu R, Molla S, Llopis I, Fernandez MJ, Salavert M, Acosta B, Gobernado M, Sanz MA. Early infections in adult patients undergoing unrelated donor cord blood transplantation. Bone Marr Transpl 2002; 30:937–943.
12. Berkowitz RJ, Hughes C, Rudnick M, Gordon EM, Strandjord S, Cheung NK, Warkentin P, Coccia PF. Oropharyngeal *Candida prophylaxis* in pediatric bone marrow transplant patients. Am J Pediatr Hematol Oncol 1985; 7:82–86.
13. Weisdorf DJ, Bostrom B, Raether D, Mattingly M, Walker P, Pihlstrom B, Ferrieri P, Haake R, Goldman A, Woods W, et al. Oropharyngeal mucositis complicating bone marrow transplantation: prognostic factors and the effect of chlorhexidine mouth rinse. Bone Marr Transp 1989; 4:89–95.
14. McDonald GB, Sharma P, Hackman RC, Meyers JD, Thomas ED. Esophageal infections in immunosuppressed patients after marrow transplantation. Gastroenterology 1985; 88:1111–1117.
15. Wu D, Hockenberry DM, Brentnall TA, Baehr PH, Ponec RJ, Kuver R, Tzung SP, Todaro JL, McDonald GB. Persistent nausea and anorexia after marrow transplantation: a prospective study of 78 patients. Transplantation 1998; 66:1319–1324.
16. Slavin MA, Osborne B, Adams R, Levenstein MJ, Schoch HG, Feldman AR, Meyers JD, Bowden RA. Efficacy and safety of fluconazole prophylaxis for fungal infections after marrow transplantation—a prospective, randomized, double-blind study. J Infect Dis 1995; 171:1545–1552.

17. Goodman JL, Winston DJ, Greenfield RA, Chandrasekar PH, Fox B, Kaizer H, Shadduck RK, Shea TC, Stiff P, Friedman DJ, Powderly WG, Silber JL, Horowitz H, Lichtin A, Wolff SN, Mangan SF, Silver SM, Weisdorf D, Ho WG, Gilbert G, Buell D. A controlled trial of fluconazole to prevent fungal infections in patients undergoing bone marrow transplantation. New Engl J Med 1992; 326:845–851.

18. Redding SW, Kirkpatrick WR, Dib O, Fothergill AW, Rinaldi MG, Patterson TF. The epidemiology of non-*albicans* Candida in oropharyngeal candidiasis in HIV patients. Spec Care Dentist 2000; 20:178–181.

19. Redding SW. The role of yeasts other than *Candida albicans* in oropharyngeal candidiasis. Curr Opin Infect Dis 2001; 14:673–677.

20. White TC, Marr KA, R.A. B. Clinical, cellular and molecular factors that contribute to antifungal drug resistance. Clin Microbiol Rev 1998; 11:382–402.

21. Nolte FS, Parkinson T, Falconer DJ, Dix S, Williams J, Gilmore C, Geller R, Wingard JR. Isolation and characterization of fluconazole- and amphotericin B-resistant *Candida albicans* from blood of two patients with leukemia. Antimicrob Agents Chemother 1997; 41:196–199.

22. Marr KA, White TC, van Burik JAH, Bowden RA. Development of fluconazole resistance in *Candida albicans* causing disseminated infection in a patient undergoing marrow transplantation. Clin Infect Dis 1997; 25:908–910.

23. Verfaillie C, Weisdorf D, Haake R, Hostetter M, Ramsay NK, McGlave P. *Candida* infections in bone marrow transplant recipients. Bone Marr Transpl 1991; 8:177–184.

24. Goodrich JM, Reed C, Mori M, et al. Clinical features and analysis of risk factors for invasive candidal infection after marrow transplantation. J Infect Dis 1991; 164: 731–740.

25. Marr KA, Seidel K, White TC, Bowden RA. Candidemia in allogeneic blood and marrow transplant recipients: evolution of risk factors after the adoption of prophylactic fluconazole. J Infect Dis 2000; 181:309–316.

26. Guiot HF, Fibbe WE, van Wout JW. Risk factors for fungal infection in patients with malignant hematologic disorders: implications for empirical therapy and prophylaxis [see comments]. Clin Infect Dis 1994; 18:525–532.

27. Sparrelid E, Hagglund H, Remberger M, et al. Bacteremia during the aplastic phase after allogeneic bone marrow transplantation is associated with early death from invasive fungal infection. Bone Marr Transpl 1998; 22:795–800.

28. Samonis G, Anaissie EJ, Bodey GP. Effects of broad-spectrum antimicrobial agents on yeast colonization of the gastrointestinal tracts of mice. Antimicrob Agents Chemother 1990; 34:2420–2422.

29. Maraki S, Mouzas IA, Kontoyiannis DP, Chatzinikolaou I, Tselentis Y, Samonis G. Prospective evaluation of the impact of amoxicillin, clarithromycin and their combination on human gastrointestinal colonization by *Candida* species. Chemotherapy 2001; 47:215–218.

30. Mavromanolakis E, Maraki S, Cranidis A, Tselentis Y, Kontoyiannis DP, Samonis G. The impact of norfloxacin, ciprofloxacin and ofloxacin on human gut colonization by *Candida albicans*. Scand J Infect Dis 2001; 33:477–478.

31. Laursen AL, Mogensen SC, Andersen HM, Andersen PL, Ellermann-Eriksen S. The impact of CMV on the respiratory burst of macrophages in response to *Pneumocystis carinii*. Clin Exp Immunol 2001; 123:239–246.

32. Nichols W, Corey L, Gooley T, Davis C, Boeckh M. High risk of death due to bacterial and fungal infection among CMV seroponegative recipients of stem cell transplantation from seropositive donors (D+/R−): evidence for "indirect" effects of primary CMV infection. J Infect Dis 2002; 185:273–282.

33. Pfaller M, Jones R, Doern G, Sader H, Messer S, Houston A, Coffrnan S, Hollis R, Group TSP. Bloodstream infections due to *Candida* species: SENTRY antimicrobial surveillance program in North American and Latin American, 1997–1998. Antimicrob Agents Chemother 2000; 44:747–751.

34. Pfaller M, Jones R, Doern G, Fluit A, Verhoef J, Sader H, Messer S, Houston A, Coffman S, Hollis F, SENTRY. Participants Group International surveillance of blood stream infections due to *Candida* species in the European SENTRY program: species distribution and antifungal susceptibility including the investigational triazole and echinocandin agents. Diagn Microbiol Infect Dis 2000; 35:19–25.

35. Pfaller M, Jones R, Doern G, Sader H, Hollis R, Messer S. International surveillance of bloodstream infections due to *Candida* species: frequency of occurrence and antifungal susceptibilities of isolates collected in 1997 in the United States, Canada, and South America for the SENTRY program. J Clin Microbiol 1998; 36:1886–1889.

36. van Burik JH, Leisenring W, Myerson D, Hackman RC, Shulman HM, Sale GE, Bowden RA, McDonald GB. The effect of prophylactic fluconazole on the clinical spectrum of fungal diseases in bone marrow transplant recipients with special attention to hepatic candidiasis. Medicine 1998; 77:246–254.

37. Safdar A, Perlin DS, Armstrong D. Hematogenous infections due to *Candida parapsilosis*: changing trends in fungemic patients at a comprehensive cancer center during the last four decades. Diagn Microbiol Infect Dis 2002; 44:11–16.

38. Pfaller M, Cabezudo I, Koontz F, Bale M, Gingrich R. Predictive value of surveillance cultures for systemic infection due to *Candida* species. Eur J Clin Microbiol 1987; 6: 628–633.

39. Hoppe JE, Klausner M, Klingebiel T, Niethammer D. Retrospective analysis of yeast colonization and infections in paediatric bone marrow transplant recipients. Mycoses 1997; 40:1–2.

40. Hoppe JE, Klingebiel T, Niethammer D. Selection of *Candida glabrata* in pediatric bone marrow transplant recipients receiving fluconazole. Pediatr Hematol Oncol 1994; 11: 207–210.

41. Chandrasekar P, Gatny C, Team at BMT. The effect of fluconazole prophylaxis on fungal colonization in neutropenic cancer patients. J Antimicrob Chemother 1994; 33: 309–318.

42. Meis J, Ruhnke M, DePauw B, Odds F, Siegert W, Verweij P. *Candida dubliniensis* candidemia in patients with chemotherapy-induced neutropenia and bone marrow transplantation. Emerg Infect Dis 1999; 5:150–153.

43. Fotedar R, Banerjee U. Changing pattern of *Candida* species in a bone marrow transplant patient. J Infect 1996; 32:243–245.

44. Wingard JR. Importance of *Candida* species other than *C. albicans* as pathogens in oncology patients. Clin Infect Dis 1995; 20:115–125.

45. Wingard JR, Merz WG, Rinaldi MG, Miller CB, Karp JE, Saral R. Association of *Torulopsis glabrata* infections with fluconazole prophylaxis in neutropenic bone marrow transplant patients. Antimicrob Agents Chemother 1993; 37:1847–1849.

46. Wingard JR, Merz WG, Rinaldi MG, Johnson TR, Karp JE, Saral R. Increase in *Candida krusei* infection among patients with bone marrow transplantation and neutropenia treated prophylactically with fluconazole. New Engl J Med 1991; 325:1274–1277.

47. Vazquez JA, Lundstrom T, Dembry L, Chandrasekar P, Boikov D, Parri MB, Zervos MJ. Invasive *Candida guilliermondii* infection: in vitro susceptibility studies and molecular analysis. Bone Marr Transpl 1995; 16:849–853.

48. Cancelas JA, Lopez J, Cabezudo E, Navas E, Garcia Larana J, Jimenez Mena M, Diz P, Perez de Oteyza J, Villalon L, Sanchez-Sousa A, et al. Native valve endocarditis due to *Candida parapsilosis*: a late complication after bone marrow transplantation-related fungemia. Bone Marr Transpl 1994; 13:333–334.

49. Sanchez V, Vazquez JA, Barth-Jones D, Dembry L, Sobel JD, Zervos MJ. Epidemiology of nosocomial acquisition of *Candida lusitaniae*. J Clin Microbiol 1992; 30: 3005–3008.

50. Minari A, Hachem R, Raad I. *Candida lusitaniae*: a cause of breakthrough fungemia in cancer patients. Clin Infect Dis 2001; 32:186–190.

51. D'Antonio D, Romano F, Pontieri E, Fioritoni G, Caracciolo C, Bianchini S, Olioso P, Staniscia T, Sferra R, Boccia S, Vetuschi A, Federico G, Gaudio E, Carruba G. Catheter-related candidemia caused by *Candida lipolytica* in a patient receiving allogeneic bone marrow transplantation. J Clin Microbiol 2002; 40:1381–1386.

52. D'Antonio D, Violante B, Mazzoni A, Bonfini T, Capuani MA, D'Aloia F, Iacone A, Schioppa F, Romano F. A nosocomial cluster of *Candida inconspicua* infections in patients with hematological malignancies. J Clin Microbiol 1998; 36:792–795.

53. Marr K, Carter R, Crippa F, Wald A, Corey L. Epidemiology and outcome of mould infections in hematopoietic stem cell transplant recipients. Clin Infect Dis 2002; 34: 909–917.

54. Catalano L, Picardi M, Anzivino D, Insabato L, Notaro R, Rotoli B. Small bowel infarction by *Aspergillus*. Haematologica 1997; 82:182–183.

55. van Burik JA, Colven R, Spach DH. Cutaneous aspergillosis. J Clin Microbiol 1998; 36:3115–3121.

56. Peterson PK, McGlave P, Ramsay NK, Rhame F, Cohen E, Perry GS 3rd, Goldman AI, Kersey J. A prospective study of infectious diseases following bone marrow transplantation: emergence of *Aspergillus* and Cytomegalovirus as the major causes of mortality. Infect Control 1983; 4:81–89.

57. Young JA, Hopkin JM, Cuthbertson WP. Pulmonary infiltrates in immunocompromised patients: diagnosis by cytological examination of bronchoalveolar lavage fluid. J Clin Pathol 1984; 37:390–397.

58. Pannuti C, Gingrich R, Pfaller MA, Kao C, Wenzel RP. Nosocomial pneumonia in patients having bone marrow transplant. Attributable mortality and risk factors. Cancer 1992; 69:2653–2662.

59. Pannuti C, Gingrich R, Pfaller M, et al. Nosocomial pneumonia in patients having bone marrow transplantation. Cancer 1991; 69:2653–2662.

60. Morrison V, Haake R, Weisdorf D. Non-*Candida* fungal infections after bone marrow transplantation: risk factors and outcome. Am J Med 1993; 96:497–503.

61. McWhinney P, Kibbler C, Hamon M, Smith O, Gandhi L, Berger L, Walesby R, Hoffbrand A, Prentice H. Progress in the diagnosis and management of aspergillosis in bone marrow transplantation: 13 years' experience. Clin Meet Dis 1993; 17:397–404.

62. Saugier-Veber P, Devergie A, Sulahian A, et al. Epidemiology and diagnosis of invasive pulmonary aspergillosis in bone marrow transplant patients: results of a 5 year retrospective study. Bone Marr Transpl 1993; 12:121–124.

63. Hoyle C, Goldman JM. Life-threatening infections occurring more than 3 months after BMT. 18 UK Bone Marrow Transplant Teams. Bone Marr Transpl 1994; 14:247–252.

64. Wald A, Leisenring W, van Burik J, Bowden RA. Epidemiology of *Aspergillus* infections in a large cohort of patients undergoing bone marrow transplantation. J Infect Dis 1997; 175:1459–1466.

65. Jantunen E, Ruutu P, Niskanen L, Volin L, Parkkali T, KoukilaKahkola P, Ruutu T. Incidence and risk factors for invasive fungal infections in allogeneic BMT recipients. Bone Marr Transpl 1997; 19:801–808.

66. Grow W, Moreb J, Roque D, Manion K, Leather H, Reddy V, Khan S, Finiewicz K, Nguyen H, Clancy C, Mehta P, Wingard J. Late onset of invasive aspergillus infection in bone marrow transplant patients at a university hospital. Bone Marr Transpl 2002; 29:15–19.

67. Baddley J, Stroud T, Salzman D, Pappas P. Invasive mold infections in allogeneic bone marrow transplant recipients. Clin Infect Dis 2001; 32:1319–1324.

68. Soubani AO, Qureshi MA. Invasive pulmonary aspergillosis following bone marrow transplantation: risk factors and diagnostic aspect. Haematologia (Budap) 2002; 32:427–437.

69. Soubani AO, Miller KB, Hassoun PM. Pulmonary complications of bone marrow transplantation. Chest 1996; 109:1066–1077.

70. Kruger W, Russmann B, Kroger N, Salomon C, Ekopf N, Eisner HA, Kaulfers PM, Mack D, Fuchs N, Durken M, Kabisch H, Erttmann R, Zander AR. Early infections in patients undergoing bone marrow or blood stem cell transplantation—a 7 year single centre investigation of 409 cases. Bone Marr Transpl 1999; 23:589–597.
71. Anaissie EJ, Stratton SL, Dignani MC, Summerbell RC, Rex JH, Monson TP, Spencer T, Kasai M, Francesconi A, Walsh TJ. Pathogenic *Aspergillus* species recovered from a hospital water system: a 3-year prospective study. Clin Infect Dis 2002; 34:780–789.
72. Crippa F, Holmberg L, Carter RA, Hooper H, Marr KA, Bensinger W, Chauncey T, Corey L, Boeckh M. Infectious complications after autologous CD34-selected peripheral blood stem cell transplantation. Biol Blood Marr Transpl 2002; 8:281–289.
73. Holmberg L, Boeckh M, Hooper H, Leisenring W, Rowley S, Heimfeld S, Press O, Maloney D, McSweeney P, Corey L, Maziarz R, Appelbaum F, Bensinger W. Increased incidence of cytomegalovirus disease after autologous CD34-selected peripheral blood stem cell transplantation. Blood 1999; 94:4029–4035.
74. Bacigalupo A, Mordini N, Pitto A, Piaggio G, Podesta M, Benvenuto F, van Lint MT, Valbonesi M, Lercari G, Carlier P, Lamparelli T, Gualandi F, Occhini D, Bregante S, Figari O, Soracco M, Vassallo F, De Stefano G. Transplantation of HLA-mismatched CD34+ selected cells in patients with advanced malignancies: severe immunodeficiency and related complications. Br J Haematol 1997; 98:760–766.
75. Fauser AA, Basara N, Blau IW, Kiehl MG. A comparative study of peripheral blood stem cell vs bone marrow transplantation from unrelated donors (MUD): a single center study. Bone Marr Transpl 2000; 25(Suppl 2):S27–S31.
76. Blau IW, Basara N, Lentini G, Guenzelmann S, Kirsten D, Schmetzer B, Bischoff M, Roemer E, Kiehl MG, Fauser AA. Feasibility and safety of peripheral blood stem cell transplantation from unrelated donors: results of a single-center study. Bone Marr Transpl 2001; 27:27–33.
77. Williamson EC, Millar MR, Steward CG, Cornish JM, Foot AB, Oakhill A, Pamphilon DH, Reeves B, Caul EO, Warnock DW, Marks DI. Infections in adults undergoing unrelated donor bone marrow transplantation. Br J Haematol 1999; 104:560–568.
78. Daly A, McAfee S, Dey B, Colby C, Schulte L, Yeap B, Sackstein R, Tarbell NJ, Sachs D, Sykes M, Spitzer TR. Nonmyeloablative bone marrow transplantation: infectious complications in 65 recipients of HLA-identical and mismatched transplants. Biol Blood Marr Transpl 2003; 9:373–382.
79. Cenci E, Mencacci A, Spreca A, Montagnoli C, Bacci A, Perruccio K, Velardi A, Magliani W, Conti S, Polonelli L, Romani L. Protection of killer antiidiotypic antibodies against early invasive aspergillosis in a murine model of allogeneic T-cell-depleted bone marrow transplantation. Infect Immun 2002; 70:2375–2382.
80. Cenci E, Mencacci A, Bacci A, Bistoni F, Kurup VP, Romani L. T cell vaccination in mice with invasive pulmonary aspergillosis. J Immunol 2000; 165:381–388.
81. Cenci E, Mencacci A, Fe d'Ostiani C, Del Sero G, Mosci P, Montagnoli C, Bacci A, Romani L. Cytokine- and T helper-dependent lung mucosal immunity in mice with invasive pulmonary aspergillosis. J Infect Dis 1998; 178:1750–1760.
82. Hebart H, Bollinger C, Fisch P, Sarfati J, Meisner C, Baur M, Loeffler J, Monod M, Latge JP, Einsele H. Analysis of T-cell responses to *Aspergillus fumigatus* antigens in healthy individuals and patients with hematologic malignancies. Blood 2002; 100:4521–4528.
83. Husni R, Gordon S, Longworth D, Arroglia A, Stillwell P, Avery R, Maurer J, Mehta A, Kirby T. Cytomegalovirus is a risk factor for invasive aspergillosis in lung transplant recipients. Clin Infect Dis 1998; 26:753–755.
84. Bartz H, Turkel O, Hoffjan S, Rothoeft T, Gonschorek A, Schauer U. Respiratory syncytial virus decreases the capacity of myeloid dendritic cells to induce interferon-gamma in naive T cells. Immunol 2003; 109:49–57.

85. Bartz H, Buning-Pfaue F, Turkel O, Schauer U. Respiratory syncytial virus induces prostaglandin E2, IL-10 and IL-11 generation in antigen presenting cells. Clin Exp Immunol 2002; 129:438–445.

86. Falk CS, Mach M, Schendel DJ, Weiss EH, Hilgert I, Hahn G. NK cell activity during human cytomegalovirus infection is dominated by US2–11-mediated HLA class I down-regulation. J Immunol 2002; 169:3257–3266.

87. Miller SA, Bia FJ, Coleman DL, Lucia HL, Young KR Jr, Root RK. Pulmonary macrophage function during experimental cytomegalovirus interstitial pneumonia. Infect Immunol 1985; 47:211–216.

88. Aoyagi M, Shimojo N, Sekine K, Nishimuta T, Kohno Y. Respiratory syncytial virus infection suppresses IFN-gamma production of gammadelta T cells. Clin Exp Immunol 2003; 131:312–317.

89. Perfect JR, Cox GM, Lee JY, Kauffman CA, de Repentigny L, Chapman SW, Morrison VA, Pappas P, Hiemenz JW, Stevens DA. The impact of culture isolation of *Aspergillus* species: a hospital-based survey of aspergillosis. Clin Infect Dis 2001; 33:1824–1833.

90. Latge JP. *Aspergillus fumigatus* and aspergillosis. Clin Microbiol Rev 1999; 12:310–350.

91. Lass-Florl C, Rath P, Niederwieser D, Kofler G, Wurzner R, Krezy A, Dierich MP. *Aspergillus terreus* infections in haematological malignancies: molecular epidemiology suggests association with in-hospital plants. J Hosp Infect 2000; 46:31–35.

92. Lai KK. A cluster of invasive aspergillosis in a bone marrow transplant unit related to construction and the utility of air sampling. Am J Infect Control 2001; 29:333–337.

93. Alberti C, Bouakline A, Ribaud P, Lacroix C, Rousselot P, Leblanc T, Derouin F. Relationship between environmental fungal contamination and the incidence of invasive aspergillosis in haematology patients. J Hosp Infect 2001; 48:198–206.

94. Richardson MD, Rennie S, Marshall I, Morgan MG, Murphy JA, Shankland GS, Watson WH, Soutar RL. Fungal surveillance of an open haematology ward. J Hosp Infect 2000; 45:288–292.

95. Hahn T, Cummings KM, Michalek AM, Lipman BJ, Segal BH, McCarthy PL Jr. Efficacy of high-efficiency particulate air filtration in preventing aspergillosis in immunocompromised patients with hematologic malignancies. Infect Control Hosp Epidemiol 2002; 23:525–531.

96. Symoens F, Burnod J, Lebeau B, Viviani MA, Piens MA, Tortorano AM, Nolard N, Chapuis F, Grillot R. Hospital-acquired *Aspergillus fumigatus* infection: can molecular typing methods identify an environmental source?. J Hosp Infect 2002; 52:60–67.

97. Leenders A, vanBelkum A, Behrendt M, Luijendijk A, Verbrugh H. Density and molecular epidemiology of *Aspergillus* in air and relationship to outbreaks of *Aspergillus* infection. J Clin Microbiol 1999; 37:1752–1757.

98. Hospenthal DR, Kwon-Chung KJ, Bennett JE. Concentrations of airborne *Aspergillus* compared to the incidence of invasive aspergillosis: lack of correlation. Med Mycol 1998; 36:165–168.

99. Morris G, Kokki MH, Anderson K, Richardson MD. Sampling of *Aspergillus* spores in air. J Hosp Infect 2000; 44:81–92.

100. Thio CL, Smith D, Merz WG, Streifel AJ, Bova G, Gay L, Miller CB, Perl TM. Refinements of environmental assessment during an outbreak investigation of invasive aspergillosis in a leukemia and bone marrow transplant unit. Infect Control Hosp Epidemiol 2000; 21:18–23.

101. Laurel VL, Meier PA, Astorga A, Dolan D, Brockett R, Rinaldi MG. Pseudoepidemic of *Aspergillus niger* infections traced to specimen contamination in the microbiology laboratory. J Clin Microbiol 1999; 37:1612–1616.

102. Bouakline A, Lacroix C, Roux N, Gangneux JP, Derouin F. Fungal contamination of food in hematology units. J Clin Microbiol 2000; 38:4272–4273.

103. Warris A, Gaustad P, Meis J, Verweij P, Abrahamsen T. Water as a source of filamentous fungi in a childhood bone marrow transplantation unit. In: International Conference on Antimicrobial Agents and Chemotherapy, San Francisco, CA, 1999.

104. Anaissie EJ, Costa SF. Nosocomial aspergillosis is waterborne. Clin Infect Dis 2001; 33:1546–1548.

105. Anaissie E, Stratton S, Summerbell R, Monson T, Rex J, Walsh T. *Aspergillus* species aerosols in hospitals: showering as a potential mode of exposure. International Conference of Antimicrobial Agents and Chemotherapy, San Francisco, CA, 1999.

106. Warns A, Voss A, Abrahamsen TG, Verweij PE. Contamination of hospital water with *Aspergillus fumigatus* and other molds. Clin Infect Dis 2002; 34:1159–1160.

107. Warns A, Gaustad P, Meis JF, Voss A, Verweij PE, Abrahamsen TG. Recovery of filamentous fungi from water in a paediatric bone marrow transplantation unit. J Hosp Infect 2001; 47:143–148.

108. Panagopoulou P, Filioti J, Petrikkos G, Giakouppi P, Anatoliotaki M, Farmaki E, Kanta A, Apostolakou H, Avlami A, Samonis G, Roilides E. Environmental surveillance of filamentous fungi in three tertiary care hospitals in Greece. J Hosp Infect 2002; 52:185–191.

109. Lyon GM, Smilack JD, Komatsu KK, Pasha TM, Leighton JA, Guarner J, Colby TV, Lindsley MD, Phelan M, Warnock DW, Hajjeh RA. Gastrointestinal basidiobolomycosis in Arizona: clinical and epidemiological characteristics and review of the literature. Clin Infect Dis 2001; 32:1448–1455.

110. Zavasky DM, Samowitz W, Loftus T, Segal H, Carroll K. Gastrointestinal zygomycotic infection caused by *Basidiobolus ranarum*: case report and review. Clin Infect Dis 1999; 28:1244–1248.

111. Pasha TM, Leighton JA, Smilack JD, Heppell J, Colby TV, Kaufman L. Basidiobolomycosis: an unusual fungal infection mimicking inflammatory bowel disease. Gastroenterology 1997; 112:250–254.

112. Jaffey PB, Haque AK, el-Zaatari M, Pasarell L, McGinnis MR. Disseminated Conidiobolus infection with endocarditis in a cocaine abuser. Arch Pathol Lab Med 1990; 114:1276–1278.

113. Walsh TJ, Renshaw G, Andrews J, Kwon-Chung J, Cunnion RC, Pass HI, Taubenberger J, Wilson W, Pizzo PA. Invasive zygomycosis due to *Conidiobolus incongruus*. Clin Infect Dis 1994; 19:423–430.

114. Ribes J, Vanover-Sams C, Baker D. Zygomycetes in human disease. Clin Microbiol Rev 2000; 13:236–301.

115. Kontoyiannis D, Wessel V, Bodey G, Rolston K. Zygomycosis in the 1990s in a tertiary care center. Clin Infect Dis 2000; 30:851–856.

116. Cohen-Abbo A, Bozeman PM, Patrick CC. Cunninghamella infections: review and report of two cases of *Cunninghamella pneumonia* in immunocompromised children. Clin Infect Dis 1993; 17:173–177.

117. Rickerts V, Bohme A, Viertel A, Behrendt G, Jacobi V, Tintelnot K, Just-Nubling G. Cluster of pulmonary infections caused by *Cunninghamella bertholletiae* in immunocompromised patients. Clin Infect Dis 2000; 31:910–913.

118. Darrisaw L, Hanson G, Vesole DH, Kehl SC. *Cunninghamella* infection post bone marrow transplant: case report and review of the literature. Bone Marr Transpl 2000; 25:1213–1216.

119. Kontoyianis DP, Vartivarian S, Anaissie EJ, Samonis G, Bodey GP, Rinaldi M. Infections due to *Cunninghamella bertholletiae* in patients with cancer: report of three cases and review. Clin Infect Dis 1994; 18:925–928.

120. Oliver M, Voorhis WV, Boeckh M, Mattson D, Bowden R. Hepatic mucormycosis in a bone marrow transplant recipient who ingested naturopathic medicine. Clin Infect Dis 1996; 22:521–524.

121. Anaissie EJ, Kuchar RT, Rex JH, Francesconi A, Kasai M, Muller FM, Lozano-Chiu M, Summerbell RC, Dignani MC, Chanock SJ, Walsh TJ. Fusariosis associated with

pathogenic fusarium species colonization of a hospital water system: a new paradigm for the epidemiology of opportunistic mold infections. Clin Infect Dis 2001; 33: 1871–1878.

122. Boutati E, Anaissie E. Fusarium, a significant emerging pathogen in patients with hematologic malignancy: ten years' experience at a cancer center and implications for management. Blood 1997; 90:999–1008.

123. Girmenia C, Pagano L, Corvatta L, Mele L, del Favero A, Martino P. The epidemiology of fusariosis in patients with haematological diseases. Gimema infection programme. Br J Haematol 2000; 111:272–276.

124. Raad I, Tarrand J, Hanna H, Albitar M, Janssen E, Boktour M, Bodey G, Mardani M, Hachem R, Kontoyiannis D, Whimbey E, Rolston K. Epidemiology, molecular mycology, and environmental sources of *Fusarium* infection in patients with cancer. Infect Control Hosp Epidemiol 2002; 23:532–537.

125. Cimon B, Carrere J, Vinatier JF, Chazalette IP, Chabasse D, Bouchara JP. Clinical significance of *Scedosporium apiospermum* in patients with cystic fibrosis. Eur J Clin Microbiol Infect Dis 2000; 19:53–56.

126. Eckburg PB, Zolopa AR, Montoya JG. Invasive fungal sinusitis due to *Scedosporium apiospermum* in a patient with AIDS. Clin Infect Dis 1999; 29:212–213.

127. Maertens J, Lagrou K, Deweerdt H, Surmont I, Verhoef GE, Verhaegen J, Boogaerts MA. Disseminated infection by *Scedosporium prolificans*: an emerging fatality among haematology patients. Case report and review. Ann Hematol 2000; 79:340–344.

128. Idigoras P, Perez-Trallero E, Pineiro L, Larruskain J, Lopez-Lopategui MC, Rodriguez N, Gonzalez JM. Disseminated infection and colonization by *Scedosporium prolificans*: a review of 18 cases, 1990–1999. Clin Infect Dis 2001; 32:E158–E165.

129. Ortoneda M, Pastor FJ, Mayayo E, Guarro J. Comparison of the virulence of *Scedosporium prolificans* strains from different origins in a murine model. J Med Microbiol 2002; 51:924–928.

130. Guerrero A, Torres P, Duran MT, Ruiz-Diez B, Rosales M, Rodriguez-Tudela JL. Airborne outbreak of nosocomial *Scedosporium prolificans* infection. Lancet 2001; 357:1267–1268.

131. Perfect JR, Marr KA, Walsh TJ, Greenberg RN, DuPont B, de la Torre-Cisneros J, Just-Nubling G, Schlamm HT, Lutsar I, Espinel-Ingroff A, Johnson E. Voriconazole treatment for less-common, emerging, or refractory fungal infections. Clin Infect Dis 2003; 36:1122–1131.

132. Goodman D, Pamer E, Jakubowski A, Morris C, Sepkowitz K. Breakthrough trichosporonosis in a bone marrow transplant recipient receiving caspofungin acetate. Clin Infect Dis 2002; 35:E35–E36.

133. Morrison VA, Weisdorf DJ. The spectrum of *Malassezia* infections in the bone marrow transplant population. Bone Marr Transpl 2000; 26:645–648.

134. Erer B, Galimberti M, Lucarelli G, Giardini C, Polchi P, Baronciani D, Gaziev D, Angelucci E, Izzi G. Trichosporon beigelii: a life-threatening pathogen in immunocompromised hosts. Bone Marr Transpl 2000; 25:745–749.

135. Krcmery V Jr, Mateicka F, Kunova A, Spanik S, Gyarfas J, Sycova Z, Trupl J. *Hematogenous trichosporonosis* in cancer patients: report of 12 cases including 5 during prophylaxis with itraconazol. Support Care Cancer 1999; 7:39–43.

136. Kunova A, Krcmery V. Fungaemia due to thermophilic cryptococci: 3 cases of *Cryptococcus laurentii* bloodstream infections in cancer patients receiving antifungals. Scand J Infect Dis 1999; 31:328.

137. Krcmery V Jr, Kunova A, Mardiak J. Nosocomial *Cryptococcus laurentii* fungemia in a bone marrow transplant patient after prophylaxis with ketoconazole successfully treated with oral fluconazole. Infection 1997; 25:130.

138. Miniero R, Nesi F, Vai S, De Intinis G, Papalia F, Targhetta R, Busca A, Vassallo E, Giacchino M. Cryptococcal meningitis following a thrombotic microangiopathy in an

unrelated donor bone marrow transplant recipient. Pediatr Hematol Oncol 1997; 14:469–474.

139. Vail G, Young R, Wheat L, Filo R, Cornetta K, Goldman M. Incidence of histoplasmosis following allogeneic bone marrow transplantation or solid organ transplant in a hyperendemic area. Transpl Infect Dis 2002; 4(3):148–151.

140. Boeckh M, Leisenring W, Riddell SR, Bowden RA, Huang ML, Myerson D, Stevens-Ayers T, Flowers ME, Cunningham T, Corey L. Late cytomegalovirus disease and mortality in recipients of allogeneic hematopoietic stem cell transplants: importance of viral load and T-cell immunity. Blood 2003; 101:407–414.

4

Assessment of the Risk for Invasive Fungal Infection Among Oncology Patients

E. J. Bow
Sections of Infectious Diseases and Hematology/Oncology, Department of Internal Medicine, University of Manitoba, Department of Medical Oncology and Hematology, Infection Control Services, Cancer Care Manitoba, and Health Sciences Center, Winnipeg, Manitoba, Canada

I. INTRODUCTION

The prevalence of patients living with cancer is rising (1) particularly as the spectrum and sophistication of available anticancer treatment strategies expands. Malignant disease and treatments thereof have profound negative effects upon the ability of the system of human host defenses to successfully engage and deflect a plethora of opportunistic pathogens met in the course of daily living. Superficial and invasive fungal infections have assumed a much more prominent role in the supportive care planning for patients undergoing intensive treatment for malignant disease.

The risk of invasive fungal infection in cancer patients varies with the underlying diagnosis, the cytotoxic or immunosuppressive regimen administered to treat the underlying cancer, and the circumstances of responsiveness of the underlying neoplasm for which the treatments are administered (2). A number of categories of predictors have been identified that have been associated with the risk of fungal infection-related morbidity. These include advanced age (3,4), advanced underlying disease (5,6), myelosuppression (7–9), immunosuppression (5–10), colonization of epithelial surfaces (6,11–14), environmental exposure (15–25), and physical damage to the integumental surfaces (6,26). Table 1 lists these variables. This chapter focuses upon the epidemiology of invasive fungal infection among cancer patient populations and reviews the relevant information pertaining to risk factors and predictors for invasive fungal infections related to cancer treatment.

II. EPIDEMIOLOGY OF INVASIVE FUNGAL INFECTION OBSERVED AT AUTOPSY

The prevalence of invasive fungal infection has been rising since the earliest descriptions among autopsied patients with cancer (8,27–30). A total of 8 (0.15%) invasive

Table 1 Principal Risk Factor Categories for Superficial and Invasive Fungal Infections in Patients Receiving Antineoplastic Therapy

Category	Principal risk factors
Myelosuppression	• Neutropaenia ▶ANC $< 0.5 \times 10^9$/L ▶Prolonged aplasia > 10–14 days • Monocytopenia ▶AMC $< 0.2 \times 10^9$/L
Immunosuppression	• Lymphopenia ▶ALC $< 0.7 \times 10^9$/L • CD4$^+$ T-lymphocytopenia ▶ALC CD4$^+$ $< 0.2 \times 10^9$/L • CD19$^+$ B-lymphocytopenia: ▶ALC CD19$^+$ $< 0.1 \times 10^9$/L • Therapies that augment immunosuppression ▶Corticosteroid therapy: Prednisone dose equivalent of 20 mg/day over 30 days or at least 700 mg cumulative dose over 30 days ▶Monoclonal antibody reagents such as rituxumab and alemtuzumab ▶Purine analogs including fludarabine, cladribine, and deoxycorfomycin
Colonization	• Multiple sites ▶Colonization index > 0.25 • *Candida* spp. ▶Oropharynx, nasopharynx, rectum, urine ▶*C. tropicalis, C. glabrata, C. krusei* • *Aspergillus* spp. ▶Nasopharynx • Administration of broad-spectrum antibacterial therapy ▶Antianaerobic activity ▶Biliary excretion • Administration of quinolone-based antibacterial prophylaxis ▶Colonization by opportunistic yeasts • Administration of azole-based antifungal prophylaxis ▶Selection for colonization by *C. glabrata, C. krusei*
Exposure	• Health care worker-related transmission ▶Transmission of opportunistic yeast on HCW hands • Fomites ▶Transmission of opportunistic yeast on equipment • Environment ▶Institutional demolition, construction, and maintenance ▶High conidial counts per unit time ▶Duration of stay in risk environments

(Continued)

Table 1 Principal Risk Factor Categories for Superficial and Invasive Fungal Infections in Patients Receiving Antineoplastic Therapy (*Continued*)

Category	Principal risk factors

Integumental damage	▶Transport routes
	▶High-efficiency particulate air-handling protective environments
	• Cytotoxic therapy
	  ▶Local irradiation vs. systemic chemotherapy
	  ▶Class of cytotoxic agent
	    Antimetabolites
	    Anthracyclines / anthraquinone
	    Topoisomerase inhibitors
	    Alkylating agents
	    Anti-CD33 monoclonal antibody reagents
	  ▶Mucositis
	    Infection risk and the mucositis score
	    Infection risk and permeability changes
	• Indwelling venous access devices
	  ▶Interaction with gut colonization
	• Urinary catheters
	  ◀Interaction with antimicrobial use and colonization
	• Ventilation assistance devices
	  ▶Interaction with antimicrobial use and colonization
	• Surgical wounds
	  ▶Interaction with antimicrobial use and colonization

Abbreviations: ANC, absolute neutrophil count; AMC, absolute monocytes count; ALC, absolute lymphocyte count; ALC CD4$^+$, absolute CD4$^+$ T-lymphocyte count; ALC CD19$^+$, absolute CD19$^+$ B-lymphocyte count.

mycoses were noted among 5530 autopsies performed between 1919 and 1936, 3 (0.1%) in 2879 performed between 1937 and 1941, 9 (0.26%), and 50 (1.2%) in 4167 performed between 1948 and 1955 (27). The prevalence of invasive mycoses at autopsy continued to rise from 1948 onwards, particularly among patients with leukemia and lymphoma in whom the rate increased from 5% in 1947–1948 to 20% in 1954–1955 (Fig. 1). Co-incident with this increase was the introduction of several new antineoplastic agents effective in these diseases including nitrogen mustard in 1945, aminopterin in 1948, prednisone in 1949, and mercaptopurine in 1952. Moreover, the introduction of penicillin in 1941, streptomycin in 1944, and the tetracyclines in 1948 provided physicians prescribing these agents with the antibacterial tools to manage the consequent, otherwise, fatal febrile neutropenic episodes.

The combination of the new antineoplastic and antibacterial agents arguably permitted leukemia and lymphoma patients to survive sufficiently long enough to become colonized and infected by opportunistic fungi. Figure 2 illustrates the continued rise in prevalence of invasive mycoses at autopsy as reported between 1948 and 1980 (8,27,29). The reduction in the incidence of invasive fungal infection noted in the international autopsy study of Bodey et al. (28) in Figure 2 corresponds

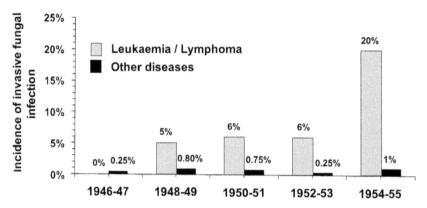

Figure 1 Increase in incidence of invasive fungal infection observed at autopsy in a hospitalized patient population.

to the time during which the empirical use of amphotericin B deoxycholate for suspected but unproven fungal infection became a standard of practice (31–33).

In more recent analysis of data from 4096 patients autopsied between 1980 and 1988 from centers in Europe, Canada, and Japan demonstrated that the prevalence of invasive mycoses was highest among acute leukemia patients (25%), followed by lymphoma (12%), and solid tumor patients (5%), respectively (28). The proportionate frequency of invasive fungal infection by underlying diagnosis was 5:2.5:1 for leukemia, lymphoma, and solid tumor, respectively (28). A single center study from Germany reporting on 8124 patients autopsied between 1978 and 1992 demonstrated the highest prevalence of invasive mycoses among patients with acute leukemia (55 of 176, 31.3%), followed by patients with the human immunodeficiency virus-mediated acquired immunodeficiency syndrome (AIDS, 60 of 314, 19.1%), organ

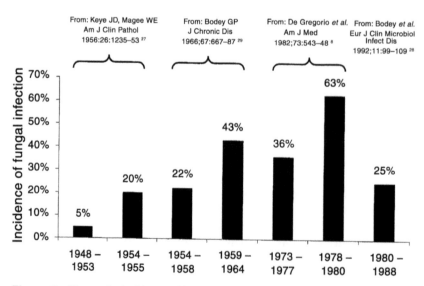

Figure 2 Change in incidence of invasive fungal infection from 1948 to 1988 as reported in different autopsy series.

transplantation (9 of 61, 14.8%), lymphoma (57 of 442, 12.9%), and solid tumors (37 of 2356, 1.6%) (30). In that study, a pattern of increasing prevalence over time was also observed from 2.2% in 1978–1982, 3.2% in 1983–1987, to 5.1% in 1988–1992 (30) similar to that observed previously (27–29).

 Candida spp. has been the pathogen most commonly associated with invasive fungal infection found postmortem in cancer patients, accounting for 66% (range 42–78%) of cases in a large international autopsy review (28). *Aspergillus* spp. accounted for 34% (range 22–55%). Cryptococcosis was identified only infrequently (2%, range 0–4%). Among 57 autopsied patients with acute leukemia, invasive fungal infection was demonstrable in 32 (56%). *Candida* spp. accounted for 17 (29.8%), *Aspergillus* spp. for 7 (12.3%), *Candida* spp. and *Aspergillus* spp. for 7 (12.3%), and Mucor spp. for 1 (1.7%) (8). In this study, molds accounted for over one-quarter (26.3%) of the infections.

 As in the older series, the most common pathogens observed at autopsy in the German series (30) were *Candida* spp. and *Aspergillus* spp.; however, the proportion of *Candida* spp. in these autopsies decreased from 77.3% to 24.6% and molds increased from 22.7% to 66.7% from 1978 to 1992. This stands in contrast to the results of the National Nosocomial Infections Surveillance System (NNISS) study in the United States, wherein *Candida* spp. accounted for 78% of nosocomial fungal infections and *Aspergillus* spp. for only 1.3% (34). While it is clear that there is a limited ability to reliably establish premortem diagnoses of invasive mold infections (35), it seems likely that the declining prevalence of *Candida* spp. at autopsy data may be a function of increased awareness by physicians of the possibility of invasive fungal infection in high-risk groups, and the more aggressive use of effective antifungal therapy (36–39).

III. SUPERFICIAL AND INVASIVE CANDIDIASIS

Oropharyngeal and esophageal candidiasis are relatively common among patients receiving immunosuppressive or myelosuppressive anticancer therapy (40,41). Superficial infection with opportunistic yeasts involves tissues of the skin, genitourinary tract, and gastrointestinal tract predominantly, the oropharynx, esophagus, and bowel. Predisposing factors include protracted courses of antibacterial therapy, irradiation to the mediastinum and area of the head and neck, and immunosuppression due to the underlying cancer and its treatment. Corticosteroids have long been recognized as a factor predisposing patients to oropharyngeal candidiasis, OPC (7).

 OPC is an important problem affecting 17% to 53% of patients undergoing involved-field irradiation for head and neck cancer (42–47). One of the major risk factors appears to be compromised salivary gland function, secondary to the destruction of glandular tissue, as a function of the local cytotoxic irradiation (42–44,46,48). The serous acini of the parotids are very sensitive to the cytoxic effects of irradiation (49–54). Moreover, cytotoxic effects of irradiation on the oral mucosal epithelium may reduce the anti-candidal activity of mucosal membrane-associated carbohydrate moieties (55). While oropharyngeal colonization with *Candida* spp. is present in almost three-quarters of patients beginning a course of irradiation therapy, more than one in four patients undergoing a course of irradiation will develop signs and symptoms of OPC (47). The incidence of OPC has been based upon the recognition of signs and symptoms that include oral pain, and/or burning associated with oral plaques, or pseudomembranes from which budding yeasts may be recognized in 10% potassium hydroxide microscopical preparations, and/or grown in microbiological culture (45,47). It is very difficult to ascribe pathogenetic significance to a pre-existing colonizing yeast isolate such as *C. albicans* in the presence of oropharyngeal inflammatory change with pseudomembrane formation that can be due to either cytotoxic therapy-related tissue damage or to the microorganism. For this reason, many clinicians opt to treat the microorganism with agents such as fluconazole.

Amifostine, an agent known to concentrate in the salivary glands (49), has been used as a cytoprotectant to reduce the cytotoxic effects of the irradiation (53,56–59). In one non-randomized, no treatment-controlled study, amifostine reduced the incidence of OPC by 48% (OR 0.32, 95% CI 0.09–1.06) and xerostomia by 75% (OR 0.05, 95% CI 0.04–0.063); however, the incidence of grade II to III mucositis was unaffected (OR 0.21, 95% CI 0.03–1.86) (53). Investigators from Duke University reported similar observations in a randomized, untreated-controlled trial in which 303 subjects were allocated to receive amifostine prior to each irradiation treatment for squamous cell head and neck cancer (58). Grade II or more acute xerostomia was reduced by 35% (OR 0.29, 95% CI 0.18–0.46), but mucositis was unaffected (58). Although OPC was not an end-point of this study, it seems possible that the magnitude of the amifostine-related xerostomia treatment effect could have permitted the recognition of a protective effect in this outcome as well. These studies have underscored the importance of cytotoxic therapy-related xerostomia in the pathogenesis of OPC in cancer patients (60).

OPC can be a marker for esophageal candidiasis (61), which in turn may increase the risk for invasive bloodstream infection (62,63). OPC has been studied among patients with HIV/AIDS (64–66); however, the relationship between OPC and esophageal candidiasis has not been as extensively analyzed in cancer patients other than those with head and neck carcinoma (44–47). Approximately 90% of HIV/AIDS patients will develop OPC at some point in the course of the illness; however, only approximately 10% will develop esophageal candidiasis (67). In one recent study from Crete, 21 of 22 cancer patients with OPC had endoscopic evidence of esophageal candidiasis and in 14 of 22 (64%), histological evidence of mucosal invasion was also present (61). This relationship may be stronger than heretofore thought.

The NNISS reported and increase in nosocomial invasive fungal infections from 2.0/1000 hospital discharges in 1980 to 3.8/1000 hospital discharges in 1990 (34). The American Society for Microbiology identified the threat posed by antimicrobial resistance as sufficiently important to recommend the development of on-going surveillance programs to detect emerging resistance, to monitor resistance rates, and to guide infection control and formulary intervention programs (68). Surveillance programs reporting on 5095 isolates from candidemia patients between 1992 and 2001 have provided a rank order of species distribution: *C. albicans* (45–58%), *C. glabrata* (12–24%), *C. parapsilosis* (7–21%), *C. tropicalis* (10–12%), *C. krusei* (0–4%), other non-*albicans Candida* spp. (1–4%) (69–83). There has been an increase in the proportion of candidemia due to non-*albicans Candida* spp., in particular *C. glabrata* that now ranks second in frequency at approximately 20% overall in the United States (71,75,77–80), Of note, centers in South America have reported a predominance of *C. parapsilosis* over *C. glabrata* (Fig. 3) (74). Wingard reported a rise in the prevalence of invasive infection in cancer patients due to non-*albicans Candida* spp., particularly *C. glabrata* (from 6.4% to 14.5%), and *C. krusei* (from 1.6% to 13%), since the introduction of fluconazole in the early 1990s (84). This observation has been made by others (85,86) and has important implications for the treatment of suspected invasive fungal infection due to *Candida* spp.

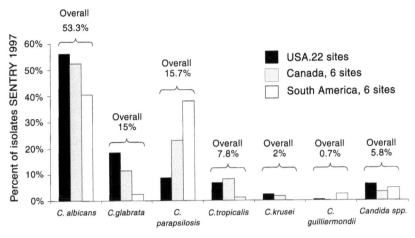

Figure 3 Percentage of Candidal isolates by species from 22 centers in the United States, six centers in Canada, and six centers in South America.

The incidence of *C. glabrata* bloodstream infection appears to be higher among older patients (70,80) who are more likely to have cancer.

Invasive fungal infection is observed more often among patients with hematological malignancies such as leukemia or lymphoma than among patients with solid tissue malignancies; however, the Invasive Fungal Infection Group (IFIG), of the European Organization for Research and Treatment of Cancer (EORTC), demonstrated species differences among candidemic patients according to whether the diagnosis was a hematological malignancy or a solid tissue malignancy (Fig. 4). Previous studies have demonstrated the gastrointestinal tract including the esophagus, stomach, and bowel as the likely sources for invasive candidiasis (30,87). *Candida albicans* accounted for 70% and 36% of the candidemias among patients with solid tissue and hematological malignancies, respectively (4). In contrast, *C. glabrata* and *C. tropicalis* accounted for only 4% and 7% of solid tumor patients as compared

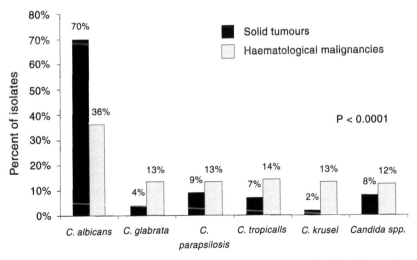

Figure 4 Percentage of Candidal isolates by species and underlying diagnosis.

to 13% and 14% of hematological malignancy patients, respectively (4). Others have made similar observations (88).

The major risk factors that have been identified among cancer patients for fungemia include neutropenia, hematopoietic stem cell transplantation, corticosteroid therapy, broad-spectrum antibacterial therapy (12), receipt of mucosal toxic chemotherapy regimens containing high-dose cytarabine (26) or etoposide (89,90), and indwelling venous access devices (85,91). Non-*albicans Candida* spp. have predominated among candidemic patients with hematological malignancies in Europe, whereas *C. albicans* has predominated among patients with solid tissue malignancies (4).

One of the non-*albicans Candida* spp., *C. parapsilosis,* has a characteristic epidemiology. The incidence of bloodstream infection because of this species has increased in the United States, Europe, Latin America, and South America (74,92–94). This is in exogenously acquired opportunistic yeast that has the propensity to colonize indwelling venous access devices, particularly in cancer patients (85,95–97), and grow in the presence of high concentrations of glucose (98). The lower attributable mortality of *C. parapsilosis* compared to *C. albicans* has been linked to its overall lower virulence (4,84,92,98,99) and is susceptibility to fluconazole.

Candida krusei has emerged as an important pathogen in neutropenic leukemia patients largely because of its intrinsic resistance to fluconazole (85,100,101). Compared to patients with *C. albicans* bloodstream infections, patients with *C. krusei* are more likely to have an underlying hematological malignancy, severe neutropenia (ANC $< 0.5 \times 10^9$/L), had a hematopoietic stem cell transplant, and received fluconazole prophylaxis (85,102). In one study, only 22% of patients with *C. krusei* fungemia compared to 79% of patients with *C. albicans* fungemia treated with fluconazole responded (102); however, these observations were not controlled for the presence or severity of neutropenia. Others have demonstrated a reduced susceptibility of *C. krusei* to polyenes, thus, accounting for the observation of breakthrough fungemia due to this species among patients receiving amphotericin B deoxycholate (69,102). Invasive *C. glabrata* infections have been associated with higher mortality rates in cancer patients (4). It has been argued that invasive *C. tropicalis* infections have a more virulent course because of more prolonged fungemia (88), higher APACHE II physiological scores (85), and longer critical care unit stays (84,85,103).

Fluconazole has been recommended as the agent of choice for the prevention of susceptible *Candida* spp. infections in hematopoietic stem cell transplant recipients (104,105). Others have shown a prophylactic treatment effect among other groups including acute myeloid leukemia patients undergoing primary or salvage remission–induction therapy (106) and those with prolonged (> 14 days) severe neutropenia (absolute neutrophils $< 0.5 \times 10^9$/L) (107). Such patients, however, are at risk of invasive bloodstream infections due to opportunistic fungi less susceptible to azole-based antifungal prophylaxis (107,108); that is, the problem of breakthrough candidemia.

Breakthrough candidemia has been defined as candidemia observed during the administration of systemic antifungal therapy for prophylaxis, empirical treatment of prolonged fever during persistent severe neutropenia, or for treatment of possible, probable, or proven invasive fungal infection for more than 3 days prior to the index blood culture (109–111). The occurrence of candidemia among patients receiving systemic antifungal therapy with amphotericin B deoxycholate (32,112) or fluconazole (112) was previously unusual. The incidence appears to be on the rise (113). Blumberg and Reboli (69) reported 11 neutropenic cancer patients with candidemia among whom five (45%; *Candida albicans*, two, and *C. krusei*, three) occurred during therapy with amphotericin B deoxycholate at doses $\geq$0.6 mg/kg/day. The presence of a hematological malignancy (109,110,113), mucositis (114), inadequate antifungal agent serum levels (115), indwelling central venous access devices (114,116), steroid therapy (more than 20 mg of prednisone equivalent daily for more than 30 days or a cumulative dose of 700 mg within 30 days) (109,111), broad-spectrum antibacterial therapy (109,111), prophylaxis with oral fluoroquinolones (114), and prolonged neutropenia (111,114) have been reported as risk factors for breakthrough candidemia. Whereas, the aetiology of de novo candidemia has been predominantly *C. albicans*, *C. tropicalis*, and *C. parapsilosis*, the isolates in breakthrough candidemia have been *C. albicans*, *C. glabrata*, and *C. krusei*, particularly among azole recipients (109,110,114). Other non-*Candida* spp. also have been reported including *Trichosporon* spp. and *Fusarium* spp. (114). A multivariate analysis of the risk factors for breakthrough candidemia identified the presence of neutropenia at the time of the index blood culture (OR 5.35, 95% CI 2.01–14.23), being in a critical care unit at the time of the index blood culture (OR 2.60, 95% CI 1.28–5.29), duration of neutropenia before the index blood culture (OR 1.02, 95% CI 1.00–1.04), and previous corticosteroid therapy (OR 2.50, 95% CI 1.23–5.15) as independent predictors (109).

IV. INVASIVE FILAMENTOUS FUNGAL INFECTION

The first case of disseminated aspergillosis was described in 1953 in a 45-year old window cleaner treated with multiple antibacterial agents, including chloramphenicol, who subsequently developed agranulocytosis (117). Filamentous fungi such as *Aspergilius* spp. are ubiquitous in the environment and have been isolated from the air, dust, furniture, soil of potted plants, ground coffee, spices, powdered milk, water condensation from refrigerators, and from moisture around bathtubs and sinks (118–122).

Acquisition is primarily through the inhalation of conidia; accordingly, it is not surprising that the commonest sites of infection involve the sinopulmonary tree (27). The small particle size (2.5–3.5 μm) *of Aspergilius* spp. conidia is conducive to transportation through the air currents to the distal airways in the lung (123). The respiratory mucosal surfaces with the alveolar macrophages constitute the first line of host defense against the inhaled conidia, and following germination into the hyphal phase, the circulating neutrophil provides the most important line of defense against dissemination from the primary pulmonary or paranasal site of inoculation (124–126) Angioinvasion by hyphae is the mechanism by which hematogenous dissemination occurs to distal sites such as the brain, skin, kidneys, or liver.

The accurate identification of the offending fungus from tissue is problematic. Fungi recognized in histological examination are not isolated in microbiological cultures in 40–60% of cases (127–130). it is nearly impossible to differentiate microscopically the hyphae *of Aspergillus* spp. from those of *Scedosporium* spp., *Fusarium* spp., or *Penicillium* spp. (131). In the absence of culture-based identification, investigators have classified hyphae that are small (3–6 μm wide), uniform, dichotomously branching, and regularly septate as *Aspergillus* spp. and hyphae that are broad (5–25 μm wide), thin-walled, irregularly shaped, and infrequently septate as Zygomycetes (27,30,132). Accordingly, the true prevalence and incidence of specific pathogens may be overestimated. In rank order, the majority of filamentous fungal infections are caused by *Aspergillus* spp. [including in rank order in invasive aspergillosis *A. fumigatus* (67%), *A. flavus* (16%), *A. niger* (5%), *A. terreus* (3%), and *A. nidulans*

($\sim$1%)] (133,134), Fusarium spp. (including *F. solani, F. oxysporum,* and *F. moniliforme*), *Scedosporium* spp. (including *S. prolificans* and *S. apiospermum,* the asexual phase of *Pseudallescheria boydii*), the Zygomycetes (including *Rhizopus* spp., *Mucor* spp., *Rhizomucor* spp., *Absidia* spp., and *Cunninghamella bertholetiae*), and the dematiaceous molds (including *Alternaria* spp., *Bipolaris* spp., *Curvularia* spp., and *Wangiella* spp.) (135). A simplified approach to classification of clinically important molds has been described by Segal et al. (136). Molds may be categorized as *Aspergillus* spp. vs. non-*Aspergillus* spp. wherein *Aspergillus* spp. may be subdivided as *A. fumigatus* or non-fumigatus *Aspergillus* spp., and non-*Aspergillus* spp. may be subdivided into *Fusarium* spp., the Zygomycetes, *Scedosporium* spp., and the dematiacious fungi.

The prevalence of invasive mold infection observed at autopsy is increasing (30,137). In a study of 8124 autopsies in Germany, there was an increase in the prevalence of invasive molds from 0.5% in 1978–1982 to 3.4% in 1988–1992, a proportional increase of 580% (30). Invasive aspergillosis is much more often associated with neoplastic (47.1–69.8%) than with non-neoplastic conditions such as solid organ transplant (4.2–10.3%), AIDS (9.2–31.1%), or other immunodeficiency states (10.7–17.6%) (30,138,139). Among neoplastic diseases, the hematological malignancies [acute leukemia (48.5%), chronic leukemia (19.1%), lymphoma (14.1%), myelodysplasia (7%), multiple myeloma (3.8%), and fanconi's syndrome (2%)] have accounted for 96.1% of cases compared to solid tumors (3.8%) (139). The incidence in patients with acute myeloid leukemia is 2-fold higher than patients with acute lymphoblastic leukemia (139). In addition, the incidence of invasive aspergillosis among allogeneic hematopoietic stem cell transplant recipients has increased between 1990 and 1998 from approximately 5% to approximately 12% (5,140). Of note, there was an increase among autologous hematopoietic stem cell transplant recipients over this period from 1.1% to 5.3%, a phenomenon conceivably linked to low doses of CD34$^+$ stem cells (141).

The development of invasive mold infection, particularly with aspergillosis, is associated with significant ramifications with regard to health care resources. Fraser predicted a 2-fold increase in the number of aspergillosis-related hospitalizations between 1970 and 1976 (137). In the 20 year period since that report, the number of hospitalizations for this diagnosis have increased nearly 8-fold (142). A report based upon the National Hospital Discharge Survey from 1980 to 1994 demonstrated an annual increase of 5.7% in the incidence of hospitalization for fungal disease in the United States (143). Patients with cancer or leukemia who develop secondary aspergillosis utilized 3.7 times the number of hospital days, incurred 6.7 times the cost, and was associated with 3.3 times the mortality rate than patients with similar diagnoses, but without aspergillosis (142).

These observations provide ample rationale for the development of effective strategies of prevention and treatment.

The understanding of the pathogenesis of aspergillosis has provided some insight into the factors that predispose susceptible patients to this infection. Outbreaks of aspergillosis have been linked to high concentrations of conidia in the environment where patients with hematological malignancies are under treatment (5,16,19,20,22,144–149). The relationship between increased ambient conidial concentrations and invasive mycoses has been difficult to demonstrate (23,150–153). However, the institution of infection control measures that reduce patient exposure to airborne conidia have been associated with reductions in the incidence of invasive aspergillosis (19,20,22,25,149,154). Recent studies have implicated stairwells as a means of conveyance of airborne conidia (24). A recent study from the International Bone Marrow Transplant Registry was able to demonstrate a treatment effect high-efficiency particulate air filtration (HEPA) with or without laminar airflow (LAF) on reducing transplant-related mortality and increasing overall survival (155). The probability of fungal pneumonia among patients undergoing allogeneic unrelated or mismatched donor hematopoietic stem cell transplant was 6% among those managed in HEPA/LAF facilities as compared to 23% among patients managed in conventional isolation, thus, a 74% risk reduction (155). Others have also been able to demonstrate a protective effect of HEPA $\pm$ LAF (156). In a retrospective cohort study, Hahn et al. (149) reported the development of invasive aspergillosis due to *A. flavus* in 9 of 35 (26%) of patients (of whom 7 of 9, 78%, died) managed in a non-HEPA/LAF unit as compared to 1 of 20 patients (5%, OR 6.58, 95% CI 0.77–56.41) managed in a HEPA/LAF unit. The non-HEPA/LAF unit was associated with high *Aspergillus* spp. conidia counts, >150 colony-forming units, CFU/m^3 compared to <4 CFU/m^3 in the HEPA/LAF unit (149). These observations have formed the basis of recommendations by the American Society of Blood and Marrow Transplantation, the Infectious Diseases Society of America, and the Centers for Disease Control and Prevention to use HEPA/LAF for the management of hematopoietic stem cell transplant in patients at highest risk for aspergillosis (104,105). Evidence suggests that other patients such as those undergoing intensive cytotoxic therapy for acute myeloid leukemia may also benefit from HEPA-based strategies (149).

In addition, increases in ambient concentrations of conidia may be generated from construction and demolition activities outside the hospital environment (157). Conidia may enter the hospital, particularly if the ambient air pressure is negative relative to the outside and be transported on air currents associated with stairwells and elevator shafts (24). Measures such as the use of N95 masks, wet buffing, and closing stairwells can reduce the risk to patients of encountering airborne conidia (24).

V. COLONIZATION

Colonization of the intestinal mucosal surfaces is thought to be the initial step in the pathogenesis of invasive infections due to opportunistic yeasts (26,87,158,159). Surveillance cultures have been used to examine colonization profiles in the study of the epidemiology of infection and the impact of infection prevention strategies in high-risk patient population (160). Although surveillance cultures have had limited value in predicting the etiology of invasive infection (161), low yeast colonization indices (162) of less than 0.25 have a high negative predictive value for invasive fungal infection (13). The risk of invasive infection increases with the number of anatomic sites colonized (162,163) and with the particular fungal species (11,163,164). Serial surveillance cultures of the nasopharynx, oropharynx, and rectum may be useful in high-risk cancer patients undergoing intensive cytotoxic therapy for acute myeloid leukemia or hematopoietic stem cell transplant receiving azole-based antifungal prophylaxis (106) to monitor the emergence of azole-resistant yeasts (165). Such a program should only be engaged after appropriate communication and agreement with the clinical microbiology laboratory (160).

Gut decontamination using oral absorbable or non-absorbable antimicrobial agents has been studied as a strategy to prevent invasive infection among neutropenic cancer patients. Manipulation of the gut microflora through use of antibacterial agents, particularly those with activity against the normal anaerobic "colonization resistance" microflora (166), has increased the likelihood of colonization of the gut by resistant microorganisms, particularly with the use of antibacterial agents with significant antianaerobic activity (167,168). A survey of antimicrobial use in a tertiary care hospital found that 58% of patients beginning a course of antibacterial therapy received agents that were inappropriate, and in 59% of the patients in this group the unnecessary agents included those with significant antianaerobic activity (169). Febrile neutropenic cancer patients who receive empirical antibacterial regimens that suppresses both the normal aerobic and anaerobic intestinal microflora have a significantly higher risk of colonization by opportunistic yeasts and invasive fungal infection (OR 3.56, 95% CI 1.24–10.23) (170). A similar quantitative study from the MD Anderson Cancer Center correlated yeast colonization with use of antibacterial regimens with antianaerobic activity, such as ticarcillin-clavulanate, or high biliary excretion rates, such as ceftriaxone (171). Augmentation of fluoroquinolone-based antibacterial prophylaxis in neutropaenic cancer patients with the administration of rifampin resulted in increased yeast colonization of the gut (172). Another prophylaxis study from Essen, Germany, sought to reduce the incidence of acute graft-vs.-host disease (GVHD) among allogeneic hematopoietic stem cell transplant recipients through suppression of the anaerobic gut microflora by the co-administration of metronidazole with prophylactic ciprofloxacin plus fluconazole (173). In comparison to the control patients receiving ciprofloxacin plus fluconazole, the study group had a 50% reduction in grades II–IV GVHD, particularly involving the liver or intestine. However, there was also a 58% increase in intestinal colonization by yeasts in the study group (odds ratio 1.94, 95% CI 1.46–2.58) and, despite the relatively limited sample size, there was an associated increase in the incidence of candidemia from 1.5% to 4.4% (OR 3.1, 95% CI 0.3–30.5) also noted (174).

The administration of multiple antibiotics has been long recognized as being associated from a 1.7- to 25.1- fold risk for colonization and infection by opportunistic fungi (91,175,176). Many agents used for the empirical management of fever in the neutropenic patient have significant suppressive effects upon the normal enteric gut microflora. Such agents, including the carbapenems (imipenem/cilastatin and meropenem), cefipime, and piperacillin/tazobactam or ticarcillin/clavulanate have been associated with suppression of the anaerobic intestinal microflora and increase in colonization by opportunistic yeasts. These examples illustrate that the choice of antibacterial agents has a significant impact upon the risk for fungal colonization and, perhaps, the risk of invasive fungal infection in neutropaenic cancer patients.

VI. MYELOSUPPRESSION AND IMMUNOSUPPRESSION

The potential anticancer therapeutic benefit of cytotoxic therapy dose-intensification, defined by the amount of drug administered per unit time (177), has been limited by myelotoxicity primarily affecting the absolute neutrophil count and the platelet count. The inverse relationship between the absolute neutrophil count and the risk of pyogenic bacterial infection has been well established (178,179). Improvements in the management of the febrile neutropenic patient (33) and the availability of platelet transfusions have ameliorated some of the dose-limiting problems. The addition of hematopoietic growth factors (granulocyte colony stimulating factor or granulocyte/macrophage colony stimulating factor) have also been important in reducing the duration of cytotoxic therapy-induced neutropenia [relative risk (RR), 0.64, 95% CI 0.55–0.75], the incidence of febrile neutropenic episodes (RR 0.74, 95% CI 0.62–0.89), and documented infection (RR 0.74, 95% CI 0.64–0.85) (180); however, there has been no observable treatment effect with regards to the prescription of antibacterial therapy (RR 0.82, 95% CI 0.57–1.18), infection-related mortality (RR 2.07, 95% CI 0.81–5.34), tumor response (RR 1.06, 95% CI 0.96–1.16), freedom from treatment failure (hazard ratio 1.22, 95% CI 0.83–1.80), or overall survival (hazard ratio 0.98, 95% CI 0.81–1.18) (180).

The use of peripheral blood as the source of stem cells for hematopoietic reconstitution has been associated with earlier neutrophil and platelet engraftment (181). Moreover, the dose of $CD34^+$ stem cells of 3×10^6/kg or more recipient body weight has been associated with faster engraftment of neutrophils, lymphocytes, monocytes, and platelets (141) and this has been associated with a reduced risk of invasive fungal infection from 26.3% to 12.2% (a 54 % reduction, hazard ratio 0.41, 95% CI 0.21–0.79, $P = 0.008$) (141).

The absolute monocyte count (AMC) has also been studied as a useful predictor of infection in cancer patients receiving cytotoxic therapy. Previous studies have examined the relationship of monocytopenia (AMC $< 0.2 \times 10^9$/L) and the risk of bacterial infection, predominantly in pediatric patient populations (182–188). One study in patients with aplastic anemia addressed the correlation between monocytopenia and invasive fungal infection (189); however, the analysis was confounded by the effects of concomitant neutropenia. Among cancer patients receiving myelosuppressive cytotoxic therapy resulting in pancytopenia, the ability to discriminate the relative contributions of monocytopenia and neutropenia to infection risk is very difficult. This question is better addressed among patients with normal absolute neutrophil counts and monocytopenia. More recently, Storek (190) reported an inverse relationship between persistent B-lymphocytopenia or monocytopenia and the risk of fungal infection following engraftment among allogeneic hematopoietic stem cell transplant recipients that appeared to be independent of the influence of neutropenia. These observations are consistent with the known role of mononuclear phagocytes in host defence against inhaled conidia and with the observed therapeutic effects of hematopoietic growth factors that affect the mononuclear phagocyte in patients with invasive fungal infection (191–194). Accordingly, monocytopenia in the absence of significant neutropenia (ANC $< 0.5 \times 10^9$/L) may be more important as a risk factor for invasive infection than heretofore thought.

The inverse relationship between the circulating $CD4^+$ T-lymphocyte count and opportunistic infections, such as those due to *Candida* spp. and *Aspergillus* spp. in HIV/AIDS patients has been well established (10,66,195,196). Little attention has been paid to cancer chemotherapy-induced reduction of the absolute lymphocyte count (ALC) and its related subsets with regard to infection risk (198). Reports published in the early 1980s drew attention to the relative lymphopenia produced in women receiving adjuvant chemotherapy with chlorambucil, methotrexate, and fluorouracil for breast cancer (198). Moreover, the late 1980s and early 1990s brought reports of lymphoma patients receiving intensive multiagent chemotherapy, and breast cancer patients receiving adjuvant chemotherapy following breast conserving lumpectomy and irradiation developing pulmonary pneumocystosis associated with profound $CD4^+$ lymphopenia (199,200). Kontoyiannis and colleagues (201) at the MD Anderson Cancer Center noted that the majority (61%) of cancer patients with invasive cryptococcosis were significantly lymphopenic with absolute lympho-cyte counts of less than 0.5×10^9/L whereas only 16% were neutropenic (absolute neutrophil count $< 0.5 \times 10^9$/L).

The recognition of early lymphopenia may be helpful in predicting those reci-pients of cytotoxic therapy who are at highest risk of a febrile neutropenic episode. Blay and colleagues (202) observed a correlation between an ALC of less than 0.7×10^9/L on day 5 of cytotoxic therapy, approximately 4 days before the ANC had fallen, and subsequent infection (OR 7.17, 95% CI 2.52–20.35). Moreover, the administration of high-dose chemotherapy (defined by the receipt of at least one of the following regimens: doxorubicin, > 90 mg/m^2; cisplatin, >100 mg/m^2; cyclo-phosphamide, >1000 mg/m^2; ifosfamide, >9000 mg/m^2; etoposide, >500 mg/m^2; or cytarabine, >1000 mg/m^2) also proved to be a useful predictor independent of other variables including patient age, performance status, tumour extension, bone marrow involvement, number of previous chemotherapy sites, and corticosteroid therapy. The odds ratio for a febrile neutropenic episode for patients with both predictors, high-dose chemotherapy and a day 5 ALC of $< 0.7 \times 10^9$/L, was 48.4 (95% CI 10.7–219.7) (202). The day 1 ALC of $< 0.7 \times 10^9$/L has also been of value as a predictor of severe thrombocytopenia (203) and severe anaemia requiring red cell transfusion (204).

While it seems clear that suppression of the circulating absolute neutrophil count, the absolute monocyte count, and the absolute lymphocyte count correlate with the risk for infection in general, it is less clear as to how this influences the risk for fungal infection in cancer patient populations. Among 35,252 HIV-infected sub-jects contained in a national HIV surveillance database, the incidence of invasive aspergillosis was 3.5 cases (95% CI 3.0–4.0) per 1000 patient-years. However, as the CD4$^+$ T-lymphocyte count fell, the incidence increased significantly from 1.0 case/1000 patient-years (95% CI 0.6–1.4) associated with a CD4$^+$ ALC of $\geq0.2 \times 10^9$/L, to 1.0 (95% CI 0.2–1.7) with a CD4$^+$ ALC of 0.1–0.199 $\times 10^9$/L, 5.1 (95% CI 2.8–7.3) with a CD4$^+$ ALC of 0.05–0.099 $\times 10^9$L, and 10.2 (95% CI 8.0–12.2) with a CD4$^+$ ALC of 0–0.049 $\times 10^9$/L (10).

Irinotecan, a topoisomerase I inhibitor is in wide use alone and in combination for metastatic colorectal malignancy. The major toxicities have been associated with neutropenia and diarrhea. More recently, significant reductions in circulating CD19$^+$ B-lymphocytes, CD4$^+$ T-lymphocytes and monocytes have been reported (205). Till date, no unexpectedly high incidence of superficial or invasive fungal infection has been reported with the use of this agent.

Purine analog therapy has increased in the treatment of lymphoreticular malig-nancies (206–209), acute myeloid leukemia (210) and in conditioning therapy of non-myeloablative allogeneic hematopoietic stem cell transplantation (211). These agents include fludarabine, cladribine (2-chlorodeoxyadenosine or CdA), and pen-tostatin (2^1-deoxycorfomycin or DCF). The infectious complications associated with the use of these agents have been reviewed extensively elsewhere (207,208). There are predictable immunological sequelae of the use of this class of agents including a reduction in the total absolute lymphocyte counts, prolonged suppression of circu-lating CD19$^+$ and CD20$^+$ B-lymphocyte counts and CD4$^+$ T-lymphocyte counts, less prolonged suppression of CD8$^+$ T-lymphocytes, transient monocytopenia and CD16$^+$ NK lymphocyte counts, and variable effects upon immunoglobulin levels. As a consequence of these effects, it is not surprising that since the early 1990s an increased incidence of opportunistic infections due to *Listeria monocytogenes*, *Herpes zoster*, and fungi including *Pneumocystis jiroveci* (formerly *carinii*), *Candida* spp., *Aspergillus* spp., and *Cryptococcus neoformans* reminiscent of those observed in the acquired immunodeficiency syndrome (212,213) has been reported among CLL patients receiving these agents (207,214,215).

$CD4^+$ T-cell numbers fall to levels similar to those observed in advanced HIV infection (207). $CD4^+$ and $CD8^+$ T-cell counts among recipients of fludarabine administered for untreated chronic lymphocytic leukemia (CLL) decreased over three courses of treatment from medians of 1.562×10^9/L and 0.510×10^9/L, respectively, to 0.172×10^9/L and 0.138×10^9/L, an 89% and 73% reduction, respectively (216). Despite this, no association between $CD4^+$ T-cell count at the end of fludarabine therapy and infection was observed (216). The $CD4^+$ T-lymphopenic effects of fludarabine among CLL patients may last a year or more (217). In a recent randomized study of 518 previously untreated CLL patients, the overall infection risk among fludarabine monotherapy recipients was higher than that among chlorambucil monotherapy recipients (9% vs. 16%, OR 1.91, 95% CI 0.99–3.69); however, recipients of the combination of fludarabine and alkylating agent had an increased risk than that of fludarabine monotherapy (16% vs. 28%, OR 2.05, 95% CI 1.17–3.60) (218). Infections due to *P. jiroveci* were seen during that study in only 0.9% of 329 fludarabine recipients (219). No cases of invasive aspergillosis infection were observed despite expectations otherwise (217,220,221) The incidence of major candidal infections (defined by the need for hospitalization for treatment) was 0%, 2%, and 5% for the chlorambucil, fludarabine, and chlorambucil plus fludarabine groups, respectively ($P = 0.01$) (219). While the incidence of invasive fungal infection among CLL patients appears relatively low, combination therapy with fludarabine in addition to an alkylating agent does increase the risk.

The incidence of invasive fungal infection among purine analog recipients has been difficult to glean from the brief descriptions available in published reports (207). Among the 2213 subjects enrolled in the 60 studies of purine therapy in patients with hematological malignancies reported by Cheson, only 51 (2.3%) examples of invasive fungal infection were sufficiently delineated to estimate the rate including invasive candidiasis ($n = 22$), pulmonary pneumocystosis ($n = 10$), invasive aspergillosis ($n = 17$), and cryptococcosis ($n = 2$). The invasive fungal infection rates seemed to be higher among CdA recipients (3.9% of 823 subjects) as compared to fludarabine (1.6% of 739 subjects, OR 2.45, 95% CI 1.25–4.79) or DCF (1.1% of 644 subjects, OR 3.72, 95% CI 1.63–8.49) recipients (207). These observations are consistent with subsequent reports wherein among CdA recipients fungal pneumonias were observed in 4% of 184 pretreated subjects and 7% of 194 untreated subjects (222).

CdA produces a predictable acute monocytopenia, the nadir of which occurs by day 7 from beginning treatment (223,224) with recovery to baseline levels by day 17 (223). Moreover, there is also significant lymphopenia, initially more pronounced for $CD8^+$ T-lymphocytes and $CD20^+$ B-lymphocytes than for $CD4^+$ T-lymphocytes and $CD16^+$ NK lymphocytes (225). Prolonged monocytopenia and $CD19^+$ B-lymphocytopenia have been linked to the risk of invasive fungal infection among hematopoietic stem cell transplant recipients (190), particularly wherein bone marrow was the source of stem cell reconstitution (226). The effect of CdA on monocytes and B-lymphocytes may independent of its effects upon the absolute neutrophil count and have a pathogenetic relationship to the greater risk for invasive fungal infection observed among the very heterogeneous population of CdA recipients reported by Cheson (207).

Alemtuzumab (Campath-IH) is an anti-CD52$^+$ monoclonal antibody with activity in lymphoreticular malignancies such as chronic lymphocytic leukemia (227–230) and for the purposes of T-cell depletion in peripheral blood stem cell transplantation (231,232). The use of this product has been associated with profound reductions in CD19$^+$ B-lymphocytes, CD4$^+$ and CD8$^+$ T-lymphocytes, and CD16$^+$ natural killer cells (227,228,230) Many reports of infectious morbidity associated with the use of alemtuzumab have focused upon DNA viral infections (231,233–238). Reports of fungal infection-related morbidity have been relatively few and vague (219,239–241). Among 24 subjects with advanced CLL progressing after fludarabine therapy, there was almost 100% reduction in circulating CD19$^+$ B-lymphocytes that lasted beyond 28 weeks of the study. In this group, 10 (42%) experienced opportunistic infections of which eight (80%) were pneumonias and seven (70%) were fungal (*P. jiroveci*, four, *Candida* spp., one, *Aspergillus* spp. with or without *Candida* spp. two) (230).

Rituximab is a humanized chimeric anti-CD20 monoclonal antibody product with activity in CD20$^+$ B-cell lymphoreticular malignancies such as diffuse large cell lymphoma (242–245). Administration of this product leads to circulating B-lymphocyte depletion lasting 6–9 months (246). However, this does not result in a significant reduction in circulating immunoglobulin levels or an increase in opportunistic infections. There is, however, an effect upon primary and secondary immune responsiveness. Van der Kolk and colleagues (247) challenged patients with progressive low-grade non-Hodgkin's lymphoma with two primary antigens and two recall antigens before and after rituximab treatment (375 mg/m^2/week intravenously for 4 weeks). All subjects had a depletion of the circulating B cells within 73 hr of administration but the quanitative immunoglobulin levels (IgG, IgA, and IgM) remained stable throughout the course of treatment. The response to recall antigens was significantly lower after rituximab therapy compared to baseline suggesting a depletion in memory B cells. However, none of the subjects developed a primary response, either before or after rituximab therapy, suggesting that the underlying disease status may have played a role in the unresponsiveness. Some investigators have observed a higher risk for late onset opportunistic viral infections due to CMV and JC papovavirus among CD34-selected peripheral blood stem cell autograft recipients of peritransplant rituximab-mediated residual lymphoma disease reduction (OR 38, 95% CI 2–729) in association with delays in CD4$^+$ T-cell recovery (248,249). To date, there has been very little to implicate a relationship between rituximab and an increased risk for invasive fungal infection.

Paclitaxel, an enhancer of tubulin polymerization leading to mitotic arrest used for the treatment of non-small cell lung cancer (NSCLC), has been associated with dose-dependent leukopenia and neutropenia when used as monotherapy in daily doses of 135–175 mg/m (2,250,251), Lower doses, 50–86 mg/m^2, administered in association with involved field irradiation has been associated with lowered CD4$^+$, CD8$^+$, NK cell, and CD19$^+$ lymphocyte counts (252). Such changes have been linked to the development of a syndrome of interstitial pneumonitis (252) among recipients of paclitaxel and involved field irradiation for NSCLC. This syndrome differs from the more commonly observed occurring outside the irradiation field in that the latter is a T-cell-mediated hypersensitivity, which is bilateral and associated with normal or elevated absolute lymphocyte counts (253).

VII. CYTOTOXIC THERAPY-INDUCED MUCOSAL INJURY AND INVASIVE FUNGAL INFECTION

Modern cytotoxic anticancer treatments, whether chemical or ionizing irradiation, exert their effects on tissues, either directly or indirectly, through the activation of cellular apoptotic pathways. The groups of cells most susceptible to the effects of these agents are those associated with cell renewal and differentiation: including hair, gonadal tissues, hematopoietic stem cells, and the committed epithelial progenitor cells. The clinical manifestation of damage to the latter group of progenitors is mucositis. Elaborate systems of scoring the severity of mucositis have been developed and direct correlations between mucositis scores and infection risk have been observed (254,255). Pseudomembranous candidiasis co-exists with mucositis in over half of patients receiving cytotoxic therapy for solid tumors (256). Mucosal colonization with *Candida* spp. in the presence of severe mucositis after high-dose cytarabine therapy has been linked to an increased risk of invasive candidiasis (26,257), The choice of cytotoxic regimen and its relative cytotoxic intensity are the most important determinants of mucosal damage (2,26,258).

A series of phases of mucosal damage have been recognized and described (259). An early inflammatory and vascular phase consists of nonspecific injury to mucosal basal cells or intestinal crypt cells in association with the release of interleukin 1, increased blood flow with consequent superficial erythema. Thereafter, an epithelial phase is recognized, wherein cytotoxic agents such as cytarabine induce apoptosis in the intestinal crypts leading to a reduction in crypt length and mitotic index, loss of villus area and reduced enterocyte height, and increased opening of intestinal mucosal tight junctions (259,261). This leads to mucosal thinning and atrophy detectable by day 4 or 5 from the start of the cytotoxic regimen. This is followed at day 7 to 10 by an ulcerative phase due to functional trauma, the cellular debris from which is recognized clinically as pseudomembrane formation (259). Micro-organisms such as opportunistic yeasts colonizing these damaged surfaces and their associated metabolic and structural lipopolysaccharide-like products may then translocate via the now incompetent cellular tight juctions. They may interact with submucosal host defences such as mononuclear phagocytes resulting in a cascade of inflammatory cytokine production that becomes associated with tissue damage. This process can be sequentially measured over time using molecular probes e.g., monosaccharides such as manitol or D-xylose, disaccharides such as lactulose, or radiolabelled products such as ethylenediamine tetraacetic acid (EDTA). Such studies have demonstrated that the time of maximum cytotoxic therapy-induced damage to the intestinal occurs at approximately 14 days following the beginning of the cytotoxic regimen, and at the same time as the neutrophil nadir (262–264). The pathogenesis of hepatosplenic fungal infection in acute leukemia patients is thought to be related to translocation of colonizing yeasts from the gut to the portal circulation and then to the liver (129,130,159,265–268). Despite the fact that hepatosplenic candidiasis in acute leukemia patients is most often diagnosed after neutrophil recovery late in the fourth week of therapy (267–269), the development of this infectious complication has been shown to correlate with malabsorption of D-xylose in week 2 of cytotoxic therapy at the time when most invasive bloodstream infections are observed (263). While difficult to demonstrate in patients, these observations support a pathogenetic model wherein candidemia develops in week 2 in following translocation across maximally damaged epithelial mucosal surfaces with seeding of viscera such as the liver and spleen. This process can only be recognized with the recovery of the host inflammatory response with neutrophil recovery (270,271).

Chemotherapeutic regimens based on agents such as irinotecan, paclitaxel, doxorubicin, etoposide, cytarabine, high-dose melphelan, or busulfan are more likely to be associated with more severe mucositis (26,256,258), Careful selection of regimen components based on an understanding of the associated mucosal toxicity can be helpful in identifying patients at risk of invasive fungal infection and for targeted application of antifungal prophylaxis regimens (107).

REFERENCES

1. Kliewer EV, Wajda A, Blanchard JF. The Increasing Cancer Burden: Manitoba Cancer Projections 1999–2005. Winnipeg: Cancer Care Manitoba/Manitoba Health, 2001:9–24.
2. Bow EJ. Invasive fungal infection in patients receiving intensive cytotoxic therapy for cancer. Br J Haematol 1998; 101:1–4.
3. Karabinis A, Hill C, Leclercq B, Tancrede C, Baume D, Andremont A. Risk factors for candidemia in cancer patients: a case-control study. J Clin Microbiol 1988; 26:429–432.
4. Viscoli C, Girmenia C, Marinus A, Collette L, Martino P, Vandercam B, et al. Candidemia in cancer patients: a prospective, multicentre surveillance study by the Invasive Fungal Infection Group (IFIG) of the European Organization for Research and Treatment of Cancer (EORTC). Clin Infect Dis 1999; 28:1071–1079.
5. Wald A, Leisenring W, van Burik JA, Bowden RA. Epidemiology of *Aspergillus* infections in a large cohort of patients undergoing bone marrow transplantation. J Infect Dis 1997; 175:1459–1466.
6. Safdar N, Maki DG. The commonality of risk factors for nosocomial colonization and infection with antimicrobial-resistant *Staphylococcus aureus*, enterococcus, gram-negative bacilli, *Clostridium difficile*, and *Candida*. Ann Intern Med 2002; 136:834–844.
7. Bodey GP. Fungal infections in the cancer patient. S Afr Med J 1977; 52:1009–1015.
8. DeGregorio MW, Lee WMF, Linker CA, Jacobs RA, Ries CA. Fungal infections in patients with acute leukemia. Am J Med 1982; 73:543–548.
9. Gerson SL, Talbot GH, Hurwitz S, Strom BL, Lusk EJ, Cassileth PA. Prolonged granulocytopenia: the major risk factor for invasive pulmonary aspergillosis in patients with acute leukemia. Ann Intern Med 1984; 100:345–351.
10. Holding KJ, Dworkin MS, Wan PC, Hanson DL, Klevens RM, Jones JL, et al. Aspergillosis among people infected with human immunodeficiency virus: incidence and survival. Adult and Adolescent Spectrum of HIV Disease Project. Clin Infect Dis 2000; 31:1253–1257.
11. Aisner J, Murillo J, Schimpff SC, Steere AC. Invasive aspergillosis in acute leukemia: correlation with nose cultures and antibiotic use. Ann Intern Med 1979; 90:4–9.
12. Jarvis WR. Epidemiology of nosocomial fungal infections, with emphasis on *Candida* species. Clin Infect Dis 1995; 20:1526–1530.
13. Laverdiere M, Rotstein C, Bow EJ, Roberts RS, Ioannou S, Carr D, et al. Impact of fluconazole prophylaxis on fungal colonization and infection rates in neutropenic patients. The Canadian Fluconazole Study. J Antimicrob Chemother 2000; 46:1001–1008.
14. Marr KA, Seidel K, White TC, Bowden RA. Candidemia in allogeneic blood and marrow transplant recipients: evolution of risk factors after the adoption of prophylactic fluconazole. J Infect Dis 2000; 181:309–316.
15. Aisner J, Schimpff SC, Bennett JE, Young VM, Wiernik PH. *Aspergillus* infections in cancer patients. Association with fireproofing materials in a new hospital. JAMA 1976; 235:411–412.

16. Arnow PM, Andersen RL, Mainous PD, Smith EJ. Pumonary aspergillosis during hospital renovation. Am Rev Respir Dis 1978; 118:49–53.
17. Sarubbi FA Jr, Kopf HB, Wilson MB, McGinnis MR, Rutala WA. Increased recovery of *Aspergillus flavus* from respiratory specimens during hospital construction. Am Rev Respir Dis 1982; 125:33–38.
18. Lentino JR, Rosenkranz MA, Michaels JA, Kurup VP, Rose HD, Rytel MW. Nosocomial aspergillosis: a retrospective review of airborne disease secondary to road construction and contaminated air conditioners. Am J Epidemiol 1982; 116:430–437.
19. Opal SM, Asp AA, Cannady PB, Morse PL, Burton LJ, Hammer PG. Efficacy of infection control measures during a nosocomial outbreak of disseminated aspergillosis associated with hospital construction. J Infect Dis 1986; 153:634–637.
20. Sherertz RJ, Belani A, Kramer BS, Elfenbein GJ, Weiner RS, Sullivan ML, et al. Imact of air filtration on nosocomial *Aspergillus* infections. Unique risk of bone marrow transplant recipients. Am J Med 1987; 83:709–718.
21. Gerson SL, Parker P, Jacobs MR, Creger R, Lazarus HM. Aspergillosis due to carpet contamination. Infect Control Hosp Epidemiol 1994; 15:221–223.
22. Loo VG, Bertrand C, Dixon C, Vityé D, Eng B, DeSalis B, et al. Control of construction-associated nosocomial aspergillosis in an antiquated hematology unit. Infect Control Hosp Epidemiol 1996; 17:360–364.
23. Cornet M, Levy V, Fleury L, Lotholary J, Barquins S, Coureul M-H, et al. Efficacy of prevention by high-efficiency particulate air filtration or laminar airflow against *Aspergillus* airborne contamination during hospital renovation. Infect Control Hosp Epidemiol 1999; 20:508–513.
24. Thio CL, Smith D, Merz WG, Streifel AJ, Bova G, Gay L, et al. Refinements of environmental assessment during an outbreak investigation of invasive aspergillosis in a leukemia and bone marrow transplant unit. Infect Control Hosp Epidemiol 2000; 21: 18–23.
25. Oren I, Haddad N, Finkelstein R, Rowe JM. Invasive pulmonary aspergillosis in neutropenic patients during hospital construction: before and after chemoprophylaxis and institution of HEP A filters. Am J Hematol 2001; 66:257–262.
26. Bow EJ, Loewen R, Cheang MS, Schacter B. Invasive fungal disease in adults undergoing remission–induction threapy for acute myeloid leukemia: the pathogenetic role of the antileukemic regimen. Clin Infect Dis 1995; 21:361–369.
27. Keye JD, Magee WE. Fungal diseases in a general hospital—a study of 88 patients. Am J Clin Pathol 1956; 26:1235–1253.
28. Bodey G, Bueltmann B, Duguid W, Gibbs D, Hanak H, Hotchi M, et al. Fungal infections in cancer patients: an international autopsy survey. Eur J Clin Microbiol Infect Dis 1992; 11:99–109.
29. Bodey GP. Fungal infections complicating acute leukemia. J Chronic Dis 1966; 19: 667–687.
30. Groll AH, Shah PM, Mentzel C, Schneider M, Just-Nuebling G, Huebner K. Trends in the postmortem epidemiology of invasive fungal infections at a university hospital. J Infect 1996; 33:23–32.
31. Pizzo PA, Robichaud KJ, Gill FA, Witebsky FG. Empiric antibiotic and antifungal therapy for cancer patients with prolonged fever and granulocytopenia. Am J Med 1982; 72:101–111.
32. EORTC International Antimicrobial Therapy Cooperative Project Group. Empiric antifungal therapy in febrile granulocytopenic patients. Am J Med 1989; 86:668–672.
33. Hughes WT, Armstrong D, Bodey GP, Bow EJ, Brown AE, Calandra T, et al. Guidelines for the use of antimicrobial agents in neutropenic patients with cancer. Clin Infect Dis 2002; 34:730–751.
34. Beck-Sague C, Jarvis WR. Secular trends in the epidemiology of nosocomial fungal infections in the United States, 1980–1990. National Nosocomial Infections Surveillance System. J Infect Dis 1993; 167:1247–1251.

35. Pagano L, Girmenia C, Mele L, Ricci P, Tosti ME, Nosari A, et al. Infections caused by filamentous fungi in patients with hematologic malignancies. A report of 391 cases by GIMEMA Infection Program. Haematologica 2001; 86:862–870.

36. Rex JH, Bennet JE, Sugar AM, Pappas PG, van der Horst CM, Edwards JE, et al. A randomized trial comparing fluconazole with amphotericin B for the treatment of candidemia in patients without neutropenia. N Engl J Med 1994; 331:1325–1330.

37. Walsh TJ, Finberg RW, Arndt C, Hiemenz J, Schwartz C, Bodensteiner D, et al. Liposomal amphotericin B for empirical therapy in patients with persistent fever and neutropenia. N Engl J Med 1999; 340:764–771.

38. Herbrecht R, Denning DW, Patterson TF, Bennett JE, Greene RE, Oestmann JW, et al. Voriconazole versus amphotericin B for primary therapy of invasive aspergillosis. N Engl J Med 2002; 347:408–415.

39. Mora-Duarte J, Betts R, Rotstein C, Colombo AL, Thompson-Moya L, Smietana J, et al. Comparison of caspofungin and amphotericin B for invasive candidiasis. N Engl J Med 2002; 347:2020–2029.

40. Roseff SA, Sugar AM. Oral and esophageal candidiasis. In: Bodey GP, ed. Candidiasis: Pathogenesis, diagnosis, and treatment. New York: Raven Press, 1993:185–203.

41. Laine PO, Lindqvist JC, Pyrhonen SO, Teerenhovi LM, Syrjanen SM, Meurman JH. Lesions of the oral mucosa in lymphoma patients receiving cytostatic drugs. Eur J Cancer B Oral Oncol 1993; 29:291–294.

42. Silverman S Jr, Luangjarmekorn L, Greenspan D. Occurrence of oral Candida in irradiated head and neck cancer patients. J Oral Med 1984; 39:194–196.

43. Fotos PG, Hellstein JW. Candida and candidosis. Epidemiology, diagnosis and therapeutic management. Dent Clin North Am 1992; 36:857–878.

44. Ramirez-Amador V, Silverman S Jr, Mayer P, Tyler M, Quivey J. Candidal colonization and oral candidiasis in patients undergoing oral and pharyngeal radiation therapy. Oral Surg Oral Med Oral Pathol Oral Radiol Endod 1997; 84:149–153.

45. Nicolatou-Galitis O, Dardoufas K, Markoulatos P, Sotiropoulou-Lontou A, Kyprianou K, Kolitsi G, et al. Oral pseudomembranous candidiasis, herpes simplex virus-1 infection, and oral mucositis in head and neck cancer patients receiving radiotherapy and granulocyte-macrophage colony-stimulating factor (GM-CSF) mouthwash. J Oral Pathol Med 2001; 30:471–480.

46. Epstein JB, Freilich MM, Le ND. Risk factors for oropharyngeal candidiasis in patients who receive radiation therapy for malignant conditions of the head and neck. Oral Surg Oral Med Oral Pathol 1993; 76:169–74.

47. Redding SW, Zellars RC, Kirkpatrick WR, McAtee RK, Caceres MA, Fothergill AW, et al. Epidemiology of oropharyngeal Candida colonization and infection in patients receiving radiation for head and neck cancer. J Clin Microbiol 1999; 37:3896–900.

48. Rossie KM, Taylor J, Beck FM, Hodgson SE, Blozis GG. Influence of radiation therapy on oral Candida albicans colonization: a quantitative assessment. Oral Surg Oral Med Oral Pathol 1987; 64:698–701.

49. Pratt NE, Sodicoff M, Liss J, Davis M, Sinesi M. Radioprotection of the rat parotid gland by WR-2721: morphology at 60 days post-irradiation. Int J Radiat Oncol Biol Phys 1980; 6:431–435.

50. Cheng VS, Downs J, Herbert D, Aramany M. The function of the parotid gland following radiation therapy for head and neck cancer. Int J Radiat Oncol Biol Phys 1981; 7: 253–258.

51. Shannon IL, Starcke EN, Wescott WB. Effect of radiotherapy on whole saliva flow. J Dent Res 1977; 56:693.

52. Markitziu A, Zafiropoulos G, Tsalikis L, Cohen L. Gingival health and salivary function in head and neck-irradiated patients. A five-year follow-up. Oral Surg Oral Med Oral Pathol 1992; 73:427–433.

53. Nicolatou-Galitis O, Sotiropoulou-Lontou A, Velegraki A, Pissakas G, Kolitsi G, Kyprianou K, et al. Oral candidiasis in head and neck cancer patients receiving radiotherapy with amifostine cytoprotection. Oral Oncol 2003;39:397–401.

54. Valdez IH, Atkinson JC, Ship JA, Fox PC. Major salivary gland function in patients with radiation-induced xerostomia: flow rates and sialochemistry. Int J Radiat Oncol Biol Phys 1993; 25:41–47.

55. Steele C, Leigh J, Swoboda R, Ozenci H, Fidel PL Jr. Potential role for a carbohydrate moiety in anti-*Candida* activity of human oral epithelial cells. Infect Immun. 2001; 69: 7091–7099.

56. McDonald S, Meyerowitz C, Smudzin T, Rubin P. Preliminary results of a pilot study using WR-2721 before fractionated irradiation of the head and neck to reduce salivary gland dysfunction. Int J Radiat Oncol Biol Phys 1994; 29:747–754.

57. Buntzel J, Kuttner K, Frohlich D, Glatzel M. Selective cytoprotection with amifostine in concurrent radiochemotherapy for head and neck cancer. Ann Oncol 1998; 9: 505–509.

58. Brizel DM, Wasserman TH, Henke M, Strnad V, Rudat V, Monnier A, et al. Phase III randomized trial of amifostine as a radioprotector in head and neck cancer. J Clin Oncol 2000; 18:3339–3345.

59. Wasserman T, Mackowiak JI, Brizel DM, Oster W, Zhang J, Peeples PJ, et al. Effect of amifostine on patient assessed clinical benefit in irradiated head and neck cancer. Int J Radiat Oncol Biol Phys 2000; 48:1035–1039.

60. Guggenheimer J, Moore PA. Xerostomia: etiology, recognition and treatment. J Am Dent Assoc 2003; 134:61–69.

61. Samonis G, Skordilis P, Maraki S, Datseris G, Toloudis P, Chatzinikolaou I, et al. Oropharyngeal candidiasis as a marker for esophageal candidiasis in patients with cancer. Clin Infect Dis 1998; 27:283–286.

62. Samonis G, Rolston K, Karl C, Miller P, Bodey GP. Prophylaxis of oropharyngeal candidiasis with fluconazole. Rev Infect Dis 1990; 12(suppl 3):S369–S373.

63. Tumbarello M, Tacconelli E, de Gaetano DK, Morace G, Fadda G, Cauda R. Candidemia in HIV-infected subjects. Eur J Clin Microbiol Infect Dis 1999; 18:478–483.

64. Chiou CC, Groll AH, Gonzalez CE, Callender D, Venzon D, Pizzo PA, et al. Esophageal candidiasis in pediatric acquired immunodeficiency syndrome: clinical manifestations and risk factors. Pediatr Infect Dis J 2000; 19:729–734.

65. Abgrall S, Charreau I, Joly V, Bloch J, Reynes J. Risk factors for esophageal candidiasis in a large cohort of HIV-infected patients treated with nucleoside analogues. Eur J Clin Microbiol Infect Dis 2001; 20:346–349.

66. Chiou CC, Groll AH, Mavrogiorgos N, Wood LV, Walsh TJ. Esophageal candidiasis in human immunodeficiency virus-infected pediatric patients after the introduction of highly active antiretroviral therapy. Pediatr Infect Dis J 2002; 21:388–392.

67. Vazquez JA. Therapeutic options for the management of oropharyngeal and esophageal candidiasis in HIV/AIDS patients. HIV Clin Trials 2000; 1:47–59.

68. American Society for Microbiology. Report of the ASM task force on antibiotic resistance. Antimicrob Agents Chemother 1995; (suppl):1–23.

69. Blumberg EA, Reboli AC. Failure of systemic empirical treatment with amphotericin B to prevent candidemia in neutropenic patients with cancer. Clin Infect Dis 1996;22: 462–466.

70. Diekema DJ, Messer SA, Brueggemann AB, Coffman SL, Doern GV, Herwaldt LA, et al. Epidemiology of candidemia: 3-year results from the emerging infections and the epidemiology of Iowa organisms study. J Clin Microbiol 2002; 40:1298–302.

71. Diekema DJ, Pfaller MA, Messer SA, Houston A, Hollis RJ, Doern GV, et al. In vitro activities of BMS-207147 against over 600 contemporary clinical bloodstream isolates of Candida species from the SENTRY Antimicrobial Surveillance Program in North America and Latin America. Antimicrob Agents Chemother 1999; 43:2236–2239.

72. Edmond MB, Wallace SE, McClish DK, Pfaller MA, Jones RN, Wenzel RP. Nosoco-
    mial bloodstream infections in United States hospitals: a three-year analysis. Clin Infect
    Dis 1999; 29:239–244.
73. Kao AS, Brandt ME, Pruitt WR, Conn LA, Perkins BA, Stephens DS, et al. The epi-
    demiology of candidemia in two United States cities: results of a population-based
    active surveillance. Clin Infect Dis 1999; 29:1164–1170.
74. Pfaller MA, Jones RN, Doern GV, Sader HS, Hollis RJ, Messer SA. International sur-
    veillance of bloodstream infections due to *Candida* species: frequency of occurrence and
    antifungal susceptibilities of isolates collected in 1997 in the United States, Canada, and
    South America for the SENTRY Program. The SENTRY Participant Group. J Clin
    Microbiol 1998;36:1886–1889.
75. Pfaller MA, Jones RN, Messer SA, Edmond MB, Wenzel RP. National surveillance of
    nosocomial blood stream infection due to species of *Candida* other than *Candida albi-
    cans*: frequency of occurrence and antifungal susceptibility in the SCOPE Program.
    SCOPE Participant Group. Surveillance and Control of Pathogens of Epidemiologic.
    Diagn Microbiol Infect Dis 1998; 30:121–129.
76. Pfaller MA, Messer SA, Houston A, Rangel-Frausto MS, Wiblin T, Blumberg HM,
    et al. National epidemiology of mycoses survey: a multicenter study of strain variation
    and antifungal susceptibility among isolates of *Candida* species. Diagn Microbiol Infect
    Dis 1998; 31:289–296.
77. Pfaller MA, Jones RN, Doern GV, Sader HS, Messer SA, Houston A, et al. Blood-
    stream infections due to *Candida* species: SENTRY antimicrobial surveillance program
    in North America and Latin America, 1997–1998. Antimicrob Agents Chemother 2000;
    44:747–751.
78. Pfaller MA, Diekema DJ, Jones RN, Sader HS, Fluit AC, Hollis RJ, et al. International
    surveillance of bloodstream infections due to *Candida* species: frequency of occurrence
    and in vitro susceptibilities to fluconazole, ravuconazole, and voriconazole of isolates
    collected from 1997 through 1999 in the SENTRY antimicrobial surveillance program.
    J Clin Microbiol 2001; 39:3254–3259.
79. Pfaller MA, Jones RN, Doern GV, Fluit AC, Verhoef J, Sader HS, et al. International
    surveillance of blood stream infections due to *Candida* species in the European SEN-
    TRY Program: species distribution and antifungal susceptibility including the investiga-
    tional triazole and echinocandin agents. SENTRY Participant Group (Europe). Diagn
    Microbiol Infect Dis 1999; 35:19–25.
80. Pfaller MA, Diekema DJ. Role of sentinel surveillance of candidemia: trends in species
    distribution and antifungal susceptibility. J Clin Microbiol 2002; 40:3551–3557.
81. Rangel-Frausto MS, Wiblin T, Blumberg HM, Saiman L, Patterson J, Rinaldi M, et al.
    National epidemiology of mycoses survey (NEMIS): variations in rates of bloodstream
    infections due to *Candida* species in seven surgical intensive care units and six neonatal
    intensive care units. Clin Infect Dis 1999; 29:253–258.
82. Saiman L, Ludington E, Pfaller M, Rangel-Frausto S, Wiblin RT, Dawson J, et al. Risk
    factors for candidemia in Neonatal Intensive Care Unit patients. The National Epide-
    miology of Mycosis Survey study group. Pediatr Infect Dis J 2000; 19:319–324.
83. Trick WE, Fridkin SK, Edwards JR, Hajjeh RA, Gaynes RP. Secular trend of hospital-
    acquired candidemia among intensive care unit patients in the United States during
    1989–1999. Clin Infect Dis 2002; 35:627–630.
84. Wingard JR. Importance of *Candida* species other than *C. albicans* as pathogens in
    oncology patients. Clin Infect Dis 1995; 20:115–125.
85. Abi-Said D, Anaissie E, Uzun O, Raad I, Pinzcowski H, Vartivarian S. The epidemiol-
    ogy of hematogenous candidiasis caused by different *Candida* species. Clin Infect Dis
    1997; 24:1122–1128.
86. Girmenia C, Martino P. Fluconazole and the changing epidemiology of candidemia.
    Clin Infect Dis 1998; 27:232–234.

87. Nucci M, Anaissie E. Revisiting the source of candidemia; skin or gut? Clin Infect Dis 2001; 33:1959–1967.

88. Kontoyiannis DP, Vaziri I, Hanna HA, Boktour M, Thornby J, Hachem R, et al. Risk factors for *Candida tropicalis* fungemia in patients with cancer. Clin Infect Dis 2001; 33:1676–1681.

89. Bishop JF, Lowenthal RM, Joshua D, Matthews JP, Todd D, Cobcroft R, et al. Etoposide in acute nonlymphocytic leukemia. Australian Leukemia Study Group. Blood 1990; 75:27–32.

90. el Mahallawy HA, Attia I, Ali-el-Din NH, Salem AE, Abo-el-Naga S. A prospective study on fungal infection in children with cancer. J Med Microbiol 2002; 51:601–605.

91. Bross J, Talbot GH, Maislin G, Hurwitz S, Strom BL. Risk factors for nosocomial candidemia: a case-control study in adults without leukemia. Am J Med 1989; 87:614–620.

92. Girmenia C, Martino P, De Bernardis F, Gentile G, Boccanera M, Monaco M, et al. Rising incidence of *Candida parapsilosis* fungemia in patients with hematologic malignancies: clinical aspects, predisposing factors, and differential pathogenicity of the causative strains. Clin Infect Dis 1996; 23:506–514.

93. Krcmery V Jr, Mrazova M, Kunova A, Grey E, Mardiak J, Jurga L, et al. Nosocomial candidaemias due to species other than *Candida albicans* in cancer patients. Aetiology, risk factors, and outcome of 45 episodes within 10 years in a single cancer institution. Support Care Cancer 1999; 7:428–431.

94. Safdar A, Perlin DS, Armstrong D. Hematogenous infections due to *Candida parapsilosis*: changing trends in fungemic patients at a comprehensive cancer center during the last four decades. Diagn Microbiol Infect Dis 2002; 44:11–16.

95. Nucci M, Anaissie E. Should vascular catheters be removed from all patients with candidemia? An evidence-based review. Clin Infect Dis 2002; 34:591–599.

96. Walsh TJ, Rex JH. All catheter-related candidemia is not the same: assessment of the balance between the risks and benefits of removal of vascular catheters. Clin Infect Dis 2002; 34:600–602.

97. Levin AS, Costa SF, Mussi NS, Basso M, Sinto SI, Machado C, et al. *Candida parapsilosis* fungemia associated with implantable and semi-implantable central venous catheters and the hands of healthcare workers. Diagn Microbiol Infect Dis 1998; 30:243–249.

98. Weems JJ Jr. *Candida parapsilosis*: epidemiology, pathogenicity, clinical manifestations, and antimicrobial susceptibility. Clin Infect Dis 1992; 14:756–766.

99. Nucci M, Colombo AL, Silveira F, Richtmann R, Salomao R, Branchini ML, et al. Risk factors for death in patients with candidemia. Infect Control Hosp Epidemiol 1998; 19:846–850.

100. Wingard JR, Merz WG, Rinaldi MG, Johnson TR, Karp JE, Saral R. Increase in *Candida krusei* infection among patients with bone marrow transplantation and neutropenia treated prophylactically with fluconazole. N Engl J Med 1991; 325:1274–1277.

101. Wingard JR. Infections due to resistant *Candida* species in patients with cancer who are receiving chemotherapy. Clin Infect Dis 1994; 19(suppl 1):S49–S53.

102. Abbas J, Bodey GP, Hanna HA, Mardani M, Girgawy E, Abi-Said D, et al. *Candida krusei* fungemia. An escalating serious infection in immunocompromised patients. Arch Intern Med 2000;160:2659–2664.

103. Wingard JR, Merz WG, Saral R. *Candida tropicalis*: a major pathogen in immunocompromised patients. Ann Intern Med 1979; 91:539–543.

104. Dykewicz CA, Jaffe HA, Kaplan JE. Guidelines for preventing opportunistic infections among hematopoietic stem cell transplant recipients. Biol Blood Marr Transpl 2000; 6:659–713.

105. Dykewicz CA. Summary of the guidelines for preventing opportunistic infections among hematopoietic stem cell transplant recipients. Clin Infect Dis 2001; 33:139–144.

106. Rotstein C, Bow EJ, Laverdiere M, Ioannou S, Carr D, Moghaddam N. Randomized placebo-controlled trial of fluconazole prophylaxis for neutropenic cancer patients:

benefit based on purpose and intensity of cytotoxic therapy. The Canadian Fluconazole Prophylaxis Study Group. Clin Infect Dis 1999; 28:331–340.

107. Bow EJ, Laverdiere M, Lussier N, Rotstein C, Cheang MS, Ioannou S. Antifungal prophylaxis for severely neutropenic chemotherapy recipients: a meta analysis of randomized-controlled clinical trials. Cancer 2002; 94:3230–3246.

108. Girmenia C, Martino P, Cassone A. Breakthrough candidemia during antifungal treatment with fluconazole in patients with hematologic malignancies. Blood 1996; 87: 838–839.

109. Uzun O, Ascioglu S, Anaissie EJ, Rex JH. Risk factors and predictors of outcome in patients with cancer and breakthrough candidemia. Clin Infect Dis 2001; 32:1713–1717.

110. Kontoyiannis DP, Reddy BT, Hanna H, Bodey GP, Tarrand J, Raad II. Breakthrough candidemia in patients with cancer differs from de novo candidemia in host factors and *Candida* species but not intensity. Infect Control Hosp Epidemiol 2002; 23:542–545.

111. Nucci M, Colombo AL. Risk factors for breakthrough candidemia. Eur J Clin Microbiol Infect Dis 2002; 21:209–211.

112. Powderly WG, Kobayashi GS, Herzig GP, Medoff G. Amphotericin B-resistant yeast infection in severely immunocompromised patients. Am J Med 1988; 84:826–832.

113. Krcmery V Jr, Spanik S, Kunova A, Trupl J. Breakthrough fungemia appearing during empiric therapy with amphotericin B. Chemotherapy 1997; 43:367–370.

114. Krcmery V Jr, Oravcova E, Spanik S, Mrazova-Studena M, Trupl J, Kunova A, et al. Nosocomial breakthrough fungaemia during antifungal prophylaxis or empirical antifungal therapy in 41 cancer patients receiving antineoplastic chemotherapy: analysis of aetiology risk factors and outcome. J Antimicrob Chemother 1998; 41:373–380.

115. Glasmacher A, Hahn C, Leutner C, Molitor E, Wardelmann E, Losem C, et al. Breakthrough invasive fungal infections in neutropenic patients after prophylaxis with itraconazole. Mycoses 1999; 42:443–451.

116. Rex JH. Editorial response: catheters and candidemia. Clin Infect Dis 1996; 22:467–470.

117. Rankin NE. Disseminated aspergillosis and moniliasis associated with agranulocytosis and antibiotic therapy. Br Med J 1953; 183:918–919.

118. Nolard N, Detand M, Beguin H. *Aspergillus* species in the environment. In: Vanden Bosche H, Mackenzie DWR, Cauwenbergh G, eds. *Aspergillus* and Aspergillosis. New York: Plenum Press, 1998:35–41.

119. Anaissie EJ, Stratton SL, Dignani MC, Lee CK, Mahfouz TH, Rex JH, et al. Cleaning patient shower facilities: a novel approach to reducing patient exposure to aerosolized *Aspergillus* species and other opportunistic molds. Clin Infect Dis 2002; 35:E86–E88.

120. Anaissie EJ, Stratton SL, Dignani MC, Summerbell RC, Rex JH, Monson TP, et al. Pathogenic *Aspergillus* species recovered from a hospital water system: a 3-year prospective study. Clin Infect Dis 2002; 34:780–789.

121. Anaissie EJ, Kuchar RT, Rex JH, Francesconi A, Kasai M, Muller FM, et al. Fusariosis associated with pathogenic fusarium species colonization of a hospital water system: a new paradigm for the epidemiology of opportunistic mold infections. Clin Infect Dis 2001; 33:1871–1878.

122. Anaissie EJ,.Costa SF. Nosocomial aspergillosis is waterborne. Clin Infect Dis 2001; 33:1546–1548.

123. Walsh TJ, Dixon DM. Nosocomial aspergillosis: environmental microbiology, hospital epidemiology, diagnosis and treatment. Eur J Epidemiol 1989; 5:131–142.

124. Diamond RD, Krzesicki R, Epstein B, Jao W. Damage to hyphal forms of fungi by human leukocytes in vitro. A possible host defense mechanism in aspergillosis and mucormycosis. Am J Pathol 1978; 91:313–328.

125. Schafmer A, Douglas H, Braude A. Selective protection against conidia by mononuclear and against mycelia by polymorphonuclear phagocytes in resistance to *Aspergillus*. Observations on these two lines of defense in vivo and in vitro with human and mouse phagocytes J Clin Invest 1982; 69:617–631.

126. Latge JP. The pathobiology of *Aspergillus* fumigatus. Trends Microbiol 2001; 9: 382–389.

127. Meyer RD, Young LS, Armstrong D, Yu B. Aspergillosis complicating neoplastic disease. Am J Med 1973; 54:6–15.

128. Masur H, Rosen PP, Armstrong D. Pulmonary disease caused by *Candida* species. Am J Med 1977; 63:914–925.

129. Anttila VJ, Ruutu P, Bondestam S, Jansson SE, Nordling S, Farkkila M, et al. Hepatosplenic yeast infection in patients with acute leukemia: a diagnostic problem. Clin Infect Dis 1994; 18:979–981.

130. Anttila VJ, Elonen E, Nordling S, Sivonen A, Ruutu T, Ruutu P. Hepatosplenic candidiasis in patients with acute leukemia: incidence and prognostic implications. Clin Infect Dis 1997; 24:375–380.

131. Anaissie E, Bodey GP, Kantarjian H, Ro J, Vartivarian SE, Hopfer R, et al. New spectrum of fungal infections in patients with cancer. Rev Infect Dis 1989; 11:369–378.

132. Schwarz J. The diagnosis of deep mycoses by morphologic methods. Hum Pathol 1982; 13:519–533.

133. Paterson DL, Singh N. Invasive aspergillosis in transplant recipients. Medicine (Baltimore) 1999; 78:123–138.

134. Perfect JR, Cox GM, Lee JY, Kauffman CA, de Repentigny L, Chapman SW, et al. The impact of culture isolation of *Aspergillus* species: a hospital-based survey of aspergillosis. Clin Infect Dis 2001; 33:1824–1833.

135. Perea S, Patterson TF. Invasive *Aspergillus* infections in hematologic malignancy patients. Semin Respir Infect 2002; 17:99–105.

136. Segal BH, Bow EJ, Menichetti F. Fungal infections in nontransplant patients with hematologic malignancies. Infect Dis Clin North Am 2002; 16:935–964, vii.

137. Fraser DW, Ward JL, Ajello L, Plikaytis BD. Aspergillosis and other systemic mycoses. The growing problem. JAMA 1979; 242:1631–1635.

138. Patterson TF, Kirkpatrick WR, White M, Hiemenz JW, Wingard JR, Dupont B, et al. Invasive aspergillosis. Disease spectrum, treatment practices, and outcomes. I3 *Aspergillus* Study Group. Medicine (Baltimore) 2000;79:250–260.

139. Cornet M, Fleury L, Maslo C, Bernard JF, Brucker G. Epidemiology of invasive aspergillosis in France: a six-year multicentric survey in the Greater Paris area. J Hosp Infect 2002; 51:288–296.

140. Marr KA, Carter RA, Crippa F, Wald A, Corey L. Epidemiology and outcome of mold infections in hematopoietic stem cell transplant recipients. Clin Infect Dis 2002; 34: 909–917.

141. Bittencourt H, Rocha V, Chevret S, Socie G, Esperou H, Devergie A, et al. Association of CD34 cell dose with hematopoietic recovery, infections, and other outcomes after HLA-identical sibling bone marrow transplantation. Blood 2002; 99:2726–2733.

142. Dasbach EJ, Davies GM, Teutsch SM. Burden of aspergillosis-related hospitalizations in the United States. Clin Infect Dis 2000; 31:1524–1528.

143. Simonsen L, Conn LA, Pinner RW, Teutsch S. Trends in infectious disease hospitalizations in the United States, 1980–1994. Arch Intern Med 1998; 158:1923–1928.

144. Weems JJ Jr, Davis BJ, Tablan OC, Kaufman L, Martone WJ. Construction activity: an independent risk factor for invasive aspergillosis and zygomycosis in patients with hematologic malignancy. Infect Control 1987; 8:71–75.

145. Perraud M, Piens MA, Nicoloyannis N, Girard P, Sepetjan M, Garin JP. Invasive nosocomial pulmonary aspergillosis: risk factors and hospital building works. Epidemiol Infect 1987; 99:407–412.

146. Weber SF, Peacock JE Jr, Do KA, Cruz JM, Powell BL, Capizzi RL. Interaction of granulocytopenia and construction activity as risk factors for nosocomial invasive filamentous fungal disease in patients with hematologic disorders. Infect Control Hosp. Epidemiol 1990; 11:235–242.

147. Flynn PM, Williams BG, Hetherington SV, Williams BF, Giannini MA, Pearson TA. *Aspergillus terreus* during hospital renovation. Infect Control Hosp Epidemiol 1993; 14:363–365.

148. Iwen PC, Davis JC, Reed EC, Winfield BA, Hinrichs SH. Airborne fungal spore monitoring in a protective environment during hospital construction, and correlation with an outbreak of invasive aspergillosis. Infect Control Hosp Epidemiol 1994; 15: 303–306.

149. Hahn T, Cummings KM, Michalek AM, Lipman BJ, Segal BH, McCarthy PL Jr. Efficacy of high-efficiency particulate air filtration in preventing aspergillosis in immunocompromised patients with hematologic malignancies. Infect Control Hosp Epidemiol 2002; 23:525–531.

150. Humphreys H, Johnson EM, Warnock DW, Willatts SM, Winter RJ, Speller DC. An outbreak of aspergillosis in a general ITU. J Hosp Infect 1991; 18:167–177.

151. Richet HM, McNeil MM, Davis BJ, Duncan E, Strickler J, Nunley D, et al. *Aspergillus fumigatus* sternal wound infections in patients undergoing open heart surgery. Am J Epidemiol 1992; 135:48–58.

152. Loudon KW, Coke AP, Burnie JP, Lucas GS, Liu Yin JA. Invasive aspergillosis clusters and sources? J Med Vet Mycol 1994; 32:217–224.

153. Mahieu LM, De Dooy JJ, Van Laer FA, Jansens H, Ieven MM. A prospective study on factors influencing aspergillus spore load in the air during renovation works in a neonatal intensive care unit. J Hosp Infect 2000; 45:191–197.

154. Alberti C, Bouakline A, Ribaud P, Lacroix C, Rousselot P, Leblanc T, et al. Relationship between environmental fungal contamination and the incidence of invasive aspergillosis in haematology patients. J Hosp Infect 2001; 48:198–206.

155. Passweg JR, Rowlings PA, Atkinson KA, Barrett AJ, Gale RP, Gratwohl A, et al. Influence of protective isolation on outcome of allogeneic bone marrow transplantation for leukemia. Bone Marrow Transplant 1998; 21:1231–1238.

156. Marr KA, Seidel K, Slavin MA, Bowden RA, Schoch HG, Flowers MED, et al. Prolonged fluconazole prophylaxis is associated with persistent protection against candidiasis-related death in allogeneic marrow transplant recipients: long-term follow-up of a randomized, placebo-controlled trial. Blood 2000; 96:2055–2061.

157. Srinivasan A, Beck C, Buckley T, Geyh A, Bova G, Merz W, et al. The ability of hospital ventilation systems to filter *Aspergillus* and other fungi following a building implosion. Infect Control Hosp Epidemiol 2002; 23:520–524.

158. Andrutis KA, Riggle PJ, Kumamoto CA, Tzipori S. Intestinal lesions associated with disseminated candidiasis in an experimental animal model. J Clin Microbiol 2000; 38: 2317.

159. Cole GT, Halawa AA, Anaissie EJ. The role of the gastrointestinal tract in hematogenous candidiasis: from the laboratory to the bedside. Clin Infect Dis 1996; 22(suppl 2): S73–S88.

160. Schimpff SC. Oral complications of cancer therapies. Surveillance cultures. NCI Monogr 1990; 37–42.

161. de Jong PJ, de Jong MD, Kuijper ED, Van der Lelie H. The value of surveillance cultures in neutropenic patients receiving selective intestinal decontamination. Scand J Infect Dis 1993; 25:107–113.

162. Pittet D, Monod M, Suter PM, Frenk E, Auckenthaler R. *Candida* colonization and subsequent infections in critically ill surgical patients. Ann Surg 1994; 220:751–758.

163. Aisner J, Schimpff SC, Sutherland JC, Young VM, Wiernik PH. *Torulopsis glabrata* infections in patients with cancer. Increasing incidence and relationship to colonization. Am J Med 1976; 61:23–28.

164. Schimpff SC, Young VM, Greene WH, Vermeulen GD, Moody MR, Wiernik PH. Origin of infection in acute nonlymphocytic leukemia. Significance of hospital acquisition of potential pathogens. Ann Intern Med 1912; 77:707–714.

165. Schimpff SC. Surveillance cultures. J Infect Dis 1981; 144:81–84.

166. van der Waaij D. Colonization resistance of the digestive tract as a major lead in the selection of antibiotics for therapy. In: New Criteria for Antimicrobial Therapy: Maintenance of Digestive Tract Colonization Resistance, Amsterdam, 1979:271–282.

167. Louie TJ, Chubb H, Bow EJ, Conly JM, Harding GK, Rayner E, et al. Preservation of colonization resistance parameters during empiric therapy with aztreonam in the febrile neutropenic patient. Rev Infect Dis 1985; 7(suppl 4):S747–S761.

168. Vollaard EJ, Clasener HA. Colonization resistance. Antimicrob. Agents Chemother. 1994; 38:409–414.

169. Hecker MT, Aron DC, Patel NP, Lehmann MK, Donskey CJ. Unnecessary use of antimicrobials in hospitalized patients: current patterns of misuse with an emphasis on the antianaerobic spectrum of activity. Arch Intern Med 2003; 163:972–978.

170. Bow EJ, Louie TJ. Changes in endogenous microflora among febrile granulocytopenic patients receiving empiric antibiotic therapy: implications for fungal superinfection. CMAJ 1987; 137:397–403.

171. Samonis G, Gikas A, Anaissie EJ, Vrenzos G, Maraki S, Tselentis Y, et al. Prospective evaluation of effects of broad-spectrum antibiotics on gastrointestinal yeast colonization of humans. Antimicrob Agents Chemother 1993; 37:51.

172. Bow EJ, Mandell LA, Louie TJ, Feld R, Palmer M, Zee B, et al. Quinolone-based antibacterial chemoprophylaxis in neutropenic patients: effect of augmented gram-positive activity on infectious morbidity. National Cancer Institute of Canada Clinical Trials Group. Ann Intern Med 1996; 125:183–190.

173. Beelen DW, Elmaagacli A, Muller KD, Hirche H, Schaefer UW. Influence of intestinal bacterial decontamination using metronidazole and ciprofloxacin or ciprofloxacin alone on the development of acute graft-versus-host disease after marrow transplantation in patients with hematologic malignancies: final results and long-term follow-up of an open-label prospective randomized trial. Blood 1999; 93:3267–3275.

174. Trenschel R, Peceny R, Runde V, Elmaagacli A, Dermoumi H, Heintschel VH, et al. Fungal colonization and invasive fungal infections following allogeneic BMT using metronidazole, ciprofloxacin and fluconazole or ciprofloxacin and fluconazole as intestinal decontamination. Bone Marr Transpl 2000; 26:993–997.

175. Wey SB, Mori M, Pfaller MA, Woolson RF, Wenzel RP. Risk factors for hospital-acquired candidemia-a matched case-control study. Arch Intern Med 1989; 149:2349–2353.

176. Viudes A, Peman J, Canton E, Ubeda P, Lopez-Ribot JL, Gobernado M. Candidemia at a tertiary-care hospital: epidemiology, treatment, clinical outcome and risk factors for death. Eur J Clin Microbiol Infect Dis 2002; 21:767–774.

177. Hryniuk W, Levine MN. Analysis of dose intensity for adjuvant chemotherapy trials in stage II breast cancer. J Clin Oncol 1986; 4:1162–1170.

178. Bodey GP, Buckley M, Sathe YS, Freireich EJ. Quantitative relationships between circulating leukocytes and infection in patients with acute leukemia. Ann Intern Med 1966; 64:328–340.

179. Bodey GP, Rodriguez V, Chang HY, Narboni. Fever and infection in leukemic patients: a study of 494 consecutive patients. Cancer 1978; 41:1610–1622.

180. Bohlius J, Reiser M, Schwarzer G, Engert A. Granulopoiesis-stimulating factors in the prevention for adverse effects in the therapeutic treatment of malignant lymphoma. Cochrane Database Syst Rev 2002; CD003189.

181. Couban S, Simpson DR, Barnett MJ, Bredeson C, Hubesch L, Howson-Jan K, et al. A randomized multicenter comparison of bone marrow and peripheral blood in recipients of matched sibling allogeneic transplants for myeloid malignancies. Blood 2002; 100: 1525–1531.

182. Jones GR, Konsler GK, Dunaway RP, Gold SH, Cooper HA, Wells RJ. Risk factors for recurrent fever after the discontinuation of empiric antibiotic therapy for fever and neutropenia in pediatric patients with a malignancy or hematologic condition. J Pediatr 1994; 124:703–708.

183. Rackoff WR, Gonin R, Robinson C, Kreissman SG, Breitfeld PB. Predicting the risk of bacteremia in childen with fever and neutropenia. J Clin Oncol 1996; 14:919–924.

184. Klaassen RJ, Goodman TR, Pham B, Doyle JJ. "Low-risk" prediction rule for pediatric oncology patients presenting with fever and neutropenia. J Clin Oncol 2000; 18: 1012–1019.

185. Baorto EP, Aquino VM, Mullen CA, Buchanan GR, DeBaun MR. Clinical parameters associated with low bacteremia risk in 1100 pediatric oncology patients with fever and neutropenia. Cancer 2001; 92:909–913.

186. Santolaya ME, Alvarez AM, Becker A, Cofre J, Enriquez N, O'Ryan M, et al. Prospective, multicenter evaluation of risk factors associated with invasive bacterial infection in children with cancer, neutropenia, and fever. J Clin Oncol 2001; 19:3415–3421.

187. Madsen K, Rosenman M, Hui S, Breitfeld PP. Value of electronic data for model validation and refinement: bacteremia risk in children with fever and neutropenia. J Pediatr Hematol Oncol 2002; 24:256–262.

188. Rosenman M, Madsen K, Hui S, Breitfeld PP. Modeling administrative outcomes in fever and neutropenia: clinical variables significantly influence length of stay and hospital charges. J Pediatr Hematol Oncol 2002; 24:263–268.

189. Weinberger M, Elattar I, Marshall D, Steinberg SM, Redner RL, Young NS, et al. Patterns of infection in patients with aplastic anemia and the emergence of *Aspergillus* as a major cause of death. Medicine (Baltimore) 1992; 71:24–43.

190. Storek J, Espino G, Dawson MA, Storer B, Flowers ME, Maloney DG. Low B-cell and monocyte counts on day 80 are associated with high infection rates between days 100 and 365 after allogeneic marrow transplantation. Blood 2000; 96:3290–3293.

191. Neumanitis J, Shannon-Dorcy K, Applebaum FR, Meyers JD, Owens A, Day R, et al. Long-term follow-up of patients with invasive fungal disease who received adjunctive therapy with recombinant human macrophage colony-stimulating factor. Blood 1993; 82:1422–1427.

192. Neumanitis J. Use of macrophage colony-stimulating factor in the treatment of fungal infections. Clin Infect Dis 1998; 26:1279–1281.

193. Leleu X, Sendid B, Fruit J, Sarre H, Wattel E, Rose C, et al. Combined anti-fungal therapy and surgical resection as treatment of pulmonary zygomycosis in allogeneic bone marrow transplantation. Bone Marr Transpl 1999; 24:417–420.

194. Richardson DS, Newland AC. Current perspectives on the use of growth factors in the therapy of acute myeloid leukaemia. Malignancy Hematol 2000; 5:189–203.

195. Masur H, Ognibene FP, Yarchoan R, Shelhamer JH, Baird BF, Travis W, et al. CD4 counts as predictors of opportunistic pneumonias in human immunodeficiency virus (HIV) infection. Ann Intern Med 1989; 111:223–231.

196. Brambilla AM, Castagna A, Nocita B, Hasson H, Boeri E, Veglia F, et al. Relation between CD4 cell counts and HIV RNA levels at onset of opportunistic infections. J Acquir Immune Defic Syndr 2001; 27:44–48.

197. Mackall CL, Fleisher TA, Brown MR, Magrath IT, Shad AT, Horowitz ME, et al. Lymphocyte depletion during treatment with intensive chemotherapy for cancer. Blood 1994; 84:2221–2228.

198. Strender LE, Blomgren H, Petrini B, Wasserman J, Forsgren M, Norberg R, et al. Immunologic monitoring in breast cancer patients receiving postoperative adjuvant chemotherapy. Cancer 1981; 48:1996–2002.

199. Browne MJ, Hubbard SM, Longo DL, Fisher R, Wesley R, Hide DC, et al. Excess prevalence of *Pneumocystis carinii* pneumonia in patients treated for lymphoma with combination chemotherapy. Ann Intern Med 1986; 104:338–344.

200. Brunvand MW, Collins C, Livingston RB, Raghu G. *Pneumocystis carinii* pneumonia associated with profound lymphopenia and abnormal T-lymphocyte subset ratios during treatment for early-stage breast carcinoma. Cancer 1991; 67:2407–2409.

201. Kontoyiannis DP, Peitsch WK, Reddy BT, Whimbey EE, Han XY, Bodey GP, et al. Cryptococcosis in patients with cancer. Clin Infect Dis 2001; 32:E145–E150.

202. Blay JY, Chauvin F, Le Cesne A, Anglaret B, Bouhour D, Lasset C, et al. Early lymphopenia after cytotoxic chemotherapy as a risk factor for febrile neutropenia. J Clin Oncol 1996; 14:636–643.
203. Blay JY, Le Cesne A, Mermet C, Maugard C, Ravaud A, Chevreau C, et al. A risk model for thrombocytopenia requiring platelet transfusion after cytotoxic chemotherapy. Blood 1998; 92:405–410.
204. Ray-Coquard I, Le Cesne A, Rubio MT, Mermet J, Maugard C, Ravaud A, et al. Risk model for severe anemia requiring red blood cell transfusion after cytotoxic conventional chemotherapy regimens. The Elypse 1 Study Group. J Clin Oncol 1999; 17: 2840–2846.
205. Melichar B, Touskova M, Vesely P. Effect of irinotecan on the phenotype of peripheral blood leukocyte populations in patients with metastatic colorectal cancer. Hepatogastroenterology 2002; 49:967–970.
206. Fidias P, Chabner BA, Grossbard ML. Purine analogs for the treatment of low-grade lymphoproliferative disorders. Oncologist 1996; 1:125–139.
207. Cheson BD. Infectious and immunosuppressive complications of purine analog therapy. J Clin Oncol 1995; 13:2431–2448.
208. Samonis G, Kontoyiannis DP. Infectious complications of purine analog therapy. Curr Opin Infect Dis 2001; 14:409–413.
209. Kay NE, Hamblin TJ, Jelinek DF, Dewald GW, Byrd JC, Farag S, et al. Chronic Lymphocytic Leukemia. Hematology 2002; 2002:193–213.
210. Estey EH, Thall PF, Cortes JE, Giles FJ, O'Brien S, Pierce SA, et al. Comparison of idarubicin + ara-C-, fludarabine + ara-C-, and topotecan + ara-C-based regimens in treatment of newly diagnosed acute myeloid leukemia, refractory anemia with excess blasts in transformation, or refractory anemia with excess blasts. Blood 2001; 98: 3575–3583.
211. Champlin R, Khouri I, Anderlini P, de Lima M, Hosing C, McMannis J, et al. Nonmyeloablative preparative regimens for allogeneic hematopoietic transplantation. Biology and current indications. Oncology (Huntingt) 2003; 17:94–100.
212. Schilling PJ, Vadhan-Raj S. Concurrent cytomegalovirus and pneumocystis pneumonia after fludarabine therapy for chronic lymphocytic leukemia. N Engl J Med 1990; 323: 833–834.
213. Anaissie E, Kontoyiannis DP, Kantarjian H, Elting L, Robertson LE, Keating M. Listeriosis in patients with chronic lymphocytic leukemia who were treated with fludarabine and prednisone. Ann Intern Med 1992; 117:466–469.
214. Morrison VA. The infectious complications of chronic lymphocytic leukemia. Semin Oncol 1998; 25:98–106.
215. Tsiodras S, Samonis G, Keating MJ, Kontoyiannis DP. Infection and immunity in chronic lymphocytic leukemia. Mayo Clin Proc 2000; 75:1039–1054.
216. Keating MJ, O'Brien S, Lerner S, Koller C, Beran M, Robertson LE, et al. Long-term follow-up of patients with chronic lymphocytic leukemia (CLL) receiving fludarabine regimens as initial therapy. Blood 1998; 92:1165–1171.
217. Wijermans PW, Gerrits WB, Haak HL. Severe immunodeficiency in patients treated with fludarabine monophosphate. Eur J Haematol 1993; 50:292–296.
218. Rai KR, Peterson BL, Appelbaum FR, Kolitz J, Elias L, Shepherd L, et al. Fludarabine compared with chlorambucil as primary therapy for chronic lymphocytic leukemia. N Engl J Med 2000; 343:1750–1757.
219. Morrison VA, Rai KR, Peterson BL, Kolitz JE, Elias L, Appelbaum FR, et al. Impact of therapy with chlorambucil, fludarabine, or fludarabine plus chlorambucil on infections in patients with chronic lymphocytic leukemia. Intergroup Study Cancer and Leukemia Group B 9011. J Clin Oncol 2001; 19:3611–3621.
220. Bergmann L, Fenchel K, Jahn B, Mitrou PS, Hoelzer D. Immunosuppressive effects and clinical response of fludarabine in refractory chronic lymphocytic leukemia. Ann Oncol 1993; 4:371–375.

221. Byrd JC, Hargis JB, Kester KE, Hospenthal DR, Knutson SW, Diehl LF. Opportunistic pulmonary infections with fludarabine in previously treated patients with low-grade lymphoid malignancies: a role for *Pneumocystis carinii* pneumonia prophylaxis. Am J Hematol 1995; 49:135–142.

222. Robak T, Blonski JZ, Kasznicki M, Konopka L, Ceglarek B, Dmoszynska A, et al. Cladribine with or without prednisone in the treatment of previously treated and untreated B-cell chronic lymphocytic leukaemia—updated results of the multicentre study of 378 patients. Br J Haematol 2000; 108:357–368.

223. Carrera CJ, Terai C, Lotz M, Curd JG, Piro LD, Beutler E, et al. Potent toxicity of 2-chlorodeoxyadenosine toward human monocytes in vitro and in vivo. A novel approach to immunosuppressive therapy. J Clin Invest 1990; 86:1480–1488.

224. Beutler E, Koziol JA, McMillan R, Sipe JC, Romine JS, Carrera CJ. Marrow suppression produced by repeated doses of cladribine. Ada Haematol 1994; 91:10–15.

225. Juliusson G, Lenkei R, Liliemark J. Flow cytometry of blood and bone marrow cells from patients with hairy cell leukemia: phenotype of hairy cells and lymphocyte subsets after treatment with 2-chlorodeoxyadenosine. Blood 1994; 83:3672–3681.

226. Storek J, Dawson MA, Storer B, Stevens-Ayers T, Maloney DG, Marr KA, et al. Immune reconstitution after allogeneic marrow transplantation compared with blood stem cell transplantation. Blood 2001; 97:3380–3389.

227. Osterborg A, Dyer MJ, Bunjes D, Pangalis GA, Bastion Y, Catovsky D, et al. Phase II multicenter study of human CD52 antibody in previously treated chronic lymphocytic leukemia. European Study Group of CAMPATH-1H Treatment in Chronic Lymphocytic Leukemia. J Clin Oncol 1997; 15:1567–1574.

228. Lundin J, Osterborg A, Brittinger G, Crowther D, Dombret H, Engert A, et al. CAMPATH-1H monoclonal antibody in therapy for previously treated low-grade non-Hodgkin's lymphomas: a phase II multicenter study. European Study Group of CAMPATH-1H Treatment in low-grade non-hodgkin's lymphoma. J Clin Oncol 1998; 16:3257–3263.

229. Keating MJ, O'Brien S, Kontoyiannis D, Plunkett W, Koller C, Beran M, et al. Results of first salvage therapy for patients refractory to a fludarabine regimen in chronic lymphocytic leukemia. Leuk Lymphoma 2002; 43:1755–1762.

230. Rai KR, Freter CE, Mercier RJ, Cooper MR, Mitchell BS, Stadtmauer EA, et al. Alemtuzumab in previously treated chronic lymphocytic leukemia patients who also had received fludarabine. J Clin Oncol 2002; 20:3891–3897.

231. Chakrabarti S, MacDonald D, Hale G, Holder K, Turner V, Czarnecka H, et al. T-cell depletion with Campath-IH "in the bag" for matched related allogeneic peripheral blood stem cell transplantation is associated with reduced graft-versus-host disease, rapid immune constitution and improved survival. Br J Haematol 2003; 121:109–118.

232. Simpson D. T-cell depleting antibodies: new hope for induction of allograft tolerance in bone marrow transplation? Bio Drugs 2003; 17:147–154.

233. Novitzky N, Rouskova A. Infectious complications following T-cell depleted hematopoietic stem-cell transplantation. Cytotherapy 2001; 3:165–173.

234. Chakrabarti S. Increased CMV infection following nonmyeloablative allogeneic stem cell transplantation: a search for the guilty. Blood 2003; 101:2071.

235. Chakrabarti S, Mackinnon S, Chopra R, Kottaridis PD, Peggs K, O'Gorman P, et al. High incidence of cytomegalovirus infection after nonmyeloablative stem cell transplantation: potential role of Campath-1H in delaying immune reconstitution. Blood 2002; 99:4357–4363.

236. Chakrabarti S, Osman H, Collingham K, Milligan DW. Polyoma viruria following T-cell-depleted allogeneic transplants using Campath-1H: incidence and outcome in relation to graft manipulation, donor type and conditioning. Bone Marr Transpl 2003; 31:379–386.

237. Cavalli-Bjorkman N, Osby E, Lundin J, Kalin M, Osterborg A, Gruber A. Fatal adenovirus infection during alemtuzumab (anti-CD52 monoclonal antibody) treatment of a

patient with fludarabine-refractory B-cell chronic lymphocytic leukemia. Med Oncol 2002; 19:277–280.

238. Crowley B, Woodcock B. Red cell aplasia due to parvovirus b19 in a patient treated with alemtuzumab. Br J Haematol 2002; 119:279–280.

239. Morrison VA. Update on prophylaxis and therapy of infection in patients with chronic lymphocytic leukemia. Expert Rev Anticancer Ther 2001; 1:84–90.

240. Lundin J, Hagberg H, Repp R, Cavallin-Stahl E, Freden S, Juliusson G, et al. Phase 2 study of alemtuzumab (anti-CD52 monoclonal antibody) in patients with advanced mycosis fungoides/Sezary syndrome. Blood 2003; 101:4267–4272.

241. Nishida S, Levi D, Kato T, Nery JR, Mittal N, Hadjis N, et al. Ninety-five cases of intestinal transplantation at the University of Miami. J Gastrointest Surg 2002; 6: 233–239.

242. King KM, Younes A. Rituximab: review and clinical applications focusing on non-Hodgkin's lymphoma. Expert Rev Anticancer Ther 2001; 1:177–186.

243. Coiffier B. Rituximab in combination with CHOP improves survival in elderly patients with aggressive non-Hodgkin's lymphoma. Semin Oncol 2002; 29:18–22.

244. Coiffier B. Immunochemotherapy: the new standard in aggressive non-Hodgkin's lymphoma in the elderly. Semin Oncol 2003; 30:21–27.

245. Akhtar S, Maghfoor I. Rituximab plus CHOP for diffuse large-B-cell lymphoma. N Engl J Med 2002; 346:1830–1831.

246. McLaughlin P, Grillo-Lopez AJ, Link BK, Levy R, Czuczman MS, Williams ME, et al. Rituximab chimeric anti-CD20 monoclonal antibody therapy for relapsed indolent lymphoma: half of patients respond to a four-dose treatment program. J Clin Oncol 1998; 16:2825–2833.

247. van der Kolk LE, Baars JW, Prins MH, van Oers MH. Rituximab treatment results in impaired secondary humoral immune responsiveness. Blood 2002; 100:2257–2259.

248. Goldberg SL, Pecora AL, Alter RS, Kroll MS, Rowley SD, Waintraub SE, et al. Unusual viral infections (progressive multifocal leukoencephalopathy and cytomegalovirus disease) after high-dose chemotherapy with autologous blood stem cell rescue and peri transplantation rituximab. Blood 2002; 99:1486–1488.

249. Matteucci P, Magni M, Di Nicola M, Carlo-Stella C, Uberti C, Gianni AM. Leukoencephalopathy and papovavirus infection after treatment with chemotherapy and anti-CD20 monoclonal antibody. Blood 2002; 100:1104–1105.

250. Rowinsky EK, Donehower RC. Paclitaxel (taxol). N Engl J Med 1995; 332:1004–1014.

251. Wiernik PH, Schwartz EL, Strauman JJ, Dutcher JP, Lipton RB, Paietta E. Phase I clinical and pharmacokinetic study of taxol. Cancer Res 1987; 47:2486–2493.

252. Reckzeh B, Merte H, Pfluger KH, Pfab R, Wolf M, Havemann K. Severe lymphocytopenia and interstitial pneumonia in patients treated with paclitaxel and simultaneous radiotherapy for non-small-cell lung cancer. J Clin Oncol 1996; 14:1071–1076.

253. Morgan GW, Breit SN. Radiation and the lung: a reevaluation of the mechanisms mediating pulmonary injury. Int J Radiat Oncol Biol Phys 1995; 31:361–369.

254. Walsh LJ, Hill G, Seymour G, Roberts A. A scoring system for the quantitative evaluation of oral mucositis during bone marrow transplantation. Spec Care Dentist 1990; 10:190–195.

255. Sonis ST, Oster G, Fuchs H, Bellum L, Bradford WZ, Edelsberg J, et al. Oral mucositis and the clinical and economic outcomes of hematopoietic stem-cell transplantation. J Clin Oncol 2001; 19:2201–2205.

256. Raber-Durlacher JE, Weijl NI, Abu SM, de Koning B, Zwinderman AH, Osanto S. Oral mucositis in patients treated with chemotherapy for solid tumors: a retrospective analysis of 150 cases. Support Care Cancer 2000; 8:366–371.

257. Sallah S, Wan JY, Nguyen NP, Vos P, Sigounas G. Analysis of factors related to the occurrence of chronic disseminated candidiasis in patients with acute leukemia in a non-bone marrow transplant setting: a follow-up study. Cancer 2001; 92:1349–1353.

258. Wardley AM, Jayson GC, Swindell R, Morgenstern GR, Chang J, Bloor R, et al. Prospective evaluation of oral mucositis in patients receiving myeloablative conditioning regimens and haemopoietic progenitor rescue. Br J Haematol 2000; 110:292–299.

259. Sonis ST. Mucositis as a biological process: a new hypothesis for the development of chemotherapy-induced stomatotoxicity. Oral Oncol 1998; 34:39–43.

260. Slavin RE, Dias MA, Saral R. Cytosine arabinoside induced gastrointestinal toxic alterations in sequential chemotherapeutic protocols: a clinical-pathologic study of 33 patients. Cancer 1978; 42:1747–1759.

261. Keefe DM, Brealey J, Goland GJ, Cummins AG. Chemotherapy for cancer causes apoptosis that precedes hypoplasia in crypts of the small intestine in humans. Gut 2000; 47:632–637.

262. Fegan C, Poynton CH, Whittaker JA. The gut mucosal barrier in bone marrow transplantation. Bone Marr Transpl 1990; 5:373–377.

263. Bow EJ, Loewen R, Cheang MS, Shore TB, Rubinger M, Schacter B. Cytotoxic therapy-induced D-xylose malabsorption and invasive infection during remission- induction therapy for acute myeloid leukemia in adults. J Clin Oncol 1997; 15:2254–2261.

264. Johansson JE, Ekman T. Gastro-intestinal toxicity related to bone marrow transplantation: disruption of the intestinal barrier precedes clinical findings. Bone Marrow Transplant 1997; 19:921–925.

265. Thaler M, Bacher J, O'Leary T, Pizzo PA. Evaluation of single-drug and combination antifungal therapy in an experimental model of candidiasis in rabbits with prolonged neutropenia. J Infect Dis 1988; 158:80–88.

266. Thaler M, Pastakia B, Shawker TH, O'Leary T, Pizzo PA. Hepatic candidiasis in cancer patients: the evolving picture of the syndrome. Ann Intern Med 1988; 108:88–100.

267. Sallah S, Semelka RC, Wehbie R, Sallah W, Nguyen NP, Vos P. Hepatosplenic candidiasis in patients with acute leukaemia. Br J Haematol 1999; 106:697–701.

268. Sallah S. Hepatosplenic candidiasis in patients with acute leukemia: increasingly encountered complication. Anticancer Res 1999; 19:757–760.

269. Woolley I, Curtis D, Szer J, Fairley C, Vujovic O, Ugoni A, et al. High dose cytosine arabinoside is a major risk factor for the development of hepatosplenic candidiasis in patients with leukemia. Leuk Lymphoma 1997; 27:469–474.

270. von Eiff M, Essink M, Roos N, Hiddemann W, Buchner T, van de LJ. Hepatosplenic candidiasis, a late manifestation of *Candida septicaemia* in neutropenic patients with haematologic malignancies. Blut 1990; 60:242–248.

271. Semelka RC, Shoenut JP, Greenberg HM, Bow EJ. Detection of acute and treated lesions of hepatosplenic candidiasis: comparison of dynamic contrast-enhanced CT and MR imaging. J Magn Reson Imaging 1992; 2:341–345.

5
Epidemiology of Fungal Infection in Patients with Human Immunodeficiency Virus

Anucha Apisarnthanarak and William G. Powderly
Division of Infectious Diseases, Washington University School of Medicine, St. Louis, Missouri, U.S.A.

I. INTRODUCTION

With the advent of highly active antiretroviral therapy (HAART), the incidence of HIV-associated opportunistic infections (OIs) has decreased substantially (Fig. 1). This trend has continued and has been reported from other countries where HAART therapy is available (1,2). Mortality associated with the acquired immunodeficiency syndrome (AIDS) has dropped precipitously and OI morbidity has declined to a rate of ~20% of that seen before the introduction of HAART (1,3–8). The decline is attributable to the efficacy of HAART, use of prophylaxis for OIs, and better all-around care of the HIV-infected individual.

Likewise, the incidence of opportunistic fungal infections is approximately 20–25% of that seen in the mid-1990s. *Pneumocystis jiroveci* pneumonia (PCP), candidal esophagitis, and cryptococcosis remain the most common opportunistic fungal infections, although fungal infections associated with advanced AIDS, such as azole-resistant candidiasis and aspergillus, are rarely seen (1,7). These findings suggest that the spectrum of disease and the relative frequencies of opportunistic fungal infections have not changed appreciably since the early years of the HIV epidemic. Despite the decline of OI incidence, opportunistic fungal infections still occur in patients who are nonadherent, who have not previously been under medical care, have never received antiretroviral therapy, or have received suboptimal therapy (1,9).

In this chapter, we review the epidemiology and risk factors for opportunistic fungal infections in HIV patients in the era of HAART. Risk factors, endemic areas, and clinical manifestations for these infections are summarized in Table 1.

II. SPECIFIC FUNGAL INFECTIONS

A. Pneumocystis jiroveci

PCP accounted for 36% of cases of the AIDS-defining OIs in the United States during 1992–1997 and continues to be a significant cause of morbidity and mortality

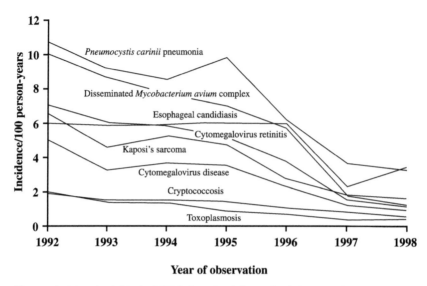

Figure 1 Trend of OIs in HIV-infected adults and adolescents from 1992 to 1998. *Source*: From Ref. 1.

despite the availability of effective prophylaxis and HAART (10). It has consistently been shown to be the most common pulmonary disease among HIV-infected patients requiring critical care (11–13). *Pneumocystis jiroveci* was previously thought to be a protozoan until 1988 when DNA analysis demonstrated it to be a fungus (14,15). Additional DNA analysis showed that *Pneumocystis* organisms in different mammals are different, and the organism that causes human PCP is now named *Pneumocystis jiroveci* (16). Although the reported incidence of PCP in the developed world has decreased significantly, the reported incidence of PCP in the developing world, especially in Africa, is increasing (17). It is not known whether the trend toward increase denotes a true increase in the prevalence of PCP, or whether the early reports from developing countries underestimated the actual prevalence. This determination is made more difficult by the lack of standardization of inclusion criteria from early studies from developing countries. On the basis of one 1997 U.S. study of patients with CD4 counts of $<100\,cells/mm^3$, the incidence of PCP at nine HIV clinic in eight cities is estimated to be 3.7 cases per 100 patient-years (3). Other epidemiological studies indicate the incidence rate to be 46 cases per 1000 patient-years according to Centers for Disease Control and Prevention surveillance in 1996 (4) and 0.22 episodes per 100 patient-years according to a 1995–1997 Swiss Study (18).

Considerable evidence supports the concept that the CD4 cell count is an accurate indicator of susceptibility to PCP even in patients who have received HAART or interleukin-2 (IL-2) (19–22). However, the nadir of the CD4 cell count prior to the institution of HAART or IL-2 does not influence the predictive value of counts substantially (22). The HIV viral load is also an independent predictor of AIDS-defining events (23,24), but it is still unclear as to how this factor is to be used as an indicator for initiating PCP prophylaxis. Clinical markers, including the wasting syndrome, the occurrence of a previous episode of pneumonia of any type, and the occurrence of previous AIDS-defining events are also independent risk factors for PCP (25). It is estimated that 15% of patients presenting with PCP have CD4 cell counts higher than $200\,cells/mm^3$, and a substantial fraction of these patients have had episodes

Table 1 Areas of Endemicity, Risk Factors, and Clinical Manifestations of Fungal Infections in Patients with AIDS

Mycosis	Areas of endemicity	Risk factors	Clinical manifestations
Pneumocystis jiroveci	Ubiquitous	CD4 < 200 cells/mm^3, clinical markers,[a] the occurrence of previous pneumonia, and AIDS-defining illnesses	Pulmonary disease,[c] dissemination
Cryptococcosis	Ubiquitous	CD4 < 100 cell/mm^3, black race, injection durg use, cigarette smoking	Meningitis, pulmonary disease,[c] skin lesions, endophthalmitis dissemination
Candidiasis	Ubiquitous	Immunosuppression, high level of HIV-1 RNA, previous colonization with *Candida* spp.	Oral thrush, esophagitis
Histoplasmosis	North American river valleys, Europe, Africa, Southeast Asia, Caribbean, Central and South Americas	Age, underlying immunosuppression	Pulmonary diseases,[c] CNS disease,[d] skin lesions, dissemination
Coccidioidomycosis	Argentina, Central America, Southwestern United States, northwestern Mexico	CD4 < 250 cells/mm^3, clinical diagnosis of AIDS	Pulmonary diseases,[c] meningitis, skin lesions, dissemination
Penicilliosis	Southern China, Hong Kong, Thailand, Vietnam	Exposure to environmental reservoirs[b]	Pulmonary diseases,[c] skin diseases, dissemination
Blastomycosis	North American river valleys, Quebec, Ontario, Manitoba	Advanced AIDS	Pulmonary diseases,[c] CNS diseases,[e] dissemination
Aspergillosis	Ubiquitous	Advanced AIDS, neutropenia, malignancy, CVC	Pulmonary diseases,[c] sinusitis, otomastoiditis, renal aspergilloma

[a]Including wasting syndrome, the occurrence of a previous episode of pneumonia of any type, the occurrence of previous AIDS-defining events.
[b]Occupational or other exposure to soil in northern Thailand.
[c]Focal and diffuse.
[d]Encephalopathy, meningitis, focal brain lesions.
[e]Meningitis, cerebral abscess.
Abbreviation: CVC, central venous catheter.
Source: Adapted from Ref. 88.

of unexplained fever or oropharyngeal candidiasis (OPC) (25,26). Therefore, it is reasonable to use these clinical indicators to initiate PCP prophylaxis before the CD4 cell count falls $<200\,\text{cells/mm}^3$. Despite the efficacy of HAART and prophylaxis regimens, patients continue to develop PCP. Risk factors for PCP in patients who received chemoprophylaxis include the use of agents other than trimethoprim–sulfamethoxazole (TMP–SMX), history of prior PCP, and a CD4 cell count of $<50\,\text{cells/mm}^3$ (27).

B. Cryptococcosis

Almost all cryptococcal infections in AIDS patients are caused by *Cryptococcus neoformans* var. *neoformans* (serotype A and D) (7,28,29). Advanced-stage AIDS patients who develop this infection usually have widely disseminated diseases with fungemia (30,31). Cryptococcal meningitis is the most frequent manifestation and is the most common life-threatening yeast infection, occurring in 5–10% of patients with AIDS in developed countries prior to the introduction of HAART (30,31). The incidence of cryptococcal meningitis in AIDS is much higher in developing countries, especially in sub-Saharan Africa, where its incidence is approaching 30% (29–31). Geographic distribution variation has not been established for cryptococcosis (32,33). The male/female ratio among AIDS patients is essentially 1:1 (32). Crypto-coccosis in children with ADDS is less common, with a prevalence of ~1.4% (34). The incidence of invasive cryptococcosis has declined in HIV-infected patients during the years since 1990 (32). However, this infection remains a significant problem in patients with limited access to health care (35). The annual incidence of invasive cryptococcosis was 1700–6600 per 100,000 persons in patients with AIDS in New York City in 1991, two per 1000 persons in the Houston area in 1994, and seven per 1000 persons in the Atlanta area in 2000 (35,36).

The only factor clearly identified to alter the risk of cryptococcal meningitis, besides low CD4 count, is fluconazole use (37). Fluconazole has been shown to be an effective means of primary prophylaxis for cryptococal infections in several studies (38–43). However, because prophylaxis has not been linked with survival benefit, the United States Public Health Service (USPHS) and Infectious Diseases Society of America (IDSA) do not endorse the routine use of primary antifungal prophylaxis in the prevention of cryptococcosis. Other risk factors that have been suggested for the development of cryptococcosis include black race, injection drug use, and cigarette smoking (32). With improvement in the treatment of HIV and increasing use of azole antifungal drugs, the survival rate of cryptococcosis in HIV-infected patients is now at 70–78% (44,45).

C. Candidiasis

Candida infection in HIV patients is almost exclusively mucosal; systemic invasion is considered rare and usually occurs as a late event (29). Mucocutaneous candidiasis occurs in three forms: OPC, esophageal, and vulvovaginal diseases. Up to 93% of persons with advanced untreated HIV develop OPC, with 60% having at least one episode per year with frequent recurrences (50–60%) (46,47). Esophageal and vulvo-vaginal diseases occur in 10–20% of patients and 30–60% of women, respectively. Rarely, invasive disease can manifest as candidemia, especially related to use of central venous catheters in patients with advanced ADDS. Candidemia has been described as a nosocomially acquired infection in patients with late-stage AIDS, with an attributable mortality rate of 31% (48). There have been few studies, mostly restricted to case series or anecdotal reports, describing the incidence and prevalence of non-esophageal invasive candidiasis in HIV-infected patients, but its incidence is probably <1% (48,49).

The widespread use of antifungal azole agents and HAART has resulted in a significant decline in the incidence of mucocutaneous candidiasis (50,51). Several factors are important in the development of mucocutaneous candidiasis including immunosuppression, high level of HIV-1 RNA, and colonization with *Candida* (46). It is notable that the relationship between the level of immunosuppression and vaginal candidiasis may not be strong. In one cross-sectional study of 833 HIV-infected and 427 HIV-uninfected women, the annual incidence of vaginal candidiasis was similar in the two groups (9%) (52).

The most common cause of mucosal candidiasis is *Candida albicans* accounting for at least 80% of clinical infections, whereas the proportion of non-C. *albicans* species has increased over time up to 20% before the advent of HAART (2,53). The most notable predisposing factor for non-C. *albicans* species is prior exposure to azole antifungals (2,53). In a multicenter prospective study of 832 persons with advanced HIV infection, fluconazole-resistant mucosal candidiasis (FRMC) occurred in 4.3% with an incidence of 4.2 per 100 patient-years follow-up (53). Prior use of TMP–SMX, prolonged high-dose fluconazole, or prior candidiasis was significantly associated with the development of FRMC. In the HAART era, studies have suggested that azole-resistant *Candida* species has been reduced to <10% (50,54,55). It is possible to hypothesize that the significant decrease in the use of azoles has caused a reduction in the selection pressure of antifungals that has contributed to the decreased percentage of resistant strains. It is estimated that at least 80% of patients with uncomplicated mucocutaneous candidiasis respond to standard treatment (topical or systemic therapy) (2). Severe recurrent infections, however, especially with azole resistance, may require short courses of amphotericin B. Candidiasis becomes more difficult to be treated with progressive loss of CD4 cells. Therefore, HAART has emerged as the most effective mode of therapy for OIs including candidiasis.

D. Histoplasmosis

Histoplasma capsulatum is a dimorphic fungus that generally causes mild and self-limited infection in immunocompetent patients, but prolonged and severe disease in immunocompromised hosts, especially those with AIDS. The mycelial form of *H. capsulatum* is found in the soil and is particularly associated with bird roosts and caves (29). Histoplasmosis is an important OI among HIV patients, which occurs in 2–5% of patients with AIDS from endemic areas and up to 25% from selected cities in the United States (Kansas City, Indianapolis, Nashville, and Memphis) (56–58). The endemic areas of histoplasma are shown in Table 1. Most cases in the endemic area are caused by exogenous exposure but less commonly resulted from reactivation of an old infection (56). Histoplasmosis occurs in <1% of patients from nonendemic areas, where reactivation of latent infection is implicated as a cause of infection (59).

Approximately 90% of cases of disseminated histoplasmosis have occurred in patients with CD4 counts <200 cells/mm^3 (median CD4 cell count <30 cells/mm^3), but localized pulmonary disease may be seen in those with high CD4 cell counts, typically >300 cells/mm^3 (56,60,61). Disseminated disease was identified at autopsy in 8% of patients with AIDS from Brazil and 44% from Venezuela whereas cutaneous involvement was more common in South America (56,62). 5 to 10% of patients with disseminated histoplasmosis have an acute septic-shock-like syndrome that includes hypotension and evidence of disseminated coagulopathy; this presentation carries a poor prognosis (29). Histoplasmosis also has been reported in Europe, Africa, and Southeast Asia (56). Infection with *H. capsulatum* var. *duboisii* has been reported in patients with AIDS in Africa (63,64).

Most knowledge about the epidemiology of histoplasmosis has been derived from outbreak investigations. As exemplified by the large outbreak in AIDS patients in Indiana between 1988 and 1993 (57), these patients serve as a sentinel markers for histoplasmosis in these areas. A review of histoplasmosis in AIDS patients in Indiana reported it to be the only OI in 22% and the first OI in 7% (57). Histoplasmosis is often the first and/or the only OI in AIDS patients. In Houston in the 1980s, it was the first OI in 75% of patients with AIDS (57). After the introduction of HAART, the incidence of histoplasmosis has declined in recent years (65). Risk factors for histoplasmosis included age and underlying immunosuppressions, especially with AIDS (66). Sex and race were not found to be associated with increased risk of disease among HIV-infected patients (66). In general, immunocompromised persons with histoplasmosis have a higher mortality rate than those who are not immunocompromised (66). In one study, the mortality rate for immunocompromised patients was 33% compared to 17% of nonimmunocompromised persons (67). If left untreated, disseminated histoplasmosis in AIDS is progressively fatal. Two multicenter studies suggested the effectiveness of itraconazole, as primary and secondary prophylaxis, in preventing histoplasmosis in patients with HIV/AIDS (61,68). This data support the use of itraconazole prophylaxis for histoplasmosis in the endemic area.

E.   Coccidioidomycosis

Coccidioides immitis was included in the surveillance case definition for AIDS in 1987 (69). It is a thermal dimorphic fungus found only in the Western hemisphere in area that marked by low annual rainfall, sandy saline soil, and periodic dust storms. The areas of highest endemicity are southern San Joaquin Valley in California and the regions encompassing Phoenix and Tucson in southern Arizona (70–73). Other areas of endemicity are shown in Table 1 .

The association between HIV disease and coccidioidomycosis is not entirely clear (74). The first case series of coccidioidomycosis occurring in HIV-infected persons suggested that seven out of 27 patients with AIDS living in southern Arizona developed symptomatic infecton with *C. immitis* (75). Six out of seven patients had diffuse nodular pulmonary infiltrates, and five had detectable anticoccidioidal antibodies in their sera; all died within 14 months of the diagnosis of coccidioidomycosis. The impact of coccidioidomycosis on patients infected with HIV is not geographically uniform, but it predominantly affects HIV-infected persons living in Arizona. In Arizona, 8.2% of all AIDS patients reporting to CDC had concomitant coccidioidomycosis compared to only 0.3% nationwide (74). The impact of HIV infection on the development of active coccidioidomycosis appears to be significantly greater in the coccidioidal endemic area within the state. Data from the California State Health Department suggested that 3.5% of patients living in Kern County (coccidioidal endemic area) were reported to have coccidioidomycosis as their AIDS-defining diagnosis compared to only 0.3% for the entire state (76). One prospective study in Arizona suggested that

13 out of 170 HIV-infected persons developed coccidioidomycosis after 41 months follow-up, yielding an estimated cumulative incidence of nearly 25% (77).

Two factors associated with the development of active coccidioidomycosis were CD4 counts <250 cells/mm^3 and the clinical diagnosis of AIDS. Length of stay in the endemic area, history of prior diagnosis of coccidioidomycosis, and a positive coccidioidal skin test were not risk factors for active disease. These data suggest that most clinical disease is due to primary infection, as opposed to reactivation of latent infection for cases outside the endemic area (70). Similar to other OIs, the incidence of coccidioidomycosis among HIV-infected persons has declined in the era of HAART (1). Retrospective study of cases of coccidioidomycosis among HIV-infected patients in the era of HAART in Arizona suggested that the number of cases of active coccidioidomycosis declined from 77 in 1995 to 61 in 1996 and 15 in 1997 (71,73,76).

F. Penicilliosis

A dimorphic fungus, *Penicillium marneffei*, has been recognized as a significant pathogen in Southeast Asia, Hong Kong, and southern China among patients in advanced stages of AIDS (78–80). In northern Thailand, this fungal infection is the third most common OI, accounting for 15–20% of all AIDS-related illnesses, a frequency rivaling tuberculosis and cryptococcal meningoencephalitis (81). Because disseminated penicilliosis is usually diagnosed in patients with CD4 cell count <100 cells/mm^3, and since it is often shortly followed by the diagnosis of more common OIs, several authors have suggested that disseminated penicilliosis should be included in the diagnostic criteria for AIDS (79–82). Infection with this organism is regarded as an AIDS-defining illness. With the further spread of HIV in Asia, disseminated *P. marneffei* infection is likely to increase in importance.

Penicillium marneffei was first isolated from Vietnamese bamboo rats in 1956, and subsequent animal and human cases have been reported from southern China, Hong Kong, Thailand, and Vietnam (83–87). In such cases, patients have either lived in or traveled to these endemic areas (88). A case–control study of risk factors of *P. marneffei* infection in HIV patients in northern Thailand suggests that a recent history of occupational or other exposure to soil in the rainy season is a significant risk factor (87). Although *P. marneffei* has been identified in bamboo, bamboo rats, their feces, and from soil obtained from their burrows, the actual reservoir and portal of entry have not been determined (88). Patients infected with *P. marneffei* have a poor prognosis without treatment (80). The mortality rate from disseminated *P. marneffei* infection is about 20% with a relapse rate of 50% after discontinuation of successful initial therapy (82,89). Two randomized controlled trials in northern Thailand suggested that itraconazole was safe, effective, and well tolerated as primary and secondary prophylaxis in penicilliosis and cryptococcosis in patients with advanced AIDS (82,90).

G. Blastomycosis

Blastomycosis is caused by the dimorphic fungus *Blastomyces dermatitidis*. It has been found in humid areas from soil with high organic content, high animal-waste component, and acid pH (91). Inhalation of conidia is the route of infection. The areas of endemicity are areas bordering the Mississippi, Missouri, and Ohio rivers and extending northward to Quebec, Ontario and Manitoba. Blastomycosis has been rarely reported in patients with AIDS and appears to occur in the later stages of HIV infections, generally with CD4 cell count <200 cells/mm^3 (29,88,92,93). In immunocompromised hosts, blastomycosis is associated with pulmonary fibrosis, pulmonary nodules, or skin infection; however, in patients with AIDS, widely disseminated infection usually occurs (94). Blastomycosis in AIDS is strongly associated with central nervous system involvement (~46%), with mortality rate of 90% (93,94).

H. Mycoses Caused by Molds

The clinical manifestations of selected mold infections in patients with AIDS are summarized in Table 2. Infection caused by molds is the least commonly encountered mycosis in AIDS (95,96). The incidence of mold infection has also decreased since the introduction of HAART (94). Although uncommon, infections caused by molds are important causes of invasive mycoses in patients with AIDS. Early recognition of these infections allows prompt diagnosis and early institution of antifungal therapy and possible surgical intervention. Their clinical manifestations can range from localized soft-tissue infections or sinusitis to widely disseminated disease. Most often, patients with mold infections have advanced AIDS with CD4 counts <200 cells/mm^3, causing widely disseminated infection (94). Other risk factors include neutropenia, use of corticosteroids, cytomegalovirus (CMV) infection, and chemotherapy (88,94). Because relapse is frequent, long-term suppressive therapy is often required. The most common routes of infection are through inhalation of conidia for dimorphic fungi, *Aspergillus* species, and various *Zygomyces*, intravenous injection of conidia via infection drug use for *Zygomyces* and *Aspergillus* species, and percutaneous inoculation for *Sporothrix schenckii* (94).

Table 2 Clinical Manifestations of Selected Mold Infections in Patients with AIDS

Organism	Clincal manifestation
Agents of hyalohyphomycosis	
Aspergillus spp.	Pulmonary, sinustits, cutaneous, focal abscess, disseminated
Pseudallescheria spp.	Pneumonia, sinustitis, endocarditis, disseminated disease, meningitis
Fusarium spp.	Fungemia, endocarditis, disseminated infection
Chrysophorium spp.	Osteomyelitis
Trichosporon spp.	Catheter-related fungemia
Geotrichum spp.	Esophageal ulcer
Pennicillium decumbens	Disseminated infection
Agents of Phaeohyphomycosis	
Alternaria spp.	Nasal soft-tissue infection, sinusitis
Exophilia spp.	Esophagitis, soft-tissue infection
Hormonema spp.	Liver abscess
Cladophialophora spp.	Brain abscess, pulmonary
Phialophora spp.	Disseminated infection
Bipolaris spp.	Endophthalmitis
Scedosporim prolificans	Disseminated infection
Agents of Zygomycosis	
Rhizopus arrhizus	Orbit, soft tissue, sinusitis
Absidia corymbifera	Renal abscesses, pharyngeal, pulmonary
Cunninghamella bertholletiae	Soft-tissue abscess
Mucor spp.	Sinusitis

Source: Adapted with permissionn from Ref. 94.

I. Dimorphic Mycoses

The dimorphic mycoses are caused by endemic mycoses, histoplasmosis, coccidioido-mycosis, paracoccidioidomycosis, blastomycosis, penicilliosis, and sporotrichosis. With the exception of sporotrichosis and paracoccidioidomyces, the epidemiology of other dimorphic fungi has been discussed in previous sections. *Sporothrix schenckii* does not occur in a specific geographic zone but occurs in the specific setting of exposure to contaminated rosebush thorns or moss (94). Disseminated *S. schenckii* had been reported in AIDS patients acquired from percutaneous inoculation (97). Paracoccidioidomyces is endemic in South America, but infection in patients with AIDS is rare (98). In contrast to immunocompetent subjects, rapid progressive paracoccidioidomyces with dissemination are usually seen in patients with AIDS and resemble disseminated histoplasmosis (94). If left untreated, these mycoses are commonly progressive and fatal.

J. Agents of Hyalohyphomycosis (*Aspergillus, Fusarium, Pseudallescheria, Chrysosporium*)

Hyalohyphomycoses is a group of lightly pigmented (hyaline) molds. These organisms have been reported occasionally in patients with advanced AIDS and uncontrolled HIV replication (99). Since the advent of HAART, these organisms have become rare in HIV patients but have become ever more common in patients with leukemia/lymphoma (100). These organisms appear similar, morphologically, to each other and require culture to confirm the specific agent (94). Risk factors for these infections include advanced AIDS with CD4 cell counts $<50\,\text{cells}/\text{mm}^3$ and other alterations in host defenses, such as neutropenia, malignancy, indwelling catheters, and comorbid conditions such as diabetes mellitus (88).

Invasive aspergillosis is not currently defined as an OI associated with AIDS. Although the incidence of these infections was increasing for some years, they have once again become uncommon. Clinical presentations may vary from sinusitis to widely disseminated infection (94,100). The course of disease may be indolent or fulminant (94). *Apsergillus* spp. colonization has been reported in ~5% of AIDS patients with the rate of proven invasive disease being <1% (101). *Aspergillus fumigatus* and *A. flavus* are the most commonly isolated species in patients with or without AIDS (88). *Aspergillus* species can be detected in soil, water, and decaying vegetation, and has been cultured from the air, dust, and environmental surfaces in hospitals (88). Outbreaks involving HIV-infected patients have not been described. Other agents of hyalohyphomycosis that have been reported to cause invasive mycoses in patients with AIDS include *Fusarium* spp., *Pseudallescheria boydii*, *Chrysosporium* species, *Geotrichum, Trichosporon beigelii*, and *Penicillium* spp. (Table 2).

K. Agents of Phaeohyphomycosis (*Cladophialophora, Alternaeria, Exophiala*)

Phaeohyphomycoses comprise a group of opportunistic molds that are dematiaceous or darkly pigmented. Although rarely occurring, these emerging pathogens cause disease in both HIV and non-HIV persons. These fungi may occur at any stage of AIDS, but a more rapid course is commonly seen with late-stage AIDS (94). Neutropenia and diabetes are risk factors for infection, whereas gardening with traumatic inoculation is a major mode of infection.

L. Zygomyces *(Rhizopus* Species, *Absidia, Mucor, Rhizomucor, Cunninghamella)*

These organisms have been reported uncommonly in patients with AIDS but may cause localized deep tissue abscesses in various organs including the kidney, liver, spleen, and stomach (102). Disseminated infection may occur and carry a poor outcome (mortality ~80%), but some of these infections progress slowly in patients with AIDS and respond well to surgery and standard antifungal therapy (103–105). Risk factors for infection include injection drug use, neutropenia, corticosteroid use, and diabetes mellitus. Contamination of injected drugs is presumed to be the most common route of infection, though inhalation of conidia is also possible (94).

III. SPECIAL CONSIDERATIONS IN HIV-INFECTED PATIENTS

A. Impact of HAART on the Clinical Presentation and Prophylaxis of OIs

Successful therapy with HAART leads to a rise in CD4 cell counts, suppression of viral replication to below detectable limits, and restoration of immune function (106–108). The increase in CD4 cell counts often occurs in two phases. The first phase (usually 2–3 months after the initiation of antiretroviral therapy) is associated with a rapid increase in CD4+ and CD8+ T cells, mainly of the memory phenotype. This phase appears to represent redistribution and expansion of pre-existing cells and may not represent true immune recovery. The second phase (starting 2–3 months after therapy) involves a more gradual rise in CD4+ T cells, mainly naïve T cells, and probably represents gradual recovery of the immune system. This may be maintained for several years and is usually adequate to protect individuals against OIs. Immune restoration not only results in significant improvement in morbidity and survival (1,3), but also results in the change in approach to prophylaxis of opportunistic mycoses.

B. Immune Reconstitution Illness

Immune reconstitution is thought to represent an inflammatory state induced by the newly restored immune system against pathogens that have previously infected the HIV-positive host. It usually occurs within the first 3 months after starting antiretroviral therapy and has been well described with *Mycobacterium avium* complex (MAC) infection, tuberculosis, CMV retinitis, Hepatitis C and Hepatitis B virus infections, fungal infections (cryptococcosis, histoplasmosis, and PCP), varicella zoster, progressive multifocal leukoencephalopathy (PML), and even malignant and noninfectious disorders (109–118). This syndrome presents with typical clinical features such as local MAC lymphadenitis without bacteremia, vitreal and extraocular disease with CMV, and PML with contrast enhancement on MRI. Fatalities have been reported in some of these cases (109–118). Along the same line, opportunistic fungal infections can be manifested with highly unusual localizations, accompanied by an intriguing spectrum of clinical findings. Five case descriptions have been reported in reference to immune reconstitution exacerbating or unveiling cryptococcal disease in 12 patients (112–114,117,118). The clinical presentations occurred from as early as 8 days to as late as 15 months after starting HAART. Remarkably, four of these patients had lymphadenitis as the primary mode of presentation (cervical

Table 3 Clinical Presentation of Specific OIs in HIV Associated with Immune Reconstitution Illness

Opportunistic infection	Clinical presentation associated with immune reconstitution illness
Mycobacterium avium complex	Focal lymphadenitis; bacteremia rare
CMV infection	Vitritis, retinitis, extraocular disease
Cryptococcosis	Pulmonary nodule, cavitary pneumonia, aseptic meningitis with elevated intracranial pressure, CSF leukocytosis, focal and necrotizing lymphadenitis, intrathoracic lymphadenopathy with hypercalcemia, supraclavicular abscess
Pneumocystis jiroveci	Granulomatous pneumonia
PML	Neurologic deficits, hypodensities with peripheral enhancement finding from magnetic resonance image
Varicella zoster	Mild, uncomplicated presentation
Hepatitis C virus (HCV) infection	Ovet hepatitis, cirrhosis, HCV-associated disorders (e.g., cryoglobulinemia)

and mediastinal). In these four patients, the diagnosis was made by histology showing cryptococcal yeast cells, and all had positive serum cryptococcal antigen at high titers but negative cerebrospinal fluid (CSF) antigen and cultures (blood, tissue, CSF). These patients were managed diversely, with continuation of antifungals or administration of corticosteroids or NSAIDS. The common denominator in all cases was the apparent enhancement of cell-mediated immunity, which paradoxically worsened the clinical outcome in response to a heavy burden of latent infections. Few cases of this novel syndrome have been reported with PCP and histoplasmosis (115,117). Because this syndrome can present with atypical clinical features, a high index of suspicion is necessary for early diagnosis. Table 3 summarizes the clinical presentations of specific OIs associated with immune reconstitution.

C. Discontinuation of Prophylatic Medications

Evidence for restoration of clinically relevant immune function has come from data on successful discontinuation of primary and secondary prophylaxis for most major IOs, when the CD4 cell count rises above a certain threshold. This has been well demonstrated for PCP, CMV retinitis, and candidiasis (119–128). There are also sufficient cohort studies to recommend appropriate prophylaxis discontinuation for toxoplasmosis, MAC, and cryptococcal meningitis (129–136). Indeed, it is probably true for all opportunistic pathogens, where the immune system is known to be capable of controlling infection. The exception is *C. immitis* infection, where cure is very difficult even in the normal host. Therefore, it is possible that specific antimicrobial prophylaxis can be stopped if viral suppression occurs and the CD4 cell counts rises above the threshold levels. Currently, the USPHS and IDSA recommend discontinuing primary prophylaxis for PCP, MAC, and toxoplasmosis in patients with sustained increases (≥ 3 months) in CD4 cell counts above thresholds (137). Secondary prophylaxis should be discontinued for PCP, MAC, toxoplasmosis, CMV retinitis, and cryptococcosis among patients with a sustained increase in CD4 cell counts (≥ 3–6 months) above the thresholds (137).

There are some reports describing breakthrough OI in patients despite a rise in CD4 cell counts (138,139). These cases are rare and represent the exception rather than the rule and suggest that immune responses to specific pathogens in some patients may not be restored satisfactorily. These cases also indicate that immune recovery may be incomplete in some patients and that close monitoring of patients is warranted. Relapse can be seen if the antiretroviral treatment fails and immuno-deficiency resumes (140). Therefore, secondary prophylaxis should be restarted if the CD4 cell count falls below threshold levels.

IV. CONCLUSION

The incidence of opportunistic mycoses has decreased significantly in developed countries as a consequence of improved treatment of HIV and prophylaxis for opportunistic mycoses. Nevertheless, HIV treatment is not optimal because of multiple factors such as adherence issues, side effects of medications, or viral resistance. Opportunistic fungal infections still occur in the developing world, where HIV treatment is still suboptimal, and in developed countries in patients who are nonadherent, who have not previously been under medical care, have never received antiretroviral therapy, or have received suboptimal therapy. Current optimism regarding the future depends on the continuing success of antiviral treatment. If treatment fails, we are likely to see the return of all OIs. Physicians who care for HIV patients in the era of HAART need to be aware of the change in clinical presentations of OIs in HIV patients and the possibility that prophylaxis medications may be discontinued in selected patients to minimize side effects and drug interactions. It appears that the future of HIV-associated mycoses is linked to the future of effective treatment of HIV itself.

REFERENCES

1.   Kaplan JE, Hanson D, Dworkin MS, Frederick T, Bertolli J, Lindegren ML, Holmberg S, Jones JL. Epidemiology of human immunodeficiency virus-associated opportunistic infections in the United States in the era of highly active antiretroviral therapy. Clin Infect Dis 2000; 30:S5–S14.
2.   Chowdhry TVH, Asaad R, Woolley I, Davis T, Davidson R, Lederman MM. The changing spectrum of HIV mortality: analysis of 249 deaths from 1995–1999. 7th Conference on Retroviruses and Opportunistic Infections, San Francisco, CA, Jan 30–Feb 2, 2000.
3.   Palella FJ, Delaney KM, Moorman AC, Loveless MO, Fuhrer J, Satten GA, Aschman DJ, Holmberg SD. Declining morbidity and mortality among patients with advanced human immunodeficiency virus infection. N Engl J Med 1998; 338:853–860.
4.   Centers for Disease Control and Prevention. Update:trends in AIDS incidence, deaths, and prevalence—United States, 1996. MMWR Morb Mortal Wkly Rep. 1997; 46:165–173.
5.   Forrest DM, Seminari E, Hogg RS, Yip B, Raboud J, Lawson R, Phillips P, Schechter MT, O'Shaughnessy MV, Montaner JS. The incidence and spectrum of AIDS-defining illnesses in persons treated with antiretroviral drugs. Clin Infect Dis 1998; 27:1379–1385.
6.   Mocroft A, Vella S, Benfield TL, Chiesi A, Miller V, Gargalianos P, d'Arminio Monforte A, Yust I, Brunn JN, Phillips AN, Lundgren JD. Changing patterns of mortality across Europe in patients infected with HIV-1. EuroSIDA Study Group. Lancet 1998; 352:1725–1730.
7.   Haddad NE, Powderly WG. The changing face of mycoses in patients with HIV/AIDS. AIDS Read 2001; 11:365–378.

8. Jain MK, Skiest DJ, Cloud JW, Jain CL, Burns D, Berggren RE. Changes in mortality related to human immunodeficiency virus infection: comparative analysis of inpatient deaths in 1995 and in 1999–2000. Clin Infect Dis 2003; 36:1030–1038.

9. Aberg JA, Koo JJ. Rate of AIDS-related opportunistic infections at San Francisco General Hospital in the era of potent antiretroviral therapy. 13th International AIDS Conference, Durban, South Africa, Jul 9–14, 2000.

10. Jones JL, Hanson DL, Dworkin MS, Alderton DL, Fleming PL, Kaplan JE, Ward S. Surveillance for AIDS-defining opportunistic illnesses, 1992–1997. MMWR CDC Surveill Summ 1999; 48:1–22.

11. Rosen MJ, Clayton K, Schneider RF, Fulkerson W, Rao AV, Stansell J, Kvale PA, Glassroth J, Reichman LB, Wallace JM, Hopewell PC. Intensive care of patients with HIV infection: utilization, critical illnesses, and outcomes; pulmonary complications of HIV Infection Study Group. Am J Respir Crit Care Med 1997; 155:67–71.

12. Nickas G, Wachter RM. Outcomes of intensive care of patients with human immunodeficiency virus infection. Arch Intern Med 2000; 28:541–547.

13. Gill JK, Greene L, Miller R, Pozniak A, Cartledge J, Fisher M, Nelson MR, Soni N. ICU admission in patients infected with the human immunodeficiency virus: a multicentre survey. Anaesthesia 1999; 54:727–732.

14. Edman JC, Kovacs JA, Masur H, Santi DV, Elwood HJ, Sogin ML. Ribosomal RNA sequence shows *Pneumocystis carinii* to be a member of the fungi. Nature 1988; 334: 519–522.

15. Stringer SL, Stringer JR, Blaser MA, Walzer PD, Cushion MT. *Pneumocystis carinii*: sequence from ribosomal RNA implies a close relationship with fungi. Exp Parasitol 1989; 68:450–461.

16. Stringer JR, Beard CB, Miller RF, Wakefield AE. A new name (*Pneumocystis jiroveci*) for pneumocystis from humans. Emerg Infect Dis 2002; 8:891–896.

17. Fisk DT, Meshnick S, Kazanjian PH. *Pneumocystis carinii* pneumonia in patients in the developing world who have acquired immunodeficiency syndrome. Clin Infect Dis 2003; 36:70–78.

18. Ledergerber B, Egger M, Erard V, Weber R, Hirschel B, Furrer H, Battegay M, Vernazza P, Bernasconi E, Opravil M, Kaufmann D, Sudre P, Francioli P, Telenti A. AIDS-related opportunistic illnesses occurring after initiation of potent antiretroviral therapy: the Swiss HIV Cohort Study. JAMA 1999; 282:2220–2226.

19. Dworkin MS, Williamson J, Jones JL, Kaplan JE. Prophylaxis with trimethoprim-sulfamethoxazole for human immunodeficiency virus-infected patients: impact on risk for infectious diseases. Clin Infect Dis 2001; 33:393–398.

20. Dworkin MS, Hanson DL, Navin TR. Survival of patients with AIDS after diagnosis of *Pneumocystis carinii* pneumonia in the United States. J Infect Dis 2001; 183:1409–1412.

21. Dworkin MS, Hanson DL, Kaplan JE, Jones JL, Ward JW. Risk for preventable opportunistic infections in persons with AIDS after antiretroviral therapy increases CD4 T lymphocyte counts above prophylaxis thresholds. J Infect Dis 2000; 182: 611–615.

22. Miller V, Mocroft A, Reiss P, Katlama C, Papadopoulos AL, Katzenstein T, van Lunzen J, Antunes F, Phillips AN, Lundgren JD. Natural history of human immunodeficiency virus type 1 viremia after seroconversion and proximal to AIDS in a large cohort of homosexual men: multicenter AIDS cohort study. Ann Intern Med 1999; 130:570–577.

23. Mellors JW, Rinaldo CR, Gupta P, White RM, Todd JA, Kingsley LA. Prognosis in HIV-1 infection predicted by the quantity of virus in plasma. Science 1996; 272: 1167–1170.

24. Lyles RH, Munoz A, Yamashita TE, Bazmi H, Detels R, Rinaldo CR, Margolick JB, Phair JP, Mellors JW. Natural history of human immunodeficiency virus type 1 viremia after seroconversion and proximal to AIDS in a large cohort of homosexual men. Multicenter AIDS Cohort Study. J Infect Dis 2000; 181:872–880.

25. Masur H. Pneumocystosis. In: Dolin R, Masur H, Sagg MS, eds. AIDS Therapy. 2d ed. Philadelphia: Churchill-Livingstone, 2003:403–418.

26. Phair J, Munoz A, Detels R, Kaslow R, Rinaldo CR, Saah A. The risk of *Pneumocystis carinii* pneumonia among men infected with HIV-1. N Engl J Med 1990; 322:161–165.

27. Moorman AC, Von Bargen JC, Palella FJ, Holmberg SD. *Pneumocystis carinii* pneumonia incidence and chemoprophylaxis failure in ambulatory HIV-infected patients. HIV Outpatient Study (HOPS) Investigators. J Acquir Immune Defic Syndr Hum Retrovirol 1998; 29:182–188.

28. Sepkowitz KA. Opportunistic infections in patients with and patients without acquired immunodeficiency syndrome. Clin Infect Dis 2002; 34:1098–1107.

29. Powderly WG. Fungal infection. In: Armstrong D, Cohen J, eds. Infectious Diseases. Vol. 2. Philadelphia: Mosby, 1999:12.1–12.6.

30. Powderly WG. Cryptococcal meningitis and AIDS. Clin Infect Dis 1993; 17:837–842.

31. Apisarnthanarak A, Powderly WG. Treatment of acute cryptococcal disease. Expert Opin Pharmacother 2001; 2:1259–1268.

32. Aberg JA, Powderly WG. Cryptococcosis. In: Dolin R, Masur H, Sagg MS, eds. AIDS Therapy. 2d ed. Philadelphia: Churchill-Livingstone, 2003:498–510.

33. Hajjeh RA, Conn LA, Stephens DS, Baughman W, Hamill R, Graviss E, Pappas PG, Thomas C, Reingold A, Rothrock G, Hutwagner LC, Schuchat A, Brandt ME, Pinner RW. Cryptococcosis: population-based multistate active surveillance and risk factors in human immunodeficiency virus-infected persons. Cryptococcal Active Surveillance Group. Clin Infect Dis 1999; 179:1412–1413.

34. Abadi J, Nachman S, Kressle AB, Pirofski L. Cryptococcosis in children with AIDS. Clin Infect Dis 1999; 28:309–313.

35. Mirza SA, Phelan M, Rimland D, Graviss E, Hamill R, Brandt ME, Gardner T, Sattah M, de Leon GP, Baughman W, Hejjeh RA. The changing epidemiology of cryptococcosis: an update from population-based active surveillance in 2 large metropolitan areas, 1992–2000. Clin Infect Dis 2003; 36:789–794.

36. Currie BP, Casadevall A. Estimation of the prevalence of cryptococcal infection among patients infected with human immunodeficiency virus in New York City. Clin Infect Dis 1994; 19:1029–1033.

37. Oursler KA, Moore RD, Chaisson RE. Risk factors for cryptococcal meningitis in HIV-infected patients. AIDS Res Hum Retroviruses 1999; 15:625–631.

38. Powderly WG, Finkelstein D, Feinberg J, Frame P, He W, van der Horst, Koletar SL, Eyster ME, Carey J, Waskin H, et al. A randomized trial comparing fluconazole with clotimazole troches for the prevention of fungal infections in patients with advanced human immunodeficiency virus infection. NIAID AIDS Clinical Trial Group. N Engl J Med 1995; 332:700–705.

39. Singh N, Barnish MJ, Berman S, Bender B, Wagener MM, Rinaldi MG, Yu VL. Low-dose fluconazole as primary prophylaxis for cryptococcal infection in AIDS patients with CD4 cell counts of $\leq 100/mm^3$: demonstration of efficacy in a positive, multicenter trial. Clin Infect Dis 1996; 23:1282–1286.

40. Quagliarello VJ, Viscoli C, Horwitz RI. Primary prevention of cryptococcal meningitis by fluconazole in HIV-infected patients. Lancet 1992; 345:548–552.

41. Ammassari A, Linzalone A, Murri R, Marasca G, Morace G, Antinori A. Fluconazole for primary prophylaxis for AIDS-associated cryptococcosis: a case–control study. Scan J Infect Dis 1995; 27:235–237.

42. Nightingale SD, Cal SX, Peterson DM, Loss SD, Gamble BA, Watson DA, Manzone CP, Baker JE, Jockusch JD. Primary prophylaxis with fluconazole against systemic fungal infections in HIV-positive patients. AIDS 1992; 6:191–194.

43. Graybill JR, Sobel JD, Saag MS, van der Horst C, Powderly WG, Cloud GA, Riser L, Hamill R, Dismukes W. Diagnosis and management of increased intracranial pressure in patients with AIDS and cryptococcal meningitis. The NIAID Mycoses Study Group and AIDS Cooperative Treatment Groups. Clin Infect Dis 2000; 30:47–54.

44. White M, Cirrincione C, Blevins A, Armstrong D. Cryptococcal meningitis: outcome in patients with AIDS and patients with neoplastic disease. J Infect Dis 1992; 165:960–963.

45. van der Horst CM, Saag MS, Cloud GA, Hamill RJ, Graybill JR, Sobel JD, Johnson PC, Tauzon CU, Kerkering T, Moskovitz BL, Powderly WG, Dismukes WE. Treatment of cryptococcal meningitis associated with the acquired immunodeficiency syndrome. National Institute of Allergy and Infectious Diseases Mycoses Study Group and AIDS Clinical Trials Group. N Engl J Med 1997; 337:15–21.

46. Fichtenbaum CJ. Candidiasis. In: Dolin R, Masur H, Saag MS, eds. AIDS Therapy. 2d ed. Philadelphia: Churchill-Livingstone, 2003:531–542.

47. Odds FC. Candida and Candidosis. London: Bailliere Tindall, 1988.

48. Launay O, Lortholary O, Bouges-Michel C, Jarrousse B, Bentata M, Guillevin L. Candidemia: a nosocomial complication in adults with late-stage AIDS. Clin Infect Dis 1998; 26:1134–1141.

49. Tumbarello M, Tacconelli E, de Gaetano Donati K, Morace G, Fadda G, Cuada R. Candidemia in HIV-infected subjects. Eur J Clin Microbiol Infect Dis 1999; 18:478–483.

50. Martins MD, Lozano-Chiu M, Rex JH. Point prevalence of carriage of fluconazole-resistant *Candida* in the oropharynx of HIV-infected patients. Clin Infect Dis 1997; 25:843–846.

51. Cauda R, Tacconelli E, Tumbarello M, Morace G, De Bernardis F, Torosantucci A, Cassone A. Role of protease inhibitors in preventing recurrent oral candidosis in patients with HIV infection: a prospective case–control study. J Acquir Immune Defic Syndr 1999; 21:20–25.

52. White MH. Is vulvovaginal candidiasis an AIDS-related illness? Clin Infect Dis 1996; 22:S124–S127.

53. Darouiche RO. Oropharyngeal and esophageal candidiasis in immunocompromised patients: treatment issues. Clin Infect Dis 1998; 26:259–272.

54. Fichtenbaum CJ, Koletar SL, Yiannoutsos C, Holland F, Pottage J, Cohn SE, Walawander A, Frame P, Feinberg J, Saag M, Van der Horst C, Powderly WG. Refractory mucosal candidiasis in advanced human immunodeficiency virus infection. Clin Infect Dis 2000; 30:749–756.

55. Tacconelli E, Bertagnolio S, Posteraro B, Tumbarello M, Boccia S, Fidda G, Cauda R. Azole susceptibility patterns and genetic relationship among oral Candida strains isolated in the era of highly active antiretroviral therapy. J Acquir Immune Defic Syndr 2002; 31:38–44.

56. Wheat J. Histoplasmosis. In: Dolin R, Masur H, Saag MS, eds. AIDS Therapy. 2nd ed. Philadelphia: Churchill-Livingstone, 2003; 33:511–521.

57. Wheat LJ, Connolly-Stringfield PA, Baker RL, Curfman MF, Eads ME, Israel KS, Norris SA, Webb DH, Zeckel ML. Disseminated histoplasmosis in the acquired immune deficiency syndrome: clinical findings, diagnosis and treatment, and review of the literature. Medicine (Baltimore) 1990; 69:361–374.

58. Marshall BC, Cox JK Jr, Carroll KC, Morrison RE. Case report: histoplasmosis as a cause of pleural effusion in the acquired immunodeficiency syndrome. Am J Med Sci 1990; 300:98–101.

59. Keath EJ, Kobayashi GS, Medoff G. Typing of *Histoplasma capsulatum* by restriction fragment length polymorphisms in a nuclear gene. J Clin Microbiol 1992; 30:2104–2107.

60. Wheat J, Hafner R, Wuifsohn M, Spencer P, Squires K, Powderly WG, Wong B, Rinaldi M, Saag M, Hamill R. Prevention of relapse of histoplasmosis with itraconazole in patients with acquired immunodeficiency syndrome. The National Institute of Allergy and Infectious Diseases Clinical Trials and Mycoses Study Group Collaborators. Ann Intern Med 1993; 118:610–616.

61. Wheat J, Hafner R, Korzun AH, Limjoco MT, Spencer P, Larsen RA, Hecht FM, Powderly WG. Itraconazole treatment of disseminated histoplasmosis in patients with the acquired immunodeficiency syndrome. AIDS Clinical Trial Group. Am J Med 1995; 98:336–342.

62. Murillo J, Castro KG. HIV infection and AIDS in Latin America. Epidemiologic features and clinical manifestations. Infect Dis Clin North Am 1994; 8:1–11.

63. Arendt V, Coremans-Pelseneer J, Gottlob R, Brit T, Bujan-Boza W, Fondu P. African histoplasmosis in a Belgian AIDS patients. Mycoses 1991; 34:59–61.

64. Carme B, Ngaporo AI, Ngolet A, Ibara JR, Ebikili B. Disseminated African histoplasmosis in a Congolese patient with AIDS. J Med Vet Mycol 1992; 30:245–248.

65. Jones JL, Hanson DL, Dworkin MS, Kaplan JE, Ward JW. Trends in AIDS-related opportunistic infections among men who have sex with men and among injecting drug users, 1991–1996. J Infect Dis 1998; 178:114–120.

66. Cano MV, Hajjeh RA. The epidemiology of histoplasmosis: a review. Semin Respir Infect 2001; 16:109–118.

67. Sathapatayavongs B, Batteiger BE, Wheat J, Salma TG, Wass JL. Clinical and laboratory features of disseminated histoplasmosis during two large urban outbreaks. Medicine (Baltimore) 1983; 62:263–270.

68. McKinsey DS, Wheat LJ, Cloud GA, Pierce M, Black JR, Bamberger DM, Goldman M, Thomas CJ, Gutsch HM, Moskovitz B, Dismukes WE, Kauffman CA. Itraconazole prophylaxis for fungal infections in patients with advanced human immunodeficiency virus infection: randomized, placebo-controlled, double-blind study. National Institute of Allergy and Infectious Diseases Mycoses Study Group. Clin Infect Dis 1999; 28:1049–1056.

69. Revision of the CDC surveillance case definition for acquired immunodeficiency syndrome. MMWR Morb Mortal Wkly Rep 1987;36(suppl 1):S1–S15.

70. Ampel NM. Coccidioidomycosis. In: Dolin R, Masur H, Saag M, eds. AIDS Therapy. 2d ed. Philadelphia: Churchill-Livingstone, 2003:522–530.

71. Pappagianis D. Epidemiology of coccidioidomycosis. In: McGinnis M, ed. Current Topics in Medical Mycology. New York: Springer-Verlag, 1988:199–238.

72. Galgiani JN. Coccidioidomycosis. West J Med 2003; 159:153–171.

73. Coccidioidomycosis—Arizona, 1990–1995. MMWR Morb Mortal Wkly Rep. 1996; 13:1069–1073.

74. Jones JL, Fleming PL, Ciesielski CA, Hu DJ, Kaplan JE, Ward JW. Coccidioidomycosis among persons with AIDS in the United States. J Infect Dis 1995; 171:961–966.

75. Bronnimann DA, Adam RD, Galgiani JN, Habib MP, Petersen EA, Porter B, Bloom JW. Coccidioidomycosis in the acquired immunodeficiency syndrome. Arm Intern Med 1987; 106:372–379.

76. Rutherford GW. Epidemiology of AIDS-related coccidioidomycosis in California. 11th International Conference on AIDS, Vancouver, 1996.

77. Ampel NM, Dols CL, Galgiani JN. Coccidioidomycosis during human immunodeficiency virus infection: results of a prospective study in a coccidioidal endemic area. Am J Med 1993; 94:235–240.

78. Hilmarsdottir I, Meynard JL, Rogeaux O, Guermonprez G, Datry A, Katlama C, Brucker G, Coutellier A, Danis M, Gentilini M. Disseminated *Penicillium marneffei* infection associated with human immunodeficiency virus: a report of two cases and a review of 35 published cases. J Acquir Immune Defic Syndr 1993; 6:466–471.

79. Supparatpinyo K, Chiewchanvit S, Hirunsri P, Uthammachai C, Nelson KE, Sirisanthana T. *Penicillium marneffei* infection in patients infected with human immunodeficiency virus. Clin Infect Dis 1992; 14:744.

80. Supparatpinyo K, Khamwan C, Baosoung V, Nelson KE, Sirisanthana T. Disseminated *Penicillium marneffei* infection in Southeast Asia. Lancet 1994; 344:110–113.

81. Supparatpinyo K, Sirisanthana T. New fungal infections in the Western Pacific. JAMA Southeast Asia 1994;10 (suppl 3):208–209.

82. Supparatpinyo K, Perriens J, Nelson KE, Sirisanthana T. A controlled trial of itraconazole to prevent relapse of *Penicillium marneffei* infection in patients infected with the human immunodeficiency virus. N Engl J Med 1998; 339:1739–1743.

83. Capponi M, Sureau P, Segretain G. Penicilliosis de *Rhizomys sinensis*. Bull Soc Pathol Exot 1956; 49:418–421.
84. Deng Z, Yun M, Ajello L. Human penicilliosis marneffei and its relation to the bamboo rat (*Rhizomys pruinosus*). J Med Vet Mycol 1986; 24:383–389.
85. Ajello L, Padhye APA, Sukroongreung S, Nilakul CH, Tamtimavanic S. Occurrence of *Penicillium marneffei* infections among wild bamboo rats in Thailand. Mycopathologia 1995; 131:1–8.
86. Chariyalertsak S, Vanittanakom P, Nelson KE, Sirisanthana T, Vanittanakom N. *Rhizomys sumatrensis Cannomys badius,* new natural animal hosts of *Penicillium marneffei*. J Med Vet Mycol 1996; 34:105–110.
87. Chariyalertsak S, Sirisanthana T, Supparatpinyo K, Praparattanapan J, Nelson KE. Case–control study of risk factors for *Penicillium marneffei* infection in human immunodeficiency virus-infected patients in Northern Thailand. Clin Infect Dis 1997; 24:1080–1086.
88. Minamoto GY, Rosenberg AS. Fungal infections in patients with acquired immunodeficiency syndrome. Med Clin North Am 1997; 81:381–409.
89. Supparatpinyo K, Nelson KE, Merz WG, Breslin BJ, Cooper CR Jr, Kamwan C, Sirisanthana T. Response to antifungal therapy by human immunodeficiency virus-infected patients with disseminated *Penicillium marneffei* infections and in vitro susceptibilities of isolates from clinical specimens. Antimicrob Agents Chemother 1993; 37:2407–2411.
90. Chariyalertsak S, Supparatpinyo K, Sirisanthana T, Nelson KE. A controlled trial of itraconazole as primary prophylaxis for systemic fungal infections in patients with advanced human immunodeficiency virus infection in Thailand. Clin Infect Dis 2002; 34:277–284.
91. Klein BS, Vergeront JM, Weeks RJ, Kumar UN, Mathai G, Varkey B, Kaufman L, Bardsher RW, Stoebig JF, Davis JP. Isolation of *Blastomyces dermatidis* in soil associated with a large outbreak of blastomycosis in Wisconsin. N Engl J Med 1986; 314:529–534.
92. Pappas PG, Pottage JC, Powderly WG, Fraser VJ, Stratton CW, McKenzie S, Tapper ML, Climel H, Bonebrake FC, Blum R. Blastomycosis in patients with the acquired immunodeficiency syndrome. Ann Intern Med 1992; 116:847–853.
93. Witzig RS, Hoadley DJ, Greer DL, Abriola KP, Hernandez RL. Blastomycosis and human immunodeficiency virus: three new cases and review. South Med J 1994; 87:715–719.
94. Graybill JR, Patterson TF. Mycoses caused by moulds. In: Dolin R, Masur H, Saag M, eds. AIDS Therapy. 2d ed. Philadelphia: Churchill-Livingstone, 2003:543–554.
95. Cunliffe NA, Denning DW. Uncommon invasive mycoses in AIDS. AIDS 1995; 9:411–420.
96. Perfect JR, Schell WA. The new fungal opportunists are coming. Clin Infect Dis 1996; 22(Suppl 2):S112–S118.
97. Donabedian H, O'Donnell E, Olszewski C, MacArthur RD, Budd N. Disseminated cutaneous and meningeal sporotrichosis in an AIDS patient. Diagn Microbiol Infect Dis 1994; 18:111–115.
98. Goldani LZ, Sugar AM. Paracoccidioidomycosis and AIDS: an overview. Clin Infect Dis 1995; 21:1275–1281.
99. Schell WA. New aspects of emerging fungal pathogens. A multifaceted challenge. Clin Lab Med 1995; 15:365–387.
100. Denning DW. Invasive aspergillosis. Clin Infect Dis 1998; 26:781–803.
101. Pursell KJ, Telzak EE, Armstrong D. Aspergillus species colonization and invasive disease in patients with AIDS. Clin Infect Dis 1992; 14:141–148.
102. Sanchez MR, Ponge-Wilson I, Moy JA, Rosenthal S. Zygomycosis and HIV infection. J Am Acad Dermatol 1994; 30(5 Pt 2):904–908.

103. Levy E, Bia MJ. Isolated renal mucormycosis: case report and review. J Am Soc Nephrol 1995; 5:2014–2019.
104. Nagy-Agren SE, Shu P, Smith GJ, Waskin HA, Altice FL. Zygomycosis (mucormycosis) and HIV infection: report of three cases and review. J Acquir Immune Defic Syndr 1995; 10:441–449.
105. Miccozzi MS, Wetli CV. Intravenous amphetamine abuse, primary cerebral mucormycosis, and acquired immunodeficiency. J Forensic Sci 1985; 30:504–510.
106. Lederman MM, Valdez H. Immune restoration with antiretroviral therapies: implications for clinical management. JAMA 2000; 284:223–228.
107. Powderly WG. Prophylaxis for opportunistic infections in an era of effective antiretroviral therapy. Clin Infect Dis 2000; 31:597–601.
108. Powderly WG. Discontinuation of secondary prophylaxis in AIDS. http://home.-mdconsult.com/das/stat/view/27796535/pers, 2002.
109. Race EM, Adelson-Mitty J, Kriegel GR, Barlam TF, Reimann KA, Letvin NL, Japour AL. Focal mycobacterial lymphadenitis following initiation of protease-inhibitor therapy in patients with advanced HIV-1 disease. Lancet 1998; 351:252–255.
110. DeSimone JA, Pomerantz RJ, Babinchak TJ. Inflammatory reactions in HIV-infected persons after initiation of highly active antiretroviral therapy. Ann Intern Med 2000; 133:447–454.
111. Woods ML II, MacGinley R, Eisen DP, Allworth AM. HIV combination therapy: partial immune reconstitution unmasking latent cryptococcal infection. AIDS 1998; 12:1491–1494.
112. Blanche P, Gombert B, Ginsburg C, Passeron A, Stubei I, Rigolet A, Salmon D, Sicard D. HIV combination therapy: immune reconstitution causing cryptococcal lymphadenitis dramatically improved by anti-inflammatory therapy. Scan J Infect Dis 1998; 30:615–616.
113. Lanzafame M, Trevenzoli M, Carretta G, Lazzarini L, Vento S, Concia E. Mediastinal lymphadenitis due to cryptococcal infection in HIV-positive patients on highly active antiretroviral therapy. Chest 1999; 116:848–849.
114. Bottaro E, Elsner B, Cassetti Y. Histoplasmosis y HAART: aparicion de andenomegalis durante el tratmiento. 3rd Argentinean Congress on AIDS, Mar del Plata, 1997.
115. Safdar A, Rubocki RJ, Horvath JA, Narayan KK, Waldron RL. Fatal immune restoration disease in human immunodeficiency virus type 1-infected patients with progressive multifocal leukoencephalopathy: impact of antiretroviral therapy-associated immune restoration. Clin Infect Dis 2002; 35:1250–1257.
116. Jenny-Avital ER, Abadi M. Immune reconstitution cryptococcosis after initiation of successful highly active antiretroviral therapy. Clin Infect Dis 2002; 35:e28–e33.
117. Shelburne SA III, Hamill RJ, Rodriguez-Barradas MC, Greenberg SB, Atmar RL, Musher DW, Gathe JC Jr, Visnegarwala F, Trautner BW. Immune reconstitution inflammatory syndrome: emergence of a unique syndrome during highly active antiretroviral therapy. Medicine (Baltimore) 2002; 82:213–227.
118. Manfredi R, Pieri F, Pileri SA, Chiodo F. The changing face of AIDS-related opportunism: cryptococcosis in the highly active antiretroviral therapy (HAART) era. Case reports and literature review. Mycopathologia 1999; 148:73–78.
119. Koletar SL, Heald AE, Finkelstein D, Finkelstein D, Hafher R, Currier JS, et al. A prospective study of discontinuing primary and secondary *Pneumocystis carinii* pneumonia prophylaxis after CD4 cell count increase to $> 200 \times 10^6$/L. AIDS 2001; 15:1509–1515.
120. Tural C, Romeu J, Sirera G, Andreu D, Conejero M, Ruiz S, Jou A, Bonjoch A, Ruiz L, Arno A, Clotet B. Long-lasting remission of cytomegalovirus retinitis without maintenance therapy in human immunodeficiency virus-infected patients. J Infect Dis 1998; 177:1080–1083.
121. Macdonald JC, Torriani FJ, Morse LS, Karavellas MP, Reed JB, Freeman WR. Lack of reactivation of cytomegalovirus retinitis after stopping CMV maintenance therapy in

AIDS patients without sustained elevations in CD4 T cells in response to highly active antiretroviral therapy. J Infect Dis 1998; 177:1182–1187.

122. Vrabec TR, Baldassano VF, Whitcup SM. Discontinuation of maintenance therapy in patients with quiescent cytomegalovirus retinitis and elevated CD4+ counts. Opthalmology 1998; 105:1259–1264.

123. Gripshover BM, Valdez H, Salata RM, Lederman MM. Withdrawal of fluconazole suppressive therapy for thrush in patients responding to combination antiviral therapy including protease inhibitors. AIDS 1998; 12:2513–2514.

124. Schneider MM, Borleffs JC, Stolk RP, Jaspers CA, Hoepelman AI. Discontinuation of *Pneumocystis carinii* pneumonia prophylaxis in HIV-1 infected patients treated with highly active antiretroviral therapy. Lancet 1999; 353:201–203.

125. Furrer H, Egger M, Opravil M, Bernasconi E, Hirsehel B, Battegay M, Telenti A, Vernazza PL, Rickenbach M, Flepp M, Malinverni R. Discontinuation of primary prophylaxis against *Pneumocystis carinii* pneumonia in HIV-1 infected adults treated with combination antiretroviral therapy. Swiss HIV Cohort Study. N Engl J Med 1999; 340:1301–1306.

126. Weverling GJ, Mocroft A, Ledergerber B, Kirk O, Gonzales-Lahoz J, d'Arminio Monforte A, Proenca R, Phillips AN, Lundgren JD, Reiss P. Discontinuation of *Pneumoncystis carinii* pneumonia prophylaxis after start of highly active antiretroviral therapy in HIV-1 infection. EuroSIDA Study Group. Lancet 1999; 353:1293–1298.

127. Lopez JC, Miro JM, Pena JM, Podzamczer D, and the GESIDA 04/98 Study Group. A randomized trial of the discontinuation of primary and secondary prophylaxis against *Pneumocystis carinii* pneumonia after HAART in patients with HIV infection. N Engl J Med 2001; 344:159–167.

128. Trikalinos TA, Loannidis JP. Discontinuation of *Pneumocystis carinii* prophylaxis in patients infected with human immunodeficiency virus: a meta-analysis and decision analysis. Clin Infect Dis 2001; 33:1901–1909.

129. Miro JM, Lopez JC, Podzamczer D, Pena JM, Alberdi C, Claramonte X, Martinez E, Cosin J, Gonzalez J, Domingo P, Casado JL. Discontinuation of toxoplasmic encephalitis prophylaxis is safe in HFV-l and *Toxoplasma gondii* co-infected patients after immunological recovery with HAART. Preliminary results of the GESIDA 04/98-B study. 7th Conference on retroviruses and opportunistic infections, San Francisco, 2000.

130. Aberg JA, Yajko DM, Jacobson MA. Eradication of disseminated *Mycobacterium avium* complex after twelve months anti-mycobacterial therapy and response to highly active retroviral therapy. J Infect Dis 1998; 178:1446–1449.

131. Martinez E, Garcia-Viejo MA, Marcos MA, Perez-Cuevas JB, Blanco JL, Mallolas J, Miro JM, Gatell JM. Discontinuation of secondary prophylaxis for cryptococcal meningitis in HIV-infected patients responding to highly active antiretroviral therapy. AIDS 2000; 14:2615–2617.

132. Aberg JA, Price RM, Heeren DM, Bredt B. A pilot study of the discontinuation of antifungal therapy for disseminated cryptococcal disease in patients with acquired immunodeficiency syndrome, following immunologic response to antiretroviral therapy. J Infect Dis 2002; 185:1179–1182.

133. Aberg JA, Williams PL, Liu T, Lederman HM, Hafner R, Torriani FJ, Lennox JL, Dube MP, MacGregor RR, Currier JS. A study of discontinuing maintenance therapy in human immunodeficiency virus-infected subjects with disseminated *Mycobacterium avium* complex: AIDS Clinical Trial Group 393 Study Team. J Infect Dis 2003; 187:1046–1052.

134. Currier JS, Williams PL, Koletar SL, Conn SE, Murphy RL, Heald AE, Hafner R, Bassily EL, Lederman HM, Knirsch C, Benson CA, Valdez H, Aberg JA, McCutchan JA. Discontinuation of *Mycobacterium avium* complex prophylaxis in patients with antiretroviral therapy-induced increases in CD4 cell count: a randomized, double-blind, placebo-controlled trial. ADDS Clinical Trial Group 362 Study Team. Ann Intern Med 2000; 133:493–503.

135. El-Sadr WM, Burman WJ, Grant LB, Matts JP, Hafner R, Crane L, Zeh D, Gallagher B, Mannheimer SB, Martinez A, Gordin F. Discontinuation of prophylaxis for *Mycobacterium avium* complex disease in HIV-infected patients who have a response to antiretroviral therapy. N Engl J Med 2000; 342:1085–1092.

136. Furrer H, Rossi M, Telenti A, Lederberger B. Discontinuing or withholding primary prophylaxis against *Mycobacterium avium* in patients on successful antiretroviral combination therapy. AIDS 2000; 14:1409–1412.

137. Masur H, Kaplan JE, Holmes KK. Guidelines for preventing opportunistic infections among HIV-infected persons—2002. Recommendations of the U.S. Public Health Service and the Infectious Diseases Society of America. Ann Intern Med 2003; 137:435–477.

138. Torriani FJ, Freeman WR, Macdonald JC, Karavellas MP, Durand DM, Jeffrey DD, Meylan PR, Schrier RD. CMV retinitis recurs after stopping treatment in virological and immunological failures of potent antiretroviral therapy. AIDS 2000; 14:173–180.

139. Johnson S, Benson C, Johnson D, Weinberg A. Recurrent CMV retinitis in a patient on highly active antiretroviral therapy despite apparent immune reconstitution. 7th Conference on Retroviruses and Opportunistic Infections, San Francisco, 2000.

140. Valentine F, Peiperi L, Chiliade P, McMeeking A. The occurrence of opportunistic infections at relatively high CD4 levels is associated with an antigen-specific absence of lymphocyte proliferative responses. 7th Conference on Retroviruses and Opportunistic Infections, San Francisco, 2000.

6

Candida Infections in the Intensive Care Unit

Joseph S. Solomkin
Department of Surgery, University of Cincinnati College of Medicine, Cincinnati, Ohio, U.S.A.

I. INTRODUCTION

There have been substantial changes in notions of prevention and management of *Candida* infection syndromes seen in critical care settings. Prospective randomized trials have been reported in the area of prophylactic therapy, and, although controversial, have legitimized the expansion of prophylactic therapy. Similarly, considerable information has come from therapeutic trials of new agents including the first echinocandin, caspofungin and an expanded spectrum imidazole, voriconazole. The availability of imidazoles and echinocandins warrant close review of the utility, if any, of continued use of amphotericin B and its derivatives in *Candida* infection. This review will focus on these particular issues.

II. PATHOGENICITY AND VIRULENCE FACTORS FOR *CANDIDA*

Four virulence factors have been demonstrated for *Candida* spp.: adherence to epithelial and endothelial cells, secretion of proteinases that degrade connective tissue proteins and facilitate invasion, production of cell-surface and shed mannans, which serve to attach the yeast to host tissues and suppress host response, and resistance to oxidative killing by neutrophils (1–5).

A. *Candida albicans*

C. albicans appears to be more virulent than other *Candida* species, and has been most closely studied. The conversion from yeast to filamentous growth is a critical step in the subsequent expression of several virulence mechanisms for *C. albicans* (2). The yeast-to-hyphal transition of *C. albicans* can be is triggered by a wide variety of factors, suggesting that hyphal growth is a response to nutrient deprivation, especially low nitrogen and that filamentous growth enables the fungus to forage for nutrients more effectively (6).

B. Adhesion, Proteases, and Mannans as Virulence Factors

C. albicans is the most common fungal pathogen of humans and has developed an extensive repertoire of virulence mechanisms that allows successful colonization and infection of the host under suitable predisposing conditions. Yeast forms adhere to various host cells and matrix elements primarily through the protein and carbohydrate elements of mannoproteins. Adherence is achieved by a combination of specific (ligand–receptor interactions) and non-specific (electrostatic charge, van der Waals forces) mechanisms which allow the yeast to attach to a wide range of tissue types and inanimate surfaces (7). Adherence for filamentous forms of *C. albicans* is mediated in part by an integrin analogue that shares antigenic, structural, and functional homologies with the β_2-integrin subunits αM and αX (8). Antibodies to the integrin $\alpha_5\beta_1$ (the fibronectin receptor on various human cell types), and antibodies specific for the integrin β_1 sub unit recognized a *C. tropicalis* membrane protein (9,10). *C. albicans* and *C. tropicalis* recognize distinct RGD ligands present at the surface of the epithelial cell (11–14).

This information supports a two-stage model for adherence of *C. albicans* to host tissues. In this model, conventional adhesins composed of a mixture of agglutinin-like cell wall proteins initiate binding to host cells. This is the followed by formation of germ tubes. The signaling that results in a switch to filamentous forms is, therefore a critical element and becomes a potential target for therapeutic intervention.

The secreted aspartic proteinases of *C. albicans* are major factors in virulence. SAP proteins fulfill a number of specialized functions during the infective process, which include the simple role of digesting molecules for nutrients, altering host cell membranes to facilitate adhesion and tissue invasion, and digesting cells and molecules of the host immune system to avoid or resist antimicrobial attack by the host (15). There are at least seven different genes that encode for secreted aspartic proteinase (16–19). SAP expression depends on the type of infection, with different SAP isogenes being activated during systemic disease as compared with mucosal infection. In addition, the activation of individual SAP genes depends on the progress of the infection; some members of the gene family being induced immediately after contact with the host whereas others are expressed only after dissemination into deep organs.

An additional element in fungal pathogenesis is cell surface mannans. These are important both for *albicans* and non-*albicans* species (20). Mannan consists of a large number of various hypermannosylated proteins that are deposited mainly at the outside of the cell wall, thereby protecting internal regions of the cell wall from large molecules like proteases. Many critical aspects of the interaction between the fungus and the host, such as adhesion, immunosurveillance, and immunomodulation, are mediated by host recognition and interaction with this mannan-rich surface of the cell wall (21).

III. THE MICROBIOLOGY, INCIDENCE, MORBIDITY, AND MORTALITY OF *CANDIDA* INFECTION

The incidence of fungal infections, particularly with *Candida* species increased substantially through the 1980s, but has since leveled off (22,23) (Fig. 1A). At many medical centers, *Candida* species remain the fourth leading cause of nosocomial bloodstream infection, preceded only by coagulase-negative staphylococci, *Staphylococcus aureus*, and enterococci (24). The prevalence of *Candida* in a particular ICU is

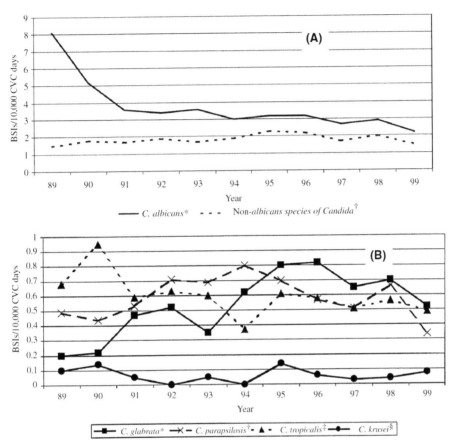

Figure 1 (**A**) Incidence of hospital-acquired bloodstream infection (BSI) due to *C. albicans* and non-*albicans* species of *Candida*, National Nosocomial Infections Surveillance system intensive care unit wards, 1989–1999. *P < 0.001 for the annual incidence of *C. albicans* BSI, determined using the χ^2 test for trend, 1989–1999. †P = 0.53 for the annual incidence of non-*albicans* species of *Candida* BSI, determined using the χ^2 test for trend, 1989–1999. CVC days, total number of days in which a central venous catheter was in place (171). (**B**) Incidence of hospital-acquired BSI with non-*albicans* species of Candida, by species, National Nosocomial Infections Surveillance system intensive care unit wards, 1989–1999. *P = 0.05 for the annual incidence of *Candida glabrata* BSI. †P = not significant for the annual incidence of *Candida parapsilosis* BSI. ‡P = 0.16 for the annual incidence of *Candida tropicalis* BSI. §P = not significant for the annual incidence of *Candida krusei* BSI. CVC days, total number of days in which a central venous catheter was in place.

dependent on the type of patients seen, their acuity, and other local factors such as fluconazole usage.

A. The Changing Microbiological Picture of *Candida* Infections

Although there are more than 100 described species of *Candida*, only four are commonly associated with infection: *C. albicans*, *C. tropicalis*, *C. parapsilosis*, and *C. glabrata*. Of these, *C. albicans* has long been the most common (>60% of infections). The other three major species are seen at rates varying from 5% to 20%.

C. tropicalis is a virulent organism and mucosal colonization by this organism frequently leads to invasive infection.

An evolution of the epidemiology of candidiasis has been recently described with a reduction in the incidence of *C. albicans* in favor of the non-*albicans* species, in particular *C. glabrata* and *C. krusei* (Fig. 1B) (25–27). This appears to have occurred because of wide usage of fluconazole, and is important because several strains of *C. glabrata* have reduced susceptibility to fluconazole. *C. krusei* is highly resistant to all triazoles.

A recent study by the NNIS group evaluated the trends in species distribution and susceptibility to fluconazole among 1579 bloodstream isolates of *Candida* spp. over a 7-year period (1992–1998) from more than 50 U.S. hospitals (26). *C. albicans* accounted for 52% of isolates, followed by *C. glabrata* 18%, *C. parapsilosis* 15%, *C. tropicalis* 11%, and *C. krusei* 2%. Since 1995, *C. glabrata* has become more prevalent than *C. parapsilosis*. The susceptibility of all *Candida* species to fluconazole remained stable, and, particularly, there was no increased level of resistance in *C. albicans*. This decrease in *C. albicans* and increase in *C. glabrata* has not been observed in all centers where fluconazole usage has increased (28). It is important for individual centers to monitor their experience, as a guide to utility of fluconazole as empiric therapy.

B. Mortality of *Candida* Infection

Observational clinical studies, either retrospective or prospective, have consistently identified a crude mortality rate of 30–60% for patients with candidemia (29–31). This is illustrated in Figure 2, where the findings of two sequential case-matched studies from the same institution are displayed (29,32). A much larger observational study involving 1447 adults at tertiary centers has recently been reported and this provides a broader survey (33). In this study, overall mortality 3 months after the

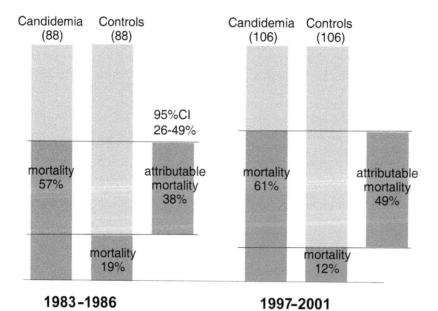

Figure 2 Attributable mortality from two case controlled retrospective studies of candidemia at the University of Iowa. *Source*: From Refs. 29,32.

initial positive blood culture result was 40%, and cause-specific mortality was 12%. Conversely, prospective therapeutic trials have found a substantially lower mortality rate, partly because of selection bias of clinical trials, which typically exclude patients with organ failure and other risk factors for mortality. As an example, a recent prospective study examining different amphotericin dosing regimens based on duration of candidemia excluded patients with renal failure (34).

C. How Does *Candida* Infection Cause Mortality?

Mortality from infectious disease occurs most commonly as a consequence of the host physiologic response to the organism. The measured severity of infection, based on acute cardiovascular, respiratory, organ function scoring, and limited blood tests, is a reliable and reproducible measure of mortality risk, and is generally regardless of the infecting microorganism, if effective antimicrobial therapy is available. The physiologic disturbance is most commonly quantified using the APACHE II or APACHE III system (35,36).

To what extent the particular infecting organism independently affects mortality resulting from specific virulence mechanisms is obvious with toxin-secreting bacteria (e.g., Group A streptococcal or clostridial infections). As *Candida* infection syndromes were being defined pathologically, death commonly resulted from untreated metastatic infection with associated organ failure. This was certainly because of organism-specific virulence factors. However, since the recognition of the virulence of these organisms, the development of less toxic antifungal agents, and more aggressive treatment of *Candida* infections, these syndromes of disseminated micro-abscesses are now rarely seen in patients without neutropenia. As this condition was obviated, outcome became primarily dependent on acute physiologic shifts and background disease.

In case-controlled studies, the controls do not experience the physiologic derangements that the candidemic patients suffer. More suitable controls might be patients with bacteremia. This has been examined in Pappas et al.'s (33) observational study (Fig. 3A), with the finding that species did not affect mortality at different severity levels. An APACHE-based analysis system was used to demonstrate outcome differences between two antifungal regimens, where a therapeutic effect appeared most notable in moderately ill patients (Fig. 3B).

IV. CLINICAL ASPECTS OF *CANDIDA* INFECTION

A. Sources of *Candida* in the Critical Care Patient

In humans, as well as in animals, the GI tract is considered to be an important portal of entry for microorganisms, including yeasts, into the bloodstream. The passage of endogenous fungi across the mucosal barrier is referred to as fungal translocation (by analogy with bacterial translocation).

Although yeast cells have no intrinsic motility, they are able to translocate across the intestinal mucosa within a few hours of ingestion, if present in high enough concentration. That *Candida* spp. can translocate from the gut into the bloodstream in humans was demonstrated in a study, where signs and symptoms of sepsis developed in a healthy volunteer 2 hr after ingestion of a suspension containing 10^{12} *C. albicans* organisms, and blood cultures taken 3 and 6 hr after ingestion were positive for *Candida* (37). That this mechanism is important in clinical disease

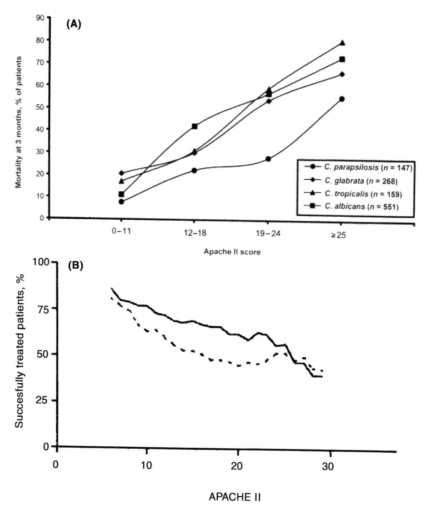

Figure 3 Effect of severity of illness, as measured by the APACHE II scoring system, on outcome from fungemia. (A) Outcome by species. *Source*: From Ref. (33). (B) Outcome by variant therapy (fluconazole vs. fluconazole + amphotericin B). Outcome by group (*solid line*, fluconazole plus amphotericin B deoxycholate; *stippled line*, fluconazole plus placebo) for subjects with the same APACHE II score ±5 points (e.g., the leftmost point of each line is the success rate for subjects having an APACHE II of 6 ± 5, or 1–11). The cell width of ±5 for this rolling stratified analysis was chosen because it placed ≥10 subjects into each cell. Qualitatively similar results were obtained for cell widths of ±3 and ±4. *Source*: From Ref. 101.

is attested by the finding of GI tract involvement and submucosal invasion in an autopsy study of patients with hematogenous candidiasis (38).

Microbial translocation has been demonstrated in several animal models, using a range of stresses. These include, most notably, malnutrition, parenteral nutrition, endotoxemia, bacterial overgrowth, and burn injury (39–42). It is enhanced by fasting (which induces complex changes in host defenses), and protein deficiency (which results in intestinal microbial overgrowth, shortened villi, increased intestinal absorption of intact proteins, and decreased intracellular killing of bacteria and fungi) (43,44).

Translocation is thought to occur as a result of flattening of the intestinal villi that results from the administration of total parenteral nutrition (45). In another animal model, bile duct ligation resulted in bacterial translocation (46). In a study involving *C. albicans*, volatile fatty acids and secondary bile salts reduced fungal adhesion to the mucosa, colonization, and dissemination in mice by causing the formation of a dense layer of bacteria in the mucosal biofilm. These bacteria success-fully competed with the yeast cells for the same adhesion sites and produced various substances that inhibited fungal growth (47). Similar results were obtained in guinea pigs and rats that had burns covering 50% of their total body surface area. After the yeast cells penetrated the lamina propria, the cells were found either free in the lymphatic vessels and in the blood vessels or engulfed by macrophages (48).

Microbial translocation is relevant in human disease. Surveillance cultures from patients with leukemia have demonstrated an association between the bacterial biotype or serotype that was most prevalent in the patient's feces, and the bacterial biotype or serotype that subsequently caused septicemia (49). Significant microbial translocation has been demonstrated in patients undergoing operation for colorectal carcinoma, intestinal obstruction, and Crohn's disease (50–52).

B. Immunosuppression of the Host Leading to Dissemination

Host defenses against *Candida* infections include T-cell immunity, important at the mucosal level in preventing colonization and superficial invasion, and phagocytic immunity. Professional phagocytes, including macrophages and neutrophils, serve to prevent deeper tissue invasion and hematogenous dissemination. Suppression of any of these arms of the immune system puts the patient at increased risk of *Candida* infection. If phagocyte function is suppressed, these cells may actually serve to trans-port microbes out of the intestine and liberate them in extraintestinal sites (53). Such settings include hematological malignancy, bone marrow, and/or organ transplanta-tion, and immunosuppressive therapy including cancer chemotherapy, corticosteroid therapy, and others. It is also worth noting that major sepsis and major injury, including burns, results in numerous defects in phagocytic function and in T-cell function (54,55). These are likely to be participatory in the emergence of *Candida* in these patient populations.

Total parenteral nutrition is a significant risk factor for *Candida* infection. This is likely to be multifactorial, including host immunosuppression and alterations in the GI tract related to absence of enteral feeding (56). In animal models, total parenteral nutrition induced macrophage suppression with decreased peritoneal macrophage superoxide production and *Candida* phagocytosis, associated with bacterial translocation to mesenteric lymph nodes (57).

C. Colonization as a Major Risk Factor for Subsequent *Candida* Infection

An important implication of this work on translocation from the intestinal tract is the potential utility of prophylaxis. The notion of an intestinal reservoir has led to a broader notion of colonization at intestinal and various extraintestinal sites as a prelude to infection. This is a central notion, suggesting points for interruption of this sequence. Clinical studies of antifungal prophylaxis in neutropenic cancer patients have shown that antifungal regimens effectively prevent hematogenous infection when they can eliminate or reduce colonization by *Candida* (58,59).

In critically ill patients, colonization with *Candida* spp. precedes and leads to infection. If multiple body sites are colonized, there will be an increased risk of severe infection in high-risk patients and the chance of invasion can be predicted by the extent of pre-existing colonization.

This notion is supported by studies demonstrating that 95% of neutropenic patients and 84% of non-neutropenic patients with documented fungal infection were infected with the same strains that had previously colonized them (60,61). Patients who were not colonized were significantly less likely to develop infection. In a study investigating the sequence of colonization and candidemia in non-neutropenic patients, Voss et al. (61) found that in patients with disseminated candidiasis, the strains recovered from the initial colonized or infected site and from the bloodstream were identical. Furthermore, nearly every patient was infected with a distinct or unique *Candida* strain. In another study involving 111 patients on bone marrow transplant and hematologic malignancy services, positive surveillance cultures were found to be highly predictive of systemic infection for *tropicalis* but not for *albicans* whereas negative surveillance cultures correlated with a low risk of candidal dissemination (62).

The density of colonization appears to be predictive of the risk of hematogenous candidiasis. In two large series of neutropenic cancer patients, hematogenous candidiasis almost never developed among noncolonized patients, compared to more than 30% infection among patients with multiple colonized sites (63,64). In another study by Richet et al. (65) among patients with acute lymphocytic leukemia, a relatively high concentration of *Candida* organisms in the stools was found to be a significant risk factor for hematogenous candidiasis. This also has been found in neonatal populations. In a study of 40 infants with very low birth weight, a value of 8×10^6 *Candida* colony-forming units (CFU)/g of stool was established as a threshold, beyond which GI symptoms (attributed to *Candida*) developed in 50% of the infants and a systemic septic response in 28.5% in the course of 1–3 weeks of heavy colonization (66,67). Fluconazole prophylaxis in this group is efficacious (68).

In general ICU populations, colonization is also a central risk factor for subsequent fungal infection. Pittet et al. (69) and colleagues performed a 6-month prospective cohort study among patients admitted to surgical and neonatal intensive care units in a 1600-bed university medical center. Routine microbiologic surveillance cultures at different body sites were performed. A *Candida* colonization index was determined daily, as the ratio of the number of distinct body sites (dbs) colonized with identical strains over the total number of dbs tested; a mean of 5.3 dbs per patient was obtained. All isolates ($n = 322$) recovered were characterized by genotyping using contour-clamped homogeneous electrical field gel electrophoresis that allowed strain delineation among these *Candida* species. Twenty-nine patients met the criteria for colonization; 11 patients (38%) developed severe infections (8 candidemia); the remaining 18 patients were heavily colonized but never required IV antifungal therapy. Among the potential risk factors for *Candida* infection, three discriminated the colonized from the infected patients— length of previous antibiotic therapy ($P < 0.02$), severity of illness assessed by APACHE II score ($P < 0.01$), and the intensity of *Candida* spp. colonization ($P < 0.01$). By logistic regression analysis, the latter two were the independent factors that predicted subsequent candidal infection.

Candida colonization always preceded infection with genotypically identical *Candida* spp. The proposed colonization indeces reached threshold values, a mean of 6 days before *Candida* infection, and demonstrated high positive predictive values

(66–100%). The intensity of *Candida* colonization assessed by systematic screening helps predicting subsequent infections with identical strains in critically ill patients.

Nolla, Leon, Roda, and colleagues performed a prospective observational study between May 1998 and January 1999 encompassing 73 ICUs in Spain. Patients were required to have stayed in the ICU for 7 or more days prior to entry. Surveillance cultures were performed weekly from tracheal aspirates, urine, and gut (oropharynx and gastric aspirates). The patients were considered *colonized* (appearance or persistence of *Candida* in surveillance cultures) or to have *invasive infection* (candidemia, endophthalmitis, peritonitis, or positive histology from an organ biopsy). *Multisite colonization* was defined as ≥2 sites positive from surveillance cultures. *Persistence* was defined as cultures of the same site revealing yeast for one or more weeks. 1766 consecutive patients were analyzed: 916 (58%) were in the colonized group, 158 with persistent multisite colonization, 359 with nonpersistent multisite colonization, 399 with single site colonization, and 107 invasive infection. Ninety-three of the 107 patients with invasive infection (87%) were previously colonized. Univariate analysis identified solid neoplasm, radiotherapy, parenteral nutrition, and hemodialysis, longer duration of ICU stay, non-*albicans*, and multisite colonization as significant risks for invasive infection. By stepwise logistic regression, persistent multisite colonization [(odds ratio {OR} 2.4, 95% confidence interval {CI} 1.3–4.2), radiotherapy OR 3.6, CI 1.1–12.3], hemodialysis (OR 2.7, CI 1.6–4.5), and colonization with non-*albicans* yeast (OR 1.8, CI 1.2–2.9) independently predicted invasive *Candida* infection.

While it is commonly stated that antibiotic administration itself is a major independent risk factor, in fact, this is not the case. In a case-controlled study, antibiotic administration was shown to be only marginally associated with candidemia and substantially less important than prior *Candida* colonization (70). There are many other factors that result in changes in the gastrointestinal flora. These include ileus, antacid therapy, and contamination with a hospital flora. The particular concern is that appropriate anti-infective therapy for a bacterial infection should not be stopped because *Candida* is identified at one or more sites. In intra-abdominal infections, mixed flora infections involving *Candida* and bacteria are the norm, rather than the exception.

V. WHO SHOULD RECEIVE ANTIFUNGAL PROPHYLAXIS IN THE ICU?

Recently, two prospective studies have been reported that add considerable clarity to this issue. Pelz and colleagues in the surgical ICU at Johns Hopkins Hospital conducted a prospective, randomized, placebo-controlled trial that entered 260 surgical patients with an anticipated length of ICU stay of at least 3 days (143). The single criteria for entry was the anticipation of 3 or more days in the ICU. The absence of any other entry criterion means that the results of the study cannot be transported to other critical care units. This unit had an extraordinarily high background incidence of *Candida* colonization and infection.

Patients were randomly assigned to receive either enteral fluconazole 400 mg/ day or placebo during their stay in the ICU. The primary end point was the time of occurrence of fungal infection during the surgical ICU stay, with planned secondary analysis of patients "on-therapy" and alternate definitions of fungal infections. The risk of candidal infection in patients receiving fluconazole was significantly less than the risk in patients receiving placebo. After adjusting for potentially confounding

Table 1 Results of a Prospective Randomized Trial of Prophylaxis with Fluconazole for *Candida* Infection in the ICU (151)

	Fluconazole ($n = 130$)	Placebo ($n = 130$)	P value
Candida infection	11 (8.5%)	20 (15%)	0.01
Peritonitis	3	8	
Candidemia	1	3	
Catheter	1	6	
C. albicans	5 (45%)	12 (60%)	NS
C. glabrata	3 (27%)	5 (25%)	NS
Mortality	14 (11%)	16 (12%)	NS

effects of the Acute Physiology and Chronic Health Evaluation (APACHE) III score, days to first dose, and fungal colonization at enrollment, the risk of fungal infection was reduced by 55% in the fluconazole group. No difference in death rate was observed between patients receiving fluconazole and those receiving placebo.

The key data elements from these studies are presented in Tables 1 and 2. It is apparent that colonization was far and away the most significant risk factor for candidemia, with a 10-fold higher likelihood of infection in colonized vs. non colonized patients. This means that of the 20 infected patients in the placebo group, only one or two were not colonized. Review of the conditions presented reveals that the main differences were in colonized catheters, a condition not believed to warrant therapy in the absence of candidemia, and in peritonitis. The benefits of antifungal prophylaxis in patients operated upon for postoperative infection have been previously identified (95).

Garbino et al. (71) performed a well-designed study to assess the effectiveness of adding fluconazole to a selective digestive decontamination regimen to prevent candidal infections. This study was a prospective, randomized, double blind, and placebo-controlled trial among medical and surgical intensive care unit patients at a large university hospital. All adult patients mechanically ventilated for at least 48 hr with an expectation to remain so for at least an additional 72 hr, and receiving selective decontamination of the digestive tract were eligible for entry. Patients were randomly assigned fluconazole 100 mg daily ($n = 103$) or placebo ($n = 101$). *Candida* infections occurred less frequently in the fluconazole group (5.8%) than in the placebo group [16%; rate ratio 0.35; 95% CI 0.11–0.94] (Tables 3 and 4). Almost all candidemia episodes occurred in the placebo group (rate ratio for fluconazole use 0.10; 95% CI 0.02–0.74). The rate of treatment failure, development of candidal

Table 2 Multivariate Analysis of Predictors of Failure in a Randomized Trial of Fluconazole 400 mg q.d. Enterally vs. Placebo (151)

	Risk ratio	95% Confidence interval
Randomization to fluconazole	0.45	0.21–0.98
Fungal colonization	10.64	1.43–78.74
APACHE III	1.02	1.01–1.04
Days to first dose of study drug	1.34	1.00–1.79

Table 3 Characteristics of 204 Patients Receiving Mechanical Ventilation and Selective Digestive Decontamination with Antibacterial Agents, Randomized to 100 mg Fluconazole Enterally or Placebo

	Fluconazole ($n = 103$)	Placebo ($n = 101$)
APACHE II	21.9	21.3
Colonized at entry	48 (47%)	50 (40%)
Newly colonized after study entry	29/55 (53%)	40/51 (78%)
Colonization index	0.56 ± 0.25	0.53 ± 0.21
Parenteral nutrition	28 (27%)	30 (30%)

Source: From Ref. 71.

infection, or increased colonization was 30% in the fluconazole group and 66% in the placebo group ($P < 0.001$). Crude in-hospital mortality was similar in the two groups (39% fluconazole vs. 41% placebo) (Fig. 4). The authors concluded that prophylactic use of fluconazole in a selected group of mechanically ventilated patients at high risk for infection reduces the incidence of *Candida* infections, in particular, candidemia.

An important feature of this study is the use of low-dose fluconazole, a 200-mg loading dose and then 100 mg/day. This lower dose (vs. that used in the Pelz study) was justified by the high incidence of *C. albicans*, 80% of identified colonizing isolates prior to study entry. Those patients who acquired yeast colonization on this dose maintained a similar species pattern, as did the infected patients. Conversely, only 45% of infecting isolates were *C. albicans* in the fluconazole-treated patients in the Pelz study, vs. 60% in the placebo-treated patients. The lower dose is preferred because of its significantly lower cost, and its clearly demonstrated efficacy; it would also appear to have less drastic effects on the pattern of colonizing and infecting isolates.

Taken together, the results of these two studies would argue that patients known to be at high risk of colonization should be placed on lower-dose fluconazole prophylaxis. The authors of the Garbino study have settled on 200 mg/day as a standard prophylaxis dose. In the case of ICU patients, it may be more cost effective to perform surveillance cultures as done in the EPCAN study on a weekly basis. These cultures are done on yeast-selective media and extensive genus and species workup are not needed.

Table 4 Outcome Results from the Study by Garbino and Colleagues (70)

	Fluconazole	Placebo	*P*
Number of patients colonized at study entry	48 (47%)	50 (49%)	0.78
Number of patients newly colonized after study entry	29/55 (53%)	40/51 (78%)	0.01
Severe infections			
Candidemia	1	9	
Peritonitis	1	1	
Pneumonia	2	0	

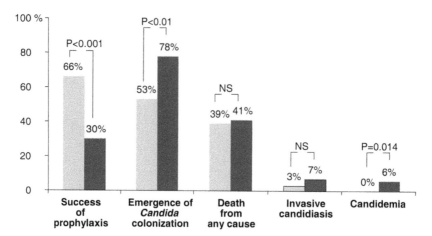

Figure 4 Results of a prospective randomized trial of low-dose fluconazole 100 mg/day ($n = 103$, light gray bar) vs. placebo ($n = 101$, black bar) in the prevention of *Candida* infection in non-neutropenic ICU patients receiving selective digestive decontamination (71).

VI. SPECIAL POPULATIONS AT RISK OF *CANDIDA* INFECTIONS AND POSSIBLY MERITING PROPHYLAXIS

A. Liver Transplantation

The incidence and mechanism of microbial entry vary in different groups of transplant recipients, depending on the organ transplanted, the donor source, the type of surgical procedure performed, and the recipient's age and general condition at the time of the procedure. Other influential factors are the conditioning regimen, the type and duration of immunosuppressive therapy, and the presence or absence of organ rejection, and graft vs. host disease. In heart transplant recipients, for example, *Aspergillus* infection is a major problem (72), whereas in other organ transplant recipients, most fungal infections are attributable to *Candida* (73). The infection is usually located at the site of the operation; an intra-abdominal abscess in liver or pancreas transplantation, the mediastinum or the lungs in heart or heart–lung transplantation, and the urinary tract in kidney transplantation; however, dissemination from the primary site is common (73–75).

Several studies have documented the efficacy of amphotericin B, liposomal amphotericin B, and fluconazole in preventing *Candida* infections (76–79). The incidence of *Candida* infection in patients not receiving prophylaxis varies between 10% and 20%, and prophylaxis is cost effective.

The results of a recently reported randomized trial illustrate the benefits of prophylaxis (80). Fungal colonization increased in patients who received placebo (from 60% to 90%) but decreased in patients who received fluconazole (from 70% to 28%). Proven fungal infection occurred in 45 of 104 placebo recipients(43%), but in only 10 of 108 fluconazole recipients (9%) ($P < 0.001$). Fluconazole prevented both superficial and invasive infection. It also prevented infection by most *Candida* species, except *C. glabrata*. Patients receiving fluconazole had higher serum cyclosporine levels and more adverse neurological events (headaches, tremors, or seizures in 13 fluconazole recipients compared to 3 placebo recipients; $P = 0.01$). Although the overall mortality rate was similar in both groups, [12 of 108 (11%) in the fluconazole group compared with

15 of 104 (14%) in the placebo group; $P > 0.2$], fewer deaths related to invasive fungal infection were seen in the fluconazole group [2 of 108 (2%) patients] than in the placebo group [13 of 104 (13%) patients] ($P = 0.003$).

Five recent studies of antifungal prophylaxis provided additional support for the use of antifungal agents to prevent serious fungal infections in patients undergoing liver transplantation (81–85).

B. Acute Necrotizing Pancreatitis

There is an increasing appreciation for the role of *Candida* in infections following acute pancreatitis (86–88). A large series of patients undergoing operation for infected pancreatic necrosis found *Candida* present in approximately 10% of the patients at their initial operation for infection (89). These patients had received prophylaxis with amoxicillin/clavulanate, a factor that might explain intestinal overgrowth and translocation of *Candida*. This is a particular issue because of the interest in the use of broad-spectrum antibiotics, especially imipenem/cilastatin, as prophylaxis for patients with necrotizing pancreatitis. Current experimental evidence favors the use of prophylactic antibiotics in severe acute pancreatitis. The results of contemporary randomized clinical trials, restricted to patients with prognostically severe acute pancreatitis, have demonstrated improvement in outcome associated with antibiotic treatment (90–92).

The incidence of fungal infection in antibiotic treated patients was demonstrated in a study of 250 consecutive patients treated with amoxicillin/clavulanate with severe acute pancreatitis treated from January 1986 to December 1998 (89). Overall mortality was 38.8% (97 patients). 182 patients (72.8%) suffered from infected necrosis. Among these patients, local *Candida* infection was observed in 31 patients whereas 23 patients (74%) suffered from local fungal infection detected at first operation. During the course of disease, 12 patients (39%) also experienced fungemia. Local *Candida* infection as compared to no *Candida* infection was associated with an increased mortality rate (84% vs. 32% $P = 0.0001$). Multivariate logistic regression analysis identified APACHE II score ($P < 0.0001$), age of the patient ($P < 0.003$), extent of pancreatic necrosis ($P < 0.002$), and local bacterial ($P < 0.04$) and fungal infection ($P < 0.004$) as independent factors significantly contributing to mortality.

It is believed that the appropriate strategy for such patients, a group similar to the population included in the Garbino study of patients receiving selective digestive decontamination, is to provide low-dose fluconazole enterally.

C. Postoperative Intra-Abdominal Infection

Because of the reported high incidence of *Candida* infection in patients with postoperative intra-abdominal infection (93,94), a randomized trial was undertaken in 49 surgical patients with recurrent gastrointestinal perforations or anastomotic leakages (95). Prophylaxis with IV fluconazole (400 mg/day) or placebo continued until resolution of the underlying surgical condition. Among patients who were not colonized at study entry, *Candida* was isolated from surveillance cultures during prophylaxis in 15% of the patients in the fluconazole group and in 62% of the patients in the placebo group (relative risk, 0.25; 95% CI 0.07–0.96; $P = 0.04$). *Candida* peritonitis occurred in 1 of 23 patients (4%) who received fluconazole, and in 7 of 20 patients (35%) who received placebo (relative risk, 0.12; 95% CI 0.02–0.93;

$P = 0.02$). Fluconazole prophylaxis prevents colonization and invasive intra-abdominal *Candida* infections in high-risk surgical patients.

VII.   MANAGEMENT OF SPECIFIC INFECTIONS

A.   Candidemia

Candidemia is defined as the isolation of any pathogenic species of *Candida* from at least one blood culture specimen. The recovery of *Candida* species from the bloodstream is a significant observation, especially if the patient is debilitated, uremic, or receiving immunosuppressive therapy.

There is a general consensus that all episodes of candidemia require therapy (96). The particular concern is the ability of at least *C. albicans* to form vegetations on previously normal heart valves and to establish metastatic abscesses. While the invasiveness of other species is lessened, it seems wisest to treat all episodes.

B.   Is Fluconazole Sufficient for Empiric Antifungal Therapy?

Fluconazole is now considered the primary treatment of choice for candidemia, particularly, if caused by *C. albicans*. This recommendation is based on several recent comparative studies of amphotericin B and fluconazole (97–100). In each of these trials, efficacy was similar, and the incidence of dose-limiting toxicities was significantly lower in persons treated with fluconazole. Therefore, fluconazole has supplanted amphotericin B as the primary treatment for uncomplicated candidemia.

The primary concern with the use of fluconazole for empiric therapy is the possibility that a resistant strain may be present, and the belief that amphotericin B, as a cidal agent, may be more efficacious in patients with shock or other evidence of a severe physiologic response to infection (96). One approach that has been recently studied in a prospective randomized trial is use of combination fluconazole/amphotericin therapy (101). This multicenter trial was conducted to compare fluconazole (800 mg/day) plus placebo with fluconazole plus amphotericin B (AmB) deoxycholate (0.7 mg/kg/day, with the placebo/AmB component given only for the first 5–6 days) as therapy for candidemia resulting from species other than *Candida krusei* in adults without neutropenia. This study addressed, inter alia, the adequacy of this combination regimen as empiric therapy. A total of 219 patients met criteria for a modified intent-to-treat analysis. The groups were similar except that those who were treated with fluconazole plus placebo had a higher mean ($\pm$standard error) APACHE II score (16.8 ± 0.6 vs. 15.0 ± 0.7; $P = 0.039$). Success rates on study day 30 by Kaplan–Meier time-to-failure analysis were 57% for fluconazole plus placebo and 69% for fluconazole plus AmB ($P = 0.08$). Overall success rates were 56% (60 of 107 patients) and 69% (77 of 112 patients; $P = 0.043$), respectively; the bloodstream infection failed to clear in 17% and 6% of subjects, respectively ($P = 0.02$). In non-neutropenic subjects, the combination of fluconazole plus AmB was not antagonistic compared to fluconazole alone, and the combination tended toward improved success and more rapid clearance from the bloodstream (101). No statistically significant difference was found by the prespecified analysis of time to failure between the two arms of the study. However, in the fluconazole plus placebo group, 44% of 107 infections had failed to respond to therapy by 30 days after the initiation of treatment, significantly more than the 31% of 112 patients who received fluconazole plus AmB. Moreover, positive blood cultures were obtained after treatment in 17% of the fluconazole plus placebo patients vs. 6% of those provided fluconazole plus AmB ($P = 0.02$). The data suggest that coadminis-tration of fluconazole plus AmB resulted in a slightly better outcome with the com-bination. It is unlikely that a study will be done comparing fluconazole to fluconazole plus an echinocandin. Since echinocandins are fungicidal, it may be par-ticularly useful to use these agents in patients with evidence of hemodynamic com-promise. Patients who have previously received fluconazole should receive an echinocandin or a polyene (amphotericin B or its lipid formulations).

As more experience has accumulated with fluconazole therapy, particularly recognition that it is efficacious for use in *Candida* infection, the issue of its adequacy as empiric therapy is raised. The answer to this depends primarily on whether or not the patient has received prior antifungal therapy (102,103). *C. albicans* has remained susceptible (26,102,103). There appears to have been a shift toward more frequent isolation of *Candida glabrata*, although this appears highly center dependent. It is also not clear that this is because of widened usage of fluconazole (104). In one large prospective observational study performed at four teaching centers, 13% of candidemias occurred in patients who were already receiving systemic antifungal agents. Candidemias developing while receiving antifungal therapy were more likely caused by non-*C. albicans* species than by *C. albicans* species ($P = 0.0005$). *C. para-psilosis* and *C. krusei* were more commonly seen with prior fluconazole therapy whereas *C. glabrata* was more commonly seen with prior amphotericin B therapy. *Candida* species isolated during episodes of breakthrough candidemia exhibited a significantly higher MIC to the antifungal agent being administered ($P < 0.001$) (105).

C. Duration of Therapy

A further issue is the notion of at least two forms of candidemia. One early study identified a group of patients with transient candidemia who had good outcomes despite receiving no antifungal therapy (106). Patients in this group had no underly-ing disease, had <1 day of documented candidemia, and had central IV catheters removed. A high percentage of these patients were found to be receiving parenteral nutrition, as compared to those patients with prolonged candidemia (66% vs. 24%; $P = 0.002$, χ^2 test). In contrast, patients with documented sustained candidemia (>2 days duration) had a mortality rate of 74%.

The authors of this study then performed a prospective trial of management based on the duration of candidemia. Patients in the transient candidemia group received a total of 200 mg of amphotericin B administered over a 5- to 7-day interval. Patients with persisting candidemia received longer-term therapy to 500 mg total dosing. There were no relapses in either group. One patient in the short course group discontinued amphotericin B prematurely because of an adverse event. Compli-cations of amphotericin B therapy were more common in the prolonged therapy group (68% vs. 38%; $P = 0.02$, χ^2 test). Hypomagnesemia (<2.0 mg/dL) was more common in the prolonged therapy group (55% vs. 7%; $P < 0.001$, χ^2 test). There was a trend toward a higher incidence of elevated creatinine levels (>50% rise from baseline) during treatment with amphotericin B in the prolonged therapy vs. short course group (34% vs. 17%; $P = 0.1$, χ^2 test). The 30-day mortality rate for patients with complicated candidemia (invasive disease and/or a significant underlying con-dition) who were not eligible for the study was 50%, vs. 19% in the two study groups combined ($P < 0.01$, χ^2 test) (34).

Duration of therapy depends on the extent and seriousness of the infection. Therapy can be limited to 7–10 days for patients with catheter-related and low-grade fungemia, without evidence of organ involvement or hemodynamic instability. On the other hand, patients with high-grade fungemia, evidence of organ involvement or hemodynamic instability need to receive antifungal therapy for 10–14 days after resolution of all signs and symptoms of infection.

VIII. CATHETER MANAGEMENT IN CANDIDEMIC PATIENTS

Candidemias seen in the intensive care unit may be catheter related. This is defined as candidemia occurring in a patient with an intravascular catheter and no other obvious site of origin of infection after careful clinical and laboratory evaluation. Several procedures have been developed to aid in the diagnosis of catheter-associated candidemia. If the catheter is removed, a quantitative culture of the tip should recover at least 15 CFU of the same *Candida* species as that found in blood culture by the roll-plate technique, or at least 100 CFU of the same *Candida* species as that found in blood culture by the sonication technique (107,108). If the catheter is not removed, a quantitative blood culture collected through a central catheter should contain at least a 10-fold greater concentration of *Candida* species than a simultaneously collected quantitative peripheral blood culture. Routine catheter tip cultures are of no value (109).

The role of central venous catheters as a factor predicting outcome in candidemia has been evaluated in recent reports. Nguyen et al. (110) reported that catheter-related candidemia had a more favorable prognosis compared to candidemia from other sources, but that prognosis was worse in patients whose catheters were retained. This was supported by a study for duration of candidemia as function of catheter removal in patients entered in a clinical trial of fluconazole vs. amphotericin B (111). A study of candidemia in Brazilian referral hospitals similarly identified only advanced age and catheter retention as significant associates of death (31).

An analysis of 363 patients who had a central venous catheter in place and received antifungal therapy revealed that catheter exchange was associated with improved outcome (80% vs. 54%, $P < 0.001$). However, the no-exchange group of patients had a higher APACHE III scores and were more likely to be neutropenic. By multivariate analysis, catheter retention was not found to significantly affect outcome.

These data suggest that catheters may play a role in perpetuating infection in non-neutropenic patients. On the other hand, the primary source of candidemia is usually the gastrointestinal tract and not the IV catheter in the setting of immunosuppression (neutropenia, corticosteroids, or other immunosuppressants); other factors such as severity of disease, visceral dissemination and recovery of neutrophils, and other immune parameters appear to have more impact on the outcome of candidemia in immunosuppressed patients.

The formation of a biofilm in these infections is likely to be an important determinant of the need to remove the catheter. Histologically, biofilms consist of a dense network of yeasts, germ tubes, pseudohyphae, and hyphae (112). The ability of a species of *Candida* to form biofilm in vitro correlates with its pathogenicity in vivo. Antifungal therapy is not highly effective in removing biofilm from catheters (113). This is particularly important in patients infected with *Candida parapsilosis* (which is more likely to be catheter-related than infection with other *Candida* species) (114).

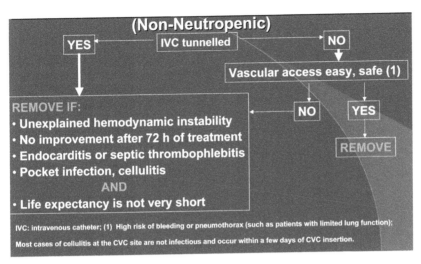

Figure 5 Management of intravascular catheter in candidemia.

The decision to remove the vascular catheter in patients with candidemia must be individualized and depends partly upon the difficulty of inserting a catheter at a new site (Fig. 5).

The use of thrombolytic therapy for infections of surgically implanted catheter has been reported with variable success, particularly, in pediatric hematology patients.

IX. DESCRIPTIONS OF SPECIFIC AGENTS

A. Imidazoles

1. Fluconazole

The mechanism of action of fluconazole is preferential inhibition of cytochrome P450 enzymes in fungal organisms. Fluconazole is active against several *Candida* species, including *C. tropicalis. C. krusei*, however, is highly resistant to this agent (25,26,115–117). Fluconazole is available in either an oral form or an IV form, both of which are rapidly and almost completely absorbed from the GI tract. The serum concentrations after oral administration are almost identical to those achieved when the drug is administered intravenously. A major advantage of fluconazole over keto-conazole is its high degree of GI absorption, which is not affected by gastric acidity or the presence of food. Steady-state serum concentrations of fluconazole are obtained within 5–10 days. An initial loading dose that is twice the usual daily dose is recommended. Fluconazole is distributed evenly in body tissues, penetrates into the vitreous humor and the aqueous humor of the eye, and crosses the blood–brain barrier. The drug is excreted largely unchanged in the urine, with only minimal liver metabolism (118–120). Consequently, dosage schedules must be adjusted in patients with renal impairment. Hemodialysis significantly reduces the serum concentrations, and the drug also appears to be removed by peritoneal dialysis. A standard dose should be given after each course of dialysis.

The toxicities of fluconazole are similar to those of other azoles and include nausea and vomiting in about 2% of patients, headache, fatigue, abdominal pain, and diarrhea; exfoliative dermatitis also occurs, but very rarely (121). Transient abnormalities of liver function have been observed in 3% of patients receiving fluconazole. In addition, fatal hepatic necrosis developed in two patients who were receiving fluconazole, but it was unclear whether the agent played a causal role in this event. No significant hormonal abnormalities have been reported after administration of fluconazole.

2. Itraconazole

Itraconazole is highly lipophilic and is tightly bound to blood cells and plasma proteins, primarily albumin, leaving only 0.2% unbound (122). It is metabolized primarily in the liver, and the single dose pharmacokinetics is not affected by renal dysfunction. The erratic absorption and reduced bioavailability of the capsule form has been overcome with the introduction of a liquid formulation in cyclodextrin (123).

Itraconazole's main metabolite, hydroxyitraconazole, reaches higher plasma concentrations than the parent compound and has in vitro antifungal activity similar to that of itraconazole (122).

Itraconazole, and to a lesser extent fluconazole (in high doses) are inhibitors of CYP3A4. Therefore, certain agents that are substrates of this enzyme, such as some of the new generation of H1-antihistamines, several HMG-CoA reductase inhibitors, and certain benzodiazepines, are contraindicated. Other drugs like cyclosporine and quinidine need careful monitoring if administered concurrently with these triazoles. Because fluconazole interacts with warfarin, phenytoin, and cyclosporine when given in a daily dose of 200 mg or more, serum concentrations of these agents should be monitored.

B. Voriconazole

Voriconazole is a second-generation azole antifungal agent that shows excellent in vitro activity against a wide variety of yeasts and molds. Voriconazole is a derivative of fluconazole that demonstrates enhanced in vitro activity against existing and emerging fungal pathogens. It can be given by either the IV or the oral route; the oral formulation has excellent bioavailability.

It has proven efficacy for treating *Candida* infections and invasive aspergillosis as well as other mould infections, such as those caused by *Fusarium* and *Scedosporium* spp. (124). Voriconazole has three important side effects that the clinician must consider: liver abnormalities, skin abnormalities, and visual disturbances. Liver abnormalities, in particular, should be monitored very carefully. The drug interaction profile of voriconazole also warrants a careful evaluation of the concomitant medications because of its inhibition of cytochrome P450. It should be noted that safety considerations related to the cyclodextrin carriers limit the IV formulation of itraconazole to administration for no longer than 14 days, and that the comparable formulation of voriconazole should not be administered to patients with a creatinine clearance of <50 mL/min (package inserts).

The side effect profile of voriconazole is unique in that transient visual disturbances that do not threaten eyesight occur in ~30% of patients given the drug. Rashes (which can manifest as photosensitivity) and hepatitis also occur. The potential for drug-drug interactions is high and requires that careful attention be given to dosage regimens, monitoring of serum levels, and effects of interacting drugs (125).

Voriconazole has been approved for the treatment of invasive aspergillosis and refractory infections with *Pseudallescheria/Scedosporium* and *Fusarium* species and will likely become the drug of choice for treatment of serious infections with those filamentous fungi.

The in vitro activities of voriconazole, posaconazole, ravuconazole, and micafungin were compared with those of fluconazole, itraconazole, ketoconazole, flucytosine, and amphotericin B against 164 candidemia isolates recovered from cancer patients in two Canadian centers (126). The MIC (50) for ravuconazole, voriconazole, posaconazole, and micafungin were 0.01, 0.03, 0.12, and 0.25 mg/L, respectively. The new antifungal agents showed substantial activity against isolates demonstrating in vitro resistance to fluconazole and itraconazole. These results suggest that the newer antifungal agents possess promising activity against invasive *Candida* isolates, particularly against those with reduced susceptibility to fluconazole and itraconazole.

C. Amphotericin B

Amphotericin B is structurally similar to membrane sterols, and its major mechanism of action is believed to be through interaction with membrane sterols and creation of pores in the fungal outer membrane (115,127). The clinical usefulness of amphotericin B is attributable to the greater affinity of amphotericin B for ergosterol (found in fungal cell membranes) than for cholesterol (the principal sterol found in mammalian cell membranes). Oxidation-dependent amphotericin B-induced stimulation of macrophages is another proposed mechanism of action (128,129). Most species of fungi that cause human infections are susceptible to amphotericin B.

Amphotericin B (AmB) is active against most systemic fungal infections. It is supplied as an AmB–deoxycholate complex suitable for IV administration. The association between AmB and deoxycholate is relatively weak; therefore, dissociation occurs in the blood. The drug itself interacts with both mammalian and fungal cell membranes to damage cells, but the greater susceptibility of fungal cells to its effects forms the basis for its clinical usefulness.

The use of AmB is associated with frequent and potentially severe side effects, including infusion-related events such as fever, rigors, and hypotension, as well as metabolic derangements such as hypokalemia and nephrotoxicity (130). The frequency of occurrence of such events may be as high as 80%. Infusion-related toxicities (e.g., fever, chills, and rigors) are likely due to AmB stimulation of cytokine and prostaglandin synthesis (131,132). Nephrotoxicity, the primary non-infusion-related toxicity, is likely to result from the nonselective cytotoxic interaction between AmB and cholesterol-containing mammalian cells (133). An acute infusion-related reaction, consisting of fever, hypotension, and tachycardia, occurs in about 20% of patients (134). Premedication regimes with, for example, acetaminophen, or hydrocortisone, are of little if any value. Meperidine (25–50 mg IV) will alleviate fevers and chills if given after they occur (135,136). Hypotension, hypertension, hypothermia, and bradycardia are other reported infusion-related toxic effects of amphotericin B deoxycholate. Ventricular arrhythmias have been associated with administration of amphotericin B deoxycholate in patients with severe hypokalemia, renal failure, or those in whom the infusion was rapidly given. Amphotericin B suppresses production of red blood cells and causes a normocytic, normochromic anemia. This is because of the inhibition of erythropoietin production is secondary to nephrotoxicity.

Common practice has been to give a 1-mg test dose and observe the patient for 1 hr in the hope of identifying patients at risk for severe acute reactions. The full dose of the drug (0.6–1 mg/kg/day) is then infused over a period of 4–6 hr, although recent data suggest that much shorter infusion times (e.g., 1 hr in patients with adequate cardiopulmonary and renal function) may be acceptable (137). The total dose depends on the extent of the infection and the patient's condition. Patients must be monitored carefully during the first day of therapy. The infusion should be discontinued if the patient becomes hemodynamically unstable.

Renal toxicity and hypokalemia are the primary toxicities of amphotericin B (138–140). Amphotericin B-induced nephrotoxicity may be glomerular (decrease in glomerular filtration rate and renal blood flow) or tubular (urinary cast, hypokalemia, hypomagnesemia, renal tubular acidosis, and nephrocalcinosis). All these abnormalities occur to varying degrees in almost all patients receiving the drug. Renal dysfunction gradually resolves after discontinuation of therapy in most patients.

Amphotericin B nephrotoxicity may be minimized by avoiding other agents with synergistic nephrotoxicity (e.g., aminoglycosides, vancomycin, cisplatin, and cyclosporine), and the administration of sodium supplementation. The latter approach consists of the IV infusion of 500 ml of 0.9% saline solution 30 min before the administration of amphotericin B and a second infusion of the same amount of saline after the amphotericin B infusion is completed (141,142).

The combined use of amphotericin B deoxycholate and other nephrotoxic agents (cyclosporine, aminoglycosides, foscarnet, and others) may result in synergistic nephrotoxicity.

D. Lipid Formulations of Amphotericin B

Newer therapeutic options have now become available with the advent of the lipid-associated formulations of amphotericin B, which are less nephrotoxic than the parent compound (143,144). So far, three lipid products of amphotericin B have been marketed in Europe and in the United States: Abelcet (amphotericin B lipid complex), Amphocil (amphotericin B colloidal dispersion), and AmBisome (liposomal amphotericin B). A prospective randomized trial has shown that Abelcet was as efficacious as conventional amphotericin B in hematogenous candidiasis (145).

Lipid formulations of amphotericin B are less nephrotoxic. These preparations differ in the amount of amphotericin B and the type of lipid used as well as in the physical form, pharmacokinetics and toxicities. Studies comparing lipid formulations of Amphotericin to the parent compound have shown a reduction in nephrotoxicity. In addition, *AmBisome* appears to reduce the incidence of acute infusion-related adverse events and hypokalemia, and to be better tolerated than amphotericin B lipid complex. However, given the great cost of these formulations and incomplete avoidance of amphotericin B toxicity, their use should be restricted to patients with significant renal impairment or patients failing on AmB therapy who cannot be treated with newer imidazoles or echinocandins.

E. The Echinocandins

The echinocandins are large lipopeptide molecules that are inhibitors of beta-(1,3)-glucan synthesis, an action that results in disruption of the fungal cell wall, in turn resulting in osmotic stress, lysis, and death of the microorganism (126,146). Two other echinocandins, anidulafungin and micafungin, are near FDA approval (146,147). In vitro and in vivo, the echinocandins are rapidly fungicidal against most *Candida* spp. and fungistatic against *Aspergillus* spp. No drug target is present in mammalian cells. The first of the class to be licensed was caspofungin, for refractory invasive aspergillosis (about 40% response rate). Adverse events are generally mild, including (for caspofungin) local phlebitis, fever, abnormal liver function tests, and mild hemolysis (148,149). Poor absorption after oral administration limits use to the IV route. Dosing is once daily and drug interactions are few. The echinocandins are widely distributed in the body and are metabolized by the liver.

Results of studies of caspofungin in candidemia and invasive candidiasis demonstrate equivalent efficacy to amphotericin B, with substantially fewer toxic effects (150). The results of a trial comparing caspofungin to amphotericin are detailed in Table 5. This study randomizes patients with invasive candidiasis (83% had candidemia and 10% had peritonitis) to receive either caspofungin (70 mg on day 1, then 50 mg q.d.) or conventional amphotericin B (0.6–1.0 mg/kg q.d.) for 14 days (149). 46% of infections were caused by *C. albicans*, 19% by *C. parapsilosis*, 16% by *C. tropicalis*, and 11% by *C. glabrata*; *C. krusei*, and *C. guilliermondii* accounted for the rest. Success was defined as both symptom resolution and microbiological clearance. By a modified intent-to-treat analysis of the 224 eligible randomized patients who received at least a single dose of their assigned therapy, success was observed in 73% of caspofungin recipients and in 62% of amphotericin B recipients ($P=0.09$). Among patients who received ≥ 5 days of therapy, success was achieved in 81% of caspofungin recipients and in 65% of amphotericin B recipients ($P=0.03$).

Table 5 Results from a Randomized Trial of Caspofungin Vs. Amphotericin B in the Management of Invasive *Candida* Infection

	Caspofungin 70/50 mg ($n=109$)		Amphotericin B, 0.6–1.0 mg/kg ($n=115$)	
	N	(%)	n	(%)
Failure (end of Rx)	29	(26.6)	44	(38.2)
Persistently (+) cultures	9	(8.3)	10	(8.7)
Persistent signs/symptoms	6	(5.5)	5	(4.3)
New lesions at distant sites	4	(3.7)	5	(4.3)
Toxicity requiring additional Rx*	3	(2.7)	19	(16.5)
Withdrawal ≤ 4 days/indeterminate	7	(6.4)	5	(4.3)
Relapse (6–8 weeks post-Rx)	7	(6.4)	8	(7.0)
Recurrent candidemia	3	(2.7)	2	(1.7)
Nonblood *Candida* infection	2	(1.8)	0	NA
Received systemic antifungal Rx	1	(0.9)	6	(5.2)
Abscess (no culture and no Rx)	1	(0.9)	0	NA

Source: From Ref. 150.
*$P = 0.028$.

Significantly, adverse events occurred more frequently among amphotericin B recipients than among caspofungin recipients; discontinuation of therapy as a result of drug-related adverse events was observed in 23% and 3% of recipients, respectively.

X. RECOMMENDATIONS FOR THERAPY—A CARE PATH

Figure 6 is an algorithm that has been developed for use at the University of Cincinnati. This algorithm is provided to aid the development of care paths for management of *Candida* infections. Therapy is divided into prophylaxis, empiric, and directed. Indications for prophylaxis in the general ICU population center upon

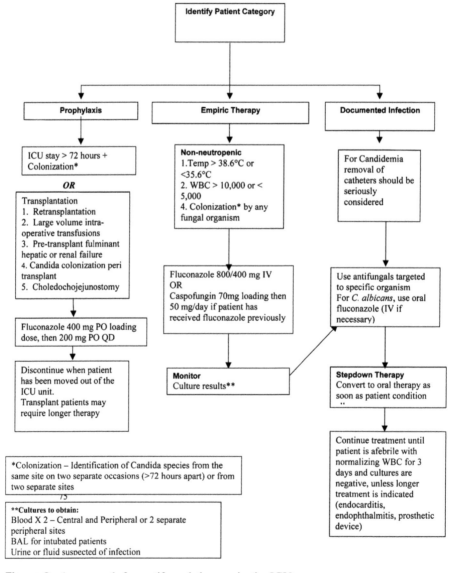

Figure 6 A care path for antifungal therapy in the ICU.

the presence of colonization. There are, nonetheless, specific conditions that mandate prophylaxis with fluconazole in the absence of colonization. These include status post-intervention for a post-operative infection (95), necrotizing pancreatitis, particularly if parenteral prophylaxis with broad-spectrum antibacterial agents is administered (89), and units with a high (>10%) incidence of yeast infections (70A). For these patients, prophylaxis with fluconazole is directed at *C. albicans*, absent evidence that fluconazole prophylaxis will decrease infections with other *Candida* species. With the high level of fluconazole activity against *C. albicans*, dosing with 400 mg load and 200 mg/day enterally with adjustments for renal failure is recommended (71). Prophylaxis is continued until the risk of infection is diminished, especially until transfer out of ICU. Prophylaxis will decrease infection by 50–70%.

The indications for empiric therapy in non-neutropenic patients center primarily on patients with sudden onset of signs of infection and documented colonization, particularly, in the absence of prior colonization. All patients with candidemia should receive antifungal therapy. If such patients have not previously received prophylaxis or therapy with fluconazole, then, therapy with fluconazole (800 mg loading dose with 400 mg daily) is indicated until speciation is available. Despite evidence that combination therapy with amphotericin B may improve outcomes, acute responses do not seem to be altered by this strategy.

If the patient has received fluconazole treatment, initial therapy should be with caspofungin or amphotericin B (or its lipid formulations). Voriconazole may be a suitable alternative but sufficient data to support this recommendation are not available.

With the availability of highly active agents, including fluconazole and caspofungin, there is now little role for amphotericin B. In the ICU, the toxicity of amphotericin B, when added to the severity of illness of patients with *Candida* infections, becomes a significant risk for increased morbidity and mortality.

XI. OTHER SITES OF *CANDIDA* INFECTIONS

A. Candida Endophthalmitis

The diagnosis of candidal endophthalmitis usually implies hematogenous spread to multiple organs and thus systemic antifungal therapy is warranted. Patients with chorioretinitis alone respond better to drug therapy than those with vitreal involvement because of the lower drug penetration in the vitreous body than in the other ocular compartments (152). Patients with vitreal involvement will require early vitrectomy in addition to antifungal therapy. Fluconazole is currently the drug of choice because of its proven efficacy and its better ocular tissue concentration including in the vitreous body (20–70% of corresponding plasma level) (153,154). A daily fluconazole dose of 800 mg is recommended until a major response has been observed at which time a reduction of the dose to 400 mg/day may be possible. While endophthalmitis due to *C. albicans* is commonly seen, more recent series have reported on the importance of endophthalmitis by non-*C. albicans* spp. If the infecting organism is potentially resistant to fluconazole (especially *C. krusei*), initiation of therapy with IV amphotericin (0.7–1.0 mg/kg/day IV) preferably in conjunction with flucytosine is recommended. Intravitreal injection of amphotericin B is also recommended in the presence of vitreal infection.

The optimal duration of therapy for endogenous endophthalmitis is not defined, but it is recommend that it be given for at least 10–14 days after complete resolution of all signs and symptoms of infection. Ophthalmologic consultation is critical in establishing the diagnosis, assessing the patient's response to therapy, detecting complications, and determining whether early vitrectomy is indicated to prevent loss of sight (155).

B. Suppurative Thrombophlebitis

A rare but serious consequence of hematogenous candidemia is suppurative thrombophlebitis, which results from infection of a vessel traumatized by prolonged catheterization. Endothelial disruption exposes the basement membrane and leads to thrombus formation and propagation. Suppurative thrombophlebitis is particularly serious because intravascular infection results in a persistent high-density fungemia. Management of this disease consists of high-dose antifungal therapy, removal of the central venous catheter, and excision of the infected vein, when possible (156,157). Typically, blood cultures remain positive for several days; sometimes, they remain positive for as long as 3–4 weeks despite appropriate antifungal therapy, if the infected vein is not excised.

C. Superficial Mucosal Infection

Oral candidiasis (thrush) appears as a whitish, patchy pseudomembrane covering an inflamed oropharynx and commonly involves the tongue, the hard and soft palates, and the tonsillar pillars. Controlled trials have documented the efficacy of nystatin suspension, clotrimazole troches, oral ketoconazole, fluconazole, or itraconazole in eradicating the clinical symptoms of oral candidiasis (158,159).

Nystatin should be given as a 10- to 30-ml suspension five times daily, and the patient should be instructed to swish it around the mouth before swallowing; alternatively, the patient may take one or two troches five times daily. Clotrimazole troches are given five times daily as a 10-mg troche that should be held in the mouth until dissolved. In surgical patients at risk for hematogenous infection, systemic therapy with ketoconazole (200–400 mg once daily), oral itraconazole solution (100–200 mg/day), or fluconazole (100 mg once daily) is preferred. Antifungal therapy should be administered for 1 week.

D. Peritonitis and Intra-Abdominal Abscess

A controversial aspect of *Candida* infectious syndromes in surgical patients is whether systemic therapy is required to eradicate *Candida* found within intra-abdominal abscesses, peritoneal fluid, or fistula drainage. *Candida* is frequently cultured from intra-abdominal infectious foci but should be considered a serious threat only in specific patient groups. Four risk factors for intra-abdominal *Candida* infection have been identified including failed treatment for intra-abdominal infection, anastomotic leakage following elective or urgent operation, surgery for acute pancreatitis, and splenectomy (93,94,160).

Systemic antifungal therapy should be provided for those patients found to have *Candida* at the site of recurrent of intra-abdominal infection or previous operation, including patients with extensive areas of communication between the abdominal cavity and the external environment via either fistulas or drain tracts. Antibacterial therapy should be provided if bacteria are identified either by Gram stain or culture. Most of these patients will have polymicrobial infection.

Occasionally, *Candida* species may cause acalculous cholecystitis or cholangitis (161,162). This problem is increasingly found in patients with percutaneously placed drainage catheters for malignancy (163). Such patients must be given systemic therapy for clinical evidence of infection, including candidemia, and the drainage catheter must be changed.

Because fluconazole is very safe and is capable of reaching high concentrations in peritoneal fluid, it is likely to be useful in the management of candidal peritonitis (164,165). Fluconazole should be given at a dosage of 100–200 mg/day orally for 2–6 weeks. Immediate removal of the peritoneal catheter has been recommended. In one study, however, seven of nine patients treated with oral flucytosine responded to therapy without catheter removal (166).

E. Urinary Tract Infection

The recovery of *Candida* species from the urinary tract most commonly results from contamination from the perirectal or the genital area. Bladder colonization is usually seen in patients who have undergone prolonged catheterization, or have diabetes mellitus, or any other disease that leads to incomplete bladder emptying. In addition, *Candida* species usually colonize in ileal conduits. Persistent candiduria in the surgical intensive care unit may, however, be an early marker of disseminated infection in critically ill high-risk patients (167). Alkalization of the urine with oral potassium–sodium hydrogen citrate is a simple and an effective method of treating candiduria in-patients with an indwelling catheter. Replacing or removing the bladder catheter is preferable. If *Candida* colonization persists, particularly, if the patient has a risk factor for cystitis (e.g., diabetes mellitus or a disease that leads to incomplete bladder emptying) or for hematogenous dissemination (e.g., immunosuppression or manipulation of the genitourinary system), antifungal therapy should be considered. Amphotericin B bladder irrigation only provides temporary clearance of funguria and systemic agents (single-dose IV amphotericin B or a 5-day course of oral fluconazole) are usually needed. Recently, a large multicenter prospective study has evaluated fluconazole vs. amphotericin B bladder irrigations for this condition (168). This study included very few ICU patients and thus was unable to specifically address the issue of progression to candidemia. Candiduria cleared by day 14 in 79 (50%) of 159 receiving fluconazole and 46 (29%) of 157 receiving placebo ($P < 0.001$). Fluconazole initially produced high eradication rates, but cultures at 2 weeks revealed similar candiduria rates among treated and untreated patients. Oral fluconazole was safe and effective for short-term eradication of candiduria, especially following catheter removal. Long-term eradication rates were disappointing and not associated with clinical benefit.

Fluconazole, 200 mg once daily, is a more attractive approach because of the convenience, cost, and very high drug concentrations achieved in the urine (169). Flucytosine is excreted in the urine in high concentrations and may be particularly useful against *C. glabrata* infection.

F. Pneumonia

Pulmonary infection remains a common and important complication of ventilator therapy. There is clear evidence that quantitative microbiology obtained by protected specimen techniques provides accurate identification of patients who have a worse prognosis than patients with negative cultures. Patients with positive cultures also appear to benefit from therapy directed specifically at the organisms identified by such techniques.

There is little information, however, regarding the significance of *Candida* species from such cultures. Until recently, *Candida* pneumonitis was considered a complication of neutropenia, with infection arising from embolism to bronchial vessels. However, this notion has more recently been challenged by data supporting the occurrence of *Candida* pneumonia in non-neutropenic patients, arising from aspiration of oropharyngeal contents. In one study involving immediate postmortem study of lung tissue in ventilated critically ill patients, 8% of such otherwise unselected patients demonstrated histologic *Candida* infection (170,171). These authors concluded, from a careful histologic study, that *Candida* colonization is uniform throughout the different lung regions, and that the presence of *Candida* in respiratory samples, independently of quantitative cultures, is not a good marker of pneumonia in critically ill, non-neutropenic, non-AIDS patients.

Nonetheless, there is little evidence of clinical or histological basis to support or recommend therapy for *Candida* obtained by tracheal or endotracheal aspirate or alveolar lavage. We believe that these techniques only document the presence of the organism in the oropharynx. While such cultures may support the use of fluconazole for antifungal prophylaxis, such cultures do not warrant therapeutic intervention.

XII. CONCLUSIONS

Continued progress in supportive care, including the development of antibiotics with increasingly broad spectra of activity has resulted in an increasing frequency of fugal infections, particularly candidiasis. Because of the inadequacy of the available knowledge base, we do not fully understand the pathophysiology of these infections in surgical patients, nor can we be always certain as to precisely when prophylaxis and therapy should be administered.

Despite these limitations, there is now sufficient information available to justify an aggressive therapeutic approach to suspected *Candida* infections. Now that less toxic agents are available (the newer triazoles, particularly fluconazole, and the lipid formulations of amphotericin B), the clinical approach to presumed fungal infections has been made far simpler.

REFERENCES

1. Yang YL. Virulence factors of Candida species. J Microbiol Immunol Infect 2003; 36(4):223–228.
2. Romani L, Bistoni F, Puccetti P. Adaptation of *Candida albicans* to the host environment: the role of morphogenesis in virulence and survival in mammalian hosts. Curr Opin Microbiol 2003; 6(4):338–343.
3. Liu H. Co-regulation of pathogenesis with dimorphism and phenotypic switching in *Candida albicans*, a commensal and a pathogen. Int J Med Microbiol 2002; 292(5–6):299–311.
4. Ibata-Ombetta S, Idziorek T, Trinel PA, Poulain D, Jouault T. *Candida albicans* phospholipomannan promotes survival of phagocytosed yeasts through modulation of bad phosphorylation and macrophage apoptosis. J Biol Chem 2003; 278(15):13086–13093.

5. Alvarez-Peral FJ, Zaragoza O, Pedreno Y, Arguelles JC. Protective role of trehalose during severe oxidative stress caused by hydrogen peroxide and the adaptive oxidative stress response in *Candida albicans*. Microbiology 2002; 148(Pt 8):2599–2606.
6. Gow NA. Germ tube growth of *Candida albicans*. Curr Top Med Mycol 1997; 8(1–2):43–55.
7. Cotter G, Kavanagh K. Adherence mechanisms of *Candida albicans*. Br J Biomed Sci 2000; 57(3):241–249.
8. Hostetter MK. Integrin-like proteins in *Candida* spp. and other microorganisms. Fungal Genet Biol 1999; 28(3):135–145.
9. Bendel CM, St Sauver J, Carlson S, Hostetter MK. Epithelial adhesion in yeast species: correlation with surface expression of the integrin analog. J Infect Dis 1995; 171(6):1660–1663.
10. DeMuri GP, Hostetter MK. Evidence for a beta 1 integrin fibronectin receptor in *Candida tropicalis*. J Infect Dis 1996; 174(1):127–132.
11. Bendel CM, Hostetter MK. Distinct mechanisms of epithelial adhesion for Candida albicans and *Candida tropicalis*. Identification of the participating ligands and development of inhibitory peptides. J Clin Invest 1993; 92(4):1840–1849.
12. Hostetter MK. Adhesion and morphogenesis in *Candida albicans*. Pediatr Res 1996; 39(4 Pt 1):569–573.
13. Hotsetter MK. Integrin-like proteins in *Candida* spp. and other micro organisms. Fungal Genet Biol 1999; 28(3):135–145.
14. Hostetter MK. Linkage of adhesion, morphogenesis, and virulence in *Candida albicans*. J Lab Clin Med 1998; 132(4):258–263.
15. Naglik JR, Challacombe SJ, Hube B. *Candida albicans* secreted aspartyl proteinases in virulence and pathogenesis [table]. Microbiol Mol Biol Rev 2003; 67(3):400–428.
16. Fallon K, Bausch K, Noonan J, Huguenel E, Tamburini P. Role of aspartic proteases in disseminated *Candida albicans* infection in mice. Infect Immun 1997; 65(2):551–556.
17. Hoegl L, Ollert M, Korting HC. The role of *Candida albicans* secreted aspartic proteinase in the development of candidoses. J Mol Med 1996; 74(3):135–142.
18. Hube B, Sanglard D, Odds FC, Hess D, Monod M, Schafer W, et al. Disruption of each of the secreted aspartyl proteinase genes SAP1, SAP2, and SAP3 of Candida albicans attenuates virulence. Infect Immun 1997; 65(9):3529–3538..
19. Sanglard D, Hube B, Monod M, Odds FC, Gow NA. A triple deletion of the secreted aspartyl proteinase genes SAP4, SAP5, and SAP6 of *Candida albicans* causes attenuated virulence. Infect Immun 1997; 65(9):3539–3546.
20. Cormack BP, Ghori N, Falkow S. An adhesin of the yeast pathogen *Candida glabrata* mediating adherence to human epithelial cells [see comments]. Science 1999; 285(5427):578–582.
21. Miyakawa Y, Kuribayashi T, Kagaya K, Suzuki M, Nakase T, Fukazawa Y. Role of specific determinants in mannan of *Candida albicans* serotype A in adherence to human buccal epithelial cells. Infect Immun 1992; 60(6):2493–2499.
22. Beck-Sague C, Jarvis WR. Secular trends in the epidemiology of nosocomial fungal infections in the United States, 1980–1990. National Nosocomial Infections Surveillance System. J Infect Dis 1993; 167(5):1247–1251.
23. National Nosocomial Infections Surveillance (NNIS) System report, data summary from January 1990–May 1999, issued June 1999. Am J Infect Control 1999; 27[6]:520–532.
24. Edmond MB, Wallace SE, McClish DK, Pfaller MA, Jones RN, Wenzel RP. Nosocomial bloodstream infections in United States hospitals: a three-year analysis. Clin Infect Dis 1999; 29(2):239–244.
25. Pfaller MA, Jones RN, Messer SA, Edmond MB, Wenzel RP. National surveillance of nosocomial blood stream infection due to species of *Candida* other than *Candida albicans*: frequency of occurrence and antifungal susceptibility in the SCOPE Program.

SCOPE Participant Group. Surveillance and Control of Pathogens of Epidemiologic. Diagn Microbiol Infect Dis 1998; 30(2):121–129.

26. Pfaller MA, Messer SA, Hollis RJ, Jones RN, Doern GV, Brandt ME, et al. Trends in species distribution and susceptibility to fluconazole among blood stream isolates of Candida species in the United States. Diagn Microbiol Infect Dis 1999; 33(4):217–222.

27. Abi-Said D, Anaissie E, Uzun O, Raad I, Pinzcowski H, Vartivarian S. The epidemiology of hematogenous candidiasis caused by different *Candida* species [see comments] [published erratum appears in Clin Infect Dis 1997 Aug;25(2):352]. Clin Infect Dis 1997; 24(6):1122–1128.

28. Garbino J, Kolarova L, Rohner P, Lew D, Pichna P, Pittet D. Secular trends of candidemia over 12 years in adult patients at a tertiary care hospital. Medicine (Baltimore) 2002; 81(6):425–433.

29. Wey SB, Mori M, Pfaller MA, Woolson RF, Wenzel RP. Hospital-acquired candidemia. The attributable mortality and excess length of stay. Arch Intern Med 1988; 148:2642–2645.

30. Nolla-Salas J, Sitges-Serra A, Leon-Gil C, Martinez-Gonzalez J, Leon-Regidor MA, Ibanez-Lucia P, et al. Candidemia in non-neutropenic critically ill patients: analysis of prognostic factors and assessment of systemic antifungal therapy. Study Group of Fungal Infection in the ICU. Intensive Care Med 1997; 23(1):23–30.

31. Nucci M, Colombo AL, Silveira F, Richtmann R, Salomao R, Branchini ML, et al. Risk factors for death in patients with candidemia. Infect Control Hosp Epidemiol 1998; 19(11):846–850.

32. Gudlaugsson O, Gillespie S, Lee K, Vande BJ, Hu J, Messer S, et al. Attributable mortality of nosocomial candidemia, revisited. Clin Infect Dis 2003; 37(9):1172–1177.

33. Pappas PG, Rex JH, Lee J, Hamill RJ, Larsen RA, Powderly W, et al. A prospective observational study of candidemia: epidemiology, therapy, and influences on mortality in hospitalized adult and pediatric patients. Clin Infect Dis 2003; 37(5):634–643.

34. Fichtenbaum CJ, German M, Dunagan WC, Fraser VJ, Medoff G, Diego J, et al. A pilot study of the management of uncomplicated candidemia with a standardized protocol of amphotericin B. Clin Infect Dis 1999; 29(6):1551–1556.

35. Knaus WA, Draper EA, Wagner DP, Zimmerman JE. APACHE II: a severity of disease classification system. Crit Care Med 1985; 13(10):818–829.

36. Knaus WA, Wagner DP, Draper EA, Zimmerman JE, Bergner M, Bastos PG, et al. The APACHE III prognostic system. Risk prediction of hospital mortality for critically ill hospitalized adults. Chest 1991; 100(6):1619–1636.

37. Krause W, Matheis H, Wulf K. Fungaemia and funguria after oral administration of *Candida albicans*. Lancet 1969; 1(7595):598–599.

38. Walsh TJ, Merz WG. Pathologic features in the human alimentary tract associated with invasiveness of *Candida tropicalis*. Am J Clin Pathol 1986; 85:498–502.

39. Deitch EA, Xu D, Naruhn MB, Deitch DC, Lu Q, Marino AA. Elemental diet and IV-TPN-induced bacterial translocation is associated with loss of intestinal mucosal barrier function against bacteria [see comments]. Ann Surg 1995; 221(3):299–307.

40. Slocum MM, Sittig KM, Specian RD, Deitch EA. Absence of intestinal bile promotes bacterial translocation. Am Surg 1992; 58(5):305–310.

41. Deitch EA, Ma WJ, Ma L, Berg R, Specian RD. Endotoxin-induced bacterial translocation: a study of mechanisms. Surgery 1989; 106(2):292–299.

42. Alexander JW, Boyce ST, Babcock GF, Gianotti L, Peck MD, Dunn DL, et al. The process of microbial translocation. Ann Surg 1990; 212:496–510; discussion.

43. DeWitt RC, Kudsk KA. The gut's role in metabolism, mucosal barrier function, and gut immunology. Infect Dis Clin N Am 1999; 13(2):465–481, x.

44. Bengmark S. Immunonutrition: role of biosurfactants, fiber, and probiotic bacteria. Nutrition 1998; 14(7–8):585–594.

45. Pappo I, Polacheck I, Zmora O, Feigin E, Freund HR. Altered gut barrier function to *Candida* during parenteral nutrition. Nutrition 1994; 10(2):151–154.

46. Deitch EA, Sittig K, Li M, Berg R, Specian RD. Obstructive jaundice promotes bacterial translocation from the gut. Am J Surg 1990; 159(1):79–84.
47. Kennedy MJ, Volz PA. Ecology of *Candida albicans* gut colonization: inhibition of *Candida* adhesion, colonization, and dissemination from the gastrointestinal tract by bacterial antagonism. Infect Immun 1985; 49(3):654–663.
48. Gianotti L, Alexander JW, Fukushima R, Childress CP. Translocation of *Candida albicans* is related to the blood flow of individual intestinal villi. Circ Shock 1993; 40(4): 250–257.
49. Tancrede CH, Andremont AO. Bacterial translocation and Gram-negative bacteremia in patients with hematological malignancies. J Infect Dis 1985; 152(1):99–103.
50. .Vincent P, Colombel JF, Lescut D, Fournier L, Savage C, Cortot A, et al. Bacterial translocation in patients with colorectal cancer [letter]. J Infect Dis 1988; 158(6):1395–1396.
51. Deitch EA. Simple intestinal obstruction causes bacterial translocation in man. Arch Surg 1989; 124(6):699–701.
52. Ambrose NS, Johnson M, Burdon DW, Keighley MR. Incidence of pathogenic bacteria from mesenteric lymph nodes and ileal serosa during Crohn's disease surgery. Br J Surg 1984; 71(8):623–625.
53. Wells CL, Maddaus MA, Simmons RL. Proposed mechanisms for the translocation of intestinal bacteria. Rev Infect Dis 1988; 10(5):958–979.
54. Lederer JA, Rodrick ML, Mannick JA. The effects of injury on the adaptive immune response. Shock 1999; 11(3):153–159.
55. Schaffer M, Barbul A. Lymphocyte function in wound healing and following injury. Br J Surg 1998; 85(4):444–460.
56. Gogos CA, Kalfarentzos F. Total parenteral nutrition and immune system activity: a review [see comments]. Nutrition 1995; 11(4):339–344.
57. Shou J, Lappin J, Minnard EA, Daly JM. Total parenteral nutrition, bacterial translocation, and host immune function. Am J Surg 1994; 167(1):145–150.
58. Goodman JL, Winston DJ, Greenfield RA, Chandrasekar PH, Fox B, Kaizer H, et al. A controlled trial of fluconazole to prevent fungal infections in patients undergoing bone marrow transplantation. N Engl J Med 1992; 326:845–851.
59. Uzun O, Anaissie EJ. Antifungal prophylaxis in patients with hematologic malignancies: a reappraisal [see comments]. Blood 1995; 86(6):2063–2072.
60. Reagan DR, Pfaller MA, Hollis RJ, Wenzel RP. Characterization of the sequence of colonization and nosocomial candidemia using DNA fingerprinting and a DNA probe. J Clin Microbiol 1990; 28(12):2733–2738.
61. Voss A, Hollis RJ, Pfaller MA, Wenzel RP, Doebbeling BN. Investigation of the sequence of colonization and candidemia in nonneutropenic patients. J Clin Microbiol 1994; 32(4):975–980.
62. Pfaller M, Cabezudo I, Koontz F, Bale M, Gingrich R. Predictive value of surveillance cultures for systemic infection due to *Candida* species. Eur J Clin Microbiol 1987; 6(6):628–633.
63. Martino P, Girmenia C, Venditti M, Micozzi A, Santilli S, Burgio VL, et al. *Candida* colonization and systemic infection in neutropenic patients. A retrospective study. Cancer 1989; 64(10):2030–2034.
64. Martino P, Girmenia C, Micozzi A, Raccah R, Gentile G, Venditti M, et al. Fungemia in patients with leukemia. Am J Med Sci 1993; 306(4):225–232.
65. Richet HM, Andremont A, Tancrede C, Pico JL, Jarvis WR. Risk factors for candidemia in patients with acute lymphocytic leukemia. Rev Infect Dis 1991; 13(2):211–215.
66. Guiot HF, Fibbe WE, van't Wout JW. Risk factors for fungal infection in patients with malignant hematologic disorders: implications for empirical therapy and prophylaxis. Clin Infect Dis 1994; 18(4):525–532.

67. Pappu-Katikaneni LD, Rao KP, Banister E. Gastrointestinal colonization with yeast species and *Candida septicemia* in very low birth weight infants. Mycoses 1990; 33(1):20–23.

68. Deresinski SC, Stevens DA. Caspofungin. Clin Infect Dis 2003; 36(11):1445–1457.

69. Pittet D, Monod M, Suter PM, Frenk E, Auckenthaler R. *Candida* colonization subsequent infections in critically ill surgical patients. Ann Surg 1994; 220(6):721–728.

70. Wey SB, Mori M, Pfaller MA, Woolson RF, Wenzel RP. Risk factors for hospital-acquired candidemia. A matched case–control study. Arch Intern Med 1989; 149: 2349–2353.

71. Garbino J, Lew DP, Romand JA, Hugonnet S, Auckenthaler R, Pittet D. Prevention of severe *Candida* infections in nonneutropenic, high-risk, critically ill patients: a randomized, double-blind, placebo-controlled trial in patients treated by selective digestive decontamination. Intensive Care Med 2002; 28(12):1708–1717.

72. Hummel M, Thalmann U, Jautzke G, Staib F, Seibold M, Hetzer R. Fungal infections following heart transplantation. Mycoses 1992; 35(1–2):23–34.

73. Castaldo P, Stratta RJ, Wood RP, Markin RS, Patil KD, Shaefer MS, et al. Clinical spectrum of fungal infections after orthotropic liver transplantation. Arch Surg 1991; 126(2):149–156.

74. Lumbreras C, Fernandez I, Velosa J, Munn S, Sterioff S, Paya CV. Infectious complications following pancreatic transplantation: incidence, microbiological and clinical characteristics, and outcome. Clin Infect Dis 1995; 20(3):514–520.

75. Rubin NE, Rubin RH. Opportunistic fungal and bacterial infection in the renal transplant recipient. J Am Soc Nephrol 1992; 2:S264–S269.

76. Lumbreras C, Cuervas-Mons V, Jara P, del Palacio A, Turrion VS, Barrios C, et al. Randomized trial of fluconazole versus nystatin for the prophylaxis of *Candida* infection following liver transplantation. J Infect Dis 1996; 174(3):583–588.

77. Mora NP, Cofer JB, Solomon H, Goldstein RM, Gonwa TA, Husberg BS, et al. Analysis of severe infections (INF) after 180 consecutive liver transplants: the impact of amphotericin B prophylaxis for reducing the incidence and severity of fungal infections. Transplant Proc 1991; 23(1 Pt 2):1528–1530.

78. Mora NP, Klintmalm G, Solomon H, Goldstein RM, Gonwa TA, Husberg BS. Selective amphotericin B prophylaxis in the reduction of fungal infections after liver transplant. Transplant Proc 1992; 24(1):154–155.

79. Tollemar J, Hockerstedt K, Ericzon BG, Jalanko H, Ringden O. Liposomal amphotericin B prevents invasive fungal infections in liver transplant recipients. A randomized, placebo-controlled study. Transplantation 1995; 59(1):45–50.

80. Winston DJ, Pakrasi A, Busuttil RW. Prophylactic fluconazole in liver transplant recipients. A randomized, double-blind, placebo-controlled trial. Ann Intern Med 1999; 131(10):729–737.

81. Winston DJ, Busuttil RW. Randomized controlled trial of oral itraconazole solution versus intravenous/oral fluconazole for prevention of fungal infections in liver transplant recipients. Transplantation 2002; 74(5):688–695.

82. Sharpe MD, Ghent C, Grant D, Horbay GL, McDougal J, David CW. Efficacy and safety of itraconazole prophylaxis for fungal infections after orthotropic liver transplantation: a prospective, randomized, double-blind study. Transplantation 2003; 76(6): 977–983.

83. Biancofiore G, Bindi ML, Baldassarri R, Romanelli AM, Catalano G, Filipponi F, et al. Antifungal prophylaxis in liver transplant recipients: a randomized placebo-controlled study. Transpl Int 2002; 15(7):341–347.

84. Singhal S, Ellis RW, Jones SG, Miller SJ, Fisher NC, Hastings JG, et al. Targeted prophylaxis with amphotericin B lipid complex in liver transplantation. Liver Transpl 2000; 6(5):588–595.

85. Singh N, Paterson DL, Gayowski T, Wagener MM, Marino IR. Preemptive prophylaxis with a lipid preparation of amphotericin B for invasive fungal infections in liver

transplant recipients requiring renal replacement therapy. Transplantation 2001; 71(7):910–913.

86. Aloia T, Solomkin J, Fink AS, Nussbaum MS, Bjornson S, Bell RH, et al. *Candida* in pancreatic infection: a clinical experience. Am Surg 1994; 60(10):793–796.

87. De Waele JJ, Vogelaers D, Blot S, Colardyn F. Fungal infections in patients with severe acute pancreatitis and the use of prophylactic therapy. Clin Infect Dis 2003; 37(2):208–213.

88. Isenmann R, Schwarz M, Rau B, Trautmann M, Schober W, Beger HG. Characteristics of infection with *Candida* species in patients with necrotizing pancreatitis. World J Surg 2002; 26(3):372–376.

89. Gotzinger P, Wamser P, Barlan M, Sautner T, Jakesz R, Fugger R. *Candida* infection of local necrosis in severe acute pancreatitis is associated with increased mortality. Shock 2000; 14(3):320–323.

90. Gumaste V. Prophylactic antibiotic therapy in the management of acute pancreatitis [in process citation]. J Clin Gastroenterol 2000; 31(1):6–10.

91. Powell JJ, Miles R, Siriwardena AK. Antibiotic prophylaxis in the initial management of severe acute pancreatitis. Br J Surg 1998; 85(5):582–587.

92. Ho HS, Frey CF. The role of antibiotic prophylaxis in severe acute pancreatitis. Arch Surg 1997; 132(5):487–492.

93. Solomkin JS, Flohr AB, Quie PG, Simmons RL. The role of *Candida* in intraperitoneal infections. Surgery 1980; 88:524–530.

94. Calandra T, Bille J, Schneider R, Mosimann F, Francioli P. Clinical significance of *Candida* isolated from peritoneum in surgical patients. Lancet 1989; 2:1437–1440.

95. Eggimann P, Francioli P, Bille J, Schneider R, Wu MM, Chapuis G, et al. Fluconazole prophylaxis prevents intra-abdominal candidiasis in high-risk surgical patients [see comments]. Crit Care Med 1999; 27(6):1066–1072.

96. Edwards JEJ, Bodey GP, Bowden RA, Buchner T, de Pauw BE, Filler SG, et al. International Conference for the Development of a Consensus on the Management and Prevention of Severe Candidal Infections [see comments]. Clin Infect Dis 1997; 25(1):43–59.

97. Rex JH, Bennett JE, Sugar AM, Pappas PG, van der Horst CM, Edwards JE, et al. A randomized trial comparing fluconazole with amphotericin B for the treatment of candidemia in patients without neutropenia. Candidemia Study Group and the National Institute [see comments]. N Engl J Med 1994; 331(20):1325–1330.

98. Anaissie EJ, Vartivarian SE, Abi-Said D, Uzun O, Pinczowski H, Kontoyiannis DP, et al. Fluconazole versus amphotericin B in the treatment of hematogenous candidiasis: a matched cohort study. Am J Med 1996; 101(2):170–176.

99. Anaissie EJ, Darouiche RO, Abi-Said D, Uzun O, Mera J, Gentry LO et al. Management of invasive candidal infections: results of a prospective, randomized, multicenter study of fluconazole versus amphotericin B and review of the literature. Clin Infect Dis 1996; 23(5):964–972.

100. Phillips P, Shafran S, Garber G, Rotstein C, Smaill F, Fong I, et al. Multicenter randomized trial of fluconazole versus amphotericin B for treatment of candidemia in non-neutropenic patients. Canadian Candidemia Study Group. Eur J Clin Microbiol Infect Dis 1997; 16(5):337–345.

101. Rex JH, Pappas PG, Karchmer AW, Sobel J, Edwards JE, Hadley S, et al. A randomized and blinded multicenter trial of high-dose fluconazole plus placebo versus fluconazole plus amphotericin B as therapy for candidemia and its consequences in nonneutropenic subjects. Clin Infect Dis 2003; 36(10):1221–1228.

102. Casasnovas RO, Caillot D, Solary E, Bonotte B, Chavanet P, Bonin A, et al. Prophylactic fluconazole and *Candida krusei* infection. N Engl J Med 1992; 326:891–892; discussion.

103. Fan Havard P, Capano D, Smith SM, Mangia A, Eng RH. Development of resistance in *Candida* isolates from patients receiving prolonged antifungal therapy. Antimicrob Agents Chemother 1991; 35:2302–2305.

104. Gleason TG, May AK, Caparelli D, Farr BM, Sawyer RG. Emerging evidence of selection of fluconazole-tolerant fungi in surgical intensive care units. Arch Surg 1997; 132(11):1197–1201.
105. Nguyen MH, Peacock JEJ, Morris AJ, Tanner DC, Nguyen ML, Snydman DR, et al. The changing face of candidemia: emergence of non-*Candida albicans* species and antifungal resistance. Am J Med 1996; 100(6):617–623.
106. Fraser VJ, Jones M, Dunkel J, Storfer S, Medoff G, Dunagan WC. Candidemia in a tertiary care hospital: epidemiology, risk factors, and predictors of mortality [see comments]. Clin Infect Dis 1992; 15(3):414–421.
107. Raad II, Sabbagh MF, Rand KH, Sherertz RJ. Quantitative tip culture methods and the diagnosis of central venous catheter-related infections. Diagn Microbiol Infect Dis 1992; 15:13–20.
108. Sherertz RJ, Raad II, Belani A, Koo LC, Rand KH, Pickett DL, et al. Three-year experience with sonicated vascular catheter cultures in a clinical microbiology laboratory. J Clin Microbiol 1990; 28:76–82.
109. Widmer AF, Nettleman M, Flint K, Wenzel RP. The clinical impact of culturing central venous catheters. A prospective study. Arch Intern Med 1992; 152:1299–1302.
110. Nguyen MH, Peacock JE Jr, Tanner DC, Morris AJ, Nguyen ML, Snydman DR, et al. Therapeutic approaches in patients with candidemia. Evaluation in a multicenter, prospective, observational study. Arch Intern Med 1995; 155(22):2429–2435.
111. Rex JH, Bennett JE, Sugar AM, Pappas PG, Serody J, Edwards JE, et al. Intravascular catheter exchange and duration of candidemia. NIAID Mycoses Study Group and the Candidemia Study Group. Clin Infect Dis 1995; 21(4):994–996.
112. Hawser SP, Douglas LJ. Biofilm formation by *Candida* species on the surface of catheter materials in vitro. Infect Immun 1994; 62(3):915–921.
113. Hawser SP, Douglas LJ. Resistance of *Candida albicans* biofilms to antifungal agents in vitro. Antimicrob Agents Chemother 1995; 39(9):2128–2131.
114. Girmenia C, Martino P, De Bernardis F, Gentile G, Boccanera M, Monaco M, et al. Rising incidence of *Candida parapsilosis fungemia* in patients with hematologic malignancies: clinical aspects, predisposing factors, and differential pathogenicity of the causative strains. Clin Infect Dis 1996; 23(3):506–514.
115. Bodey GP. Azole antifungal agents. Clin Infect Dis 1992; 14(suppl 1):S161–S169.
116. Martins MD, Rex JH. Resistance to antifungal agents in the critical care setting: problems and perspectives. New Horiz 1996; 4(3):338–344.
117. Pfaller MA, Jones RN, Doern GV, Sader HS, Hollis RJ, Messer SA. International surveillance of bloodstream infections due to *Candida* species: frequency of occurrence and antifungal susceptibilities of isolates collected in 1997 in the United States, Canada, and South America for the SENTRY Program. The SENTRY Participant Group. J Clin Microbiol 1998; 36(7):1886–1889.
118. Debruyne D. Clinical pharmacokinetics of fluconazole in superficial and systemic mycoses. Clin Pharmacokinet 1997; 33(1):52–77.
119. Oono S, Tabei K, Tetsuka T, Asano Y. The pharmacokinetics of fluconazole during haemodialysis in uraemic patients. Eur J Clin Pharmacol 1992; 42:667–669.
120. Rosemurgy AS, Markowsky S, Goode SE, Plastino K, Kearney RE. Bioavailability of fluconazole in surgical intensive care unit patients: a study comparing routes of administration. J Trauma 1995; 39(3):445–447.
121. Terrell CL. Antifungal agents. Part II. The azoles. Mayo Clin Proc 1999; 74(1):78–100.
122. De Beule K, Van Gestel J. Pharmacology of itraconazole. Drugs 2001; 61(suppl 1):27–37.
123. Pandya NA, Atra AA, Riley U, Pinkerton CR. Role of itraconazole in haematology/oncology. Arch Dis Child 2003; 88(3):258–260.
124. Donnelly JP, de Pauw BE. Voriconazole—a new therapeutic agent with an extended spectrum of antifungal activity. Clin Microbiol Infect 2004; 10(suppl 1):107–117.

125. Johnson LB, Kauffman CA. Voriconazole: a new triazole antifungal agent. Clin Infect Dis 2003; 36(5):630–637.

126. Laverdiere M, Hoban D, Restieri C, Habel F. In vitro activity of three new triazoles and one echinocandin against *Candida* bloodstream isolates from cancer patients. J Antimicrob Chemother 2002; 50(1):119–123.

127. Brajtburg J, Powderly WG, Kobayashi GS, Medoff G. Amphotericin B: current understanding of mechanisms of action. Antimicrob Agents Chemother 1990; 34:183–188.

128. Sokol-Anderson M, Sligh JEJ, Elberg S, Brajtburg J, Kobayashi GS, Medoff G. Role of cell defense against oxidative damage in the resistance of *Candida albicans* to the killing effect of amphotericin B. Antimicrob Agents Chemother 1988; 32(5):702–705.

129. Sokol-Anderson ML, Brajtburg J, Medoff G. Amphotericin B-induced oxidative damage and killing of *Candida albicans*. J Infect Dis 1986; 154(1):76–83.

130. Gallis HA, Drew RH, Pickard WW. Amphotericin B: 30 years of clinical experience. Rev Infect Dis 1990; 12:308–329.

131. Vonk AG, Netea MG, van der Meer JW, Kullberg BJ. Modulation of the pro- and anti-inflammatory cytokines by amphotericin B [letter; comment]. J Infect Dis 1999; 180(4):1408–1411.

132. Arning M, Kliche KO, Heer-Sonderhoff AH, Wehmeier A. Infusion-related toxicity of three different amphotericin B formulations and its relation to cytokine plasma levels. Mycoses 1995; 38(11–12):459–465.

133. Sabra R, Branch RA. Amphotericin B nephrotoxicity. Drug Saf 1990; 5(2):94–108.

134. Khoo SH, Bond J, Denning DW. Administering amphotericin B—a practical approach. J Antimicrob Chemother 1994; 33(2):203–213.

135. Burks LC, Aisner J, Fortner CL, Wiernik PH. Meperidine for the treatment of shaking chills and fever. Arch Intern Med 1980; 140(4):483–484.

136. Goodwin SD, Cleary JD, Walawander CA, Taylor JW, Grasela THJ. Pretreatment regimens for adverse events related to infusion of amphotericin B. Clin Infect Dis 1995; 20(4):755–761.

137. Cleary JD, Weisdorf D, Fletcher CV. Effect of infusion rate on amphotericin B-associated febrile reactions. Drug Intell Clin Pharm 1988; 22(10):769–772.

138. Miano-Mason TM. Mechanisms and management of amphotericin B-induced nephrotoxicity. Cancer Pract 1997; 5(3):176–181.

139. Sawaya BP, Briggs JP, Schnermann J. Amphotericin B nephrotoxicity: the adverse consequences of altered membrane properties [editorial]. J Am Soc Nephrol 1995; 6(2): 154–164.

140. Carlson MA, Condon RE. Nephrotoxicity of amphotericin B. J Am Coll Surg 1994; 179(3):361–381.

141. Anderson CM. Sodium chloride treatment of amphotericin B nephrotoxicity. Standard of care?. West J Med 1995; 162(4):313–317.

142. Branch RA. Prevention of amphotericin B-induced renal impairment. A review on the use of sodium supplementation. Arch Intern Med 1988; 148(11):2389–2394.

143. de Marie S, Janknegt R, Bakker-Woudenberg IA. Clinical use of liposomal and lipid-complexed amphotericin B. J Antimicrob Chemother 1994; 33(5):907–916.

144. Brajtburg J, Bolard J. Carrier effects on biological activity of amphotericin B. Clin Microbiol Rev 1996; 9(4):512–531.

145. Walsh TJ, Hiemenz JW, Seibel NL, Perfect JR, Horwith G, Lee L, et al. Amphotericin B lipid complex for invasive fungal infections: analysis of safety and efficacy in 556 cases. Clin Infect Dis 1998; 26(6):1383–1396.

146. Denning DW. Echinocandin antifungal drugs. Lancet 2003; 362(9390):1142–1151.

147. Anidulafungin: ECB, LY 303366, V-echinocandin, VEC, VER 002, VER-02. Drugs R D 2003; 4(3):167–173.

148. Johnson MD, Perfect JR. Caspofungin: first approved agent in a new class of antifungals. Expert Opin Pharmacother 2003; 4(5):807–823.

149. Ullmann AJ. Review of the safety, tolerability, and drug interactions of the new antifungal agents caspofungin and voriconazole. Curr Med Res Opin 2003; 19(4):263–271.

150. Mora-Duarte J, Betts R, Rotstein C, Colombo AL, Thompson-Moya L, Smietana J, et al. Comparison of caspofungin and amphotericin B for invasive candidiasis. N Engl J Med 2002; 347(25):2020–2029.

151. Pelz RK, Hendrix CW, Swoboda SM, Diener-West M, Merz WG, Hammond J, et al. Double-blind placebo-controlled trial of fluconazole to prevent candidal infections in critically ill surgical patients. Ann Surg 2001; 233(4):542–548.

152. Savani DV, Perfect JR, Cobo LM, Durack DT. Penetration of new azole compounds into the eye and efficacy in experimental *Candida endophthalmitis*. Antimicrob Agents Chemother 1987; 31:6–10.

153. Venditti M, De Bernardis F, Micozzi A, Pontieri E, Chirletti P, Cassone A, et al. Fluconazole treatment of catheter-related right-sided endocarditis caused by *Candida albicans* and associated with endophthalmitis and folliculitis. Clin Infect Dis 1992; 14: 422–426.

154. Laatikainen L, Tuominen M, von Dickhoff K. Treatment of endogenous fungal endophthalmitis with systemic fluconazole with or without vitrectomy [letter]. Am J Ophthalmol 1992; 113(2):205–207.

155. Martinez-Vazquez C, Fernandez-Ulloa J, Bordon J, Sopena B, de la Fuente J, Ocampo A, et al. *Candida albicans* endophthalmitis in brown heroin addicts: response to early vitrectomy preceded and followed by antifungal therapy [see comments]. Clin Infect Dis 1998; 27(5):1130–1133.

156. Yackee JM, Topiel MS, Simon GL. Septic phlebitis caused by *Candida albicans* and diagnosed by needle aspiration. South Med J 1985; 78:1262–1263.

157. Strinden WD, Helgerson RB, Maki DG. *Candida* septic thrombosis of the great central veins associated with central catheters Clinical features and management. Ann Surg 1985; 202:653–658.

158. Mascarenas CA, Hardin TC, Pennick GJ, Rinaldi MG, Graybill JR. Treatment of thrush with itraconazole solution: evidence for topical effect. Clin Infect Dis 1998; 26(5):1242–1243.

159. Crutchfield CE, Lewis EJ. The successful treatment of oral candidiasis (thrush) in a pediatric patient using itraconazole [letter]. Pediatr Dermatol 1997; 14(3):246.

160. Rantala A, Lehtonen OP, Kuttila K, Havia T, Niinikoski J. Diagnostic factors for postoperative candidosis in abdominal surgery. Ann Chir Gynaecol 1991; 80:323–328.

161. Hiatt JR, Kobayashi MR, Doty JE, Ramming KP. Acalculous *Candida cholecystitis*: a complication of critical surgical illness [review]. Am Surg 1991; 57(12):825–829.

162. Irani M, Truong LD. Candidiasis of the extrahepatic biliary tract. Arch Pathol Lab Med 1986; 110:1087–1090.

163. Khardori N, Wong E, Carrasco CH, Wallace S, Patt Y, Bodey GP. Infections associated with biliary drainage procedures in patients with cancer. Rev Infect Dis 1991; 13:587–591.

164. Levine J, Bernard DB, Idelson BA, Farnham H, Saunders C, Sugar AM. Fungal peritonitis complicating continuous ambulatory peritoneal dialysis: successful treatment with fluconazole, a new orally active antifungal agent [see comments]. Am J Med 1989; 86(6 Pt 2):825–827.

165. Corbella X, Sirvent JM, Carratala J. Fluconazole treatment without catheter removal in *Candida albicans* peritonitis complicating peritoneal dialysis [letter; comment]. Am J Med 1991; 90(2):277.

166. Eisenberg ES, Leviton I, Soeiro R. Fungal peritonitis in patients receiving peritoneal dialysis: experience with 11 patients and review of the literature [published erratum appears in Rev Infect Dis 1986; 8(5):839]. Rev Infect Dis 1986; 8(3):309–321.

167. Nassoura Z, Ivatury RR, Simon RJ, Jabbour N, Stahl WM. Candiduria as an early marker of disseminated infection in critically ill surgical patients: the role of fluconazole therapy. J Trauma 1993; 35:290–295.

168. Sobel JD, Kauffman CA, McKinsey D, Zervos M, Vazquez JA, Karchmer AW, et al. Candiduria: a randomized, double-blind study of treatment with fluconazole and placebo. The National Institute of Allergy and Infectious Diseases (NIAID) Mycoses Study Group. Clin Infect Dis 2001; 30(1):19–24.

169. Tacker JR. Successful use of fluconazole for treatment of urinary tract fungal infections. J Urol 1992; 148(6):1917–1918.

170. el-Ebiary M, Torres A, Fabregas N, de la Bellacasa JP, Gonzalez J, Ramirez J, et al. Significance of the isolation of *Candida* species from respiratory samples in critically ill, non-neutropenic patients. An immediate postmortem histologic study. Am J Respir Crit Care Med 1997; 156(2 Pt 1):583–590.

171. Trick WE, Fridkin SK, Edwards JR, Hajjeh RA, Gaynes RP. Secular trend of hospital-acquired candidemia among intensive care unit patients in the United States during 1989–1999. Clin Infect Dis 2002; 35(5):627–630.

7

Fungal Infections in Immunocompromised Hosts: Host Defenses, Risks, and Epidemiology in Special Patient Groups—Pediatrics

Charles B. Foster
Division of Pediatric Infectious Diseases, Johns Hopkins Hospital, Baltimore, Maryland, U.S.A.

Stephen J. Chanock
Section of Genomic Variation, Pediatric Oncology Branch, National Cancer Institute, National Institutes of Health, Bethesda, Maryland, U.S.A.

I. INTRODUCTION

While the basic principles with regard to identification and management of fungal infections in immunocompromised children are similar to those encountered in adult patients, there are additional considerations for pediatric patients at risk for fungal infections. Notably, the developmental immaturity of host responses to infection encountered during the first few months of life, place young infants at particularly high risk for a wide range of infectious complications, especially with fungal pathogens (1). Both term and preterm infants may be viewed as immunocompromised hosts and are at high risk for neonatal fungal infections, especially with candidiasis (2–6). However, the consequences are particularly severe in very low birth weight infants (7).

In the absence of a specific predisposing factor, the new diagnosis of an invasive or persistent fungal infection in a child should raise the possibility of an underlying defect in host defense. Indeed, most primary immunodeficiencies, such as chronic granulomatous disease (CGD) and severe combined immunodeficiency (SCID) can present in the first years of life, but are often missed until the second or third serious infection (8,9). Syndromes such as congenital cutaneous candidiasis and disseminated histoplasmosis of infancy may also be present in otherwise healthy infants (10,11). Despite significant advances in reducing the rate of perinatal HIV transmission through the use of antiretroviral therapy, previously undiagnosed HIV infection in the young child can be present with opportunistic fungal infections, such as candidiasis or in rare circumstances, cryptococcosis (12).

The clinical implications of developmental maturation of the immune system separate the child from the adult. In this regard, young children are at a high risk for primary infection with fungal pathogens, especially if there is an underlying immune deficit. At birth, the antibody repertoire is comprised of maternal IgG, which crosses the placenta easily, unlike IgM (13). Since immunoglobulin is transported across the placenta beginning in the eighth week of gestation, antibody levels in the infant reach 50% of maternal levels at 30 weeks gestation and by term are at, or above maternal levels (14). Passively acquired maternal immunoglobulin levels decline over the first months of life and reach a physiologic nadir at approximately 3–4 months of life. In term infants, the immunoglobulin levels at the nadir are frequently in the range of 400 mg/dL while in the very low birth weight infant levels may be less than 100 mg/dL (14,15). Although cell-mediated immunity in the term infant is relatively intact, infants are immunologically naïve because of a lack of exposure to complex pathogens (1). Immaturity of response to complex polysaccharide antigens (often critical components of encapsulated bacterial pathogens) is also notable in the first months of life (16). In the neonate, B-cells respond poorly to polysaccharides, and granulocytes are impaired in adhesion and in migration (17–19). Decreased granulocyte marrow reserves and mobilization are evident during severe infection or stress, rendering infants neutropenic. Together, these host factors make young infants, especially premature infants, more vulnerable to fungal colonization and also invasive disease.

Specific types of infections provide important clues to deficits in immune function. Fungal infections are more likely to occur in children with deficits of T-cell function or phagocytic defects; fungal infection in the child with a deficit in B-cell function is less common (8,9). In fact, the original descriptions of primary immune deficiencies have been partially based on the diagnosis of opportunistic infections, such as with fungal pathogens. The development of severe invasive fungal infection in childhood is distinctly rare and almost always associated with an underlying deficit in immune function. In fact, the diagnosis of an invasive mycosis should prompt a thorough examination of the immune function. Since most primary immune deficiencies are present in childhood, even the diagnosis of an atypical persistence of mucosal candidiasis should result in consideration for screening for immune function.

CD4+ T-cell lymphocyte counts vary by age; normal CD4+ T-lymphocyte counts are higher in infants and young children than in adults (20,21). Knowledge of these differences are particularly relevant when using CD4+ cell counts to evaluate an HIV-infected child's risk for opportunistic infection (Table 1) (22). Unlike adults, children with HIV infection may experience opportunistic infections at higher CD4+ levels. In evaluating a young child for evidence of immune suppression, therefore, the extent to which CD4+ counts deviate from age-specific norms should be taken into consideration. The Centers for Disease Control and Prevention (CDC)

Table 1 CD4+ T-lymphocyte Counts, Age and Risk for Opportunistic Infection in Pediatric HIV

Age	< 12 months	1–5 years	6–12 years
No evidence	> 1500	> 1000	> 500
Moderate	750–1499	500–999	200–499
Severe	< 750	< 500	< 200

1994 Revised Classification System uses age-specific norms to categorize HIV-infected children based on the degree of immunosuppression (23). The accompanying table (Table 1) summarizes the degree of immune suppression associated with age-specific CD4+ T-lymphocyte counts and percentages.

For instance, infection with *Pneumocystis carinii* arises in children with abnormal T-cell function, such as SCIDS or HIV infection (8). The spectrum of T-cell abnormalities in chromosome 22q11.2 deletion syndromes including DiGeorge syndrome are more varied than in SCIDS, but on occasions, PCP has been reported in patients with DiGeorge syndrome (24). Patients with a primary defect in phagocytic function, such as CGD are also at high risk for life-threatening infections with bacteria (*Staphylococci*, enteric-gram negatives such as *Burkholderia cepacia* and *Serratia marcescens*) and fungal (*Aspergillus* spp.) pathogens (9). Prophylaxis with trimethoprim–sulfamethoxazole and interferon gamma may reduce mortality from bacterial infection in this population by as much as 70%, but prophylaxis against fungal infection is more challenging (25,26). Recent data suggest, however, that prophylaxis with the oral antifungal agent itraconazole is well-tolerated and is effective in preventing both superficial and serious life-threatening fungal infections (27). Patients with other neutrophil disorders, such as myeloperoxidase deficiency, specific granule deficiency and leukocyte adhesion deficiency have been reported (28).

II. SPECIFIC FUNGAL INFECTIONS

A. *Candida* Species

1. Mucocutaneons Candidiasis

In immunocompetent patients, *Candida* is a commensal organism, and colonization of the skin or mucosal membranes is ubiquitous. Newborns are typically colonized during passage through the vagina (29). In healthy newborn infants, mild mucocutaneous infection is common and does not indicate the presence of a defect in host defenses. Oral candidiasis or thrush can be treated with oral nystatin and in older children with clotrimazole troches. Persistent infections may result from the continued use of colonized pacifiers or bottles. More extensive disease, involving the esophagus, for example, or infection that persists despite appropriate treatment should, however, raise the suspicion of an underlying immune defect, including both primary and acquired. For instance, mild esophagitis in the HIV-infected child can be treated with oral nystatin; however, many HIV-infected children with esophagitis have required treatment with either an azole or amphotericin B. Concurrent oral candidiasis is common and many HIV-infected children with esophagitis have a variety of associated signs and symptoms including odynophagia, retrosternal pain, drooling, fever, nausea and vomiting, dehydration, hoarseness, and occasionally upper gastrointestinal bleeding. Risk factors for *Candida* esophagitis in this population include prior oral pharyngeal candidiasis, low CD4 count and use of antibiotics (30). In neutropenic cancer patients, mucosal colonization with *Candida* may provide a portal through which dissemination and invasive infection can develop. Rarely, patients can develop necrotizing *Candida* esophagitis resulting in perforation. Management requires prompt surgical intervention and systemic antifungal therapy (31).

Chronic mucocutaneous candidiasis (CMC) is a rare inherited disease that results in severe candidal infection of the skin, nails, and mucosa. Invasive candidiasis in this syndrome, however, is distinctly uncommon. In approximately 50% of reported cases, an associated endocrine disorder is present (32). Recently, a gene for autoimmune polyglandular syndrome Type 1 has been cloned and mapped to chromosome 21q22.3 (33). This autosomal recessive disorder is characterized by autoimmune polyendocrinopathy, chronic candidiasis, and ectodermal dystrophy. The syndrome frequently presents during infancy with persistent diaper rash. Case reports and reviews from the literature suggest that other distinct types of CMC might exist and that some families have a form of CMC without polyendocrinopathy.

2. *Locally Invasive* Candida *Infection*

In healthy children, locally invasive candidal infection occurs in three settings: laryngitis, otitis externa, and vulvovaginitis. Laryngeal candidal infection develops in children treated with inhaled corticosteroids for asthma. Presentation includes a hoarse voice and the diagnosis is confirmed by direct observation of the vocal cords. Chronic otitis externa occurs in children receiving extended courses of antibacterial therapy and/or local otic drops including corticosteroids. Systemic treatment is often indicated and on rare occasion, namely extension into the mastoid, surgery is indicated. Vulvovaginitis occurs in postpubertal females. Risk factors include diabetes, corticosteroid therapy, birth control pills, or extended use of tetracycline for acne. Vaginal troches are the first line of therapy, but relapse or recurrence is not uncommon.

3. *Congenital Cutaneous Candidiasis*

In contrast to neonatal candidiasis, which generally develops in an infant colonized with *Candida*, acquired either during passage through an infected birth canal or postnatally, congenital cutaneous candidiasis is acquired in utero by ascending infection, but this is relatively uncommon with fewer than 100 cases reported (34). The pathogenesis of this disorder is incompletely understood, though it is plausible that predisposing conditions include *Candida* chorioamnionitis. While fetal membranes are generally found to be intact, a possible role for subclinical rupture of membranes has been suggested. Once the amniotic fluid becomes infected, the *Candida* infection may spread to the skin, lungs, or gastrointestinal tract. Clinically, the disorder usually presents within the first 6 days of life with generalized erythematous papules and pustules caused by *Candida* spp. In full-term infants weighing more than 2500 g, it is generally benign and self-limited; management includes topical or oral antifungal therapy. However, it is critical to be vigilant, because dissemination can develop (35,36). In contrast to the benign course observed for this disease in full-term infants, preterm neonates weighing less than 1000 g with chronic cutaneous candidiasis are at higher risk of systemic infection and death. Diagnosis in the preterm infant warrants a thorough work-up, including blood, urine, and CSF cultures. The latter is particularly important because of the severe consequences of meningitis in the neonate (37). Systemically infected infants may have clinical signs of respiratory distress together with elevated white blood cell counts and hyperglycemia. With early recognition and aggressive treatment with systemic antifungal therapy, the mortality from this condition can be reduced. At this time, conventional amphotericin B therapy is the drug of choice.

4. *Neonatal Candidiasis*

This is a common form of disseminated candidiasis in premature infants, particularly those hospitalized in the neonatal intensive care unit (NICU) for an extended period of time (2). Overall *Candida* species account for approximately 10% of infections observed in the NICU (7,38–40). Risk factors for systemic candidiasis in the NICU include gestational age (< 32 weeks), low Apgars scores, shock, disseminated intravascular coagulopathy, prior use of intralipid therapy, parenteral nutrition, H2 blockers, extended intubation, and central venous catheters (41,42). As with most infections in this setting, clinical signs and symptoms are frequently nonspecific; in some circumstances, persistent candidemia is observed (43). Severe infection can present with respiratory distress, episodes of apnea and bradycardia, hyperglycemia, or temperature instability. Other *Candida* spp. appear to be on the rise (40). There is some controversy as to whether infection with *C.albicans* carries a higher or lower risk for adverse outcomes, compared to *C.parapsilosis*. The recent trends indicate that non-*Albicans* species represent a greater percentage of blood-borne infection in the NICU (44).

The consequences of systemic infection are significant, which have led many to advocate sampling of urine and cerebrospinal fluid in addition to blood cultures (2). For instance, the risk for neurodevelopmental abnormalities is high, as is mortality. Renal ultrasound, echocardiogram, and ophthalmologic exam can reveal the presence of disease foci such as renal fungal balls or hydronephrosis, endocarditis, or endopthalmitis (45,46). Conventional amphotericin B has traditionally been the drug of choice for the treatment of neonatal candidiasis, and is generally well tolerated in this age group (47). Some investigators advocate the addition of oral 5-fluorocytosine (5-FC) to amphotericin B therapy when there is persistent candidemia, or the presence of either meningitis or endocarditis, but one should be cautious in monitoring for hematotoxicity. This has prompted investigation of fluconazole prophylaxis in preterm infants, which indicates that the prophylactic administration of fluconazole to very low birth weight infants can decrease the rate of fungal colonization (48). While larger studies are required to definitely show that prophylaxis decreases the risk of invasive *Candida*, results from one of these studies suggests that prophylaxis also decreases the risk for serious infection. While these findings are provocative, based on current data, it is premature to recommend universal adoption of fluconazole prophylaxis in all NICUs, although units with particularly high rates of fungal infection might consider this approach. The impact of prophylaxis on isolation of *Candida* species with intrinsic resistance to fluconazole will also need to be explored in detail.

5.   Catheter- and Devise-Associated Candidemia

Most children with life-threatening illness who require frequent blood sampling or infusional therapy have an indwelling venous catheter placed to facilitate venous access. However, there is risk for development of catheter-associated infection, which is usually due to bacterial pathogens, but on occasions, can be fungal, most commonly *Candida* spp. Vigorous activity often results in movement of the catheter, which can increase risk for infection. Usually lines are placed in the thoracic and neck region, but on some occasions are placed in the femoral region, which presents an especially daunting challenge for maintaining cleanliness. Given the high frequency of *Candida* diaper dermatitis in young patients, femoral lines may be at a higher risk of colonization or infection with *Candida* spp.

The diagnosis of a fungal infection associated with an indwelling device such as a vascular catheter or an intraventricular reservoir should lead to prompt removal of the infected hardware (49). Indwelling hardware infected with *Candida* or other fungal pathogens are notoriously difficult to clear with antifungal therapy and are frequently identified as a source for persistent infection. Infected catheters should be removed promptly to prevent dissemination (50–52). Following removal of the catheter, follow-up blood cultures should be performed. Patients with persistent candidemia should be evaluated for suppurative phlebitis, thrombosis, endocarditis, or other foci of residual infection (36).

Candiduria in children is a distinctly rare event and usually associated with an underlying structural abnormality or recent instrumentation (53). In the newborn, it is unusual and should be confirmed by suprapubic tap in the evaluation for possible disseminated infection. Follow-up radiographic studies, including possible CT or ultrasound as well as dynamic studies are indicated if there is evidence for persistent candiduria.

6. Neutropenia and Candidemia

Many of the original studies that established the efficacy of empiric antibiotic therapy in febrile neutropenic patients included children. The risk for serious bacterial infection is significant enough to warrant empirical antibiotics when the absolute neutrophil count (ANC) falls below 500/μL, but the risk is even higher when the ANC is below 100/μL (54). Standard algorithms for choosing antibacterial agents vary by institutional bias and experience, but should take into account local antibiotic sensitivity patterns of infection. The use of antibiotics is warranted in this setting, but a major consequence of broad spectrum antibiotics results in alteration of normal colonization patterns, favoring fungal pathogens. Like adults, children with persistent fever and neutropenia are at a high risk for serious fungal infection, especially after 5–7 days. Diagnosis of fungal infections in the neutropenic child is as challenging as in the adult; a delay can lead to disseminated disease, which is associated with increased morbidity and mortality. Studies in both children (age > 2) and adults have suggested that liposomal amphotericin B is as effective as conventional amphotericin B in patients with fever and neutropenia (55–57). However, in most institutions, the drug has primarily been reserved for children who are either refractory to or intolerant of conventional antifungal therapy. New azoles, such as voriconazole, can be administered to children for either prophylaxis or treatment of documented infection (58).

7. Hepatosplenic Candidiasis

This is a particularly difficult infectious complication observed in children and adults undergoing therapy for lymphoreticular malignancies. It is also known as chronic disseminated candidiasis, a distinct form of invasive candidiasis, primarily seen in granulocytopenic patients (59,60). The infection often becomes clinically apparent in children who remain persistently febrile despite recovery from myelosuppression, and in fact, can progress despite resolution of neutropenia. In adults with acute leukemia, the incidence has been reported to be as high as 7% (61); pediatric risks are probably comparable. Suggested risk factors include the dose intensity of chemotherapy, use of steroids, duration of neutropenia, relapsed leukemia, detection of *Candida* species on surveillance cultures, and central venous catheterization (59–61). Extended therapy with conventional amphotericin B may be required for as long as 6–12 months; treatment failures are not uncommon. Amphotericin B lipid complex (ABLC), which is highly concentrated in the reticuloendothelial system of the liver and spleen, has garnered interest in the treatment of this infection (62). In a published report, six children (ages 4–17 years) with HSC were treated with

ABLC, which was well tolerated for a short course (4–6 weeks). Sustained radiologic response of liver and spleen lesions was observed even after discontinuation of ABLC, because of loading of the reticuloendothelial system.

B. *Aspergillus* Species

1. Invasive Aspergillosis

The diagnosis and management of invasive *Aspergillus* infection is challenging in pediatric patients, for many of the same reasons observed in adults, clinical signs and symptoms can evolve slowly and come to medical attention at a critical juncture. Presentation can be insidious or acute. In children, invasive *Aspergillus* infection is generally associated with defects in host defenses such as CGD, HIV infection, Job's Syndrome, neutropenia, aplastic anemia, corticosteroids, T-cell abnormalities, and indwelling foreign bodies such as catheters or vascular grafts (28,63). The most common site is the respiratory tract, especially the lungs. Children with CGD also present with sinus infection and osteomyelitis, which underscore the two routes of infection—direct inoculation and dissemination of infection, probably via the blood stream. Outbreaks of aspergillosis have been described in pediatric oncology wards, transplant centers and NICUs, often associated with nearby construction work (64). Aerosolization of spores results in colonization of the sinopulmonary tract and skin, which can be the source of infection.

Aspergillus pulmonary infection in the pediatric patient can be detected by radiographic studies, in particular, computerized tomography studies of the chest (65). The diagnosis of aspergillosis in children is established on the basis of sampling of tissue or body fluids. With the advent of modern bronchoscopic techniques suitable for small children, bronchoalveolar lavage is routinely performed in children, but not always neonates. *Aspergillus* species are commonly isolated from the upper respiratory tract, even among healthy individuals, In this regard, isolation of *Aspergillus* from bronchoalveolar lavage specimens will provide suggestive evidence of infection. Definitive diagnosis of *Aspergillus* requires histopathologic evidence or a positive sterile site culture as well as clinical or radiologic evidence of infection.

New antifungal agents with activity against aspergillosis, such as voriconazole, have been quickly introduced into the pediatric setting. The efficacy and toxicity profiles do not appear to differ between adult and child. Already, several pediatric studies have established its safety in neutropenic children and ongoing studies are investigating its utility in primary immunodeficiencies, such as CGD, as well as in the oncology and transplant setting.

2. Hypersensitivity Aspergillosis

Older children are also prone to develop allergic hypersensitivity aspergillosis, especially if there is a strong history for reactive airway disease. Occasionally, children with chronic lung disease, such as those with cystic fibrosis, can develop manifestations consistent with hypersensitivity aspergillosis. This condition develops most likely in the setting of asthma, recurrent cough with positive culture for *Aspergillus* species, chest radiogram with fleeting infiltrates, IgE, and *Aspergillus* precipitants. Therapy is long term and includes at least one course of corticosteroids and antifungal therapy, though frequent relapse often requires repeated courses of therapy.

C. Other Fungal Infections

Critically ill children and neonates are at risk for nosocomial and endemic fungal infections. In the NICU, the risk for acquisition of a severe fungal infection is high and can be related to catheters, especially for candidal infection as detailed above. Infection with *Malassezia* spp. can occur in children receiving lipid supplementation or from colonized health care workers (66–68). Like adults, infection with *Alternaria-Fusarium*, or *Trichosporon* spp. occurs in immunocompromised children, particularly in transplant, oncology, or NICU environments.

Most children exposed to *Histoplasma capsulation* in an endemic region, namely the central United States, do not develop clinical symptoms, In a healthy child, infection with *Histoplasma capsulation* is often a mild illness with few clinical manifestations. Symptoms of acute localized pulmonary histoplasmosis may resemble those of influenza and resolve within days. A unique manifestation of the disease occurs among infants and young children, generally between the ages of 5 and 25 months (11). Following exposure to a large inoculum of *Histoplasma capsulatum,* these otherwise healthy infants may develop an overwhelming primary infection with disseminated histoplasmosis. This syndrome has a case fatality rate as high as 40–50% if not diagnosed expeditiously. Major clinical features include fever, failure to thrive, hepatosplenomegaly, and pancytopenia. The diagnosis is established by isolation or visualization of the organism in samples obtained from one or more of the following sites: bone marrow, spleen, liver, lymph node, cerebral spinal fluid, or bronchoalveolar lavage fluids. In children with a defect in cellular immunity, such as those observed with the acquired immunodeficiency syndrome (AIDS), or with solid organ transplants, acute disseminated histoplasmosis can occur, and is associated with significant morbidity and mortality.

In regions endemic for *Blastomyces dermatididis* (Ohio, Mississippi, and Missouri River Basins) both pulmonary and extrapulmonary manifestations can develop in healthy children. Illness is usually mild, but on occasion, respiratory distress has been described. Chronic infection can present with night sweats and failure to thrive (i.e., failure to develop and gain weight). Radiographic changes in the lung are often more significant than the clinical manifestations. Long-term therapy with azoles can be given, but many still recommend amphotericin B (69).

Infection with *Coccidioides immitis* occurs most frequently in the southwest United States. Most children do not have clinical manifestations following primary exposure, but less than 5% develop severe pulmonary disease. Disseminated infection is rare in older children, but more common in neonates and young children. Immunocompromised children are at risk for disseminated infection, which includes both pulmonary and extrapulmonary disease (e.g., osteomyelitis, meningitis, and cutaneous disease). Extended therapy is required to eradicate infection.

Zygomycetes infections are distinctly uncommon in children, but when encountered are usually observed in the setting of immunosuppression or an underlying metabolic disorder (e.g., diabetes or acidemia). Additional predisposing factors for rhinocerebral mucormycosis include environmental exposure and extended use of corticosteroids. Amphotericin B is typically used for treatment as the azoles and echinocandins are frequently inactive, but the cornerstone of therapy is surgical debridement.

Children rarely develop meningitis due to *Cryptococcus neoformans,* a ubiquitous yeast-like fungus. Infection with *C. neoformans* occurs through inhalation of the acapsular yeast cells. Although depression of cell-mediated immunity has been identified as a major factor predisposing individuals for invasive cryptococcal disease, humoral factors, such as specific antibodies may also be important in immunity. In the pre-HAART era, the prevalence of cryptococcal infection in HIV-1-infected children was about 1%. Infection in the neonate is very uncommon (70).

D. Therapeutic Considerations

Similar to the adult population, the development of new antifungal agents, such as the liposomal amphotericins, echinocandins, and voriconazole, represent important advances for the management of invasive fungal infections in children. Parallel studies in children have shown comparable toxicity profiles for lipid formulations of amphotericin, voriconazole, and the echinocandins. For example, based on data from adult studies, many pediatric centers now use voriconazole as first-line therapy for invasive pulmonary aspergillosis.

A particular note of caution, however, is warranted with regard to the use of newer antifungals agents in the treatment of children, especially neonates, with invasive fungal infection. While these agents may well become the standard of care for children, the experience with many of these agents in children is limited and often is extrapolated from the experience in adult populations (71,72). This concern is particularly true among neonates and preterm infants, in whom toxicity profiles and pharmacokinetic parameters differ substantially from adults and even older children. The pharmacokinetics of antifungal agents can differ between children and adults, and in fact, between children and infants (73). Many advocate a judicious and careful dosing schedule for amphotericin B and its lipid formulations in the neonate (74–76). Generally, increased excretion of compounds is observed in older children; for instance, fluconazole should be given at higher doses or twice a day to older children (77).

It is likely that most serious fungal infections will lead to consultation with infectious disease consultants with expertise in pediatric issues, such as diagnosis and pharmacology. The importance of future research to establish the safety, efficacy, and pharmacokinetics of these agents among pediatric patients cannot be overemphasized. The value of enrolling children with life-threatening diseases on clinical trials is illustrated by the major advances that have been made in the management of pediatric cancers through participation in co-operative clinical trials.

REFERENCES

1. Tosi MF, Cates KL. Immunologic and pathologic responses to infection. In: Feigin RD, Cherry JD, eds. Textbook of Pediatric infectious Diseases. Philadelphia: W.B. Saunders Company, 1998:14–53.
2. Benjamin DK Jr, Garges H, Steinbach WJ. *Candida* bloodstream infection in neonates. Semin Perinatol 2003; 27:375–383.
3. Cates KL, Rowe JC, Ballow M. The premature infant as a compromised host. Curr Probl Pediatr 1983; 13:1–63.
4. Leibovitz E. Neonatal candidiasis: clinical picture, management controversies and consensus, and new therapeutic options. J Antimicrob Chemother 2002; 49:69–73.
5. Lopez Sastre JB, Coto Cotallo GD, Fernandez Colomer B. Neonatal invasive candidiasis: a prospective multicenter study of 118 cases. Am J Perinatol 2003; 20:153–163.
6. Rowen JL, Tate JM. Management of neonatal candidiasis. Neonatal Candidiasis Study Group. Pediatr Infect Dis J 1998; 17:1007–1011.

7. Butler KM, Baker CJ. *Candida*: an increasingly important pathogen in the nursery. Pediatr Clin North Am 1988; 35:543–563.
8. Deerojanawong J, Chang AB, Eng PA, Robertson CF, Kemp AS. Pulmonary diseases in children with severe combined immune deficiency and DiGeorge syndrome. Pediatr Pulmonol 1997; 24:324–330.
9. Winkelstein JA, Marino MC, Johnston RB Jr, Boyle J, Curnutte J, Gallin JI, Malech HL, Holland SM, Ochs H, Quie P, Buckley RH, Foster CB, Chanock SJ, Dickler H. Chronic granulomatous disease. Report on a national registry of 368 patients. Medicine (Baltimore) 2000; 79:155–169.
10. Darmstadt GL, Dinulos JG, Miller Z. Congenital cutaneous candidiasis: clinical presentation, pathogenesis, and management guidelines. Pediatrics 2000; 105:438–444.
11. Odio CM, Navarrete M, Carrillo JM, Mora L, Carranza A. Disseminated histoplasmosis in infants. Pediatr Infect Dis J 1999; 18:1065–1068.
12. Muller FM, Groll AH, Walsh TJ. Current approaches to diagnosis and treatment of fungal infections in children infected with human immuno deficiency virus. Eur J Pediatr 1999; 158:187–199.
13. Kohler PF, Farr RS. Elevation of cord over maternal IgG immunoglobulin: evidence for an active placental IgG transport. Nature 1966; 210:1070–1071.
14. Ballow M, Cates KL, Rowe JC, Goetz C, Desbonnet C. Development of the immune system in very low birth weight (less than 1500 g) premature infants: concentrations of plasma immuno globulins and patterns of infections. Pediatr Res 1986; 20:899–904.
15. Stiehm ER, Fudenberg HH. Serum levels of immune globulins in health and disease: a survey. Pediatrics 1966; 37:715–727.
16. Lee CJ. Bacterial capsular polysaccharides—biochemistry, immunity and vaccine. Mol Immunol 1987; 24:1005–1019.
17. Anderson DC, Hughes BJ, Smith CW. Abnormal mobility of neonatal polymorphonuclear leukocytes. Relationship to impaired redistribution of surface adhesion sites by chemotactic factor or colchicine. J Clin Invest 1981; 68:863–874.
18. Miller ME. Immune-inflammatory response in the human neonate. Am J Pediatr Hematol Oncol 1981; 3:199–203.
19. Rijkers GT, Dollekamp EG, Zegers BJ. The in vitro B-cell response to pneumococcal polysaccharides in adults and neonates. Scand J Immunol 1987; 25:447–452.
20. Bofill M, Janossy G, Lee CA, MacDonald-Burns D, Phillips AN, Sabin C, Timms A, Johnson MA, Kernoff PB. Laboratory control values for CD4 and CD8 T lymphocytes. Implications for HIV-1 diagnosis. Clin Exp Immunol 1992; 88:243–252.
21. Waecker NJ Jr, Ascher DP, Robb ML, Moriarty R, Krober M, Rickman WJ, Butzin CA, Fischer GW. Age-adjusted CD4+ lymphocyte parameters in healthy children at risk for infection with the human immunodeficiency virus. The Military Pediatric HIV Consortium. Clin Infect Dis 1993; 17:123–125.
22. Pirofski L. Fungal infections in children with human immunodeficiency virus infection. Semin Pediatr Infect Dis 2001; 12:288–295.
23. Caldwell MB, Oxtoby MJ, Simonds RJ, Rogers MF. Centers for Disease Control and Prevention. 1994 Revised classification system for human immunodeficiency virus infection in children less than 13 years of age. MMWR 1994; 43:1–10.
24. Perez E, Sullivan KE. Chromosome 22q11.2 deletion syndrome (DiGeorge and velocardiofacial syndromes). Curr Opin Pediatr 2002; 14:678–683.
25. The International Chronic Granulomatous Disease Cooperative Study Group. A controlled trial of interferon gamma to prevent infection in chronic granulomatous disease. N Engl J Med 1991; 324:509–516.
26. Margolis DM, Melnick DA, Alling DW, Gallin JI. Trimethoprim–sulfamethoxazole prophylaxis in the management of chronic granulomatous disease. J Infect Dis 1990; 162:723–726.

27. Gallin JI, Alling DW, Malech HL, Wesley R, Koziol D, Marciano B, Eisenstein EM, Turner ML, DeCarlo ES, Starling JM, Holland SM. Itraconazole to prevent fungal infections in chronic granulomatous disease. N Engl J Med 2003; 348:2416–2422.
28. Holland SM. Update on phagocytic defects. Pediatr Infect Dis J 2003; 22:87–88.
29. Vazquez JA, Sobel JD. Mucosal candidiasis. Infect Dis Clin North Am 2002; 16:793–820.
30. Chiou CC, Groll AH, Gonzalez CE, Callender D, Venzon D, Pizzo PA, Wood L, Walsh TJ. Esophageal candidiasis in pediatric acquired immunodeficiency syndrome: clinical manifestations and risk factors. Pediatr Infect Dis J 2000; 19:729–734.
31. Gaissert HA, Roper CL, Patterson GA, Grillo HC. Infectious necrotizing esophagitis: outcome after medical and surgical intervention. Ann Thorac Surg 2003; 75:342–347.
32. Ahonen P, Myllarniemi S, Sipila I, Perheentupta J. Clinical variation of autoimmune polyendocrinopathy–candidias–ectodermal dystrophy (APECED) in a series of 68 patients. N Engl J Med 1990; 322:1829–1836.
33. Aaltonen J, Bjorses P, Sandkuijl L, Perheentupa J, Peltonen L. An autosomal locus causing autoimmune disease: autoimmune polyglandular disease type I assigned to chromosome 21. Nat Genet 1994; 8:83–87.
34. Johnson DE, Thompson TR, Ferrieri P. Congenital candidiasis. Am J Dis Child 1981; 135:273–275.
35. Bendel CM, Hostetter M. Systemic candidiasis and other fungal infections in the newborn. Semin Pediatr Infect 1994; 5:35–41.
36. Benjamin DK Jr, Poole C, Steinbach WJ, Rowen JL, Walsh TJ. Neonatal candidemia and end-organ damage: a critical appraisal of the literature using meta-analytic techniques. Pediatrics 2003; 112:634–640.
37. Fernandez M, Moylett EH, Noyola DE, Baker CJ. Candidal meningitis in neonates: a 10-year review. Clin Infect Dis 2000; 31:458–463.
38. Stoll BJ, Gordon T, Korones SB, Shankaran S, Tyson JE, Bauer CR, Fanaroff AA, Lemons JA, Donovan EF, Oh W, Stevenson DK, Ehrenkranz RA, Papile LA, Verier J, Wright LL. Early-onset sepsis in very low birth weight neonates: a report from the National Institute of Child Health and Human Development Neonatal Research Network. J Pediatr 1996; 129:72–80.
39. Stoll BJ, Gordon T, Korones SB, Shankaran S, Tyson JE, Bauer CR, Fanaroff AA, Lemons JA, Donovan EF, Oh W, Stevenson DK, Ehrenkranz RA, Papile LA, Verter J, Wright LL. Late-onset sepsis in very low birth weight neonates: a report from the National Institute of Child Health and Human Development Neonatal Research Network. J Pediatr 1996; 129:63–71.
40. Kossoff EH, Buescher ES, Karlowicz MG. Candidemia in an neonatal intensive care unit: trends during fifteen years and clinical features of 111 cases. Pediatr Infect Dis J 1998; 17:504–508.
41. El-Masry FA, Neal TJ, Subhedar NV. Risk factors for invasive fungal infection in neonates. Acta Paediatr 2002; 91:198–202.
42. Saiman L, Ludington E, Pfaller M, Rangel-Frausto S, Wiblin RT, Dawson J, Blumberg HM, Patterson JE, Rinaldi M, Edwards JE, Wenzel RP, Jarvis W. Risk factors for candidemia in Neonatal Intensive Care Unit patients. The National Epidemiology of Mycosis Survey Study Group. Pediatr Infect Dis J 2000; 19:319–324.
43. Chapman Rl, Faix RG. Persistently positive cultures and outcome in invasive neonatal candidiasis. Pediatr Infect Dis J 2000; 19:822–827.
44. Faix RG. Invasive neonatal candidiasis: comparison of albicans and parapsilosis infection. Pediatr Infect Dis J 1992; 11:88–93.
45. Noyola DE, Fernandez M, Moylett EH, Baker CJ. Ophthalmologic, visceral, and cardiac involvement in neonates with candidemia. Clin Infect Dis 2001; 32:1018–1023.
46. Noyola DE, Bohra L, Paysse EA, Fernandez M, Coats DK. Association of candidemia and retinopathy of prematurity in very low birthweight infants. Ophthalmology 2002; 109:80–84.

47. Benjamin DK Jr, DeLong ER, Steinbach WJ, Cotton CM, Walsh TJ, Clark RH. Empirical therapy for neonatal candidemia in very low birth weight infants. Pediatrics 2003; 112:543–547.
48. Kaufman D, Boyle R, Hazen KC, Patrie JT, Robinson M, Donowitz LG. Fluconazole prophylaxis against fungal colonization and infection in preterm infants. N Engl J Med 2001; 345:1660–1666.
49. Montero A, Romero J, Vargas JA, Regueiro CA, Sanchez-Aloz G, De Prados F, De la Torre A, Aragon G. *Candida* infection of cerebrospinal fluid shunt devices: report of two cases and review of the literature. Acta Neurochir (Wien) 2000; 142:67–74.
50. Eppes SC, Troutman JL, Gutman LT. Outcome of treatment of candidemia in children whose central catheters were removed or retained. Pediatr Infect Dis J 1989; 8:99–104.
51. Karlowicz MG, Hashimoto LN, Kelly RE Jr, Buescher ES. Should central venous catheters be removed as soon as candidemia is detected in neonates? Pediatrics 2000; 106:E63.
52. Leibovitz E, Iuster-Reicher A, Amitai M, Mogilner B. Systemic candidal infections associated with use of peripheral venous catheters in neonates: a 9-year experience. Clin Infect Dis 1992; 14:485–491.
53. Lundstrom T, Sobel J. Nosocomial candiduria: a review. Clin Infect Dis 2001; 32: 1602–1607.
54. Lehrnbecher T, Foster C, Vazquez N, Mackall CL, Chanock SJ. Therapy-induced altterations in host defense in children receiving therapy for cancer. J Pediatr Hematol Oncol 1997; 19:399–417.
55. Cagnoni PJ, Walsh TJ, Prendergast MM, Bodensteiner D, Hiemenz S, Greenberg RN, Arndt CA, Schuster M, Seibel N, Yeldandi V, Tong KB. Pharmacoeconomic analysis of liposomal amphotericin B versus conventional amphotericin B in the empirical treatment of persistently febrile neutropenic patients. J Clin Oncol 2000; 18:2476–2483.
56. Uhlenbrock S, Zimmermann M, Fegeler W, Jurgens H, Ritter J. Liposomal namphotericin B for prophylaxis of invasive fungal infections in high-risk paediatric patients with chemotherapy-related neutropenia: interim analysis of a prospective study. Mycoses 2001; 44:455–463.
57. Walsh TJ, Finberg RW, Arndt C, Hiemenz J, Schwartz C, Bodensteiner D, Pappas P, Seibel N, Greenberg RN, Dummer S, Schuster M, Holcenberg JS. Liposomal amphotericin B for empirical therapy in patients with persistent fever and neutropenia. National Institute of Allergy and Infectious Diseases Mycoses Study Group. N Engl J Med 1999; 340:764–771.
58. Walsh TJ, Pappas P, Winston DJ, Lazarus HM, Petersen F, Raffalli J, Yanovich S, Stiff P, Greenberg R, Donowitz G, Schuster M, Reboli A, Wingard J, Arndt C, Reinhardt J, Hadley S, Finberg R, Laverdiere M, Perfect J, Garber G, Fioritoni G, Anaissie E, Lee J. Voriconazole compared with liposomal amphotericin B for empirical antifungal therapy in patients with neutropenia and persistent fever. N Engl J Med 2002; 346:225–234.
59. Walsh TJ, Whitcomb PO, Revankar SG, Pizzo PA. Successful treatment of hepatosplenic candidiasis through repeated cycles of chemotherapy and neutropenia. Cancer 1995; 76:2357–2362.
60. Klingspor L, Stintzing G, Tollemar J. Deep *Candida* infection in children with leukaemia: clinical presentations, diagnosis and outcome. Acta Paediatr 1997; 86:30–36.
61. Anttila VJ, Elonen E, Nordling S, Sivonen A, Ruutu T, Ruutu P. Hepatosplenic candidiasis in patients with acute leukemia: incidence and prognostic implications. Clin Infect Dis 1997; 24:375–380.
62. Walsh TJ, Whitcomb P, Piscitelli S, Figg WD, Hill S, Chanock SJ, Jarosinski P, Gupta R, Pizzo PA. Safety, tolerance, and pharmacokinetics of amphotericin B lipid complex in children with hepatosplenic candidiasis. Antimicrob Agents Chemother 1997; 41: 1944–1948.
63. Shetty D, Giri N, Gonzalez CE, Pizzo PA, Walsh TJ. Invasive aspergillosis in human immunodeficiency virus-infected children. Pediatr Infect Dis J 1997; 16:216–221.

64. Singer S, Singer D, Ruchel R, Mergeryan H, Schmidt U, Harms K. Outbreak of systemic aspergillosis in a neonatal intensive care unit. Mycoses 1998; 41:223–227.
65. Thomas KE, Owens CM, Veys PA, Novelli V, Costoli V. The radiological spectrum of invasive aspergillosis in children: a 10-year review. Pediatr Radiol 2003; 33:453–460.
66. Chang HJ, Miller HL, Watkins N, Arduino MJ, Ashford DA, Midgley G, Aguero SM, Pinto-Powell R, von Reyn CF, Edwards W, McNeil MM, Jarvis WR. An epidemic of *Malassezia pachydermatis* in an intensive care nursery associated with colonization of health care workers pet dogs. N Engl J Med 1998; 338:706–711.
67. Chryssanthou E, Broberger U, Petrini B. *Malassezia pachydermatis* fungaemia in a neonatal intensive care unit. Acta Paediatr 2001; 90:323–327.
68. Welbel SF, McNeil MM, Pramanik A, Silberman R, Oberle AD, Midgley G, Crow S, Jarvis WR. Nosocomial *Malassezia pachydermatis* bloodstream infections in a neonatal intensive care unit. Pediatr Infect Dis J 1994; 13:104–108.
69. Dismukes WE, Bradsher RW Jr, Cloud GC, Kauffman CA, Chapman SW, George RB, Stevens DA, Girard WM, Saag MS, Bowles-Patton C. Itraconazole therapy for blastomycosis and histoplasmosis. The National Institute for Allergy and Infectious Diseases (NIAID). Mycoses Study Group. Am J Med 1992; 93:489–497.
70. Kaur R, Mittal N, Rawat D, Mathur MD. Cryptococcal meningitis in a neonate. Scand J Infect Dis 2002; 34:542–543.
71. Kotwani RN, Gokhale PC, Bodhe PV, Kirodian BG, Kshirsagar NA, Pandya SK. A comparative study of plasma concentrations of liposomal amphotericin B (L-AMP-LRC-1) in adults, children and neonates. Int J Pharm 2002; 238:11–15.
72. Walsh TJ, Seibel NL, Arndt C, Harris RE, Dinubile MJ, Reboli A, Hiemenz J, Chanock SJ. Amphotericin B lipid complex in pediatric patients with invasive fungal infections. Pediatr Infect Dis J 1999; 18:702–708.
73. Scarcella A, Pasquariello MB, Giugliano B, Vendemmia M, de Lucia A. Liposomal amphotericin B treatment for neonatal fungal infections. Pediatr Infect Dis J 1998; 17:146–148.
74. Al Arishi H, Frayha HH, Kalloghlian A, Al Alaiyan S. Liposomal amphotericin B in neonates with invasive candidiasis. Am J Perinatol 1998; 15:643–648.
75. Juster-Reicher A, Leibovitz E, Linder N, Amitay M, Flidel-Rtmon O, Even-Tov S, Mogilner B, Barzilai A. Liposomal amphotericin B (AmBisome) in the treatment of neonatal candidiasis in very low birth weight infants. Infection 2000; 28:223–226.
76. Juster-Reicher A, Flidel-Rimon O, Amitay M, Even-Tov S, Shinwell E, Leibovitz E. High-dose liposomal amphotericin B in the therapy of systemic candidiasis in neonates. Eur J Clin Microbiol Infect Dis 2003; 22:603–607.
77. Lee JW, Seibel NL, Amantea M, Whitcomb P, Pizzo PA, Walsh TJ. Safety and pharmacokinetics of fluconazole in children with neoplastic diseases. J Pediatr 1992; 120(6): 987–993.

8
Clinical Manifestations of Invasive Fungal Infections

Ben E. de Pauw
Department of Blood Transfusion and Transplant Immunology and Mycology Research Center Nijmegen, University Medical Center, St Radboud, Nijmegen, The Netherlands

Jacques F. G. M. Meis
Department of Medical Microbiology and Infectious Diseases, and Mycology Research Center Nijmegen, Canisius-Wilhelmina Hospital, Nijmegen, The Netherlands

I. UNEXPLAINED FEVER

Invasive fungal infections are principally encountered in patients who are seriously immunosuppressed over a long period of time (1). These opportunistic infections occur particularly in those with an impaired cellular immunity and/or a severe granulocytopenia (2,3). This association has crucial repercussions for both establishing the diagnosis and instituting an appropriate therapy. Granulocytes are supposed to protect an individual against opportunistic pathogens and this reaction accounts under normal circumstances for most signs and symptoms that may accompany a serious local and, subsequently, invasive fungal infection. As a consequence of the low number of granulocytes, the inflammatory reaction is muted and the absence of infiltrating white cells around the germinating fungi prohibits an early radiological diagnosis, which has in turn consequences for the management of these diseases (4). More than one-third of patients in whom an invasive fungal infection was found at autopsy never received any antifungal therapy, which indicates that the symptoms of an active and, obviously, lethal fungal infection are neither alarming nor very typical (1). Even in non-neutropenic patients, the diagnosis of an invasive fungal infection may be problematic because the clinical presentation is nonspecific and variable, related to the organs afflicted. Moreover, sometimes patients do not appear to be seriously endangered because the accompanying symptoms are ameliorated by concomitantly administered anti-inflammatory drugs. Because of the suppression of the fever by concurrent corticosteroids, even patients suffering from chronic disseminated mycoses may feel relatively well until the infection progresses and organ failure becomes evident. The fact that a large proportion of these opportunistic infections affect critically ill patients at the extremes of age is a further explanation for the paucity of symptoms. In addition, it has to be emphasized that the clinical picture can be disturbed by coexisting other infections too; they appear to play a role in a significant proportion of patients (5). The perturbed inflammatory reaction as a result of a low number of granulocytes, often in combination with immune modulating drugs, is responsible for a very wide spectrum of diseases, especially because chemotherapy-induced granulocytopenia is not a constant factor. It is a rather dynamic process with a time-dependent increase or decrease in the number of immune reactive cells. Upon return of the granulocytes, the clinical signs and symptoms will become readily detectable but in many cases, the infection would have reached an advanced stage by then (6). As is apparent from Table 1, there are very few clinical signs that can be regarded as characteristic for a particular invasive fungal infection. Fever, being present in 99% of the episodes, appears to be the only consistent signal of a possible, acute infection. This applies not merely to common organisms such as *Candida* and *Aspergillus* species but also to endemic mycoses, as well as to the emerging, more rare fungi like zygomycetes (mucormycosis), *Fusarium*, *Scedosporium/Pseudallescheria*, *Saccharomyces*, and *Rhodotorula* species. All of these organisms have occasionally been associated with life-threatening systemic symptoms and shock, but quite commonly unexplained fever is the first manifestation (7–14).

Candidemia can manifest itself with a sudden onset of fever and a sepsis syndrome accompanied by chills, hypotension, and myalgia and skin lesions. In patients eventually diagnosed with invasive candidiasis, unexplained fever was the first indication of infection in 88% of cases, whereas clinically documented organ involvement was encountered in barely 10% (15). Life-threatening organ infections may follow episodes of unexplained fever with numerous blood cultures that remained negative in spite of the fact that the blood is probably the vehicle for transport of the organisms from the gastrointestinal tract to the deep organs (16,17). Patients who develop candidemia during prophylaxis tend to be more acutely ill at the time of presentation and have a higher rate of disseminated disease, as well as pneumonia (18). Whilst acute disseminated candidiasis can arise within a few hours, the chronic form of this infection usually takes several days or even weeks to evolve to the full picture (Fig. 1) (19,20). The initial signs and symptoms of chronic disseminated candidiasis are

Table 1 Clinical Symptoms Suggestive of an Invasive Fungal Infection

---

All fungal infections
Persisting or new fever in patients known to be colonized by a fungus
Yeast infections
Retrosternal pain, upper abdominal discomfort
Increasing alkaline phosphatase with persisting, undulating fever
Multiple small hepatosplenic lesions on ultrasound when granulocytes recover
Chorioretinal lesions when granulocytes recover
Fever in combination with unexplained rash and muscular tenderness
Growing, sometimes partly necrotic, macronodular cutaneous lesions
Unexplained pain in spine and other bones; arthralgia
Mold infections
Dry cough with persisting fever
Chest pain related to respiration movements
Single or multiple pulmonary infiltrates, particularly wedge-shaped and halo sign
Air crescent sign when granulocytes recover
Elevated antigen levels, notably increasing titers
Facial pain with abnormality on nasal sinus x-ray

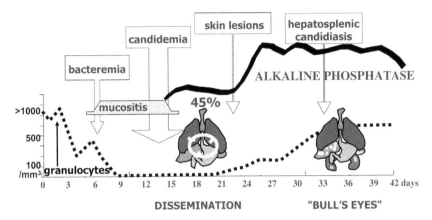

Figure 1 Sequence of events in disseminated candidiasis during neutropenia.

nonspecific, the most common presentation being persistent, sometimes intermittent, fever despite empirical broad-spectrum antibiotics with a gradual clinical deterioration and incremental dysfunction of the organs affected.

Over 30 years ago, it was shown that the diagnosis of invasive aspergillosis was not made during life in approximately two-third of patients who had evidence of disease at autopsy (21). More than three decades later, this percentage has not changed significantly. Invasive pulmonary aspergillosis in bone marrow transplant recipients often has an insidious inception such as fever unresponsive to empirical antibiotic therapy (22–24). However, the incidence of invasive aspergillosis amongst neutropenic patients with persisting fever is extremely low if other symptoms such as dyspnea, cough, and pleuritic chest pain are completely lacking. In a population without specific risk factors, which include prolonged deep granulocytopenia and exposure to moderate or high doses of corticosteroids, the frequency of invasive aspergillosis is well below 1%. In specific risk groups, such as allogeneic bone marrow transplant recipients with graft-vs.-host disease and cytomegalovirus reactivation, the incidence of invasive fungal infections may amount to more than 25%, but as a rule the persisting fever will be accompanied by another symptom indicative of a localized infection (23,24). The same is true for virtually all other mold infections.

Notwithstanding the lack of specificity of continuing fever as a trademark of invasive fungal infections, the clinicians' behavior in the prescription of systemically active antifungals is often guided by this rather aspecific early clinical sign given the dismal prognosis of a firmly established invasive fungal infection (25). In some categories of patients, it might be justifiable to start a broad-spectrum antifungal agent after 5–7 days of adequate antibacterial treatment if fever persists, provided that attempts to make a more precise diagnosis are not delayed in the false confidence that a possible mycotic infection has been covered.

II. BRONCHOPNEUMONIA

A. *Aspergillus* and *Aspergillus*-like Pulmonary Fungal Infections

Pulmonary infections, either as the primary focus or as a complication of septicemia, offer granulocytopenic patients a gloomy prospect as they have been blamed for 70%

of all fatal infections (26). Both Gram-negative and Gram-positive bacteria have been identified as causative agents of bronchopneumonia in the normal population, as well as in the immunocompromised host. However, although micro-organisms like *Pseudomonas aeruginosa* and *Mycobacterium tuberculosis* can show a strikingly similar clinical picture, a pneumonia caused by *Aspergillus fumigatus* or another mold ought to be the leading diagnostic consideration when a chest radiograph displays a gradually progressive pulmonary infiltrate in conjunction with antibacterial-refractory fever and chest pain (21–24). Mold infections are typically airborne and acquired by inhalation of spores into the airways of the sinuses and bronchial tree prior to or during immunosuppressive therapy. Particularly, smokers show a high prevalence of colonization of the airways by *Aspergillus* species.

Therefore, pneumonia, which evolves over days to weeks is by far the most common manifestation of invasive aspergillosis and other molds (21–24). Classically, the patient presents with fever, tachycardia, and new pulmonary infiltrates, preferably in the upper lobes. Pulmonary infiltrates deserve a careful work-up that encompasses all clinical, laboratory, as well as radiological findings. An example is given in Figure 2. Symptoms other than fever may be absent in the early stages of infection, while some patients with invasive aspergillosis will present with dyspnea or nonproductive cough. Suspicion should rise to a red alert zone in a patient with pleuritic pain and rubbing, or radiographic evidence of a pleural effusion or localized pulmonary infiltrates. *Aspergillus* species and other fungi have a propensity for invading blood vessels and surrounding tissue such as ribs, muscles, pericardium, and pleura, thereby causing local thrombosis, hemorrhage, and tissue damage. This behavior explains the principal symptoms because fungal invasion causes extensive necrosis and occlusion of small blood vessels that ultimately can lead to infarction of lung tissue. It is often difficult or even impossible to discriminate between a beginning invasive pulmonary fungal infection and pulmonary embolism and infarction on clinical grounds.

Typically, chest radiographs performed early in the evolution of infection fail to show infiltrates; it may take more than 3 days for the infection to generate enough

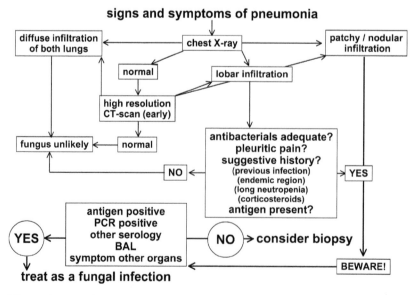

Figure 2 Algorithm for the diagnostic approach of pulmonary infiltrates.

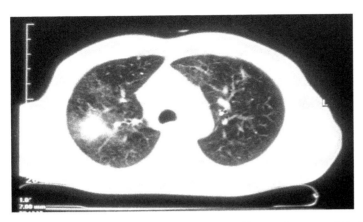

Figure 3 'Halo'-sign type of a pulmonary infiltrate. Courtesy of Dr Siem de Marie, University Medical Center Erasmus, Rotterdam, The Netherlands.

damage or for the few remaining granulocytes to concentrate around the infectious focus to allow recognition on a radiograph (6). By then, nodular patchy densities are the most prominent radiological manifestations of invasive pulmonary aspergillosis. In contrast, chest computed tomographs are already abnormal in a very early stage of development. Pulmonary nodules or areas of wedge-shaped consolidation on a chest radiograph are regarded as highly suspicious (27). The most characteristic findings on a high-resolution computed tomograph of the chest in neutropenic patients is a distinct halo of ground–glass attenuation around focal nodules (Fig. 3), which corresponds pathologically to hemorrhage around a focus of pulmonary infarction and a so-called air crescent sign (6,27). Notably upon engraftment and return of neutrophils, cavitation of the pneumonic process may occur as the normal lung previously infiltrated by fungal hyphae undergoes ischemic necrosis and separates from surrounding tissue. Under these circumstances, a so-called mycotic lung sequestrum may evolve with a risk of fatal massive hemoptysis that is exceptional in other patients.

While computerized tomography of the chest has shown to be an important aid to an early diagnosis, the pattern of the pulmonary infiltrate is merely suggestive of and not specific for a fungal infection. Unfortunately, cultures of specimens from bronchoalveolar lavage or bronchoscopic biopsy, if obtained at all, are often inconclusive or negative. On the other hand, nonculture techniques may assist in the interpretation of the radiographic findings. Serial serological monitoring of fungal antigens such as galactomannan or glucan, as well as screening for the possible presence of fungal nucleic acid sequences in blood or bronchoalveolar material by means of PCR assays may help to identify the origin of a lung infiltrate (28–31). Conversely, a positive test may indicate the necessity to perform a high-resolution computerized tomography. Efforts to establish a microbiological diagnosis should be vigorously pursued. It remains to be emphasized that it is impossible to distinguish pulmonary infections caused by *Aspergillus* species from infections with other molds such as *Rhizopus, Absidia,* and *Mucor* without cultures or histology. This also applies to *Bipolaris, Exserohilum,* and *Alternaria* species and, to a lesser extent, to increasingly encountered *Fusarium, Scopulariopsis,* and *Scedosporium* species (12,32,33). Pulmonary aspergillosis in immunocompromised patients has many faces (2,21,34). In patients with only mild abnormalities of their immune system, a more slowly progressive form of invasive pulmonary aspergillosis may develop. Among lung transplant recipients, the spectrum of disease encompasses bronchitis, both ulcerative and pseudomembranous, invasive pneumonia, empyema, disseminated infection, bronchocentric granulomatosis, aspergilloma, surgical wound infection, and allergic bronchopulmonary aspergillosis (35). Ulcerative tracheobronchitis is a form of invasive aspergillosis characteristically found in lung transplant recipients. It is usually seen within 1 month after transplant on routine bronchoscopy. While patients are asymptomatic and chest radiographs generally unchanged from baseline, the bronchoscopic picture reveals a pattern of severe tracheobronchitis progressing to multiple ulcers at the site of anastomosis. Possible sequelae vary from superficial scarring to bronchial necrosis with anastomotic dehiscence and invasive pulmonary disease. Endobronchial aspergillosis occurs rarely in bone marrow transplant recipients.

B. Other Pathogens

Primary pulmonary candidiasis without evidence of other systemic candidal infection is extremely exceptional, although incidentally isolated bronchopneumonia and lung abscesses have been reported (36). *Candida glabrata* apparently causing pneumonia has been reported in patients with longstanding IV catheters who were treated with broad-spectrum antibiotics after cytotoxic chemotherapy and long-term corticosteroid therapy (37).

Occasionally, *Cryptococcus neoformans* stays confined to the lungs, presenting with dull chest pain, dyspnea, and cough; a chest x-ray will show miliary or nodular shadows in these cases (38).

Fever, cough, and chest pain and bilateral infiltrates visible on chest radiographs are rather germane signs and symptoms, which, however, can be caused by an array of fungal organisms. In the respective endemic areas, *Histoplasma capsulatum, Coccidioides immitis*, and *Paracoccidioides brasiliensis* (Fig. 4) have been held responsible for debilitating and even life-threatening pulmonary infections (39,40). A segmental pneumonia can be seen in approximately half of patients, whereas pleural effusions, nodules, or intrapulmonary cavities remain limited to a small number of cases. Symptomatic patients infected with *Blastomyces dermatitidis* usually have an influenza-like syndrome with fever, chills, arthralgias, cough, pleuritic chest pain, and hemoptysis (41). In acute blastomycosis, chest radiographs may

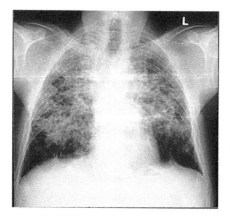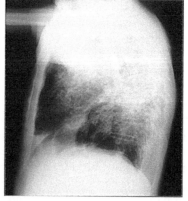

Figure 4 Pulmonary pattern of a *Paracoccidioides* infection.

show massive lobar or segmental consolidation that resembles a pulmonary malignancy, whereas the chronic form may mimic tuberculosis. Pleural thickening and small pleural effusions do occur but large pleural effusions are uncommon. Miliary disease and diffuse pneumonitis, often associated with respiratory failure, have been reported and are associated with a high mortality. *Pneumocystis carinii/jerovici*, now classified as a fungus, is the predominant cause of opportunistic interstitial pneumonia in transplant recipients. Typically, a patient becomes increasingly dyspneic with fever and malaise followed by nonproductive cough in association with the chest radiography exhibiting bilateral infiltrates or asymmetric abnormalities.

Management of pulmonary infiltrates is complex. Many infiltrates do have a noninfectious etiology and can be due to adverse effects of cytotoxic therapy, irradiation or pulmonary hemorrhage. Furthermore, it has to be emphasized that conditions favorable for development of fungal infections also facilitate other pathogenic micro-organisms. Alangaden et al. (5) described a survey on 88 bone marrow or peripheral stem cell recipients who suffered from graft-versus-host disease. From this group, 12 had to be readmitted to the hospital with a suspected pulmonary infection. Cough and fever had been the initial symptoms in the majority of cases; 10 out of 12 were shown to have pulmonary aspergillosis, although Gram-negative pathogens, including *P. aeruginosa* and *Enterobacter cloacae,* were concurrently isolated from the sputum or blood of 6 out of 10 patients. Moreover, for 5 of the 6 patients, not only the initial presentation but also the chest radiographic findings had been compatible with bacterial pneumonia. Without a computerized scan of the chest, half of the patients might have been treated as pure bacterial pneumonia and the coexisting pulmonary aspergillosis might have been missed. This observation indicates the complexity of the problem, as well as the urge to maximize the diagnostic efforts. The critical decision faced by the clinician at the bedside of patients with pulmonary infiltrates is whether or not to undertake invasive procedures. Sputum cultures are rarely diagnostic and the yield of bronchoscopy with bronchoalveolar lavage is disappointingly low. Percutaneous needle aspiration appears a better method to obtain adequate specimens for histological examination and/or culture, but this procedure is frequently considered precluded because of a concurrent thrombocytopenia. The exact role of these diagnostic approaches for the optimal management of patients remains controversial because the yield depends on the collaboration and skills of various specialists.

III. SKIN LESIONS

Mycotic infections of the skin have a rather common occurrence. However, sometimes skin lesions reflect serious, often life-threatening underlying fungal infections. Fungi that are known to involve the skin are listed in Table 2. In about 10% of patients, acute invasive candidiasis is accompanied by severe myalgia and typical pinkish-purple, painless subcutaneous nodules that may arise anywhere on the body (36). *Candida* species may also produce lesions that resemble ecthyma gangrenosum or purpura fulminans, but such a distinctive appearance is more common in disseminated fusariosis (Fig. 5). The clinical signs and symptoms of infections by *Saccharomyces cerevisiae*, also known as baker's yeast, *Rhodotorula*, and *Malassezia furfur*, the causative agent of pityriasis versicolor, are in essence not different from those encountered in acute disseminated candidiasis. The correct diagnosis of these more rare fungi is seldom suspected before the organism is recovered from blood, urine,

Table 2 Differential Diagnosis of Skin Lesions in Febrile Immunosuppressed Patients

Maculo-papulomatous lesions
Drug allergy (allopurinol, cotrimoxazole, penicillins, cephalosporins, etc.)
Reaction to blood transfusion
Fungi (*Candida* species, *Malassezia furfur*, *Cryptococcus neoformans*, *Trichosporon*,
    Histoplasma, *Coccidioides immitis*, *Penicillium marneffei*)
Viral (measles, rubeola)
Graft-versus-host disease
Pustulae, folliculitis
Fungi (*Candida* species, *Malassezia furfur*, *Fusarium* species, *Blastomyces*, *Penicillium*
    marneffei)
Bacterial (staphylococci, streptococci)
Viral (Herpes viruses)
Ulcerative lesions and necrosis
Bacterial (staphylococci, streptococci, enterococci, *Pseudomonas aeruginosa*, etc.)
Anaerobic organisms (*Clostridium perfringens*, *Actinomyces*)
Fungi (*Trichosporon*, *Blastomyces*, *Aspergillus*, *Alternaria*, and *Scedosporium* species)
Erythema
Drug allergy (allopurinol, cotrimoxazole, penicillins, cephalosporins, etc.)
Fungi (*Candida* species, particularly in skin folds, *Coccidioides immitis*)
Viral (measles, rubeola)
Graft-versus-host disease
Overheating

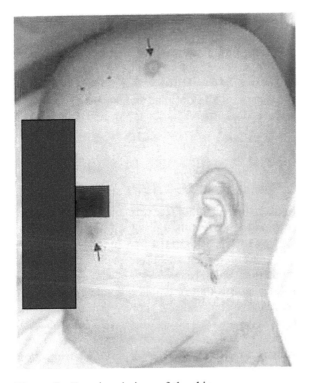

Figure 5 Fusarium lesions of the skin.

or a cutaneous lesion. *Penicillium marneffei*, endemic in South-East Asia can cause disseminated infections with papular skin lesions in immunocompromised patients (42).

Cutaneous disease accounts for 75–80% of cases of sporotrichosis. *Trichosporon beigelii* and *Sporothrix schenckii* naturally gain access to the body through minor injuries of fingers and hands. Subsequently small, erythematous papules or subcutaneous nodules at a site of injury may emerge. These lesions often wax and wane for months or years but eventually the organism will reach the local lymph nodes. If IV catheters are the porte d'entree for *T. beigelii*, an overwhelming disseminated infection may ensue in patients with neutrophil defects (43).

In blastomycosis, skin disease usually occurs in conjunction with pulmonary disease (41). The well-demarcated and indurated lesions tend to appear on sunlight-exposed parts of the body, notably the face and distal extremities. In the early phase, a small papule or pustule is seen that gradually enlarges over a period of weeks or months, becoming elevated, verrucous, and crusted. Removal of the crust reveals a granulomatous base with numerous small abscesses that exude purulent material. Sometimes, central healing and scarring go together with active expansion at the outer border of the lesion.

Within the first days of onset of an infection with *C. immitis*, a fine, generalized maculopapular rash, sometimes urticarial in appearance develops in 10–40% of patients (39). The development of cutaneous hypersensitivity may be manifest as erythema nodosum or erythema multiforme, which occurs in less than 25% of infected individuals.

Nonspecific skin lesions, usually firm nodules, are suggestive but uncommon in neutropenic patients with disseminated histoplasmosis.

A. fumigatus and *A. flavus* have been described as the cause of necrotizing infections at the insertion site of long-standing central venous catheters (2,21,24). Involvement of the skin with Mucorales like *Rhizopus arrhizus* may be primary or secondary, following dissemination from another site (7,10). Other fungi with a *Aspergillus*-like behavior such as *Fusarium, Curvularia, Pseudallescheria*, and *Alternaria* species have also been held responsible for similar cutaneous infections in the compromised host (Fig. 5) (8,13,44). Moreover, *Pseudallescheria boydii* is a well-recognized cause of mycetoma—a localized noncontagious infection that can progress very slowly and involves cutaneous tissue, fascia, and bone (12). Mycetoma may be caused by either various other fungi or actinomycetes and generally follows a local trauma.

IV. SINUSITIS AND CENTRAL NERVOUS SYSTEM DISEASE

Hematogenous spread of *Aspergillus* species from the lung to the brain can occur. Differential diagnostic considerations are summarized in Table 3. As a rule, affected patients develop headache, seizures, or other focal neurological signs, depending on the localization of the infection. Aspergillosis of the central nervous system may also originate from an aggressive *Aspergillus* sinusitis with or without a pulmonary infection (2,21). Presenting symptoms include fever, orbital swelling, facial pain, and nasal congestion. In bone marrow transplant recipients and other severely immunocompromised patients, *Aspergillus* sinusitis is frequently destructive, extending beyond the sinuses to the orbit or brain. The clinical picture of zygomycosis, fusariosis, and alternariosis resembles aspergillosis. However, in zygomycosis, the

Table 3 Differential Diagnosis Central Nervous System Disease in Febrile
Immunosuppressed Patients

Meningitis/encephalitis-like
Bacteria (meningococcus, pneumococus. *Listeria monocytogenes*)
Fungi (*Candida* species and other yeasts, *Cryptococcus neoformans*, endemic fungi)
Viral (cytomegalovirus, herpes)
Graft-versus-host disease
Radiotherapy- and chemotherapy-induced tissue damage
Cyclosporin toxicity
Intracerebral
Bacterial (staphylococci, streptococci, *Pseudomonas aeruginosa*, etc.)
Fungi (mainly molds like *Aspergillus* species, zygomycetes, blastomycosis)
Parasites (*Toxoplasma gondii*)
Lymphoma, including post-transplant lymphoma
Cyclosporin toxicity
Primary brain tumor

---

rhinocerebral form is more pronounced and aggressive than in aspergillosis, featuring painful unilateral facial swelling, ptosis, proptosis, and dilation or fixation of the pupil, together with a dark, serosanguinous nasal discharge (Fig. 5) (7,10). Drainage of black material from the eye is sometimes seen. Local symptoms of sinusitis and palatal or orbital cellulitis may be encountered or in more advanced disease ulceration of the nasal septum with even necrosis or perforation. The nasal turbinate bones are often black and necrotic. Neurologic sequelae evolve after a few days and usually are rapidly progressive and include blindness, cranial nerve involvement, and finally, contralateral hemiplegia because of thrombosis of the carotid artery or cerebral abscesses. Progressive lethargy develops and coma follows. Severe myalgias, sinusitis, ocular symptoms, and multiorgan system involvement are distinctive symptoms of disseminated fusariosis. *Pseudallescheria boydii* may also infect the eye and central nervous system, particularly in severely immunosuppressed patients and after accidents (45,46).

In cases of acute disseminated candidiasis, involvement of the central nervous system, presenting with headache, lethargy, and disorientation as a manifestation of meningitis, encephalitis, abscess, or hemorrhage is not an uncommon feature in children (47,48). It is frustrating that in fewer than 50% of such cases, examination of cerebrospinal fluid will reveal yeast cells.

Central nervous system involvement is reported in less than 5% of cases of blastomycosis. Abscesses presenting as massive lesions are most common; meningitis is usually a late complication and frequently associated with multiorgan disease. Short-term mortality rates associated with fungal infections of the central nervous system are extremely high, with exception of cryptococcal meningitis. Usually *C. neoformans* spreads from the lungs to central nervous system causing a highly variable clinical pattern of signs and symptoms. The most common signs and symptoms include headache, fever, nucheal rigidity, cranial nerve palsies, impaired memory and judgment, lethargy, obtundation, and coma (38). Patients may present with acute symptoms of only a few days' duration, particularly when they are immunosuppressed, whereas others may have subtle symptoms for weeks or months before the diagnosis is made.

V. DISSEMINATED DISEASE AND MISCELLANEOUS ISSUES

Many fungi may trigger serious, acute disseminated infections with potential invasion of many vital organs. *Candida* species, *Aspergillus* species, *Fusarium* species, and *Pseudallescheria boydii* have been incriminated in a wide range of clinical syndromes, varying from esophagitis to disseminated sepsis-like infections. Severe myalgias and polyarthralgias, with or without disseminated ecthyma gangrenosum-like skin lesions, and multiorgan system involvement are starting symptoms of an acute disseminated infection by any of these organisms.

Alternatively, a disseminated fungal infection may mimic a single organ infection, but in most cases, a limited number of organs seem to be infected; in these cases, the clinical and laboratory symptomatology is determined by the affected organ. Ophthalmologic examination is a valuable tool for monitoring patients at risk of disseminated candidiasis and can establish infection in patients with negative blood cultures and no detectable colonization at other sites. Fundoscopic abnormalities, either early or mature, are present at baseline in approximately 10–20% of patients (49,50). The characteristic fluffy exudates may precede a loss of visual acuity and, if inadequately treated, blindness. *Candida* endophthalmitis seldom occurs in neutropenic patients since the lesions are the result of an inflammatory response that requires granulocytes. Other organs that serve as favorite destinations of a disseminated *Candida* infection or other fungi are the bones and the heart. Arthritis and osteomyelitis usually have an insidious onset, the long bones, vertebrae, hip or knee being most commonly affected (16). Endocarditis is associated with indwelling intravascular catheters and the typical, large vegetations may subsequently be shed as fungal emboli all over the body. Surgical replacement of the valve is essential but patients are often not able to undergo open heart surgery.

Since the introduction of mucosa damaging chemotherapy, chronic disseminated candidiasis is being recognized rather frequently (20,51). A schematic course of the evolution of such an infection is depicted in Figure 1. Typically, the patient has an irregular fever, complaints of abdominal discomfort with anorexia, vomiting, right upper quadrant tenderness, and elevation of alkaline phosphatase levels with or without hepatosplenomegaly (52). After recovery from neutropenia, an abdominal ultrasound or CT scan will demonstrate rather unique multiple abscesses in the liver and/or spleen, known as "bull's eyes." Intra-abdominal abscesses or peritonitis caused by *Candida* species are serious complications of recurrent surgery for acute pancreatitis or of continuous ambulatory peritoneal dialysis.

Patients with candidal esophagitis typically complain of a burning retrosternal pain that becomes worse on swallowing. The diagnosis of oropharyngeal candidiasis is often made clinically but it has to be taken into account that it is impossible to distinguish between *Candida* and other infections, particularly Herpes simplex. Blastomyces can be found in painless osteolytic lesions. This organism can also infect the prostate and epididymis, whereas the kidney is usually spared. Patients note a painful swelling of the testis or epididymis, a perineal ache, or symptoms of urinary obstruction.

By virtue of the organism's propensity for vascular invasion, inadequately treated pulmonary aspergillosis often disseminates to other sites, including the pericardium (Fig. 6) and myocardium, brain, eyes, kidneys, and gastrointestinal tract. *Pseudallescheria boydii* may also infect the eye, sinuses, ear, lungs, heart, bone, joints, and skin, particularly in the immunosuppressed patient. In addition, *Fusarium, Curvularia, Bipolaris, Exserohilum*, and *Alternaria* species have been held responsible for

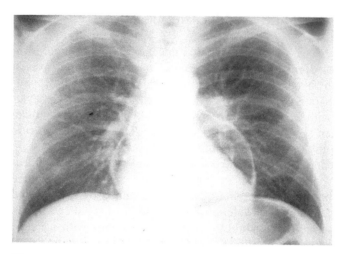

Figure 6 Pneumopericardium due to aspergillosis.

disseminated infections very similar to those caused by *Aspergillus* species. In fact, often only on the basis of culture and histology, the distinction between the various fungi can be made.

REFERENCES

1. Bodey GP, Bueltmann B, Duguid W, Gibbs D, Hanak H, Mall G, Martino P, Meunier F, Milliken S, Naoe S, Okudaira M, Scevola D, van't Wout J. Fungal infections in cancer patients: an international autopsy survey. Eur J Clin Microbiol Infect Dis 1992; 11: 99–109.
2. Denning DW. Invasive aspergillosis. Clin Infect Dis 1998; 26:781–805.
3. Gerson SL, Talbot GH, Hurwitz S, Strom BL, Lusk EJ, Cassileth PA. Prolonged granulocytopenia: the major risk factor for invasive pulmonary aspergillosis in patients with acute leukemia. Ann Intern Med 1984; 100:345–351.
4. Sickles EA, Greene WH, Wiernik PH. Clinical presentation of infection in granulocytopenic patients. Arch Intern Med 1975; 135:715–719.
5. Alangaden GJ, Wahiduzzaman M, Chandrasekar PH, the Bone Marrow Transplant Group. Aspergillosis: the most common community-acquired pneumonia with Gram-negative bacilli as copathogens in stem cell transplant recipients with graft-versus-host-disease. Clin Infect Dis 2002; 35:659–564.
6. Caillot D, Couaillier J-F, Bernard A, Casasnovas O, Denning DW, Mannone L, Lopez J, Couillault G, Pirard F, Vagner O, Guy H. Increasing volume and changing characteristics of invasive pulmonary aspergillosis on sequential thoracic computed tomography scans in patients with neutropenia. J Clin Oncol 2001; 19:253–259.
7. Anaissie E. Opportunistic mycoses in the immunocompromised host: experience at a cancer center and review. Clin Infect Dis 1992; 14 (suppl 1):S43–S53.
8. Boutati EI, Anaissie EJ. Fusarium, a significant emerging pathogen in patients with hematologic malignancy: ten years' experience at a cancer center and implications for management. Blood 1997; 90:999–1008.
9. Girmenia C, Pagano L, Corvatta L, Mele L, Del Favero A, Martino P for the Gimema Infection Programme. The epidemiology of fusariosis in patients with haematological diseases. Br J Haematol 2000; 111:272–276.
10. Kontoyiannis DP, Wessel VC, Bodey GP, Rolston KVI. Zygomycosis in a tertiary care center. Clin Infect Dis 2000; 30:851–856.

11. Lyke KE, Miller NS, Towne L, Merz WG. A case of cutaneous ulcerative alternariosis: rare association with diabetes mellitus and unusual failure of itraconazole treatment. Clin Infect Dis 2001; 32:1178–1187.

12. Mesnard R, Lamy T, Dauriac C, Le Prise PY. Lung abscess due to *Pseudallescheria boydii* in the course of acute leukaemia. Report of a case and review of the literature. Acta Haematol 1992; 87:78–82.

13. Nucci M, Anaissie E. Cutaneous infection by *Fusarium* species in healthy and immuno-compromised hosts: implications for diagnosis and management. Clin Infect Dis 2002; 35:909–920.

14. Revankar SG, Patterson JE, Sutton DA, Pullen R, Rinaldi MG. Disseminated phaeohy-phomycosis: review of an emerging mycosis. Clin Infect Dis 2002; 34:467–476.

15. Viscoli C, Girmenia C, Marinus A, Collette L, Martino P, Vandercam B, Doyen C, Lebeau B, Spence D, Krcmery V, De Pauw B, Meunier F, the Invasive Fungal Infection Group of EORTC. Candidemia in cancer patients: a prospective, multicenter surveillance study by the Invasive Fungal Infection Group (IFIG) of the European Organization for Research and Treatment of Cancer (EORTC). Clin Infect Dis 1999; 28:1071–1079.

16. Gathe JC, Harris RL, Garland B, Bradshaw MW, Williams TW. *Candida* osteomyelitis. Report of five cases and review of the literature. Am J Med 1987; 82:927–937.

17. Goodrich JM, Reed EC, Mori M, Fisher LD, Skerrett S, Dandliker PS, Klis B, Counts GW, Meyers JD. Clinical features and analysis of risk factors for invasive candidal infection after marrow transplantation. J Infect Dis 1991; 164:731–740.

18. Uzun O, Ascioglu S, Anaissie EJ, Rex JH. Risk factors and predictors of outcome in patients with cancer and breakthrough candidemia. Clin Infect Dis 2001; 32:1713–1717.

19. Vincent J-L, Anaissie E, Bruining H, Demajo W, El-Ebiary M, Haber J, Hiramatsu Y, Nitenberg G, Nyström P-O, Pettit D, Rogers T, Sandven P, Sganga G, Schaller M-D, Solomkin J. Epidemiology, diagnosis and treatment of systemic *Candida* infection in surgical patients under intensive care. Intensive Care Med 1998; 24:206–216.

20. Sallah S, Semelka RC, Wehbie R, Sallah W, Nguyen NP, Vos P. Hepatosplenic candidia-sis in patients with acute leukaemia. Br J Haematol 1999; 106:697–701.

21. Young RC, Bennett JE, Vogel CL, Carbone PP, DeVita VT. Aspergillosis. The spectrum of the disease in 98 patients. Medicine 1970; 49:147–173.

22. Denning DW, Marinus A, Cohen J, Spence D, Herbrecht R, Pagano L, Kibbler C, Krcmery V, Offher F, Cordonnier F, Jehn U, Ellis M, Collette L, Sylvester R, the EORTC Invasive Fungal Infections Cooperative Group. An EORTC multicentre prospective survey of invasive aspergillosis in haematological patients. Diagnosis and therapeutic outcome. J Infect 1998; 37:173–180.

23. Paterson DL, Singh N. Invasive aspergillosis in transplant recipients. Medicine 1999; 78:123–138.

24. Patterson TF, Kirkpatrick WR, White M, Hiemenz J, Wingard JR, Dupont B, Rinaldi MG, Stevens DA, Graybill JR for the 3 Aspergillus Study Group. Invasive aspergillosis. Disease spectrum, treatment practices, and outcomes. Medicine 2000; 79:250–260.

25. Pizzo PA, Robichaud KJ, Gill FA, Witebsky FG. Empiric antibiotic and antifungal therapy for cancer patients with prolonged fever and granulocytopenia. Am J Med 1984; 72:101–107.

26. Novakova IRO, Donnelly JP, De Pauw BE. Potential sites of infections that develop in febrile neutropenic patients. Leuk Lymph 1993; 10:461–467.

27. Kuhlman JE, Fishman EK, Siegelman SS. Invasive pulmonary aspergillosis in acute leukemia: characteristic findings on CT, the CT halo sign, and the role of CT in early diagnosis. Radiology 1985; 157:611–614.

28. Verweij PE, Stynen D, Rijs AJMM, de Pauw BE, Hoogkamp-Korstanje JA, Meis JF. Sandwich enzyme-linked immunosorbent assay compared with Pastorex latex agglutina-tion test for diagnosing invasive aspergillosis in immunocompromised patients. J Clin Microbiol 1995; 33:1912–1914.

29. Obayashi T, Yoshida M, Mori T, et al. Plasma $(1\rightarrow3)$-beta-D-glucan measurement in the diagnosis of invasive deep mycosis and fungal febrile episodes. Lancet 1995; 345:17–20.
30. Van Burik JA, Meyerson D, Schrecklise RW, Bowden RA. Panfungal PCR assay for the detection of fungal infection in human blood specimens. J Clin Microbiol 1998; 36: 1169–1175.
31. Kami M, Fukui T, Ogawa S, Kazuyama Y, Machida U, Tanaka Y, Kanda Y, Kashima T, Yamazaki Y, Hamaki T, Mori S, Akiyama H, Mutou Y, Sakamaki H, Osumi K, Kimura S, Hirai H. Use of real-time PCR on blood samples for diagnosis of invasive aspergillosis. Clin Infect Dis 2001; 33:1504–1512.
32. Morrison VA, Haake RJ, Weisdorf DJ. Non-candidal fungal infections after bone marrow transplantation: risk factors and outcome. Am J Med 1994; 96:497–503.
33. Marr KA, Carter RA, Crippa F, Wald A, Corey L. Epidemiology and outcome of mold infections in hematopoietic stem cell transplant recipients. Clin Infect Dis 2002; 34: 909–917.
34. Baddley JW, Stroud TP, Salzman D, Pappas PG. Invasive mold infections in allogeneic bone marrow transplant recipients. Clin Infect Dis 2001; 32:1319–1324.
35. Gordon SM, Avery RK. Aspergillosis in lung transplantation: incidence, risk factors, and prophylactic strategies. Transpl Infect Dis 2001; 3:161–166.
36. Meunier F. Candidiasis. Eur J Clin Microbiol Infect Dis 1989; 8:438–447.
37. Kontoyiannis DP, Reddy BT, Torres HA, Luna M, Lewis RE, Tarrand J, Bodey GP, Raad II. Pulmonary candidiasis in patients with cancer: an autopsy study. Clin Infect Dis 2002; 33:400–403.
38. Saag MS, Graybill RJ, Larsen RA, Pappas PG, Perfect JR, Powderley WG, Sobel JD, Dismukes WE for the Mycosis Study Group Cryptococcal subproject. Practice guidelines for management of cryptococcal disease. Clin Infect Dis 2000; 30:710–718.
39. Galgiani JN, Ampel NM, Cantanzaro A, Johnson RH, Stevens DA, Williams PL. Practice guidelines for the treatment of coccidioidomycosis. Clin Infect Dis 2000; 30:653–657.
40. Wheat J, Sarosi G, McKinsey D, Hamill R, Bradsher R, Johnson P, Loyd J, Kauffman C. Practice guidelines for the management of patients with histoplasmosis. Clin Infect Dis 2000; 30:688–695.
41. Chapman SW, Bradsher RW Jr, Campbell GD, Pappas PG, Kauffman CA. Practice guidelines for the treatment of blastomycosis. Clin Infect Dis 2000; 30:679–683.
42. Supparatpinyo K, Chiewchanvit S, Hirunsri P, Uthammachai C, Nelson KE, Sirisanthana T. Penicillium marneffei infection in patients infected with human immunodeficiency virus. Clin Infect Dis 1992; 14:871–874.
43. Kauffman CA, Hajjeh R, Chapman SW for the Mycosis Study Group. Practice guidelines for the management of patients with sporotrichosis. Clin Infect Dis 2000; 30: 684–687.
44. Shearer C, Chandrasekar PH. Cutaneous alternariosis and regional lymphadenitis during allogeneic BMT. Bone Marrow Transplant 1993; 11:497–499.
45. Safdar A, Papadopoulos EB, Young JW. Breakthrough *Scedosporium apiospermum* (*Pseudallescheria boydii*) brain abscess during therapy for invasive pulmonary aspergillosis following high-risk allogeneic hematopoietic stem cell transplantation. Scedosporiasis and recent advances in antifungal therapy. Transpl Infect Dis 2002; 4:212–217.
46. Ruchel R, Wilichowski E. Cerebral *Pseudallescheria mycosis* after near-drowning. Mycosis 1995; 38:473–475.
47. Lipton SA, Hickey WF, Morris JH, Loscalzo J. Candidal infection in the central nervous system. Am J Med 1984; 76:101–108.
48. McCullers JA, Vargas SL, Flynn PM, Razzouk I, Shenep J. Candidal meningitis in children with cancer. Clin Infect Dis 2000; 31:451–457.
49. Rex J, Bennett J, Sugar A, et al. A randomised trial comparing fluconazole with amphotericin B for the treatment of candidemia in patients without neutropenia. N Eng J Med 1994; 331:1325–1330.

50. Philips P, Safran S, Garber G, Rostein C, Smaill F, Fong I, Salit I, Miller M, Williams K, Conly JM, Ioannou S, for the Canadian Candidemia Study Group. Multicenter randomized trial of fluconazole versus amphothericin B for the treatment of candidemia in non-neutropenic patients. Eur J Clin Microbiol Infect Dis 1997; 16:337–345.
51. Blijlevens NMA, Donnelly JP, De Pauw BE. Impaired gut function as risk factor for invasive candidiasis in neutropenic patients. Brit J Haematol 2002; 117:259–264.
52. Haron E, Feld R, Tuffnell P, Patterson B, Hasselback B, Matlow A. Hepatic candidiasis: an increasing problem in immunocompromised patients. Am J Med 1987; 83:17–26.

9

Clinical Syndromes by *Candida* Species

María Cecilia Dignani
Head Infectious Diseases FUNDALEU (Foundation for the Fight Against Leukemia),
Uriburu, Buenos Aires, Argentina

I. INTRODUCTION

Candidiasis refers to infections caused by any of the >150 species of the genus *Candida*, mainly *Candida albicans*. The history of candidiasis dates back to the fourth century B.C. Since the 1940s, the frequency and severity of these infections have been increasing sharply as a result of the widespread use of broad spectrum antibiotics, steroids, and other immunosuppressive drugs (1). *Candida* species are ubiquitous human commensals. They become pathogens in situations where the host's resistance to infection is lowered locally or systemically. In such circumstances, *Candida* spp. can cause superficial, locally invasive, or disseminated infection. *Candida* spp. are the fourth most common cause of bloodstream infections in the United States (2). These bloodstream infections are associated with an estimated annual national cost that ranges from US$200 million to $1 billon (3,4).

II. THE PATHOGEN

Candida spp. are thin-walled, small yeasts (4–6 μm) that reproduce by budding. The genus *Candida* belongs to the order Saccharomycetales, family Saccharomycetaceae.

Seven species in the genus *Candida* are well-known opportunistic causes of infection (Table 1), while many others have been described as pathogens in individual case reports or short case series (5).

In 1995, a new species, *C. dubliniensis*, was defined. Morphologically and physiologically, the phenotype of *C. dubliniensis* resembles *C. albicans*. Germ tubes formed by *C. dubliniensis* are indistinguishable from those of *C. albicans*. *Candida dubliniensis* colonies sometimes appear as a darker green hue than those of *C. albicans* on a commercial differential isolation medium (6). It differs from *C. albicans* principally by the nonreactivity of its DNA with a *C. albicans*-specific molecular probe (7), but the presence of intracellular β-glucosidase activity in *C. dubliniensis* is otherwise the only phenotypic difference found with high consistency (6).

Candida albicans can grow over a very wide pH range, from below 2.0 to almost 8.0 and under aerobic, microaerophilic, and even anaerobic conditions of incubation.

Table 1 List of *Candida* spp. that are Opportunistic Human Pathogens

Species commonly implicated in human infections	Species uncommonly implicated in human infections
C. albicans	*C. catelunata*
C. glabrata	*C. chiropterorum*
C. guilliermondii	*C. ciferrii*
C. krusei	*C. dubliniensis*
C. lusitaniae	*C. famata*
C. parapsilosis	*C. haemulonii*
C. tropicalis	*C. humicola*
	C. inconspicua
	C. kefyr
	C. lambica
	C. lipolytica
	C. norvegensis
	C. pelliculosa
	C. pintolopesii
	C. pulcherrima
	C. rugosa
	C. utilis
	C. zeylanoides

III. EPIDEMIOLOGY

The *Candida* spp. colonize primarily the gastrointestinal tract, and can also be found in the vagina, urethra, skin, and under the finger nails. *Candida albicans* has been recovered from different environmental sources that include fresh and seawater, soil, and any items that have contact with humans directly, such as clothing, bedding, and toothbrushes. Places where *C. albicans* is found are almost invariably the result of human and animal contamination (1,8,9).

   Candida spp. can be part of the normal oral flora in 25–50% of healthy subjects (10). In hospitalized patients, the oral carriage rates are higher (50–70%) (11). Oral carriage rates are also higher in certain settings, such as HIV-infected patients (12), denture users with denture stomatitis (13), diabetic patients (14), patients on chemotherapy for malignant conditions (15,16), and children (17). The species that predominate in skin samples are *C. guilliermondii* and *C. parapsilosis*, rather than *C. albicans*.

   Colonization at a specific site by more than one species of *Candida* can be as high as 44% (11,12,18–21). Simultaneous *Candida* colonization of more than one site may involve the same or different *Candida* strains. Concurrent isolation of similar species is the most common finding when the sites are anatomically related. More than 90% of *Candida* strains isolated simultaneously from vagina, urethra, and anus represent the same species. By contrast, only 61–75% of simultaneously isolated anal and oral *Candida* strains were the same (18,22).

   The predominant source of infection in all types of candidiasis is the patient himself or herself. Transmission of *Candida* spp. from the gastrointestinal tract to the bloodstream requires prior overgrowth of the number of yeasts in their commensal habitat (23), and is favored by loss of the integrity of the gastrointestinal mucosa (24,25).

Exogenous transmission of *Candida* also occurs. Outbreaks of *Candida* spp. infection resulting from contaminated materials have been described (26–29). Transmission of *Candida* species from staff to patient and from patient to patient has been demonstrated (30,31), mainly in specialized, relatively closed settings, such as burn (32), geriatric (21), hematology (33,34), intensive care (medical, surgical, adult, and neonatal) (35–37), and transplantation units (38,39).

The acquisition of *Candida* spp. by neonates can be the result of two mechanisms. Most newborn babies acquire a *Candida* flora from the maternal vagina at the time of birth or during gestation. However, nonperinatal nosocomial transmission can also occur (40). The hands of the hospital personnel may be a potential reservoir for nosocomial *Candida* spp. acquisition by neonates (41).

The survival of clinical isolates of five species of *Candida* was determined on the palms of human volunteers (42). Transmission from one hand to a second and to a third hand was observed in 69% and 38% of the experiments, respectively. *Candida albicans* was able to survive for 24 hr on inanimate surfaces, and transmission to and from inanimate surfaces was successful in 90% of the experiments.

Although most women who suffer from *Candida* spp. vulvovaginitis are infected with an endogenous commensal strain, there is a possibility of sexual transmission between partners (43,44), especially in the setting of receptive oral sex (45,46). Most cases of recurrence of vaginal *Candida* spp. infection have been ascribed to relapse with the same strain (47), rather than to infection with a new strain.

Among heroin abusers, hematogenous candidiasis (48) is usually acquired through the IV injection of a solution of heroin dissolved in contaminated lemon juice. The lemon juice originally becomes contaminated most probably with yeasts from the heroin users themselves an example of indirect transmission of an endogenous strain (49–51).

Candida albicans is the most commonly implicated organism in human candidiasis (52). The most frequent nonalbicans species regarded as pathogens are *C. dublinensis, C. glabrata, C. guilliermondii, C. krusei, C. lusitaniae, C. parapsilosis, C. pseudotropicalis*, and *C. tropicalis*.

The widespread use of the antifungal agent fluconazole for therapy and prophylaxis in HIV-infected patients has been associated with the appearance of fluconazole-resistant strains of *C. albicans* (53,54) and increasing frequency of non-*albicans Candida* strains in the oral mucosa (55,56). However, since the time the highly active antiretroviral therapy (HAART) became available, the rate of carriage of fluconazole-resistant *C. albicans* has significantly declined as a function of he host's immune status (57).

Candida spp. are now the fourth most common organism isolated from blood of hospitalized patients in the United States (58). A survey of 1591 cases of hematogenous candidiasis found that the prevalence of non-*albicans Candida* species was 46% and was largely unchanged from 1952 to 1992 (59). However, more recent data suggest that in certain settings a reduction in the rates of *C. albicans* in favor of the non-*albicans* spp., may be occurring (60–63). These changes may be a consequence of increased immunosuppression, the use of prophylactic antifungal treatments, or the lack of adequate infection control measures. The use of prophylactic antifungal treatments with azoles has been associated with the likelihood of infections by *C. glabrata* and *C. krusei* (64,65), not *C. parapsilosis* (62). A strong association between *C. parapsilosis* and IV catheters has been suggested (66).

IV. PATHOGENESIS

The pathogenicity of *Candida* spp. relies mainly on the state of the host. *Candida* spp. are considered opportunistic pathogens because they are usually benign colonizers of mucosal surfaces, and disease occurs when there is a breakdown in the host defense.

Factors associated with the organism also contribute to its ability to cause disease. The most relevant virulence factors for *Candida* spp. include adherence to a wide range of tissue types and inanimate surfaces, dimorphism, enzyme production, phenotypic switching, and modulation of cytokine production by human monocytes.

Candida albicans adheres more strongly to epithelial cells than *C. tropicalis*, followed by *C. parapsilosis*. These findings are in agreement with the virulence ranking of these species (67). The different ability of each *Candida* species or strains to produce biofilm in vitro may be considered a virulence factor responsible for catheter-related candidemia in patients receiving total parenteral nutrition. Non-*albicans Candida* species are more likely to produce biofilm than *Candida albicans* strains (68).

Candida albicans is able to grow in a variety of cell shapes and forms. These range from spheroidal, budding blastoconidia through short and long pseudohyphal forms, to true hyphae and refractile chlamydospores. This phenomenon is commonly referred to as "dimorphism," although the term "pleomorphism" would be more appropriate. Pleomorphism appears to be important (but not essential) in causing disease (69), while hyphal forms may be more virulent. Both forms (yeasts and hyphae) can penetrate host tissues and express virulence attributes (70).

One of the most extensively studied groups of *Candida* enzymes are the secreted aspartyl proteinases produced by *C. albicans*, *C. dublinensis* (71), *C. guillermondii* (72), *C. parapsilosis* (73), and *C. tropicalis* (74). These enzymes produce nonspecific proteolysis of host proteins involved in defenses against infection. *C. albicans*, *C. dublinensis C. glabrata*, *C. krusei*, *C. lusitaniae*, *C. parapsilosis*, and *C. tropicalis* (75–77) also produce phospholipases. Such enzymes are important in invasion through hydrolysis of phospholipids of the host tissues (78,79). Phospholipase B has proved to be essential for *C. albicans* virulence (77).

Colonies of *C. albicans* grown on agar media sometimes show variations in form, particularly after long periods of incubation. This is the expression of a phenomenon called phenotypic switching, which may be related to the relative virulence of the species (80). The rate of phenotype switching is higher among strains of *C.albicans* from patients with invasive infections than among those colonizing superficial sites (81). Phenotypic switching contributes to the virulence of *C. albicans* by facilitating its ability to survive, invade tissues, and escape from host defenses (80). On the other end, neutrophils can augment the switching process toward a more susceptible strain (82).

Virulence of *C. albicans* may also be related to its ability to induce secretion of Interleukin 10 (IL-10) by monocytes, with selective inhibition of IL-12 and interferon gamma resulting in impaired immune response to *Candida* (83).

V. SYNDROMES

A. Disseminated candidiasis

Incidence: Hematogenous infections with a *Candida* spp. can be chronic or acute in nature, and the pattern of disease varies in different types of patients.

The overall incidence of candidemia has increased persistently worldwide during the last few decades. This increase is the consequence of increasing populations of individuals who are immunosuppressed as a result of their underlying disease (malignancy, AIDS, and newborns with very low weight birth) or as a consequence of their immunosuppressive treatment (chemotherapy, radiation, transplantation, prophylaxis, and treatment of graft rejection or graft versus host disease). Data from the United States showed an 11-fold increase in incidence of hematogenous *Candida* infections between 1980 and 1989, from 0.013 to 0.15 cases per 1000 admissions (84) and an increase from 2.0 to 3.8 fungal infections per 1000 hospital discharges, with *Candida* species accounting for 78.3% of the 30,477 fungal infections reported (85). In a population based surveillance, the average annual incidence of candidemia in two cities in the United States from 1992 to 1993 was 8 per 100,000 population (86). Currently in the United States, *Candida* species represent approximately 8% of all organisms isolated in blood cultures and *Candida* spp. are the fourth leading cause of bloodstream infection (58). The magnitude of the increase in the incidence of candidemia may vary in different medical settings and geographic areas. For examples, in Finland, *Candida* spp. are the eighth leading cause of bloodstream infections (87). As another example, the rate of candidemia increased >11-fold (2.5–28.5 cases/1000 admissions) from 1981 to 1995 in a neonatal intensive care unit in the United States (63), while the rate of candidemia only doubled to 0.71/10,000 patients/days between 1987 and 1995 in five Dutch University hospitals (88).

The increased incidence of candidemia probably achieved its maximum in the 1990s and is starting to decline after the availability and widespread use of fluconazole. In a study where the characteristics of candidemia before and after the newer antifungal triazoles were compared in a tertiary care community hospital, the incidence of candidemia dropped from 13% (1986–1989) to as low as 0.06% after the introduction of fluconazole (1994–1997) (89). In another study that included cancer patients, the incidence of candidemia decreased from 7.1% (1972–1973) to 3.4% (1998) (90).

The incidence of candidemia in patients receiving total parenteral nutrition has been reported to be as high as 22% (91), similar to the one observed among burn patients colonized with *Candida* strains (12–21%) (92–94).

Morbidity and mortality: The mortality attributable to hematogenous candidiasis was estimated to be 38% among a group of patients hospitalized during the 1983–1986 period (95). A second analysis done in the same institution during the 1997–2001 period showed a comparably high (49%) attributable mortality (96). In another institution, the mortality of patients with candidemia in1998 was reduced (33%) compared to the one observed during the 1974–1982 period (77%) (90). The crude mortality of disseminated candidiasis ranges from 26% to 75% (63,97–104). Candidemia is also associated with a 30 day prolongation of hospital stay (95).

The most important prognostic factors for outcome of hematogenous candidiasis include: older age, poor performance status, presence and persistence of neutropenia, corticosteroid therapy, extensive organ involvement with candidiasis, and lack of antifungal treatment (101,102,105,106). Central venous catheter retention appears to play a limited role if any (107–110). Different species of *Candida* have been associated with different attributable mortality, lowest with *C. parapsilosis*, and highest with *C. tropicalis* and *C. glabrata* (40–70%). *Candida krusei* has similar mortality to *C. albicans* (15–35%) (111).

The reported response rate of chronic disseminated candidiasis has varied from 54% to 90% series and does not seem to be improved by splenectomy (60%) (112–115).

Table 2 Risk Factors for Hematogenous Candidiasis

Increased colonization	Increased translocation	Increased invasion of deep tissues

Endogenous
• Broad spectrum
  antibiotics
Exogenous
• Heroin users[a]
• Hospital stay
• Contaminated TPN
	• Intestinal graft-vs
	  host disease
	• Malnutrition
	• Mucositis
	• Surgery
	• Severe burns
	• TPN
		Immunosupression
		• Cancer
		• Corticosteroid treatment
		• Hemodialysis
		• Neutropenia
		• Premature neonates (<32
		  weeks, 5′ Apgar <5)
		• TPN
		• Transplantation
		• Severe burns

Abbreviations: TPN, total parenteral nutrition.
[a]In the case of heroin abusers with hematogenous candidiasis, the infection may be transmitted through IV injection of a solution of heroin dissolved in contaminated lemon juice (48).

Risk factors: Colonization with *Candida* spp. (mainly in the gastrointestinal tract) seems to be an essential step for the development of invasive candidiasis (23). This is supported by studies that show colonization of the gut by the same strain that subsequently causes candidemia (116–119). A higher density of colonization was associated with a higher risk of infection among patients with acute lymphocytic leukemia (120), other hematological cancers (121), infants with very low birth weight (122), and patients admitted to surgical intensive care units (123). Hematogenous candidiasis developed in > 30% of neutropenic cancer patients colonized with *Candida* spp. at multiple sites compared with no infection among those who were not colonized (124–126).

Several other factors also contribute to the development of hematogenous candidiasis through one or more mechanisms (see Table 2). The presence of central venous catheters has been found to be a risk factor for candidemia in some but not all series. The mechanism by which the catheter can be a risk factor for candidiasis is thought to be through contamination of the skin leading to catheter infection and subsequent dissemination. However, in contrast to the gut colonization by *Candida* spp. as a source for candidemia, published data do not fully support skin colonization by *Candida* spp. as a source of catheter-related candidemia (127). It is possible that the presence of CVC represented more a marker of severity of illness (in the studies that identified the CVC as risk factors) rather than a risk factor for the development of candidiasis. On the other hand, CVCs are associated with an increased incidence of thrombophlebitis. These thrombi may get seeding in the setting of hematogenous candidiasis and thus become a source of persistent infection (128–130).

Clinical Presentation

Acute disseminated: The clinical presentation of hematogenous candidiasis varies in different patient populations. In neonates, the clinical picture of hematogenous candidiasis is similar to that of bacterial sepsis, and spread of the infection to different organs is a common event. The most frequent sites of *Candida* involvement are the skin (66%) (131), followed by the central nervous system (CNS) (up to 64%)

(132), and retina (50%) (133). Respiratory dysfunction and apnea are the most common presenting signs (70% of cases) (104,134).

The most common pattern of disseminated *Candida* infection in adults is the acute type seen typically in non-neutropenic patients in intensive care units, or in patients with hematologic malignancies during chemotherapy-induced neutropenia. Fever unresponsive to antibacterial drugs is the usual presenting symptom. However, other manifestations may include those of sepsis (135). Disseminated candidiasis can involve any organ in the body. Endophthalmitis is a common result of *Candida* dissemination. *Candida* spp. gain access to the eye via the capillaries of the choroid and the retina, where they proliferate and induce focal inflammation and abscess formation. The frequency of ocular involvement by *Candida* spp. varies from 3% (136) to 78% (137–141) depending on the patient population (less in neutropenic patients probably because of their inability to develop an inflammatory response), the diagnostic criteria used, the study design (prospective versus retrospective), and the physician who performed the ophthalmologic examination (ophthalmologist vs. nonophthalmologist). A recent prospective study conducted among 31 patients with candidemia showed a 26% rate of ocular candidiasis. Of note, only five patients were found to have ocular involvement at the time of diagnosis of candidemia, while the remaining three patients had documented chorioretinitis within 2 weeks of diagnosis (141). This study suggests that patients with candidemia should have an ophthalmologic evaluation at baseline and 2 weeks after diagnosis. Another recent prospective study conducted among patients with candidemia found that 20 of 180 patients (15%) had retinal lesions. Most of these lesions were nonspecific; even though they could have been because of candidiasis, other etiologies could not be ruled out (142). None of the patients with retinal lesions had ocular symptoms at the time of the ophthalmologic exam.

Skin lesions may be present in 10–15% of patients with hematogenous candidiasis in neutropenic patients along with myalgias. These lesions may present like pink nodules (143,144), ecthyma gangrenosum (145), or other nonspecific lesions that resemble a drug rash (135,146).

IV heroin users who suffer from disseminated candidiasis develop a unique pattern of organ involvement. They acquire the infection by IV injection of contaminated drug solutions (48,147). The initial symptoms may last from a few hours to even a month, and the patients complain of fever, shivering, sweating, asthenia, or headache (148). Within 1–4 days of candidemia, 75–80% of patients will develop nodular cutaneous lesions affecting mainly the scalp (147,149). Fifty percent of patients may develop ocular involvement (chorioretinitis, hyalitis, episcleritis, anterior uveitis, and endophtalmitis) within a few days to up to 3 weeks after onset of the infection (147,150). At a later time (from 15 days to 5 months after the infection), osteoarticular lesions (mainly costochondritis and vertebral lesions) (147) may develop in up to 42% of patients.

Chronic disseminated candidiasis: Less common than the acute disseminated disease, chronic disseminated candidiasis (CDC) (previously known as hepatosplenic candidiasis) is almost always associated with recovery from neutropenia and may arise subsequent to a treated episode of acute hematogenous candidiasis. The condition occurs mainly among patients with acute leukemia undergoing cytotoxic chemotherapy, and those undergoing allogeneic bone marrow transplant, and is characterized by persistent fever nonresponsive to broad-spectrum antibiotics, negative blood cultures, abdominal pain (mainly right upper quadrant pain), increased liver function tests, in particular serum alkaline phosphatase, and multiple abscesses in the liver, spleen, lungs, and kidneys. Hepatomegaly and/or splenome-galy detected by abdominal examination is found in half of patients with CDC while abdominal tenderness is found in about two-third of these patients (113). Response to treatment is low. The median number of days for disappearance of fever among patients who will have a favorable outcome ranges from 4 to 26 days (median 19) (114). Usually, only a minority of patients with CDC (20–30%) develop positive blood cultures for *Candida* spp. (113–115).

Candida abscesses are usually detectable on ultrasonography, computed tomo-graphic scan (CT), or magnetic resonance imaging (MRI) (151). Four patterns of CDC have been described by ultrasonography. Early in the disease, the *Candida* microabscesses may show a "wheel within a wheel" image (first pattern) or a "typical bull's eye" (second pattern) and/or uniformly hypoechoic lesions (third pattern). Late in the course of the disease, fibrosis or calcification of the lesions may show as echogenic foci with variable degrees of acoustic shadowing (fourth pattern). On CT, only the third and fourth patterns are commonly seen. MRI imaging is more sensitive than CT for the detection of the presence and number of CDC lesions (152) and is accurate for assessing different stages of the disease (153). Three patterns of CDC have been described by MRI imaging. The acute pattern (within 2 weeks of therapy) consists of lesions < 1cm in diameter appearing as well-defined-high-intensity foci on T2-weighted images. The subacute pattern (from 2 weeks to 3 months of therapy) shows similar size lesions that are mildly hyperintense on T1-weighted images, along with a perilesional ring. The chronic pattern reveals lesions (1–3 cm in diameter) with irregular margins, with decreased enhancement on images obtained after gadolinium injection.

Catheter-associated candidemia: The term catheter-related candidemia implies that a catheter can have a role in the pathogenesis of candidemia, either as a primary source of the organism (primary catheter-related candidemia as a result of CVC colonization from skin) or as a factor that can perpetuate candidemia originating from another site (secondary catheter-related candidemia as a result of CVC seeding from blood).

Primary catheter-associated candidemia: This is a rather uncommon entity, because as mentioned earlier under the section of risk factors, the gut, and not the skin, appears to be the primary source of hematogenous candidiasis (127). Further complicating this issue are the widely varying definitions of catheter-related candide-mia used by different authors. Examples of definitions used include: candidemia in a patient with: (a) central venous catheter in place (154); (b) central venous catheter in place without any other source of infection (155,156); (c) central venous catheter in place with positive CVC tip culture for the same *Candida* spp. causing fungemia (154–157) or positive catheter-related thrombus for the same *Candida* spp. (155); (d) central venous catheter in place with CVC exit site positive for the same *Candida* spp. causing candidemia (155).

The lack of a standard definition (including lack of established methodology for catheter culture) makes understanding the pathogenesis, clinical features, and outcome of this entity very difficult.

Bodey et al. (158) defined catheter-related candidemia as candidemia that occurs in a patient with an intravascular catheter, and no other obvious origin for the infection after careful clinical and laboratory evaluation. If the catheter is removed, a quantitative culture of the tip should recover ≥15 CFU of the same *Candida* spp. by the roll plate or ≥100 CFU by the sonication technique. If the cathe-ter is not removed, a quantitative blood culture collected through a CVC should contain at least a 10-fold greater concentration of *Candida* spp. than a simultaneously collected quantitative peripheral blood culture.

To be more precise, there are two issues that should be included in the definition of catheter-related candidemia: (a) lack of recovery of the same *Candida* spp. from other colonizing sites (because of the high likelihood that sources other than CVC such as gut, contaminated TPN solution, or other are the primary source of candidemia in a large proportion of patients) and (b) presence of molecular relatedness between colonizing (skin or CVC tip) and infecting strains (blood), as the mere recovery of the same species of *Candida* does not necessarily mean that the organisms are genotypically related (159).

Secondary catheter-associated candidemia: In this entity, the primary source of the candidemia is not the catheter, but the catheter can become a secondary source. This is the case of patients with candidemia of other origin. *Candida* spp. adheres to a CVC-related thrombus, the vessel walls and the CVC, and these infected sites become a source for subsequent candidemia. This is the case of septic venous thrombophlebitis.

Candida thrombophlebitis of the central veins is rare (130,160,161) and occurs mainly in severely ill patients. Risk factors include CVC in place, treatment with multiple antibiotics and TPN, admission to ICU, and abdominal surgery. The most common sites of thrombophlebitis include the subclavian, the innominate, and the superior cava vein. In most cases, *C. albicans* is the causative pathogen. Clinical presentation includes fever, edema of the area involved, and persistent candidemia (2–3 weeks), even after removal of the CVC and appropriate antifungal chemotherapy (130).

Candida thrombophlebitis of the peripheral veins is also a rare entity. Risk factors are the same as those for thrombophlebitis of the central veins. Patients usually present with fever or sepsis. Locally, symptoms may range from a noninflamed thrombosed vein, to a warm, tender, erythematous vein with or without purulent drainage (128,129,162–164).

B. Local Infections

Local infections by *Candida* spp. can be divided in two groups: mucocutaneous infections and locally invasive ones. The most common mucocutaneous forms of candidiasis involve the female genitalia, the skin and nails, and the oral cavity (thrush) (sometimes with concomitant esophageal invasion). Locally invasive candidiasis involving deep tissues are almost always the result of hematogenous spread of a *Candida* organism from an endogenous or, less often, an exogenous site. Table 3 summarizes the recognized forms of local *Candida* infection and lists the settings in which they are most commonly encountered.

1. Mucocutaneous Infections

Oral candidiasis: Oral *Candida* infections occur predominantly among immunosuppressed patients or from populations at risk exposed to other factors that favor the overgrowth, and invasiveness of this fungus include immunosuppressed individuals such as newborns with birth asphyxia, diabetic patients, patients infected with HIV, patients receiving corticosteroid or cytotoxic chemotherapy particularly for hematological malignancies, patients undergoing maxillofacial radiotherapy, and recipients of organ and/or stem cell transplantation. Oral *Candida* infections also

Table 3 Overview of Types of *Candida* Infections and Their Predisposing Factors

Type of disease	Major predisposing/risk factors
Oropharyngeal infection	Age extremes
	Denture wearers
	Diabetes mellitus
	Antibiotic use
	Radiotherapy for head and neck cancer
	Inhaled and systemic corticosteroids
	Cytotoxic chemotherapy
	HIV infection
	Hematologic malignancies
	Stem cell or solid organ transplantation
Esophagitis	Systemic corticosteroids
	AIDS
	Cancer
	Stem cell or solid organ transplantation
Lower gastrointestinal infection	Cancer
	Surgery
Vulvovaginal infection	Oral contraceptives
	Pregnancy
	Diabetes mellitus
	Systemic corticosteroids
	Antibiotic use
Infections of the skin and nails	Local moisture and occlusion
	Inmersion of hands in water
	Peripheral vascular disease
Cutaneous congenital candidiasis	Intrauterine foreign body
	Prematurity
Chronic mucocutaneous candidiasis	T-lymphocyte defects
Urinary tract infection	Indwelling urinary catheter
	Urinary obstruction
	Urinary tract procedures
	Diabetes mellitus
Pneumonia	Aspiration
Endocarditis	Major surgery
	Previous bacterial endocarditis or valvular disease
	IV drug abuse
	Long-term central venous catheter
Pericarditis	Thoracic surgery
	Immunosuppression
Central nervous system (CNS) infection	CNS surgery
	Ventricular-peritoneal shunt
Ocular infection	Ocular surgery
	Trauma
Bone and joint infection	Surgery
	Trauma
	Intra articular injections
	Diabetic foot
Abdominal infection	Recurrent perforation
	Repeat abdominal surgery
	Anastomotic leaks
	Pancreatitis
	Continuous ambulatory peritoneal dialysis
	Solid organ transplantation

develop in nonimmunosuppressed individuals exposed to prolonged antibiotic treatment (165,166), inhaled steroids (167), and those who wear dentures (166).

The prevalence of oral *Candida* infection (thrush) in association with AIDS approaches 100%, when CD4 counts decrease below 200/μL. The improvement of the immune system of HIV-infected patients associated with the administration of HAART has resulted in a significant decrease in the incidence of oropharyngeal candidiasis (57,168). Thrush can be present in 28–38% of cancer patients undergoing therapy with corticosteroids or cytotoxic agents (169,170).

Esophageal candidiasis: This accounts for up to 15% of the AIDS-defining illnesses (171). Of note, up to 30% of patients with *Candida* esophagitis may not have oral thrush (172,173), while 64–88% of patients with thrush have concomitant esophageal candidiasis (172,174).

The usual presentation of oral and esophageal infections is in the form of white "cottage cheese" patches. Other presentations include the pseudomembranous type ("thrush") that reveal a raw bleeding surface when scraped; the erythematous type, which are flat, red, sometimes sore areas; the candidal leukoplakia, consisting of nonremovable white thickening of epithelium because of *Candida* spp., and angular cheilitis, presenting as sore fissures at corners of mouth. In addition to all of these, median rhomboid glossitis, an abnormality of tongue associated with ovoid, denuded area in median posterior portion of the tongue, can be associated with candidiasis. In elderly patients, particularly those who wear dentures, a more chronic form of disease is seen that is characterized principally by areas of non-specific erythema, often beneath denture surfaces (9).

Other gastrointestinal sites: Candidiasis can involve any site of the gastrointestinal tract with the esophagus and the small bowel as most common sites. These lesions may be clinically significant and may progress to hematogenous infection. The pathology of infection of the lower GI tract by *Candida* spp. ranges from mucosal ulceration with or without pseudomembrane to exophytic lesions. In deep invasive lesions, pseudohyphae may extend beyond the muscular layer and reach the serosa (175). Direct vascular invasion through the bowel wall has been reported only in patients receiving immunosuppressive chemotherapy (175,176). These patients may have extensive involvement of the GI tract from mouth to anus, while non-neutropenic surgical patients exhibit a more localized involvement (177). The histologic criteria for diagnosing this form of the disease include the presence of budding yeast forms, mycelial forms, or both on KOH smears or culture; a disrupted epithelium; and a submucosal inflammatory reaction.

Candida infections of the genitalia: *Candida* vulvovaginitis (CVV) is the second most frequent genital complaint in women, with around 75% experiencing at least one episode of CVV in their life time, and half by 25 years of age (178). Several risk factors have been associated with CVV including oral contraceptives, corticosteroids and antibiotics (179), diabetes (180), and pregnancy (181). Sexual transmission of *Candida* strains may occur after receptive oral sex. CVV does not appear to correlate with vaginal intercourse (43,46).

In most cases, the presentation is acute, the symptoms are not severe, and the condition responds readily to treatment. However, around 5% of women develop a chronic or recurrent form of *Candida* vulvovaginitis (RCVV) resistant to antifungal treatment (182). The majority of women with RCVV do not suffer any obvious underlying immune deficit or illness. A local change in vaginal immune defenses appears to increase the susceptibility to this infection (183). Most cases of RCVV are caused by the same strain of *Candida* that developed subtle genetic variations (47). Drug resistance does not seem to be an important factor in RCVV (183).

Genital infections in males are less common than in females and can be caused by the yeast itself or by an allergic reaction to the presence of *Candida* antigen after unprotected intercourse. *Candida* balanoposthitis is a recognized entity, usually presenting only as mild irritation with focal signs of erythema but sometimes becoming severe, even leading to phimosis in rare instances (184). Although *Candida* yeasts can be sexually transmitted, it is practically impossible to differentiate between transmission from a sexual partner and that from the patient's own flora via the anus. Among partners of patients with RVCC, strain typing of the infecting *Candida* strains have shown identity or near identity between strains recovered from both partners (47).

Candida *infections of the skin and nails: Candida* spp. inhabits the skin and mucus membranes in around 75% of the population without causing harm (185). In occluded sites of the body where the surface remains moist (typically the groins and the armpits, or the spaces between toes and the breastfolds) *Candida* infections can occur. These infections present as a pruritic rash with a poorly defined edge and abundant erythematous vesiculo-pustular lesions. Fissures may occur in interdigital spaces (186).

Invasive infections of the fingernails (onychomycosis) are mainly caused by *C. albicans* and *C. parapsilosis* (less commonly *C. glabrata* and *C. guilliermondii*) (187–189). *Candida* spp. are the most common etiology of onychomycosis of the fingernails while dermatophytes are the most common cause of onychomycosis of the toenails (190,191).

Chronic swelling and inflammation of the nail fold (paronychia) is a condition characterized by the presence under the fold of a mixed microbial flora of normally commensal organisms, including yeast flora and the most common species is *C. albicans* (186,192).

Neonates may develop a rare entity referred to as cutaneous congenital candidiasis. Among neonates weighing >1000 g, the condition usually presents with a generalized macular erythematous rash that may become pustular, papular, or vesicular, with subsequent desquamation. Among premature neonates weighing <1000 g, this entity presents with a widespread desquamating or erosive dermatitis that can evolve to hematogenous candidiasis and increased risk of death. Presence of intrauterine foreign body is considered a major risk factor for the development of this infection (193).

Skin lesions by *Candida* spp. can also represent a manifestation of hematogenous candidiasis. They are lesions of major diagnostic value in the immunocompromised host.

Chronic mucocutaneous candidiasis: In rare cases, individuals are chronically susceptible to superficial *Candida* infections, as a result of a defect in T-lymphocyte responsiveness to the fungus. However, the defect varies from case to case with no single predominant deficiency in cellular immunity.

Through childhood and into adulthood, such patients suffer from unremitting mucocutaneous *Candida* lesions, including severe nail and skin involvement and vaginitis. The lesions sometimes develop into a gross, disfiguring granulomatous appearance (194,195).

2. Locally Invasive Infections

The most common situation when deep tissues are infected with *Candida* spp. is in the setting of hematogenous candidiasis. In this setting we may have the impression that only one organ is involved when any of these possibilities occur: (1) all tissues except one eradicate the yeast; or (2) one tissue succumbs to infection more rapidly and extensively than the others. The physician should therefore be alert to the possibility of disseminated infection even in cases where only a single organ shows signs of disease. Some examples of single-organ *Candida* infections without concomitant disseminated disease are certainly known, but these are greatly outnumbered by instances of disseminated disease.

Urinary tract infections: *Candida* micro-organisms frequently exist as saprophytes on the external genitalia or urethra; however, yeasts in measurable quantities are present in <1% of clean voided urine specimens (196). The isolation of *Candida* specimens from a urine sample may represent contamination, colonization, or lower or upper urinary tract infection. Contamination is more common in female patients with vulvovaginal candidiasis, and it can be excluded by repeating the urine sample with proper collection techniques.

Colonization (asymptomatic candiduria) and infection occurs only in patients with local or systemic predisposing risk factors (Table 4) (197,198).

Asymptomatic candiduria: The incidence of asymptomatic candiduria has increased dramatically during the last decade among hospitalized patients, especially those with indwelling bladder or drainage devices. The prevalence of candiduria varies considerably in the same hospital and ranges from 2% to 11% and is more prevalent among patients with leukemia, bone marrow transplantation, and in those patients admitted to ICU (199).

Although *C. albicans* is the most common species recovered in candiduria (50%), non-*albicans* species are common particularly with *C. glabrata*. (200,201).

Distinguishing colonization from infection may be difficult. In catheterized patients, the presence of pyuria and a high colony count (10^3 cfu/mL) may not help in the diagnosis of infection, while a high colony count in urine suggests infection among non-catheterized patients.

Asymptomatic candiduria in nonseverely immunocompromised patients usually follows a benign course (198,201). In a series of 316 patients, none developed complications (urinary tract infection or candidemia) (201), while in another series of 816 patients, only 1% (six patients) developed candidemia (198). No antifungal therapy is required for asymptomatic candiduria. This condition is usually transient and associated with very low morbidity. Antifungal treatment resulted in a comparable

Table 4 Predisposing Factors for Colonization or Infection of the Urinary Tract by *Candida* Species (338)

Predisposing factors	Candiduria	Lower UTI	Upper UTI
Extreme age	X	X	
Female sex	X	X	
Broad-spectrum antibiotics	X	X	X
Indwelling bladder catheter in place	X	X	
Diabetes mellitus	X	X	X
Immunosuppression	X	X	X
Renal transplantation	X	X	X
Urinary tract obstruction	X	X	X
Urinary tract instrumentation	X	X	X
Surgery	X	X	X

rate of, eradication of candiduria 2 weeks after discontinuation of the antifungal agent (201). Discontinuation of the predisposing factors when possible is the recommended strategy. In catheterized subjects, removal of the catheter and discontinuation of broad-spectrum antibiotics eliminates candiduria in 40% of patients, while catheter exchange alone resolves candiduria in 20% of patients (201).

The favorable outcome of asymptomatic candiduria does not, however, apply to severely immunosuppressed patients (such as those with prolonged neutropenia) and recipients of renal transplantation, in whom the development of urinary tract infection and candidemia is more likely to occur. Asymptomatic candiduria in renal transplant recipients requires antifungal treatment. Candiduria in the neutropenic and the critically ill patient has been of controversial value as a marker of hematogenous candidiasis (202–204) and certainly implies a site of *Candida* colonization that as such contributes to the likelihood of invasive infection. Although candiduria alone cannot predict hematogenous candidiasis with accuracy, persistent candiduria in a severely immunocompromised patient with fever should lead to the investigation of disseminated candidiasis and evaluation for empiric antifungal treatment.

Eradication of candiduria is also recommended for patients undergoing urologic instrumental procedures caused by the high risk of disseminated candidiasis (205,206).

Lower urinary tract infections: Symptoms are comparable to those observed in patients with bacterial cystitis. If a cystoscopy is performed, it reveals soft, pearly white elevated patches with hyperemic and friable mucosa underneath. Emphysematous cystitis and prostatic abscess are occasional complications of *Candida* cystitis (207). Antifungal treatment is always indicated and the outcome is usually favorable. Oral fluconazole (200 mg/day × 7–14 days) is the recommended treatment because of its efficacy, high urine concentration, and low toxicity. For fluconazole resistant *Candida* species, intravenous (IV) amphotericin B (0.3–1 mg/kg/day for 1–7 days) is also effective (208). Of note, even a single dose of IV amphotericin B, 0.3 mg/kg, has been shown to be highly efficacious in lower urinary tract candidiasis (209). Other effective but less used alternatives include bladder instillation with Amphotericin B 50–200 µg/mL and oral flucytosine 25 mg/kg qid (208). Amphotericin B instillation is not recommended because it requires an indwelling catheter and hospitalization. Monotherapy with oral flucytosine cannot be used in patients with renal failure but may be very useful for treating *C. glabrata* infections.

Upper urinary tract infections: Ascending pyelonephritis and urosepsis by *Candida* species are indistinguishable from bacterial pyelonephritis and urosepsis. These infections occur mainly among patients with urinary obstruction and stasis. Complications include pyonephrosis, focal abscesses, development of fungal balls (bezoars) resulting in obstruction and renal colic, and papillary necrosis. Fungal bezoars are rare and develop mainly in the pelvis and upper ureters. Candidemia is also an uncommon complication of ascending infection and occurs mainly among patients with obstruction, or following urologic procedure or manipulation. Ultrasonography and CT scanning are useful in the diagnosis of fungal balls, hydronephrosis, and intrarenal and perinephric abscesses (207). These infections require systemic antifungal treatment, typically with fluconazole. The duration of the treatment will depend on the severity of the infection. Failures of medical treatment are usually because of obstruction, and resolution of the obstruction may require percutaneous nephrostomy, drainage, placement of ureteral stents, or surgical removal of bezoars.

Renal candidiasis: This infection is usually secondary to the hematogenous spread of *Candida* species. It is accompanied by fever and other constitutional manifestations of *Candida* sepsis. These patients may develop candiduria without any other symptom of renal involvement other than variable reduction in renal function (207). This entity is described in detail in the section on hematogenous candidiasis.

A clinical approach to the patient with candiduria is described in Figure 1.

Pneumonia: *Candida* pneumonia is classified as primary in the absence of other manifestations of hematogenous candidiasis. The infection is very rare and results from aspiration of food contents. Secondary *Candida* pneumonia, the most frequent presentation, is associated with hematogenous candidiasis (210).

Cardiovascular infections: Cardiovascular infections caused by *Candida* spp. can present as endocarditis, myocarditis, or pericarditis.

Endocarditis: *Candida* spp. are responsible for 65% of fungal endocarditis (9,211). *Candida* spp. cause 2–10% of prosthetic valve endocarditis (212), and among patients with prosthetic valve, those who develop candidemia have a 25% risk of developing *Candida* endocarditis (213). Fourteen percent of infective endocarditis among IV drug abusers are caused by *Candida* spp. (9,211,214,215).

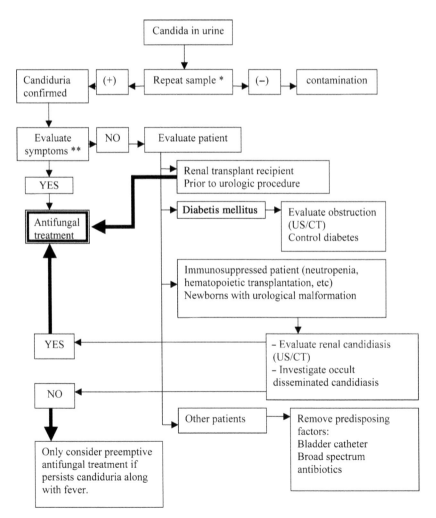

Figure 1 Clinical approach to the patient with candiduria. *Also check for genital candidiasis. **Lower, upper or systemic symptoms that cannot be associated to other etiology.

Reported risk factors for *Candida* endocarditis include: (1) major surgery (cardiac and others), (2) pre-existent bacterial endocarditis or valvular disease; (3) in situ pacemaker, or long-term CVC. Other populations that also reported cases of *Candida* endocarditis include neonates and occasionally immunosuppressed patients. Among neonates, *Candida* endocarditis is a less common event than hematogenous infection and seems to affect mainly the right side of the heart (216).

The clinical presentation of *Candida* endocarditis resembles bacterial endocarditis with fever at presentation (75%), new or changing heart murmur (50%), and/or heart failure (25%). Unlike bacteria endocarditis, however, the risk of embolization of major arteries is very high ($\geq 2/3$ patients). Embolic lesions are usually detected in brain, kidneys, spleen, liver, skin, eyes, and the coronary arteries. Classic signs of infective endocarditis like finger clubbing, Osler's nodes, splinter hemorrhage Roth's spot, and splenomegaly are uncommon (214,217–219). The most commonly involved valves are the aortic and mitral valves, even among IV drug abusers and among patients with a central venous catheter in place (218).

Myocarditis: This infection almost always occurs in the setting of hematogenous dissemination, mainly among immunocompromized patients (220,221), and is associated with conduction disturbances, hypotension, and shock (222).

Pericarditis: Pericarditis is a rare condition that is associated with serious complications, including hematogenous spread and tamponade (9,211,223). The infection is associated with immunosuppression (including AIDS), previous antibiotic therapy, pericardiectomy, thoracic surgery, and hematogenous *Candida* infection (224).

Central nervous system infections: CNS infections by *Candida* spp. are rare and can present as meningitis or abscesses. *Candida* infections of the CNS are usually secondary to hematogenous disease or associated with CNS surgery or ventricular-peritoneal shunt (9). In the setting of hematogenous disease, meningitis is more frequent in neonates (64%) (131) than among adults (225). Prematurity is one of the principal risk factors for neonatal meningitis (226). *Candida* meningitis usually presents as an acute infection among neonates, while its course may be indolent or chronic in adults. Neurosurgery-related candidiasis can present with the features of bacterial meningitis in adults (227,228).

Although the pathogenesis of *Candida* meningitis is unclear, recent data suggest that *C. albicans* is able to adhere, invade, and trancytose across human brain microvascular endothelial cells without affecting the monolayer integrity (229).

Ocular infections: Ocular *Candida* infections include keratitis, chorioretinitis, and endophthalmitis. Most cases of chorioretinitis and endophthalmitis are secondary to hematogenous spread and may be the earliest manifestation of hematogenous candidiasis. A few of these infections are secondary to trauma (mainly after ocular surgery), while keratitis is usually associated with local trauma.

Bone and joint infections: Most cases of bone and joint *Candida* infections are secondary to hematogenous candidiasis. Primary *Candida* osteitis and arthritis are rare and result from accidental implantation of the fungus by traumatic means (e.g., surgery, intra-articular injection of corticosteroids) or by contiguity in patients with infected diabetic foot ulcers. The infection typically involves a single joint or bone. Diagnosis is best achieved by culturing the organism from the joint fluid.

Abdominal infections: *Candida* spp. are frequently cultured from intra-abdominal material but should be considered significant only in certain subsets of patients, such as those receiving TPN or broad-spectrum antibiotics, patients with recurrent perforations or abdominal infections, necrotizing pancreatitis, and anastomotic leak (230–233).

Primary biliary candidiasis (infection of gallbladder and/or the biliary tree by *Candida* spp.) is very rare. In the only series of biliary candidiasis, risk factors included candidemia (3 of 27 patients), and the known risk factors for hematogenous candidiasis, including colonization and poor physiologic scores, suggest that in most of these patients the biliary involvement was secondary to hematogenous spread (234). The diagnosis is usually made with pure or persistent growth of *Candida* spp. from the biliary tract and response to antifungal treatment. Histopathological documentation of tissue invasion is desirable but not always feasible.

There is an increasing appreciation for the role of *Candida* in infections following acute necrotizing pancreatitis (235).

Liver, gallbladder, and subphrenic abscesses have been described in cancer patients with percutaneously placed drainage catheters (236).

Candida peritonitis is seen in patients on continuous ambulatory peritoneal dialysis (CAPD). A review of 105 cases of peritonitis in patients undergoing CAPD indicated that fungi accounted for 8% of all infections (237). Another series of 20 cases of CAPD-related fungal peritonitis revealed that 75% of these infections were caused by *Candida* spp, mostly *C. albicans* (238). *Candida* peritonitis has also been reported in a patient with liver cirrhosis (239) and in patients with intra-abdominal malignancies (240). In *Candida* peritonitis, the infection tends to remain localized and presents with low grade fever, abdominal pain and tenderness. The peritoneal dialysate is usually cloudy and contains more than 100 neutrophils/mm^3. If untreated, *Candida* peritonitis may lead to hematogenous candidiasis (232).

Wound infections: The diagnosis of candida wound infections is difficult. Recovering *Candida* spp. from wounds does not necessarily imply that this organism is causing tissue infection and should not compel physicians to use systemic antifungal therapy. However, such therapy should be considered in those patients whose wound infections do not respond to appropriate antibacterial therapy, particularly if the same *Candida* spp. is repeatedly isolated from the wound site. In a recent survey *C. albicans* was found in 0.43% of 2458 wound swabs in patients at a teaching hospital (241). Patients undergoing coronary artery bypass grafting may develop deep sternal wound infections by *Candida* spp. with or without concomitant sternal osteomyelitis. This infection may present up to 150 days after surgery and is characterized by a chronic, indolent course, requiring surgery and prolonged antifungal treatment (median 6 months) and may recur (242). *Candida* spp. have been also reported to cause ostomy wound infections (243), necrotizing fascitis following renal transplantation (244), and postlaminectomy wound infection (245).

VI. DIAGNOSIS

A. Direct Microscopy

Direct microscopy is a simple and economic approach to the detection of *Candida* spp.; however, negative results from microscopy should not be regarded as definitive. Yeast cells (and pseudohyphal or hyphal forms when present) are easily visualized by phase-contrast microscopy of any wet specimen. Like all fungi, *Candida* spp. are Gram-positive and can usually be visualized with a Gram stain. They do not show up well with hematoxylin–eosin or Giemsa stains, and are better evaluated by periodic acid-Schiff's reaction and Gomori's methenamine silver stains. The presence of *Candida* spp. in the urine is often detectable by direct microscopy. In cases of suspected hematogenous *Candida* infection, microscopic examination of blood smears will occasionally reveal the fungal cells.

B. Isolation Methods

Blood cultures with hematogenous candidiasis are negative in one-quarter to one-third of patients. Biphasic blood culture media and vented culture bottles are optimal for the detection of *Candida* yeasts. Pretreating blood samples by cell lysis and centrifugation enhances the yield of blood cultures (246). Combination of lysis-centrifugation and the automated BACTEC® system for identification offers an average time to detection of around 3–4 days. *Candida albicans, C. parapsilosis*, and *C. tropicalis* usually appear within 3 days in blood cultures, whereas *C. krusei* and *C. glabrata* often take longer to grow.

The *Candida* spp. are all able to grow on standard mycologic isolation media at 35°C. Sabouraud agar pH 5.6 with chloramphenicol and gentamicin added to minimize bacterial contamination is widely used for the culture of *Candida* organisms from clinical samples. Note that cycloheximide ("Actidione") should *not* be incorporated in isolation media for *Candida* yeasts because it inhibits the growth of some species. Most pathogenic *Candida* spp. also grow on many bacteriologic isolation media, including blood agar, brain–heart infusion agar and tryptose agar.

One commercial product, CHROMagar Candida®, allows the rapid presumptive identification of *C. albicans, C. tropicalis*, and *C. krusei* at the time of isolation, and may distinguish colonies of *C. dubliniensis* from those of *C. albicans* (6). However, the shelf life of the medium in a refrigerator is short (maximally 2 months), and the volume of medium poured in the Petri plate must be sufficient (at least 20 mL) to ensure formation of the correct colony color.

C. Identification Methods

The methods currently adopted in most routine clinical laboratories remain those based on morphologic and physiologic testing.

The most common strategy for identification of yeasts is to use rapid, simple, and specific tests to identify isolates of *C. albicans*. For non-*C. albicans* species, a battery of physiologic tests combined with scrutiny of microscopic morphology will ensure correct identification of all but a few of the yeasts recovered from clinical material.

The preliminary identification of *C. albicans* can most easily be done by recognition of its characteristic colony color on a suitable differential isolation medium. An alternative specific test for *C. albicans* is its ability to produce germ tubes (short hyphal outgrowths) in serum after 3 h at 37°C (more than 90% of *C. albicans* isolates produce positive germ tube) and detection of its N-acetyl-β-D-galactosaminidase and L-proline aminopeptidase activities: only *C. albicans* among *Candida* spp. expresses both enzymes (247,248). Commercial systems based on this property are also available. The newly described species *C. dubliniensis* closely resembles *C. albicans* in all of these screening tests. Testing of apparent *C. albicans* isolates for the absence of β-glucosidase activity (6) can confirm the identity of an isolate as *C. albicans*.

Isolates that cannot be recognized as *C. albicans* or *C. dubliniensis* at this prescreening stage should be examined for the morphology of their blastoconidia and for their ability to produce pseudohyphae and chlamydospores on suitable semistarvation media such as corn meal or cream of rice–Tween agars, and their carbohydrate assimilation profiles should be determined. Several commercial kits are available, of which the API 20C kit is very widely used internationally. A recently developed kit (ID 32C) in the API series offers more rapid yeast identification and the possibility of automated reading.

To establish unequivocally that two strains are identical would theoretically require determination of the entire DNA base sequence from both isolates.

D. Serological Methods of Detection

1. Antibody Detection

A plethora of test methods have been tried, including agglutination of coated latex particles, immunodiffusion and immunoelectrophoretic test systems, radioimmunoassay and enzyme immunoassay, often with sophisticated refinements (249). Unfortunately, detection of *Candida* antibodies, falls short of discriminative specificity and sensitivity for prospective diagnostic purposes regardless of the detection method used.

2. Antigen Detection

Methods for antigen detection failed to achieve satisfactory diagnostic results in a routine prospective diagnostic setting. Three groups of antigens have been studied: (1) Mannan, (2) (1–3)-β-D-glucan, and (3) *Candida* enolase.

3. Polymerase Chain Reaction

Amplification of DNA of *Candida* spp. appears to be a quick and specific diagnostic tool. While multiple approaches have been pursued, several limitations still need to be overcome before this methodology can be routinely used.

4. Detection of Metabolites

Another approach to diagnosis of *Candida* infections is the detection of specific *Candida* metabolites by chemical methods. D-arabinitol is the most promising metabolite in terms of its near unique specificity as a *Candida* product. Because levels of the metabolite may become elevated in patients with impaired renal function, results of D-arabinitol testing are usually expressed as a serum D-arabinitol: creatinine (Ara/Cre) ratio. However, serial Ara/Cre determinations for detection of *Candida* infection and for monitoring therapeutic responses among patients at risk of such infections did not perform better than blood culture (250).

D-arabinitol/L-arabinitol ratio was evaluated among urine samples of 61 patients undergoing treatment for hematologic malignancies (251) and 117 neonates (252), but was found to be of limited diagnostic value.

Mannose is another metabolite of *Candida* spp. that could be useful for the early detection of candidal infection. This test however requires a complicated gas–liquid chromatography system and suffers low sensitivity (39%) (253).

VII. THERAPY

A. Disseminated Candidiasis

1. Acute Disseminated

Hematogenous candidiasis is associated with significant mortality and morbidity (see earlier section Morbidity and Mortality). As a result, all patients with positive blood cultures for *Candida* spp. should receive antifungal treatment (254).

Fluconazole, a well-tolerated triazole, has good activity against *Candida* spp. Five studies compared fluconazole to IV amphotericin B. These studies were randomized (156,255,256) prospective observational (99) and matched cohort (257). Fluconazole dosages were generally around 400 mg/day (range 200–800) orally or intravenously, while IV amphotericin B was given at doses of 0.3–1.2 mg/kg. All these studies showed that fluconazole was as effective as and better tolerated than amphotericin B. It is currently recommended that fluconazole, be administered at 600–800 mg/day IV for 3 days, particularly if the infecting organism is known to be or is likely to be *C. albicans*. If the patient responds rapidly to this regimen, the dosage may be decreased to 400 mg/day and the drug given orally (258).

Itraconazole therapy for hematogenous candidiasis has not been adequately evaluated mainly because of the low bioavailability of the itraconazole capsules. A new solution of itraconazole has been recently developed. This formulation has improved the solubility of itraconazole, leading to enhanced absorption and bioavailability compared with the original capsule formulation and making this formulation potentially suitable for the treatment of hematogenous candidiasis. An IV formulation of itraconazole is now available and was found to be effective against hematogenous candidiasis in animal models (259). Clinical data are not available yet.

Voriconazole is a new azole that has been recently marketed. Its spectrum includes *Candida* spp. (including some that are fluconazole-resistant strains). and the drug has shown good clinical activity in the treatment of esophageal candidiasis (260). It is likely that voriconazole will be effective in candidal bloodstream infections.

Lipid-associated formulations of amphotericin B are less nephrotoxic than the parent compound. Three lipid products of amphotericin B are available: amphotericin B colloidal dispersion (ABCD) (Amphocil), amphotericin B lipid complex (ABLC) (Abelcet), and liposomal amphotericin B (L-AMB) (AmBisome). Several studies have evaluated the utility of the lipid amphotericin B preparations for hematogenous candidiasis. A large prospective randomized trial has shown that ABLC at a dose of 5 mg/kg/day was as effective as, and probably less nephrotoxic than 0.7–1 mg/kg/day of, conventional amphotericin B in hematogenous candidiasis (261). Data regarding the treatment of hematogenous candidiasis with ABCD are Vlimited to trials where the drug was used because of intolerance to, or failure of conventional amphotericin B. In such studies, the response rate was 70% among evaluable patients (no. 107), and 50% among the intent-to-treat-population (no. 239) (262). The efficacy of L-AMB in hematogenous candidiasis has been studied in the neonatal population with response rates ranging between 72 and 100% (263,265) Among 52 adults who were intolerant to or failed to respond to conventional Amphotericin B, 83% responded to L-AMB (266). Among the three lipid formulations of amphotericin B, L-AMB (AmBisome) is the least nephrotoxic and appears to result in significantly less infusion-related reactions (267,268). There is no consensus about optimal dosing of the lipid formulations of amphotericin B. However, doses of L-AMB as low as 1–3 mg/kg/day and those of ABLC and ABCD of 5 mg/kg/day seem to be adequate for the treatment of *Candida* infections. The substantial cost of the lipid formulation of amphotericin B limits their use to patients at risk for renal failure and those intolerant to conventional amphotericin B who are infected by an azole-resistant strain and are unable to receive caspofungin (see later).

A new class of antifungal agents called echinocandin has been developed, and caspofungin is the first marketed agent of this class. Caspofungin is approved for treating candidemia and invasive candidiasis and was as effective as and better tolerated than amphotericin B in a randomized, double-blind trial that enrolled 239 (mainly non-neutropenic) patients (269). Caspofungin is better tolerated than the lipid formulations amphotericin B for the treatment of Fluconazole-resistant *Candida* infections. Micafungin and anidulafungin, other members of the Echinocandins class, are currently being evaluated under study for the treatment of candidemia (270).

Therapeutic recommendations: For patients who are hemodynamically unstable and those with high-grade persistent fungemia, two-drug antifungal regimens may be considered for faster clearance of the infection (258). Recently, a randomized, blinded, multicenter trial in 219 non-neutropenic subjects with candidemia showed that the combination of fluconazole plus amphotericin B was not antagonistic when compared to fluconazole, and resulted in more rapid clearance of the organism from the bloodstream (197).

Duration of therapy depends on the extent and seriousness of the infection. Therapy can be limited to 7–10 days for patients with low-grade fungemia, without evidence of organ involvement or hemodynamic instability. On the other hand, patients with high-grade fungemia, organ involvement, or hemodynamic instability should receive antifungal therapy for 10–14 days after resolution of all signs and symptoms of infection (258).

2. Chronic Disseminated Candidiasis (CDC)

Amphotericin treatment of 23 patients with CDC (median 112 days, mean total dose 4.5 g) resulted in a response rate of 82% (114). Alternative agents included fluconazole with a response rate of 88% ($n = 20$) (113) to 100% ($n = 5$) (271), and the lipid formulations of amphotericin B. ABLC has been used in 11 patients as primary treatment in doses ranging from 2.5 mg/kg day for 6 weeks (272) to 5 to 11 mg/kg/day for a median of 4 months (273). L-AMB has been successfully used in two patients who failed to respond conventional amphotericin B (274,275).

Treatment duration is usually prolonged until 1–2 months after complete resolution of clinical findings of infection (258,276).

Patients with candidemia and CVCs in place: Removing all CVCs in patients with candidemia is considered standard practice (208,277), based on the belief that the CVC is the primary source of candidemia and that its removal reduces the morbidity and mortality associated with candidemia. However, arguments against removal of all CVCs in patients with candidemia include: (1) the gastrointestinal origin of most candidemias (see section on hematogenous candidiasis, risk factors); (2) the cost, difficulties, and complications associated with CVC replacement in certain settings (patients with difficult venous access, multiple CVCs in place, high risk for bleeding or pneumothorax, others); and (3) the lack of randomized trials designed to specifically answer the question of CVC removal or retention among patients with candidemia.

In a recent evidence-based review, Nucci and Anaissie (110) showed that among 203 candidemia studies, only 14 evaluated outcome in relation to CVC removal or retention, and among those, only four performed multivariate analysis and included confounding variables such as severity of illness. Analysis of these four studies showed that the beneficial effect of CVC removal on mortality was not present in one study, was marginal in two studies, and was only significant in a subset of 21 neutropenic patients in the fourth study.

Removal of CVC is recommended when its access is no longer needed, or when its replacement is easy and safe (nontunneled, nonimplanted CVC). In addition, the CVCs should be removed in the presence of high-grade fungemia, hemodynamic instability, organ infection (endophtalmitis and other) or pocket site infection, or when the patient remains with a pyrexia of unknown etiology despite 72 hr of adequate antifungal treatment (appropriate dose of an agent usually active against the infecting *Candida* strain). Removal of all CVCs in infections by *Candida parapsilosis* is also recommended unless other sources such as contaminated TPN are responsible for the candidemia. In patients with candidemia and implantable or semi-implantable CVCs, medical antifungal treatment without CVC removal should be considered first, especially in the absence of any of the clinical settings mentioned above. A detailed approach to managing CVC in candidemia is presented in Figure 2 (258).

In the setting of secondary CVC-related candidemia (septic thrombophlebitis or endocarditis), removal of the CVC in all patients should be done. Excision of the infected vein, when possible, may shorten the duration of the bloodstream infection. Duration of antifungal therapy in the setting of thrombophlebitis should be determined by the clinical response. Patients should continue to receive therapy until 2 weeks after resolution of all signs and symptoms of infection (129,162). Repeat surgery may be needed if the vein excision was not complete and blood cultures remain positive (163). Patients with thrombophlebitis of the central veins are not surgical candidates. In those cases, aggressive medical treatment alone has been reported to be successful in 8 of 10 patients (130).

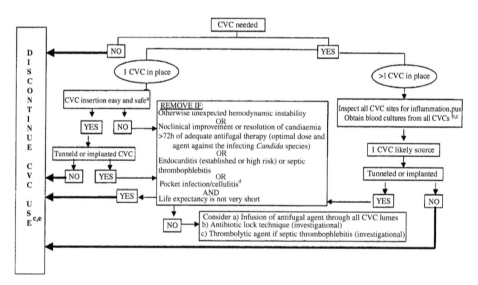

Figure 2 Proposed management of central venous catheters (CVCs) in nonneutropenic patients with candidemia. [a]High risk of bleeding or pneumothorax; serious complication with bleeding or pneumothorax (susch as patients with limited lung function). [b]Value of quantitative blood cultures not established. [c]Especially in patients with *Candida parapsilosis* (typically associated with CVC-related candidemia). [d]Most cases of cellulitis at the CVC site are not infectious and occur within a few days of CVC insertion. Patients with severe neutropenia and mucositis are unlikely to benefit from CVC removal. [e]Candidemia caused by contaminated IV fluids and total parenteral nutrition may occur. Removal of CVC recommended in addition to elimination of source of contamination. *Source*: Vascular catheters and candidemia, CID, 2002; 34(1 March):597. (Figure is from Clin Infect Dis 34(5): 591–599).

The average total dose of amphotericin B given to patients who survived was 2 g. Despite CVC removal and appropriate antifungal therapy, blood cultures may remain positive for up to 3 weeks (278).

3. Cytokine Therapy for Hematogenous Candidiasis

The immune status of the host plays a predominant role in the pathogenesis of opportunistic fungal infections, including hematogenous candidiasis (279). Polymorphonuclear leukocytes and macrophages are the predominant host defenses against candidal infections. Four cytokines, granulocyte colony stimulating factor (G-CSF), granulocyte-macrophage stimulating factor (GM-CSF), macrophage-stimulating factor (M-CSF), and interferon gamma, seem to be promising as adjuvant therapy for proven fungal infections including candidiasis (270,271).

Interferon gamma enhances the candidacidal activity of phagocytes probably through increased production of reactive oxygen radicals and modulates the phagocytosis of *Candida albicans* by endothelial cells. Both G-CSF and GM-CSF activate phagocytic cells and restrict the growth of *C. albicans*. Despite the promising in vitro and experimental data, the clinical experience with cytokines for the treatment of fungal infections remains limited. Anecdotal reports showed favorable outcome of cytokine therapy (interferon-gamma plus G- or GM-CSF) in three patients with hematologic malignancies and refractory chronic disseminated candidiasis (unpublished, Anaissie EJ et al. in press).

B. Local Infections

1. Mucocutaneous Infections

Oropharyngeal candidiasis: In general, systemic treatments with fluconazole, itraconazole, amphotericin B, and caspofungin are more effective than the topical treatments with nystatin or clotrimazole (282).

Elimination of the colonization of the denture by extensive and regular cleaning is also recommended in denture-related oropharyngeal candidiasis. (283).

Esophageal candidiasis: Randomized studies showed that caspofungin and voriconazole were as effective as fluconazole (200 mg/day) (260,284) or amphotericin B (0.5 mg/kg/day) (285) for the treatment of esophageal candidiasis. Duration of therapy is at least 10 to 14 days.

Lower gastrointestinal candidiasis: Because stool cultures do not differentiate between colonization and infection, candidiasis in the lower gastrointestinal tract is usually a postmortem diagnosis; hence, there are no reliable criteria governing when and how to treat this condition. Patients with diarrhea caused by heavy colonization with *Candida* spp. may respond dramatically to two to four days of nystatin therapy (286).

Candida infections of the genitalia: In uncomplicated cases, most cases of vulvovaginal candidiasis can be successfully treated with topical azoles, a single day treatment of oral fluconazole (150 mg) or itraconazole capsules (200 mg bid), or 5 days of ketoconazole (400 mg/day) (287). A recent randomized double-blind study showed that fluconazole 150 mg single dose was as effective as 3 days of itraconazole 200 mg/day (288). In cases of recurrent vulvovaginal candidiasis (defined as more than four episodes per year), acute severe attacks, or failure to conventional therapy, treatment (fluconazole, itraconazole, or ketoconazole) should be prolonged for 14 days, followed by a maintenance regimen (fluconazole 150 or 100 mg weekly for 6 months). *Candida balanitis* responds quickly with twice-a-day application of miconazole, clotrimazole, or other topical antifungal agents. Relief is almost immediate, but treatment should be continued for 10 days. Preparations containing topical steroids give temporary relief by suppressing inflammation, but the eruption rebounds and worsens, sometimes even before the steroid cream has been discontinued.

Candida infections of the skin and nails: Oral fluconazole (50 mg/day, or 150 mg/week) (289), itraconazole (100 or 200 mg/day), ketoconazole (200 mg/day), or terbinafine (125–250 mg bid) can be effective (290,291). Terbinafine seems to be more active against infections caused by *C. parapsilosis* and *C. albicans* (292). Treatment also includes adequate hygiene and measures directed at promoting dryness and avoidance of occlusion.

Congenital cutaneous candidiasis may resolve with topical and oral nystatin treatment. However, in patients with burnlike dermatitis, or positive cultures for *Candida* spp. from any site, respiratory distress, or laboratory finding consistent with sepsis, systemic antifungal treatment is recommended because of the high likelihood of developing hematogenous infection (196).

Topical treatments for onychomycosis by *Candida* spp. are usually of little value and oral therapy should be used. Topical antifungal agents may have a role in preventing relapse of the infection after successful oral therapy. Oral treatment options include: itraconazole (200 bid × 7 day per month × 3 pulses), terbinafine (250 mg/day × 12 weeks), and fluconazole (150 mg/week × 9–18 months) (293).

Antifungal treatments can ameliorate the morbidity of patients suffering of chronic mucocutaneous candidiasis. Effective agents include itraconazole (200 mg/day) and fluconazole (50–200 mg/day) given for months continuously or intermittently (294–296). Relapses will occur because of persistence of the immune defect.

2. Locally Invasive Infections

Urinary tract infections: Treatment of urinary tract infections usually require the same treatment given for hematogenous candidiasis. Release of obstruction when present is essential for successful outcome (see earlier section Urinary tract infections).

Pneumonia: The recommended treatment for *Candida* pneumonia is the one that applies to hematogenous candidiasis.

Cardiovascular infections Candida: endocarditis is associated with high mortality and high frequency of relapse. In two reports of fungal endocarditis mostly caused by *C. albicans*, the 5-year survival ranged from 67% to 75%, with a relapse of 19–33%. Relapses may develop up to 9 years after the first episode (214,297).

Treatment of *Candida* endocarditis includes surgery and antifungal chemotherapy given prior (1–2 weeks), during, and after (6–8 weeks) surgery followed by prolonged (1–2 years) suppressive antifungal therapy for periods as along as 2 years after surgery. The recommended drugs include amphotericin B or its lipid formulation, and fluconazole for suppressive therapy. Doses and standard duration of therapy have not been established (211,218). Caspofungin is a less toxic option than amphotericin B but has not been investigational in this setting.

The rationale for valve replacement in *Candida* endocarditis relies on the fact that antifungal agents are fungistatic and may penetrate poorly into the vegetations. Furthermore, candidal vegetations tend to be large, leading to a higher rate of embolic complications compared to bacterial endocarditis. Successful outcome with medical treatment alone has been reported even in the setting of prosthetic valve endocarditis (298).

Candida myocarditis is usually treated like an acute condition; therefore, there are no standard recommendations for treatment. The same treatment that applies to hematogenous candidiasis is recommended, because 62% of cases of hematogenous candidiasis have myocardial involvement without valvulitis (222,258).

Candida pericarditis is best treated with a combined surgical and medical approach, including pericardial drainage or/and pericardiectomy and prolonged antifungal therapy (224,299). Amphotericin B has been the most commonly used antifungal agent and achieves high concentration within pericardium (50% of the serum concentration) (300). Other antifungal agents such as fluconazole, caspofungin, and the lipid formulations of amphotericin B are also likely to be effective.

Central nervous system infections: Standard therapy for *Candida* meningitis is amphotericin B plus flucytosine (301). The combination of high-dose fluconazole (800 mg/day) and flucytosine (50 mg/kg/day) is a particularly attractive approach because of the high cerebral spinal fluid concentrations achieved with both agents (302,303). Therapy should be given until all signs and symptoms of infection have resolved.

Ocular infections: The management of *Candida* endophthalmitis consists of prompt initiation of antifungal therapy (to prevent blindness) with an agent that has high intraocular penetration and surgical consultation. Fluconazole is currently the drug of choice because of its proven efficacy and its higher concentration in ocular tissue. It is recommended to give 800 mg/day of fluconazole until a major response is observed at which time it may be possible to reduce the dose to 400 mg/day. If the infecting organism is potentially resistant to fluconazole, then high-dose amphotericin B (0.7–1 mg/kg/day) should be given, preferably in conjunction with flucytosine because of the poor intraocular penetration of amphotericin B. Therapy should be continued for at least 10–14 days after resolution of all signs and symptoms of infection. In the presence of vitreal or severe ocular infection, amphotericin B may have to be administered intraocularly (258).

Bone and joint infections: Early diagnosis of *Candida* arthritis and systemic anti-fungal therapy are important to prevent destruction of the cartilage or loosening of the prosthesis. For the treatment of *Candida* osteomyelitis, surgical drainage of pus is essential for a good response; however, debridement of bony lesions may not be needed. Fluconazole 400–800 mg/day or amphotericin B for 6 months is recommended (304–308).

Abdominal infections: Because fluconazole (400–800 mg/day for 2–6 weeks) is safe and achieves high concentration in the peritoneal fluid, it is likely to be useful in the management of candidal peritonitis and other intra-abdominal infections. The use of peritoneal amphotericin B is discouraged because of the local toxicity (local irritation and fibrosis). Liver, gallbladder, or subphrenic abscesses have been reported in patients with percutaneously placed drainage catheters for malignancy (236). Catheter exchange or removal may be indicated in this setting.

Patients with candidal peritonitis after long-term ambulatory peritoneal dialysis should receive therapy with systemic antifungal agents and the peritoneal catheter may need to be removed (309,310).

VIII. PREVENTION

The strategies for the prevention of severe candidal infections should be effective and safe, and not associated with a high likelihood of development of resistance to antifungal agents. The best strategy should focus on identification of the target population (those at highest risk for developing severe candidiasis), implementing simple but effective infection control measures and, when needed, providing antifungal chemoprophylaxis.

A. Identification of Patients at Risk

As mentioned earlier, patients at highest risk for severe candidal infections include those who are colonized with *Candida* spp. at two or more sites, who have or likely to have significant disruption of the integrity of the gut mucosa (leading to increased translocation of *Candida* spp.), and who are immunosuppressed (either locally such as after organ transplantation or systemically following immunosuppressive therapy). The patient populations at risk include neonates; critically ill adults (surgical, burn, hemodialysis patients, among others); cancer patients; bone marrow/stem cell, and solid organ transplantation recipients; and advanced stages of AIDS.

B. Infection Control Measures

Handwashing: Up to 58% of health care workers can carry *Candida* spp. on their hands, and transmission from staff to patients and from patient to patient has been documented in several studies (see section on epidemiology). Strict handwashing remains the simplest and most effective measures to prevent the acquisition of organisms by patients. The use of artificial fingernails should be discouraged in areas housing high-risk patients as artificial fingernails may harbor yeasts (245,311).

    Equipment, devices, and IV solutions: Cleaning, sterilization, and disinfection of all medical equipment and care of intravascular devices should follow the Centers for Diseases Control and Prevention guidelines for the prevention of nosocomial infections. Preparation of TPN infusates should follow strict aseptic techniques to avoid exogenous contamination.

C. Antifungal Chemoprophylaxis

Chemoprophylaxis with systemic antifungal agents should be limited to high-risk patients.

    Hematologic and bone marrow (BMT)/stem cell transplant (HSCT) patients: Patients with acute leukemia and/or bone marrow/stem cell transplantation and any patients with anticipated prolonged neutropenia are more likely to benefit from antifungal chemoprophylaxis. Fluconazole has been the most commonly used agent for prophylaxis because of its excellent safety profile. Two randomized, prospective, double-blinded, placebo controlled trials that enrolled HSCT recipients showed that prophylactic Fluconazole given in doses of 400 mg/day significantly reduced the incidence of superficial and invasive candidiasis (312,313), improved overall survival (312), and was associated with fewer fungal-related deaths (313). Continuation of Fluconazol to day 75 after transplant was shown to improve survival in one study of high-risk allogeneic patients (314). Similar studies were also conducted among patients with acute leukemia. Fluconazol was effective in reducing colonization and superficial infection, but studies did not show a decrease in invasive fungal infections (315–317). In a recent randomized placebo-controlled study, fluconazole 400 mg/day was as effective as 200 mg/day for prophylaxis of yeast infections in recipients of bone marrow transplantation (318). This study also shows no major benefit of prolonging fluconazole prophylaxis beyond day 100 after transplantation. Another randomized trial showed that fluconazole 200 mg/day was as effective as low dose amphotericin B (0.2 mg/kg/day) for prophylaxis of fungal infections in HSCT recipients (319).

Itraconazole capsules (200 mg/day) (320) and solution (5 mg/kg/day) (321,322) are also effective in reducing documented fungal infections (mostly hematogenous candidiasis) in these patients. In a nonblinded randomized study that compared Itraconazole solution (5 mg/kg/day) to Fluconazole suspension (100 mg/day), a trend favoring Itraconazole was observed albeit at the cost of additional gastrointestinal toxicity (323).

Conventional amphotericin B is not an adequate drug for prophylaxis because of its high toxicity. Among the lipid formulations of amphotericin B, L-AMB (AmBisome) is the least toxic (267,268) and, therefore, the most appropriate for prophylaxis when prophylaxis with an azole is not possible. This agent has been used in doses of 1 mg/kg/day (324) to 2 mg/kg/day thrice weekly (325), although the incidence of fungal infections was too low in the placebo groups to detect any statistically significant benefit from this agent. The high cost of the lipid formulations of Amphotericin B, the lack of data that support significant reduction in morbidity and mortality, and the availability of new and safer antifungal agents such as the Echinocandins, and the new azole voriconazole, limit the use of lipid formulations of amphotericin B for prophylaxis of invasive candidiasis.

Patients who develop chronic disseminated candidiasis may need to undergo further cytotoxic chemotherapy or bone marrow transplantation while radiological findings may not have been completely resolved. In this setting, two reports suggest that keeping patients on antifungal therapy (secondary prophylaxis) during subsequent periods of neutropenia, including after myeloablative chemotherapy and stem cell transplantation, may result in a successful outcome in $\geq 80\%$ of the patients (326,327).

Surgical and critically ill patients: A prospective randomized, double-blind, placebo-controlled study showed that IV Fluconazole (400 mg/day) significantly reduced colonization, and intra-abdominal infections by *Candida* spp. among patients undergoing surgery for recurrent gastrointestinal perforation or anastomotic leaks (328). Among 260 critically ill surgical patients with a length of ICU stay of at least three days, Fluconazole 400 mg/day reduced the risk of fungal infection by 55%, although there was no difference in death between the Fluconazole and the placebo group (329).

Liver transplant patients: Prophylaxis with liposomal Amphotericin B (AmBisome) was evaluated in a prospective randomized, double-blind, placebo-controlled study. This study showed that a dose of 1 mg/kg/day for 5 days after transplantation was effective in preventing fungal infections in this patient population. This benefit was still present even one year after transplantation (11% incidence of fungal infections in the AmBisome group versus 29% in the placebo group, $p < 0.05$) (330).

Fluconazole is also effective for prophylaxis of fungal infections in this patient population. One study compared Fluconazole 100 mg/day with nystatin from days 3 to 28 after transplantation. The incidence of fungal infections was significantly lower in the fluconazole group (13%) than in the nystatin group (34%) (331). In a prospective randomized, double-blind, placebo-controlled study, fluconazole (400 mg/day until 10 weeks after transplantation), significantly reduced colonization, and superficial and invasive fungal infections (332). Of note, no patient had to discontinue Fluconazole because of hepatotoxicity.

Very low birth weight infants: A randomized trial designed to look at rectal colonization of infants by *Candida* spp. compared placebo to fluconazole (6 mg/kg every 72 hr during the first 7 days, and every 24 hr from days 8 to 28 of life) and showed a significant reduction of rectal colonization by *Candida* spp. through day 28 of life among infants of all weights randomized to fluconazole. This effect persisted through day 56 among infants weighing $< 1.250\,g$ (333). This study suggested but did not demonstrate that fluconazole may be useful in reducing candidal infections among infants weighing $< 1.250\,g$. Later, another prospective, randomized, double-blind clinical trial conducted in 100 preterm infants with birth weights $<1000\,g$ showed that Fluconazole given during the first 6 weeks of life was effective in preventing fungal colonization and invasive fungal infection. Invasive fungal infections developed in 20% and in none of the infants that belonged to the placebo and Fluconazole group, respectively (334).

D. Preemptive Antifungal Therapy

Systemic antifungal chemoprophylaxis can be associated with toxicity, cost, and emergence of resistance. An alternative approach is give pre-emptive antifungal therapy which consists of limiting antifungal therapy only to those patients at high risk for serious candidal infections and who also exhibit evidence of significant colonization with *Candida* spp. at two or more sites. This strategy has been proposed in the setting of cancer chemotherapy (335) and surgery (336,337).

REFERENCES

1. Anaissie Book Candidiasis. In: Kwon-Chung KJ, Bennett JE, eds. Medical Mycology. Malvern, Pennsylvania: Lea & Febiger, 1992:280–336.
2. Edmond MB, et al. Nosocomial bloodstream infections in United States hospitals: a three-year analysis. Clin Infect Dis 1999; 29(2):239–244.
3. Miller LG, Hajjeh RA, Edwards JE Jr. Estimating the cost of nosocomial candidemia in the United States [comment]. Clin Infect Dis 2001; 32(7):1110.
4. Rentz AM, Halpern MT, Bowden R. The impact of candidemia on length of hospital stay, outcome, and overall cost of illness [comment]. Clin Infect Dis 1998; 27(4): 781–788.
5. Hazen KC. New and emerging yeast pathogens. Clin Microbiol Rev 1995; 8:462–478.
6. Schoofs A, et al. Use of specialised isolation media for recognition and identification of *Candida dubliniensis* isolates from HIV-infected patients. Eur J Clin Microbiol Infect Dis 1997; 16(4):296–300.
7. Sullivan DJ, et al. *Candida dubliniensis* spp. nov.: phenotypic and molecular characterization of a novel species associated with oral candidosis in HIV-infected individuals. Microbiology 1995; 141(Pt 7):1507–1521.
8. James CW, Anaissie Book. Epidemiology of *Candida* infections. In: Bodey GP, ed. Candidiasis: Pathogenesis, Diagnosis and Treatment. New York: Raven Press, 1993:85–107.
9. Edwards JE. *Candida spp.* In: Principles and Practice of Infectious Diseases. Mandell D, Bennett JE, ed. New York: Churchill Livingstone, 2000:2656–2674.
10. Odds FC. *Candida* and Candidosis. 2nd ed. London: Bailliere Tindall, 1998.
11. Odds FC. *Candida* infections an overview. Crit Rev Microbiol1987; 15:1–5.
12. Sangeorzan JA, et al. Epidemiology of oral candidiasis in HIV-infected patients: colonization, infection, treatment, and emergence of fluconazole resistance. Am J Med 1994; 97(4):339–346.
13. Budtz-Jorgensen E, Stenderup A, Grabowski M. An epidemiological study of yeasts in elderly denture wearers. Comm Dental Oral Epidemiol 1975; 3:115–119.

14. Tapper-Jones LM, et al. Candidal infections and populations of *Candida albicans* in mouths of diabetics. J Clin Pathol 1981; 34:706–711.

15. Samaranayake LP, et al. The oral carriage of yeasts and coliforms in patients on cytotoxic therapy. J Oral Pathol 1984; 13(4):390–393.

16. Main BE, et al. The effect of cytotoxic therapy on saliva and oral flora. Oral Surg Oral Med Oral Pathol 1984; 58(5):545–548.

17. Martin MV, Wilkinson GR. The oral yeast flora of 10-year-old schoolchildren. Sabouraudia 1983; 21(2):129–135.

18. Odds FC, et al. Carriage of *Candida* species and *C. albicans* biotypes in patients undergoing chemotherapy or bone marrow transplantation for haematological disease. J Clin Pathol 1989; 42(12):1259–1266.

19. Fisher BM, et al. Carriage of *Candida* species in the oral cavity in diabetic patients: relationship to glycaemic control. J Oral Pathol 1987; 16(5):282–284.

20. Leung WK, et al. Oral colonization, phenotypic, and genotypic profiles of *Candida* species in irradiated, dentate, xerostomic nasopharyngeal carcinoma survivors. J Clin Microbiol 2000; 38(6):2219–2226.

21. Fanello S, et al. Nosocomial *Candida albicans* acquisition in a geriatric unit: epidemiology and evidence for person-to-person transmission. J Hosp Infect 2001; 47:46–52.

22. Odds FC, et al. *Candida* species and *C. albicans* biotypes in women attending clinics in genitourinary medicine. J Med Microbiol 1989; 29(1):51–54.

23. Krause W, Matheis H, Wulf K. Fungaemia and funguria after oral administration of *Candida albicans.* Lancet 1969; i(Mar 22):598–599.

24. Stone HH, et al. *Candida sepsis*: pathogenesis and principles of treatment. Ann Surg 1974; 179(5):697–711.

25. Pappo I, et al. Altered gut barrier function to *Candida* during parenteral nutrition. Nutrition 1994; 10(2):151–154.

26. McCray E, et al. Outbreak of *Candida parapsilosis* endophthalmitis after cataract extraction and intraocular lens implantation. J Clin Microbiol 1986; 24:625–628.

27. Plouffe JF, et al. Nosocomial outbreak of *Candida parapsilosis* fungemia related to intravenous infusions. Arch Intern Med 1977; 137:1686–1689.

28. Weems JJ Jr, et al. *Candida parapsilosis* fungemia associated with parenteral nutrition and contaminated blood pressure transducers. J Clin Microbiol 1987; 25(6):1029–1032.

29. Welbel SF, et al. *Candida parapsilosis* bloodstream infections in neonatal intensive care unit patients: epidemiologic and laboratory confirmation of a common source outbreak. Pediatr Infect Dis J 1996; 15(11):998–1002.

30. Pfaller MA. Nosocomial candidiasis: emerging species, reservoirs, and modes of transmission. Clin Infect Dis 1996; 22(suppl 2):S89–S94.

31. Vincent JL, et al. Epidemiology, diagnosis and treatment of systemic *Candida* infection in surgical patients under intensive care. Intens Care Med 1998; 24(3):206–216.

32. Robert F, et al. Use of random amplified polymorphic DNA as a typing method for *Candida albicans* in epidemiological surveillance of a burn unit. J Clin Microbiol 1995; 33(9):2366–2371.

33. Doi M, et al. Strain relatedness of *Candida albicans* strains isolated from children with leukemia and their bedside parents. J Clin Microbiol 1994; 32:2253–2259.

34. Berger C, et al. A *Candida krusei* epidemic in a hematology department. Schweiz Med Wochenschr 1988; 118(2):37–41.

35. Rangel-Frausto MS, et al. National Epidemiology of Mycoses Survey (NEMIS): Variations in rates of bloodstream infections due to *Candida* species in seven surgical intensive care units and six neonatal intensive care units. Clin Infect Dis 1999; 29(2):253–258.

36. Huang YC, et al. Outbreak of *Candida albicans* fungaemia in a neonatal intensive care unit. Scand J Infect Dis 1998; 30(2):137–142.

37. Rodero L, et al. Nosocomial transmission of *Candida albicans* in newborn infants. Rev Argentina Microbiol 2000; 32(4):179–184.

38. Sanchez V, et al. Epidemiology of nosocomial acquisition of *Candida lusitaniae*. J Clin Microbiol 1992; 30(11):3005–3008.

39. Sanchez V, et al. Nosocomial acquisition of *Candida parapsilosis*: an epidemiologic study. Am J Med 1993; 94(6):577–582.

40. Reef SE, et al. Nonperinatal nosocomial transmission of *Candida albicans* in a neonatal intensive care unit: prospective study. J Clin Microbiol 1998; 36(5):1255–1259.

41. Finkelstein R, et al. Outbreak of *Candida tropicalis* fungemia in a neonatal intensive care unit. Infect Control Hosp Epidemiol 1993; 14(10):587–590.

42. Rangel-Frausto MS, et al. An experimental model for study of *Candida* survival and transmission in human volunteers. Eur J Clin Microbiol Infect Dis 1994; 13(7):590–595.

43. Geiger AM, Foxman B, Gillespie BW. The epidemiology of vulvovaginal candidiasis among university students. Am J Public Health 1995; 85(8 Pt 1):1146–1148.

44. Foxman B. The epidemiology of vulvovaginal candidiasis: risk factors. Am J Public Health 1990; 80(3):329–331.

45. Geiger AM, Foxman B. Risk factors for vulvovaginal candidiasis: a case–control study among university students. Epidemiology 1996; 7(2):182–187.

46. Reed BD, et al. Sexual behaviors and other risk factors for *Candida vulvovaginitis*. J Womens Health Gender-Based Med 2000; 9(6):645–655.

47. Lockhart SR, et al. Most frequent scenario for recurrent Candida vaginitis is strain maintenance with "substrain shuffling": demonstration by sequential DNA fingerprinting with probes CA3, C1, and CARE2. J Clin Microbiol 1996; 34:767–777.

48. Mellinger M, et al. Epidemiological and clinical approach to the study of candidiasis caused by *Candida albicans* in heroin addicts in the Paris region: analysis of 35 observations. Bull Narcotics 1982; 34(3–4):61–81.

49. Newton-John HF, Wise K, Looke DF. Role of the lemon in disseminated candidiasis of heroin abusers. Med J Aust 1984; 140(13):780–781.

50. Elbaze P, et al. The skin as the possible reservoir for *Candida albicans* in the oculocutaneous candidiasis of heroin addicts. Acta Derm Venereol (Stockh) 1992; 72:180–181.

51. Bougnoux ME, et al. Mixed *Candida glabrata* and *Candida albicans* disseminated candidiasis in a heroin addict. Eur J Clin Microbiol Infect Dis 1997; 16(8):598–600.

52. Pfaller MA, et al. International surveillance of blood stream infections due to *Candida* species in the European SENTRY Program: species distribution and antifungal susceptibility including the investigational triazole and echinocandin agents. SENTRY Participant Group (Europe). Diagn Microbiol Infect Dis 1999; 35(1):19–25.

53. Martins MD, Lozano-Chiu M, Rex JH. Point prevalence of oropharyngeal carriage of fluconazole-resistant *Candida* in human immunodeficiency virus-infected patients. Clin Infect Dis 1997; 25(4):843–846.

54. Rex JH, Rinaldi MG, Pfaller MA. Resistance of *Candida* species to fluconazole. Antimicrob Agents Chemother 1995; 39:1–8.

55. Canuto MDM, et al. Epidemiology of oropharyngeal colonization and infection due to non-*Candida albicans* species in HIV-infected patients. Med Clin 1999; 112(6):211–214.

56. Redding SW, et al. The epidemiology of non-*albicans Candida* in oropharyngeal candidiasis in HIV patients. Special Care Dent 2000; 20(5):178–181.

57. Martins MD, Lozano-Chiu M, Rex JH. Declining rates of oropharyngeal candidiasis and carriage of *Candida albicans* associated with trends toward reduced rates of carriage of fluconazole-resistant *C. albicans* in human immunodeficiency virus-infected patients. Clin Infect Dis 1998; 27(5):1291–1294.

58. Pfaller MA, et al. National surveillance of nosocomial blood stream infection due to *Candida albicans*: frequency of occurrence and antifungal susceptibility in the SCOPE Program. Diagn Microbiol Infect Dis 1998; 31(1):327–332.

59. Wingard JR. Importance of *Candida* species other than *C. albicans* as pathogens in oncology patients. Clin Infect Dis 1995; 20:115–125.

60. Yamamura DL, et al. Candidemia at selected Canadian sites: results from the Fungal Disease Registry, 1992–1994. Fungal Dis Reg Can Infect Dis Soc Cmaj 1999; 160(4):493–499.

61. Nguyen MH, et al. The changing face of candidemia: emergence of non-*Candida albicans* species and antifungal resistance. Am J Med 1996; 100(6):617–623.

62. Abi-Said D, et al. The epidemiology of hematogenous candidiasis caused by different *Candida* species [published erratum appears in Clin Infect Dis 1997; 25(2):352]. Clin Infect Dis 1997; 24(6):1122–1128.

63. Kossoff EH, Buescher ES, Karlowicz MG. Candidemia in a neonatal intensive care unit: trends during fifteen years and clinical features of 111 cases. Pediatr Infect Dis J 1998; 17:504–508.

64. Wingard JR, et al. Increase in *Candida krusei* infection among patients with bone marrow transplantation and neutropenia treated prophylactically with fluconazole. New Engl J Med 1991; 325(18):1274–1277.

65. Wingard JR, et al. Association of *Torulopsis glabrata* infections with fluconazole prophylaxis in neutropenic bone marrow transplant patients. Antimicrob Agents Chemother 1993; 37(9):1847–1849.

66. Levin AS, et al. *Candida parapsilosis* fungemia associated with implantable and semi-implantable central venous catheters and the hands of healthcare workers. Diagn Microbiol Infect Dis 1998; 30:243–249.

67. Vartivarian S, Smith CB. Anaissie Book. Pathogenesis, Host Resistance and Predisposing Factors. In: Bodey GP, ed. Candidiasis: Pathogenesis, Diagnosis and Treatment. New York: Raven Press, 1993:59–84.

68. Shin JH, et al. Biofilm production by isolates of *Candida* species recovered from non-neutropenic patients: comparison of bloodstream isolates with isolates from other sources. J Clin Microbiol 2002; 40(4):1244–1248.

69. Sobel JD, Muller G, Buckley HR. Critical role of germ tube formation in the pathogenesis of candidal vaginitis. Infect Immun 1984; 44(3):576–580.

70. Mitchell AP. Dimorphism and virulence in *Candida albicans*. Curr Opin Microbiol 1998; 1(6):687–692.

71. Gilfillan GD, et al. *Candida dubliniensis*: phylogeny and putative virulence factors. Microbiology 1998; 144(Pt 4):829–838.

72. Monod M, et al. Multiplicity of genes encoding secreted aspartic proteinases in *Candida* species. Mol Microbiol 1994; 13(2):357–368.

73. De Bernardis F, et al. Biotyping and virulence properties of skin isolates of *Candida parapsilosis*. J Clin Microbiol 1999; 37(11):3481–3486.

74. Zaugg C, et al. Secreted aspartic proteinase family of *Candida tropicalis*. Infect Immun 2001; 69(1):405–412.

75. Hannula J, et al. Comparison of virulence factors of oral *Candida dubliniensis* and *Candida albicans* isolates in healthy people and patients with chronic candidosis. Oral Microbiol Immunol 2000; 15(4):238–244.

76. de Oliveira EE, et al. Killer toxin and enzyme production by *Candida albicans* isolated from buccal mucosa in patients with cancer. Rev Soc Bras Med Trop 1998; 31(6):523–527.

77. Ghannoum MA. Potential role of phospholipases in virulence and fungal pathogenesis. Clin Microbiol Rev 2000; 13(1):122–143,CP3.

78. Barrett-Bee K, et al. A comparison of phospholipase activity, cellular adherence and pathogenicity of yeasts. J Gen Microbiol 1985; 131(Pt 5):1217–1221.

79. Ghannoum MA, Abu-Elteen KH. Pathogenicity determinants of *Candida*. Mycoses 1990; 33:265–282.

80. Odds EC. Switch of phenotype as an escape mechanism of the intruder. Mycoses 1997; 40(suppl 2):9–12.

81. Jones S, White G, Hunter PR. Increased phenotypic switching in strains of *Candida albicans* associated with invasive infections. J Clin Microbiol 1994; 32(11):2869–2870.

82. Kolotila MP, Diamond RD. Effects of neutrophils and in vitro oxidants on survival and phenotypic switching of *Candida albicans* WO-1. Infect Immun 1990; 58(5):1174–1179.

83. Xiong JB, et al. *Candida albicans* and *Candida krusei* differentially induce human blood mononuclear cell interleukin-12 and gamma interferon production. Infect Immun 2000; 68(5):2464–2469.

84. Fisher-Hoch SP, Hutwagner L. Opportunistic candidiasis: an epidemic of the 1980s. Clin Infect Dis 1995; 21:897–904.

85. Beck-Sague C, Jarvis WR. Secular trends in the epidemiology of nosocomial fungal infections in the United States, 1980–1990. National Nosocomial Infections Surveillance Syst. J Infect Dis 1993; 167:1247–1251.

86. Kao AS, et al. The epidemiology of candidemia in two United States cities: results of a population-based active surveillance. Clin Infect Dis 1999; 29(5):1164–1170.

87. Lyytikainen O, et al. Nosocomial bloodstream infections in Finnish hospitals during 1999–2000. Clin Infect Dis 2002; 35(2):e14–e19.

88. Voss A, et al. Occurrence of yeast bloodstream infections between 1987 and 1995 in five Dutch university hospitals. Eur J Clin Microbiol Infect Dis 1996; 15(12):909–912.

89. Baran J Jr, Muckatira B, Khatib R. Candidemia before and during the fluconazole era: prevalence, type of species and approach to treatment in a tertiary care community hospital. Scand J Infect Dis 2001; 33(2):137–139.

90. Safdar A, Perlin DS, Armstrong D. Hematogenous infections due to *Candida parapsilosis*: changing trends in fungemic patients at a comprehensive cancer center during the last four decades. Diagn Microbiol Infect Dis 2002; 44(1):11–16.

91. Montgomerie JZ, Edwards JE Jr. Association of infection due to *Candida albicans* with intravenous hyperalimentation. J Infect Dis 1978; 137(2):197–201.

92. Spebar MJ, Pruitt BA Jr. Candidiasis in the burned patient. J Trauma-Injury Infect Crit Care 1981; 21(3):237–239.

93. Sheridan RL, et al. Candidemia in the pediatric patient with burns. J Burn Care Rehabil 1995; 16(4):440–443.

94. Desai MH, et al. *Candida* infection with and without nystatin prophylaxis. A 11-year experience with patients with burn injury. Arch Surg 1992; 127(2):159–162.

95. Wey SB, et al. Hospital-acquired candidemia. The attributable mortality and excess length of stay. Arch Intern Med 1988; 148(12):2642–2645.

96. Gudlaugsson O, Gillerpie S, Lee K, Vande Berg J, Hu J, Messer S, et al. Attributable mortality of nosocomial candidemia, revisited.Clin Infect Dis 2003; 37(9):1172–1177.

97. Fraser VJ, et al. Candidemia in a tertiary care hospital: epidemiology, risk factors, and predictors of mortality [see comments]. Clin Infect Dis 1992; 15(3):414–421.

98. Meunier F, Aoun M, Bitar N. Candidemia in immunocompromised patients. Clin Infect Dis 1992; 14(suppl 1):S120–S125.

99. Nguyen MH, et al. Therapeutic approaches in patients with candidemia. Evaluation in a multicenter, prospective, observational study. Arch Intern Med 1995; 155(22):2429–2435.

100. Nolla-Salas J, et al. Candidemia in non-neutropenic critically ill patients: analysis of prognostic factors and assessment of systemic antifungal therapy. Study Group of Fungal Infection in the ICU. Intens Care Med 1997; 23(1):23–30.

101. Viudes A, et al. Candidemia at a tertiary-care hospital: epidemiology, treatment, clinical outcome and risk factors for death [comment]. Eur J Clin Microbiol Infect Dis 2002; 21(11):767–774.

102. Uzun O, Anaissie EJ. Predictors of outcome in cancer patients with candidemia. Ann Oncol 2000; 11(12):1517–1521.

103. Kazama I, Furukawa K. A study for candidemia during the six year period from 1993 to 1999 in St. Luke's International Hospital. Kansenshogaku Zasshi—J Japan Assoc Infect Dis 2003; 77(3):158–166.

104. Chapman RL. *Candida* infections in the neonate. Curr Opin Pediatr 2003; 15(1):97–102.

105. Pappas PG, et al. A prospective observational study of candidemia: epidemiology, therapy, and influences on mortality in hospitalized adult and pediatric patients. Clin Infect Dis 2003; 37(5):634–643.

106. Uzun O, et al. Risk factors and predictors of outcome in patients with cancer and breakthrough candidemia. Clin Infect Dis 2001; 32(12):1713–1717.

107. Nucci M, et al. Risk factors for death among cancer patients with fungemia. Clin Infect Dis 1998; 27(1):107–111.

108. Viscoli C, et al. Candidemia in cancer patients: a prospective, multicenter surveillance study by the Invasive Fungal Infection Group (IFIG) of the European Organization for Research and Treatment of Cancer (EORTC). Clin Infect Dis 1999; 28(5):1071–1079.

109. Anaissie EJ, et al. Predictors of adverse outcome in cancer patients with candidemia. Am J Med 1998; 104(3):238–245.

110. Nucci M, Anaissie E. Should vascular catheters be removed from all patients with candidemia? An evidence-based review [comment]. Clin Infect Dis 2002; 34(5):591–599.

111. Krcmery V, Barnes AJ. Non-*albicans Candida* spp. causing fungaemia: pathogenicity and antifungal resistance. J Hosp Infect 2002; 50(4):243–260.

112. Maksymiuk AW, et al. Systemic candidiasis in cancer patients. Am J Med 1984; 77(4D):20–27.

113. Anaissie E, et al. Fluconazole therapy for chronic disseminated candidiasis in patients with leukemia and prior amphotericin B therapy. Am J Med 1991; 91:142–150.

114. Sallah S, et al. Hepatosplenic candidiasis in patients with acute leukaemia. Br J Haematol 1999; 106(3):697–701.

115. Pagano L, et al. Chronic disseminated candidiasis in patients with hematologic malignancies. Clinical features and outcome of 29 episodes. Haematologica 2002; 87(5):535–541.

116. Voss A, et al. Investigation of the sequence of colonization and candidemia in nonneutropenic patients. J Clin Microbiol 1994; 32(4):975–980.

117. Saiman L, et al. Risk factors for candidemia in Neonatal Intensive Care Unit patients. The National Epidemiology of Mycosis Survey study group. Pediatr Infect Dis J 2000; 19(4):319–324.

118. Reagan DR, et al. Characterization of the sequence of colonization and nosocomial candidemia using DNA fingerprinting and a DNA probe. J Clin Microbiol 1990; 28:2733–2738.

119. Klempp-Selb B, Rimek D, Kappe R. Karyotyping of *Candida albicans* and *Candida glabrata* from patients with *Candida* species. Mycoses 2000 43:159–163.

120. Richet HM, et al. Risk factors for candidemia in patients with acute lymphocytic leukemia. Rev Infect Dis 1991; 13(2):211–215.

121. Guiot HF, Fibbe WE, van't Wout JW. Risk factors for fungal infection in patients with malignant hematologic disorders: implications for empirical therapy and prophylaxis [see comments]. Clin Infect Dis 1994; 18(4):525–532.

122. Pappu-Katikaneni LD, Rao KP, Banister E. Gastrointestinal colonization with yeast species and *Candida septicemia* in very low birth weight infants. Mycoses 1990; 33(1):20–23.

123. Pittet D, et al. *Candida* colonization and subsequent infections in critically ill surgical patients. Ann Surg 1994; 220:751–758.

124. Pfaller M, et al. Predictive value of surveillance cultures for systemic infection due to *Candida* species. Eur J Clin Microbiol Infect Dis 1987; 6:628–633.

125. Martino P, et al. *Candida* colonization and systemic infection in neutropenic patients. A retrospective study. Cancer 1989; 64(10):2030–2034.

126. Martino P, et al. Prospective study of *Candida* colonization, use of empiric amphotericin B and development of invasive mycosis in neutropenic patients. Eur J Clin Microbiol Infect Dis 1994; 13(10):797–804.

127. Nucci M, Anaissie E. Revisiting the source of candidemia: skin or gut? Clin Infect Dis 2001; 33(12):1959–1967.
128. Torres-Rojas JR, et al. Candidal suppurative peripheral thrombophlebitis. Ann Intern Med 1982; 96(4):431–435.
129. Walsh TJ, et al. Candidal suppurative peripheral thrombophlebitis: recognition, prevention, and management. Infect Control 1986; 7(1):16–22.
130. Benoit D, et al. Management of candidal thrombophlebitis of the central veins: case report and review. Clin Infect Dis 1998; 26:393–397.
131. Faix RG, et al. Mucocutaneous and invasive candidiasis among very low birth weight (less than 1,500 grams) infants in intensive care nurseries: a prospective study. Pediatrics 1989; 83(1):101–107.
132. Faix RG. Systemic *Candida* infections in infants in intensive care nurseries: high incidence of central nervous system involvement. J Pediatr 1984; 105:616–622.
133. Baley JE, Annable WL, Kllegman RM. *Candida endophthalmitis* in the premature infant. J Pediatr 1981; 98:458–461.
134. van den Anker JN, van Popele NM, Sauer PJ. Antifungal agents in neonatal systemic candidiasis. Antimicrob Agents Chemother 1995; 39:1391–1397.
135. Louria DB, Stiff DP, BB. Disseminated moniliasis in the adult. Medicine 1962; 41: 307–333.
136. Scherer WJ, Lee K. Implications of early systemic therapy on the incidence of endogenous fungal endophthalmitis. Ophthalmology 1997; 104(10):1593–1598.
137. Edwards JE Jr, et al. Ocular manifestations of *Candida septicemia*: review of seventy-six cases of hematogenous *Candida endophthalmitis*. Medicine 1974; 53:47–75.
138. Brooks RG. Prospective study of *Candida endophthalmitis* in hospitalized patients with candidemia. Arch Intern Med 1989; 149(10):2226–2228.
139. Henderson DK, Edwards JEJ, Montgomerie JZ. Hematogenous *Candida endophthalmitis* in patients receiving parenteral hyperalimentation fluids. J Infect Dis 1981; 143: 655–661.
140. Parke DW, Jones DB, Gentry LO. Endogenous endophthalmitis among patients with candidemia. Ophthalmology 1982; 89:789–796.
141. Krishna R, et al. Should all patients with candidaemia have an ophthalmic examination to rule out ocular candidiasis? Eye 2000; 14:30–34.
142. Rodriguez-Adrian LJ, et al. Retinal lesions as clues to disseminated bacterial and candidal infections: frequency, natural history, and etiology. Medicine 2003; 82(3):187–202.
143. Bodey GP, Luna M. Skin lesions associated with disseminated candidiasis. JAMA 1974; 229(11):1466–1468.
144. Kressel B, Szewczyk C, Tuazon CU. Early clinical recognition of disseminated candidiasis by muscle and skin biopsy. Arch Intern Med 1978; 138(3):429–433.
145. Fine JD, et al. Cutaneous lesions in disseminated candidiasis mimicking ecthyma gangrenosum. Am J Med 1981; 70(5):1133–1135.
146. Balandran L, et al. A cutaneous manifestation of systemic candidiasis. Ann Intern Med 1973; 78(3):400–403.
147. Bisbe J, et al. Disseminated candidiasis in addicts who use brown heroin: report of 83 cases and review. Clin Infect Dis 1992; 15(6):910–923.
148. Dupont B, Drouhet E. Cutaneous, ocular, and osteoarticular candidiasis in heroin addicts: new clinical and therapeutic aspects in 38 patients. J Infect Dis 1985; 152(3):577–591.
149. Bielsa I, et al. Systemic candidiasis in heroin abusers. Cutaneous findings. Int J Dermatol 1987; 26(5):314–319.
150. Sorrell TC, et al. Exogenous ocular candidiasis associated with intravenous heroin abuse. Br J Ophthalmol 1984; 68(11):841–845.
151. Samuels BI, Pagani JJ, Libshitz HI. Radiologic features of *Candida* infections. In: Bodey GP, ed. Candidiasis: Pathogenesis, Diagnosis and Treatments. New York: Raven Press, 1993:137–157.

152. Semelka RC, et al. Detection of acute and treated lesions of hepatosplenic candidiasis: comparison of dynamic contrast-enhanced CT and MR imaging. J Magn Reson Imag 1992; 2(3):341–345.

153. Semelka RC, et al. Hepatosplenic fungal disease: diagnostic accuracy and spectrum of appearances on MR imaging. AJR. Am J Roentgenol 1997; 169(5):1311–1316.

154. Lecciones JA, et al. Vascular catheter-associated fungemia in patients with cancer: analysis of 155 episodes. Clin Infect Dis 1992; 14(4):875–883.

155. Dato VM, Dajani AS. Candidemia in children with central venous catheters: role of catheter removal and amphotericin B therapy. Pediatr Infect Dis J 1990; 9(5):309–314.

156. Rex JH, et al. A randomized trial comparing fluconazole with amphotericin B for the treatment of candidemia in patients without neutropenia. Candidemia Study Group and the National Institute [see comments]. N Engl J Med 1994; 331(20):1325–1330.

157. Rose HD. Venous catheter-associated candidemia. Am J Med Sci 1978; 275(3):265–269.

158. Bodey GP, Anaissie EJ, Edwards JE. Definitions of *Candida* infections. In: Bodey GP, ed. Candidiasis: Pathogenesis, Diagnosis, and Treatment. New York: Raven Press, 1993:407–408.

159. Xu JP, et al. Species and genotypic diversities and similarities of pathogenic yeasts colonizing women. J Clin Microbiol 1999; 37(12):3835–3843.

160. Wiley EL, Hutchins GM. Superior vena cava syndrome secondary to *Candida* thrombophlebitis complicating parenteral alimentation. J Pediatr 1977; 91(6):977–979.

161. Garcia E, et al. Surgical management of *Candida* suppurative thrombophlebitis of superior vena cava after central venous catheterization. Intensive Care Med 1997; 23(9):1002–1004.

162. Malfroot A, et al. Suppurative thrombophlebitis with sepsis due to *Candida albicans*: an unusual complication of intravenous therapy in cystic fibrosis. Pediatr Infect Dis 1986; 5(3):376–377.

163. Hauser CJ, et al. Surgical management of fungal peripheral thrombophlebitis. Surgery 1989; 105(4):510–514.

164. Khan EA, Correa AG, Baker CJ. Suppurative thrombophlebitis in children: a ten-year experience. Pediatr Infect Dis J 1997; 16(1):63–67.

165. Rossie K, Guggenheimer J. Oral candidiasis: clinical manifestations, diagnosis, and treatment. Pract Periodont Aesth Dent 1997; 9(6):635–641; quiz 642.

166. Hedderwick S, Kauffman CA. Opportunistic fungal infections: superficial and systemic candidiasis. Geriatrics 1997; 52(10):50–54, 59.

167. Toogood JH. Complications of topical steroid therapy for asthma. Am Rev Respir Dis 1990; 141(2 Pt 2):S89–S96.

168. Greenspan D, et al. Effect of highly active antiretroviral therapy on frequency of oral warts. Lancet, 2001. 357(9266):1411–1412.

169. Samonis G, et al. Prophylaxis of oropharyngeal candidiasis with fluconazole. Rev Infect Dis 1990; 12(Suppl 3):S369–S373.

170. Yeo E, et al. Prophylaxis of oropharyngeal candidiasis with clotrimazole. J Clin Oncol 1985; 3(12):1668–1671.

171. Mocroft A, et al. The incidence of AIDS-defining illnesses in 4883 patients with human immunodeficiency virus infection. Royal Free/Chelsea and Westminster Hospitals Collaborative Group. Arch Intern Med 1998; 158(5):491–497.

172. Porro GB, Parente F, Cernuschi M. The diagnosis of esophageal candidiasis in patients with acquired immune deficiency syndrome: is endoscopy always necessary? [see comments]. Am J Gastroenterol 1989; 84(2):143–146.

173. Holt PM. Candida infection of the esophagus. Gut 1968; 9:227–231.

174. Samonis G, et al. Oropharyngeal candidiasis as a marker for esophageal candidiasis in patients with cancer. Clin Infect Dis 1998; 27:283–286.

175. Luna MA, Tortoledo ME. Histologic identification and pathologic patterns of disease caused by *Candida*. In: Bodey GP, ed. Candidiasis: Pathogensis, Diagnosis, and Treatment. New York: Raven Press, 1993:21–42.

176. Walsh TJ, Merz WG. Pathologic features in the human alimentary tract associated with invasiveness of *Candida tropicalis*. Am J Clin Pathol 1986; 85(4):498–502.
177. Solomkin JS, Simmons RL. *Candida* infection in surgical patients. World J. Surg 1980; 4:381–394.
178. Sobel JD, et al. Vulvovaginal candidiasis: epidemiologie, diagnostic, and therapeutic considerations. Am J Obstet Gynecol 1998; 178(2):203–211.
179. Oriel JD, Waterworth PM. Effects of minocycline and tetracycline on the vaginal yeast flora. J Clin Pathol 1975; 28(5):403–406.
180. Vazquez JA, Sobel JD. Fungal infections in diabetes. Infect Dis Clin N Am 1995; 9(1):97–116.
181. Morton RS, Rashid S. Candidal vaginitis: natural history, predisposing factors and prevention. Proc R Soc Med 1977; 70(suppl 4):3–6.
182. Hurley R. Recurrent *Candida* infection. Clin Obstetrics Gynaecol 1981; 8(1):209–214.
183. Fidel PL, Sobel JD. Immunopathogenesis of recurrent vulvovaginal candidiasis. Clin Microbiol Rev 1996; 9(3):335–348.
184. Mayser P. Mycotic infections of the penis. Andrologia 1999; 31(suppl 1):13–16.
185. Appleton SS. Candidiasis: pathogenesis, clinical characteristics, and treatment. J Calif Dent Assoc 2000; 28(12):942–948.
186. Zuber TJ, Baddam K. Superficial fungal infection of the skin. Where and how it appears help determine therapy. Postgrad Med 2001; 109(1):117–120, 123–126, 131–132.
187. Haneke E, Roseeuw D. The scope of onychomycosis: epidemiology and clinical features. Int J Dermatol 1999; 38(suppl 2):7–12.
188. Ng KP, et al. Onychomycosis in Malaysia. Mycopathologia 1999; 147(1):29–32.
189. Segal R, et al. The frequency of *Candida parapsilosis* in onychomycosis. An epidemiological survey in Israel. Mycoses 2000; 43(9–10):349–353.
190. Ginter G, et al. Increasing frequency of onychomycoses—is there a change in the spectrum of infectious agents? Mycoses 1996; 39(suppl 1):118–122.
191. Rigopoulos D, et al. Epidemiology of onychomycosis in southern Greece. Int J Dermatol 1998; 37(12):925–928.
192. Rockwell PG. Acute chronic paronychia. Am Fam Physician 2001; 63(6):1113–1116.
193. Darmstadt GL, Dinulos JG, Miller Z. Congenital cutaneous candidiasis: clinical presentation, pathogenesis, and management guidelines. Pediatrics 2000; 105(2):438–444.
194. Kirkpatrick CH. Chronic mucocutaneous candidiasis. Eur JI clin Microb Infect Dis Dermatol 1989; 8:448–456.
195. Kirkpatrick CH. Chronic mucocutaneous candidiasis. J Am Acad Dermatol 1994; 31(suppl 2):S14–S17.
196. Schonebeck J, Steen L, Tarnvik A. 5-fluorocytosine treatment of *Candida* infections of the urinary tract and other sites. Scand J Urol Nephrol 1972; 6(1):37–45.
197. Rex JH, et al. A randomized and blinded multicenter trial of high-dose fluconazole plus placebo versus fluconazole plus amphotericin B as therapy for candidemia and its consequences in nonneutropenic subjects [comment]. Clin Infect Dis 2003; 36(10):1221–1228.
198. Kauffman CA, et al. Prospective multicenter surveillance study of funguria in hospitalized patients. Clin Infect Dis 2000; 30(1):14–18.
199. Rivett AG, Perry JA, Cohen J. Urinary candidiasis: a prospective study in hospital patients. Urol Res 1986; 14:183–186.
200. Sobel JD, et al. Candiduria: a randomized, double-blind study of treatment with fluconazole and placebo. The National Institute of Allergy and Infectious Diseases (NIAID) Mycoses Study Group [comment]. Clin Infect Dis 2000; 30(1):19–24.
201. Sobel JD, et al. Candiduria: a randomized, double-blind study of treatment with fluconazole and placebo. Clin Infect Dis 2000; 30(1):19–24.
202. Chakrabarti A, Reddy TC, Singhi S. Does candiduria predict candidaemia?. Indian J Med Res 1997; 106:513–516.
203. Huang CT, Leu HS. Candiduria as an early marker of disseminated infection in critically ill surgical patients. J Trauma-Injury Infect Crit Care 1995; 39(3):616.

204. Nassoura Z, et al. Candiduria as an early marker of disseminated infection in critically ill surgical patients: the role of fluconazole therapy. J Trauma 1993; 35:290–295.

205. Ang BS, et al. Candidemia from a urinary tract source: microbiological aspects and clinical significance. Clin Infect Dis 1993; 17(4):662–666.

206. Gross M, et al. Unexpected candidemia complicating ureteroscopy and urinary stenting. Eur J Clin Microbiol Infect D 1998; 17(8):583–586.

207. Lundstrom T, Sobel J. Nosocomial candiduria: a review. Clin Infect Dis 2001; 32(11):1602–1607.

208. Rex JH, et al. Practice guidelines for the treatment of candidiasis. Infectious Diseases Society of America. Clin Infect Dis 2000; 30(4):662–678.

209. Fisher, Efficacy of a single intravenous dose of Amphotericin B in urinary tract infections caused by *Candida*. J Infect Dis 1987; 156:685–686.

210. Haron E, et al. Primary *Candida pneumonia*. Experience at a large cancer center and review of the literature [Review] [33 refs]. Medicine 1993; 72(3):137–142.

211. Bayer AS, Scheld WM. Endocarditis and intravascular infections. In: Mandell GL, Bennett JE, Dolin R, eds. In Mandell: Principles and Practice of Infectious Diseases. Philadelphia, Pensulvania: Churchill Livingstone, 2000:857–884.

212. Melgar GR, et al. Fungal prosthetic valve endocarditis in 16 patients. An 11-year experience in a tertiary care hospital. Medicine (Baltimore) 1997; 76(2):94–103.

213. Nasser RM, et al. Incidence and risk of developing fungal prosthetic valve endocarditis after nosocomial candidemia. Am J Med 1997; 103(1):25–32.

214. Rubinstein E, et al. Fungal endocarditis: analysis of 24 cases and review of the literature. Medicine (Baltimore) 1975; 54(4):331–334.

215. Weems JJ. Candida parapsilosis: epidemiology, pathogenicity, clinical manifestations, and antimicrobial susceptibility. Clin Infect Dis 1992; 14(3):756–766.

216. Pacheco-Rios A, et al. Candida endocarditis in the first year of life. Bol Med Hosp Infantil Mex 1993; 50(3):157–161.

217. Hallum JL, Williams TWJ. *Candida* endocarditis. In: Candidiasis: Pathogenesis, Diagnosis, and Treatment, Bodey GP. ed. New York: Raven, 1993:357–369.

218. Ellis ME, et al. *Fungal endocarditis: evidence in the world literature, 1965–1995*. Clin Infect Dis 2001; 32(1):50–62.

219. Berbari EF, Cockerill FR, 3rd, Stecjekverg JM. Infective endocarditis due to unusual or fastidious microorganisms. Mayo Clin Proc 1997; 72(6):532–542.

220. Atkinson JB, et al. Cardiac fungal infections: review of autopsy findings in 60 patients. Hum Pathol 1984; 15(10):935–942.

221. Atkinson JB, et al. Cardiac infections in the immunocompromised host. Cardiol Clin 1984; 2(4):671–686.

222. Franklin WG, Simon AB, Sodeman TM. *Candida myocarditis* without valvulitis. Am J Cardiol 1976; 38(7):924–928.

223. Karchmer WE. Infective endocarditis. In: Braunwald E, ed. Braunwald: Heart Disease: A Textbook of Cardiovascular Medicine. 6th ed. : W. B. Saunders Company, 2001:1723–1750.

224. Rabinovici R, et al. Candida pericarditis: clinical profile and treatment. Ann Thorac Surg 1997; 63:1200–1204.

225. Lipton SA, et al. Candidal infection in the central nervous system. Am J Med 1984; 76:101–108.

226. Moylett EH. Neonatal *Candida meningitis*. Seminars in Pediatric Infectious Diseases 2003; 14(2):115–122.

227. Geers TA, Gordon SM. Clinical significance of *Candida* species isolated from cerebrospinal fluid following neurosurgery. Clin Infect Dis 1999; 28(5):1139–1147.

228. Sanchez-Portocarrero J, et al. *Candida* cerebrospinal fluid shunt infection. Report of two new cases and review of the literature. Diagn Microbiol Infect Dis 1994; 20(1):33–40.

229. Jong AY, et al. Traversal of *Candida albicans* across human blood–brain barrier in vitro. Infect Immun 2001; 69(7):4536–4544.

230. Rutledge R, Mandel SR, Wild RE. *Candida* species Insignificant contaminant or pathogenic species. Am Surg 1986; 52(6):299–302.
231. Calandra T, et al. Clinical significance of *Candida* isolated from peritoneum in surgical patients. Lancet 1989; 2(8677):1437–1440.
232. Solomkin JS, et al. The role of *Candida* in intraperitoneal infections. Surgery 1980; 88:524–530.
233. Rantala A, et al. Diagnostic factors for postoperative candidosis in abdominal surgery. Ann Chir Gynaecol 1991; 80:323–328.
234. Diebel LN, et al. Gallbladder and biliary tract candidiasis. Surgery 1996; 120(4):760–764; discussion 764–765.
235. Aloia T, et al. *Candida* in pancreatic infection: a clinical experience. Am Surg 1994; 60(10):793–796.
236. Khardori N, et al. Infections associated with biliary drainage procedures in patients with cancer. Rev Infect Dis 1991; 13(4):587–591.
237. Echeverria MJ, et al. Microbiological diagnosis of peritonitis in patients undergoing continuous ambulatory peritoneal dialysis. Review of 5 years at the Hospital de Galdakao. Enferm Infecc Microbiol Clin 1993; 11(4):178–181.
238. Michel C, et al. Fungal peritonitis in patients on peritoneal dialysis. Am J Nephrol 1994; 14(2):113–120.
239. Suarez A, et al. Ascitic peritonitis due to *Candida albicans*. Rev Espan Enferm Dig 1994; 86(3):691–693.
240. Kopelson G, Silva-Hutner M, Brown J. Fungal peritonitis and malignancy: report of two patients and review of the literature. Med Pediatr Oncol 1979; 6(1):15–22.
241. Wariso BA, Nwachukwu CO. A survey of common pathogens in wound in patients at the University of Port Harcourt Teaching Hospital (U.P.T.H), Port Harcourt. W Afr J Med 2003; 22(1):50–54.
242. Malani PN, et al. *Candida albicans* sternal wound infections: a chronic and recurrent complication of median sternotomy. Clin Infect Dis 2002; 35(11):1316–1320.
243. Ratliff CR, Donovan AM. Frequency of peristomal complications. Ostomy Wound Manage 2001; 47(8):26–29.
244. Wai PH, et al. Candida fasciitis following renal transplantation. Transplantation 2001; 72(3):477–479.
245. Parry MF, et al. Candida osteomyelitis and diskitis after spinal surgery: an outbreak that implicates artificial nail use. Clin Infect Dis 2001; 32(3):352–357.
246. Berenguer J, et al. Lysis-centrifugation blood cultures in the detection of tissue-proven invasive candidiasis. Disseminated versus single-organ infection. Diagn Microbiol Infect Dis 1993; 17:103–109.
247. Perry JL, Miller GR, Carr DL. Rapid, colorimetric identification of *Candida albicans*. J Clin Microbiol 1990; 28:614–615.
248. Heelan JS, Siliezar D, Coon K. Comparison of rapid testing methods for enzyme production with the germ tube method for presumptive identification of *Candida albicans*. J Clin Microbiol 1996; 34:2847–2849.
249. Bougnoux ME, et al., Comparison of antibody, antigen, and metabolite assays for hospitalized patients with disseminated or peripheral candidiasis. J Clin Microbiol 1990; 28:905–909.
250. Walsh TJ, et al., Diagnosis and therapeutic monitoring of invasive candidiasis by rapid enzymatic detection of serum D-arabinitol. Am J Med 1995. 99(2): p. 164–172.
251. Christensson B, Sigmundsdottir G, Larsson L. D-arabinitol—a marker for invasive candidiasis. Med Mycol 1999; 37(6):391–396.
252. Sigmundsdottir G, et al. Urine D-arabinitol/L-arabinitol ratio in diagnosis of invasive candidiasis in newborn infants. J Clin Microbiol 2000; 38(8):3039–3042.
253. de Repentigny L, et al. Comparison of enzyme immunoassay and gas–liquid chromatography for the rapid diagnosis of invasive candidiasis in cancer patients. J Clin Microbiol 1985; 21(6):972–979.

254. Edwards JE Jr, et al. International conference for the development of a consensus on the management and prevention of severe candidal infections. Clin Infect Dis 1997; 25:43–59.

255. Anaissie EJ, et al. Management of invasive candidal infections: results of a prospective, randomized, multicenter study of fluconazole versus amphotericin B and review of the literature. Clin Infect Dis 1996; 23(5):964–972.

256. Kujath P, et al. Comparative study of the efficacy of fluconazole versus amphotericin B/flucytosine in surgical patients with systemic mycoses. Infection 1993; 21(6):376–382.

257. Anaissie EJ, et al. Fluconazole versus amphotericin B in the treatment of hematogenous candidiasis: a matched cohort study. Am J Med 1996; 101(2):170–176.

258. Dignani M, Solomkin J, Anaisse EJ. Candida, In: Clinical Mycology. Anaisse EJ, McGinnis MR, P MA, eds. Philadelphia, PA: Churchill Livingston, 2003:195–239.

259. Odds FC, et al. Activities of an intravenous formulation of itraconazole in experimental disseminated Aspergillus, Candida, and Cryptococcus infections. Antimicrob Agents Chemother 2000; 44(11):3180–3183.

260. Ally R, et al. A randomized, double-blind, double-dummy, multicenter trial of voriconazole and fluconazole in the treatment of esophageal candidiasis in immunocompromised patients. Clin Infect Dis 2001; 33(9):1447–1454.

261. Anaissie E, et al. Amphotericin B lipid complex (ABLC) versus amphotericin B for treatment of hematogenous and invasive candidiasis: a prospective, randomized, multicenter trial. In: 35th Interscience Conference on Antimicrobial Agents and Chemotherapy, Washington, DC, 1995.

262. Dupont B. Clinical efficacy of amphotericin B colloidal dispersion against infections caused by Candida spp. Chemotherapy 1999; 45:27–33.

263. Scarcella A, et al. Liposomal amphotericin B treatment for neonatal fungal infections. Pediatr Infect Dis J 1998; 17(2):146–148.

264. Juster-Reicher A, et al. Liposomal amphotericin B (AmBisome) in the treatment of neonatal candidiasis in very low birth weight infants. Infection 2000; 28(4):223–226.

265. Weitkamp JH, et al. Candida infection in very low birth-weight infants: outcome and nephrotoxicity of treatment with liposomal amphotericin B (AmBisome). Infection 1998; 26:15–19.

266. Ringden O, et al. Efficacy of amphotericin B encapsulated in liposomes (AmBisome) in the treatment of invasive fungal infections in immunocompromised patients. J Antimicrob Chemother 1991; 28(suppl B):73–82.

267. Wingard JR, et al. A randomized, double-blind comparative trial evaluating the safety of liposomal amphotericin B versus amphotericin B lipid complex in the empirical treatment of febrile neutropenia. L Amph/ABLC Collaborative Study Group. Clin Infect Dis 2000; 31(5):1155–1163.

268. White MH, et al. Randomized, double-blind clinical trial of amphotericin B colloidal dispersion vs. amphotericin B in the empirical treatment of fever and neutropenia. Clin Infect Dis 1998; 27(296–302).

269. Mora-Duarte J, et al. Comparison of caspofungin and amphotericin B for invasive candidiasis [comment]. N Engl J Med 2002; 347(25):2020–2029.

270. Schranz J, et al. Efficacy of anidulafungin for the treatment of candidemia. in Interscience Conference on Antimicrobial Agents and Chemotherapy, Chicago, IL, 2003.

271. Kauffman CA, et al. Hepatosplenic candidiasis: successful treatment with fluconazole. Am J Med 1991; 91(2):137–141.

272. Walsh TJ, et al. Safety, tolerance, and pharmacokinetics of amphotericin B lipid complex in children with hepatosplenic candidiasis. Antimicrob Agents Chemother 1997; 41(9):1944–1948.

273. Sallah S, et al. Amphotericin B lipid complex for the treatment of patients with acute leukemia and hepatosplenic candidiasis. Leuk Res 1999; 23(11):995–999.

274. Sharland M, Hay RJ, Davies EG. Liposomal amphotericin B in hepatic candidosis. Arch Dis Childhood 1994; 70(6):546–547.

275. Bjorkholm M, et al. Successful treatment of hepatosplenic candidiasis with a liposomal amphotericin B preparation. J Intern Med 1991; 230(2):173–177.

276. Oude Lashof AM, et al. Duration of antifungal treatment and development of delayed complications in patients with candidaemia. Eur J Clin Microbiol Infect Dis 2003; 22(1):p. 43–48.

277. Mermel LA, et al. Guidelines for the management of intravascular catheter-related infections. Clin Infect Dis 2001; 32:1249–1272.

278. Strinden WD, Helgerson RB, Maki DG. Candida septic thrombosis of the great central veins associated with central catheters. Clinical features and management. Ann Surg 1985; 202(5):653–658.

279. Roilides E, et al. The role of immunoreconstitution in the management of refractory opportimistic fungal infections. Med Mycol 1998; 36:12–25.

280. Kullberg BJ, Anaissie EJ. Cytokines as therapy for opportunistic fungal infections. Res Immunol 1998; 149(4–5):478–488; discussion 515.

281. Rodriguez Adrian LJ, et al., The potential role of cytokine therapy for fungal infections in patients with cancer is recovery from neutropenia all that is needed? Clin Infeet Dis 1998; 26(6):1270–1208.

282. Arathoon EG, et al. Randomized, double-blind, multicenter study of caspofungin versus amphotericin B for treatment of oropharyngeal and esophageal candidiases. Antimicrob Agents Chemother 2002; 46(2):451–457.

283. Webb BC, et al. Candida-associated denture stomatitis. Aetiology and management: a review. Part 1. Factors influencing distribution of Candida species in the oral cavity. Aust Dent J 1998; 43(1):45–50.

284. Villanueva A, et al. A randomized double-blind study of caspofungin versus fluconazole for the treatment of esophageal candidiasis. Am J Med 2002; 113(4):294–299.

285. Villanueva A, et al., A randomized double blind study of caspofungin versus amphotericin for the treatment of candidal esophagitis [comment]. Clin Infect Dis 2001; 33(9):1529–1535.

286. Gupta TP, Ehrinpreis MN. Candida-associated diarrhea in hospitalized patients. Gastroenterology 1990; 98:780–785.

287. Sobel JD, et al. Single oral dose fluconazole compared with conventional clotrimazole topical therapy of Candida vaginitis. Am J Obstet Gynecol 1995; 172:1263–1268.

288. De Punzio C, et al. Fluconazole 150 mg single dose versus itraconazole 200 mg per day for 3 days in the treatment of acute vaginal candidiasis: a double-blind randomized study. 2003; (Feb 10): 193–197.

289. Nozickova M, et al. A comparison of the efficacy of oral fluconazole, 150 mg/week versus 50 mg/day, in the treatment of tinea corporis, tinea cruris, tinea pedis, and cutaneous candidosis. Int J Dermatol 1998; 37(9):703–705.

290. Villars V, Jones TC. Clinical efficacy and tolerability of terbinafine (Lamisil)—a new topical and systemic fungicidal drug for treatment of dermatomycoses. Clin Exp Dermatol 1989; 14(2):124–127.

291. Jung EG, et al. Systemic treatment of skin candidosis: a randomized comparison of terbinafine and ketoconazole. Mycoses 1994; 37(9–10):361–365.

292. Ryder NS, Wagner S, Leitner I. In vitro activities of terbinafine against cutaneous isolates of Candida albicans and other pathogenic yeasts. Antimicrob Agents Chemother 1998; 42:1057–1061.

293. Habif TP. Clinical Dermatology: A Color Guide to Diagnosis Therapy. 3rd ed. St. Louis, MO: Mosby-Year Book, 1996.

294. Rybojad M, et al. Familial chronic mucocutaneous candidiasis associated with autoimmune polyendocrinopathy. Treatment with fluconazole: 3 cases. Ann Dermatol Venereol 1999; 126(1):54–56.

295. Hay RJ. Overview of studies of fluconazole in oropharyngeal candidiasis. Rev Infect Dis 1990; 12(suppl 3):S334–S337.

296. Tosti A, et al. Itraconazole in the treatment of two young brothers with chronic mucocutaneous candidiasis. Pediatr Dermatol 1997; 14(2):146–148.

297. Muehrcke DD, Lytle BW, Cosgrove DM. III. Surgical and long-term antifungal therapy for fungal prosthetic valve endocarditis. Ann Thorac Surg 1995; 60(3):538–543.

298. Nguyen MH, et al. Candida prosthetic valve endocarditis: prospective study of six cases and review of the literature. Clin Infect Dis 1996; 22(2):262–267.

299. Kraus WE, Valenstein PN, Corey GR. Purulent pericarditis caused by Candida: report of three cases and identification of high-risk populations as an aid to early diagnosis. Rev Infect Dis 1988; 10(1):34–41.

300. Eng RH, et al. Candida pericarditis. Am J Med 1981; 70(4):867–869.

301. Smego RA Jr, Perfect JR, Durack DT. Combined therapy with amphotericin B and 5-fluorocytosine for Candida meningitis. Rev Infect Dis 1984; 6:791–801.

302. Nguyen MH, Yu VL. Meningitis caused by *Candida* species: an emerging problem in neurosurgical patients. Clin Infect Dis 1995; 21:323–327.

303. Shapiro S, Javed T, Mealey J Jr. Candida albicans shunt infection. Pediatr Neurosci 1989; 15(3):125–130.

304. Sugar AM, Saunders C, Diamond RD. Successful treatment of Candida osteomyelitis with fluconazole. A noncomparative study of two patients. Diagn Microbiol Infect Dis 1990; 13:517–520.

305. Tang C. Successful treatment of Candida albicans osteomyelitis with fluconazole. J Infect 1993; 26:89–92.

306. El-Zaatari MM, et al. Successful treatment of Candida albicans osteomyelitis of the spine with fluconazole and surgical debridement: case report. J Chemother 2002; 14(6):627–630.

307. Wang YC, Lee ST. *Candida* vertebral osteomyelitis: a case report review of the literature. Chang Gung Med 2001; 24(12):810–815.

308. Petrikkos G, et al. Case report. Successful treatment of two cases of post-surgical sternal osteomyelitis, due to Candida krusei and Candida albicans, respectively, with high doses of triazoles (fluconazole, itraconazole). Mycoses 2001; 44(9–10):422–425.

309. Bren A. Fungal peritonitis in patients on continuous ambulatory peritoneal dialysis. Eur J Clin Microbiol Infect Dis 1998; 17(12):839–843.

310. Cheng IK, et al. Fungal peritonitis complicating peritoneal dialysis: report of 27 cases and review of treatment. Quart J Med 1989; 71(265):407–416.

311. Hedderwick SA, et al. Pathogenic organisms associated with artificial fingernails worn by healthcare workers. Infect Control Hosp Epidemiol 2000; 21(8):505–509.

312. Slavin MA, et al. Efficacy and safety of fluconazole prophylaxis for fungal infections after bone marrow transplantation—A prospective, randomized, double-blind study. J Infect Dis 1995; 171:1545–1542.

313. Goodman JL, et al. A controlled trial of fluconazole to prevent fungal infections in patients undergoing bone marrow transplantation [see comments]. N Engl J Med 1992; 326(13):845–851.

314. Marr KA, et al. Prolonged fluconazole prophylaxis is associated with persistent protection against candidiasis-related death in allogeneic marrow transplant recipients: long-term follow-up of a randomized, placebo-controlled trial. Blood 2000; 96(6):2055–2061.

315. Rotstein C, et al. Randomized placebo-controlled trial of fluconazole prophylaxis for neutropenic cancer patients: benefit based on purpose and intensity of cytotoxic therapy. The Canadian Fluconazole Prophylaxis Study Group. Clin Infect Dis 1999; 28(2):331–340.

316. Schaffner A, Schaffner M. Effect of prophylactic fluconazole on the frequency of fungal infections, amphotericin B use, and health care costs in patients undergoing intensive chemotherapy for hematologic neoplasias. J Infect Dis 1995; 172(4):1035–1041.

317. Winston DJ, et al. Fluconazole prophylaxis of fungal infections in patients with acute leukemia. Results of a randomized placebo-controlled, double-blind, multicenter trial. Ann Intern Med 1993; 118(7):495–503.

318. MacMillan ML, et al. Fluconazole to prevent yeast infections in bone marrow transplantation patients: a randomized trial of high versus reduced dose, and determination of the value of maintenance therapy. Am J Med 2002; 112(5):369–79.

319. Koh LP, et al. Randomized trial of fluconazole versus low-dose amphotericin B in prophylaxis against fungal infections in patients undergoing hematopoietic stem cell transplantation. Am J Hematol 2002; 71(4):260–267.

320. Nucci M, et al. A double-blind, randomized, placebo-controlled trial of itraconazole capsules as antifungal prophylaxis for neutropenic patients. Clin Infect Dis 2000; 30(2):300–305.

321. Menichetti F, et al. Itraconazole oral solution as prophylaxis for fungal infections in neutropenic patients with hematologic malignancies: a randomized, placebo-controlled, double-blind, multicenter trial. GIMEMA Infection Program. Gruppo Italiano Malattie Ematologiche dell' Adulto. Clin Infect Dis 1999; 28(2):250–255.

322. Harousseau JL, et al. Itraconazole oral solution for primary prophylaxis of fungal infections in patients with hematological malignancy and profound neutropenia: a randomized, double-blind, double- placebo, multicenter trial comparing itraconazole and amphotericin B. Antimicrob Agents Chemother 2000; 44(7):1887–1893.

323. Morgenstern GR, et al. A randomised controlled trial of itraconazole versus fluconazole for the prevention of fungal infections in patients with haematological malignancies. Br J Haematol 1999; 105(4):901–911.

324. Tollemar J, et al. Randomized double-blind study of liposomal amphotericin B (Ambisome) prophylaxis of invasive fungal infections in bone marrow transplant recipients. Bone Marrow Transplantation 1993; 12(6):577–582.

325. Kelsey SM, et al. Liposomal amphotericin (AmBisome) in the prophylaxis of fungal infections in neutropenic patients: a randomised, double-blind, placebo-controlled study. Bone Marr Transpl 1999; 23(2):163–168.

326. Bjerke JW, Meyers JD, Bowden RA. Hepatosplenic candidiasis—a contraindication to marrow transplantation? Blood 1994; 84(8):2811–2814.

327. Walsh T, et al. Successful treatment of hepatosplenic candidiasis through repeated episodes of neutropenia. Cancer 1995; 76:2357–2362.

328. Eggimann P, et al. Fluconazole prophylaxis prevents intra-abdominal candidiasis in high-risk surgical patients. Crit Care Med 1999; 27(6):1066–1072.

329. Pelz RK, et al. Double-blind placebo-controlled trial of fluconazole to prevent candidal infections in critically ill surgical patients. Ann Surg 2001; 233(4):542–548.

330. Tollemar J, et al. Liposomal amphotericin B prevents invasive fungal infections in liver transplant recipients. A randomized, placebo-controlled study. Transplantation 1995; 59:45–50.

331. Lumbreras C, et al. Randomized trial of fluconazole versus nystatin for the prophylaxis of Candida infection following liver transplantation. J Infect Dis 1996; 174:583–588.

332. Winston DJ, Pakrasi A, Busuttil RW. Prophylactic fluconazole in liver transplant recipients: a randomized, double-blind, placebo-controlled trial. Ann Intern Med 1999; 131:729–737.

333. Kicklighter SD, et al. Fluconazole for prophylaxis against candidal rectal colonization in the very low birth weight infant. Pediatrics 2001; 107(2):293–298.

334. Kaufman D, et al. Fluconazole prophylaxis against fungal colonization and infection in preterm infants [comment]. N Engl J Med 2001; 345(23):1660–1666.

335. Uzun O, Anaissie EJ. Antifungal prophylaxis in patients with hematological malignancies: a reappraisal. Blood 1995; 86:2063–2072.

336. Solomkin JS. Timing of treatment for nonneutropenic patients colonized with *Candida*. Am J Surg 1996; 172(6A):44S–48S.

337. Anaissie EJ, Bishara AB, Solomkin JS. Fungal infections in surgical patients.Chapter 85., in ACS Surgery: Principles and Practice., D.W. Wilmore, et al. Editors. 2002, WebMD Corp.: New York. p. 1289.

338. Sobel J. Fungal infections of the genitourinary tract. In: EJ A, McGinnis MR, Pfaller M, eds. Medicla Mycology. Philadelphia, IL: Churchill Livingston, 2003:496–508.

10
Aspergillosis

William J. Steinbach
Division of Pediatric Infectious Diseases, Duke University Medical Center, Durham, North Carolina, U.S.A.

Juergen Loeffler
Medizinische Klinik, Labor Prof. Dr. Einsele In der Hals- Nasen- Ohren- Klinik, Tübingen, Germany

David A. Stevens
Department of Medicine, Santa Clara Valley Medical Center, Stanford University Medical School, San Jose, California, U.S.A.

Aspergillosis refers to infection with any of the >150 recognized species of the genus *Aspergillus*. These are in mould form in the environment, on artificial media, and when invading tissues. Aspergilli are the second most common of the fungi infecting immunocompromised hosts, but are the most common cause of mortality caused by invasive mycoses in the USA, these infections, moreover, are increasing in frequency relative to *Candida* infections, possibly because of success with prophylactic regimens for the latter mycoses. In 1996, annual hospital costs associated with aspergillosis were estimated to be >US $633 million in the USA (1).

I. ETIOLOGY AND EPIDEMIOLOGY

Aspergilli are ubiquitous in the environment and are associated with decaying matter with growth in temperatures of 40–50°C, e.g., self-heating organic compost. They have been easily isolated from soil, air, and even swimming pools and saunas. They are also isolated from houses, particularly from basements, crawl spaces, bedding, humidifiers, ventilation ducts, potted plants, wicker or straw material, and house dust. In surveys, they have even been found in condiments, pasta, and marijuana samples. This pervasiveness should not make it surprising that they are sometimes found in normal expectorated sputa.

In tissues, Aspergilli may be seen as septate hyphae, dichotomously branched (resembling the divergence of fingers from one another), and may produce their characteristic conidia in tissues or artificial media. If the septation can be seen, they can be differentiated from the zygomycetes, but Aspergilli may be confused with *Pseudallescheria boydii unless* the characteristic terminal spores of the latter are seen.

Several putative *Aspergillus* virulence factors have been identified, including melanin and secreted proteases, toxins, and hemolysins (2). However, gene disruption studies have rarely identified prominent virulence factors, suggesting that the true virulence of *A. fumigatus* is likely multifactorial and dependent on host immune status.

Aspergillosis generally results from airborne conidia and is not contagious. The threat to hospitalized patients has been revealed in outbreaks of infection, particularly pulmonary infection in immunocompromised hosts, associated with building renovation and new construction. The suspected vector has been unfiltered air, as from inlets contaminated with bird excreta and fireproofing materials. Hospital water, which may become aerosolized during such activities as patient showering, is a newly described possible source (3).

The most common species infecting humans are *A. fumigatus* (64–67% in two series) (4,5), *A. flavus, A. niger*, and *A. terreus.* However, some patient isolates are speciated by the clinical laboratory only with difficulty, and they may be reported only as "*Aspergillus* species." Molecular biology tools will be a help in speciation in the future. For example, Rath et al. (6) have been able to identify five different *Aspergillus* species by SSCP (single-strand conformational polymorphism, a sensitive method that in conjunction with PCR, is able to distinguish amplicons that differ in sizes) using 27 culture collection strains and 55 patient isolates. *Aspergillus fumigatus* has a small spore size, enabling it to penetrate deeply into the lung alveoli (7). Most pulmonary diseases are caused by *A. fumigatus*, although isolated sinus disease is frequently caused by *A. niger* or *A. flavus* (8). *Aspergillus* terreus, which can be resistant to polyene antifungals (e.g., amphotericin B), has been reported to cause approximately 3% of cases of invasive aspergillosis (IA) (4).

Aspergillus aerosolizes conidia readily; while immunocompetent people breathe and clear conidia everyday (2,4), immunocompromised patients are at risk for the development of IA. Since the route of infection appears to be pulmonary, the first line of defense is formed by alveolar macrophages. In vitro studies with murine cells have suggested that resident pulmonary macrophages are responsible for digesting inhaled *Aspergillus* conidia (9,10). If conidia escape and germinate into hyphae, then the hyphae become susceptible to neutrophil killing through the release of toxic oxygen radicals (11). Thus, disease risk is associated with neutropenia, challenge with overwhelming microbial doses, and/or corticosteroid suppression of macrophage conidiacidal activity (12). More recent studies have shown that CD4 T-cell responses are important for both protection against and effective therapy of invasive infection (13–15). The mechanism by which T-cells function to protect against invasive aspergillosis is not clear, but they may enhance phagocyte killing of conidia (14).

II. SYNDROMES

A. Invasive Aspergillosis

Invasive aspergillosis is generally a problem of immunocompromised hosts, while more aggressive immunosuppression and anticancer therapy are the most important factors contributing to the rise of *Aspergillus* infections. Usually, several of the following factors are present: leukopenia, glucocorticoid therapy, cytotoxic chemotherapy, and broad-spectrum antibacterials. Neutropenia is the time-honored risk factor for invasive mold infections; the risk of IA is calculated to increase from 1% per day after the first 3 weeks of neutropenia to 4–5% per day after 5 weeks (16). The incidence of IA can be as high as 70% if neutropenia exceeds 34 days (17). Repeated cycles of neutropenia may be an added risk factor. Corticosteroids suppress the ability of monocytes/macrophages to kill conidia through inhibition of nonoxidative processes and impairment of lysosomal activity, and also inhibit polymorphonuclear neutrophils in their chemotaxis, oxidative burst, and antifungal activity against hyphae (18). The results of one in vitro study suggest that corticosteroids may actually accelerate the growth of *A. fumigatus* (19).

Some series have reported an incidence as high as 41% at autopsy in patients with acute leukemia, and notably in 89% of these cases it played a significant role in the death of the patient. Pulmonary involvement was present in 97% of patients, and the infection was widely disseminated to various organs in 25% of patients. In patients with leukemia, there is particularly an association with relapses of the malignancy. In heart transplant patients, the incidence of infection goes up to 28%. The incidence in bone marrow transplant patients ranges from 5% to 20%, with a higher frequency in certain groups, such as patients undergoing allogeneic transplantation or suffering from graft-versus-host disease (GVHD), and mortality is 68 to >95% in various series. Numerous studies have repeatedly identified the risk factors for IA as older age, receipt of a hematopoietic stem cell transplant (HSCT) from an HLA-mismatched or unrelated donor, and underlying disease, and infections are more common in the summer (8,20). Pediatric patients undergoing transplantation are generally less vulnerable to infections than their adult counterparts (21), although recent reviews have reported substantial incidences of IA, ranging from 6% to 19% after HSCT (22,23).

The primary risk periods for invasive mould infections are during the early, preengraftment time period, and then again later during therapy of GVHD. Over the last decade, the late time period has become increasingly significant, with most mould infections occurring during GVHD therapy (20,24,25) while in the outpatient setting. In reviews of patients undergoing allogeneic HSCT, IA was diagnosed at a median of 88–115 days post-transplant (26–29), with mortality exceeding 80% (30). Recent studies that focused on the risks for infection late after allogeneic HSCT identified GVHD, corticosteroid exposure, secondary neutropenia and lymphopenia, and CMV disease as important variables (8). It is unknown whether CMV represents a risk in itself or signifies an underlying immune defect that is not well controlled in multivariable analyses. IA is also commonly seen in lung and liver transplant recipients (in the former also associated with CMV), and other steroid-treated patients. Mortality in solid organ transplant patients ranges from 70% to 93% (31). IA is also a problem in patients with the neutrophil defect of chronic granulomatous disease and in patients with the cell-mediated immunity depression seen in AIDS (32).

Radiographic presentation varies from single nodular lesions to bilateral diffuse pulmonary infiltrates. The classic picture is that of fever and pulmonary infiltrates or nodules, especially progressing to a cavity (usually when granulocytopenia is reversed), or wedge-shaped densities resembling infarcts. The pulmonary pathology in all these entities is that of hemorrhagic infarction and pneumonia. Pulmonary emboli are common because of the organism's tendency to invade blood vessel walls. These processes often combine to produce a "target lesion" pathologically, consisting of a necrotic center surrounded by a ring of hemorrhage.

As with most invasive mould infections, the clinical signs and symptoms are very nonspecific. The most common clinical symptom triggering evaluation is

unremitting fever (26), but high fever may be absent in those patients receiving corticosteroid therapy (33). Other early symptoms of pulmonary disease include dry
cough and possibly chest pain. The chest pain may be misinterpreted as esophagitis
or viral pleuritis. Dyspnea is more common is patients with diffuse disease, and the
presentation in some patients is similar to a pulmonary embolism. Hemoptysis can
occur and may be fatal with the first presenting episode (34), while in neutropenic
patients a pneumothorax is also an occasional presenting feature (7).

B. Invasive Tracheobronchitis

Invasive airway disease with ulcerative, pseudomembranous, or plaque-like tracheobronchitis occurs, particularly in immunocompromised hosts, and may presage parenchymal invasion. Cases of infection of the larynx, trachea, or epiglottis have been
reported. Localized infection that has commonly been limited to the anastomotic site
has been described in heart–lung and lung transplant recipients (35).

C. Disseminated Aspergillosis

Mycelia invading blood vessels may produce a microangiopathic hemolytic anemia.
Dissemination can result in Budd–Chiari syndrome, myocardial infarction, gastrointestinal disease, or skin lesions. Esophageal ulcers may produce gastrointestinal
bleeding. Abscesses are common in the kidney, liver, and myocardium.

A frequent target of disseminated disease is the central nervous system (CNS),
where hematogenous spread results in occlusion of intracranial vessels and infarction
(36). This may manifest as the characteristic single or multiple cerebral abscesses, or
meningitis, an epidural abscess, or a subarachnoid hemorrhage (37). Cerebral aspergillosis has been noted in 25–40% of patients with invasive pulmonary disease
(8,26,28,38). The classical presenting features of abscesses such as headache, nausea,
and vomiting are rare (<10% of cases). More frequently, presenting signs and symptoms include altered mental status, confusion, hemiparesis, and cranial nerve palsies
(39). Computed tomography (CT) of the head often reveals one or multiple
hypodense, well-demarcated lesions. Hemorrhage and mass effect are unusual, but
for patients with adequate peripheral white blood cell counts, ring enhancement
and surrounding edema are frequent (7). The cerebrospinal fluid (CSF) glucose level
is normal, and cultures of the CSF are negative. Biopsy of these lesions, if feasible,
is warranted to differentiate *Aspergillus* infections from those caused by other fungi,
such as *Pseudallescheria*, dematiaceous fungi, Mucorales or *Fusarium*, which may
alter one's choice of antifungal therapy. A surgical approach leads to laboratory
characterization of the causative agent together with removal of nonviable tissue,
which may not be well penetrated by systemic antifungals (40,41). Stereotactic procedures for abscess drainage have also been used (42). However, systemic antifungal
therapy is used in almost every case. Meningitis is unusual, cases have been reported
in neutropenic patients or those on prolonged corticosteroid therapy. It may present
as an extension of paranasal sinus disease. Intrathecal therapy (via a reservoir) has
been used as an adjunct to systemic therapy. Epidural abscesses are usually secondary to a contiguous site of infection, such as in a vertebral body. Surgical drainage
along with systemic therapy is indicated. The published literature suggests that
mortality in CNS infection exceeds 90% (43).

D. Locally Invasive Aspergillosis

Examples of locally invasive disease abound and are usually severe. These include invasion of burn wounds, focal rhinitis (particularly in immunosuppressed and/or granulocytopenic hosts), sinusitis (in these hosts or following dental procedures), and osteomyelitis or endophthalmitis (after fungemia, trauma, or surgery).

E. Invasive Sinusitis

Invasive *Aspergillus* sinusitis is likely underdiagnosed because of lack of detailed examination, but patients can present with sinus congestion, facial pain or swelling, orbital swelling, headache, or epistaxis (7,33). A high index of suspicion is necessary in immunocompromised patients. These infections are characterized by mucosal invasion with infarction and spread of infection in centrifugal fashion to contiguous structures. Early diagnosis is imperative, and the onset of new local symptoms, such as epistaxis, naso-orbital pain, a positive nasal swab culture in a febrile, susceptible host, or an abnormal sinus radiographic finding should lead to immediate otolaryngologic evaluation, including careful inspection of the nasal turbinates. Rhinoscopic examination may reveal insensitive areas with decreased blood flow, localized pallor of the nasal septum or turbinate mucosa, frank crusting or ulceration, or blackened necrotic foci. Although surveillance nasal cultures are of questionable value, baseline sinus radiographs or limited CT should be considered in these high-risk patients. T_2-weighted magnetic resonance imaging (MRI) images may show decreased signal intensity compared to those of bacterial sinusitis, which show increased signal intensity (7). The maxillary sinus is most commonly involved, followed by the ethmoid, sphenoid, and frontal sinuses (44). Biopsy and subsequent fungal culture of suspicious lesions are important not only to demonstrate mucosal invasion but also to differentiate *Aspergillus* infections from those caused by other fungi, such as Mucorales or *Alternaria* species. Mortality is high, ranging from 20% in patients with leukemia in remission who are undergoing maintenance therapy, up to 100% in patients with relapsed leukemia or those undergoing HSCT (45,46).

F. Cutaneous Aspergillosis

This can be either primary, resulting from skin injury or traumatic inoculation, or secondary, from contiguous extension or hematogenous dissemination. The majority of cutaneous infections are caused by *A. fumigatus*, *A. flavus*, or *A. terreus*, but *A. chevalieri* has recently been reported to cause morphologically distinct skin lesions (47). In general, primary infection is most common in burn victims, neonates, and solid organ transplant recipients, whereas skin lesions in HSCT recipients usually result from contiguous extension of infected structures under the skin or from hematogenous dissemination (48). Recent reviews have reported that skin lesions may occur in 4–11% of patients with documented pulmonary aspergillosis, and may be the first presenting sign of disease (49–51).

Cutaneous aspergillosis often begins as an area of raised erythema which progresses from red to purple, then pustulates, developing a central ulceration with an elevated border covered by a black eschar, and may ulcerate (7,52,53). These lesions may be single or multiple, may not be tender, and occur most commonly on the extremities. Although the late stages are characteristic of *Aspergillus* infections, a skin biopsy with fungal culture is indicated to rule out other infections that may manifest in a similar fashion. Infections arising at the site of an IV catheter puncture typically begin with erythema and induration and progress to necrosis that extends radially (53). The *A. chevalieri* lesions are erythematous, hyperkeratotic, and vesiculopapular. Cutaneous disease has been associated with the use of adhesive tape; erythematous indurated plaque-like lesions progress to necrotic ulcers.

G. Other Sites

Vertebral osteomyelitis or diskitis is the most common bone infection, with joint infections being distinctly uncommon (43,54). Surgical debridement is generally required in addition to systemic antifungal therapy.

Urinary tract infections are generally a consequence of hematogenous spread. Infections that involve the renal parenchyma are more common in immunocompromised hosts. The appearance of a fungus ball usually represents renal papillary necrosis; prostatic abscesses with or without a fungus ball also occur (55). For management of abscesses and fungus balls, surgical removal is usually indicated as an adjunct to systemic antifungal therapy. Local irrigation has also been used for urinary bladder and renal pelvis infections.

III. DIAGNOSIS

Diagnosis is difficult because aspergilli are frequently contaminants in sputum and even in other cultures during handling. Despite many efforts developing new and exciting detection tools, such as PCR assays, the diagnosis of IA still remains very difficult (Table 1). Several reasons are responsible for these limitations. First, IA often shows nonspecific and variable clinical signs, the manifestations are subtle and occur late in the course of disease. Second, IA occurs in many different patient cohorts, those at risk for a short period of time or for years. Because of residual defects and tissue infarcts, the disease has a potential to reactivate, mainly during prolonged or continuous immunosuppression and it may occur as a subacute or chronic infection. Third, no unique universally applicable test with sufficient sensitivity and specificity exists yet, and in consequence, IA is often diagnosed late leading to a delayed initiation of antifungal therapy, with a fatal outcome.

A. Microscopy, Culture, and Histopathology

Direct microscopy can be useful for the detection of *Aspergillus* spp. in bronchoalveolar lavage (BAL) or endotracheal aspirates. This method is a relatively fast, moderately sensitive tool with good specificity for fungal infection. Microscopy might be considered with material aspirated from pulmonary lesions. In wound aspergillosis, sometimes fruiting bodies can be seen. However, in the absence of these, microscopy does not allow an unequivocal diagnosis of IA, because other moulds, such as *Fusarium*, *Pseudallescheria*, and *Scopulariopsis* species may have identical appearances in microscopy and histology. The use of stains, such as calcofluor white, may be helpful in achieving a greater sensitivity. Combining microscopy and culture increases the diagnostic yield for IA in pulmonary specimens by 15–20% (56–58).

The yield of premortem and even autopsy cultures in autopsy-proven IA is extremely low (59). Culture of respiratory secretions from patients with IA is also often negative (57), and the predictive value of cultures for *Aspergillus* spp. in

Table 1 Diagnosis of Invasive Aspergillosis

Authors	Method of detection	Study population	Type of clinical specimen	Sensitivity	Specificity
Tomee et al. (91)	Antibodies	LungTx	Serum	100% (4 patients)	n.d.
Chan et al. (71)	Antibodies	BMT	Serum	100% for aspergilloma, 33.3% for IA	n.d.
Haynes et al. (72)	Antibodies	Neutropenic	Urine	100%	n.d.
Weig et al. (73)	Antibodies	Various	Urine	64%	n.d.
Ribaud et al. (26)	Galactoman (Platelia)	BMT	Serum	55%	81%
Maertens et al. (78)	Galactoman (Platelia)	Hematological	Serum	92.6%	95.4%
Fortun et al. (92)	Galactoman (Platelia)	Liver Tx	Serum	55.6%	93.3%
Sulahian et al. (93)	Galactoman (Platelia)	BMT (pediatric)	Serum	90.6%	94%
Salonen et al. (94)	Galactoman (Platelia)	Hematological	Serum	100% (with proven IA)	n.d.
Herbrecht et al. (95)	Galactoman (Platelia)	Hematological	Serum	64.5% (with proven IA), 16.4% (probable)	94.8%
Lass-Florl et al. (96)	Panfungal PCR	Hematological	Whole blood	75%	96%
Hebart et al. (97)	Panfungal PCR	SCT	Whole blood	100%	65%
Buchheidt et al. (98)	*Aspergillus*-specific nested PCR	Immunosuppressed	Whole blood BAL	91.7% 100%	81.3% 90.2%
Jones et al. (99)	*Aspergillus* mitochondrial	Neutropenic	BAL	100%	100%
Raad et al. (100)	*Aspergillus* mitochondrial	Cancer	Whole blood	100% (with proven IA)	100% (with proven IA)
Ferns et al. (101)	*Aspergillus* mitochondrial	Leukemia/BMT	Whole blood	86%	n.d.
Buchheidt et al. (102)	*Aspergillus*-specific nested PCR	Hematological	BAL	93.9%	94.4%
Raad et al. (103)	*Aspergillus* mitochondrial	Cancer	BAL	80%	93%
Hayette et al. (104)	*Aspergillus* protease	Intensive care	BAL	100%	96%
Einsele et al. (105)	Panfungal	BMT	Whole blood	100% (2 specimens)	98%

Abbreviations: TX, transplanation; n.d., not determined; BMT, bone marrow transplantation; IA, invasive aspergillosis; Galactoman, Galactomannan antigen assay; SCT, stem cell transplanation; BAL bronchoalveolar lavage.

IA varies widely from 40% to 100% (60). The sputum culture, while having good positive predictive value in the appropriate setting (especially, neutropenic patients, particularly if febrile), is positive in only 8–34% of cases, and obtaining tissue is advisable to make the diagnosis. Prospective culturing of the nose of granulocytopenic patients has been of some value, because a positive nasal culture (and particularly the presence of nasal *Aspergillus* lesions) has led to the early diagnosis of concurrent pulmonary or sinus disease. However, negative nasal cultures are common in pulmonary aspergillosis.

Culture or cytology of BAL fluid may also be useful in diagnosis of invasive disease. However, BAL samples may only be positive in 30–50% of IA patients (61). A positive culture of *Aspergillus* from an otherwise sterile site provides proof of the disease. However, culture may have a reduced ability to detect *Aspergillus* at an advanced stage of the disease, owing to necrosis occupying a large portion of a lesion. *Aspergillus* species are very rarely isolated from blood (62). *Aspergillus*-positive blood cultures very frequently represent environmental contamination, especially when taken from a nonsterile site (63). The invasion of blood vessels, resulting in thrombosis and distal infarction, may possibly account for the low sensitivity of blood or tissue cultures, as blood flow through the affected areas may be reduced thereby. Additionally, immune responses of the host, such as cytotoxic effects, may reduce viability of the fungal cells.

Although *Aspergillus* species are able to grow on blood agar and other agar media, the sensitivity is higher when specific fungal media are used (64). Modifications of blood culture systems, such as aeration by shaking or adding hydrogen peroxide to prevent low oxygen pressure, have not been associated with increased isolation rates of *Aspergillus*.

B. Antibodies

Although almost all persons carry anti-*Aspergillus* antibodies because of environmental exposure, the titers are low (except in certain patient cohorts such as patients with cystic fibrosis) and infection might correlate with an increasing number of antibodies (65–68). Data from the more commonly reported techniques suggest a high degree of sensitivity in allergic disease or aspergillomas, but generally a low sensitivity in invasive disease. Because the frequency of false-positive reactions, even in the presence of other mycoses, is low, a positive test in invasive disease may be useful. In immunocompromised patients, the presence of anti-*Aspergillus* antibodies is often not a result of an acute invasive infection, and it is likely that antibodies have been present before the onset of immunosuppression. Growth of *A. fumigatus* in tissues of these patients is not correlated with an increase of the antibody titer. Thus, the use of antibody detection in immunosuppressed patients might be limited.

Sridhar et al. (69) reported a retrospective analysis of 10 cases of confirmed IA. Serology performed by gel diffusion precipitin test was positive in only one case of sinonasal aspergillosis. The presence of serum IgG or IgA antibodies against seven *Aspergillus* recombinant antigens was assessed in patients with IA (70). Superoxide dismutase and a 94 kDa antigen were the most immunogenic for IgA, while the IgG pattern varied from patient to patient. The authors conclude from their study that the detection of antibodies against these antigens should not be used as a diagnostic method.

More recently, Chan et al. (71) presented data from an antibody assay with a purified recombinant antigenic cell wall galactomannoprotein of *A. fumigatus*, Afmplp. Clinical evaluation revealed that the test was 100% sensitive for patients with aspergilloma and 33% sensitive for patients with IA. No false-positive results were found for serum samples from 80 healthy persons and 39 patients infected with other fungi or bacteria indicating a high specificity. This new antibody assay lends hope for the future of antibody testing in IA.

Haynes et al. (72) reported the presence of an immunodominant antigen, a 18-kDa protein in urine samples from patients with IA, whereas urine samples from patients without evidence of IA were unreactive. They proposed that these antigens should play a valuable role in the diagnosis of IA. Over a decade later, Weig et al. (73) showed in their study using serum samples that recombinant mitogillin (the 18-kDa protein studied by Haynes et al.) improves the serodiagnosis of *A. fumigatus* infection. They detected positive IgG-titers in 31 out of 42 sera from patients with pulmonary IA, but only in 1% of the serum samples of healthy persons.

C. Antigens

Serological tests are an important tool for rapid diagnosis of IA. Except for the study of Haynes et al. (72) mentioned above, the use of these assays has focused on the *Aspergillus* galactomannan (GM) antigen. GM is a polysaccharide with a linear mannan core containing 1–2- and 1–6-linked residues. The antigenic side chains that branch from 1–2-linked mannose residues are composed of 1–5-galactofuranosyl residues (74). GM was the first antigen detected in animal models as well as in patients with IA (75–77). Two commercially available kits are available for the detection of GM in clinical samples.

The latex agglutination kit is commercially available in Europe (Pastorex® *Aspergillus*, Sanofi Diagnostics Pasteur, Marnes La Coquette, France) and has a detection threshold of 15 ng/mL (2,78). The early latex agglutination tests showed only a low sensitivity (79) but a high specificity. The detection threshold of the Pastorex assay was reported to be 15 ng of GM per mL with a sensitivity of 25–70% and a specificity of 90–100%. However, Kappe et al. (80) reported that the antibody used in this assay cross-reacted with *Penicillium* and *Acremonium* species and *Alternaria alternata*, which are all potential laboratory contaminants.

Later, an enzyme-linked immunosorbent assay (ELISA) technique was introduced using a rat anti-GM monoclonal antibody, EB-A2, which recognizes the 1→5-β-D-galactofuranoside side chains of the GM molecule. The threshold of detection with ELISA improved to 5 ng/mL (78). A sandwich ELISA technique was introduced in 1995 (81) and by using the same antibody as both a capture and detector antibody in the sandwich ELISA (Platelia® *Aspergillus*, Bio-Rad, France), the threshold for detection can be lowered to 1 ng/mL. The Platelia assay was approved for use in the United States in May 2003. The sandwich ELISA, Platelia *Aspergillus*, is widely available and has a sensitivity of 50–90% and a specificity of 81–93% when serum is used (26,78). However, when samples were serially analyzed, both the sensitivity (93%) and the specificity (95%) were higher (78). GM was detected in 63% of the patients before onset of clinical disease (82,83). The sandwich ELISA was able to detect GM at least 2 weeks earlier than the latex agglutination test (84–86). For patients receiving empiric antifungals, the sensitivity of GM detection appears to be lower, but specificity is preserved. Administration of some antibacterials can lead to false positive results.

Antigenemia can be observed from 1 week up to 2 months, depending on the type of patient (85,87,88). Furthermore, a decrease of the antigen titer in serum is indicative of treatment efficacy (83,85,89,90). Animal models suggest a decline in titer with echinocandin therapy appears less common. There have been several clinical studies utilizing the GM assays in various populations (Table 1), generally with useful sensitivities and specificities. One continued debate is the exact cut-off value used in serum vs. urine, as well as adult vs. pediatric patients.

Another major component of the *Aspergillus* cell wall is the polysaccharide 1–3-glucan. An ELISA-based assay (G-test) has been established for the detection of 1–3-glucan (106). The components of this assay are purified from a lysate of the horseshoe crab, *Limulus polyphemus* (107), including factor G, which triggers the 1–3-glucan-sensitive hemo-lymph-clotting pathway. The detection threshold of the assay is 10–20 pg/mL serum. The G-test has been used for the detection of 1–3-glucan during various systemic fungal infections (108–110) in humans and animals (108). Unlike the GM assays, this assay is not able to distinguish amongst fungi.

D. Biochemical Methods

Francis et al. (111) reported a study detecting the hexitol D-mannitol in BAL by gas–liquid chromatography–mass spectroscopy, in rabbits with pulmonary IA. Measuring d-mannitol levels was significantly more diagnostically sensitive than culture and levels were significantly elevated in lavage of infected rabbits compared to controls. Serum concentrations were not useful because of high-background levels. Wong et al. (112) described a rat model of IA and postulated that *A. fumigatus* can produce and release sufficient D-mannitol in the tissues of infected animals to raise serum D-mannitol levels. The value of this diagnostic marker seems to remain limited and further investigation in patients with IA is mandatory.

E. Radiological Signs

Different radiological tools, such as chest radiography, ultrasonography, CT, and MR imaging, are available. The appearance of IA on chest radiographs is extremely heterogenous. The most distinctive appearances are cavitations and pleural-based, wedge-shaped lesions. In addition, nodular shadows with and without cavitation and thin- or thick-walled cavities (especially in patients with AIDS) are typical signs of IA. However, pulmonary IA often results in false-negative chest radiographs. Therefore, high-resolution CT scans often play an important role in the detection of IA (113–119). Early lesions in the lung of neutropenic patients are small nodules with the so-called halo sign: small, often pleural-based lesions with surrounding low attenuation. These nodules may further cavitate leading to the air crescent sign. Both signs are highly distinctive for IA of the lung, probably representing radiographic correlates of edema or hemorrhage, and infarction, related to the organism's vasculotropism. The duration of the halo sign is short and demonstrates the value of early CT.

Miaux et al. (120) reviewed imaging data of five patients with cerebral aspergillosis. They concluded that lesions are often located in the basal ganglia and demonstrate an intermediate signal intensity within surrounding high-signal areas on long-repetition-time MR scans. These lesions were multiple and more numerous on MR images than on CT scans.

F. Nucleic Acid-Based Diagnosis in Clinical Materials

Since the first presentation of the polymerase chain reaction (PCR) by Saiki et al. (121) in 1988, several hundred papers have been published dealing with the detection of fungal DNA. However, no PCR kit system is currently on the market.

The critical and important issues for the detection of fungal DNA by PCR from clinical material are the type of clinical material and its sampling, the DNA extraction protocol, the PCR design, the detection and specification of the amplicon, the need for appropriate controls, especially to exclude contamination, and the question whether quantitative PCR assays are beneficial.

G. Choice of Clinical Material

The kind of clinical specimen that should be analyzed depends on the disease entity and the condition of the patient. Blood and blood fractions can be easily collected and this material contains circulating leukocytes with phagocytized conidia and hyphae, free fungal cell elements, as well as free circulating fungal DNA. Examination of the detection limit of plasma and whole blood samples shows that the assay is more sensitive when performed on whole blood rather than on plasma. Three patients with documented IA were negative with plasma PCR but positive when whole blood specimens were analyzed. Bronchoalveolar lavages are more difficult to obtain, and PCR from BAL has not yet been able to distinguish infection from contamination (122). Sputum shows a very low specificity. CSF fluid cannot be used in routine diagnosis based on weekly screening. Hendolin et al. (123) developed a panfungal PCR for the detection of *Aspergillus* DNA in tissue specimens from the paranasal sinuses. Jaeger et al. (124) described an assay based on a nested PCR for fungal endophthalmitis.

H. DNA Extraction

The essentials of successful fungal DNA extraction are an enrichment of fungal DNA, the elimination of potential *Taq*-inhibitors and the avoidance of contamination with airborne spores.

The release of fungal DNA can either be managed using an enzymatic or a mechanical approach. Many protocols rely on the enzymes zymolase and lyticase, 1,3-glucanases that generate fungal spheroplasts (125). However, an efficient release of DNA from many molds, such as *A. niger*, *A. terreus*, Mucorales, and *Fusarium* species, requires additional treatment, including boiling of the samples with NaOH (126), high-speed cell disruption, grinding with mortar and pestle, or repeated freeze-thawing using liquid nitrogen (127).

I. Target Genes

The selection of a target gene, and the design of the primers and probes are the most important issues when creating a PCR assay. Single or multicopy genes could be selected. Assays that amplify single copy genes are often highly specific (species-specific) but might not be sensitive enough to detect a low fungal load, whereas multicopy genes show high sensitivity but low specificity because of many highly conserved gene regions. In contrast to *Candida* species where a variety of PCR protocols based on single copy genes (lanosterol-14-α-demethylase, actin, chitin synthase) exist, the detection of mold DNA is limited to multicopy gene analysis. Recently, Kanbe et al. (128) described a nested PCR assay using a mixture of specific primers binding to the DNA topoisomerase II gene. Primers targeting multicopy genes bind to the 18S or 28S subunits of the ribosomal DNA (97,98,129) or to the highly variable intergenic transcribed spacer regions (ITS 1–4) that flank the riboso- mal gene regions (130–132). Furthermore, mitochondrial genes have been used for the design of primers for diagnostic assays (99). Recently, Luo et al. (132) described a multiplex PCR with five sets of species-specific primers binding to the ITS1 and ITS2 regions. They found that this multiplex PCR method provided 100% sensitivity and specificity testing a total of 242 fungal isolates. Raad et al. (100) performed a study on whole blood specimens from 54 patients with cancer and pulmonary infil- trates. PCR was performed by amplifying *Aspergillus* mitochondrial DNA. The sensitivity, specificity, positive and negative predictive value were 100% for proven IA and 57%, 100%, 100%, and 92%, respectively, for the probable and possible IA cases, indicating the high sensitivity of their PCR assay. Furthermore, Ferns et al. (101) described a PCR assay based on the amplification by nested PCR of a 135 bp fragment in the mitochondrial region of *A. fumigatus* or *A. flavus* (121 bp). They were able to detect 1 CFU/2 mL of blood. Six of seven patients with clinical evidence of IA were PCR positive. Buchheidt et al. (102) developed a two-step PCR assay ena- bling the authors to detect 10 fg of *Aspergillus* DNA, corresponding to 1–5 CFU/mL of spiked samples in vitro.

J. Amplicon Detection

After amplification of fungal DNA by PCR, species or genera can be distinguished by different techniques. The traditional methods involve gel electrophoresis followed by hybridization protocols. These techniques include Southern blots, Slot blots, or PCR-ELISA using species- or genus-specific probes. This step is especially important when using panfungal primer sets that recognize conserved gene regions in many pathogenic fungi. Southern blot assays were successfully applied to the detection of different *Aspergillus* species (103,133). An assay based on the commercially avail- able PCR-ELISA format from Roche is able to specifically detect *Aspergillus* DNA extracted from 10 CFU (126). Fletcher et al. (134) compared the sensitivity of a plate hybridization assay with Southern blotting. They conclude that both assays showed an identical sensitivity of 1.5 pg; however, by plate assay, results were obtained within 3 hr Willinger et al. (135). analyzed maxillary sinus samples from patients with histologically proven fungal infections by PCR and culture. For identification and speciation of the fungi, three different techniques were studied. By sequence analysis of the amplicon, identification of the fungal DNA was successful in 90%; by hybridization, fungal DNA could be speciated in 77%, whereas culture was positive in only 52% of the analyzed samples. The differentiation of fungi by sequencing ana- lysis has also been successfully explored by Turenne et al. (130), performing an automated fluorescent capillary electrophoresis system.

K. Real-Time PCR

These recently developed PCR assays combine rapid in vitro amplification of DNA with real-time speciation and quantification of DNA load. However, the number of protocols for the detection of *Aspergillus*-DNA by real-time PCR tests is very limited. The Tubingen group established a quantitative PCR protocol for the detec- tion of *A. fumigatus* (136). The sensitivity of the assay was comparable to previously described PCR protocols (5 CFU/mL). The Light Cycler allowed a quantification of fungal load in a limited number of clinical specimens from patients with hematological malignancies and histologically proven invasive fungal infection. Five out of nine positive samples showed a fungal load between 5 and 10 CFU/mL, 2/9 samples between 10 and 100 CFU/mL, and 2/9 samples were positive with more than 100 CFU/mL blood. Three additional quantitative PCR assays based on the TaqMan technology were described recently. Bowman et al. (137) developed a PCR to monitor disease progression and measure the efficacy of caspofungin acetate in a murine model of disseminated aspergillosis. They conclude that because of its much larger dynamic range and its higher sensitivity, the quantitative PCR assay is superior to traditional CFU determination. Costa et al. (138). developed two Taq-Man PCR tests, targeting the mt gene and the FKS gene of *A. fumigatus*, including a quantification of the fungal DNA load in spiked blood samples. Finally, Pham et al. (139) report the design and evaluation of a real-time PCR assay for the detection of mould DNA in serum. The test has a lower limit of sensitivity of 110 fg (three genomes). Quantitative analysis of the positive serum samples showed a mean fungal load of 1.6×10^5 genomes and a maximum fungal load of 4.2×10^7 genomes.

L. Diagnostic Conclusions

In severe disease, an aggressive, invasive approach, as well as making a tissue diagnosis early in the illness, appears to be a key to survival. In the appropriate clinical setting, such as an immunocompromised host with fever and a pulmonary infiltrate, repeated isolation of the same species in culture, and particularly a BAL or other endobronchial culture, correlates with invasive disease. Sometimes, even a single sputum culture (especially with heavy growth) may have to be the stimulus for therapy if invasive procedures cannot be done. Negative cultures do not rule out invasive disease. CT scanning of the chest done at the earliest suspicion of this diagnosis initially may reveal a halo sign or, later, a lesion with an air crescent, which is highly predictive of this diagnosis. These are the situations where a positive galactomannan, PCR, or glucan test could be particularly helpful, in prompting therapy even if a specific microbiologic diagnosis from tissue is not possible.

IV. THERAPY

A. Prevention

Prophylaxis of susceptible patients, such as immunocompromised hosts, using intranasal, inhaled, or systemic antifungals, is an approach to avoid disease and the need for therapy. One strategy for this would be to identify the highest risk patients, such as those identified by screening respiratory cultures as colonized, or those with HSCT and GVHD, and targeting prophylaxis to them. Reducing airborne spores, such as by filtering hospital air, keeping patients in rooms with positive pressure relative to the corridor, and with frequent air changes and high unidirectional air flow in the room; reducing activities that increase spore counts, such as room maintenance, when the patient is in the room, separating patients from areas of construction, preventing bird access to ductwork, preventing dust, avoiding carpeting in patient areas, wet mopping, substituting sponge baths for showers and bottled water for tap water, and restricting contaminated materials (e.g., potted plants, sterilization of spices), are believed to be worthwhile efforts for patients who will be transiently immunosuppressed or neutropenic.

B. Therapy—Overview

In invasive disease, prompt, aggressive chemotherapy has produced superior survival statistics at some institutions, although recovery from neutropenia is a necessary accompaniment of recovery in almost every success. Therapy may need to be initiated on only a high degree of suspicion. Surgical excision has an important role in the invasion of bone, burn wounds, epidural abscesses, and vitreal disease. It may have a function in invasive pulmonary disease for which chemotherapy has failed or where disease impinges on major vascular structures, and there is a heightened risk of sudden, fatal exsanguination. In pleural disease, locally instilling antifungals may be useful.

Therapy should be continued after lesions resolve, cultures are negative, and reversible underlying predispositions have abated. Reinstating therapy, in patients who have responded, should be considered if immunosuppression is reinstituted or neutropenia recurs.

There is little agreement on the best systemic chemotherapy for IA, and the optimal therapy remains elusive. Amphotericin B deoxycholate (AmB) has been the "gold standard" since its approval in 1958 and a guideline-recommended treatment choice (140); but now after years of limited therapeutic options there are several new exciting possibilities. There has been a recent surge in the development of newer antifungals for treating IA, including new formulations of older drugs (amphotericin B lipid products, cyclodextrin–itraconazole) and entirely new classes of drugs (echinocandins) with novel targets (141) (Table 2). Newer strategies have also been explored with combination antifungal therapies as well as cytokine therapy to augment the host response system.

C. Amphotericin B Formulations

Amphotericin B has been the treatment of choice for IA as well as the standard of comparison for all newer antifungal agents for over 40 years. However, the fact that AmB remained at such a post is not by virtue of its effectiveness, but rather because of the lack of alternatives until recently (142).

Table 2 Selected Antifungal Agents with Activity Against *Aspergillius*

Drug Class	Drug Name (Brand / Investigational name)	Formulation
Polyene	[a]Amphotericin B Deoxycholate (Fimgizone®)	IV
	[a]Amphotericin B Lipid Complex (Abelcet®)	IV
	[a]Amphotericin B Colloidal Dispersion (Amphocil®; Amphotec®)	IV
	[a]Liposomal Amphotericin B (AMBisome®)	IV
Triazole	[a]Itraconazole (Sporanox®)	PO, IV
	[a]Voriconazole (VFend®)	PO, IV
	Posaconazole (SCH 56592)	PO
	Ravuconazole (BMS-207147; ER-30346)	PO, IV
Echinocandin	[a]Caspofimgin (MK-0991)	IV
	Anidulafungin (VER-002; LY303366)	IV
	[a]Micafungin (FK463)	IV

[a]Licensed for clinical use in the united states.

In addition to conventional AmB, three fundamentally different lipid-associated formulations have been developed that offer the advantage of an increased daily dose of the parent drug, better delivery to the primary reticuloendothelial organs (lungs, liver, spleen) (141–144), and reduced toxicity. ABLC (Abelcet®, Enzon, Bridgewater, New Jersey, U.S.A.) is a tightly packed ribbon-like structure of a bilayered membrane formed by combining dimyristoyl phosphatidylcholine, dimyrisotyl phosphatidylglycerol, and amphotericin B in a ratio of 7:3:3. ABCD (Amphocil®, AstraZeneca, London; or Amphotec®, Intermune Pharmaceuticals, Brisbane, California, U.S.A.) is composed of disk-like structures of cholesteryl sulfate complexed with amphotericin B in an equimolar ratio. L-AmB (AmBisome®, Fujisawa Healthcare, Inc., Deerfield, Ilinois, U.S.A.), the only "true liposomal" product, consists of small uniformly sized unilamellar vesicles of a lipid bilayer of hydrogenated soy phosphatidylcholine–distcaryl phosphatidylglycerol–cholesterol–amphotericin B in the ratio 2:0.8:1:0.4. There are no data or consensus opinions among authorities indicating improved efficacy of any new AmB lipid formulation over conventional AmB (143,145,146). This leaves the clearest indication for a lipid formulation over AmB to be reducing glomerular toxicity.

Animal studies clearly indicate that on a similar dosing schedule the lipid products are almost always not as potent as AmB, but that the ability to safely administer higher daily doses of the parent drug improves their efficacy (147). Experimental in vitro and in vivo studies support concentration-dependent killing with a prolonged postantifungal effect, suggesting large daily doses will be most effective and achieving optimal peak concentrations is important (148). A multicenter maximum tolerated dose study of liposomal AmB including 39 patients with IA using doses from 7.5 to 15 mg/kg/day found no demonstrable dose-limiting nephrotoxicity or infusion-related toxicity, but the study was not statistically powered for dose-dependent efficacy (149). Other authors point out the scant support for higher doses of AmB (150), emphasizing the varying experimental conditions in published studies and no evidence of a clinical dose effect to support higher doses of AmB.

D. Itraconazole

First publicly described in 1983 (151) and available for treatment of *Aspergillus* in 1990, itraconazole (Sporanox®, Ortho-Biotech, Raritan, New Jersey, U.S.A.) adopted a triazole nucleus with higher specificity for the fungal cytochrome enzyme system over the older imidazoles. Historically, there have been several constraints with itraconazole: no parenteral formulation, erratic oral absorption in high-risk patients, and significant drug interactions. Azole–drug interactions may lead to decreased plasma concentration of the azole, related to either decreased absorption or increased metabolism, or increased concentration of coadministered drugs (152).

To overcome problems with variable capsule absorption, itraconazole has now been solubilized in cyclodextrin with substantial improvement as an oral solution (153,154). A new IV formulation of itraconazole was also approved in the US for pulmonary and extrapulmonary aspergillosis in patients who are intolerant of or refractory to AmB (155). The IV formulation can rapidly achieve high and steady-state plasma concentrations (156) as opposed to the 7–10 day period needed for the capsule or oral formulation (157). The IV formulation was shown to be effective in experimental IA with dose-dependent survival (158).

A multicenter open-label study performed in 31 patients with pulmonary IA who received 14 days of IV itraconazole followed by 12 weeks of capsules showed that target therapeutic concentrations were obtained within 2 days in 91% of patients and these levels were also maintained after switching to oral therapy. A complete or partial response was seen in 48% (15/31) of patients (156). These two new itraconazole formulations will allow better pharmacokinetics, especially in high-risk patients in whom capsules might be difficult to use because of mucositis, vomiting, or GVHD. While guidelines generally dictate a logical approach to include itraconazole as oral therapy after disease progression is arrested with parenteral AmB (140), in some studies itraconazole is a useful alternative therapy to AmB with comparable response rates (159,160).

E. Voriconazole

Voriconazole (Vfend®, Pfizer Pharmaceuticals, New York, New York, U.S.A.) is a new second generation triazole synthetic derivative of fluconazole. Both fungicidal (161–163) activity and fungistatic (163) activity against *Aspergillus* have been demonstrated and voriconazole also inhibits 24-methylene dehydrolanosterol demethylation and *Aspergillus* conidiation and pigmentation (162).

In vitro studies have generally shown greater activity of voriconazole over AmB and itraconazole (164–167), whereas other studies have shown itraconazole had superior activity over voriconazole (168). In an analysis of 413 *Aspergillus* clinical isolates from phase III clinical trials, voriconazole was generally equivalent in vitro to itraconazole and superior to AmB (169). Additionally, whereas *A. terreus* is known to be frequently refractory to AmB (170), in vitro testing has shown greatly increased susceptibility to voriconazole (171).

Animal model studies of voriconazole for IA have mirrored the excellent in vitro efficacy against *Aspergillus*, including superior survival rates over itraconazole and equivalence to AmB (172). In guinea pig models, voriconazole approximated the ability of AmB to reduce tissue burden and showed increased survival over AmB (173) and itraconazole (174). In another guinea pig model, voriconazole performed markedly better than itraconazole in cyclodextrin against *Aspergillus* endocarditis (175), but in a rabbit model AmB was significantly more effective than voriconazole at decreasing tissue burdens (176).

There are a growing number of anecdotal clinical publications of voriconazole success against IA, often after failing another therapy. The largest prospective clinical trial of voriconazole involved 392 patients at 92 centers in 19 countries over 3 years and compared initial randomized therapy with voriconazole versus AmB followed by other licensed antifungal therapy. Patients who initially received voriconazole had statistically significantly better complete or partial response (53%) vs. those initially receiving AmB (32%). Survival also improved to 71% for voriconazole vs. 58% for those initially receiving AmB (177). Analysis in an open, noncomparative multicenter study of 116 patients treated with voriconazole as primary therapy (60 patients) or salvage therapy (56 patients) also yielded encouraging results as 14% had a complete and 34% had a partial response (178). Additionally, a review of 42 children with IA treated with voriconazole showed the drug was well tolerated and had an overall response rate of 43% (179).

The comparator in the pivotal prospective randomized study was AmB, and this raises the question whether better tolerated therapy, such as a lipid formulation of AmB, might have produced a better result. Although voriconazole has not been compared in a randomized trial to other modalities, such as itraconazole, echinocandin, or combination therapy, the superiority of voriconazole demonstrated over the reference standard, initial therapy with AmB, makes it for many clinicians the current first choice for primary therapy for IA.

F. Other Triazoles: Posaconazole and Ravuconazole

Posaconazole (Schering-Plough Research Institute, Kenilworth, New Jersey, U.S.A.) is a second-generation triazole and closely related to itraconazole. In vitro testing has shown posaconazole had superior activity over itraconazole and AmB against *Aspergillus* species (180–183) and was also active against itraconazole-resistant isolates (184). In vitro comparison against voriconazole and several of the other second-generation triazoles has shown posaconazole had the greatest activity (185–190), as well as superior activity against echinocandins (191). Posaconazole also had similar activity to itraconazole against an AmB-resistant isolate of *A. fumigatus*, but superior activity against a voriconazole-resistant isolate (188,192).

Animal models have shown efficacy with posaconazole (181), including survival and antifungal efficacy in clearing tissue burden superior (193) or equal to AmB and superior to itraconazole (194). In another rabbit model, posaconazole significantly prolonged survival compared to itraconazole or AmB (195), and in a murine model posaconazole showed a significant reduction in mortality over AmB (196). In a multicenter study including 25 patients with IA to evaluate "salvage" therapy in patients who are refractory to invasive fungal infections, posaconazole was well tolerated and effective in 53% (8/15) at week 4 and 85% (6/7) at week 8 (197).

Ravuconazole (Eisai Medical Research, Inc., Ridgefield Park, New Jersey, U.S.A.) is structurally more similar to fluconazole and voriconazole, containing a thiazole instead of a second triazole. In vitro studies have demonstrated fungicidal activity comparable to other azole compounds as well as general superiority over AmB against various *Aspergillus* species, including activity against *A. terreus* (198,199). Another study found ravuconazole activity slightly less than itraconazole or AmB, but no ravuconazole-resistant isolates were detected (200).

One murine study revealed that both ravuconazole and itraconazole led to decreased lung fungal burden in a dose-dependent fashion (201). Other murine models revealed ravuconazole superior to itraconazole or AmB (202). Using a guinea pig model of disseminated aspergillosis, ravuconazole was also more effective in reducing positive organ cultures compared to AmB or itraconazole (203). A rabbit model showed survival efficacy as well as a decrease in tissue fungal burden comparable to AmB, and only AmB and ravuconazole consistently eliminated *A. fumigatus* from organ tissues (204).

G. Caspofungin

Caspofungin (Cancidas®; Merck, Whitehouse Station, New Jersey, U.S.A.) is a fungistatic water-soluble semisynthetic derivative of the natural product pneumocandin B_o (205). There is in vitro activity against *Aspergillus* (206), and fluorescent dyes have demonstrated the focus of caspofungin killing is the apical and subapical branching cells (207). Caspofungin activity against *A. fumigatus* was also markedly increased with the in vitro addition of human sera (208). Caspofungin has shown an additive effect with monocytes and monocyte-derived macrophages, but not neutrophils, on *Aspergillus* hyphal growth (209). Animal models have shown that despite dose-dependent hyphal damage, there was no reduction in residual fungal burden or galactomannan antigenemia, unlike AmB (210). Other animal models have demonstrated equivalent efficacy with caspofungin and AmB (137,211), and in a murine disseminated aspergillosis model caspofungin showed 50% effective doses (ED$_{50}$), using daily dosing, comparable to AmB (212).

In a pivotal clinical study leading to US approval, 56 patients with acute IA underwent "salvage" therapy after failing primary therapy for more than a week or developing significant nephrotoxicity. Recipients generally tolerated caspofungin well and had better outcome that historic controls; 41% (22/54) had a favorable response with caspofungin (213). A recent update on all 90 patients enrolled in that trial revealed 45% had a complete or partial response, and the drug was generally well tolerated (214). A Spanish study before licensure revealed a 67% (8/12) favorable response rate among patients with proven or probable IA (215).

H. Other Echinocandins: Micafungin and Anidulafungin

Micafungin (Fujisawa Healthcare, Inc., Deerfield, Illinois, U.S.A.) is an echinocandin lipopeptide compound (216–218) and like all echinocandins is fungistatic in vitro vs. *Aspergillus* (219). In vitro micafungin compared favorably with AmB or itraconazole (219–222), including activity against AmB-resistant isolates (223). Animal models have shown efficacy (224,225), including a murine pulmonary aspergillosis model where micafungin caused hyphal damage and in a neutropenic rabbit model where micafungin caused dose-dependent damage of hyphal structures in the lung tissues of animals, and a significant improvement in animal survival rates comparable to those treated with liposomal AmB (226). One murine model showed that based on the ED$_{50}$ and survival, micafungin was 1.7–2.3 times inferior to AmB (227), while another murine study yielded a similar survival rate and ED$_{50}$ compared to AmB (228).

In an open-label, multicenter study of micafungin monotherapy that included 10 patients with IA, overall clinical response was 60% with no safety-related issues (229). A recent study of micafungin combined with an existing antifungal agent in pediatric and adult bone marrow transplant patients with IA revealed an overall complete or partial response of 39%, including 40% in allogeneic transplant patients (230).

Anidulafungin (Vicuron, King of Prussia, Pennsylvania, U.S.A.) in some in vitro studies was more active than caspofungin against *Aspergillus* species (191,231), and both drugs were considerably more active than AmB (232) or itraconazole (231) but generally less active than posaconazole (191). Favorable antifungal interactions with anidulafungin and neutrophils or monocytes have been demonstrated (233), similar to work with caspofungin (209). Survival in several rabbit models of IA was comparable to AmB; however, tissue fungal burden was not reduced and was actually quite higher compared to untreated controls (204,234). For instance, while anidulafungin did yield dose-dependent damage of hyphal elements, tissues from the AmB-treated rabbits seldom revealed any hyphal elements (234). In another mouse model, AmB was superior to anidulafungin in reducing renal tissue fungal load, but anidulafungin was effective using an AmB-resistant isolate (235).

I. Combination Therapy

While each individual antifungal agent has limitations, combinations might prove more effective and create a widened spectrum of drug activity, more rapid antifungal effect, synergy, lowered dosing of toxic drugs, or a reduced risk of antifungal resistance (236). An extensive review of combination antifungal therapy for IA is presented elsewhere and showed a two-third clinical improvement rate (237). Before newer antifungals became available, many combinations involved agents not historically viewed as effective anti-Aspergillus drugs, singly. For instance, while 5-fluorocytosine (5-FC) has little inherent anti-Aspergillus activity (238), the fungistatic 5-FC might enhance the antifungal activity of AmB, especially in anatomical sites where AmB penetration is often suboptimal, such as CSF, heart valves, and the vitreous (43). In vitro combination studies for *Aspergillus* demonstrate synergy and antagonism occur with about equal frequency (239). Animal models followed (240–242) and case series indicated clinical improvement (243–245). The only published prospective clinical study of combination therapy for pulmonary IA (246) compared AmB monotherapy to AmB + 5-FC, but the study was terminated early because of poor outcomes in both arms.

Similarly, although rifampin and its analogs alone have no inherent antifungal activity, it is postulated that AmB increases the permeability of the fungal membrane to allow increased penetration of rifampin, which then inhibits the fungal RNA polymerase (247,248). In vitro studies show synergy (249,250) as well as animal models (251) but there are also reports of antagonism (241). However, coadministration of rifampin with azoles, although almost consistently demonstrating enhanced activity in vitro, should be discouraged in humans because of the potent P450 enzyme-inducing properties of rifampin that can result in clinically ineffective azole concentrations (140,152,252,253). There are some successful clinical reports with rifampin, but the potential for drug interactions is too high to recommend its combination use.

The most debated combination scheme for treatment of IA is AmB + itraconazole, and the theoretical risks of antagonism with this combination have been reviewed (254). The concern is that the polyene AmB, which functions by binding to ergosterol in the cell membrane, will be antagonized with an azole, which inhibits a late enzyme step in ergosterol synthesis. Therefore, instead of attacking the fungal membrane at two different steps for a synergistic interaction, the concern is the azole will alter the target for the polyene. Pretreatment with itraconazole would be expected to have a much more deleterious effect than concurrent treatment, and this has been demonstrated in vitro (255).

Clinical therapy with AmB and azoles has been extensively reviewed (254). Despite continuously heard concerns of AmB with azoles, AmB + itraconazole for IA is used (5). One retrospective clinical case series of 21 patients examining concurrent therapy of AmB + itraconazole demonstrated no clinical antagonism and a statistically non-significant improvement in mortality over monotherapy (256). Other studies reached the same conclusion (5).

Unfortunately, there is less available information regarding combinations including the newer antifungals and it is clear more testing needs to be done. In vitro testing of caspofungin with various other antifungals showed positive interactions, especially AmB + caspofungin (257,258), and there were also in vitro positive interactions with micafungin and AmB (259,260). In animal models, there was an additive effect with AmB + caspofungin (261), and murine models have shown significantly higher survival with micafungin + AmB compared to monotherapy with each drug (262,263). Other models showed neither micafungin + itraconazole nor micafungin + AmB resulted in significant improvement over monotherapy with itraconazole or AmB, but no antagonism was seen with any combination (224). In vitro studies with voriconazole and an echinocandin were additive, whereas voriconazole + AmB was indifferent (259).

J. Sequential Therapy

There are reports of various patterns of sequential antifungal therapy, which raises another issue other than concomitant therapy: the appropriate and safe sequence of agents. Confounding matters is the long half-life of AmB; hence, even sequential use has an element of concurrent therapy (264). The most practical experience is with the sequence of AmB followed by itraconazole. The consensus seems to be that there are many instances of initial therapy with AmB followed by itraconazole with generally no harm seen (5,159,160,264). A widely accepted regimen uses AmB to treat a patient's acute disease until neutropenia recovers, and then itraconazole maintenance antifungal coverage (5,265). While this sequence appears safe and is recommended in recent guidelines (140), the most debated sequence is the reverse, with an azole followed by AmB. Antagonism is once again postulated because of azole inhibition of fungal ergosterol synthesis and subsequent exhaustion of the target for AmB, with loss of antifungal effect of AmB (266).

There has been in vitro antagonism with sequential azole than AmB, whereas concurrent administration showed minimal antagonism (255,267–269). Clinical reports do support this sequential antagonism (270) but also can show clinical improvement with itraconazole then changed to AmB (271,272).

K. Immunomodulatory Therapy

Host defense is paramount as IA generally only develops in certain subsets of severely imrnunocompromised patients. Few patients with persistent neutropenia and IA survive, and indeed resolution of IA has followed neutrophil recovery in most cases. Immunotherapy is designed to increase the number of phagocytic cells, shorten the duration of neutropenia, modulate the kinetics or actions of those cells at the site of infection, and/or activate the fungicidal activity of phagocytes to kill fungal cells more efficiently (2,273).

Protective immunity is associated with CD4+ Th-1 cells producing interferon-γ (IFN-γ), interleukin (IL)-2, IL-15, macrophages producing IL-12, or those mice treated with antagonism of IL-4 or IL-10. Disease progression is seen in mice producing Th-2 cytokines IL-4, IL-10, IL-13, or mice treated with neutralizing antibody to INF-γ or IL-12 (14,145,274). IL-4 deficient mice were more resistant than wild-type mice to infections (275), and a murine model demonstrated decreased fungal burden and increased survival of IL-10 knockout mice compared to wild type (276). Th-1 resistance was also impaired upon IL-12 neutralization and in IL-12 deficient mice (275); however, administration of recombinant IL-12 failed to increase protective effects in mice (15). One in vitro study found that anti-IL-10 antibody, IFN-γ, and GM-CSF administration counteracted the suppressive host defense effects of IL-10 on phagocyte hyphal damage and oxygen radical production (277).

Prophylaxis with human recombinant granulocyte colony-stimulating factor (G-CSF) + AmB or itraconazole showed some additive effect in neutropenic animal models of IA but not in those immunosuppressed with cortisone, which has a greater effect against macrophages. In a neutropenic murine model, human G-CSF alone was ineffective but with AmB showed synergy in survival greater than with itraconazole + G-CSF (278). G-CSF administered to human volunteers increased the fungicidal activity against *Aspergillus* conidia through enhanced respiratory bursts of their PMNs by 4-fold (279). However, there is no clear evidence G-CSF benefits patients with aspergillosis. One review found no significant reduction in fungal infections in acute myelocytic leukemia patients treated with G-CSF (280).

GM-CSF and macrophage colony-stimulating factor (M-CSF) treated human macrophages exhibit enhanced conidial phagocytosis, oxygen radical production, and hyphal damage (281,282). In a murine model, the antifungal activity of bronchoalveolar macrophages treated with dexamethasone was significantly less than macrophages from dexamethasone + GM-CSF treated mice (283–285). Additionally, GM-CSF administered before dexamethasone blocked the deleterious effects, but if given after dexamethasone, GM-CSF could not reverse the effect on macrophages (283). This confirmed earlier in vitro work demonstrating bronchoalveolar macrophage coincubation with GM-CSF followed by adding dexamethasone significantly prevented the conidiacidal suppression. Also, bronchoalveolar macrophage coincubation with dexamethasone and subsequent GM-CSF addition removed the deleterious effect if the dexamethasone was discontinued, but if the dexamethasone pretreatment continued despite GM-CSF use, the anticonidiacidal effects persisted (286). In another study, both murine and human GM-CSF can counteract dexamethasone suppression of murine macrophage function (287).

There are case reports of GM-CSF as part of a treatment regimen with success (288–290). GM-CSF has been shown to offer some protection against IA in one clinical trial in patients with acute myelogenous leukemia, decreasing the fungal infection-related mortality from 19% to 2% (291). A small pilot study of GM-CSF in combination with AmB for treatment of proven fungal infection included two patients with refractory aspergillosis, with one showing a partial response and the other failing therapy (292). A neutropenic rabbit model demonstrated that prophylactic administration of M-CSF 3 days prior to inoculation and then throughout neutropenia augmented pulmonary host defenses against IA, leading to increased survival and greater numbers of activated pulmonary alveolar macrophages compared to controls (293). A phase I trial of M-CSF in patients suggested some benefit in patients with *Aspergillus* infections, but an insufficient number of patients were treated to show a statistical benefit (282,294). However, the use of GM-CSF is not without its concerns, as bone marrow recovery may lead to liquefaction of pulmonary foci and to potential erosive bleeding caused by an increased inflammatory response, especially in the first week following cavitation (295,296).

In vitro TNF-α appears to enhance early host defense against *Aspergillus* invasion as well as a late defense with increased PMN hyphal damage by oxygen radical production (297,298). In vitro GM-CSF and TNF-α administration have been shown to counteract dexamethasone-induced immunodeficiency (299). Animal model depletion of TNF-α results in increased fungal burden and mortality (300) and resistance is further impaired in IFN-γ deficient mice (275). Treatment of mice with neutralizing antibodies to TNF-α and GM-CSF reduces the influx of PMNs into the lungs and delays fungal clearance (301). Intratracheal administration of a TNF-α agonist resulted in survival benefits when given 3 days before *A. fumigatus* inoculation but not when given concomitantly with conidia, suggesting that pretreatment may provide macrophage priming (300). However, excessive toxicities in doses required to have a biologically useful effect preclude safe administration in humans (297,302).

IFN-γ and G-CSF can each enhance the oxidative bursts and fungicidal activity in vitro of human PMNs against *A. fumigatus* hyphae, with the combination of the two cytokines showing an additive effect (303). IFN-γ can also restore the corticosteroid-suppressed fungicidal activity of human PMN and elutriated monocytes (281,299,304), and IFN-γ-treated human monocytes show enhanced oxygen radical production and damage to *A. fumigatus* hyphae (281).

Exogenous administration of IFN-γ and TNF-α has resulted in protective effects in a murine model of IA (305). Conversely, IFN-γ and TNF-α neutralization resulted in increased disease and increased expression of IL-10. Although IFN-γ is better than G-CSF or GM-CSF at enhancing PMN hyphal damage and both IFN-γ and GM-CSF treatment result in enhanced hyphal damage by PMNs in vitro (306), combination treatment does not increase damage (281). In vitro IFN-γ augments PMNs of CGD patients by an undetermined mechanism (307), although previous work demonstrated a myeloperoxidase-dependent oxidative process (308). IFN-γ has been proven to help prevent IA in CGD patients (310), and there are case reports of the successful use of antifungals with IFN-γ for treatment in CGD patients (310,311).

GM-CSF treatment of neutrophils with voriconazole increases activity against hyphae compared to control neutrophils and voriconazole, but no comparable effect was seen on monocytes (264,304). An in vivo additive effect was also found with G-CSF and posaconazole in one study (312), and no antagonism in another in vivo study (313). Anecdotally, granulocyte transfusions have been helpful in treating patients with IA (314–317). G-CSF-primed donor granulocyte transfusion was used to treat 15 patients with neutropenia-related fungal infections refractory to AmB, including seven patients with IA and the favorable responses appeared to be mainly because of the granulocyte transfusion (318). Another study showed infections cleared in five of nine patients with IA (319). A review of granulocyte transfusions in treating fungal infections in neutropenic patients following bone marrow transplantation showed no improvement in infections; however, this was before the use of G-CSF to prime donors (320,321).

REFERENCES

1. Dasbach EJ, Davies GM, et al. Burden of aspergillosis-related hospitalizations in the United States. Clin Infect Dis 2000; 31:1524–1528.
2. Latge JP. *Aspergillus fumigatus* and aspergillosis. Clin Microbiol Rev 1999; 12:310–350.
3. Anaissie EJ, Stratton SL, et al. Pathogenic *Aspergillus* species recovered from a hospital water system: a 3-year prospective study. Clin Infect Dis. 2002; 34(6):780–789.
4. Perfect JR, Cox GM, et al. The impact of culture isolation of *Aspergillus* species: a hospital-based survey of aspergillosis. Clin Infect Dis 2001; 33:1824–1833.
5. Patterson TF, Kirkpatrick WR, et al. Invasive aspergillosis. Disease spectrum, treatment practices, and outcomes. Medicine 2000; 79:250–260.
6. Rath PM, Ansorg R. Identification of medically important *Aspergillus* species by single strand conformational polymorphism (SSCP) of the PCR-amplified intergenic spacer region. Mycosis 2000; 43:381–386.
7. Denning D. Invasive aspergillosis. Clin Infect Dis 1998; 26:781–805.
8. Marr KA, Carter RA, et al. Epidemiology and outcome of mould infections in hematopoietic stem cell transplant recipients. Clin Infect Dis 2002; 34:909–917.

9. Schaffner A, Douglas H, et al. Selective protection against conidia by mononuclear and against mycelia by polymorphonuclear phagocytes in resistance to *Aspergillus:* Observations on these two lines of defense *in vivo* and *in vitro* with human and mouse phagocytes. J Clin Invest 1982; 69:617–631.
10. Schaffner A. Macrophage–*Aspergillus* interactions. Immunol Ser 1994; 60:545–552.
11. Schneemann M, Schaffner A. Host defense mechanism in *Aspergillus fumigatus* infections. In: Brakhage AA, Jahn B, Schmidt A, eds. *Aspergillus fumigatus.* Vol. 2. Contributions to Microbiology, 1999:57–68.
12. Dixon DM, Polak A, et al. Fungus dose-dependent primary pulmonary aspergillosis in immunosuppressed mice. Infect Immun 1989; 75:1452–1456.
13. Hebart H, Daginik S, et al. Sensitive detection of human cytomegalovirus peptide-specific cytotoxic T-lymphocyte responses by interferon-gamma-enzyme-linked immunospot assay and flow cytometry in healthy individuals and in patients after allogeneic stem cell transplantation. Blood 2002; 99:3830–3837.
14. Cenci E, Mencacci A, et al. Cytokine- and T helper-dependent lung mucosal immunity in mice with invasive pulmonary aspergillosis. J Infect Dis 1998; 178:1750–1760.
15. Cenci E, Perito S, et al. Tand Tcytokines in mice with invasive aspergillosis. Infect Immun 1997; 65:564–570.
16. Schwartz RS, Mackintosh FR, et al. Multivariate analysis of factors associated with invasive fungal disease during remission induction therapy for acute myelogenous leukemia. Cancer 1984; 53:411–419.
17. Gerson SI, Talbot GH, et al. Prolonged granulocytopenia: the major risk factor for invasive pulmonary aspergillosis in patients with acute leukemia. Ann Intern Med 1984; 100:345–351.
18. Duong M, Ouellet N, et al. Kinetic study of host defense and inflammatory response to *Aspergillus fumigatus* in steroid-induced immunosuppressed mice. J Infect Dis 1998; 178:1472–1482.
19. Ng TTC, Robson GD, et al. Hydrocortisone-enhanced growth *of Aspergillus* spp.: implications for pathogenesis. Microbiology 1994; 140:2475–2479.
20. Wald A, Leisenring W, et al. Epidemiology *of Aspergillus* infection in a large cohort of patients undergoing bone marrow transplantation. J Infect Dis 1997; 175:1459–1466.
21. Engelhard D. Bacterial and fungal infections in children undergoing bone marrow transplantation. Bone Marrow Transplant 1998; 21:S78–S80.
22. Benjamin DKJ, Miller WC, et al. Infections diagnosed in the first year after pediatric stem cell transplantation. Pediatr Infect Dis J 2002; 21:227–234.
23. Busca A, Saroglia EM, et al. Analysis of early infectious complications in pediatric patients undergoing bone marrow transplantation. Support Care Cancer 1999; 7:253–259.
24. Jantunen E, Ruutu P, et al. Incidence and risk factors for invasive fungal infections in allogeneic BMT recipients. Bone Marrow Transplant 1997; 19:801–808.
25. Grow WB, Moreb JS, et al. Late onset of invasive aspergillus infection in bone marrow transplant patients at a university hospital. Bone Marrow Transplant 2002; 29:15–19.
26. Ribaud P, Chastang C, et al. Survival and prognostic factors of invasive aspergillosis after allogeneic bone marrow transplantation. Clin Infect Dis 1999; 28:322–330.
27. Ninin E, Milpied N, et al. Longitudinal study of bacterial, viral, and fungal infections in adult recipients of bone marrow transplants. Clin Infect Dis 2001; 33:41–47.
28. Saugier-Veber P, Devergie A, et al. Epidemiology and diagnosis of invasive pulmonary aspergillosis in bone marrow transplant patients: results of a 5 year retrospective study. Bone Marrow Transplant 1993; 12:121–124.
29. Martino R, Subira M, et al. Invasive fungal infections after allogeneic peripheral blood stem cell transplantation: incidence and risk factors in 395 patients. Br J Haematol 2002; 116:475–482.
30. Baddley JW, Stroud TP, et al. Invasive mold infections in allogeneic bone marrow transplant recipients. Clin Infect Dis 2001; 32:1319–1324.

31. Denning DW. Therapeutic outcome in invasive aspergillosis. Clin Infect Dis 1996; 23:608–615.
32. Denning DW, Follansbee S, et al. Pulmonary aspergillosis in AIDS. Patterns of disease, predisposing factors and therapeutic outcome. N Engl J Med 1991; 324:654–662.
33. Ho PL, Yuen KY. Aspergillosis in bone marrow transplant recipients. Crit Rev Oncol Hematol 2000; 34:55–69.
34. Meyers JD. Fungal infections in bone marrow transplant patients. Semin Oncol 1990; 3:10–13.
35. Kramer MR, Denning DW, et al. Ulcerative tracheobronchitis after lung transplantation. Am Rev Respir Dis 1991; 144:552–556.
36. Young RC, Bennett JE, et al. Aspergillosis. The spectrum of the disease in 98 patients. Medicine 1970; 49:147–173.
37. Walsh TJ, Caplan LR, et al. *Aspergillus* infections of the central nervous system: a clinicopathological analysis. Ann Neurol 1985; 18:574–582.
38. Wingard JR, Beals SU, et al. *Aspergillus* infections in bone marrow transplant recipients. Bone Marrow Transplant 1987; 2:175–181.
39. Maschke M, Dietrich U, et al. Opportunistic CNS infection after bone marrow transplantation. Bone Marrow Transplant 1999; 23:1167–1176.
40. Venugopal PV, Venugopal TV, et al. Cerebral aspergillosis. Report of two cases. Sabouraudia 1977; 15:225–230.
41. Henze G, Aldenhoff P, et al. Successful treatment of pulmonary and cerebral aspergillosis in an immunosuppressed child. Eur J Pediatr 1982; 138:263–265.
42. Goodman ML, Coffey RJ. Stereotactic drainage of *Aspergillus* brain abscess with long-term survival: case report and review. Neurosurgery 1989;24:96–99.
43. Denning DW, Stevens DA. Antifungal and surgical treatment of invasive aspergillosis: review of 2121 published cases. Rev Infect Dis 1990; 26:1147–1201.
44. Drakos PE, Nagler A, et al. Invasive fungal sinusitis in patients undergoing bone marrow transplantation. Bone Marrow Transplant 1993; 12:203–208.
45. Kavanagh KT, Hughes WT, et al. Fungal sinusitis in immunocompromised children with neoplasms. Ann Oto Rhinol 1991; 100:331–336.
46. Iwen PC, Rupp ME, et al. Invasive mold sinusitis: 17 cases in immunocompromised patients and review of the literature. Clin Infect Dis 1997; 24:1178–84.
47. Naidu J, Singh SM. *Aspergillus* chevalieri (Mangin) Thorn Church: a new opportunistic pathogen of human cutaneous aspergillosis. Mycoses 1994; 37:271–274.
48. Van Burik JH, Colven R, et al. Cutaneous aspergillosis. J Clin Microbiol 1998; 36:3115–3121.
49. D'Antonio D, Pagano L, et al. Cutaneous aspergillosis in patients with haematological malignancies. Eur J Clin Micriobiol Infect Dis 2000; 19:362–365.
50. Watsky KL, Eisen RN, et al. Unilateral cutaneous emboli of *Aspergillus* Arch Dermatol 1990; 126:1214–1217.
51. Schimmelpfenning C, Naumann R, et al. Skin involvement as the first manifestation of systemic aspergillosis in patients after allogeneic hematopoietic cell transplantation. Bone Marrow Transplant 2001; 27:753–755.
52. Walmsley S, Devi S, et al. Invasive *Aspergillus* infections in a pediatric hospital: A ten year review. Pediatr Infect Dis J 1993; 12:673–682.
53. Allo MA, Miller J, et al. Primary cutaneous aspergillosis associated with Hickman intravenous catheters. N Engl J Med 1987; 317:1105–8.
54. Mawk JR, Erickson DL, et al. Aspergillus infections of the lumbar disc spaces. JNeurosurg 1983; 58:270–274.
55. Bibler MR, Gianis JT. Acute ureteral colic from an obstructing renal aspergilloma. Rev Infect Dis 1987; 9:790–794.
56. Levy H, Horak DA, et al. The value of bronchoalveolar Iavage and bronchial washings in the diagnosis of invasive pulmonary aspergillosis. Respir Med 1992; 86:243–248.
57. Kahn FW, Jones JM, et al. The role of bronchoalveolar lavage in the diagnosis of invasive pulmonary aspergillosis. Am J Clin Pathol 1986; 86:518–23.

58. Fischler DF, Hall GS, et al. Aspergillus in cytology specimens: a review of 45 specimens from 36 patients. Diagn Cytopathol 1997; 25:37–42.

59. Bartlett JG. Aspergillosis update. Medicine 2000; 79:281–282.

60. Treger TR, Vissher DW, et al. Diagnosis of pulmonary infections caused by *Aspergillus*: usefulness of respiratory cultures. J Infect Dis 1985; 152:572–576.

61. Wong K, Waters CM, et al. Surgical management of invasive pulmonary aspergillosis in imniuno-compromised patients. Eur J Cardiothorac Surg 1993; 6:138–143.

62. Duthie R, Denning DW. *Aspergillus* fungaemia: report of two cases review. Clin Infect Dis 1995; 20:598–605.

63. Kontoyiannis DP. Significance of aspergillemia in patients with cancer. A 10-year study. Clin Infect Dis 2000; 31:188–189.

64. Horvath JA, Dummer S. The use of respiratory-tract cultures in the diagnosis of invasive pulmonary aspergillosis. Am J Med 1996; 100:171–178.

65. Igea JM, Cuevas M, et al. IgG subclass response to *Aspergillus fumigatus*. Int Arch Allergy Appl Immunol 1993; 101:277–282.

66. Knutsen AP, Mueller KR, et al. Serum anti-*Aspergillus fumigatus* antibodies by immunoblot and ELISA in cystic fibrosis with allergic bronchopulmonary aspergillosis. J Allergy Clin Immunol 1994; 93:926–931.

67. Kurup VP, Resnick A, et al. Antibody isotype responses in *Aspergillus*-induced diseases. J Lab Clin Med 1990; 115:298–303.

68. van Rens MTM, Vernooy-Jeras R, et al. Detection of immunoglobulins G and A to *Aspergillus fumigatus* by immunoblot analysis for monitoring *Aspergillus*-induced lung disease. Eur Respir J 1998; 11:1274–1280.

69. Sridhar H, Jayshree RS, et al. Invasive aspergillosis in cancer. Mycoses 2002; 45:358–363.

70. Centeno-Lima S, de Lacerda JM, et al. Follow-up of anti-*Aspergillus* IgG and IgA antibodies in bone marrow transplanted patients with invasive aspergillosis. J Clin Lab Anal 2002; 16:156–162.

71. Chan CM, Woo PC, et al. Detection of antibodies specific to an antigenetic cell wall galactomannoprotein for serodiagnosis of *Aspergillus fumigatus* aspergillosis. J Clin Microbiol 2002; 40:2041–2045.

72. Haynes KA, Latgé JP, et al. Detection of Aspergillus antigens associated with invasive infection. J Clin Microbiol 1990; 28:2040–2044.

73. Weig M, Frosch M, et al. Use of recombinant mitogillin for improved serodiagnosis of *Aspergillus fumigatus*-associated diseases. J Clin Microbiol 2001; 39:1721–1730.

74. Latgé JP, Kobayashi H, et al. Chemical and immunological characterization of the extracellular galactomannan secreted by *Aspergillus fumigatus*. Infect Immun 1994; 62:5424–33.

75. Andrews CP, Weiner MH. Immunodiagnosis of invasive pulmonary aspergillosis in rabbits. Fungal antigens detected by radioimmunoassay in bronchoalveolar lavage fluid. Am Rev Respir Dis 1981; 124:60–64.

76. Dupont B, Huber M, et al. Galactomannan antigenemia and antigenuria in aspergillosis: studies in patients and experimentally infected rabbits. J Infect Dis 1987; 155:1–11.

77. Richard C, Romon I, et al. Invasive pulmonary aspergillosis prior to BMT in acute leukernia patients does not predict a poor outcome. Bone Marrow Transplant. 1993; 12:237–241.

78. Maertens J, Verhaegen J, et al. Autopsy-controlled prospective evaluation of serial screening for circulating galactomannan by a sandwich enzyme- linked immunosorbent assay for hematological patients at risk for invasive aspergillosis. J Clin Microbiol 1999; 37:3223–3228.

79. Verweij PE, Denning DW. Diagnostic and therapeutic strategies for invasive aspergillosis. Semin Resp Crit Care Med 1997; 18:203–215.

80. Kappe R, Schulze-Berge A. New cause for false-positive results with the Pastorex *Aspergillus* antigen latex agglutination test. J Clin Microbiol 1993; 31:2489–2490.

81. Stynen D, Goris A, et al. A new sensitive sandwich enzyme-linked immunosorbent assay to detect galactofuran in patients with invasive aspergillosis. J Clin Microbiol 1995; 33:497–500.

82. Williamson EC, Oliver DA, et al. Aspergillus antigen testing of bone marrow transplant recipients. J Clin Pathol 2000; 53:362–366.

83. Bretagne S, Marmorat-Khuong A, et al. Serum Aspergillus galactomannan antigen testing by sandwich ELISA : practical use in neutropenic patients. J Infect 1997; 35:7–15.

84. Haynes KA, Rogers TR. Retrospective evaluation of a latex agglutination test for diagnosis of invasive aspergillosis in immunocompromised patients. Eur J Clin Microbiol Infect Dis 1994; 13:670–674.

85. Rohrlich P, Sarfati J, et al. Prospective sandwich ELISA galactomannan assay: early predictive value and clinical use in invasive aspergillosis. Pediatr Infect. Dis J 1996; 15:321–327.

86. Verweij PE, Stynen D, et al. Sandwich enzyme-linked immunosorbent assay compared with Pastorex latex agglutination test for diagnosing invasive aspergillosis in immunocompromised patients. J Clin Microbiol 1995; 33:1912–1914.

87. Sulahian A, Tabouret M, et al. Comparison of an enzyme immunoassay and latex agglutination test for detection of galactomannan in the diagnosis of invasive aspergillosis. Eur J Clin Microbiol Infect Dis 1996; 15:139–145.

88. Verweij PE, Dompeling EC, et al. Serial monitoring of Aspergillus antigen in the early diagnosis of invasive aspergillosis with two examples. Infection 1997; 25:86–89.

89. Patterson TF, Miniter P, et al. Effect of immunosuppression and amphotericin B on *Aspergillus* antigenemia in an experimental model. J Infect Dis 1988; 158:415–422.

90. Van Cutsem, Meulemans JL, et al. Effect of tissue invasion and treatment with itraconazole or amphotericin B on galactomannan levels in plasma of guinea-pigs with experimental invasive aspergillosis. J Med Vet Mycol 1993; 31:315–324.

91. Tomee JF, Mannes GP, et al. Serodiagnosis and monitoring of Aspergillus infections after lung transplantation. Ann Intern Med 1996; 125:197–201.

92. Fortun J, Martin-Davila P, et al. The Ramon y Cajal Hospital's Liver Transplant Group. Aspergillus antigenemia sandwich- enzyme immunoassay test as a serodiagnostic method for invasive aspergillosis in liver transplant recipients. Transplantation 2001; 71:145–149.

93. Sulahian A, Boutboul F, et al. Value of antigen detection using an enzyme immunoassay in the diagnosis and prediction of invasive aspergillosis in two adult and pediatric hematology units during a 4-year prospective study. Cancer 2001; 91:311–318.

94. Salonen J, Lehtonen OP, et al. Aspergillus antigen in serum, urine and bronchoalveolar lavage specimens of neutropenic patients in relation to clinical outcome. Scand J Infect Dis 2000; 32:485–490.

95. Herbrecht R, Letscher-Bru V, et al. Aspergillus galactomannan detection in the diagnosis of invasive aspergillosis in cancer patients. J Clin Oncol 2002; 20:1898–1906.

96. Lass-Florl C, Aigner J, et al. Screening for Aspergillus spp. using polymerase chain reaction of whole blood samples from patients with haemato logical malignancies. Br J Haematol 2001; 113:180–184.

97. Hebart H, Loeffler J, et al. Early detection of Aspergillus infection after allogeneic stem cell transplantation by polymerase chain reaction screening. J Infect Dis 2000; 181:1713–1719.

98. Buchheidt D, Baust C, et al. Detection of *Aspergillus* species in blood and bronchoalveolar lavage samples from immunocompromised patients by means of 2-step polymerase chain reaction: clinical results. Clin Infect Dis 2001; 33:428–435.

99. Jones ME, Fox AJ, et al. PCR-ELISA for the early diagnosis of invasive pulmonary *Aspergillus* infection in neutropenic patients. J Clin Pathol 1998; 51:652–650.

100. Raad I, Hanna H, et al. Polymerase chain reaction on blood for the diagnosis of invasive pulmonary aspergillosis in cancer patients. Cancer 2002; 94:1032–1036.

101. Ferns RB, Fletcher H, et al. The prospective evaluation of a nested polymerase chain reaction assay for the early detection of *Aspergillus* infection in patients with leukaemia or undergoing allograft treatment. Br J Haematol 2002; 119:720–725.
102. Buchheidt D, Baust C, et al. Clinical evaluation of a polymerase chain reaction assay to detect Aspergillus species in bronchoalveolar lavage samples of neutropenic patients. Br J Haematol 2002; 116:803–811.
103. Raad I, Hanna H, et al. Diagnosis of invasive pulmonary aspergillosis using polymerase chain reaction-based detection of *Aspergillus* in BAL. Chest 2002; 121:1171–1176.
104. Hayette MP, Vaira D, et al. Detection of *Aspergillus* species by PCR in bronchoalveolar lavage fluid. J Clin Microbiol 2001; 39:2338–2340.
105. Einsele H, Hebart H, et al. Detection and identification of fungal pathogens in blood by using molecular probes. J Clin Microbiol 1997; 35:1353–1360.
106. Miyazaki T, Kohno S, et al. Plasma (l-3)-β-D-glucan and fungal antigenemia in patients with candidemia, aspergillosis and cryptococcosis. J Clin Microbiol 1995; 33:3115–3118.
107. Miyazaki T, Kohno S, et al. (l-3)-β-D-glucan in culture fluid of fungi activates factor *G*, a limulus coagulation factor. J Clin Lab Anal 1995; 9:334–339.
108. Mitsutake K, Kohno S, et al. Detection of (l-3)-β-D-glucan in a rat model of aspergillosis. J Clin Lab Anal 1995; 9:119–122.
109. Obayashi T, Yoshida M, et al. Plasma (1-3)-β-D-glucan measurement in diagnosis of invasive deep mycosis and fungal febrile episodes. Lancet 1995; 345:17–20.
110. Yuasa K, Goto H, et al. Evaluation of the diagnostic value of the measurement of (1-3)-β-D-glucan in patients with pulmonary aspergillosis. Respiration 1996; 63:78–83.
111. Francis P, Lee JW, et al. Efficacy of unilamellar liposomal amphotericin B in treatment of pulmonary aspergillosis in persistently granulocytopenic rabbits: the potential role of bronchoalveolar lavage D-mannitol and galactomannan as markers of infection. J Infect Dis 1994; 169:356–368.
112. Wong B, Brauer KL, et al. Increased amounts of the *Aspergillus* metabolite D-mannitol in tissue and serum of rats with experimental aspergillosis. J Infect Dis 1989; 160:95–103.
113. Caillot D, Casasnpvas O, et al. Improved management of invasive pulmonary aspergillosis in neutropenic patients using early thoracic computed tomographic scan and surgery. J Clin Oncol 1997; 15:139–147.
114. Moro M, Galvin JR, et al. Fungal pulmonary infections after bone marrow transplantation: evaluation with radiography and CT. Radiology 1991; 178:721–726.
115. Staples CA, Kang EY, et al. Invasive pulmonary aspergillosis in AIDS: radiographic, CT and pathologic findings. Radiology 1995; 196:409–414.
116. Kuhlman JE, Fishman EK, et al. Invasive pulmonary aspergillosis in acute leukemia: characteristic findings on CT, the CT halo sign and the role of CT in early diagnosis. Radiology 1985; 157:611–614.
117. Blum U, Windfuhr M, et al. Invasive pulmonary aspergillosis. MRI, CT and plain radiographic findings and their contribution for early diagnosis. Chest 1994; 106:1156–1167.
118. Taccone A, Occhi M, et al. CT of invasive pulmonary aspergillosis in children with cancer. Pediatr Radiol 1993; 23:177–180.
119. Primack SL, Hartman TE, et al. Pulmonary nodules and the CT halo sign. Radiology 1994; 190:513–515.
120. Miaux Y, Ribaud P, et al. MR of cerebral aspergillosis in patients who have had bone marrow transplantation. Am J Neuroradiol 1995; 16:555–562.
121. Saiki RK, Gelfand DH, et al. Primer-directed enzymatic amplification of DNA with a thermostable DNA polymerase. Science 1988; 239:487–491.
122. Kawazu M, Kanda Y, et al. Rapid diagnosis of invasive pulmonary aspergillosis by quantitative polymerase chain reaction using bronchial lavage fluid. Am J Hematol 2003; 72:27–30.

123. Hendolin PH, Paulin L, et al. Panfungal PCR and multiplex liquid hybridization for detection of fungi in tissue specimens. J Clin Microbiol 2000; 38:4186–4192.

124. Jaeger EE, Carroll NM, et al. Rapid detection and identification of *Candida*, *Aspergillus*, and *Fusarium* species in ocular samples using nested PCR. J Clin Microbiol 2000; 38:2902–2908.

125. Scott J, Schekman R. Lyticase: endoglucanase and protease activities that act together in yeast cell lysis. J Bacteriol 1980; 142:414–423.

126. Loeffler J, Hebart H, et al. Detection of PCR-amplified fungal DNA by using a PCR-ELISA system. Med Mycol 1998; 36:275–279.

127. Hopfer RL, Walden P, et al. Detection and differentiation of fungi in clinical specimens using polymerase chain reaction (PCR) amplification and restriction enzyme analysis. J Med Ved Mycol 1993; 31:65–75.

128. Kanbe T, Yamaki K, et al. Identification of the pathogenic Aspergillus species by nested PCR using a mixture of specific primers to DNA topoisomerase II gene. Microbiol Immunol 2002; 46:841–848.

129. Melchers WJG, Verweij PE, et al. General primer-mediated PCR for the detection of Aspergillus species. J Clin Microbiol 1994; 32:1710–1717.

130. Turenne CY, Sanche SE, et al. Rapid identification of fungi by using the ITS2 genetic region and an automated fluorescent capillary electrophoresis system. J Clin Microbiol 1999; 37:1846–1851.

131. Zhao J, Kong F, et al. Identification of *Aspergillus fumigatus* and related species by nested PCR targeting ribosomal DNA internal transcribed spacer regions. J Clin Microbiol 2001; 39:2261–2266.

132. Luo G, Mitchell TG. Rapid identification of pathogenic fungi directly from cultures by using multiplex PCR. J Clin Microbiol 2002; 40:2860–2865.

133. Kappe R, Okeke CN, et al. Molecular probes for the detection of pathogenic fungi in the presence of human tissue. J Med Microbiol 1998; 47:811–820.

134. Fletcher HA, Barton RC, et al. Detection of *Aspergillus fumigatus* PCR produces by a microtitre plate based DNA hybridisation assay. J Clin Pathol 1998; 51:617–620.

135. Willinger B, Obradovic A, et al. Detection and identification of fungi from fungus balls of the maxillary sinus by molecular techniques. J Clin Microbiol 2003; 41:581–585.

136. Loeffler J, Henke N, et al. Quantification of fungal DNA by using fluorescence resonance energy transfer and the Light Cycler system. J Clin Microbiol 2000; 38:586–590.

137. Bowman JC, Abruzzo GK, et al. Quantitative PCR assay to measure *Aspergillus fumigatus* burden in a murine model of disseminated aspergillosis: demonstration of efficacy of caspofungin acetate. Antimicrob Agents Chemother 2001; 45:3474–3481.

138. Costa C, Vidaud D, et al. Development of two real-time quantitative TaqMan PCR assays to detect circulating *Aspergillus fumigatus* DNA in serum. J Microbiol Methods 2001; 38:3478–3480.

139. Pham AS, Tarrand JJ, et al. Diagnosis of invasive mould infection by real-time quantitative PCR. Am J Clin Pathol 2003; 119:38–44.

140. Stevens DA, Kan VL, et al. Practice guidelines for diseases caused by *Aspergillus* Clin Infect Dis 2000; 30:696–709.

141. Steinbach WJ, Stevens DA. Review of newer antifungal and immunomodulatory strategies for invasive aspergillosis. Clin Infect Dis 2003; 37(Suppl. 3):S157–S187.

142. Kullberg BJ, de Pauw BE. Therapy of invasive fungal infections. Neth J Med 1999; 55:118–127.

143. Wong-Beringer A, Jacobs RA, et al. Lipid formulations of amphotericin B: clinical efficiacy and toxicities. Clin Infect Dis 1998; 27:603–618.

144. Hiemenz JW, Walsh TJ. Lipid formulations of amphotericin B: Recent progress and future directions. Clin Infect Pis 1996; 22:S133–S144.

145. Graybill JR, Tollemar J, et al. Antifungal compounds: controversies, queries and conclusions. Med Mycol 2000; 38:323–333.

146. Dix SP, Andriole VT. Lipid formulations of amphotericin B. Curr Clin Top Infect Dis 2000; 20:1–23.
147. Luna B, Drew RH, et al. Agents for treatment of invasive fungal infections. Otolaryngol Clin North Am 2000; 33:277–299.
148. Groll AH, Piscitelli SC, et al. Antifungal pharmacodynamics: concentration-effect relationships *in vitro* and *in vivo* Pharmacotherapy 2001; 21:133S-148S.
149. Walsh TJ, Goodman JL, et al. Safety, tolerance, and pharmacokinetics of high-dose liposomal amphotericin B (AmBisome) in patients infected with *Aspergillus* species and other filamentous fungi: maximum tolerate dose study. Antimicrob Agents Chemother 2001; 45:3487.
150. Ellis M. Amphotericin B preparations: a maximum tolerated dose in severe invasive fungal infections? Transpl Inf Dis 2000; 2:51–61.
151. Van Cutsem J, Van Gerven F, et al. Itraconazole, a new triazole that is orally active against *Aspergillus* Antimicrob Agents Chemother 1984; 26:527–534.
152. Tucker RM, Denning DW, et al. The interaction of azoles with rifampin, phenytoin, and carbamazepine: in vitro and clinical observations. Clin. Infect. Dis. 1992; 14:165–174.
153. Stevens DA. Itraconazole in cyclodextrin solution. Pharmacotherapy 1999; 19:603–611.
154. De Beule K, Van Gestel J. Pharmacology of itraconazole. Drugs 2001; 61:27–37.
155. Slain D, Rogers PD, et al. Intravenous itraconazole. Ann Pharmacother 2001; 35:720–729.
156. Caillot D, Bassaris H, et al. Intravenous itraconazole followed by oral itraconazole in the treatment of invasive pulmonary aspergillosis in patients with hematologic malignancies, chronic granulomatous disease, or AIDS. Clin Infect Dis 2001; 33:e83–90.
157. Chiller TM, Stevens DA. Treatment strategies for *Aspergillus* infections. Drug Res Update 2000; 3:89–97.
158. Odds FC, Oris M, et al. Activities of an intravenous formulation of itraconazole in experimental disseminated *Aspergillus*, *Candida*, and *Cryptococcus* infections. Antimicrob Agents Chemother 2000; 44:3180–3183.
159. Denning DW, Lee JY, et al. NIAID Mycoses Study Group multicenter trial of oral itraconazole therapy for invasive aspergillosis. Am J Med 1994; 97:135–144.
160. Stevens DA, Lee JY. Analysis of compassionate use itraconazole therapy for invasive aspergillosis by the NIAID Mycoses Study Group criteria. Arch Intern Med 1997; 157:1857–1862.
161. Manavathu EK, Cutright JL, et al. Organism-dependent fungicidal activity of azoles. Antimicrob Agents Chemother 1998; 42:3018–3021.
162. Sabo JA, Abdel-Rahman SM. Voriconazole: a new triazole antifungal. Ann Pharmacother 2000; 34:1032–1043.
163. Johnson EM, Szekely A, et al. In vitro activity of voriconazole, itraconazole and amphotericin B against filamentous fungi. J Antimicrob Chemother 1998; 42:741–745.
164. Cuenca-Estrella M, Rodriquez-Tudela JL, et al. Comparison of the in-vitro activity of voriconazole (UK-109,496), itraconazole and amphotericin B against clinical isolates of *Apergillusfumigatus* J Antimicrob Chemother 1998; 42:531–533.
165. Clancy C, Nguyen N. In vitro efficacy and fungicidal activity of voriconazole against *Aspergillus* and *Fusarium* species. Eur J Clin Microbiol Infect Dis 1998; 17:573–575.
166. Espinel-Ingroff A. In vitro activity of the new triazole voriconazole (UK-109,496) against opportunistic filamentous and dimorphic fungi and common and emerging yeast pathogens. J Clin Microbiol 1998; 36:198–202.
167. Espinel-Ingroff A, Boyle K, et al. In vitro antifungal activities of voriconazole and reference agents as determined by NCCLS methods: review of the literature. Mycopathologia 2001; 150:101–115.

168. Verweij PE, Mensink M, et al. In vitro activities of amphotericin B, itraconazole and voriconazole against 150 clinical and environmental *Aspergillus fumigatus* isolates. J Antimicrob Chemother 1998; 42:389–392.

169. Espinel-Ingroff A, Johnson E, et al. Activity of voriconazole, itraconazole and amphotericin B in vitro against 577 molds from the voriconazole phase III clinical studies. Program and abstracts of the 42nd Interscience Conference on Antimicrobial Agents and Chemotherapy, San Diego, CA, (Abstract M-1518, Washington, DC), 2002.

170. Iwen PC, Rupp ME, et al. Invasive pulmonary aspergillosis due to *Aspergillus terreus:* 12-year experience and review of the literature. Clin Infect Dis 1998; 26:1092–1097.

171. Sutton DA, Sanchie SE, et al. In vitro amphotericin B resistance in clinical isolates *of Aspergillus terreus,* with a head-to-head comparison to voriconazole. J Clin Microbiol 1999; 37:2343–2345.

172. Murphy M, Bernard EM, et al. Activity of voriconazole (UK-109,496) against clinical isolates of *Aspergillus* species and its effectiveness in an experimental model of invasive pulmonary aspergillosis. Antimicrob Agents Chemother 1997; 41:696–698.

173. Chandrasekar PH, Cutright J, et al. Efficacy of voriconazole against invasive pulmonary aspergillosis in a guinea-pig model. J Antimicrob Chemother 2000; 45:673–676.

174. Kirkpatrick WR, McAtee RK, et al. Efficacy of voriconazole in a guinea pig model of disseminated invasive aspergillosis. Antimicrob Agents Chemother 2000; 44:2865–2868.

175. Martin MV, Yates J, et al. Comparison of voriconazole (UK-109,496) and itraconazole in prevention and treatment of *Aspergillus fumigatus* endocarditis in guinea pigs. Antimicrob Agents Chemother 1997; 41:13–16.

176. George D, Miniter P, et al. Efficacy of UK-109,496, a new azole antifungal agent, in an experimental model of invasive aspergillosis. Antimicrob Agents Chemother 1996; 40:86–91.

177. Herbrecht R, Denning DW, et al. Voriconazole versus amphotericin B for primary therapy of invasive aspergillosis. N Engl J Med 2002; 347:408–415.

178. Denning DW, Ribaud P, et al. Efficacy and safety of voriconazole in the treatment of acute invasive aspergillosis. Clin Infect Dis 2002; 34:563–571.

179. Walsh TJ, Lutsar I, et al. Voriconazole in the treatment of aspergillosis, scedosporiosis and other invasive fungal infections in children. Pediatr Infect Dis J 2002; 21:240–248.

180. Marco F, Pfaller MA, et al. *In vitro* activity of a new triazole antifungal agent, SCH56592, against clinical isolates of filamentous fungi. Mycopathologia 1998; 141:73–77.

181. Cacciapuoti A, Loebenberg D, et al. *In vitro* and *in vivo* activities of SCH 56592 (Posaconazole), a new triazole antifungal agent, against *Aspergillus* and *Candida* Antimicrob Agents Chemother 2000; 44:2017–2022.

182. Uchida K, Yokota N, et al. *In vitro* antifungal activity of posaconazole against various pathogenic fungi. Int J Antimicrob Agents 2001; 18:167–172.

183. Tortorano AM, Dannaoui E, et al. Effect of medium composition on static and cidal activity of amphotericin B, itraconazole, voriconazole, posaconazole and terbinafine against *Aspergillus fumigatus*: a multicenter study. J Chemother 2002; 14:246–252.

184. Oakley KL, Moore CB, et al. *In vitro* activity of SCH-56592 and comparison with activities of amphotericin B and itraconazole against *Aspergillus* spp. Antimicrob Agents Chemother 1997; 41:1124–1126.

185. Espinel-Ingroff A, Rezusta A. E-test method for testing susceptibilities of *Aspergillus* spp. to the new triazoles voriconazole and posaconazole and to established antifungal agents: comparison with NCCLS broth microdilution method. J Clin Microbiol 2002; 40:2101–2107.

186. Espinel-Ingroff A, Bartlett M, et al. Optimal susceptibility testing conditions for detection of azole resistance in *Aspergillus* spp.: NCCLS collaborative evaluation. Antimicrob Agents Chemother 2001; 45:1828–1835.

187. Chandrasekar PH, Cutright JL, et al. *Aspergillus:* Rising frequency of clinical isolation and continued susceptibility to antifungal agents, 1994–1999. Diagn Microbiol Infect Dis 2001; 41:211–214.

188. Manavathu EK, Cutright JL, et al. A comparative study of in vitro susceptibilities of clinical and laboratory-selected resistant isolates of *Aspergillus* spp. to amphotericin B, itraconazole, voriconazole and posaconazole (SCH 56592). J Antimicrob Chemother 2000; 46:229–234.

189. Pfaller MA, Messer SA, et al. Antifungal activities of posaconazole, ravuconazole, and voriconazole compared to those of itraconazole and amphotericin B against 239 clinical isolates of *Aspergillus* spp. and other filamentous fungi: Report from SENTRY antimicrobial surveillance program, 2000. Antimicrob Agents Chemother 2002; 46:1032–1037.

190. Espinel-Ingroff A, Fothergill A, et al. Testing conditions for determination of minimum fungicidal concentrations of new and established antifungal agents *fox Aspergillus* spp.: NCCLS collaborative study. J Clin Microbiol 2002; 40:3204–3208.

191. Espinel-Ingroff A. Comparison of in vitro activities of the new triazole SCH56592 and the echinocandins MK-0991 (L-743,872) and LY303366 against opportunistic filamentous and dimorphic fungi and yeasts. J Clin Microbiol 1998; 36:2950–2956.

192. Manavathu EK, Abraham OC, et al. Isolation and *in vitro* susceptibility to amphotericin B, itraconazole and posaconazole of voriconazole-resistant laboratory isolates of *Aspergillus fumigatus* Clin Microbiol Infect 2001; 7:130–137.

193. Graybill JR, Bocanegra R, et al. SCH56592 treatment of murine invasive aspergillosis. J Antimicrob Chemother 1998; 42:539–542.

194. Petraitiene R, Petraitis V, et al. Antifungal activity and pharmokinetics of posaconazole (SCH 56592) in treatment and prevention of experimental invasive pulmonary aspergillosis: correlation with galactomannan antigenemia. Antimicrob Agents Chemother 2001; 45:857–869.

195. Kirkpatrick WR, McAtee RK, et al. Efficacy of SCH56592 in a rabbit model of invasive aspergillosis. Antimicrob Agents Chemother 2000; 44:780–782.

196. Oakley KL, Morrissey G, et al. Efficacy of SCH-56592 in a temporarily neutropenic murine model of invasive aspergillosis with an itraconazole-susceptible and an itraconazole-resistant isolate of *Aspergillus fumigatus*. Antimicrob Agents Chemother 1997; 41:1504–1507.

197. Hachem RY, Raad II, et al. An open, non-comparative multicenter study to evaluate efficacy and safety of posaconazole (SCH 56592) in the treatment of invasive fungal infections refractory to or intolerant to standard therapy. Program and abstracts of the 40th Interscience Conference on Antimicrobial Agents and Chemotherapy, Toronoto, Ontario, 2000. (Abstract 1109, Washington, DC).

198. Fung-Tomc JC, Huczko E, et al. *In vitro* activity of a new oral triazole, BMS-207147 (ER-30346). Antimicrob Agents Chemother 1998; 42:313–318.

199. Espinel-Ingroff A. Germinated and nongerminated conidial suspensions for testing of susceptibilities of *Aspergillus* spp. to amphotericin B, itraconazole, posaconazole, ravueonazole, and voriconazole. Antimicrob Agents Chemother 2001; 45:605–607.

200. Moore CB, Walls CM, et al. In vitro activity of the new triazole BMS-207147 against *Aspergillus* species in comparison with itraconazole and amphotericin B. Antimicrob Agents Chemother 2000; 44:441–443.

201. Hata K, Kimura J, et al. Efficacy of ER-30346, a novel oral triazole antifungal agent, in experimental models of aspergillosis, candidiasis, and cryptococcosis. Antimicrob Agents Chemother 1996; 40:2243–2247.

202. Hata K, Kimura J, et al. *In vitro* and *in vivo* antifungal activities of ER-30346, a novel oral triazole with a broad antifungal spectrum. Antimicrob Agents Chemother 1996; 40:2237–2242.

203. Kirkpatrick W, Perea S, et al. Efficacy of ravueonazole (BMS-207147) in a guinea pig model of disseminated aspergillosis. J Antimicrob Chemother 2002; 49:353–357.

204. Roberts J, Schock K, et al. Efficacies of two new antifungal agents, the triazole ravueo-nazole and the echinocandin LY-303366, in an experimental model of invasive aspergil-losis. Antimicrob Agents Chemother 2000; 44:3381–3388.
205. Deresinski SC, Stevens DA. Caspofungin. Clin Infect Dis 2003; 36:1445–1457.
206. Arikan S, Paetznick V, et al. Comparative evaluation of disk diffusion with microdilu-tion assay in susceptibility testing of caspofungin against *Aspergillus* and *Fusarium* iso-lates. Antimicrob Agents Chemother 2002; 46:3084–3087.
207. Bowman JC, Hicks S, et al. The antifungal echinocandin caspofungin acetate kills growing cells *of Aspergillus fumigatus* in vitro. Antimicrob Agents Chemother 2002; 46:3001–3012.
208. Chiller T, Farrokhshad K, et al. Influence of human sera on the *in vitro* activity of the echinocandin caspofungin (MK-0991) against *Aspergillus fumigatus* Antimicrob Agents Chemother 2000; 44:3302–3305.
209. Chiller T, Farrokhshad K, et al. The interaction of human monocytes, monocyte-derived macrophages, an polymorphonuclear neutrophils with caspofungin (MK-0991), an echinocandin, for antifungal activity against *Aspergillus fumigatus* Diagn Microbiol Infect Dis 2001; 39:99–103.
210. Petraitiene R, Petraitis V, et al. Antifungal efficacy of caspofungin (MK-0991) in experi-mental pulmonary aspegillosis in persistently neutropenic rabbits: pharmacokinetics, drug deposition, and relationship to galactomannan antigenemia. Antimicrob Agents Chemother 2002; 46:12–23.
211. Abruzzo GK, Gill CJ, et al. Efficacy of the echinocandin caspofungin against dissemi-nated aspergillosis and candidiasis in cyclophosphamide-mduced immunosuppressed mice. Antimicrob Agents Chemother 2000; 44:2310–2318.
212. Abruzzo GK, Flattery AM, et al. Evaluation of the echinocandin antifungal MK-0991 (L-743,872): efficacies in mouse models of disseminated aspergillosis, candidiasis, and cryptococcosis. Antimicrob Agents Chemother 1997; 41:2333–2338.
213. Maertens J, Raad I, et al. Multicenter, noncomparative study to evaluate safety and effi-cacy of caspofungin in adults with invasive aspergillosis refractory or intolerant to amphotericin, amphotericin B lipid formulations, or azoles. Program and abstracts of the 40th Interscience Conference on Antimicrobial Agents and Chemotherapy, Tor-onto, Ontario, 2000. Abstract J-l 103. Washington, DC.
214. Maertens J, Raad I, et al. Update on the multicenter noncomparative study of caspo-fungin in adults with invasive aspergillosis refractory or intolerant to other antifungal agents: analysis of 90 patients. Program and abstracts of the 42nd Interscience Confer-ence on Antimicrobial Agents and Chemotherapy, San Diego, CA, 2002. Abstract M-868. Washington, DC.
215. Sanz-Rodriguez C, Aguado JM, et al. Caspofungin therapy in documented fungal infec-tions: Spanish experience before licensure of the drug. Program and abstracts of the 42nd Interscience Conference on Antimicrobial Agents and Chemotherapy, San Diego, CA, 2002. Abstract M-895. Washington, DC.
216. Walsh TJ, Viviani MA, et al. New targets and delivery systems for antifungal therapy. Med Mycol 2000; 38:335–347.
217. Mikamo H, Sato Y, et al. *In vitro* antifungal activity of FK463, a new water-soluble echinocandin-like lipopeptide. J Antimicrob Chemother 2000; 46:485–487.
218. Hatano K, Morishita Y, et al. Antifungal mechanism of FK463 against *Candida albi-cans* and *Aspergillus fumigatus* J Antibiot (Tokyo) 2002; 55:219–222.
219. Tawara S, Ikeda F, et al. *In vitro* activities of a new lipopeptide antifungal agent, FK463, against a variety of clinically important fungi. Antimicrob Agents Chemother 2000; 44:57–62.
220. Uchida K, Nishiyama Y, et al. *In vitro* antifungal activity of a novel lipopeptide anti-fungal agent, FK463, against various fungal pathogens. J Antibiot (Tokyo) 2000; 53:1175–1181.
221. Tomishima M, Ohki H, et al. FK463, a novel water-soluble echinocandin lipopeptide: synthesis and antifungal activity. J Antibiot (Tokyo) 1999; 52:674–676.

222. Nakai T, Uno J, et al. *In vitro* activity of FK463, a novel lipopeptide antifungal agent, against a variety of clinically important molds. Chemotherapy 2002; 48:78–81.

223. Stevens DA. Susceptitbility to micafungin of isolates from clinical trials. Program and abstract of the 42nd interscience Conference on Antimicrobial Agents and Chemotherapy, San Diego, CA, 2002. [Abstract M-1520, Washington, DC.]

224. Capilla Luque J, Clemons KV, et al. Efficacy of micafungin alone and in combination against systemic murine aspergillosis. Antimicrob. Agents Chemother. 2003; 47:1452–1455.

225. Clemons KV, Stevens DA. Efficacy of micafungin alone or in combination against experimental pulmonary aspergillosis. Program and abstracts of the Focus on Fungal Infections 12, Phoenix, AZ, 2002. [Abstract 10.]

226. Nakai T, Hatano K, et al. Electron microscopic findings for micafungin-treated pulmonary aspergillosis in mice. Program and abstracts of the 42nd Interscience Conference on Antimicrobial Agents and Chemotherapy, San Diego, CA, 2002. Abstract M-1511. Washington, DC.

227. Ikeda F, Wakai Y, et al. Efficacy of FK463, a new lipopeptide antifungal agent, in mouse models of disseminated candidiasis and aspergillosis. Antimicrob Agents Chemother 2000; 44:614–618.

228. Matsumoto S, Wakai Y, et al. Efficacy of FK463, a new lipopeptide antifungal agent, in mouse models of pulmonary aspergillosis. Antimicrob Agents Chemother 2000; 44:619–621.

229. Kohno S, Masaoka T, et al. A multicenter, open-label clinical study of FK463 in patients with deep mycoses in Japan. Program and abstracts of the 41st Interscience Conference on Antimicrobial Agents and Chemotherapy, Chicago, IL, 2001. Abstract J-834. Washington, DC.

230. Ratanatharathorn V, Flynn P, et al. Micafungin in combination with systemic antifungal agents in the treatment of refractory aspergillosis in bone marrow transplant patients. Program and abstracts of the American Society of Hematology 44th Annual Meeting, Philadelphia, 2002. Abstract 2472. Washington, DC.

231. Pfaller MA, Marco F, et al. *In vitro* activity of two echinocandin derivatives, LY303366, and MK-0991 (L-743,792), against clinical isolates of *Aspergillus*, *Fusarium*, *Rhizopus*, and other filamentous fungi. Diagn Microbiol Infect Dis 1998; 30:251–255.

232. Zhanel GG, Karlowsky JA, et al. *In vitro* activity of a new semisynthetic echinocandin, LY-303366, against syernstic isolates of *Candida* species, *Cryptococcus neoformans*, *Blastomyces dermatitidis*, and *Aspergillus* species. Antimicrob Agents Chemother 1997; 41:863–865.

233. Brummer E, Chauhan SD, et al. Collaboration of human phagocytes with LY303366 for antifungal activity against *Aspergillus fumigatus* J Antimicrob Chemother 1999; 43:491–496.

234. Petraitis V, Petraitiene R, et al. Antifungal efficacy, safety, and single-dose pharmacokinetics of LY303366, a novel echinocandin B, in experimental pulmonary aspergillosis in persistently neutropenic rabbits. Antimicrob Agents Chemother 1998; 42:2898–2905.

235. Verweij PE, Oakley KL, et al. Efficacy of LY303366 against amphotericin B-susceptible and -resistant *Aspergillus fumigatus* in a murine model of invasive aspergillosis. Antimicrob Agents Chemother 1998; 42:873–878.

236. Lewis RE, Kontoyiannis DP. Rationale for combination antifungal therapy. Pharmacotherapy 2001; 21:149S–164S.

237. Steinbach WJ, Stevens, DA, et al. Combination and sequential antifungal therapy for invasive aspergillosis: review of published in vitro and in vivo interactions and 6,281 clinical cases from 1966–2001. Clin Infect Dis, 2003; 37(Suppl. 3):S188–S224.

238. Firkin FC. Therapy of deep-seated fungal infections with 5-fluorocytosine. Aust N Z J Med 1974; 4:462–467.

239. Denning DW, Hanson LH, et al. In vitro susceptibility and synergy studies of *Aspergillus* species to conventional and new agents. Diag Micro Infect Dis 1992; 15:21–34.

240. Carrizosa J, Kohn C, et al. Experimental *Aspergillus* endocarditis in rabbits. J Lab ClinMed 1975; 86:746–753.

241. Schmitt HJ, Bernard EM, et al. Combination therapy in a model of pulmonary aspergillosis. Mycoses 1991; 34:281–285.

242. George D, Kordick D, et al. Combination therapy in experimental invasive aspergillosis. Clin Infect Dis 1993; 168:692–698.

243. Brincker H, Christensen BE, et al. Itraconazole treatment of pulmonary aspergillosis in leukemia patients during a nosocomial epidemic associated with indoor building renovation. Mycoses 1991; 34:395–400.

244. Burch PA, Karp JE, et al. Favorable outcome of invasive aspergillosis in patients with acute leukemia. J Clin Oncol 1987; 5:1985–1993.

245. Denning D, Williams A. Invasive pulmonary aspergillosis diagnosed by blood culture and successfully treated. Br J Dis Chest 1987; 81:300–304.

246. Verweij PE, Donnelly JP, et al. Amphotericin B versus amphotericin B plus 5-flucytosine: poor results in the treatment of proven systemic mycoses in neutropenic patients. Infection 1994; 22:81–85.

247. Beggs WH, Sarosi LA, et al. Synergistic action of amphotericin B and rifampin on *Candida albicans* Am Rev Respir Dis 1974; 110:671–673.

248. Medoff G. Antifungal actions of rifampin. Rev Infect Dis 1983; 5:614–619.

249. Kitahara M, Seth VK, et al. Activity of amphotericin B, 5-fluorocytosine, and rifampin against six clinical isolates of *Aspergillus* Antimicrob Agents Chemother 1976; 9:915–919.

250. Hughes CE, Harris C, et al. *In vitro* activities of amphotericin B in combination with four antifungal agents and rifampin against *Aspergillus* spp, Antimicrob Agents Chemother 1984; 25:560–562.

251. Arroyo J, Medoff G, et al. Therapy of murine aspergillosis with amphotericin B in combination with rifampin or 5-fluorocytosine. Antimicrob Agents Chemother 1977; 11:21–25.

252. Lewis RE, Klepser ME, et al. Combination systemic antifungal therapy for cryptococcosis, candidiasis, and aspergillosis. J Infect Dis Pharmacother 1999; 3:61–83.

253. Denning DW. Treatment of invasive aspergillosis. J Infect 1994; 28:25–33.

254. Sugar AM. Use of amphotericin B with azole antifungal drugs: what are we doing? Antimicrob Agents Chemother 1995; 39:1907–1912.

255. Kontoyiannis DP, Lewis RE, et al. Itraconazole- amphotericin B antagonism in *Aspergillus fumigatus:* an E-test based strategy. Antimicrob Agents Chemother 2000; 44:2915–2918.

256. Popp AI, White MH, et al. Amphotericin B with and without itraconazole for invasive aspergillosis: a three-year retrospective study. Int J Infect Dis 1999; 3:157–160.

257. Arikan S, Lozano-Chiu M, et al. In vitro synergy studies with caspofungin and amphotericin B against *Aspergillus* and *Fusarium* spp. Antimicrob Agents Chemother 2002; 46:245–247.

258. Bartizal K, Gill CJ, et al. In vitro preclinical evaluation studies with the echinocandin antifungal MK-0991 (L-743,872). Antimicrob Agents Chemother 1997; 41:2326–2332.

259. Manavathu EK, Ganesan LT, et al. *In vitro* antifungal activity of voriconazole in two-drug combination with micafungin, caspofungin, and amphotericin B. Program and abstracts of the 41st Interscience Conference on Antimicrobial Agents and Chemotherapy, Chicago, IL, (Abstract J-125, Washington, DC.) 2001.

260. Stevens DA. Drug interaction in vitro between a polyene (AmBisome) and an echinocandin (FK463) vs. *Aspergillus* species. 39th Interscience Conference on Antimicrobial Agents and Chemotherapy, San Francisco, CA, 1999. [Abstract 151, Washington, DC.]

261. Douglas CM, Bowman JC, et al. Use of a novel real-time PCR assay to demonstrate efficacy of caspofungin, alone and in combination with amphotericin B, in reducing *Aspergillus fumigatus* tissue burden in chronically immunosuppressed mice with dissemi-

nated infection. Program and abstracts of the 41st Interscience Conference on Antimicrobial Agents and Chemotherapy, Chicago, IL, 2001. (Abstract J-1836, Washington, DC.).

262. Kohno S, Maesaki S, et al. Synergistic effects of combination of FK463 with amphotericin B: enhanced efficacy in a murine model of invasive pulmonary aspergillosis. Program and abstracts of the 40th Interscience Conference on Antimicrobial Agents and Chemotherapy, Toronto, Ontario, 2000. (Abstract 1686, Washington, DC.).

263. Nakajima M, Tamada S, et al. Pathological findings in a murine pulmonary aspergillosis model: treatment with FK463, amphotericin B and a combination of FK463 and amphotericin B. Program and abstracts of the 40th Interscience Conference on Antimicrobial Agents and Chemotherapy, Toronto, Ontario, 2000. (Abstract 1685, Washington, DC.).

264. Stevens DA, Kullberg B, et al. Combined treatment: antifungal drugs with antibodies, cytokines or drugs. Med Mycol 2000; 38:305–315.

265. Nucci M, Pulcheri W, et al. Amphotericin B followed by itraconazole in the treatment of disseminated fungal infections in neutropenic patients. Mycoses 1994; 37:433–437.

266. Sud IJ, Feingold DS. Effect of ketoconazole on the fungicidal action of amphotericin B in *Candida albicans*. Antimicrob Agents Chemother 1983; 23:185–187.

267. Schaffner A, Frick PG. The effect of ketoconazole on amphotericin B in a model of disseminated aspergillosis. J Infect Dis 1985; 151:902–910.

268. Maesaki S, Kohno S, et al. Effects of antifungal agent combinations administered simultaneously and sequentially against *Aspergillus fumigatus* Antimicrob Agents Chemother 1994; 38:2843–2845.

269. Pahls S, Schaffner A. *Aspergillus fumigatus* pneumonia in neutropenic patients receiving fluconazole for infection due to *Candida* species: is amphotericin B combined with fluconazole the appropriate answer? Clin Infect Dis 1994; 18:484–485.

270. Schaffner A, Bohler A. Amphotericin B refractory aspergillosis after itraconazole: evidence for significant antagonism. Mycoses 1993; 36:421–424.

271. Nanas JN, Saroglou G, et al. Itraconazole for the treatment of pulmonary aspergillosis in heart transplant recipients. Clin Transplant 1998; 12:30–34.

272. Galimberti R, Kowalczuk A, et al. Cutaneous aspergillosis: a report of six cases. Br J Dermatol 1998; 139:522–526.

273. Roilides E, Pizzo PA. Modulation of host defenses by cytokines: evolving adjuncts in prevention and treatment of serious infections in immunocompromised hosts. Clin Infect Dis 1992; 15:508–524.

274. Saxena S, Bhatnagar PK, et al. Effect of amphotericin B lipid formulation on immune response in aspergillosis. Int J Pharm 1999; 188:19–30.

275. Cenci E, Mencacci A, et al. Interleukin-4 causes susceptibility to invasive pulmonary aspergillosis through suppression of protective type I response. J Infect Dis 1999; 180:1957–1968.

276. Clemons KV, Grunig G, et al. Role of IL-10 in invasive aspergillosis: increased resistance of IL-10 gene knockout mice to lethal systemic aspergillosis. Clin Exp Immunol 2000; 122:186 191.

277. Roilides E, Dimitriadou A, et al. L-10 exerts suppressive and enhancing effects on antifungal activity of mononuclear phagocytes against *Aspergillus fumigatus* J Immunol 1997; 158:322–329.

278. Polak-Wyss A. Protective effect of human granulocyte colony-stimulating factor (hG-CSF) on *Cryptococcus* and *Aspergillus* infections in normal and immunosuppressed mice. Mycoses 1991; 34:205–215.

279. Liles WC, Huang JE, et al. Granulocyte colony-stimulating factor administered *in vivo* augments neutrophil-mediated activity against opportunistic fungal pathogens. J Infect Dis 1997; 175:1012–1015.

280. Geller RB. Use of cytokines in the treatment of acute myelocytic leukemia: a critical review. J Clin Oncol 1996; 14:1371–1382.

281. Roilides E, Holmes A, et al. Antifungal activity of elutriated human monocytes against *Aspergillus fumigatus* hyphae: enhancement by granulocyte-macrophage colony stimulating factor and interferon-gamma. J Infect Dis 1994; 170:894–899.

282. Nemunaitis J. Use of macrophage colony-stimulating factor in the treatment of fungal infections. Clin Infect Dis 1998; 26:1279–1281.

283. Brummer E, Maqbool A, et al. In vivo GM-CSF prevents dexamethasone suppression of killing *of Aspergillus fumigatus* conidia by bronchoalveolar macrophages. J Leukoc Biol 2001; 70:868–872.

284. Brummer E, Kamberi M, et al. Regulation by granulocyte–macrophage colony-stimulating factor and/or steroids given in vivo of proinfiammatory cytokine and chemokine production by bronchoalveolar macrophages in response to *Aspergillus* conidia. J Infect Dis 2003; 187:705–709 286.

285. Kamberi, M, Brummer, E, et al. Regulation of bronchoalveolar macrophage proinfiammatory cytokine production by dexamethasone and granulocyte-macrophage colony-stimulating factor after stimulation by *Aspergillus* conidia or lipopolysaccharide. Cytokine 2002; 19:14–20.

286. Brummer E, Maqbool A, et al. Protection of bronchoalveolar macrophages by granulocyte–macrophage colony-stimulating factor against dexamethasone suppression of fungicidal activity for *Aspergillus fumigatus* conidia. Med Mycol 2001; 39:509–515.

287. Brummer E, Maqbool A, et al. Protection of peritoneal macrophages by granulocyte/macrophage colony-stimulating factor (GM-CSF) against dexamethasone suppression of killing of *Aspergillus,* and the effect of human GM-CSF. Microbes Infect 2002; 4:133–138.

288. Abu Jawdeh L, Haidar R, et al. *Aspergillus* vertebral osteomyelitis in a child with a primary monocyte killing defect: response to GM-CSF therapy. J Infect 2000; 41:97–100.

289. Bodey GP. The potential role of granulocyte-macrophage colony stimulating factor in therapy of fungal infections: a commentary. Eur J Clin Microbiol Infect Dis 1994; 13:363–366.

290. Boots RJ, Paterson DL, et al. Successful treatment of post-influenza pseudomembranous necrotising bronchial aspergillosis with liposomal amphotericin, inhaled amphotericin B, gamma interferon and GM-CSF. Thorax 1999; 54:1047–1049.

291. Rowe JM, Andersen JW, et al. A randomized, placebo-controlled phase III study of granulocyte-macrophage colony-stimulating factor in adult patients (> 55 to 70 years of age) with acute myelogenous leukemia: a study of the Eastern Cooperative Oncology Group (E1490). Blood 1995; 86:457–462.

292. Bodey GP, Anaissie E, et al. Role of granulocyte macrophage colony-stimulating factor as adjuvant therapy for fungal infections in patients with cancer. Clin Infect Dis 1993; 17:705–707.

293. Gonzalez CE, Lyman CA, et al. Recombinant human macrophage colony-stimulating factor augments pulmonary host defences against *Aspergillus fumigatus* Cytokine 2001; 15:87–95.

294. Nemunaitis J, Meyers JD, et al. Phase I trial of recombinant human macrophage colony-stimulating factor (rhM-CSF) in patients with invasive fungal infections. Blood 1991; 78:907–913.

295. Albelda SM, Talbot GH, et al. Pulmonary cavitation and massive hemoptysis in invasive pulmonary aspergillosis. Influence of bone marrow recovery in patients with acute leukemia. Am Rev Respir Dis 1985; 131:115–120.

296. Groll A, Renz S, et al. Fatal haemoptysis associated with invasive pulmonary aspergillosis treated with high-dose amphotericin B and granulocyte–macrophage colony-stimulating factor (GM-CSF). Mycoses 1992; 35:67–75.

297. Roilides E, Dimitriadou-Georgiadu A, et al. Tumor necrosis factor alpha enhances antifungal activities of polymorphonuclear and mononuclear phagocytes against *Aspergillus fumigatus* Infect Immun 1998; 66:5999–6003.

298. Roilides E, Dignani MC, et al. The role of immunoreconstitution in the management of refractory opportunistic fungal infections. Med Mycol 1998; 36:12–25.
299. Roilides E, Blake C, et al. Granulocyte–macrophage colony-stimulating factor and interferon-gamma prevent dexamethasone-induced immunosuppression of antifungal monocyte activity against *Aspergillus fumigatus* hyphae. J Med Vet Mycol 1996; 34:63–69.
300. Mehrad B, Strieter RM, et al. Role of TNF-alpha in pulmonary host defense in murine invasive aspergillosis. J Immunol 1999; 162:1633–1640.
301. Schelenz S, Smith DA, et al. Cytokine and chemokine responses following pulmonary challenge with *Aspergillus fumigatus:* obligatory role of TNF-alpha and GM-CSF in neutrophil recruitment. Med Mycol 1999; 37:183–194.
302. Rodriguez-Adrian LJ, Grazziutti ML, et al. The potential role of cytokine therapy for fungal infections in patients with cancer: is recovery from neutropenia all that is needed? Clin Infect Dis 1998; 26:1270–1278.
303. Roilides E, Uhlig K, et al. Enhancement of oxidative response and damage caused by human neutrophils to *Aspergillus fumigatus* hyphae by granulocyte colony-stimulating factor and gamma interferon. Infect Immun 1993; 61:1185–1193.
304. Vora S, Chauhan S, et al. Activity of voriconazole combined with neutrophils or monocytes against *Aspergillus fumigatus:* Effects of granulocyte colony-stimulating factor and granulocyte–macrophage colony-stimulating factor. Antimicrob Agents Chemother 1998; 42:2299–2303.
305. Nagai H, Guo J, et al. Interferon-gamma and tumor necrosis factor-alpha protect mice from invasive aspergillosis. J Infect Dis 1995; 172:1554–1560.
306. Gaviria JM, van Burik JH, et al. Comparison of interferon-gamma, granulocyte colony-stimulating factor, and granulocyte-macrophage colony-stimulating factor for priming leukocyte-mediated hyphal damage of opportunistic fungal pathogens. J Infect Dis 1999; 179:1038–1041.
307. Rex JH, Bennett J, et al. In vivo interferon-gamma therapy augments the *in vitro* ability of chronic granulomatous disease neutrophils to damage *Aspergillus* hyphae. J Infect Dis 1991; 163:849–852.
308. Rex JH, Bennett JE, et al. Normal and deficient neutrophils can cooperate to damage *Aspergillus fumigatus* hyphae. J Infect Dis 1990; 162:523–529.
309. Group TICGDCS. A controlled trial of interferon gamma to prevent infection in chronic granulomatous disease. N Engl J Med 1991; 324:609–516.
310. Saulsbury FT. Successful treatment of *Aspergillus* brain abscess with itraconazole and interferon-gamma in a patient with chronic granulomatous disease. Clin Infect Dis 2001; 32:e137–e139.
311. Bernhisel-Broadbent J, Camargo EE, et al. Recombinant human interferon-gamma as adjunct therapy for *Aspergillus* infection in a patient with chronic granulomatous disease. J Infect Dis 1991; 163:908–911.
312. Graybill JR, Bocanegra R, et al. Granulocyte colony-stimulating factor and azole antifungal therapy in murine aspergillosis: Role of immune suppression. Antimicrob Agents Chemother 1998; 42:2467–2473.
313. Menzel Jr F, Jackson C, et al. Combination treatment of posaconazole and granulocyte colony-stimulating factor against *Aspergillus* in a mouse pulmonary infection model. Program and abstracts of the 42nd Interscience Conference on Antimicrobial Agents and Chemotherapy, San Diego, CA, 2002.(Abstract M-858. Washington, DC.).
314. Swerdlow B, Deresinski S. Development of *Aspergillus* sinusitis in a patient receiving amphotericin B. Am J Med 1984; 76:162–166.
315. Ozsahin H, von Planta M, et al. Successful treatment of invasive aspergillosis in chronic granulomatous disease by bone marrow transplantation, granulocyte colony-stimulating factor-mobilized granulocytes, and liposomal amphotericin B. Blood 1998; 92:2719–2724.

316. Bielori B, Toren A, et al. Successful treatment of invasive aspergillosis in chronic gran-
      ulomatous disease by granulocyte transfusions followed by peripheral blood stem cell
      transplantation. Bone Marrow Transplant 2000; 26:1025–1028.
317. Catalano L, Fontana R, et al. Combined treatment with amphotericin-B and granulo-
      cyte transfusion from G-CSF-stimulated donors in an aplastic patient with invasive
      aspergillosis undergoing bone marrow transplantation. Haematologia 1997; 82:71–72.
318. Dignani MC, Anaissie EJ, et al. Treatment of neutropenia-related fungal infections with
      granulocyte colony-stimulating factor-elicited white blood cell transfusions: a pilot
      study. Leukemia 1997; 11:1621–1630.
319. Peters C, Minkov M, et al. Leucocyte transfusions from rhG-CSF or prednisolone sti-
      mulated donors for treatment of severe infections in immunocompromised neutropenic
      patients. Br JHaematol 1999; 106:689–696.
320. Bhatia S, McCullough J, et al. Granulocyte transfusions: efficacy in treating fungal
      infections in neutropenic patients following bone marrow transplantation. Transfusion
      1994; 34:226–232.
321. Hubel K, Carter RA, et al. Granulocyte transfusion therapy for infections in candidates
      and recipients of HPC transplantation: a comparative analysis of feasibility and out-
      come for community donors versus rselated donors. Transfusion 2002; 42:1414–1421.

11

Endemic Mycoses Fungal Infections in Immunocompromised Patients

Robert W. Bradsher
Division of Infectious Diseases, University of Arkansas for Medical Sciences and Central Arkansas Veterans Health Care System, Little Rock, Arkansas, U.S.A.

I. INTRODUCTION

The epidemiology patterns of fungal infections are opportunistic and endemic. The opportunistic fungi include *Candida*, *Aspergillus*, *Fusarium*, and *Rhizopus* species. *Histoplasma*, *Blastomyces*, and *Coccidioidomyces* are the fungi more traditionally characterized as endemic fungi; these endemic mycoses may also be present in an opportunistic fashion in the immunocompromised patient. These three endemic organisms are acquired by inhalation of spores, which then transform into yeast phase at the body temperature and are found in distinctive geographical locales. However, the organisms considered as opportunistic fungi (*Aspergillus*, *Candida*, *Fusarium*, and *Rhizopus*) do not cause endemic or geographically localized diseases as they are ubiquitous throughout nature and found worldwide.

The epidemiology features, including the risk factors, for the endemic fungal infections tend to fall into geographical patterns. Persons with each of these fungi are likely to live in fairly remote parts of the world with specific ecologic and climatic conditions. However, with the frequency of national and international travel, patients may present with a fungus infection obtained in a remote location of the world; travel history is an essential part of the diagnostic evaluation. Likewise, certain job or recreation related activities might put a person at risk for these endemic fungi. The vast majority of persons infected with these fungi have adequate host defenses. Therefore, many of these infections will cause few or no symptoms at the time of infection, but may later reactivate to cause systemic disease as the person ages or if the human host becomes immune suppressed. The chapter gives a brief summary of the geographical niches for the three common endemic mycoses in the United States and reviews the historical and clinical aspects of these selected endemic fungal infections and two other endemic infections outside the United States.

A. Histoplasmosis

Histoplasma capsulatum is the cause of the endemic mycosis histoplasmosis and was first found as a cause of disease in humans by Darling in 1906 from autopsies in

Panama (1). This is of interest because further cases were not described in Panama for decades. The history of histoplasmosis shifted to the center of the United States where histoplasmosis is now recognized to be very common. As described by Sell (2), Nashville Tennessee became the focus for investigation of this fungus. In 1934, the blood smear from an infant was found have organisms that were similar to the description from Darling's original case. Cultures of specimen of bone marrow and blood from an autopsy revealed a fungus, *Histoplasma capsulatum*. Over the next several years, 70 or so cases of histoplasmosis were summarized in a review by Meleney (3); all were of the disseminated form and were uniformly fatal. A filtrate of the mycelial form of the fungus was used as a skin test to identify subclinical or asymptomatic cases of infection. This led to a pioneering article by Christie and Peterson in 1945 (4) that allowed greater understanding of interactions of fungi with human hosts. Children with pulmonary calcifications that had been thought to be because of tuberculosis were skin tested with Histoplasmin and found to have been infected with the fungus, even though they never had symptoms. Studies of military recruits and others subsequently confirmed that large numbers of normal persons are infected with *H. capsulatum* early in life, with resultant pulmonary calcifications but little or no clinical illness (5). These studies found that the majority of cases of histoplasmosis occur in the central section of the United States. However, there have been reports of cases throughout the eastern half of the United States and through-out Latin America (6). Infections have also been reported, albeit less commonly, in Asia, including Malaysia, Thailand, India, and Indonesia (6). There is also an African form of histoplasmosis (7). The organisms appear the same as in the mycelial form, but the yeast form is considerably larger. This strain is known as the *H. duboisii* form or large-form African histoplasmosis; a similar pattern of illness is seen in this African histoplasmosis form.

In the United States, there were estimates of 200,000 new cases of histoplasmo-sis per year in 1968 (8) that accounts for the 80–95 percent positive skin test rates for children in some highly endemic areas. In the presence of a depressed immune system, such as with HIV infection, corticosteroid therapy, organ transplantation, or, sometimes, for no obvious reason, progressive disseminated histoplasmosis may occur (6). In some endemic areas of the country, histoplasmosis is the most frequent opportunistic infection that leads to a diagnosis of AIDS.

The best, and perhaps the only, way to make a diagnosis of acute symptomatic pulmonary histoplasmosis, which is manifest with fever, chills, myalgia, dyspnea, and hypoxia, is to obtain a history of exposure (9). Careful attention should be placed to occupational or recreational exposure to bird droppings or bat guano, since either of these can act as a growth nutrient for *H. capsulatum* (6). Activities such as cutting down trees that had been known to be bird roosts, destroying chicken coops, which had remained unused for long periods of time, or spelunking in caves known to have large bat populations might prompt the consideration of histoplasmosis.

The vast majority of cases of histoplasmosis are asymptomatic and self-limited. The classification system used by Goodwin and Des Prez remains the most useful (6). In the normal host with a moderate to minimal exposure history, usual histoplasmo-sis was considered to be subclinical or asymptomatic in the vast majority of persons. Infection could either be from primary inoculation or could occur as reinfection with a subsequent exposure to the fungus, particularly, if continuous exposure did not occur in the endemic area. For example, those who left the endemic area for histoplasmosis for a number of years could develop a clinical or subclinical infection again upon return to the geographical areas in which *H. capsulatum* was found (6).

In normal hosts, acute pulmonary histoplasmosis with symptomatic disease manifest by fever, chills, myalgia, dyspnea, and hypoxia was described, but usually in patients with a significant exposure history. As with the asymptomatic form of the infection, the acute pulmonary histoplasmosis could be seen in both primary and reinfection scenarios (6).

Histoplasmosis was also described in the abnormal host. In those with excessive fibrotic response to the fungus, mediastinal fibrosis and retroperitoneal fibrosis were described (6). A solitary pulmonary nodule called a histoplasmoma can also be caused by excessive fibrosis, but with less severe manifestations of excessive scarring and collagen production than mediastinal fibrosis (6). In these cases, growth of the fungus is not considered to be the primary factor but the assumption is that too much fibrosis occur in response to the fungal antigens.

In other abnormal hosts, *H. capsulatum* can act as an opportunistic pathogen. In those with structural defects of the lung due to centrilobular or bullous emphysema, chronic pulmonary histoplasmosis may occur (6). Usually found in middle aged to older cigarette smokers, this condition consists of cavitary lesions on chest radiographs, symptoms of fever, and copious sputum production. Antifungal treatment can reduce symptoms and signs, but the relapse rate is high (6,9). It is thought that growth of the fungus is not as much of the problem as is the inability of host defenses to clear the organism because of the structural defects of the emphysema. Finally, in the abnormal host with cellular immune deficiency, progressive disseminated histoplasmosis may occur. Currently, the usual clinical setting for this severe and often fatal condition is HIV infection with depression of the CD_4 lymphocyte counts below 150–200/mm^3 (9). The clinical manifestations of histoplasmosis in AIDS patients have been extensively reviewed (10). Prior to the AIDS epidemic, patients with lymphoreticular neoplasms (e.g., Hodgkins disease), immunosuppressant chemotherapy (e.g., for organ transplantation or rheumatic diseases), sarcoidosis, or steroid-treated patients were the more commonly diagnosed with progressive disseminated histoplasmosis (6). Infection of the reticuloendothelial system with focal destructive granulomatous lesions in reaction to the hematogenously disseminated fungi accounts for the majority of signs in progressive disseminated histoplasmosis rather than findings in the lung (6). Bone marrow involvement is very common with thrombocytopenia, anemia, and/or leukopenia frequently found. Because of this localization, samples of bone marrow for culture and histology are appropriate methods of diagnosis of this condition. Symptoms and signs of fever, hepatosplenomegaly, and oropharyngeal or intestinal ulceration are commonly seen. Gastrointestinal bleeding in AIDS patients who reside or have resided in the *Histoplasma* endemic area should prompt a search for this fungus (9). Less commonly, Addison's disease, meningitis, or endocarditis may be diagnosed secondary to histoplasmosis (6).

The diagnosis of histoplasmosis has been reviewed extensively by Wheat (11). For cases of acute pulmonary histoplasmosis or the mild clinical cases of usual histoplasmosis, a history of exposure is essential to make the diagnosis. In the other manifestations, culture of clinical specimens is helpful and will generally take 2–3 weeks. Histopathology also allows a secure diagnosis with either Wright staining of bone marrow, peripheral blood smears, or Gomori methenamine silver stains of tissue specimens. Wheat has reported success in diagnosis of primary histoplasmosis, as well as relapse, with detection of *Histoplasma* polysaccharide antigen in the urine of infected individuals (12); commercial testing for this antigen is available. Even though skin testing with histoplasmin allowed understanding of the epidemiology of this infection, the usefulness of skin testing for diagnosis is low (11). In the endemic areas, skin tests simply mean prior infection and do not indicate if the histoplasmosis is responsible for the clinical signs and symptoms of the patient. The same is the case for *Histoplasma* serology. Both complement fixation and immuno-diffusion precipitin bands for antibodies have sufficiently high rates of both false-positivity and false-negativity to limit their usefulness (11). Positive serologic studies should prompt even greater efforts to locate tissue material for culture and histo-pathology.

Antifungal treatment of histoplasmosis has been summarized in guidelines from the Infectious Diseases Society of America (13). In asymptomatic primary (usual histoplasmosis) cases of histoplasmosis, treatment is not necessary. In acute pulmonary histoplasmosis, supportive care with supplemental oxygen and even ventilatory support may be more important than the specific antifungal therapy. Typically, in a severely ill patient with this diagnosis, amphotericin B is administered to a total of 500 mg dose over a period of 2–3 weeks in the adult patient; some recommend concomitant corticosteroids (6). Lipid formulations of Amphotericin B can be used in this setting as clinically indicated. After discharge from he hospital, itraconazole, 200 mg twice daily, should be used to complete a 6 months course. For patients who are not sufficiently ill to require hospitalization, itraconazole alone, 200 mg once or twice daily for 6 months could be used (13).

In progressive disseminated histoplasmosis, amphotericin B is considered the drug of choice for life-threatening infection, and after stabilization, followed by itra-conazole 200 mg twice daily for 6–18 months would be appropriate according to the immune status of the host and the speed of response to therapy. The first oral agent, ketoconazole, was associated with successful outcomes in those without AIDS (13) but ketoconazole was found to have an unacceptably high failure rate, both, for initial therapy and chronic suppressive therapy of this fungus in AIDS patients (9). Itraco-nazole has been effective in primary treatment of histoplasmosis in AIDS patients (13) as well as chronic suppression (13). In addition, in non-AIDS associated progres-sive disseminated histoplasmosis, itraconazole has been shown to be effective (13).

In chronic pulmonary histoplasmosis, itraconazole and amphotericin B have been shown to be effective although both have a relatively high relapse rate (13). An initial course of amphotericin B (0.7 mg/kg/d), followed by itraconazole 200 mg, twice daily for 12 to 24 months is suggested. Fluconazole has not been well studied in chronic pulmonary histoplasmosis but it does not appear to be as effective as itraconazole in AIDS patients; this agent or voriconazole might be considered in a patient who is unable to tolerate itraconazole (13).

For central nervous system disease, amphotericin B or liposomial amphotericin B ((Ambisome) 3 mg/kg/d) are recommended until stabilization, followed by fluco-nazole (800 mg/d) or voriconazole. Ambisome may achieve higher brain tissue levels than amphotericin B and it appears to have a better safety profile.

For granulomatous mediastinitis with obstruction, the treatment of choice is amphotericin B followed by itraconazole for 6–12 months for more severe disease. Although clinical trials have not been done, itraconazole alone is typically effective in moderate to mild disease.

1. Treatment of Special Populations

For pregnant women, amphotericin B is the drug of choice because of the potential of embryotoxicity of azoles. AIDS patients need suppressive therapy for life or until immune reconstitution after HAART (CD4 count sustained $\geq 200/\mu L$). Because of limited trials with azoles, children with severe disease might be best treated with amphotericin B (1 mg/kg/d for 40 days); itraconazole 200 mg/d for 6 months might be expected to be effective.

B. Blastomycosis

The first reported case of blastomycosis was by Gilchrist in 1894 with subsequent isolation of a fungus, *Blastomyces dermatitidis* (14). This dimorphic fungus has a characteristic geographic niche in a similar area as the endemic area for histoplasmosis, but perhaps a bit more restricted, and includes states surrounding the Mississippi and Ohio Rivers in the United States (15). The majority of cases have been reported from Arkansas, Kentucky, Mississippi, North Carolina, Tennessee, Louisiana, Illinois, Minnesota, and Wisconsin (15). Most are endemic or isolated infections, but a few epidemics of infection from point sources have also been described. Cases have also been reported in Canada in the provinces of Manitoba, Ontario, Alberta, and Saskatchewan (15). Blastomycosis has been described in Africa and in India, and extremely rarely from Israel, Lebanon, Saudi Arabia, and Mexico. There had been previous reports of blastomycosis in South America and Central America; most likely, these cases are of paracoccidioidomycosis, which were once known as South America blastomycosis. This terminology has been abandoned since it is preferable to use the term that identifies the infecting fungus, *Paracoccidioides brasiliensis,* and since the infection from *B. dermatitidis* has been documented to occur outside of North America (16).

The epidemiology of blastomycosis is not as fully characterized as that of histoplasmosis because there are no reliable skin test or in vitro markers of prior asymptomatic infection. Records of infection are dependent on clinical diagnosis. Some epidemiologic clues are noted. Occupational or recreational exposures that have been important in blastomycosis are ones that lead to contact with soil (16). Specifically, this includes fishing, hunting, farming, construction work, or other activities that involve disturbances of moist earth (15). In several of the epidemics of infection, soil near bodies of water was thought to be responsible (17–19). Therefore, exposure to outdoor activities is a frequent historical cause in patients with blastomycosis.

Infections with this fungus begin with inhalation of spores into the lung. If the organism escapes nonspecific host defense mechanisms, the fungus undergoes phase transition from mycelia to yeast cells with increased numbers in the parenchyma of the lung and spread to other organs through the bloodstream. With the development of immunity, inflammatory pyogranulomatous reactions occur at the initial pulmonary site and at the widespread foci of infection. The initial response to the fungus is suppurative followed by granuloma formation. This mixed neutrophilic and mononuclear cell response is distinctive of blastomycosis, although necrosis or fibrosis may also be found (16). Typically, the granuloma of blastomycosis does not caseate, as found in tuberculosis. Despite spontaneous resolution of the pneumonia in some cases, endogenous reactivation may occur at either pulmonary or extrapulmonary sites with or without previous therapy (15).

The clinical manifestations of blastomycosis are variable. Weight loss, fever, malaise, fatigue, and other nonspecific complaints are fairly common but offer little diagnostic help in blastomycosis. The typical patient is a young to middle-aged male who works or recreates outdoors. Apart from an epidemic, it is very rare for children to be diagnosed with blastomycosis (16). The male-to-female ratio has been reported from 4:1 to 15:1 in series of endemic cases (15). However, some of these studies were from Veterans Administration medical centers, which conspicuously add bias to the ratio.

Many patients with blastomycosis will have a delay in diagnosis since it is uncommon even in endemic areas and because the illness can mimic other disease processes. The different types of clinical presentations in pulmonary blastomycosis include acute pneumonia and chronic pneumonia. Patients with acute pneumonia may appear to have acute bacterial pneumonia with fever, chills, and a productive purulent cough with or without hemoptysis. Chronic pneumonia because blastomy-cosis exists 2–6 months prior to diagnosis with weight loss, night sweats, fever, cough with sputum production, and chest pain. Many such patients are thought to have malignancy or tuberculosis. A pulmonary infiltrate is the most common presentation of clinical blastomycosis with the majority of patients showing either an alveolar or mass-like infiltrate. Miliary or reticulonodular patterns are the next most frequent pattern. Although cavitary disease may occur, this pattern is not found commonly as in chronic pulmonary histoplasmosis or tuberculosis. Because of the mass lesions on chest roentenograms, many blastomycosis patients are initially thought to have lung cancer.

Skin lesions are the most common manifestation of extrapulmonary blastomy-cosis and almost always originate from dissemination from a lung focus, rather than from cutaneous inoculation. The skin typically has either verrucous or ulcera-tive lesions. The verrucous or fungating form is raised with a sharp but irregular border, that may suggest a diagnosis of cancer, unless specific examination for fungus is made with stains, such as Gomori's methenamine silver stain. Ulcers because of blastomycosis have the same histologic changes as the verrucous, form but are different in that the subcutaneous abscess has drained to the surface. The borders are heaped-up, and the base usually contains exudate. Osteomyelitis due to *B. dermatitidis* infection is reported in the vertebrae, pelvis, sacrum, skull, ribs, or long bones more commonly, but almost every bone has had involvement reported (16). The genitourinary system is next most likely in frequency of involvement, and because males are more likely to have extrapulmonary manifestations than females, prostatitis and epididymo-orchitis have been reported most commonly (15). Urine collected after prostatic massage will improve the detection of genitourinary involve-ment. Typically, as with skin or bone infection, the organism will cause concurrent presentations in the lung as well as the prostate or testicle; chest radiographs should be performed in every case of this infection to aid the diagnosis. Meningitis, or even more commonly, epidural or cranial abscesses are the manifestations of neurologic involvement of blastomycosis (15). Both may be difficult to diagnose, and require biopsy or evaluation of ventricular fluid for higher positive culture rates than lumbar spinal fluid. Lesions of blastomycosis have been reported to cause disease in virtually every organ. Widely disseminated or miliary blastomycosis may occur with adult respiratory distress syndrome (ARDS) as the presenting feature (20,21). The majority of patients, but not all, with this pattern of diffuse infiltrates, noncardiac pulmonary edema, and refractory hypoxemia die very quickly.

Immunocompromised patients have been reported with blastomycosis, includ-ing patients with AIDS and sarcoidosis, transplantation patients, and those being trea-ted with corticosteroids. This infection has not been frequently diagnosed in the cancer patient with neutropenia; cellular immunity is a more important host defense than leu-kocytes. A number of immunosuppressed patients with blastomycosis have been reported with an increased percentage of cases in the patient population from 1978 through 1991 as compared to the cases from 1956 through 1977 (22). Although this could have been from a bias in referral patterns of patients, the speculation was that this more likely reflected the continually enlarging population of patients with complicated immune compromising illnesses, who have lived in the endemic area of this fungus (22). A number of cases of adult respiratory distress syndrome were described in these immunocompromised hosts, as has been described with blastomycosis in AIDS patients (23). Although blastomycosis may cause infections in immunocompromised patients, other fungal infections such as progressive disseminated histoplasmosis or cryptococcal meningitis are more likely to be opportunistic than blastomycosis. Immunosuppressed patients are thought to develop infection following exposure in the environment or through subsequent reactivation, just like immunocompetent patients. Unlike similar fungi, *B. dermatitidis* has been reported a significant pathogen following infection with human immunodeficiency virus (HIV) in only a relatively small number of cases (23,24).

The diagnosis of blastomycosis is made by either seeing the fungus in tissue, exudates, or by growing the organism by culture. As with *H. capsulatum*, *B. dermatitidis* is relatively easy to detect in both smears and cultures and, since colonization does not occur, this discovery is reliable for a secure diagnosis (16). In addition to examinations of sputum by potassium hydroxide preparations, cytology preparations can be used for a dependable diagnosis. Cytology is commonly performed since blastomycosis often looks radiographically like carcinoma of the lung. Many cases will be diagnosed only after one or more invasive procedures such as bronchoscopy or open biopsy. Other diagnostic tests including complement fixation (CF) antibodies, immunodiffusion precipitin bands, and delayed hypersensitivity skin testing with blastomycin are, unfortunately, unreliable for diagnosis. Therefore, a serodiagnosis of blastomycosis is problematic owing to potential low sensitivity and low specificity rates. In the future, newer antibody detection systems may be useful, as might newly described antigens such as a surface protein of *B. dermatitidis,* which may allow more consistent detection of antibody in patients (15,25). Skin testing with blastomycin is, unfortunately, no better than serology as a diagnostic procedure. This mycelial phase antigen does not provide suitable specificity or sensitivity for reliable patient assessment, and blastomycin is no longer obtainable clinically. Until antigen testing is available for *B. dermatitidis*, as had been described for *H. capsulatum* (11), the diagnosis of blastomycosis will depend on visualization of the fungus on smear, in tissue, or in culture.

Antifungal therapy for blastomycosis has been summarized by the Infectious Diseases Society of America (26). The first consideration for the patient diagnosed with blastomycosis is whether or not to use an antifungal agent. Subclinical disease occurs with this infection just as with *H. capsulatum* and *Coccidioides immitis*. This approach of observation should be limited to mild pulmonary blastomycosis in the normal host. If the patient has deterioration or progression of the pneumonia, antifungal therapy should begin. The presence of pleural disease or any extrapulmonary manifestations during the course of illness means that antifungal treatment should be given.

IV amphotericin B in a dosage of at least 1.0 g resulted in cure without relapse in up to 90% of treated patients in various series (15) and a dosage of 2 g has been associated with cure rates of up to 97% (27). However, this high degree of antifungal activity of amphotericin B is associated with a relatively large amount of toxicity. In a group of patients with blastomycosis reported by Abernathy (27), almost three-fourths experienced a decline in renal function and a number of other toxicities were also reported including anemia, anorexia and nausea, fever, hypokalemia, and thrombophlebitis. Interruption of therapy during some point of the course was required in 41% of patients and termination of therapy with amphotericin B before reaching the desired amount was mandatory because of toxicity in 14% of the patients (27).

Azole antifungal agents have been used in blastomycosis; orally absorbed agents of ketoconazole, itraconazole, and fluconazole are generally well tolerated with itraconazole being the most useful for blastomycosis. Itraconazole is preferred to ketoconazole because of a high cure rate and lower rates of toxicity (26), particularly with regards to endocrine abnormalities associated with ketoconazole. Itraconazole is regarded as the primary oral agent (26).

There has been some experience in *B. dermatitidis* infections treated with fluconazole at doses of 200–800 mg per day (28). This agent, which is approved by the FDA only for cryptococcal infection and *Candida* infections, should not be considered equivalent to itraconazole for blastomycosis; it might be considered so when itraconazole is not tolerated, or in the case of central nervous system involvement when amphotericin B cannot be utilized. There have been no clinical trials of voriconazole in blastomycosis.

In the very ill and in the immunocompromised patient, amphotericin B remains the treatment of choice (26). For life-threatening disease, a cumulative dose of 1.5–2.5 g, is recommended. Lipid formulations of amphotericin B can be used in patients who cannot tolerate conventional amphotericin B. Itraconazole, at a dose of 200 mg twice daily for 6 months, should replace amphotericin B as therapy in compliant patients who do not have overwhelming or life-threatening blastomycosis, and to those who have had rapid response over 1–2 months to amphotericin B treatment (26). However, for a person with life-threatening manifestation of infection, such as the appearance of adult respiratory distress syndrome (ARDS), or the person with central nervous system involvement with blastomycosis, amphotericin B remains the treatment of choice.

In addition to antifungal therapy, surgery is indicated in some patients with large abscesses, empyema, bronchopleural fistula, bone debridement, or in cases of osteomyelitis that are poorly responsive to azole antifungal agents.

C. Coccidioidomycosis

Like histoplasmosis, coccidioidomycosis was described first in Latin America in the Southern Hemisphere. In 1891, a medical student named Alejandro Posadas working in the pathology laboratory of Robert Wernicke diagnosed a patient with an unusual skin tumor in Buenos Aires. In 1892, the patient's illness was described in Argentina (29) with Wernicke reporting the same case in Germany (30). Four years later, Rixford and Gilchrist reported the first North American case from a Portuguese immigrant patient in California (31,32). There is a rich history of the mycology and ecology of this fungus in the first three decades of the 20th century (33).

With a disease pattern like histoplasmosis, there are probably similar numbers of cases of coccidioidomycosis as histoplasmosis diagnosed annually in the United States (33). The majority of patients have minimal to mild disease with only 1% of infected persons developing progressive disease (33,34). Persons of Filipino or other Asian descent and African-Americans have a much greater risk of disseminated coccidioidomycosis (33,34). In addition, any immunosuppression, including the mild form of immunosuppression associated with pregnancy, will lead to an increased risk of dissemination (33).

Coccidioidomycosis occurs in the Lower Sonoran Life Zone (33). This corresponds to central California, Arizona, Nevada, Utah, Texas, and New Mexico. In Central America, Guatemala, Honduras and Mexico can possibly be endemic foci for this fungus. In South America, cases are diagnosed in Argentina, Paraguay, Bolivia, Venezuela, Uruguay, and Ecuador (33). These endemic areas for coccidioidomycosis have hot summers and mild winters, alkaline soil and little rainfall.

Exposure to dust, dirt, or disturbed soil in the endemic area raises the potential for infection;hence recreational or occupational risks exist for coccidioidomycosis. Construction workers, excavation workers, or military personnel have an increased propensity for infection (33,35). An earthquake in the late 1990s in Los Angeles led to increases in the cases (36). The potential of even larger number of new cases of coccidioidomycosis with increasing population movement into coccidioidomycosis endemic areas has been noted (37).

Like histoplasmosis, many patients infected with *C. immitis* have no clinical symptoms. The pneumonia that occurs may be associated with immunologic manifestations of erythema nodosa as well as fever, sweats, cough, and sputum production. Disseminated disease of coccidioidomycosis involves the skin and soft tissues, bones and joints, and the meninges. The disease is also more likely to be severe in immunocompromised patients. Typically, this would include those with altered T-lymphocyte function such as renal transplants or AIDS patients.

Diagnosis is made with either isolation of the fungus or by serology. Of the endemic fungi, coccidioidomycosis has the most reliable antibody testing for diagnosis. As with histoplasmosis, positive skin tests for fungal antigens of coccidioidomycosis are frequently found in children and adults. In the San Joaquin Valley, prevalence rates of 50–70% have been documented. Long-term exposure in these areas is not required for infection however. There are reports of infection far outside of the endemic area after having been exposed to dust from the coccidioidomycosis region (33). Persons may have only briefly visited an endemic area before returning home with their incubating infection (34).

Antifungal therapy for coccidioidomycosis has been summarized by the Infectious Diseases Society of America (38). This therapy is recommended for patients with severe forms of the disease and for patients with immunosuppression. More than 90% of acute episodes of coccidiodomycosis resolve without antifungal therapy. However, some authors recommend antifungal therapy for patients with symptomatic uncomplicated acute respiratory infection. A follow up of 1–2 years of these patients is recommended for the early identification of chronic pulmonary or extrapulmonary disease. The length of therapy ranges from 1 year to lifelong suppression in immunocompromised patients.

In the absence of immunosuppression, asymptomatic solitary pulmonary nodules do not require antifungal therapy or surgical resection. Asymptomatic pulmonary cavities may resolve with time. Resection may be indicated if the cavity is still detectable after 2 years, if it shows enlargement or if it is located adjacent to pleura, with risk of pyopneumothorax. Symptomatic or ruptured cavities usually will require surgical intervention and antifungal therapy.

Progressive or chronic pulmonary, disseminated and extrapulmonary disease require antifungal therapy and in, diagnosis of coccidiodomycosis during the 3rd trimester of pregnancy or immediately during the postpartum period. Antifungal agents for coccidioidomycosis include IV amphotericin B (0.5–0.7 mg/kg/d, fluconazole

(400–800 mg/d po or IV once daily), and itraconazole (200 mg po twice daily). Amphotericin B is the drug of choice for pregnant women and for patients with rapidly progressive or life-threatening disease, while azoles are used in cases of sub-acute or chronic presentations or after stabilization of more severe disease. In a recent randomized, double-blind trial that included 198 patients, fluconazole (400 mg/d) and itraconazole (200 mg twice daily) were comparable in efficacy for the treatment of progressive nonmeningeal coccidioidomycosis, although a trend toward greater efficacy with itraconazole was observed (39). Despite the availability of antifungal agents, relapse is frequent after discontinuation of therapy. In the above-mentioned trial, relapse rates occurred among 28% and 18% of patients randomized to flucona-zole and itraconazole, respectively.

For the treatment of meningeal disease, fluconazole is currently preferred in doses from 400–1000 mg/d. Itraconazole (400–600 mg/d) may also be effective. Patients who do not respond to azoles are candidates for intrathecal amphotericin B (0.01–1.5 mg, from daily to weekly dosing). Patients who respond to azoles should continue this treatment indefinitely. Hydrocephalus may develop regardless of the type therapy and does not necessarily indicate failure of antifungal therapy.

Newly available antifungal agents appear to be promising for the treatment of coccidioidomycosis. Voriconazole has been shown to be effective in a patient with meningeal disease refractory to fluconazole (40). Caspofungin and posaconazole appear to be active in experimental infections but no clinical data are available yet (41,42). Liposomal amphotericin B (Ambisome) was effective in a patient with disseminated disease who could not receive conventional amphotericin B (43). AmBisome has been shown to be more effective than conventional amphotericin B and fluconazole in an experimental model of coccidioidal meningeal disease in rabbits (44), and might be an attractive option for the treatment of meningeal disease when patients cannot tolerate conventional amphotericin B.

D. Paracoccidioidomycosis

Paracoccidioidomycosis is due to the fungus *Paracoccidioides brasiliensis* and is the only fungal infection geographically restricted to Latin America (45). Humans and armadillos are the only known susceptible hosts to natural infection (46). The pattern of infection is similar to that of histoplasmosis or coccidioidomycosis in that primary infection is thought to be pulmonary and is most commonly asymptomatic. Later in life, the previously asymptomatic infection can reactivate into systemic disease. In paracoccidioidomycosis, this usually occurs in middle-aged to older-aged adult males who present with either pneumonia, mucocutaneous lesions, or skin lesions (47).

Paracoccidioidomycosis has been diagnosed in patients in the United States, Canada, Europe, and Asia. However, some of these patients are individuals who had lived in Latin America at some point before the diagnosis (45). The endemic area for paracoccidioidomycosis ranges from Mexico to Argentina with the largest number of cases being reported from Brazil, followed by Venezuela, Colombia, and Ecuador (45). As with histoplasmosis and blastomycosis, there are probably hyperendemic sub-regions within these countries. The infection remains relatively rare even in endemic areas and why one individual develops disease from the infection while the next person does not is not clear.

There are gender differences in this infection. Children and young adults are unlikely to develop systemic disease. Skin tests with an antigen of *P. brasiliensis* (paracoccidioidin) have similar positive results of around 60–70% in normal healthy children and adults of both sexes (45). However, clinical disease is found almost exclusively in men. This may be secondary to hormonal differences relating to fungal growth, but the explanation is not fully understood (45).

Severe and progressive disease is known as subacute infection or juvenile form. The progressive adult form is more likely to be seen in older men with chronic disease (45). This is the only fungal infection that responds to sulfonamide therapy, although azole or amphotericin therapy is more reliable (45).

Since the infection may remain dormant with later activation and subsequent disease up to three to four decades after primary infection, the major way to make the diagnosis outside of Latin America is a history of travel or residence previously in Central or South America (45,47). Diagnosis is confirmed by observations of the characteristic numerous buds with the refractile cell wall of the fungal elements on KOH examination of sputum or pus, by culture, or by histologic examination of tissue.

Paracoccidioidomycosis can be a fatal disease if left untreated. Effective agents include the sulfa drugs, ampohotericin B, and the azoles. Treatment is usually very long and relapses are frequent. Sulfa drugs include sulfadiazine (4 g/d in 4 doses for adults) or trimethoprima-sulfamethoxazole (1 double strength tablet twice a day) among others. However, sulfa treatments require maintenance of 3–5 years to avoid relapse.

Currently, the drug of choice is itraconazole (100–200 mg/d) for 6 months. This therapy is associated with a response rate of 98% and a relapse rate of < 5% (48,49). Of note, although itraconazole can effectively control active disease, the pulmonary fibrosis present at the onset of treatment may not clear, and could even worsen, as fibrosis correlates with the severity of pulmonary infiltrates at diagnosis (50) *Amphotericin b* (0.7–1.5 mg/kg) is reserved for severe refractory disease (total dose 1.5–3 g). Initial amphotericin B treatment should be followed by maintenance with azoles or sulfas. This sequential therapy has been associated with a 75% response and 15–25% of relapse (48). Ketoconazole (200–400 mg/d) for 6 months is also ineffective, but is associated with a higher toxicity and relapse rate (11%) than itraconazole. Fluconazole is not recommended because of a very high relapse rate (50%) (48).

One randomized study compared itraconazole (50–100 mg/d) to ketoconazole (200–400 mg/d) and sulfadiazine (100–150 mg/kg/d up to 6g) for 4–6 months for the treatment of active paracoccidioidomycosis in 42 patients and failed to show superiority of any of these agents (51). However, the small sample size, the low dose of intraconazole use, and the lack of follow up represent serious limitations for this study.

Voriconazole is active in vitro against *P. brasiliensis* (52), but no clinical data exist to support its use. Terbinafine is an allylamine active in vitro against *P. brasiliensis* (53) and was effective, at a dose of 250 mg twice a day for 6 months, in a patient refractory to trimethoprima-sulphametoxazol (54).

E. Penicilliosis

The only dimorphic fungus of the genus *Penicillium* is *Penicillium marneffei*. This fungus has been described as a cause of systemic illness in HIV-infected individuals who resided in Southeast Asia and residents of southern China (55). The organism was first isolated in 1956 from bamboo rats in Vietnam (56). The first case in a human was described in 1959 after the author had accidentally inoculated the organism into his finger; he treated himself with oral nystatin successfully (56), but this agent has not been associated with cure subsequently. The next case was described by DiSalvo et al. (57) in a minister who had worked in Vietnam and later developed Hodgkin's disease requiring a splenectomy. The spleen grew *P. marneffei*. Prior to the surge in the HIV epidemic in Southeast Asia, penicilliosis was extremely uncommon. However, since 1988, the infection has been diagnosed much more frequently; Supparatpinyo et al. (58) report that 15–20% of all AIDS-related illnesses are due to this fungal infection. It is the third most common opportunistic infection in this patient group in Thailand following tuberculosis and cryptococcosis (60).

The organism grows as a mold at 25°C and as yeast at 37°C. Unlike *Histoplasma*, which divides by budding, *P. marneffei* divides by fission. The histology is similar to that seen in blastomycosis in that both suppuration and granulomatous changes in the tissue may be found in response to the fungus.

The majority of cases of penicilliosis in Thailand have been in males with the vast majority being immunosuppressed by HIV infection (55,59). In contrast, cases in southern China were reported in persons with normal immune systems (55). A handful of cases have been in persons from the USA or Europe, but all had exposure to Southeast Asia or China.

The manifestations of *P. marneffei* have been systemic illness with skin lesions, cough, lymphadenopathy, and weight loss (55,59). The disease has been considered to be very similar to the manifestations of histoplasmosis in HIV-infected individuals. Amphotericin has been associated with improvement, but relapse is common once the antibiotic is stopped; itraconazole as maintenance therapy has been successful in preventing relapse (61).

As with paracoccidioidomycosis, it is unlikely that a diagnosis of *P. marneffei* will be made in the Western world unless a careful history of exposure is obtained. Culture and/or histology would identify the organism once the diagnosis has been considered.

Disseminated penicilliosis is usually fatal if left untreated and the outcome is very poor when treatment is delayed. By contrast, timely and appropriate therapy are associated with a high survival rate. Relapses after the end of treatment are frequent among immunocompromised patients. Amphotericin B, itraconazole, and fluconazole have all been used for treatment of penicilliosis.

The current treatment for severe disease consists of amphotericin B (0.6 mg/kg/d) for 2 weeks, followed by itraconazole 200 mg twice a day for 10 weeks. This strategy was effective in 97% of 74 HIV positive patients with disseminated disease (61). For mild to moderate disease, itraconazole or ketoconazole is recommended.

Continued suppressive therapy is recommended in HIV-infected patients to prevent relapses (62). Primary prophylaxis with itraconazole 200 mg/d should also be considered for HIV infected patients, who live in endemic areas of penicilliosis especially if their CD4 is < 200 cells/μL.

II. SUMMARY

There are a number of systemic fungal infections that has a specific and characteristic geographic niche. Careful historical questioning may be the only means to make the diagnosis. Many of these endemic fungi will cause asymptomatic primary infection in a portion of the population that lives in the endemic area. Either at the time of primary infection or much later, the disease may progress with lymphohematogenous dissemination to various organs. Skin, nodes, bone marrow, lungs, or the central nervous system are the most common sites of progressive infection. Culture and histologic examination of tissue will confirm the diagnosis of fungal infection and treatment with either amphotericin B or an azole, such as itraconazole or fluconazole, may well cure the infection.

REFERENCES

1. Darling ST. A protozoon general infection producing pseudotubercles in the lungs and focal necroses in the liver, spleen and lymph nodes. JAMA 1906; 46:1283–1285.
2. Sell SH. Appreciation of histoplasmosis: the Vanderbilt story. South Med J 1989; 82: 238–242.
3. Meleney HE. Histoplasmosis (reticulo-endothelial cytomycosis): a review with mention of thirteen unpublished cases. Am J Trop Med 1940; 20:3–16.
4. Christie A, Peterson JC. Pulmonary calcification in negative reactors to tuberculin. Am J Public Health 1945; 35:1131–1147.
5. Edwards LB, Acquaviva FA, Livesay VT, Cross FW, Palmer CE. An atlas of sensitivity of tuberculin, PPD-B, and histoplasmin in the United States. Am Rev Respir Dis 1969; 99(4):1–132.
6. Goodwin RA Jr, Des Prez RM. Histoplasmosis. Am Rev Respir Dis 1978; 117:929–956.
7. Duncan JT. Tropical African histoplasmosis. Trans R Soc Trop Med Hyg 1958; 52: 468–474.
8. US National Communicable Disease Center: Morbidity and Mortality Weekly Report, Annual Supplement, Summary 1968, MMWR 1969; 7.
9. Bradsher RW. Histoplasmosis and blastomycosis. Clin Infect Dis 1996; 22(suppl 2): S102–S111.
10. Wheat LJ, Slama TG, Zeckel ML. Histoplasmosis in the acquired immune deficiency syndrome. Am J Med 1985; 78:203–210.
11. Wheat LJ. Diagnosis and management of histoplasmosis. Eur J Clin Microbiol Infect Dis 1989; 8:480–490.
12. Wheat LJ, Kohler RB, Tewari RP. Diagnosis of disseminated histoplasmosis by detection of *Histoplasma capsulatum* antigen in serum and urine specimens. N Engl J Med 1986; 314:83–88.
13. Wheat J, Sarosi G, McKinsey D, Hammill R, Bradsher R, Johnson P, Loyd J, Kauffman C. Treatment Guidelines for histoplasmosis for the Infectious Diseases Society of America. Clin Infect Dis 2000; 30:688–695.
14. Gilchrist TC, Stokes WR. A case of pseudo-lupus vulgaris caused by a *blastomyces*. J Exp Med 1898; 3:53–78.
15. Bradsher RW. Blastomycosis. Infect Dis Clin North Am 1988; 2:877–898.
16. Sarosi GA, Davies SF. Blastomycosis. Am Rev Respir Dis 1979; 120:911–938.
17. Klein BS, Vergeront JM, Weeks RJ, et al. Isolation of *Blastomyces dermatitidis* in soil associated with a large outbreak of blastomycosis in Wisconsin. N Engl J Med 1986; 314:529–534.
18. Klein BS, Vergeront JM, DiSalvo AF, Kaufman L, Davis JP. Two outbreaks of blastomycosis along rivers in Wisconsin: isolation of *Blastomyces dermatitidis* from riverbank soil and evidence of its transmission along waterways. Am Rev Respir Dis 1987; 136:1333–1338.
19. Dismukes WD. Blastomycosis: leave it to beaver. N Engl J Med 1986; 314:575–577.
20. Meyer KC, McManus EJ, Maki DG. Overwhelming pulmonary blastomycosis associated with the adult respiratory distress syndrome. N Engl J Med 1993; 329:1231–1236.

21. Evans ME, Haynes JB, Atkins JB, Atkinson JB, Delvaux TC Jr, Kaiser AB. *Blastomyces dermatitidis* and the adult respiratory distress syndrome. Am Rev Respir Dis 1982; 126:1099–1102.
22. Pappas PG, Threlkeld MG, Bedsole GD, Cleveland KO, Gelfand MS, Dismukes WE. Blastomycosis in immunocompromised patients. Medicine 1993; 72:311–325.
23. Pappas PG, Pottage JC, Powderly WG, et al. Blastomycosis in patients with the acquired immunodeficiency syndrome. Ann Intern Med 1992; 116:847–853.
24. Witzig RS, Hoadley DJ, Greer DL, Abriola KP, Hernandez RL. Blastomycosis and HIV. South Med J 1994; 87:715–719.
25. Klein BS, Jones JM. Isolation, purification, and radiolabeling of a novel 120-kD surface protein on Blastomyces dermatitidis yeasts to detect antibody in infected patients. J Clin Invest 1990; 85:152–161.
26. Chapman SE, Bradsher RW, Campbell GD, Pappas PG, Kauffman CA. Practice guidelines for the management of patients with blastomycosis. Clin Infect Dis 2000; 30:679–683.
27. Abernathy RS. Amphotericin therapy of North American blastomycosis. Antimicrob Agents Chemother 1967; 3:208–211.
28. Pappas PG, Bradsher RW, Kauffman CA, Cloud GA, Thomas CJ, Campbell GD Jr, Chapman SW, Newman C, Dismukes WE, and the National Institute of Allergy and Infectious Diseases Mycoses Study Group: Treatment of blastomycosis with higher doses of fluconazole. Clin Infect Dis 1997; 25:200–205.
29. Posadas A. Un nuevo caso de micosis fungiodea con psoiospermias. An Cir Med Argent 1892; 15:585–597.
30. Wernicke R. Ueber einen Protozoenbefund bei Mycosis fungoides. Zentralbl Bakeriol 1892; 12:859–861.
31. Rixford E. A case of protozoic dermatitis. Occidental M Times 1894; 8:704–707.
32. Rixford E, Gilchrist TC. Two cases of protozoan (coccidioidal) infection of the skin and other organs. Johns Hopkins Hosp Rep 1896; 1:209–268.
33. Drutz DJ, Catanzaro A. Coccidioidomycosis. Am Rev Respir Dis 1978; 117:559–585, 727–771.
34. Stevens DA. Coccidioidomycosis. N Engl J Med 1995; 332:1077–1082.
35. Standaert SM, Schaffner W, Galgiani JN, et al. Coccidioidomycosis among visitors to a *Coccidioides immitis* endemic area: an outbreak in a military reserve unit. J Infect Dis 1995; 171:1672–1675.
36. Schneider E, Hajjeh RA, Spiegel RA, et al. A coccidioidomycosis outbreak following the Northridge, California, earthquake. JAMA 1997; 277:904–908.
37. Galgiani JN. Coccidioidomycosis: a regional disease of national importance. Ann Intern Med 1999; 130:293–300.
38. Galgiani JN, et al. Practice guideline for the treatment of coccidioidomycosis. Infectious Diseases Society of America. Clin Infect Dis 2000; 30(4): 658–661.
39. Galgiani JN, et al. Comparison of oral fluconazole and itraconazole for progressive, nonmeningeal coccidioidomycosis. A randomized, double-blind trial. Mycoses Study Group. Ann Intern Med, 2000; 133(9):676–686.
40. Cortez KJ, Walsh TJ, Bennett JE. Successful treatment of coccidioidal meningitis with voriconazole. Clin Infect Dis 2003; 36(12):1619–1622.
41. Deresinski SC. Coccidioidomycosis: efficacy of new agents and future prospects. Curr Opin Infect Dis 2001; 14(6):693–696.
42. Gonzalez GM, et al. Correlation between antifungal susceptibilities of Coccidioides immitis in vitro and antifungal treatment with caspofungin in a mouse model. Antimicrob Agents Chemother 2001; 45(6):1854–1859.
43. Antony S, Dominguez DC, Sotelo E. Use of liposomal amphotericin B in the treatment of disseminated coccidioidomycosis. J Nat Med Assoc 2003; 95(10):982–985.
44. Clemons KV, et al. Efficacy of intravenous liposomal amphotericin B (AmBisome) against coccidioidal meningitis in rabbits. Antimicrob Agents Chemother 2002; 46(8):2420–2426.

45. Restrepo A. Paracoccidioides brasiliensis. In: Mandell GL, Douglas RG, Bennett JE, eds. Principles and Practice of Infectious Diseases. Philadelphia: Churchill Livingstone, 2000:2768–2772.

46. Gagagli E, Sano A, Coelho KI, et al. Isolation of *Paracoccidioides brasiliensis* from armadillo in an endemic area for paracoccidioidomycosis. Am J Trop Med Hyg 1998; 58: 505–512.

47. Manns BJ, Baylis BW, Urbanski SJ, Gibb AP, Rabin HR. Paracoccioidomycosis: case report and review. Clin Infect Dis 1996; 23:1026–1032.

48. Restrepo-Moreno, A. *Paracoccidiodomycosis.* In: Dismukes WE, Pappas PG, Sobel JD, eds. Clinical Mycology. New York: Oxford University Press, 2003:328–345.

49. Naranjo MS, et al. Treatment of paracoccidioidomycosis with itraconazole. J Med Vet Mycology 1990; 28(1):67–76.

50. Tobon AM, et al. Residual pulmonary abnormalities in adult patients with chronic paracoccidioidomycosis: prolonged follow-up after itraconazole therapy. Clin Infect Dis 2003; 37(7):898–904.

51. Shikanai-Yasuda MA, et al. Randomized trial with itraconazole, ketoconazole and sulfadiazine in paracoccidioidomycosis. Medical Mycology 2002; 40(4):411–417.

52. Kappe R, Antifungal activity of the new azole UK-109, 496 (voriconazole). Mycoses, 1999; 42:83–86.

53. Hahn RC, et al. In vitro comparison of activities of terbinafine and itraconazole against Paracoccidioides brasiliensis. J Clin Microb 2002; 40(8):2828–2831.

54. Ollague JM, de Zurita AM, Calero G. Paracoccidioidomycosis (South American blastomycosi successfully treated with terbinafine: first case report. Br J Dermatol 2000; 143(1):188–191.

55. Duong RA. Infection due to *Penicillium marneffei*, an emerging pathogen: review of 155 reported cases. Clin Infect Dis 1996; 23:125–130.

56. Segretain G. *Penicillium marneffei* n. sp., agent d'une mycose du systeme reticuloendothelial. Mycopathol Mycol Appl. 1959; 11:327–353.

57. DiSalvo AF, Fickling AM, Ajello L. Infection caused by *Penicillium marneffei*: Description of first natural infection in man. Am J Clin Pathol 1973; 59:259–263.

58. Supparatpinyo K, Sirisanthana T. New fungal infections in the Western Pacific. JAMA Southeast Asia 1994; 10(suppl 3):208–209.

59. Supparatpinyo K, Khamwan C, Baosoang V, Nelson KE, Sirisanthana T. Disseminated *Penicillium marneffei* infection in Southeast Asia. Lancet 1994; 344:110–113.

60. Supparatpinyo K, Perrieus J, Nelson KE, Sirisanthana T. A controlled trial of itraconazole to prevent relapse of *Penicillium marneffe* infection in patients infected with the human immunodeficiency virus. N Engl J Med 1998; 339:1739–1743.

61. Sirisanthana T, et al. Amphotericin B and itraconazole for treatment of disseminated Penicillium marneffei infection in human immunodeficiency virus-infected patients. Clin Infect Dis 1998; 26(5):1107–1110.

62. Supparatpinyo K, et al. A controlled trial of itraconazole to prevent relapse of Penicillium marneffei infection in patients infected with the human immunodeficiency virus. New Engl J Med 1998; 339(24):1739–1743.

12

Emerging Fungal Infections

Rhonda V. Fleming
Division of Infectious Diseases, Texas Tech University Health Sciences Center, El Paso, Texas, U.S.A.

Elias J. Anaissie
The University of Arkansas for Medical Sciences, Myeloma and Transplantation Research Center, Little Rock, Arkansas, U.S.A.

I. INTRODUCTION

An increased number of fungal pathogens are arising as a result of novel therapies in the field of oncology and transplantation. *Candida* spp. constitutes the fourth most common cause of nosocomial bloodstream infection (1). *Candida albicans* is by far the most common cause of candidemia, however, emerging antifungal resistance in non-*albicans* species has become a common problem in high-risk population. Parallel to the emergence of non-*albicans' Candida* infections, increasingly recognized pathogenic yeasts have emerged as a cause of invasive infections, which include *Trichosporon* species, *Malassezia* species, *Hansenula anomala,* and *Wangiella dermatitidis.*

Aspergillus fumigatus is the leading cause of pneumonia in hematopoietic transplant recipients. However, non-*Aspergillus* filamentous fungi now account for 27% of mold infections in transplant recipients (2). Characteristically, filamentous fungi including *Fusarium* spp., *Scedosporium* spp., *Acremonium* spp., and *Paecilomyces* species cause clinical infection that is indistinguishable from that of invasive aspergillosis and are associated with poorer outcome (3).

The increasing importance of these emerging pathogens mandates familiarity with the pathogenesis and options for therapeutic and preventive measures. The epidemiology, microbiology, clinical presentation, and treatment of these uncommon fungi is discussed in this review.

II. EMERGING YEASTS

A. *Trichosporon* species

1. Epidemiology

Trichosporon species are pathogenic yeasts that are known to colonize the normal human skin, as well as respiratory, gastrointestinal, and urinary tracts. *Trichosporon* infections are rare but have been associated with a wide spectrum of clinical manifestations, ranging from superficial involvement in immunocompetent patients to deep invasive and disseminated disease in immunosuppressed individuals (4,5). Superficial infection of hair shafts caused by *Trichosporon* is known as white piedra (6). White piedra presents as a soft white nodule on hairs in the axillae, scalp, and genital region. In contrast, a deep localized or disseminated infection is seen in immunocompromised patients. *Trichosporon* is also responsible for the summer-type hypersensitivity pneumonitis described in Japan (7–9). Risk factors for *Trichosporon* fungemia include acute leukemia, neutropenia, itraconazole prophylaxis, and the presence of a central venous catheter (10). The three most common portals of entry for *Trichosporon* infections are the respiratory tract, gastrointestinal tract, and skin (4,5,11).

2. Microbiology

Trichosporon is a yeast-like, rapid growing, and characteristically a producer of urease enzyme. On cornmeal tween agar, *Trichosporon* species are distinguished by the presence of hyphae, pseudohyphae, blastoconidia, and arthroconidia. All the clinical manifestations were previously attributed to *Trichosporon beigelii*; however, recent taxonomic revisions of the genus *Trichosporon* suggested that *T. beigelii* consists of 17 species with five varieties (12–15). The new taxonomy suggests that *T. asahii* and *T. mucoides* are associated with deep invasive infections, *T. asteroids* and *T. cutaneum* cause superficial infections, and *T. ovoides* and *T. inkin* cause white piedra of the scalp and pubic hair, respectively. *Trichosporon pullulans* has also been associated with invasive infection in immunocompromised hosts (10,16,17). *Trichosporon asahii,* a major cause of deep-seated trichosporonosis, is also associated with summer-type hypersensitivity pneumonitis (18).

3. Pathogenesis and Clinical Manifestations

Trichosporon expresses glucuronoxylomannan (GXM) in its cell wall that is antigenically and biochemically similar to GXM in *Cryptococcus neoformans* (19,20). This antigen may be detected in sera from patients with disseminated *Trichosporon* infection by the cryptococcal latex agglutination assay (21,22). The GXM-like polysaccharide antigen *of Trichosporon* was shown to inhibit phagocytosis by monocytes (20). Reduced phagocytic response and microbicidal activity may be attenuated by GXM-mediated immunosuppression (23). The clinical manifestation of invasive trichosporonosis is similar to that of disseminated candidiasis. Widespread infection occurs because of hematogenous dissemination resulting in azotemia, pulmonary infiltrates, characteristic chorioretinitis, and fungemia with septic shock. Multiple cutaneous lesions occur in 30% of patients with trichosporonosis (4). Characteristically, the skin lesions are described as purpuric papules and nodules with central necrosis or ulceration. Fungal cultures of cutaneous lesions yield *Trichosporon* in 90% of the cases (24). A chronic hepatic trichosporonosis following recovery from neutropenia is also described with *Trichosporon* (4,5,25).

4. Treatment

Disseminated trichosporonosis in neutropenic patients carries an unfavorable outcome, because *Trichosporon* is known to be resistant to the fungicidal effects of amphotericin B (11). Previous attempts to treat invasive trichosporonosis with amphotericin B were unsuccessful, reporting a mortality rate approaching 80% in cancer patients (5,10). A neutropenic rabbit model of disseminated trichosporonosis at the National Cancer Institute suggested better activity of the triazoles superior to that of amphotericin B against *Trichosporon* (11). Antifungal triazoles have demonstrated the best activity in clearing *Trichosporon* infection (26). In vitro data confirm superiority of triazoles compared with amphotericin B against *Trichosporon* infections (27). Fluconazole alone has been considered the best first line of therapy. The new triazoles voriconazole, posaconazole, and ravuconazole exhibit more activity in vitro against *Trichosporon* than fluconazole (27). Treatment relies on rapid diagnosis of trichosporonosis and differentiation from more common *Candida* species. Echinocandins have poor activity against *Trichosporon* (28,29) and should not be recommended for treatment.

B. *Wangiella dermatitidis*

1. *Epidemiology*

Wangiella dermatitidis (also known as *Exophiala dermatitidis*) is a black yeast that inhabits the soil and plants and has been mainly associated with infection of skin and subcutaneous tissue. *Wangiella dermatitidis* is an occasional agent of mycetoma and phaeohyphomycosis in humans; however, it has also been reported as the etiologic agent in cases of keratitis, otitis externa, peritonitis, endophthalmitis, and fungemia associated with central venous catheters. *Wangiella* is a neurotropic fungus and infections of the central nervous system have been reported predominantly in Asia (30,31). These infections occur in both immunocompetent and immunosuppressed patients; however, disseminated infections tend to occur in immunosuppressed patients. Environmental factors also play a role in the transmission of *Wangiella*. Epidemiologic data from an outbreak of *Wangiella* meningitis in patients receiving injectable steroids have recently been reported (32). In this outbreak, five patients receiving epidural or intra-articular injections of methylprednisolone that were prepared by an index pharmacy developed meningitis. Microbiologic cultures from unopened vials yielded isolates of *W. dermatitidis*.

2. *Microbiology*

Wangiella dermatitidis grows slowly on potato dextrose agar and displays black colonies from the front and reverse. Colonies are initially mucoid but after 3–4 weeks develop aerial hyphae. *Wangiella* is characterized by septate, brown hyphae, conidiophores, and yeast cells. Unlike *Exophiala species, W. dermatitidis* produces phialides but not annelids.

3. *Pathogenesis and Clinical Manifestations*

Wangiella is darkly pigmented because of melanin. The fungal pigments dihydroxyphenylalanine melanin and dihydroxynaphthalene melanin have recently been linked to virulence in some human pathogenic fungi. Although the function of melanin in human pathogenic fungi is not clearly defined, its role in protecting fungal cells has clearly been shown (33,34). In a murine model of disseminated *W. dermatitidis* infection, longer survival was demonstrated in the melanin-deficient mutant (35). The most common clinical manifestation of *Wangiella* is subcutaneous phaeohyphomycosis. The infection develops after traumatic implantation of the fungus through the skin. Dissemination is more commonly seen in immunocompromised patients.

4. Treatment

Treatment of *Wangiella* infections commonly involves amphotericin B and response to therapy is variable. Limited data are available on treatment, however, in vitro data suggest activity of amphotericin B, miconazole, terbinafine, itraconazole, posaconazole, voriconazole, and anidulafungin against *Wangiella* (36–38). Voriconazole exhibited higher antifungal activity in vitro when compared with itraconazole (39). In a murine model of disseminated *Wangiella* infections, posaconazole prolonged survival and significantly reduced brain *W. dermatitidis* counts (38). In vitro data suggest modest activity of the echinocandin anidulafungin against *W. dermatitidis* (37). Response to antifungal therapy in *Wangiella* infections depends on the extent of the infection. For localized infections, the treatment is variable, but generally a combination of both medical and surgical intervention is recommended (40). hi cases of fungemia, removal of central venous access, along with systemic antifungal therapy, remains the mainstay of treatment.

C. *Malassezia* species

1. Epidemiology

Malassezia are lipophilic yeasts that colonize the human skin and body surfaces. It has been shown that *Malassezia* colonize the skin as early as the neonatal period (41). Factors that predispose for *Malassezia* colonization in neonates differ from those factors that predispose to invasive infection. Pathogens of the genus *Malassezia* comprise seven known species including *Malassezia furfur* and *M. pachydermatis.* *Malassezia furfur* is the causative agent of *Pityriasis versicolor* and has also been implicated in seborrheic dermatitis and dandruff. It has also been recovered in blood cultures from newborns and adult patients receiving lipid-replacement therapy through central venous catheters (42,43). These infections are not associated with neutropenia. *Malassezia pachydermatis* is an emerging pathogen increasingly reported to cause infections in neonates, is also a recognized cause of canine, feline, and equine dermatitis, and may lead to zoonosis. *Malassezia pachydermatis* has been reported to spread from dogs to humans via the unwashed hands of a healthcare worker causing a nosocomial outbreak in a neonatal intensive care unit (44).

2. Microbiology

Malassezia species are lipophilic yeasts that comprise seven species involved in pathogenic disease, which include *M. furfur* and *M. pachydermatis.* Other lipid-requiring species, known as *M. furfur complex*, include *M. sympodialis, M. globosa, M. obtuse, M. restricta,* and *M. slooffiae.* Lipid dependency differentiates among *Malassezia* species; *M. furfur* is obligately lipophilic and requires long chain fatty acids for growth, but *M. pachydermatis* does not. Culture of *M. furfur* from blood is best achieved with isolator tubes and planting onto a solid medium supplemented with a lipid source (45). The laboratory diagnosis of *M. pachydermatis* can be complicated by the fact that this organism can be misidentified as *Candida lipolytica* by some conventional systems (46).

3. Pathogenesis and Clinical Manifestations

Exposure *of Malassezia* to lipid emulsions in parenteral hyperalimentation solution enhances growth of this organism. Hematogenous infection with multiple tissue invasions has been described in neonates. Massive lung involvement is characteristic. Fever is the predominant feature of *Malassezia* infection, but bradycardia, respiratory failure, thrombocytopenia, and catheter blockage have been described in several cases (47). In immunocompromised patients, the infection presents as folliculitis and catheter-related fungemia. Isolated folliculitis in neutropenic patients resembles the lesions of acute disseminated candidiasis. IV lipid infusion was not shown to be a risk factor for *M. pachydermatis* infection. The overall outcome for this infection is more favorable when compared with the infections of other uncommon fungi.

4. Treatment

Treatment of *Malassezia* fungemia requires prompt removal of IV central catheters and discontinuation of the fat emulsion therapy followed by systemic antifungal therapy (48). *Malassezia* species are usually susceptible to antifungal azoles but exhibit variable activity to amphotericin B and resistance to flucytosine (49). Recent reports suggest better in vitro activity of voriconazole compared with that of itraconazole and amphotericin B *against Malassezia* spp.(50). In vitro data demonstrate better activity of the new azoles voriconazole and albaconazole (ABC) against *Malassezia* species (51,52). The same reports demonstrated variable susceptibilities to terbinafine against *Malassezia* species. Strains of *M. furfur, M. globosa*, and *M. obtusa* were more tolerant to terbinafine.

D. *Pichia* species

1. Epidemiology

Pichia species belong to the ascomycetous class and are increasingly recognized as human pathogens. The genus *Pichia* has several species, but clinically important species include *P. anomala, P. guillermondii, P. norvegensis*, and *P. ohmeri*. Infections caused by *Pichia* are rare but have been increasingly reported among children and preterm neonates (53,54). Several outbreaks of *P. anomala* were reported especially from intensive care unit settings (54–57). Cross-transmission from healthcare worker hands was thought to contribute to the spread of the organism in one outbreak (54). Other risk factors identified included acute leukemia, use of broad-spectrum antibiotics, use of central venous catheters, endotracheal intubation, and high colonization rate with *P. anomala* (56,58).

2. Microbiology

Pichia anomala (formerly *H. anomala)* is a free-living environmental yeast, which grows well in a high-sugar containing medium. In the majority of cases, the organism presents in its teleomorphic form and less commonly in the anamorphic form of *C. pelliculosa.* Colony morphology of *Pichia* is similar to that of *Candida* species. Ascospores production is the distinctive feature that differentiates *Pichia* from *Candida* species.

3. Clinical Manifestations

The spectrum of disease ranges from asymptomatic fungemia to severe disseminated life-threatening infection. Fungemia is the most common manifestation of this infection, however, ventriculitis, endocarditis, pneumonia, lymphadenitis, and enteritis have also been described (53,55,56).

4. Treatment

Pichia anomala is susceptible to all currently by available antifungal agents, however, two cases of breakthrough fungemia have been described in patients receiving fluconazole (59). One study demonstrated comparable or higher activity of voriconazole against *P. anomala* compared with that of amphotericin B, fluconazole, and itraconazole (60). In contrast, other in vitro data have demonstrated resistance of P. *ohmeri* to fluconazole, itraconazole, and ketoconazole (61). There is a paucity of data regarding in vitro antifungal susceptibility *of Pichia* species to newly developed antifungals. Response rate because of *Pichia* fungemia is high when early therapy is instituted and central venous catheter is removed.

III. EMERGING FILAMENTOUS FUNGI

Hyalohyphomycosis is the term used for infections caused by colorless septate fungal hyphae (nondematiaceous) in infected tissue (Table 1). *Non-Aspergillus* filamentous fungi account now for 27% of mold infections in organ-transplant recipients (2). A similar increase was also reported among recipients of hematopoietic stem-cell transplants (62). These molds are likely to be associated with disseminated infection and poorer outcome, than is aspergillosis. These filamentous fungi including species of *Fusarium, Scedosporium, Acremonium,* and *Paecilomyces* cause clinical infection indistinguishable from that of invasive aspergillosis. A remarkable feature of some of these hyaline molds is the ability to cause fungemia and disseminate hematogenously causing numerous embolic skin lesions. In histologic sections, they appear as hyaline, septate, branching filamentous organisms that can mimic aspergillosis. Definitive identification in hyalohyphomycosis requires isolation of the fungal organism. Although hyaline hyphae represent the distinctive feature of the hyalohyphomycosis, it is the identification of conidia and phialides that makes the distinction of non-*Aspergillus* hyalohyphomycosis.

A. *Fusarium* species

1. Epidemiology

Fusarium species recently emerged as a cause of disseminated infections in neutropenic patients and those undergoing transplantation (62–65). *Fusarium* represents the second most common fungal pathogen, after *Aspergillus,* as the cause of life-threatening invasive infection in recipients of hematopoietic transplant. *Fusarium* is a ubiquitous fungus commonly found in soil, water, and plants, and is a well-recognized plant pathogen that may cause extensive crop destruction and contamination. *Fusarium* species are causative agents of superficial and localized infections in immunocompetent hosts and deep invasive or disseminated infections in severely immunocompromised hosts (64). Risk factors for invasive fusariosis include acute leukemia, hematopoietic transplant, neutropenia, and use of corticosteroids (63,66). Specific portals of entry are the respiratory tract and skin. Trauma constitutes the major predisposing factor for development of cutaneous infections caused by *Fusarium* in immunocompetent hosts (65). Similarly, the skin is predominantly the primary source of infection, especially in patients with onychomycosis.

Table 1 Overall Characteristics of Emerging Hyaline Fungi

Genus	Portal entry	Clinical presentation	Diagnosis	Treatment
Fusarium spp.	Skin, respiratory	Skin lesion, disseminated	Culture of blood, tissue	VRC
Acremonium spp.	Cutaneous, respiratory, gastrointestinal	Endophthalmitis, keratitis, disseminated	Culture of blood, tissue	VRC, surgery
Scedosporium spp.	Trauma, respiratory tract	CNS[a], subcutaneous, bone, disseminated	Culture of blood, tissue	VRC: *S. apiospermum* Surgery: *S. prolificans*
Paecilomyces spp.	Skin, respiratory tract	Localized and disseminated Peritonitis in CAPD	Culture of blood, tissue, sterile fluids	VRC: *P. lilacinus* AmB, VRC: *P. variotii* Surgery, catheter removal
Trichoderma spp.	Respiratory and gastrointestinal tract	Peritonitis in CAPD, localized, disseminated	Culture of blood, tissue, sterile fluids	Catheter removal Optimal anti fungal unclear
Zygomycetes	Percutaneous, respiratory tract	Rhinocerebral in DM, localized, disseminated	Tissue culture	Medical and surgical High-dose AmB

[a]Scedosporium in CNS seen in both immunocompetent and immunosuppressed hosts.
Abbreviations: VRC, voriconazole; AmB, amphotericin B; CNS, central nervous system; CAPD, continuous ambulatory peritoneal dialysis; DM, diabetes mellitus.

2. Microbiology

Fusarium species are septate filamentous fungi that produce conidiophores, phialides, macroconidia, and microconidia. In the early phase of growth where only microconidia are apparent, some *Fusarium* spp. may resemble *Acremonium* spp. In the later phases of growth, the more characteristic sickle-shaped multiseptate macroconidia are used in identifying the genus and species *of Fusarium*. Three species causing human disease are more commonly seen in the genera *Fusarium: F. solani*, *F. oxysporum*, and *F. moniliforme*. Molecular methods such as 28S rRNA gene sequencing may also be used for rapid identification of *Fusarium* to the species level (67).

3. Pathogenesis and Clinical Manifestations

Human fusariosis in immunocompetent patients results as a consequence of trauma, burn, or foreign body and include keratitis, onychomycosis, and occasionally cellulitis (68). In immunocompromised patients, inhalation of conidia of *Fusarium* through the respiratory tract after high-dose chemotherapy or transplantation may lead to sinopulmonary infection with subsequent hematogenous dissemination. Breakdown of the skin or trauma appears to be a common portal of entry, especially in the setting of onychomycosis with associated cellulitis (65). Similar to *Aspergillus*, this organism is highly angioinvasive and leads to tissue infarction in severely immunocompromised patients. In contrast, *Fusarium* continuously releases spores into the bloodstream and is frequently isolated from blood in disseminated infections. The pathogenesis of this phenomenon is caused by the occurrence in vivo of intravascular adventitious forms (69). The clinical picture resembles invasive aspergillosis characterized by fever unresponsive to broad-spectrum antibiotics, and nodular cutaneous lesions. Skin lesions occur in 70% of the infections and are commonly seen in extremities and occasionally in trunk and face (65). Evolution from painful subcutaneous lesions to erythematous induration followed by ecthyma gangrenosum-like necrotic lesion surrounded by a rim of erythema is characteristic of fusarial infection (64,65).

4. Treatment

The outcome of disseminated fusariosis in neutropenic patients remains poor despite aggressive antifungal therapy. Mortality rates for disseminated infection are variable and approach 100% in the absence of neutrophil recovery. A combined approach of surgical debridement, excision of localized infections (sinuses, eye, soft tissue, bone), and removal of infected intravascular catheters is required for patients with localized infections. Treatment options have been limited by the lack of activity of available antifungal agents against *Fusarium* spp., and higher doses of amphotericin B (1.0–1.5 mg/kg) or its lipid formulations (5 mg/kg/day) were required (70,71). The antifungal agents fluconazole and itraconazole are not active against *Fusarium* species. The new azoles voriconazole and posaconazole introduce a treatment option that demonstrates both in vitro and in vivo activity against some *Fusarium* spp. and represent a less toxic alternative to amphotericin B (72). New antifungal agents exhibit variable activity against *Fusarium* isolates depending on the species and rapid identification at the species level is required (50,60,73). There is no reported clinical or in vitro activity of caspofungin against *Fusarium* species.

B. *Acremonium* species

1. *Epidemiology*

Acremonium species are saprophytic filamentous fungi commonly isolated from the environment. Unlike other filamentous fungi, many cases of human disease occur in immunocompetent hosts. A reported outbreak involving four cases of *Acremonium* endophthalmitis was reported from an ambulatory surgery center where colonization of humidifier water in the ventilator system was thought to be the source of the infection (74). *Acremonium* is one of the causative agents of white mycetoma and usually presents after trauma. Keratomycosis caused by *Acremonium* usually develops in contact lens wearers. Invasive disease, however, is almost exclusively seen in immuno-compromised patients with neutropenia and transplantation (75,76).

2. *Microbiology*

The genus *Acremonium* (also known as *Cephalosporium*) contains 100 species, however, species implicated in human infections include *A. falcifome*, *A. kiliense*, *A. strictum*, and *A. recifei*. Recently, it was demonstrated by DNA sequence analysis that *A. strictum* displays a broad genetic polymorphism (77). Like other hyaline molds, septate colorless hyphae are found in tissue. Variation in the diameter of the hyphae and both 45° and 90° branching are usually present (69).

3. *Pathogenesis and Clinical Manifestations*

The respiratory and gastrointestinal tracts are considered portals of entry of deep infection caused by *Acremonium* species. Similar to *Fusarium* and *Paecilomyces* species, *Acremonium* can invade vascular structures resulting in thrombosis, tissue infarction, and necrosis. In vivo sporulation can occur facilitating dissemination and may explain the high rate of hematogenous disseminated cutaneous lesions, as well as positive blood cultures. The spectrum of invasive disease ranges from sinusitis, endophthalmitis, osteomyelitis, arthritis, peritonitis, pneumonia, meningitis, esophagitis, subcutaneous infections, and disseminated infections (75,76,78,79).

4. *Treatment*

Optimal treatment of invasive infections caused by *Acremonium* has not been established given the rarity of this disease. *Acremonium* species have little susceptibility to available antifungal agents; however, recent reports suggest higher in vitro activities of the new azoles and caspofungin against *Acremonium* (28,80). In vitro activity of amphotericin B against *Acremonium* is variable (75,81). Anecdotal cases of invasive infections suggested some benefit with the use of amphotericin B and surgical excision of the infected tissue. Successful treatment of *Acremonium strictum* pneumonia with posaconazole has recently been reported in a patient with leukemia who failed amphotericin B treatment (82), suggesting that the second-generation triazoles may be effective antifungals against *Acremonium* infections.

C. *Scedosporium* species

1. *Epidemiology*

Scedosporium species are common fungi found in soil and stagnant or polluted water that were previously associated with asymptomatic colonization and now have emerged as an important cause of deep infection in immunocompromised patients and accidentally injured people. Two medically significant species of *Scedosporium* include *S. apiospermum* (teleomorph: *Pseudallescheria boydii*) and *S. prolificans*. *Scedosporium apiospermum* is associated with three distinct clinical entities: mycetoma, deeply invasive infection known as pseudallescheriasis, and saprophytic colonization. Mycetoma, previously termed "Madura foot," is the most common manifestation in normal hosts, usually occurs after penetrating injury, and presents as tumor-like swelling with draining sinuses. It most commonly involves the lower extremities resulting in arthritis and osteomyelitis. Other manifestations include mycotic keratitis and nonmycetoma-like cutaneous and subcutaneous infections. Deeply invasive infection caused by *S. apiospermum* is usually seen in immunocompromised patients with the lung being the most frequent site of infection. Central nervous system infection is seen in both immunosuppressed and healthy population. Noninvasive colonization of the lower respiratory tract in patients with cystic fibrosis and bronchiectasis, as well as fungus-ball formation in preformed cavities, is similar to those seen with *Aspergillus* (83,84). *Scedosporium prolificans* causes localized infection usually restricted to bone and soft tissue in immunocompetent patients and causes deeply invasive infection in immunocompromised hosts (85,86). *Scedosporium prolificans* has been documented to cause disseminated infection exclusively in immunocompromised patients with neutropenia and after hematopoietic transplantation (87,88). The portal of entry in disseminated disease is by inhalation of conidia through the lungs and further hematogenous spread. Recent reports of nosocomial outbreaks of *S. prolificans* in hematology–oncology units have been reported (88,89). The organism was thought to be aerially transmitted in both outbreaks. Invasive deep infection caused by *S. prolificans* has also been reported among AIDS patients (90,91).

2. Microbiology

The anamorph genus *Scedosporium* contains two medically important pathogens: *S. apiospermum,* the asexual state of *P. boydii,* and *S. prolificans* (formerly *S. inflatum).* The species are distinguished by their terminal annelloconidia with an inflated base in *S. prolificans,* whereas those of *S. apiospermum* are cylindrical. In histologic sections, the genus *Scedosporium* appears as a septate hyaline mold that cannot be reliably distinguished from *Aspergillus* species or *Fusarium* species unless conidia are present (92). The sexual stage of *S. prolificans* is *Petriella* species.

3. Pathogenesis and Clinical Manifestations

Phagocytic host defenses against conidia of P. *boydii* depend upon monocytes and macrophages, whereas the defense against hyphae depends upon PMNs. In healthy individuals, localized infection result from penetrating trauma and dissemination is rarely seen. Only one fatal report of a healthy man with *S. apiospermum* osteomyelitis of the foot developed CNS infection and died (93). Mycetoma develops after trauma causing destruction of the muscle, tendons, and bone. A chronic infection with draining sinus tract is characteristic of mycetoma. Similar to invasive aspergillosis, the route of entry *of Scedosporium* spp. is through inhalation of conidia leading to sinopulmonary infection and subsequent hematogenous dissemination. The clinical hallmark of disseminated infection includes multiple skin lesions, characterized by cutaneous nodules with a tender eschar and surrounding erythema accompanied by neurologic symptoms suggestive of CNS involvement (83,87). Compared to

Aspergillus, Scedosporium maybe isolated from bloodstream with a reported rate of fungemia of 75% (87). Fever is a prominent feature that should prompt the performance of a CT scan of the chest that may demonstrate nonspecific bronchopneumonia, nodular densities, wedge-shape infiltrates, or halo sign. Like *Aspergillus,* a crescent sign may be evident in patients recovering from neutropenia. Disseminated infection is seen in both species *of Scedosporium.* CNS infection caused by *S. apiospermum* is clinically and pathologically indistinguishable from CNS aspergillosis. Frequently, it manifests as either multiple or solitary parenchymal brain abscesses; the majority of cases are fatal even when early and aggressive therapy is instituted. A recent review of CNS scedosporiosis identified medical immunosuppression and near-drowning as risk factors for the acquisition of CNS infection (94).

4. Treatment

Disseminated infections caused by *Scedosporium* spp. in immunocompromised patients often carry a poor outcome. Until recently, administration of high-dose amphotericin B has been the initial approach to the treatment of invasive pseudallescheriasis; however, response rate has been dismal in immunocompromised hosts. In vitro studies have shown amphotericin B and its lipid formulations to have poor activity on either *S. apiospermum* or *S. prolificans* (95). The echinocandins may have inhibitory in vitro activity against *S. apiospermum* (80,96), but fluconazole has no activity against *Scedosporium* species. Recent in vitro studies demonstrated superiority of voriconazole compared with other conventional antifungal agents, against *Scedosporium* spp.(97–99). The same studies demonstrated fungistatic but not fungicidal activity of voriconazole and itraconazole against *S. apiospermum.* The combination of the azoles voriconazole, itraconazole, and posaconazole with human PMN leukocytes exhibited synergy or additive effects against hyphae of *S. apiospermum* and *S. prolificans* in vitro (100). These data suggest that recovery of host defense is essential for treatment response. In vitro, *S. prolificans* is more resistant to treatment compared with *S. apiospermum* (97); this observation was confirmed with clinical experience. The overall response of voriconazole to *S. apiospermum* infection in pediatric patients with invasive scedosporiosis was 83%; however, patients with *S. prolificans* infection remained refractory to voriconazole monotherapy (101). In an immunocompetent rabbit model of invasive *S. prolificans* infection, the investigational azole ABC was superior to amphotericin B to reduce the tissue burden (102). Recent in vitro studies demonstrated that the combination of the antifungal allylamine terbinafine with azoles was synergistic against *S. prolificans* (103,104). In addition, there are increased number of anecdotal successes with the combination of voriconazole plus terbinafine as therapy against invasive *S. prolificans* (105,106). Surgical resection remains the only definite therapy for infection caused by *S. prolificans.*

D. *Paecilomyces* species

1. Epidemiology

Paecilomyces spp are saprophytic fungi that are distributed worldwide in soil, decaying plants, and food products. *Paecilomyces* spp. have been shown to survive well on commonly used fabrics and plastics and is frequently found as airborne contaminant in clinical specimens and resistant to most sterilizing techniques. Human infections caused by *Paecilomyces* are rare but devastating in immunocompromised patients with neutropenia. Human cases include cutaneous disease, onychomycosis, catheter-related fungemia, pneumonia, peritonitis, osteomyelitis, and prosthetic-valve endocarditis. Other infections reported in immunocompetent hosts include keratitis in contact lens wearers, skin infection, sinusitis, pneumonia, and rarely vaginitis. Several outbreaks have been attributed to *Paecilomyces* in the last two decades. The first surgical outbreak reported 13 cases of *P. lilacinus* endophthalmitis after insertion of intraocular lens that were manipulated with the same neutralizing solution (107). A nosocomial outbreak caused by *P. lilacinus* was also reported in two hematology–oncology units after administration of a contaminated skin lotion (108,109). Risk factors for invasive infection are neutropenia, use of corticosteroids, diabetes, and transplantation.

2. Microbiology

Paecilomyces is a genus of hyaline filamentous fungi closely related to *Penicillium*, from which it is distinguished by the characteristic of the phialides. There are two medically significant species of the genus *Paecilomyces* responsible for human disease: *P. variotii* and *P. lilacinus*. Both species differ morphologically, clinically, and in their in vitro susceptibility to antifungal therapy.

3. Pathogenesis and Clinical Manifestations

The portal of entry for this fungus includes respiratory tract, indwelling catheters, and the skin resulting in hematogenous dissemination. Similar to *Fusarium* and *Acremonium* species, the development of adventitious forms in tissue may explain its propensity for dissemination (69). Clinical manifestations of this infection are variable; in immunocompetent hosts, infections caused by *Paecilomyces* have been documented as keratitis associated with the use of contact lens, sporothrichosis-like skin infection, sinusitis, and lung abscess. In immunocompromised patients, disseminated disease has been reported, but other manifestations include onychomycosis, catheter-related fungemia, pneumonia, peritonitis, osteomyelitis, and prosthetic-valve endocarditis.

4. Treatment

All cases of infection caused by *Paecilomyces* should be identified to the species level. Previous studies have demonstrated that *P. variotii* and *P. lilacinus* show significant differences in their in vitro susceptibilities to the commonly used antifungals. *Paecilomyces variotii* is susceptible to amphotericin B and the azole antifungals including itraconazole and voriconazole (110), whereas *P. lilacinus* often shows variable resistance to amphotericin B, flucytosine, and the azole antifungals (111). However, voriconazole has recently been shown to have in vitro activity against *P. lilacinus* (112). Despite predicted resistance, high dosage of amphotericin B deoxycholate (1 mg/kg/day) with surgical intervention for localized disease has been recommended and remains a therapeutic option for *P. lilacinus* infection. The use of lipid formulations of amphotericin B (5 mg/kg/day) or voriconazole may allow for less toxic alternatives in primary therapy.

E. *Trichoderma* species

1. Epidemiology

Members of the genus *Trichoderma* are the main components of the soil micro flora, but they are also encountered in air. *Trichoderma* is a filamentous fungus that was previously regarded as nonpathogenic to humans and has emerged as an important fungal pathogen in immunocompromised patients and peritoneal dialysis patients. Twenty cases of *Trichoderma* infections in humans have been reported so far. The first report describes a case of *T. viride* isolated from a pulmonary mycetoma in a patient with chronic lung disease (113). Eight cases of peritonitis were documented in patients undergoing continuous ambulatory peritoneal dialysis by different species of *Trichoderma* (114–121). Four cases of disseminated infection by *Trichoderma* were reported in two patients receiving bone marrow transplant (122,123), one in a renal transplant (124), and one in a neutropenic patient with lymphoma (125). Other infections caused by *Trichoderma* include endocarditis, sinusitis, liver abscess, pneumonia, infected perihepatic hematoma, and skin infection (126–130).

2. Microbiology

Trichoderma is a filamentous fungus species, member of the class Hyphomycetes. *Trichoderma* species are rapid-growing organisms and form colonies that are initially smooth or translucent and later become floccose, forming concentric white and green rings. A characteristic sweet or "coconut" odor is produced by some species. Microscopically, it is characterized by smooth-walled hyaline, septate, and branched hyphae. Five species of the genus *Trichoderma* have been identified as human pathogens: *T. longibrachiatum*, *T. harzianum*, *T. koningii*, *T. pseudokoningii*, and *T. viride*. Teleomorphs *of Trichoderma* are species of the ascomycete genus *Hypocrea*.

3. Pathogenesis and Clinical Manifestations

The lack of pathogenicity of *Trichoderma* species in immunocompetent hosts was evident after the report of an inadvertent infusion of *T. viride* in a contaminated IV solution. This patient received a single dose of amphotericin B and remained well (131). Suggested portals of entry for *Trichoderma* infection include the respiratory and gastrointestinal tract, and skin. *Trichoderma* infections appear mainly in immunocompromised patients as nodular pulmonary infiltrates, peritonitis complicating peritoneal dialysis, localized cutaneous lesions, endocarditis, and disseminated infection.

4. Treatment

Most isolates of *Trichoderma* demonstrate resistance to fluconazole and flucytosine but found susceptible to and intermediate to amphotericin B, itraconazole, ketoconazole, and miconazole (124,130). In vitro, voriconazole showed better activity against *T. longibrachiatum* than amphotericin B and itraconazole (112). Likewise, good in vitro activity against species of *Trichoderma* was demonstrated with terbinafine and posaconazole (110,132). Although data are limited, the activity of two echinocandins' derivatives anidulafungin and caspofungin appears promising in vitro (80). Mortality associated with disseminated infection approaches 100%. Previous reports of *Trichoderma* infections associated favorable outcome when the administration of amphotericin B was coupled with surgical resection (127,130,133). Complete response after surgical drainage alone was reported in a liver-transplant recipient with *T. pseudokoningii* liver abscess (128). Favorable outcome of *Trichoderma* spp. peritonitis was associated with catheter removal (115,118,119). Surgical resection of localized infection is recommended whenever feasible.

F. Zygomycetes

There are two orders of Zygomycetes containing organisms that cause human disease: the Mucorales and Entomophthorales. The majority of human infections are caused by the Mucorales. *Rhizopus* spp. is the most common genera to cause human infection; however, other genera associated with human infection include *Mucor, Rhizomucor, Absidia, Apophysomyces, Saksenaea, Cunninghamella, Cokeromyces,* and *Syncephalastrum* species. Described herein are the most relevant characteristics of these organisms in immunocompromised hosts.

1. Epidemiology

Members of the class Zygomycetes are filamentous fungi found in soil, decaying fruit and vegetables, and old bread. Commonly, zygomycosis develops in patients with diabetic ketoacidosis, immunocompromised patients with neutropenia, and recipients of solid-organ or hematopoietic stem-cell transplant (134,135). Other populations at risk include high-risk newborns, burned patients, trauma, and patients receiving deferoxamine therapy. The major mode of transmission is presumed to be the inhalation route, however, percutaneous route of infection plays a significant role, particularly in surgery, trauma, burns, needle sticks, and tattooing. Apart from the risk incurred by cutaneous breakdown, burned wounds have the additional risk for zygomycosis because of the administration of sulfamylon cream and broad-spectrum antibiotics to prevent infections caused by *Pseudomonas aeruginosa.* The development of zygomycosis in areas of skin breakdown has been associated with a variety of environmental factors such as contaminated adhesive products, elastic bandages, and tongue depressors used in the hospital setting. Gastrointestinal zygomycosis occurs in the setting of diabetes mellitus or organ transplant.

2. Microbiology

The *Mucorales* grow rapidly and well on both fungal selective and nonselective media. Characteristically, in tissue sections, the Zygomycetes display wide, hyaline, aseptate hyphae in a setting of extensive necrosis. The width of the hyphae varies substantially and generally branches at 90°. Better recovery in culture media is obtained in minimally manipulated tissue placed onto the culture medium or baited with breads to promote mycelial growth (136).

3. Pathogenesis and Clinical Manifestations

Neutrophils constitute the major host defense mechanism against zygomycosis. Alteration in the number or quality of neutrophils, monocytes, or macrophages results in increased risk for invasive zygomycosis. Ketoacidosis plays an important role in predisposing diabetic patients to zygomycosis. Low serum pH impairs the phagocytic and chemotactic ability of neutrophils (137). The interaction between transferrin, iron molecules, and fungus has been associated as promoting fungal growth. Resembling invasive aspergillosis, Zygomycetes are angioinvasive resulting in thrombosed vessels and tissue necrosis. The clinical manifestations of disease have evolved from primarily rhinocerebral infection in diabetic patients to pulmonary and disseminated disease including gastrointestinal, subcutaneous, cutaneous, allergic disease, and even asymptomatic colonization.

Rhinocerebral infection represents one-third to one-half of all cases of zygomycosis. Following inhalation of fungal spores, the infection originates in the sinuses, resulting in sinus pain, drainage, and soft-tissue swelling. The disease becomes rapidly progressive with local extension including periorbital tissues. Extension into the mouth is manifested by necrotic ulceration in the hard palate. Involvement of the ethmoid sinuses may be associated with cavernous sinus thrombosis (138).

Pulmonary involvement occurs in severely neutropenic patients and manifests as solitary nodular, lobar or segmental, cavitary, and bronchopneumonic lesions. Angioinvasion may result in thrombosis of pulmonary vessels and subsequent pulmonary infarction. Cutaneous infection may result from primary inoculation or secondary to disseminated disease. The lesions appear red and indurated that often develop in black eschars. Extension to the subjacent bone and development of necrotizing fasciitis may result from cutaneous or subcutaneous zygomycosis.

4. Treatment

Disseminated zygomycosis carries a high-mortality rate despite antifungal therapy. A combined approach with medical and surgical treatment is required to obtain a favorable outcome. Medical therapy consists in correction of the immune status and antifungal therapy. High doses of amphotericin B remain the first-line therapy for most cases of zygomycosis. Lipid formulations of amphotericin B with or without the use of cytokines demonstrated activity in patients' refractory to therapy with amphotericin B (139,140). The currently available triazoles including voriconazole and the echinocandins are considered inactive when given as monotherapy. The combination of voriconazole and terbinafine demonstrated in vitro synergy against Zygomycetes in 44% of the isolates (141). The experimental azole posaconazole has shown in vitro activity in animal models and in some patients with refractory zygomycosis (142–144).

Surgical debridement is considered an integral part of treatment for localized disease. Surgical resection for localized pulmonary lesions improved survival compared with medical therapy alone (145).

IV. DEMATIACEOUS MOLDS

Dematiaceous fungi represent a group of heterogeneous fungal organisms characterized by the presence of pale brown to dark melanine-like pigment in their cell wall. Clinical entities related to dematiaceous fungi are chromoblastomycosis and phaeohyphomycosis. Black-grained mycetoma is also associated with dematiaceous fungi. The description of localized, subcutaneous infections caused by dematiaceous fungi is not described in this chapter. Focus is on the salient aspects of invasive disease in immunocompromised hosts.

1. Epidemiology

Darkly pigmented fungi are widely distributed in the environment and occasionally cause human infections. In the past two decades, there has been an increasing report of dematiaceous fungi as causative of invasive infection in patients with cancer and hematopoietic or organ transplant (2,146). Invasive disease has also been reported in patients with AIDS, diabetes, and chronic granulomatous disease and is increasingly reported in patients undergoing peritoneal dialysis. The number of dematiaceous molds that have been documented as agent of phaeohyphomycosis continues to increase. A recognized group of these organisms seems to be neurotropic, where they localize in the CNS causing one or multiple brain lesions. Dematiaceous fungi that are known to be neurotropic include *Cladophialophora bantiana*, *Wangiella* (*Exophiala*) *dermatitidis*, *Ramichloridium obovoideum*, *Xylohypha* (*Cladosporium*), *Fonsecaea pedrosoi*, *Chaetomium atrobrunneum*, and *Dactylaria* (*Ochrochonis*) *gallopavum*. In addition, *Bipolaris* spp. and *Exserohilum rostratum* most commonly cause sinusitis and invade the CNS via extension from the paranasal sinuses. Other fungal pathogens, known as etiologic agents of sinusitis, include *Curvularia* and *Alternaria* spp. In addition to causing invasive disease, these dark molds are also etiologic agents of allergic reactions manifested by sinusitis and pulmonary disease. In a recent prospective multicenter study of mycelial non-*Aspergillus* infections in organ transplant, phaeohyphomycosis represented 9.4% (5/53) of all the infections (2). Suggested portals of entry for phaeohyphomycosis include not only the direct inoculation by penetrating injury but also the inhalation route, ingestion of contaminated food or water, and breakdown of skin barrier with the use of vascular catheters. Although most of the pathogens have a worldwide distribution, *R. obovoideum* is a well-known cause of sinusitis and CNS infection in the Middle East.

2. Microbiology

Phaeohyphomycosis is characterized by dark-walled fungal elements consisting of yeast-like cells, pseudohyphae, and hyphae. Despite the dematiaceous nature of these fungi, the brown pigment is not always present (147). Some of them produce various amounts of melanin pigment in their cell walls under different conditions. In vivo, melanin production may be minimal and fungal elements appear colorless; however, in culture, increasing melanin production leads to darker pigmentation. In histologic sections, confirmation of the presence of dematiaceous mold can be achieved by using a melanin-specific stain as the Fontana–Mason stain (148).

3. Pathogenesis and Clinical Manifestations

Melanin plays an important role in evasion of host defense by dematiaceous molds. Melanins have attracted interest as virulence factors in fungi. Among the mechanisms proposed is quenching of oxidative metabolites, which reduces susceptibility to antifungal and enzymatic degradation (149,150). Unlike chromoblastomycosis and mycetoma, phaeohyphomycosis invades deep structures and elicits a variety of inflammatory responses. Subcutaneous phaeohyphomycosis usually presents as a single lesion, but multiple lesions have been occasionally described. The clinical manifestations of CNS disease commonly include headache, low-grade fever, and eventual development of focal neurologic signs. Patient may have no history of mold exposure, no obvious portals of entry, or distant dissemination. The clinical spectrum also includes sinusitis, pneumonia, ocular disease, arthritis, osteomyelitis, fungemia, endocarditis, peritonitis, and gastrointestinal disease. In the spectrum of sinus infection, *Bipolaris* or *Exserohilum* may occur as an allergic sinusitis or asthma. *Bipolaris hawaiiensis* is associated with a more aggressive behavior, frequently leading to bone erosion or tissue necrosis (151,152).

4. Treatment

Cerebral phaeohyphomycosis has a high degree of mortality requiring early and aggressive therapy. There are no trials that assess and compare the different strategies for the treatment of phaeohyphomycosis. Historically, early treatment with amphotericin B and complete surgical resection has been recommended until new alternatives are found. Treatment depends on the extent and location of the infection. Surgical excision is the first choice of treatment for subcutaneous and cutaneous phaeohyphomycosis resulting in cure in the majority of cases. The in vitro activity of amphotericin B, itraconazole, and voriconazole was demonstrated against 25 strains of dematiaceous fungi. Overall, the fungicidal activity of the three agents was similar, with the exception of decreased activity of the azoles against *B. spicifera* and *Dactylaria constricta* var. *gallopava* (112). Few clinical data are available with the use of echinocandins in the treatment of phaeohyphomycosis; however, micafungin demonstrated in vitro activity against the dematiaceous fungi *Cladosporium trichoides*, *E. spinifera*, *F. pedrosoi*, and *E. dermatitidis* (153). As a class, the antifungal triazoles may have superior activity against many dematiaceous molds and offer less toxic alternatives to amphotericin B. The duration of treatment has not been established; however, long-term therapy may prevent recurrences.

Whenever possible, surgical resection is recommended for lesions in other organs, coupled with systemic antifungal therapy. Reduction in immunosuppressive agents may be attempted if feasible.

V. *CRYPTOCOCCUS* SPP.

1. Epidemiology

Cryptococcosis is an infection caused by the encapsulated yeast-like fungus *C. neoformans*. Cryptococcal infections occur worldwide without any defined endemic areas, but the environmental distribution of the serotypes shows some differences. Antigenic specificity of the capsular polysaccharide defines four different serotypes of *C. neoformans*: A, B, C, and D. Serotype D constitutes the majority of clinical isolates of *C. neoformans* var. *neoformans*. In contrast, serotype A describes the newly recognized *C. neoformans* var. *grubii* (154). The overwhelming majority of isolates from serotypes A and D are recovered from AIDS patients. The less common serotypes B and C are classified as *C. neoformans* var. *gattii*. Accompanying the increase in cryptococcosis after the HIV epidemic is the recognition that non-*neoformans* *Cryptococcus* strains are now reported with increasing frequency. Focus in this section, is on the less common strains of *Cryptococcus* that cause human disease.

Cryptococcus neoformans var. *gattii* is largely restricted to tropical and subtropical areas where the infection occurs in otherwise healthy individuals. The only known environmental source of *C. neoformans* var. *gattii* is the river gum tree (*Eucalyptus camaldulensis*), as well as the forest red gum (*Eucalyptus tereticornis*), which grows in rural Australia. The role of Eucalyptus tree and the occurrence of human infections caused by *Cryptococcus* cannot be established. In a surveillance study of cryptococcosis in Australia, all the *C. neoformans* var. *gattii* infections occurred in healthy hosts (155). In the same study, meningitis was the commonest manifestation, and focal CNS and pulmonary lesions were found primarily in patients with *C. neoformans* var. *gattii*. Another study conducted in Taiwan (156) identified 21 (35.6%) cryptococcal infections caused by *C. neoformans* var. *gattii*. Infection tended to occur predominantly during the months of July and August.

Infections with cryptococci other than *C. neoformans* are rare; however, several cases of infections with non-*neoformans* species have been reported (Table 2). *Cryptococcus laurentii* has emerged as an important cause of fungemia in neutropenic patients and peritonitis in a setting of continuous ambulatory peritoneal dialysis.

Table 2 Non-*neoformans* Cryptococcal Human Infections Reported in the Literature

Species	Year	Patients	Clinical diagnosis	Treatment	Outcome	Reference
Cryptococcus. laurentii	2002	Ganglioneuroblastoma	Fungemia	AmB	Response	164
	2001	VLBW	Fungemia	AmB	Favorable	165
	1999	Cancer	Fungemia	FLC	Favorable	166
	1999	Cancer	Fungemia	AmB	Favorable	166
	1999	Cancer	Fungemia	Not stated	Death	166
	1998	AIDS	Meningitis	AmB	Favorable	167
	1998	VLBW	Fungemia	AmB+FC	Favorable	168
	1998	IVDU	Fungemia	FLU	Favorable	168
	1998	DM	Keratitis	AmB+FC	Enucleation	169
	1997	BMT	Fungemia	FLC	Favorable	170
	1995	Immunocompetent	Uveitis	FLC	Favorable	171
	1989	CAPD	Peritonitis	Cath removal	Favorable	172
	1989	CAPD	Peritonitis	AmB	Favorable	173
	1981	Dermatomyositis	Lung abscess	AmB	Favorable	174
	1977	Immunocompetent	Cutaneous	AmB	Favorable	175
Cryptococcus albidus	2004	HSCT, neutropenia	Fungemia	AmB,ITC	Favorable	176
	2004	Renal transplant	Disseminated	FLC	Favorable	177
	2000	Sezary syndrome	Cutaneous	FLC	Favorable	178
	1998	AIDS	Fungemia	AmB+FC	Death	167
	1998	ALL, neutropenia	Fungemia	AmB	Favorable	179
	1996	HIV	Fungemia	FLC	Death	180
	1993	Hemodialysis	Empyema	AmB	Favorable	181
	1987	Leukemia,	Fungemia	AmB+FC	Death	182
	1980	RA	Meningitis	AmB	Death	183
	1973	Immunocompetent	Meningitis	AmB	Favorable	184
	1972	Immunocompetent	Pneumonia	AmB	Favorable	185
Cryptococcus curvatus	1995	AIDS	Myeloradiculitis	AmB	Favorable	186
Cryptococcus luteolus	1955	Measles	Pneumonia	None	Favorable	187
Cryptococcus uniguttulatus	2001	SHA	Ventriculitis	AmB	Death	188

Abbreviations: ALL, acute lymphocytic leukemia; AmB, amphotericin B; BMT, bone marrow transplant; CAPD, continuous ambulatory peritoneal dialysis; DM, diabetes mellitus; FC, flucytosine; FLC, fluconazole; HIV, human immunodeficiency virus; HSCT, hematopoietic stem-cell transplant; IVDU, intravenous drug use; RA, rheumatoid arthritis; SHA, subarachnoid hemorrhage; VLBW, very low birth weight.

There are also reports on *C. albidus* sepsis and meningitis, *C. curvatus* myeloradiculitis, and *C. humicola* meningitis, all reported in immunosuppressed patients with AIDS or cancer.

2. Pathogenesis and Clinical Manifestations

The major virulence factors identified in *C. neoformans* and non-*neoformans* are capsule formation and melanin synthesis. However, those factors are less expressed in the non-*neoformans* species (157). There is a distinct characteristic between infections and *C. neoformans* variety. *Cryptococcus neoformans* var. *gattii* is common in immunocompetent hosts. Early manifestations of meningoencephalitis for both varieties include headache, nausea, unsteady gait, dementia, irritability, confusion, and blurred vision. When compared with *C. neoformans* var. *neoformans*, infections caused by var. *gattii* are associated with cerebral or pulmonary cryptococcomas, papilledema, high CSF, and serum cryptococcal antigen titers (158). Hypodense lesions and hydrocephalus are common radiologic findings in cranial CT in cases of meningitis caused by *C. neoformans* var. *gattii*, and CSF analysis consists of mild pleocytosis with elevated protein level (159).

3. Treatment

Most isolates of *C. neoformans* remain susceptible to amphotericin B, flucytosine, and fluconazole (160). The standard regimen of amphotericin B (0.7 mg/kg/day) in combination with flucytosine (100 mg/kg/day) for 2 weeks of induction followed by fluconazole (400 mg/d) for 8 weeks is recommended for both HIV-infected and healthy hosts with cryptococcal meningitis (161,162). Infections caused by *C. neoformans* var. *gattii* demonstrate slower response to antifungal therapy. Anecdotal reports suggested longer induction with amphotericin B combined with flucytosine for 2–7 months (159). Worse prognosis is usually associated with var. *gattii*. Neurologic sequela is often present despite prolonged amphotericin B therapy and intraventricular shunt. Ocular complications are common. Visual loss accompanies var. *gattii* infections in 50% of the cases (159,163) and is associated with optic atrophy following optic disc swelling. Limited data on in vitro susceptibilities of non-*neoformans* cryptococci demonstrate higher resistance to fluconazole and flucytosine of these species compared with *C. neoformans* var. *neoformans*.

VI. CONCLUSION

Infections caused by these newly recognized pathogens represent an increasing problem in the immunocompromised host. These infections are difficult to diagnose and can present to the clinicians caring for high-risk patients with a serious challenge. Because of the uncommon occurrence of these infections, clinical trials focusing on optimal antifungal therapy are almost impossible to perform, further complicating the choice of antifungal agent and the complete understanding of the role of adjunctive measures such as surgery, cytokines, etc. The recent availability of several new antifungal agents, some with promising in vitro and experimental activity against these pathogens, may result in an improved outcome.

REFERENCES

1. Pfaller MA, Diekema DJ, Jones RN, Sader HS, Fluit AC, Hollis RJ, Messer SA. International surveillance of bloodstream infections due to *Candida* species: frequency of occurrence and in vitro susceptibilities to fluconazole, ravueonazole, and voriconazole of isolates collected from 1997 through 1999 in the SENTRY antimicrobial surveillance program. J Clin Microbiol 2001; 39:3254–3259.

2. Husain S, Alexander BD, Munoz P, Avery RK, Houston S, Pruett T, Jacobs R, Dominguez EA, Tollemar JG, Baumgarten K, Yu CM, Wagener MM, Linden P, Kusne S, Singh N. Opportunistic mycelial fungal infections in organ transplant recipients: emerging importance of non-*Aspergillus* mycelial fungi. Clin Infect Dis 2003; 37:221–229.

3. Fleming RV, Walsh TJ, Anaissie EJ. Emerging and less common fungal pathogens. Infect Dis Clin North Am 2002; 16:915–933, vi–vii.

4. Walsh TJ. Trichosporonosis. Infect Dis Clin North Am 1989; 3:43–52.

5. Hoy J, Hsu KC, Rolston K, Hopfer RL, Luna M, Bodey GP. *Trichosporon beigelii* infection: a review. Rev Infect Dis 1986; 8:959–967.

6. Therizol-Ferly M, Kombila M, Gomez de Diaz M, Duong TH, Richard-Lenoble D. White piedra and *Trichosporon* species in equatorial Africa. I. History and clinical aspects: an analysis of 449 superficial inguinal specimens. Mycoses 1994; 37:249–253.

7. Nishiura Y, Nakagawa-Yoshida K, Suga M, Shinoda T, Gueho E, Ando M. Assignment and serotyping of *Trichosporon* species: the causative agents of summer-type hypersensitivity pneumonitis. J Med Vet Mycol 1997; 35:45–52.

8. Ando M, Arima K, Yoneda R, Tamura M. Japanese summer-type hypersensitivity pneumonitis. Geographic distribution, home environment, and clinical characteristics of 621 cases. Am Rev Respir Dis 1991; 144:765–769.

9. Ando M, Suga M, Nishiura Y, Miyajima M. Summer-type hypersensitivity pneumonitis. Intern Med 1995; 34:707–712.

10. Krcmery V Jr, Mateicka F, Kunova A, Spanik S, Gyarfas J, Sycova Z, Trupl J. Hematogenous trichosporonosis in cancer patients: report of 12 cases including 5 during prophylaxis with itraconazole. Support Care Cancer 1999; 7:39–43.

11. Walsh TJ, Lee JW, Melcher GP, Navarro E, Bacher J, Callender D, Reed KD, Wu T, Lopez-Berestein G, Pizzo P. Experimental *Trichosporon* infection in persistently granulocytopenic rabbits: implications for pathogenesis, diagnosis, and treatment of an emerging opportunistic mycosis. J Infect Dis 1992; 166:121–133.

12. Gueho E, de Hoog GS, Smith MT. Neotypification of the genus *Trichosporon*. Antonie Van Leeuwenhoek 1992; 61:285–288.

13. Gueho E, Smith MT, de Hoog GS, Billon-Grand G, Christen R, Batenburg-van der Vegte WH. Contributions to a revision of the genus *Trichosporon*. Antonie Van Leeuwenhoek 1992; 61:289–316.

14. Gueho E, Faergemann J, Lyman C, Anaissie EJ. *Malassezia* and *Trichosporon:* two emerging pathogenic basidiomycetous yeast-like fungi. J Med Vet Mycol 1994; 32 (suppl 1):367–378.

15. Kemker BJ, Lehmann PF, Lee JW, Walsh TJ. Distinction of deep versus superficial clinical and nonclinical isolates of *Trichosporon beigelii* by isoenzymes and restriction fragment length polymorphisms of rDNA generated by polymerase chain reaction. J Clin Microbiol 1991; 29:1677–1683.

16. Kunova A, Godal J, Sufliarsky J, Spanik S, Kollar T, Krcmery V Jr. Fatal *Trichosporon pullulans* breakthrough fungemia in cancer patients: report of three patients who failed on prophylaxis with itraconazole [letter]. Infection 1996; 24:273–274.

17. Moylett EH, Chinen J, Shearer WT. *Trichosporon pullulans* infection in 2 patients with chronic granulomatous disease: an emerging pathogen and review of the literature. J Allergy Clin Immunol 2003; 111:1370–1374.

18. Sugita T. Intraspecies diversity of *Trichosporon asahii* as the causative agent of opportunistic fungal infection and summer-type hypersensitivity pneumonitis. Nippon Ishinkin Gakkai Zasshi 2003; 44:7–12.

19. Melcher GP, Reed KD, Rinaldi MG, Lee JW, Pizzo PA, Walsh TJ. Demonstration of a cell wall antigen cross-reacting with cryptococcal polysaccharide in experimental disseminated trichosporonosis. J Clin Microbiol 1991; 29:192–196.

20. Lyman CA, Devi SJ, Nathanson J, Frasch CE, Pizzo PA, Walsh TJ. Detection and quantitation of the glucuronoxylomannan-like polysaccharide antigen from clinical and nonclinical isolates of *Trichosporon beigelii* and implications for pathogenicity. J Clin Microbiol 1995; 33:126–130.

21. McManus EJ, Bozdech MJ, Jones JM. Role of the latex agglutination test for cryptococcal antigen in diagnosing disseminated infections with *Trichosporon beigelii*. J Infect Dis 1985; 151:1167–1169.

22. McManus EJ, Jones JM. Detection of a *Trichosporon beigelii* antigen cross- reactive with *Cryptococcus neoformans* capsular polysaccharide in serum from a patient with disseminated *Trichosporon* infection. J Clin Microbiol 1985; 21:681–685.

23. Lyman CA, Garrett KF, Pizzo PA, Walsh TJ. Response of human polymorphonuclear leukocytes and monocytes to *Trichosporon beigelii*: host defense against an emerging opportunistic pathogen. J Infect Dis 1994; 170:1557–1565.

24. Nahass GT, Rosenberg SP, Leonardi CL, Penneys NS. Disseminated infection with *Trichosporon beigelii*. Report of a case and review of the cutaneous and histologic manifestations. ArchDermatol 1993; 129:1020–1023.

25. Walsh TJ, Newman KR, Moody M, Wharton RC, Wade JC. Trichosporonosis in patients with neoplastic disease. Medicine (Baltimore) 1986; 65:268–279.

26. Anaissie E, Gokaslan A, Hachem R, Rubin R, Griffin G, Robinson R, Sobel J, Bodey G. Azole therapy for trichosporonosis: clinical evaluation of eight patients, experimental therapy for murine infection, and review. Clin Infect Dis 1992; 15:781–787.

27. Paphitou NI, Ostrosky-Zeichner L, Paetznick VL, Rodriguez JR, Chen E, Rex JH. In vitro antifungal susceptibilities of *Trichosporon* species. Antimicrob Agents Chemother 2002; 46:1144–1146.

28. Espinel-Ingroff A. Comparison of in vitro activities of the new triazole SCH56592 and the echinocandins MK-0991 (L-743,872) and LY303366 against opportunistic filamentous and dimorphic fungi and yeasts. J Clin Microbiol 1998; 36:2950–2956.

29. Uchida K, Nishiyama Y, Yokota N, Yamaguchi H. In vitro antifungal activity of a novel lipopeptide antifungal agent, FK463, against various fungal pathogens. J Antibiot (Tokyo) 2000; 53:1175–1181.

30. Ajanee N, Alam M, Holmberg K, Khan J. Brain abscess caused by *Wangiella dermatitidis*: case report. Clin Infect Dis 1996; 23:197–198.

31. Matsumoto T, Matsuda T, McGinnis MR, Ajello L. Clinical and mycological spectra of *Wangiella dermatitidis* infections. Mycoses 1993; 36:145–155.

32. CDC. *Exophiala* infection from contaminated injectable steroids prepared by a compounding pharmacy—United States, July–November 2002. MMWR 2003;51(49): 1109–1112.

33. Langfelder K, Streibel M, Jahn B, Haase G, Brakhage AA. Biosynthesis of fungal melanins and their importance for human pathogenic fungi. Fungal Genet Biol 2003; 38:143–158.

34. Peltroche-Llacsahuanga H, Schnitzler N, Jentsch S, Platz A, De Hoog S, Schweizer KG, Haase G. Analyses of phagocytosis, evoked oxidative burst, and killing of black yeasts by human neutrophils: a tool for estimating their pathogenicity? Med Mycol 2003; 41:7–14.

35. Dixon DM, Polak A, Szaniszlo PJ. Pathogenicity and virulence of wild-type and melanin-deficient *Wangiella dermatitidis*. J Med Vet Mycol 1987; 25:97–106.

36. Meletiadis J, Meis JF, de Hoog GS, Verweij PE. In vitro susceptibilities of 11 clinical isolates of *Exophiala* species to six antifungal drugs. Mycoses 2000; 43:309–312.

37. Odabasi Z, Paetznick VL, Rodriguez JR, Chen E, Ostrosky-Zeichner L. In vitro activity of anidulafungin against selected clinically important mold isolates. Antimicrob Agents Chemother 2004; 48:1912–1915.
38. Graybill JR, Najvar LK, Johnson E, Bocanegra R, Loebenberg D. Posaconazole therapy of disseminated phaeohyphomycosis in a murine model. Antimicrob Agents Chemother 2004; 48:2288–2291.
39. McGinnis MR, Pasarell L, Sutton DA, Fothergill AW, Cooper CR Jr, Rinaldi MG. In vitro activity of voriconazole against selected fungi. Med Mycol 1998; 36:239–242.
40. Gold WL, Vellend H, Salit IE, Campbell IE, Summerbell R, Rinaldi M, Simor AE. Successful treatment of systemic and local infections due to *Exophiala* species. Clin Infect Dis 1994; 19:339–341.
41. Ashbee HR, Leek AK, Puntis JW, Parsons WJ, Evans EG. Skin colonization by *Malassezia* in neonates and infants. Infect Control Hosp Epidemiol 2002; 23:212–216.
42. Hruszkewycz V, Holtrop PC, Batton DG, Morden RS, Gibson P, Band JD. Complications associated with central venous catheters inserted in critically ill neonates. Infect Control Hosp Epidemiol 1991; 12:544–548.
43. Sizun J, Karangwa A, Giroux JD, Masure O, Simitzis AM, Alix D, De Parscau L. *Malassezia furfur*-related colonization and infection of central venous catheters. A prospective study in a pediatric intensive care unit. Intensive Care Med 1994; 20:496–499.
44. Chang HJ, Miller HL, Watkins N, Arduino MJ, Ashford DA, Midgley G, Aguero SM, Pinto-Powell R, von Reyn CF, Edwards W, McNeil MM, Jarvis WR. An epidemic of *Malassezia pachydermatis* in an intensive care nursery associated with colonization of health care workers' pet dogs. N Engl J Med 1998; 338:706–711.
45. Marcon MJ, Powell DA, Durrell DE. Methods for optimal recovery of *Malassezia furfur* from blood culture. J Clin Microbiol 1986; 24:696–700.
46. Larone D. Medically Important Fungi: A Guide to Identification. Washington, DC: ASM press, 1995.
47. Dankner WM, Spector SA, Fierer J, Davis CE. *Malassezia fungemia* in neonates and adults: complication of hyperalimentation. Rev Infect Dis 1987; 9:743–753.
48. Marcon MJ, Powell DA. Epidemiology, diagnosis, and management of *Malassezia furfur* systemic infection. Diagn Microbiol Infect Dis 1987; 7:161–175.
49. Marcon MJ, Durrell DE, Powell DA, Buesching WJ. In vitro activity of systemic antifungal agents against *Malassezia furfur*. Antimicrob Agents Chemother 1987; 31:951–953.
50. Ghannoum MA, Kuhn DM. Voriconazole—better chances for patients with invasive mycoses. Eur J Med Res 2002; 7:242–256.
51. Gupta AK, Kohli Y, Li A, Faergemann J, Summerbell RC. In vitro susceptibility of the seven *Malassezia* species to ketoconazole, voriconazole, itraconazole and terbinafine. Br J Dermatol 2000; 142:758–765.
52. Garau M, Pereiro M Jr, del Palacio A. In vitro susceptibilies of *Malassezia* species to a new triazole, albaconazole (UR-9825), and other antifungal compounds. Antimicrob Agents Chemother 2003; 47:2342–2344.
53. Murphy N, Buchanan CR, Damjanovic V, Whitaker R, Hart CA, Cooke RW. Infection and colonisation of neonates by *Hansenula anomala*. Lancet 1986; 1:291–293.
54. Chakrabarti A, Singh K, Narang A, Singhi S, Batra R, Rao KL, Ray P, Gopalan S, Das S, Gupta V, Gupta AK, Bose SM, McNeil MM. Outbreak of *Pichia anomala* infection in the pediatric service of a tertiary-care center in Northern India. J Clin Microbiol 2001; 39:1702–1706.
55. Kalenic S, Jandrlic M, Vegar V, Zuech N, Sekulic A, Mlinaric-Missoni E. *Hansenula anomala* outbreak at a surgical intensive care unit: a search for risk factors. Eur J Epidemiol 2001; 17:491–496.
56. Thuler LC, Faivichenco S, Velasco E, Martins CA, Nascimento CR, Castilho IA. Fungaemia caused by *Hansenula anomala*—an outbreak in a cancer hospital. Mycoses 1997; 40:193–196.

57. Aragao PA, Oshiro IC, Manrique El, Gomes CC, Matsuo LL, Leone C, Moretti-Branchini ML, Levin AS. *Pichia anomala* outbreak in a nursery: exogenous source? Pediatr Infect Dis J 2001; 20:843–848.

58. Haron E, Anaissie E, Dumphy F, McCredie K, Fainstein V. *Hansenula anomala* fungemia. Rev Infect Dis 1988; 10:1182–1186.

59. Krcmery V Jr, Oravcova E, Spanik S, Mrazova-Studena M, Trupl J, Kunova A, Stopkova-Grey K, Kukuckova E, Krupova I, Demitrovicova A, Kralovicova K. Nosocomial breakthrough fungaemia during antifungal prophylaxis or empirical antifungal therapy in 41 cancer patients receiving antineoplastic chemotherapy: analysis of aetiology risk factors and outcome. J Antimicrob Chemother 1998; 41:373–380.

60. Espinel-Ingroff A. In vitro activity of the new triazole voriconazole (UK-109,496) against opportunistic filamentous and dimorphic fungi and common and emerging yeast pathogens. J Clin Microbiol 1998; 36:198–202.

61. Garcia-Martos P, Dominguez I, Marin P, Garcia-Agudo R, Aoufi S, Mira J. Antifungal susceptibility of emerging yeast pathogens. Enferm Infecc Microbiol Clin 2001; 19: 249–256.

62. Marr KA, Carter RA, Crippa F, Wald A, Corey L. Epidemiology and outcome of mould infections in hematopoietic stem cell transplant recipients. Clin Infect Dis 2002; 34:909–917.

63. Anaissie E, Kantarjian H, Ro J, Hopfer R, Rolston K, Fainstein V, Bodey G. The emerging role of *Fusarium* infections in patients with cancer. Medicine (Baltimore) 1988; 67:77–83.

64. Boutati EI, Anaissie EJ. *Fusarium*, a significant emerging pathogen in patients with hematologic malignancy: ten years' experience at a cancer center and implications for management. Blood 1997; 90:999–1008.

65. Nucci M, Anaissie E. Cutaneous infection by *Fusarium* species in healthy and immunocompromised hosts: implications for diagnosis and management. Clin Infect Dis 2002; 35:909–920.

66. Nucci M, Anaissie EJ, Queiroz-Telles F, Martins CA, Trabasso P, Solza C, Mangini C, Simoes BP, Colombo AL, Vaz J, Levy CE, Costa S, Moreira VA, Oliveira JS, Paraguay N, Duboc G, Voltarelli JC, Maiolino A, Pasquini R, Souza CA. Outcome predictors of 84 patients with hematologic malignancies and *Fusarium* infection. Cancer 2003; 98:315–319.

67. Hennequin C, Abachin E, Symoens F, Lavarde V, Reboux G, Nolard N, Berche P. Identification of *Fusarium* species involved in human infections by 28S rRNA gene sequencing. J Clin Microbiol 1999; 37:3586–3589.

68. Dignani MC, Anaissie E. Human fusariosis. Clin Microbiol Infect 2004; 10(suppl 1):67–75.

69. Liu K, Howell DN, Perfect JR, Schell WA. Morphologic criteria for the preliminary identification of *Fusarium*, *Paecilomyces*, and *Acremonium* species by histopathology. Am J Clin Pathol 1998; 109:45–54.

70. Walsh TJ, Hiemenz JW, Seibel NL, Perfect JR, Horwith G, Lee L, Silber JL, DiNubile MJ, Reboli A, Bow E, Lister J, Anaissie EJ. Amphotericin B lipid complex for invasive fungal infections: analysis of safety and efficacy in 556 cases. Clin Infect Dis 1998; 26:1383–1396.

71. Walsh TJ, Goodman JL, Pappas P, Bekersky I, Buell DN, Roden M, Barrett J, Anaissie EJ. Safety, tolerance, and pharmacokinetics of high-dose liposomal amphotericin B (AmBisome) in patients infected with *Aspergillus* species and other filamentous fungi: maximum tolerated dose study. Antimicrob Agents Chemother 2001; 45: 3487–3496.

72. Perfect JR, Marr KA, Walsh TJ, Greenberg RN, DuPont B, de la Torre-Cisneros J, Just-Nubling G, Schlamm HT, Lutsar I, Espinel-Ingroff A, Johnson E. Voriconazole treatment for less-common, emerging, or refractory fungal infections. Clin.Infect Dis 2003; 36:1122–1131.

73. Gallagher JC, Dodds Ashley ES, Drew RH, Perfect JR. Antifungal pharmacotherapy for invasive mould infections. Expert Opin Pharmacother 2003; 4:147–164.

74. Fridkin SK, Kremer FB, Bland LA, Padhye A, McNeil MM, Jarvis WR. *Acremonium kiliense* endophthalmitis that occurred after cataract extraction in an ambulatory surgical center and was traced to an environmental reservoir. Clin Infect Dis 1996; 22: 222–227.

75. Fincher RM, Fisher JF, Lovell RD, Newman CL, Espinel-Ingroff A, Shadomy HJ. Infection due to the fungus *Acremonium* (*Cephalosporium*). Medicine (Baltimore) 1991; 70:398–409.

76. Krcmery V Jr, Kunova E, Jesenska Z, Trupl J, Spanik S, Mardiak J, Studena M, Kukuckova E. Invasive mold infections in cancer patients: 5 years' experience with *Aspergillus*, *Mucor*, *Fusarium* and *Acremonium* infections. Support Care Cancer 1996; 4:39–45.

77. Novicki TJ, LaFe K, Bui L, Bui U, Geise R, Marr K, Cookson BT. Genetic diversity among clinical isolates of *Acremonium strictum* determined during an investigation of a fatal mycosis. J Clin Microbiol 2003; 41:2623–2628.

78. Koc AN, Utas C, Oymak O, Sehmen E. Peritonitis due to *Acremonium strictum* in a patient on continuous ambulatory peritoneal dialysis [letter]. Nephron 1998; 79: 357–358.

79. Kouvousis N, Lazaros G, Christoforatou E, Defteros S, Petropoulou-Milona D, Lelekis M, Zacharoulis A. Pacemaker pocket infection due to *Acremonium* species. Pacing Clin Electrophysiol 2002; 25:378–379.

80. Pfaller MA, Marco F, Messer SA, Jones RN. In vitro activity of two echinocandin derivatives, LY303366 and MK-0991 (L-743,792), against clinical isolates of *Aspergillus*, *Fusarium*, *Rhizopus*, and other filamentous fungi. Diagn Microbiol Infect Dis 1998; 30:251–255.

81. Guarro J, Gams W, Pujol I, Gene J, review. *Acremonium* species: new emerging fungal opportunists—in vitro antifungal susceptibilities and review. Clin Infect Dis 1997; 25:1222–1229.

82. Herbrecht R, Letscher-Bru V, Fohrer C, Campos F, Natarajan-Ame S, Zamfir A, Waller J. *Acremonium strictum* pulmonary infection in a leukemic patient successfully treated with posaconazole after failure of amphotericin B. Eur J Clin Microbiol Infect Dis 2002; 21:814–817.

83. Castiglioni B, Sutton DA, Rinaldi MG, Fung J, Kusne S. *Pseudallescheria boydii* (Anamorph *Scedosporium apiospermum*). Infection in solid organ transplant recipients in a tertiary medical center and review of the literature. Medicine (Baltimore) 2002; 81:333–348.

84. Cimon B, Carrere J, Vinatier JF, Chazalette JP, Chabasse D, Bouchara JP. Clinical significance of *Scedosporium apiospermum* in patients with cystic fibrosis. Eur J Clin Microbiol Infect Dis 2000; 19:53–56.

85. Wood GM, McCormack JG, Muir DB, Ellis DH, Ridley MF, Pritchard R, Harrison M. Clinical features of human infection with *Scedosporium inflatum*. Clin Infect Dis 1992; 14:1027–1033.

86. Idigoras P, Perez-Trallero E, Pineiro L, Larruskain J, Lopez-Lopategui MC, Rodriguez N, Gonzalez JM. Disseminated infection and colonization by *Scedosporium prolificans*: a review of 18 cases, 1990–1999. Clin Infect Dis 2001; 32:E158–E165.

87. Berenguer J, Rodriguez-Tudela JL, Richard C, Alvarez M, Sanz MA, Gaztelurrutia L, Ayats J, Martinez-Suarez JV. Deep infections caused by *Scedosporium prolificans*. A report on 16 cases in Spain and a review of the literature. Scedosporium Prolificans Spanish Study Group. Medicine (Baltimore) 1997; 76:256–265.

88. Alvarez M, Lopez Ponga B, Rayon C, Garcia Gala J, Roson Porto MC, Gonzalez M, Martinez-Suarez JV, Rodriguez-Tudela JL. Nosocomial outbreak caused by *Scedosporium prolificans* (*inflatum*): four fatal cases in leukemic patients. J Clin Microbiol 1995; 33:3290–3295.

89. Guerrero A, Torres P, Duran MT, Ruiz-Diez B, Rosales M, Rodriguez-Tudela JL. Airborne outbreak of nosocomial *Scedosporium prolificans* infection. Lancet 2001; 357: 1267–1268.

90. Nenoff P, Gutz U, Tintelnot K, Bosse-Henck A, Mierzwa M, Hofmann J, Horn LC, Haustein UF. Disseminated mycosis due to *Scedosporium prolificans* in an AIDS patient with Burkitt lymphoma. Mycoses 1996; 39:461–465.

91. Hopwood V, Evans EG, Matthews J, Denning DW. *Scedosporium prolificans*, a multi-resistant fungus, from a U.K. AIDS patient. J Infect 1995; 30:153–155.

92. Tadros TS, Workowski KA, Siegel RJ, Hunter S, Schwartz DA. Pathology of hyalohyphomycosis caused by *Scedosporium apiospermum* (*Pseudallescheria boydii*): an emerging mycosis. Hum Pathol 1998; 29:1266–1272.

93. Horre R, Feil E, Stangel AP, Zhou H, Gilges S, Wohrmann A, de Hoog GS, Meis JF, Marklein G, Schaal KP. Scedosporiosis of the brain with fatal outcome after traumatization of the foot, case report. Mycoses 2000; 43(suppl 2):33–36.

94. Nesky MA, McDougal EC, Peacock JE Jr. *Pseudallescheria boydii* brain abscess successfully treated with voriconazole and surgical drainage: case report and literature review of central nervous system pseudallescheriasis. Clin Infect Dis 2000; 31:673–677.

95. Carrillo-Munoz AJ, Quindos G, Tur C, Ruesga M, Alonso R, del Valle O, Rodriguez V, Arevalo MP, Salgado J, Martin-Mazuelos E, Bornay-Llinares FJ, del Palacio A, Cuetara M, Gasser I, Hernandez-Molina JM, Peman J. Comparative in vitro antifungal activity of amphotericin B lipid complex, amphotericin B and fluconazole. Chemotherapy 2000; 46:235–244.

96. Del Poeta M, Schell WA, Perfect JR. In vitro antifungal activity of pneumocandin L-743,872 against a variety of clinically important molds. Antimicrob Agents Chemother 1997; 41:1835–1836.

97. Carrillo AJ, Guarro J. In vitro activities of four novel triazoles against *Scedosporium* spp. Antimicrob Agents Chemother 2001; 45:2151–2153.

98. Cuenca-Estrella M, Ruiz-Diez B, Martinez-Suarez JV, Monzon A, Rodriguez-Tudela JL. Comparative in-vitro activity of voriconazole (UK-109,496) and six other antifungal agents against clinical isolates of *Scedosporium prolificans* and *Scedosporium apiospermum*. J Antimicrob Chemother 1999; 43:149–151.

99. Radford SA, Johnson EM, Warnock DW. In vitro studies of activity of voriconazole (UK-109,496), a new triazole antifungal agent, against emerging and less-common mold pathogens. Antimicrob Agents Chemother 1997; 41:841–843.

100. Gil-Lamaignere C, Roilides E, Mosquera J, Maloukou A, Walsh TJ. Antifungal triazoles and polymorphonuclear leukocytes synergize to cause increased hyphal damage to *Scedosporium prolificans* and *Scedosporium apiospermum*. Antimicrob Agents Chemother 2002; 46:2234–2237.

101. Walsh TJ, Lutsar I, Driscoll T, Dupont B, Roden M, Ghahrarnani P, Hodges M, Groll AH, Perfect JR. Voriconazole in the treatment of aspergillosis, scedosporiosis and other invasive fungal infections in children. Pediatr Infect Dis J 2002; 21:240–248.

102. Capilla J, Yustes C, Mayayo E, Fernandez B, Ortoneda M, Pastor FJ, Guarro J. Efficacy of albaconazole (UR-9825) in treatment of disseminated *Scedosporium prolificans* infection in rabbits. Antimicrob Agents Chemother 2003; 47:1948–1951.

103. Meletiadis J, Mouton JW, Meis JF, Verweij PE. Combination chemotherapy for the treatment of invasive infections by *Scedosporium prolificans*. Clin Microbiol Infect 2000; 6:336–337.

104. Meletiadis J, Mouton JW, Meis JF, Verweij PE. In vitro drug interaction modeling of combinations of azoles with terbinafme against clinical *Scedosporium prolificans* isolates. Antimicrob Agents Chemother 2003; 47:106–117.

105. Gosbell IB, Toumasatos V, Yong J, Kuo RS, Ellis DH, Perrie RC. Cure of orthopaedic infection with *Scedosporium prolificans*, using voriconazole plus terbinafine, without the need for radical surgery. Mycoses 2003; 46:233–236.

106. Howden BP, Slavin MA, Schwarer AP, Mijch AM. Successful control of disseminated *Scedosporium prolificans* infection with a combination of voriconazole and terbinafine. Eur J Clin Microbiol Infect Dis 2003; 22:111–113.

107. Pettit TH, Olson RJ, Foos RY, Martin WJ. Fungal endophthalmitis following intraocular lens implantation. A surgical epidemic. Arch Ophthalmol 1980; 98:1025–1039.

108. Itin PH, Frei R, Lautenschlager S, Buechner SA, Surber C, Gratwohl A, Widmer AF. Cutaneous manifestations of *Paecilomyces lilacinus* infection induced by a contaminated skin lotion in patients who are severely immuno suppressed. J Am Acad Dermatol 1998; 39:401–409.

109. Orth B, Frei R, Itin PH, Rinaldi MG, Speck B, Gratwohl A, Widmer AF. Outbreak of invasive mycoses caused by *Paecilomyces lilacinus* from a contaminated skin lotion. Ann Intern Med 1996; 125:799–806.

110. Garcia-Effron G, Gomez-Lopez A, Mellado E, Monzon A, Rodriguez-Tudela JL, Cuenca-Estrella M. In vitro activity of terbinafine against medically important non-dermatophyte species of filamentous fungi. J Antimicrob Chemother 2004; 53:1086–1089.

111. Aguilar C, Pujol I, Sala J, Guarro J. Antifungal susceptibilities of *Paecilomyces* species. Antimicrob Agents Chemother 1998; 42:1601–1604.

112. Espinel-Ingroff A. In vitro fungicidal activities of voriconazole, itraconazole, and amphotericin B against opportunistic moniliaceous and dematiaceous fungi. J Clin Microbiol 2001; 39:954–958.

113. Escudero Gil MR, Pino Corral E, Munoz Munoz R. Pulmonary mycoma cause by *Trichoderma viride*. Acta Dermosifiliogr 1976; 67:673–680.

114. Esel D, Koc AN, Utas C, Karaca N, Bozdemir N. Fatal peritonitis due to *Trichoderma* sp. in a patient undergoing continuous ambulatory peritoneal dialysis. Mycoses 2003; 46:71–73.

115. Bren A. Fungal peritonitis in patients on continuous ambulatory peritoneal dialysis. Eur J Clin Microbiol Infect Dis 1998; 17:839–843.

116. Guiserix J, Ramdane M, Finielz P, Michault A, Rajaonarivelo P. *Trichoderma harzianum* peritonitis in peritoneal dialysis [letter]. Nephron 1996; 74:473–474.

117. Loeppky CB, Sprouse RF, Carlson TV, Everett ED. *Trichoderma viride* peritonitis. South Med J 1983; 76:798–799.

118. Rota S, Marchesi D, Farina C, de Bievre C. *Trichoderma pseudokoningii* peritonitis in automated peritoneal dialysis patient successfully treated by early catheter removal [letter]. Perit Dial Int 2000; 20:91–93.

119. Ragnaud JM, Marceau C, Roche-Bezian MC, Wone C. Infection peritoneale a *Trichoderma koningii* sur dialyse peritoneale continue ambulatorie. Med Malad Infect 1984; 7:402–405.

120. Campos-Herrero M, Bordes A, Perera A, Ruiz M, Fernandez A. *Trichoderma koningii* peritonitis in a patient undergoing peritoneal dialysis. Clin Microbiol Newslett 1996; 18:150–152.

121. Tanis BC, van der Pijl H, van Ogtrop ML, Kibbelaar RE, Chang PC. Fatal fungal peritonitis by *Trichoderma longibrachiatum* complicating peritoneal dialysis. Nephrol Dial Transplant 1995; 10:114–116.

122. Richter S, Cormican MG, Pfaller MA, Lee CK, Gingrich R, Rinaldi MG, Sutton DA. Fatal disseminated *Trichoderma longibrachiatum* infection in an adult bone marrow transplant patient: species identification and review of the literature. J Clin Microbiol 1999; 37:1154–1160.

123. Gautheret A, Dromer F, Bourhis JH, Andremont A. *Trichoderma pseudokoningii* as a cause of fatal infection in a bone marrow transplant recipient [letter]. Clin Infect Dis 1995; 20:1063–1064.

124. Guarro J, Antolin-Ayala MI, Gene J, Gutierrez-Calzada J, Nieves-Diez C, Ortoneda M. Fatal case of *Trichoderma harzianum* infection in a renal transplant recipient. J Clin Microbiol 1999; 37:3751–3755.

125. Myoken Y, Sugata T, Fujita Y, Asaoku H, Fujihara M, Mikami Y. Fatal necrotizing stomatitis due to *Trichoderma longibrachiatum* in a neutropenic patient with malignant lymphoma: a case report. Int J Oral Maxillofac Surg 2002; 31:688–691.

126. Bustamante-Labarta MH, Caramutti V, Allende GN, Weinschelbaum E, Torino AF. Unsuspected embolic fungal endocarditis of an aortic conduit diagnosed by transesophageal echocardiography. J Am Soc Echocardiogr 2000; 13:953–954.

127. Furukawa H, Kusne S, Sutton DA, Manez R, Carrau R, Nichols L, Abu-Elmagd K, Skedros D, Todo S, Rinaldi MG. Acute invasive sinusitis due to *Trichoderma longibrachiatum* in a liver and small bowel transplant recipient. Clin Infect Dis 1998; 26:487–489.

128. Chouaki T, Lavarde V, Lachaud L, Raccurt CP, Hennequin C. Invasive infections due to *Trichoderma* species: report of 2 cases, findings of in vitro susceptibility testing, and review of the literature. Clin Infect Dis 2002; 35:1360–1367.

129. Jacobs F, Byl B, Bourgeois N, Coremans-Pelseneer J, Florquin S, Depre G, Van de Stadt J, Adler M, Gelin M, Thys JP. *Trichoderma viride* infection in a liver transplant recipient. Mycoses 1992; 35:301–303.

130. Munoz FM, Demmler GJ, Travis WR, Ogden AK, Rossmann SN, Rinaldi MG. *Trichoderma longibrachiatum* infection in a pediatric patient with aplastic anemia. J Clin Microbiol 1997; 35:499–503.

131. Robertson MH. Fungi in fluids—a hazard of intravenous therapy. J Med Microbiol 1970; 3:99–102.

132. Marco F, Pfaller MA, Messer SA, Jones RN. In vitro activity of a new triazole antifungal agent, Sch 56592, against clinical isolates of filamentous fungi. Mycopathologia 1998; 141:73–77.

133. Seguin P, Degeilh B, Grulois I, Gacouin A, Maugendre S, Dufour T, Dupont B, Camus C. Successful treatment of a brain abscess due to *Trichoderma longibrachiatum* after surgical resection. Eur J Clin Microbiol Infect Dis 1995; 14:445–448.

134. Gonzalez CE, Rinaldi MG, Sugar AM. Zygomycosis. Infect Dis Clin North Am 2002; 16:895–914, vi.

135. Ribes JA, Vanover-Sams CL, Baker DJ. Zygomycetes in human disease. Clin Microbiol Rev 2000; 13:236–301.

136. Rinaldi MG. Zygomycosis. Infect Dis Clin North Am 1989; 3:19–41.

137. Chinn RY, Diamond RD. Generation of chemotactic factors by *Rhizopus oryzae* in the presence and absence of serum: relationship to hyphal damage mediated by human neutrophils and effects of hyperglycemia and ketoacidosis. Infect Immun 1982; 38:1123–1129.

138. de Medeiros CR, Bleggi-Torres LF, Faoro LN, Reis-Filho JS, Silva LC, de Medeiros BC, Loddo G, Pasquini R. Cavernous sinus thrombosis caused by zygomycosis after unrelated bone marrow transplantation. Transpl Infect Dis 2001; 3:231–234.

139. Gonzalez CE, Couriel DR, Walsh TJ. Disseminated zygomycosis in a neutropenic patient: successful treatment with amphotericin B lipid complex and granulocyte colony-stimulating factor. Clin Infect Dis 1997; 24:192–196.

140. Wehl G, Hoegler W, Kropshofer G, Meister B, Fink FM, Heitger A. Rhinocerebral mucormycosis in a boy with recurrent acute lymphoblastic leukemia: long-term survival with systemic antifungal treatment. J Pediatr Hematol Oncol 2002; 24:492–494.

141. Dannaoui E, Afeltra J, Meis JF, Verweij PE. In vitro susceptibilities of zygomycetes to combinations of antimicrobial agents. Antimicrob Agents Chemother 2002; 46:2708–2711.

142. Sun QN, Najvar LK, Bocanegra R, Loebenberg D, Graybill JR. In vivo activity of posaconazole against *Mucor* spp. in an immunosuppressed-mouse model. Antimicrob Agents Chemother 2002; 46:2310–2312.

143. Sun QN, Fothergill AW, McCarthy DI, Rinaldi MG, Graybill JR. In vitro activities of posaconazole, itraconazole, voriconazole, amphotericin B, and fluconazole against 37 clinical isolates of Zygomycetes. Antimicrob Agents Chemother 2002; 46:1581–1582.

144. Tobon AM, Arango M, Fernandez D, Restrepo A. Mucormycosis (zygomycosis) in a heart–kidney transplant recipient: recovery after posaconazole therapy. Clin Infect Dis 2003; 36:1488–1491.

145. Tedder M, Spratt JA, Anstadt MP, Hegde SS, Tedder SD, Lowe JE. Pulmonary mucormycosis: results of medical and surgical therapy. Ann Thorac Surg 1994; 57:1044–1050.

146. Vartivarian SE, Anaissie EJ, Bodey GP. Emerging fungal pathogens in immunocompromised patients: classification, diagnosis, and management. Clin Infect Dis 1993; 17(suppl 2):S487–S491.

147. McGinnis MR. Chromoblastomycosis and phaeohyphomycosis: new concepts, diagnosis, and mycology. J Am Acad Dermatol 1983; 8:1–16.

148. Fothergill AW. Identification of dematiaceous fungi and their role in human disease. Clin Infect Dis 1996; 22(suppl 2):S179–S184.

149. Nosanchuk JD, Casadevall A. The contribution of melanin to microbial pathogenesis. Cell Microbiol 2003; 5:203–223.

150. Gomez BL, Nosanchuk JD. Melanin and fungi. Curr Opin Infect Dis 2003; 16:91–96.

151. Fryen A, Mayser P, Glanz H, Fussle R, Breithaupt H, de Hoog GS. Allergic fungal sinusitis caused by *Bipolaris* (*Drechslera*) *hawaiiensis*. Eur Arch Otorhinolaryngol 1999; 256:330–334.

152. Saenz RE, Brown WD, Sanders CV. Allergic bronchopulmonary disease caused by *Bipolaris hawaiiensis* presenting as a necrotizing pneumonia: case report and review of literature. Am J Med Sci 2001; 321:209–212.

153. Nakai T, Uno J, Otomo K, Ikeda F, Tawara S, Goto T, Nishimura K, Miyaji M. In vitro activity of FK463, a novel lipopeptide antifungal agent, against a variety of clinically important molds. Chemotherapy 2002; 48:78–81.

154. Franzot SP, Salkin IF, Casadevall A. *Cryptococcus neoformans* var. *grubii*: separate varietal status for *Cryptococcus neoformans* serotype A isolates. J Clin Microbiol 1999; 37:838–840.

155. Speed B, Dunt D. Clinical and host differences between infections with the two varieties of *Cryptococcus neoformans*. Clin Infect Dis 1995; 21:28–34; discussion 35–36.

156. Chen Y, Chang S, Shih C, Hung C, Luhbd K, Pan Y, Hsieh W. Clinical features and in vitro susceptibilities of two varieties of *Cryptococcus neoformans* in Taiwan. Diagn Microbiol Infect Dis 2000; 36:175–183.

157. Ikceda R, Sugita T, Jacobson ES, Shinoda T. Laccase and melanization in clinically important *Cryptococcus* species other than *Cryptococcus neoformans*. J Clin Microbiol 2002; 40:1214–1218.

158. Mitchell DH, Sorrell TC, Allworth AM, Heath CH, McGregor AR, Papanaoum K, Richards MJ, Gottlieb T. Cryptococcal disease of the CNS in immunocompetent hosts: influence of cryptococcal variety on clinical manifestations and outcome. Clin Infect Dis 1995; 20:611–616.

159. Correa Mdo P, Severo LC, Oliveira Fde M, Irion K, Londero AT. The spectrum of computerized tomography (CT) findings in central nervous system (CNS) infection due to-*Cryptococcus neoformans* var. *gattii* in immunocompetent children. Rev Inst Med Trop Sao Paulo 2002; 44:283–287.

160. Brandt ME, Pfaller MA, Hajjeh RA, Hamill RJ, Pappas PG, Reingold AL, Rimland D, Wamock DW. Trends in antifungal drug susceptibility of *Cryptococcus neoformans* isolates in the United States: 1992 to 1994 and 1996 to 1998. Antimicrob Agents Chemother 2001; 45:3065–3069.

161. Pappas PG, Perfect JR, Cloud GA, Larsen RA, Pankey GA, Lancaster DJ, Henderson H, Kauffman CA, Haas DW, Saccente M, Hamill RJ, Holloway MS, Warren RM, Dismukes WE. Cryptococcosis in human immunodeficiency virus-negative patients in the era of effective azole therapy. Clin Infect Dis 2001; 33:690–699.

162. van der Horst CM, Saag MS, Cloud GA, Hamill RJ, Graybill JR, Sobel JD, Johnson PC, Tuazon CU, Kerkering T, Moskovitz BL, Powderly WG, Dismukes WE. Treatment of cryptococcal meningitis associated with the acquired immunodeficiency syndrome.

National Institute of Allergy and Infectious Diseases Mycoses Study Group and AIDS Clinical Trials Group. N Engl J Med 1997; 337:15–21.

163. Seaton RA, Verma N, Naraqi S, Wembri JP, Warrell DA. Visual loss in immunocompetent patients with *Cryptococcus neoformans* var. *gattii* meningitis. Trans R Soc Trap Med Hyg 1997; 91:44–49.

164. Averbuch D, Boekhoutt T, Falk R, Engelhard D, Shapiro M, Block C, Polacheck I. Fungemia in a cancer patient caused by fluconazole-resistant *Cryptococcus laurentii*. Med Mycol 2002; 40:479–484.

165. Cheng MF, Chiou CC, Liu YC, Wang HZ, Hsieh KS. *Cryptococcus laurentii* fungemia in a premature neonate. J Clin Microbiol 2001; 39:1608–1611.

166. Kunova A, Krcmery V. Fungaemia due to thermophilic cryptococci: 3 cases of *Cryptococcus laurentii* bloodstream infections in cancer patients receiving antifungals [letter]. Scand J Infect Dis 1999; 31:328.

167. Kordossis T, Avlami A, Velegraki A, Stefanou I, Georgakopoulos G, Papalambrou C, Legakis NJ. First report of *Cryptococcus laurentii* meningitis and a fatal case of *Cryptococcus albidus* cryptococcaemia in AIDS patients. Med Mycol 1998; 36:335–339.

168. Johnson LB, Bradley SF, Kauffman CA. Fungaemia due to *Cryptococcus laurentii* and a review of non-neoformans cryptococcaemia. Mycoses 1998; 41:277–280.

169. Ritterband DC, Seedor JA, Shah MK, Waheed S, Schorr I. A unique case of *Cryptococcus laurentii* keratitis spread by a rigid gas permeable contact lens in a patient with onychomycosis. Cornea 1998; 17:115–118.

170. Krcmery V Jr, Kunova A, Mardiak J. Nosocomial *Cryptococcus laurentii* fungemia in a bone marrow transplant patient after prophylaxis with ketoconazole successfully treated with oral fluconazole [letter]. Infection 1997; 25:130.

171. Custis PH, Haller JA, de Juan E Jr. An unusual case of cryptococcal endophthalmitis. Retina 1995; 15:300–304.

172. Mocan H, Murphy AV, Beattie TJ, McAllister TA. Fungal peritonitis in children on continuous ambulatory peritoneal dialysis. Scott Med J 1989; 34:494–496.

173. Sinnott JT 4th, Rodnite J, Emmanuel PJ, Campos A. *Cryptococcus laurentii* infection complicating peritoneal dialysis. Pediatr Infect Dis J 1989; 8:803–805.

174. Lynch JP 3rd, Schaberg DR, Kissner DG, Kauffman CA. *Cryptococcus laurentii* lung abscess. Am Rev Respir Dis 1981; 123:135–138.

175. Kamalam A, Yesudian P, Thambiah AS. Cutaneous infection by *Cryptococcus laurentii*. Br J Dermatol 1977; 97:221–223.

176. Ramchandren R, Gladstone DE. *Cryptococcus albidus* infection in a patient undergoing autologous progenitor cell transplant. Transplantation 2004; 77:956.

177. Lee YA, Kim HJ, Lee TW, Kim MJ, Lee MH, Lee JH, Ihm CG. First report of *Cryptococcus albidus*—induced disseminated cryptococcosis in a renal transplant recipient. Korean J Intern Med 2004; 19:53–57.

178. Narayan S, Batta K, Colloby P, Tan CY. Cutaneous cryptococcus infection due to *C. albidus* associated with Sezary syndrome. Br J Dermatol 2000; 143:632–634.

179. Wells GM, Gajjar A, Pearson TA, Hale KL, Shenep JL. Brief report. Pulmonary cryptosporidiosis and *Cryptococcus albidus* fimgemia in a child with acute lymphocytic leukemia. Med Pediatr Oncol 1998; 31:544–546.

180. Loison J, Bouchara JP, Gueho E, de Gentile L, Cimon B, Chennebault JM, Chabasse D. First report of *Cryptococcus albidus* septicaemia in an HIV patient. J Infect 1996; 33:139–140.

181. Horowitz ID, Blumberg EA, Krevolin L. *Cryptococcus albidus* and mucormycosis emphyema in a patient receiving hemodialysis. South Med J 1993; 86:1070–1072.

182. Gluck JL, Myers JP, Pass LM. Cryptococcemia due to *Cryptococcus albidus*. South Med J 1987; 80:511–513.

183. Melo JC, Srinivasan S, Scott ML, Raff MJ. *Cryptococcus albidus* meningitis. J Infect 1980; 2:79–82.

184. da Cunha T, Lusins J. *Cryptococcus albidus* meningitis. South Med J 1973; 66:1230.

185. Krumholz RA. Pulmonary cryptococcosis. A case due to *Cryptococcus albidus*. Am Rev Respir Dis 1972; 105:421–424.
186. Dromer F, Moulignier A, Dupont B, Gueho E, Baudrimont M, Improvisi L, Provost L, Gonzalez-Canali G. Myeloradiculitis due to *Cryptococcus curvatus* in AIDS. AIDS 1995; 9:395–396.
187. Binder L, Csillag A, Toth G. *Cryptococcus luteolus* as a cause of pulmonary mycosis. Orv Hetil 1955; 96:687–691.
188. McCurdy LH, Morrow JD. Ventriculitis due to *Cryptococcus uniguttulatus*. South Med J 2001; 94:65–66.

13

Conventional Methods for the Laboratory Diagnosis of Fungal Infections in the Immunocompromised Host

Michael A. Pfaller
Department of Pathology and Department of Epidemiology, University of Iowa College of Medicine and College of Public Health, Iowa City, Iowa, U.S.A.

Sandra S. Richter
Department of Pathology, University of Iowa College of Medicine, Iowa City, Iowa, U.S.A.

Daniel J. Diekema
Department of Pathology and Department of Medicine, University of Iowa College of Medicine, Iowa City, Iowa, U.S.A.

I. INTRODUCTION

The frequency of invasive fungal disease due to systemic and opportunistic pathogens has increased dramatically over the past two decades (1–7). This increase in infections is associated with considerable morbidity and mortality (8–10) and is largely because of expanding patient populations at risk for the development of life-threatening fungal infections, which include individuals undergoing solid-organ and blood and marrow transplantation (BMT), major surgery, those with AIDS, neoplastic disease, immunosuppressive therapy, and premature birth (2,4,6,10–13). Serious infections are being reported with an ever-increasing spectrum of pathogens including the well-known opportunistic fungal pathogens *Candida albicans*, *Cryptococcus neoformans*, and *Aspergillus fumigatus* (2,3,14,15). New and emerging pathogens include species of *Candida* and *Aspergillus* other than *C. albicans* and *A. fumigatus*, yeasts such as *Trichosporon*, *Rhodotorula*, and *Malassezia* species, hyaline hyphomycetes including *Fusarium*, *Acremonium*, and *Paecilomyces* species, and a wide variety of dematiaceous fungi (Table 1) (6,14–19). Modern medical mycology has become an extremely challenging study of infections caused by a broad range of taxonomically diverse opportunistic fungi (16). It is now quite clear that *there are no nonpathogenic fungi*; virtually any fungus can cause a lethal mycosis in an immunocompromised host.

Table 1 Spectrum of Opportunistic Fungal Pathogens[a]

Organism group	Examples of specific pathogens
Candida	*C. albicans*
	C. glabrata
	C. parapsilosis
	C. tropicalis
	C. dubliniensis
	C. krusei
	C. lusitaniae
	C. guilliermondii
	C. rugosa
Other yeasts	*Cryptococcus neoformans*
	Trichosporon
	Blastoschizomyces
	Rhodotorula
	Malassezia
	Saccharomyces
	Hansenula
Aspergillus	*A. fumigatus*
	A. flavus
	A. niger
	A. versicolor
	A. terreus
	A. nidulans
Zygomycetes	*Rhizopus*
	Rhizomucor
	Mucor
	Absidia
	Apophysomyces
	Cunninghamella
	Saksenaea
	Cokeromyces
Other hyaline molds	*Fusarium*
	Acremonium
	Scedosporium apiospermum
	S. prolificans
	Trichoderma
	Paecilomyces
	Chrysosporium
Dematiaceous molds	*Alternaria*
	Bipolaris
	Curvularia
	Exophiala
	Cladophialophora
	Phialophora
	Dactylaria
	Wangiella
Dimorphic molds	*Histoplasma*
	Coccidioides
	Blastomyces
	Paracoccidioides
	Sporothrix
	Penicillium marneffei
Other	*Pneumocystis jiroveci*

[a]List not all inclusive.

Table 2 Laboratory Diagnosis of Invasive Fungal Infections

Conventional microbiologic
  Direct microscopy (Gram, Giemsa, and Calcofluor stains)
  Culture
  Identification
  Susceptibility testing
Histopathologic
  Conventional microscopy
    Routine stains (H&E)
    Special stains (GMS, Mucicarmine, PAS)
  Direct immunofluorescence
  In situ hybridization
Immunologic
Molecular
  Direct detection
  Identification
  Strain typing
Biochemical
  Metabolites
  Cell-wall components
  Enzymes

Abbreviations: H&E, hematoxylin and eosin; GMS, Gormori's methenamine silver; PAS, periodic acid-Schiff

Owing to the complexity of the various patient groups at risk for infection and the increasing array of fungal pathogens, opportunistic mycoses pose a considerable diagnostic challenge to both clinicians and microbiologists (16,20,21). Despite recognition of the importance of the invasive mycoses, these infections remain difficult to diagnose. The current diagnostic approach includes clinical suspicion, culture of appropriate sites, histopathologic examination of tissue biopsies, and diagnostic imaging techniques (Table 2) (16,22–27). Although these approaches may suffer from a lack of diagnostic sensitivity and specificity, it is absolutely essential that individuals and institutions caring for high-risk immunocompromised patients place a high priority on maximizing their diagnostic capabilities for early diagnosis of invasive opportunistic fungal infections (16,21,23). Optimal diagnosis and treatment of mycotic infections in the compromised host are directly dependent upon a team approach involving clinicians, microbiologists, and pathologists (16,22,27).

In this chapter, the more conventional diagnostic approaches including direct microscopy, culture, and histopathology are addressed (Table 2). Diagnostic imaging and the nonculture-based methods of serology and molecular diagnostics are covered in subsequent chapters.

II. CLINICAL RECOGNITION OF FUNGAL INFECTION

The increased frequency of invasive mycoses requires that clinicians caring for immunocompromised individuals have an enhanced index of clinical suspicion and a greater appreciation of the major risk factors that predispose patients to fungal infections (2,6,11). Specific fungal infections may be associated with well-known clinical scenarios such as endophthalmitis and macronodular skin lesions (candidiasis), onychomycosis in a neutropenic patient (fusariosis), sinus infection in diabetic ketoacidosis (zygomycosis), or myalgias and myositis (candidemia caused by *C. tropicalis*). Other clinical signs and symptoms that may be associated with fungal infections include suppurative thrombophlebitis (*Candida*), cholestasis (chronic disseminated or hepatosplenic candidiasis), purpura fulminans and bullous dermatitis (*Candida*, *Aspergillus*, and *Fusarium* spp.), and osteomyelitis (*Candida*) (26,28). Although these are useful clinical clues, they are not entirely specific and often are observed rather late in the course of the infectious process. The newer serologic and molecular diagnostic tests promise to enhance the diagnostic approach to fungal infections; however, at present conventional microbiologic and histologic methods serve as the cornerstone for definitive diagnosis of the mycoses. Unfortunately, these methods may require invasive procedures (biopsy), may not exhibit optimal sensitivity or specificity, and often are too slow (culture) to provide a diagnosis in a clinically meaningful time frame.

III. SPECTRUM OF OPPORTUNISTIC FUNGAL PATHOGENS

As noted earlier, the spectrum of possible opportunistic fungal pathogens is quite broad (Table 1). However, *C. albicans* remains the most common fungal pathogen (3) and *A. fumigatus* is the commonest mold pathogen (29). Likewise, *Candida* spp., *Aspergillus* spp., and *C. neoformans* account for more than 80% of all fungal infections in BMT, solid-organ transplant, and other immunosuppressed patient populations (30).

The frequency of fungal infections, predilection for specific fungal pathogens, and the time of onset of various fungal infections differ for different patient groups (Table 3) (13). Unique risk factors, exposures, and the degree and duration of immunosuppression account likely for this variability (13). Thus, invasive aspergillosis (IA) exerts a major impact on patients following allogeneic BMT, lung and liver transplant, whereas infections caused by *Candida* spp. are most problematic among neonates, postsurgical intensive care unit (ICU) patients, and postpancreas and small-bowel transplant patients (Table 3) (2,11–13,21,31,32). Aside from *Candida* and *Aspergillus* spp., the less common and "emerging" fungal pathogens are often found in the environment and tend to cause infection in those individuals with long-term immunosuppression (6). The greater the degree and duration of immunosuppression, the broader the spectrum of possible opportunistic fungal pathogens (20,28).

IV. CONVENTIONAL METHODS FOR THE LABORATORY DIAGNOSIS OF FUNGAL INFECTIONS

The laboratory diagnosis of fungal infections begins with the proper collection and prompt transport of clinical material to the microbiology laboratory. Direct microscopic examination is useful to provide a rapid presumptive diagnosis and an aid in directing culture efforts. Culture on appropriate medium, while not rapid, provides important information regarding the identity of the etiologic agent and is necessary to provide an isolate for subsequent antifungal susceptibility testing. Histopathologic examination of biopsy material using special stains is usually done outside of the mycology laboratory but is often essential in defining the type and extent of the infection. Every step of this process is enhanced by direct communication between the clinician, the mycologist, and the pathologist. Information regarding a

Table 3 Relative Frequency of Opportunistic Mycoses Among Different Patient Groups[a]

Patient group	Asp	Can	Cryp	Tri	PCP	Hyal	Phae	Blas[b]	Hist[b]	Cocci[b]	Pmar[b]	Zygo
Transplant												
Allo. BMT	++++	+++	++	++	+++	++	+	(+)	(+)	(+)	(+)	++
Liver	+++	++++	+++	+	+	+	+	(+)	(+)	(+)	(+)	+
Lung	++++	+++	++	+	+	+	+	(+)	(+)	(+)	(+)	+
Kidney	++	+++	++	+	+	+	+	(+)	(+)	(+)	(+)	+
Heart	++++	+++	+	+	+	+	+	(+)	(+)	(+)	(+)	+
Pancreas	++	++++	+	+	+	+	+	(+)	(+)	(+)	(+)	+
Sm. Bowel	++	++++	+	+	+	+	+	(+)	(+)	(+)	(+)	+
Malignancy												
Heme	+++	++++	++	+	++	+	+	(+)	(+)	(+)	(+)	+
Solid	++	++++	++	+	++	+	+	(+)	(+)	(+)	(+)	++
HIV/AIDS	++	++	+++		++++	+	+	(++)	(++++)	(++++)	(++++)	+
Critical care												
Adult	+	++++	+	+	+	+						++
Neonate		++++	+	+	+							+

[a]Relative frequency of mycoses within each patient group indicated as ++++ (most frequent) to + (least frequent).
[b]Frequency of endemic mycoses indicated by (+) to (++++) within endemic regions only.
Abbreviations: Allo BMT., allogeneic blood and marrow transplant; Sm. bowel, small bowel; Heme, hematologic malignancy; Solid, solid tumor malignancy; Asp., aspergillosis; Can., candidiasis; Tric, trichosporonosis; Cryp., cryptococcosis; PCP., *Pneumocystis jiroveci* pneumonia; Hyal., hyalohyphomycosis; Phae., phaeohyphomycosis; Blas., blastomycosis; Hist., histoplasmosis; Cocci., coccidioidomycosis; Pmar., *Penicillium marneffei*; Zygo., zygomycosis.
For mycosis abbreviations, see Table 1 for specific examples within each group.

clinical suspicion for a specific fungus will alert the laboratory to modify routine processing (e.g., addition of olive oil to the culture to enhance detection of *Malassezia*) or to be on the alert for a biohazardous organism (e.g., *Coccidioides immitis*).

A. Specimen Collection and Processing

As in the case with all infectious diseases, the diagnosis of fungal infection is directly dependent upon the proper collection of the appropriate clinical specimen and prompt transport of specimens to the clinical laboratory (16,24,33,34). Clinical and radiographic examination, as well as consideration of the most likely fungal pathogen that may cause a specific type of infection in a given patient should drive the selection of the appropriate specimen for culture and microscopic examination (Tables 3 and 4). Specimens should be collected after proper cleaning and decontamination of the collection site and under aseptic conditions if possible. An adequate amount of suitable clinical material should be promptly submitted for culture and examination (Table 5). Unfortunately, many specimens submitted to the laboratory are either of insufficient amount or of poor quality and are inadequate to make a diagnosis. As a general rule, swab specimens are inappropriate for mycologic and microbiologic culture and microscopic examination (33).

Specimens should be placed in a sterile, leak proof container, and be properly labeled and accompanied by a relevant clinical history. As mentioned earlier, the clinical information is very important in directing specimen processing and as an aid in interpreting the culture results. The clinical information is especially important when the specimen is from a nonsterile site such as the respiratory, genitourinary, (GU) or gastrointestinal (GI) tract, and the skin.

Whenever possible, specimens should be delivered to the laboratory within 2 hr of collection to prevent overgrowth by bacteria or other commensal flora. Most fungi can be recovered from specimens submitted in bacteriologic transport medium, although direct microscopic examination may be obscured by the transport medium components. In general, most specimens for fungal culture may be safely stored at 4°C for a short time.

As with any infectious disease, there are specimens that are better than others for diagnosis of mycotic infections (Table 4). Cultures of blood, cerebrospinal fluid (CSF), and other normally sterile body fluids are usually quite useful and should be performed if clinical signs and symptoms are suggestive of hematogenous dissemination. Biopsies of skin lesions or other focal sites of infection often yield a diagnosis and should be obtained for culture and histopathologic examination whenever possible. Diagnosis of oral or vaginal thrush is often best established by clinical presentation and direct microscopic [wet mount or potassium hydroxide (KOH) preparation] examination of scrapings or secretions because culture often represents simple colonization or contamination. Similarly, fungal infections of the GI tract are better diagnosed by biopsy and histopathologic examination of the involved tissue than by culture alone. Culture of lower respiratory tract and urine specimens may be confounded by contamination with normal oral and periurethral flora, respectively, and care should be taken to minimize the possibility of such contamination when obtaining these specimens (Table 5). Twenty-four-hour collections of sputum or urine are not appropriate for mycologic examination because of overgrowth of bacterial and fungal contaminants (Table 5).

Table 4 Selection of Clinical Specimens for Detection and Isolation of Opportunistic Fungal Pathogens

Suspected pathogen	Blood	Bone marrow	Brain and cerebrospinal fluid	Joint fluid	Eye	Urine	Respiratory	Skin and mucous membranes	Multiple systemic sites
Yeasts									
Candida spp.	++++	+	++	+	+	+++	+	+++	+++
Cryptococcus neoformans	+++	+	++++		+	++	+++	+	++
Trichosporon spp.	++++					++	+++	++	+++
Malassezia spp.	++++						+	+++	+
Rhodotorula spp.	++++					+	+		+
Molds									
Aspergillus spp.	+[a]		++		+	+	++++	++	+++
Zygomycetes			+		++		++++	++	+++
Fusarium spp.	+++		++	+	+		++	++++	+++
Scedosporium apiospermum	+		++		+		+	+++	++
Scedosporium prolificans			+	+	+		+	+++	+++
Dematiaceous molds			+++	+	+		+++	++	++
Dimorphic									
Histoplasma capsulatum	+++	++	+	+	+	+	++	++	++
Blastomyces dermatitidis		+	+	+		+	++	++++	+++
Coccidioides immitis	++	+	++	+	+	+	++++	+++	+++
Paracoccidioides brasiliensis		+					++	++++	++
Penicillium marneffei	+++	++	+	++			++++	++	+++
Sporothrix schenckii	+		+	+			++	++++	+
Other									
Pneumocystis jiroveci		+					++++		+

[a] *Aspergillus terreus* only.
Source: Adapted from Ref. 16.
Note: Predominant sites for recovery are ranked in order of importance and frequency (i.e., ++++, most important or most frequent; +, Less important or less frequent) based on the most common clinical presentation.

Table 5 Collection and Processing of Clinical Specimens for Recovery of Fungi

Specimen type[a]	Collection guidelines	Comments
Blood	20–30 mL blood A variety of broth-based systems (BactT/Alert, BACTEC, ESP, Septi-Check), as well as lysis centrifugation systems Transport at room temperature within 24 hr Do not refrigerate Isolator should be processed within 16 hr	Avoid catheter draws if possible Lysis centrifugation (Isolator) preferred for dimorphics, filamentous fungi, and *C. neoformans* Subculture broth systems to blood, chocolate, and BHI agar Plate lysate (Isolator) onto blood, chocolate, and BHI agar
Sterile fluids (CSF, pleural, pericardial, peritoneal, or joint fluid)	Collect in sterile container At least 3–5 mL fluid Transport immediately to laboratory Concentrate by centrifugation, use sediment for culture and supernatant for antigen testing	May need ~30 mL CSF for chronic meningitis May inoculate all but CSF into blood-culture bottles for yeasts
Tissue biopsy	Place in sterile container with small amount of nonbacteriostatic saline Transport immediately to laboratory	Tissue should be minced rather than ground to optimize recovery of fungi
Bone marrow	Sterile collection using a lysis centrifugation pediatric tube (Isolator) or a heparin tube Transport at room temperature within 4 hr. Do not refrigerate	Useful when disseminated histoplasmosis or coccidioidomycosis is suspected
Respiratory tract	Early morning sputum collected in sterile container Minimum volume, 1 mL Induced sputum, BAL, or tissue biopsy is preferred for diagnosis of invasive fungal infection Transport to laboratory within 2 hr May refrigerate for up to 24 hr	24 hr sputum collections not acceptable Induced sputum or BAL best for *P. jiroveci* detection by microscopy Isolation of *Candida* spp. usually represents oral contamination Significance of culture positive for *Aspergillus* spp. depends on patient risk group

Site	Collection	Comments
Intravascular catheter tip	Approximately 5 cm of the distal end should be sent in a sterile dry container. Transport within 2 hr at room temperature. May refrigerate for up to 24 hr	Any number of fungal colonies may be significant
Corneal scrapings	Direct inoculation on fungal media (e.g., BHI) is optimal. May use aerobic swab transport system for conjunctival infection. Intraocular fluid should be collected in a sterile container. Transport immediately to laboratory	Skin contamination is problematic. Blood cultures should also be obtained. Consultation with laboratory personnel regarding media selection and inoculation procedures is helpful
Urine	First AM specimen collected in a sterile container. Volume > 1 mL (50–200 mL best). Transport at room temperature within 2 hr. May refrigerate for up to 24 hr	24 hr collections not acceptable. Candiduria of uncertain clinical significance. May represent colonization or contamination
Wounds and abscess	Aspirates or biopsies preferable to swabs. Place material into sterile anaerobic transport system. Transport to laboratory within 2 hr	Avoid swabs whenever possible. If surgical drainage of an abscess is performed, send both abscess material and a portion of the abscess wall

[a]Specimen collection sites are not all inclusive.
Source: Adapted from Refs. 23, 34.

B. Direct Microscopy

Direct microscopic examination of specimens submitted to the microbiology laboratory is performed routinely as a means of providing a rapid diagnosis and to guide specimen processing and culture. In contrast with histopathologic examination (see below), direct microscopy, as performed in the microbiology laboratory, does not utilize fixed tissue and relies instead on rapid examination of wet mounts, zGram, Giemsa, or Calcofluor-stained material (Table 6). Such direct microscopy is perhaps the most rapid, useful, and cost-effective means of diagnosing fungal infections (24).

Detection of fungal elements microscopically may provide a presumptive diagnosis in < 1 hr compared to days or weeks with culture. In some instances, a definitive diagnosis may be possible by direct microscopy based on the distinctive morphology of the infecting fungus (Table 7). For example, if distinctive yeast cells, spherules, or other structures are observed microscopically, an etiologic diagnosis can be made for infections caused by *Histoplasma capsulatum, Blastomyces dermatitidis, C. immitis, Pneumocystis jiroveci (carinii)*, and *Penicillium marneffei* (Table 7). In other infections, microscopy can usually yield preliminary information that a yeast or a mold is present and, in some instances, the morphologic appearance may provide a presumptive diagnosis of the type of infection (e.g., aspergillosis, fusariosis, candidiasis, and trichosporonosis) but not the actual species identification of the etiologic agent (Table 7).

All direct examinations should be confirmed by culture. Detection of fungal elements on direct examination often serves to guide the laboratory in selecting the most appropriate means as to culture the clinical material. Similarly, the direct microscopic results may aid in the interpretation of the culture results (Figs. 1 and 2). Direct examination is less sensitive than culture for most mycotic infections, and a negative microscopic examination does not rule out a fungal infection.

Direct microscopy, as performed in the microbiology laboratory, most commonly relies on the use of 10–20% KOH containing the fluorophore Calcofluor white, or staining of smears, or touch preparations with either Gram or Giemsa stains (Table 6). The Calcofluor white binds to the chitin in the fungal cell wall and fluoresces blue-white or green, providing rapid and sensitive means of detecting fungi in clinical material (24) (Fig. 3). The Gram stain is useful for detection of *Candida* and *Cryptococcus* spp. (Figs. 4–6) and also stains hyphal elements of molds such as *Aspergillus* (Fig. 7), *Fusarium*, and the Zygomycetes (Figs. 8 and 9). Fungi are typically Gram-positive but may appear speckled or Gram-negative (Figs. 4–10). The capsular material of *C. neoformans* often appears as an orange-red precipitate around the cells (Fig. 6). Many fungi will stain blue with the Giemsa stain but this stain is especially useful in detecting *H. capsulatum* intracellularly in bone marrow, peripheral blood, bronchoalveolar lavage (BAL) specimens, or touch preparations of lymph nodes or other tissues (Fig. 11).

The morphologic characteristics of fungi seen on direct microscopic examination include budding yeasts, hyphae, and pseudohyphae. The combination of budding yeast cells and pseudohyphae is characteristic of *Candida* (Figs. 1–5); however, these structures may also be seen with *Trichosporon* and *Geotrichum* (Table 7).

Among the molds, *Aspergillus* spp. typically shows hyaline dichotomous acute angle branching septate hyphae (Fig. 12); however, this appearance is also typical of other hyaline molds such as *Fusarium, Acremonium, Paecilomyces, Trichoderma*, and *Scedosporium* (Table 7). In contrast, the Zygomycetes (e.g., *Rhizopus, Mucor*)

Table 6 Methods and Stains Available for Direct Microscopic Detection of Fungal Elements

Method/stain	Use	Comments
Alcian blue stain	Detection of *C. neoformans* in CSF	Rapid (2 min); insensitive and not commonly used
Calcofluor white stain	Detection of all fungi including *P. jiroveci*	Rapid (1–2 min); detects fungal cell wall chitin by bright fluorescence. Used in combination with KOH. Requires fluorescent microscope and proper filters. Background fluorescence may make examination of some specimens difficult
Fluorescent monoclonal antibody treatment	Examination of respiratory specimens for *P. jiroveci*	Sensitive and specific method for detecting the cysts of *P. jiroveci*. Does not stain the extracystic (trophozoite) forms
Fontana–Masson Stain	Melanin stain for histologic sections	Confirms the presence of melanin in lightly pigmented cells of dematiaceous fungi when present in tissue sections. Useful for distinguishing *C. neoformans* (positive) from most other yeasts (e.g., *Candida* spp. are negative for melanin).
Giemsa stain	Examination of bone marrow, peripheral smears, touch preparations, and respiratory specimens	Detect intracellular *H. capsulatum* and both intracystic and extracystic (trophozoite) forms of *P. jiroveci*. Does not stain cysts of *P. jiroveci*. Does stain organisms other than *H. capsulatum* and *P. jiroveci*
Gram stain	Detection of bacteria and fungi	Rapid (2–3 min); commonly performed on clinical specimens. Will stain most yeasts and hyphal elements. Most fungi stain Gram-positive, but some, such as *C. neoformans*, exhibit stippling or appear Gram-negative
Hematoxylin and eosin stain	General purpose histologic stain	Best stain to demonstrate host reaction in infected tissue. Stains most fungi, but small numbers of organisms may be difficult to differentiate from background. Useful in demonstrating natural pigment in dematiaceous fungi
India ink	Detection of encapsulated yeasts	Rapid (1 min); insensitive (40%) means of detecting *C. neoformans* in CSF
KOH treatment	Clearing specimens of cellular debris to make fungi more visible	Rapid (5 min); some specimens may be difficult to clear and require an additional 5–10 min. May produce confusing artifacts. Most useful when combined with Calcofluor white
Methylene blue treatment	Detection of fungi in skin scrapings	Rapid (2 min); may be used in combination with KOH. Largely replaced by Calcofluor white (improved sensitivity and specificity)
Methenamine silver stain (GMS)	Detection of fungi in histologic sections and *P. jiroveci* cysts in respiratory specimens	Staining of tissue may take up to 1 hr. Respiratory specimens more rapid (5–10 min). Best stain for detection of all fungi. Usually performed in cytopathology laboratory
Mucicarmine stain	Histopathologic stain for mucin	Useful for demonstrating capsular material of *C. neoformans*. May also stain the cell walls of *B. dermatitidis* and *Rhinosporidium sieberi*.
Papanicolaou stain (PAP)	Cytologic stain used primarily to detect malignant cells	Stains most fungal elements; yeasts > hyphae. Allows cytologist to detect fungal elements
PAS stain	Histologic stain for detection of fungi	Stains both yeasts and hyphae in tissue. *Blastomyces dermatitidis* may appear pleomorphic. PAS-positive artifacts may resemble yeast cells
Toluidine blue stain	Examination of respiratory specimens for *P. jiroveci*	Stains *P. jiroveci* cysts a purple color. Does stains other fungi. Largely displaced by fluorescent antibody and Calcofluor white treatments
Wright stain	Examination of bone marrow, peripheral smears, and touch preparations	Similar to Giemsa stain. Detects intracellular *H. capsulatum*

Source: Adapted from Refs. 16, 24.

Table 7 Characteristic Features of Opportunistic and Pathogenic Fungi in Clinical Specimens and in Cultures

Fungus	Microscopic morphologic features in clinical specimens	Characteristic morphologic features in culture		Additional tests for identification
		Macroscopic	Microscopic	
Candida spp.	Oval, budding yeasts 2–6 μm in diameter. Pseudohyphae and hyphae may be present. (Figs. 1–5)	Variable morphology. Colonies usually pasty, white to tan, and opaque. May have smooth or wrinkled morphology. Some colonies produce fringes of pseudohyphae at periphery.	Clusters of blastoconidia, pseudohyphae, and/or terminal chlamydospores in some species	Germ-tube production by *C. albicans*, *C. dubliniensis*, and *C. stellatoidea*. Carbohydrate assimilation. Morphology on cornmeal agar. Colony color on CHROMagar
Cryptococcus neoformans	Spherical budding yeasts of variable size, 2–15 μm. Capsule may be present. No pseudohyphae or hyphae (Figs. 6 and 22)	Colonies are shiny, mucoid, dome shaped, and cream to tan in color	Budding spherical cells of varying size. Capsule present. No pseudohyphae. Cells may have multiple narrow-based buds	Tests for urease (+), phenoloxidase (+), and nitrate reductase (−). Latex agglutination or EIA test for polysaccharide antigen. Carbohydrate assimilation Mucicarmine and melanin stains in tissue
Trichosporon spp.	Hyaline arthroconidia, blastoconidia, and pseudohyphae 2–4 by 8 μm	Colonies are variably smooth and shiny to membranous, dry, and cerebriform	Hyphae, pseudohyphae, blastoconidia, and arthroconidia. No chlamydospores	Carbohydrate assimilation and biochemical tests
Malassezia spp.	Small oval budding yeasts. "Bowling pin" appearance with collarette (Fig. 23). Both hyphal and yeast forms may be seen in skin scrapings	Slow-growing colonies. May require fatty acid source (olive oil) for growth	Small oval budding cells with collarette. Rudimentary hyphae	Species may be differentiated by lipid requirement: *M. furfur* and *M. sympodialis*, positive; *M. pachydermatis*, negative. *Malassezia furfur* will grow in 10% Tween 20, whereas *M. sympodialis* will not
Aspergillus spp.	Septate, dichotomously branched hyphae of	Varies with species. Colonies of *A. fumigatus* usually blue-green to	Varies with species. Conidiophores with	Identification based on microscopic and colonial morphology

	uniform width (3–6 μm). Conidial heads may be seen in cavitary lesions (Figs. 7 and 12)	gray-green; *A. flavus* yellow-green; *A. niger* black; other species vary widely	enlarged vesicles covered with flask-shaped metulae or phialids. Hyphae are hyaline and septate	Identication based on microscopic morphologic features.
Zygomycetes	Broad, thin-walled, pauci-septate hyphae, 6–25 μm with nonparallel sides and random branches. Hyphae stain poorly with GMS stain and often stain well with H&E stain (Figs. 8, 9, and 13)	Colonies are rapid growing, wooly, and gray-brown to gray-black in color	Broad, ribbon-like hyphae with rare septa and irregular sides. Sporangium or sporangiola produced from sporangiophore. *Rhizopus* spp.: rhizoids at base of sporangiophore (Fig. 9)	
Fusarium spp.	Hyaline, septate, dichotomously branching hyphae. Angioinvasion is common. May be indistinguishable from *Aspergillus* spp. (Fig. 20)	Colonies are purple, lavender, or rose-red with rare yellow variants	Both macro- and microconidia may be present. Macroconidia are multicelled and sickle- or boat-shaped	Identification based on microscopic and colonial morphology
Scedosporium apiospermum (anamorph, asexual stage; *Pseudallescheria scheria boydii* is the teleomorph or sexual stage)	Hyaline, branching septate hyphae. Angioinvasion is common	Wooly, mouse-gray colonies	Single-celled brownish conidia produced at the tips of annellides (*S. apiospermum*). Cleistothecia containing ascospores may be produced (*P. boydii*)	Identification based on microscopic and colonial morphology. May be confused with *Aspergillus* spp. in tissue

(Continued)

Table 7 Characteristic Features of Opportunistic and Pathogenic Fungi in Clinical Specimens and in Cultures (*Continued*)

Fungus	Microscopic morphologic features in clinical specimens	Characteristic morphologic features in culture		Additional tests for identification
		Macroscopic	Microscopic	
Scedosporium prolificans	Hyaline, branching septate hyphae	Wooly, gray to dark brown. Does not grow on cycloheximide-containing medium	Inflated conidiophores	Based on morphologic appearance. *Scedosporicum prolificans* does not have a known sexual stage
Dematiaceous fungi (e.g., *Alternaria, Cladosporium, Curvularia*) (Table 1)	Pigmented (brown, tan, or black) hyphae, 2–6 µm wide. May be branched or unbranched. Often constricted at the point of septation	Colonies are usually rapidly growing, wooly, and gray, olive, black, or brown in color	Varies considerably depending on genus and species. Hyphae are pigmented. Conidia may be single or in chains, smooth or rough and dematiaceous	Identification based on microscopic and colonial morphology
Histoplasma capsulatum	Small (2–4 µm) budding yeasts within macrophages (Figs. 11 and 18)	Colonies are slow growing and white or buff-brown in color (25°C). Yeast phase colonies [37°C] are smooth, white, and pasty.	Thin septate hyphae that produce tuberculate macroconidia and smooth-walled micro conidia (25°C). Small oval budding yeasts produced at 37°C	Demonstration of temperature-regulated dimorphism by conversion from mold to yeast phase at 37°C. Exoantigen and DNA probe tests
Coccidioides immitis	Spherical, thick-walled spherules, 20–200 µm. Mature spherules contain small, 2–5 µm endo spores. Arthroconidia and hyphae may form in cavitary lesions. (Fig. 17)	Colonies initially appear moist and glabrous, rapidly becoming downy and gray-white with a tan or brown reverse	Hyaline hyphae with rectangular arthroconidia separated by empty disjunctor cells	Exoantigen and nucleic acid probe tests

Organism				
Blastomyces dermatitidis	Large (8–15 μm) thick-walled budding yeast cells. The junction between mother and daughter cells is typically broad-based. Cells may appear multinucleate (Figs. 10 and 19)	Colonies vary from membranous yeast-like colonies to cottony white mold-like colonies at 25°C. When grown at 37°C, yeast phase colonies are wrinkled, folded and glabrous	Hyaline, septate hyphae with one-celled smooth conidia (25°C). Large thick-walled budding yeast at 37°C	Demonstration of temperature-regulated dimorphism; exoantigen and DNA probe tests.
Sporothrix schenckii	Yeast-like cells of varying sizes. Some may appear elongated or "cigar-shaped". Tissue reaction forms asteroid bodies (Fig. 21)	Colonies initially smooth, moist, and yeast-like becoming velvety as aerial hyphae develop (25°C). Tan to brown pasty colonies at 37°C	Thin branching septate hyphae Conidia borne in rosette-shaped clusters at the end of the conidiophore (25°C). Variable sized budding yeast at 37°C.	Demonstration of thermal dimorphism; exoantigen and DNA probe.
Penicillium marneffei	Oval, intracellular yeast cells with septum.	Colonies produce diffusible red pigment at 25°C	Septate hyphae with metulae, phialides with chains of conidia in a "paint-brush" distribution (25°C). Yeast cells divide by fission (37°C)	Demonstration of thermal dimorphism
Pneumocystis jiroveci	Cysts are round, collapsed, or crescent shaped. Trophozoites seen on special stains. (Figs. 14–16).	Not applicable	Not applicable	Immunofluorescent stain, GMS, Giemsa, Toluidine blue stains (Table 6)

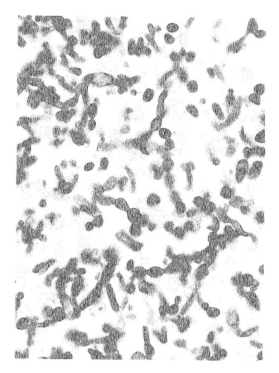

Figure 1 *Candida albicans* demonstrating budding yeasts and pseudohyphae. GMS stain. Magnification, ×1000.

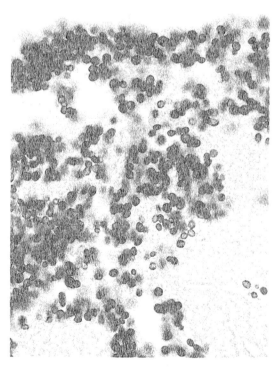

Figure 2 *Candida glabrata* demonstrating small budding yeasts without pseudohyphae. GMS stain. Magnification, ×1000.

Figure 3 *Candida tropicalis* in CSF stained with Calcofluor white. Magnification, ×1000.

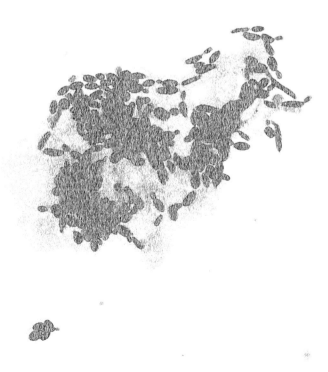

Figure 4 *Candida parapsilosis* from a central nervous system shunt. Budding yeasts and pseudohyphae visualized on Gram stain. Magnification, ×1000.

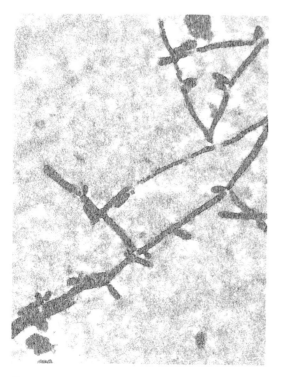

Figure 5 *Candida tropicalis* from a blood culture. Budding yeasts and hyphae seen on Gram stain. Magnification, ×1000.

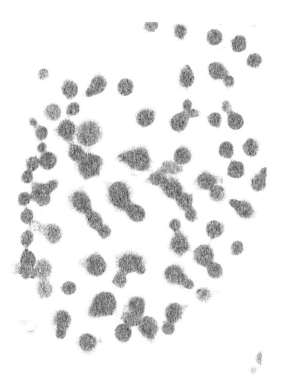

Figure 6 *Cryptococcus neoformans* in CSF. Variable-sized encapsulated budding yeasts seen on Gram stain. Note stippling because of uneven retention of crystal violet stain. Magnification, ×1000.

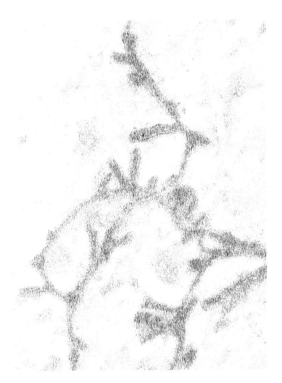

Figure 7 *Aspergillus versicolor* detected by Gram stain in a tracheal aspirate. Although often Gram-positive, this specimen did not retain the crystal violet and appears Gram-negative. Magnification, ×1000.

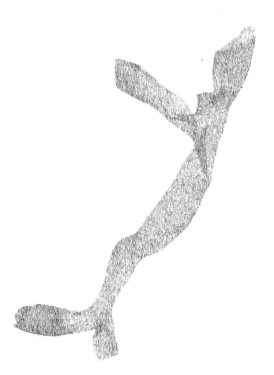

Figure 8 Hyphal fragment of *Rhizopus* spp. in pleural fluid demonstrating characteristic broad aseptate hypha that folds back on itself. Gram stain. Magnification, ×1000.

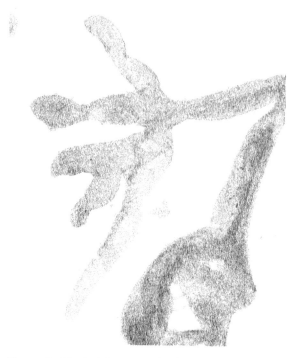

Figure 9 Hyphal fragment of *Rhizopus* spp. demonstrating root-like rhizoids. Gram stain. Magnification, ×1000.

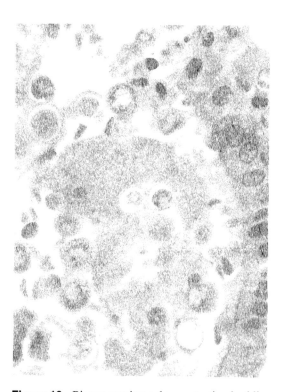

Figure 10 Biopsy specimen demonstrating budding yeast cells of *B. dermatitidis.* H&E stain. Magnification, ×1000.

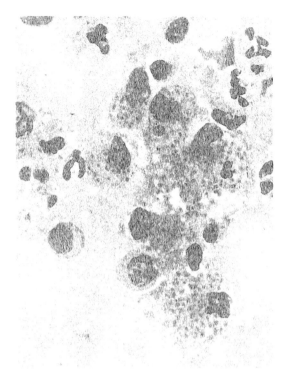

Figure 11 Macrophages containing numerous intracellular yeast forms of *H. capsulatum.* Giemsa stain. Magnification, ×1000.

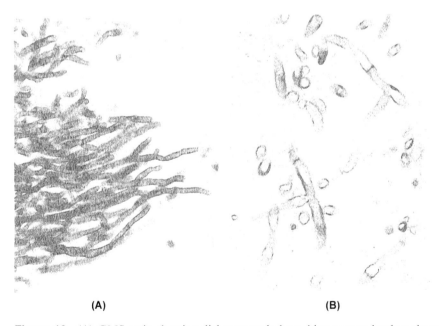

(A)   (B)

Figure 12 (A) GMS stain showing dichotomously branching septate hyphae characteristic of *Aspergillus* spp. Magnification, ×1000. (B) GMS stain showing the branching septate hyphae of *Trichoderma longibracheatum* that are indistinguishable from that of *Aspergillus* spp. Magnification, ×1000.

characteristically show broad ribbon-like sparsely septate or aseptate hyphae (Figs. 8 and 13). Finally, the dematiaceous fungi often present as darkly pigmented yeast-like and hyphal forms that may be visualized on unstained material and further characterized by the Fontana–Masson stain for melanin (Tables 6 and 7).

Although the cysts and/or intracystic bodies of *P. jiroveci* may be detected in induced sputum or BAL fluid following staining with Giemsa (Figs. 14 and 15), Gomori's methenamine silver (GMS) (Fig. 16), or toluidine blue stains, the commercial availability of fluorescent monoclonal antibody-based conjugates has enhanced the detection of this organism and provides a sensitive and highly specific diagnosis (35).

C. Histopathology

Histopathology and cytopathologic examination of tissue, fine-needle aspirates, or cytologic preparations employ a variety of stains designed to illustrate the cellular morphology of the host and any potential infecting organism invading the cells or tissues (Table 6). Among the more useful stains for detecting fungi in tissues are GMS stain and the Periodic Acid-Schiff (PAS) stain. In addition, fungi may be detected with hematoxylin and eosin (H&E) and Papanicolaou stains and further characterized using mucicarmine and Fontana–Masson stains (Table 6) (27,36–38). The H&E, GMS, and PAS stains can detect fungi such as *B. dermatitidis*, *H. capsulatum*, *C. immitis*, *Candida* spp. *Fusarium*, *Sporothrix*, *Cryptococcus*, and the hyphae of Zygomycetes (e.g., *Rhizopus, Mucor*), as well as *Aspergillus* spp. (Table 6)(Figs. 17–22). Although most fungi may be visualized in tissue stained with H&E when present in large numbers, *Candida* and *Aspergillus* species do not stain well and may be missed in H&E-stained tissue sections. In order to detect small numbers of organisms and to clearly define the morphologic features of the infecting organism, special stains such as GMS and PAS must be used. The Fontana–Masson stain is used to stain for melanin in the fungal cell wall. It is useful in highlighting lightly pigmented dematiaceous fungi and for differentiating capsule-negative strains of *C. neoformans* (positive for melanin) from other yeasts (negative for melanin) in tissue (27). The mucicarmine stain is also used to identify *C. neoformans* in tissue by staining the polysaccharide capsule of the fungus. When available, specific immunofluorescent stains may be quite helpful not only in detection of fungal elements, but also in confirming a presumptive histologic identification of fungi, such as *Aspergillus*, *Candida*, *Cryptococcus*, the dimorphic fungi, and others (39). In situ hybridization with specific molecular probes may also be used more in the future (40). Finally, histologic examination of fixed tissue serves as an aid in determining infection (deep penetration into viable tissue) vs. colonization (superficial involvement of nonviable tissue) (27). A description of the microscopic morphologic features of several of the etiologic agents is presented in Table 7.

D. Culture

The most-sensitive means of diagnosing a fungal infection is generally considered the isolation of the infecting agent on culture media. In most instances, culture is necessary to specifically identify the etiologic agent and, if indicated, to determine the susceptibility to various antifungal agents.

Multiple factors must be considered in order to optimize the recovery of fungi from clinical material. In addition to adequate specimen procurement, a combination of culture media should be used to ensure the isolation of a broad array of medi-

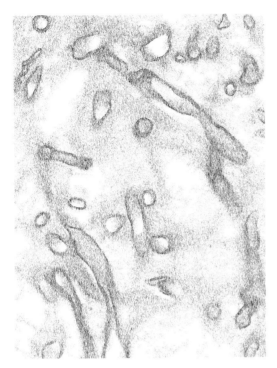

Figure 13 Tissue biopsy showing *Rhizopus* spp. stained with H&E. The variation in shape and size of hyphae is evident. Magnification, ×1000.

Figure 14 Giemsa-stained BAL cytopreparation. Mature *P. jiroveci* cysts containing intra-cystic forms with purple nuclei and light blue cytoplasm are seen. The cyst wall is unstained and appears as a clear rim. Magnification, ×1000.

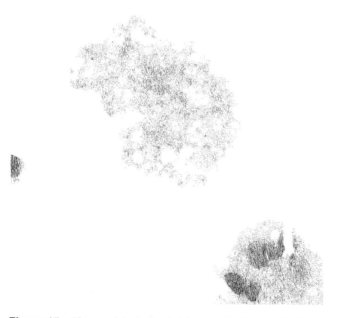

Figure 15 Clump of *P. jiroveci* stained with Giemsa. Both extracystic and intracystic forms are evident. Magnification, ×1000.

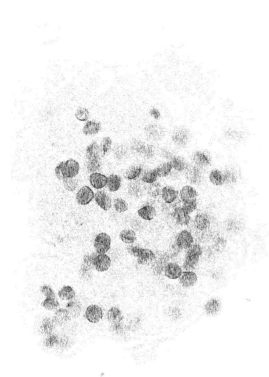

Figure 16 GMS stain of BAL fluid demonstrating cysts of *P. jiroveci (carinii)*. Both intact and collapsed cysts are present. Extracystic forms (clump) are not stained. Magnification, ×1000.

Figure 17   A mature spherule of *C. immitis* in lung tissue. PAS stain. Magnification, ×500.

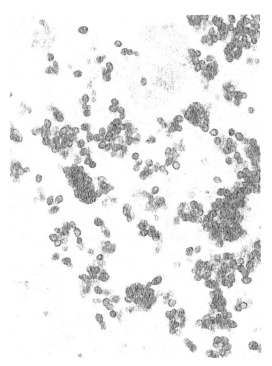

Figure 18   Silver stain demonstrating small budding yeast forms of *H. capsulatum*. Note the similarity in size and shape to *C. glabrata* shown in Figure 2.

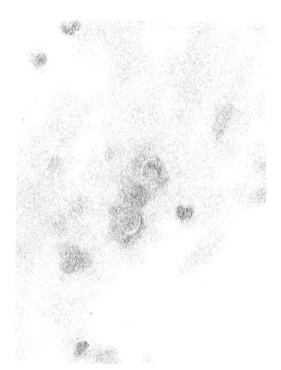

Figure 19 Broad-based budding yeasts of *B. dermatitidis* in a cytological preparation. PAS stain. Magnification, ×1000.

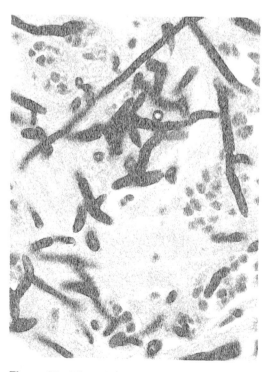

Figure 20 Tissue biopsy showing the branching septate hyphae of *Fusarium* spp. GMS stain. Magnification, ×1000.

Figure 21 PAS stain of tissue demonstrating the variable size and shape of *Sporothrix schenckii* yeast cells. Magnification, ×1000.

Figure 22 *Cryptococcus neoformans* in skin biopsy stained with PAS. Note variation in size and capsular artifact surrounding yeast cells. Magnification, ×1000.

cally important fungi. Generally, both selective and nonselective media are used for primary recovery of fungi from clinical specimens. Nonselective media such as brain heart infusion (BHI) agar or Sabouraud glucose plus BHI (SABHI) agar will permit the recovery of both rapidly growing molds and yeasts, as well as the more slowly growing, or fastidious fungi. Sabouraud glucose agar is generally considered inferior to these media for primary isolation and should not be used. Routine bacteriologic media, such as sheep blood agar and chocolate agar will support the growth of most fungi; however, growth may be slow and not detectable in the short time period (3–5 days) allowed for the incubation of most bacterial cultures. A blood-containing medium such as BHI, with 5–10% sheep blood, may be used in addition to the non-selective primary isolation media as an aid in recovering fastidious dimorphic fungi such as *H. capsulatum* and *B. dermatitidis*. Although cycloheximide is often added to BHI-blood agar to inhibit the growth of rapidly growing yeasts and molds that may "contaminate" the specimen, it is important to realize that this agent can inhibit the growth of many opportunistic pathogens that may also be the etiologic agent of the infection. For this reason, media supplemented with cycloheximide must always be complemented by the same media without the inhibitory agent. Specimens that may be contaminated with bacteria should also be cultured on a selective medium such as inhibitory mold agar, SABHI, or BHI plus antibacterial agents (e.g., genta-micin, chloramphenicol, or ciprofloxacin plus streptomycin). CHROMagar (Hardy Diagnostics, Santa Maria, California, U.S.A.) is a recently developed medium that is both selective for fungi and differential for certain *Candida* species (41,42). This medium inhibits bacterial growth and because different species of *Candida* appear as different colored colonies, it is useful in detecting mixed cultures of *Candida* and other fungi (42). In certain situations, it is necessary to utilize specialized media for recovery of specific fungi. For example, medium supplemented with olive oil is necessary for recovery of *Malassezia furfur* (Fig. 23), and the use of malt agar, or even sterile bread without preservatives, will enhance the isolation of the Zygomycetes.

Although not all serious fungal infections are marked by hematogenous disse-mination and fungemia, detection of fungemia is useful in diagnosing opportunistic infection caused by *Candida* spp., *C. neoformans*, *Trichosporon* spp., *Malassezia* spp., *Fusarium* spp., and occasionally *Acremonium* spp. (23,26,43). Blood cultures may be negative in the face of disseminated disease; however, advances in blood culture tech-nology have markedly improved the ability of laboratories to detect fungemia (43,44). The lysis centrifugation method (Isolator, Wampole, Dayton, New Jersey, U.S.A.) and the continuous monitoring automated blood culture systems are all sen-sitive methods for the detection of fungemia caused by *Candida* spp. (43). The devel-opment of specialized broth media containing lytic agents, resins, charcoal, or diatomaceous earth coupled with continuous agitation has contributed to the improved performance of the broth-based systems (43). However, recovery of *C. neoformans*, *H. capsulatum*, *M. furfur*, and *Fusarium* spp. may be inferior to broth-based methods compared with results of the lysis centrifugation method (43–45). Optimal detection of fungemia requires the collection of adequate volumes (20–30 mL) of blood and the use of both a broth-(vented, agitated) and an agar-based (lysis centrifugation) blood culture method (16,26).

Interpretation of the results of fungal cultures may be difficult because of the issues of colonization of certain body sites (e.g., respiratory, GI, and GU tracts) and contamination of specimens or cultures by environmental organisms many of which can also serve as etiologic agents of opportunistic mycoses. While most iso-lates of *Candida*, *C. neoformans*, *H. capsulatum*, and *Fusarium* obtained from blood

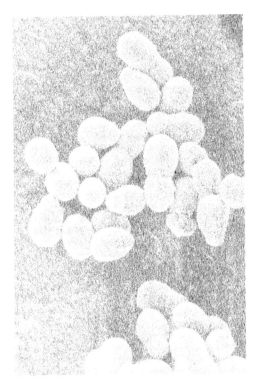

Figure 23 Scanning electron micrograph of *M. furfur* colonizing the lumen of a central venous catheter. The characteristic collarette at the junction between mother and daughter cell may be seen.

cultures are clinically significant (26,43,44), others such as *Aspergillus* spp. (not *A. terreus)* and *Penicillium* spp. (not *P. marneffei)* are most probably contaminants (46). Direct visualization of the organism in tissue helps to confirm the clinical importance of the isolation of *Aspergillus* from cultures obtained from the respiratory tract (25). However, for high-risk patients, such as allogeneic BMT recipients, individuals with hematologic malignancies, and those with neutropenia or malnutrition, a positive culture alone that yields *Aspergillus* spp. is associated with invasive disease (25) (Table 8). Specific identification of fungi isolated from culture can often

Table 8 Risk of IA Among Patients in Different Risk Categories Whose Cultures were Positive for *Aspergillus* spp.

Risk category	% Risk of IA (range)
High[a]	57 (50–64)
Intermediate[b]	15 (8–28)
Low[c]	< 1 (0–1)

[a]Includes allogeneic BMT, neutropenia, and hematologic cancer patients.
[b]Includes autologous BMT, malnutrition, corticosteroids, HIV, solid-organ transplant, diabetes, underlying pulmonary disease, and solid-organ cancer patients.
[c]Includes cystic fibrosis and connective tissue disease patients.
Source: Adapted from Ref. 25.

help in determining clinical significance: *A. niger* is rarely a pathogen, whereas *A. terreus* and *A. flavus* have been shown to be statistically associated with IA when isolated from respiratory tract cultures (25). Likewise, *H. capsulatum*, *B. dermatitidis*, and *C. immitis* are virtually always considered to be pathogens.

E. Identifying Characteristics of Fungi

Identification of fungi to genus and species is increasingly important as the spectrum of opportunistic pathogens continues to expand. Although the clinical presentation of many fungal infections may be indistinguishable, specific identification of the etiologic agent may have a direct bearing on the prognosis and therapeutic considerations. Now, more than ever it is clear that a single approach (e.g., using amphotericin B) for the management of all fungal infections is inadequate for many of the invasive mycoses (47,48). Furthermore, the identification of fungal pathogens may have additional diagnostic and epidemiologic implications. In the case of the more unusual mycoses, specific identification of the etiologic agent may provide access to the literature and the experience of others regarding the clinical course of infection and response to therapy.

The first and most basic step in the identification process is to differentiate yeasts from molds. Visual inspection of colonies growing on agar provides the first clue; yeasts usually produce pasty opaque colonies, whereas molds form large filamentous or "hairy" colonies with variations in texture, color, and topography. Microscopic examination with visualization of budding cells and pseudohyphae (yeasts) or filamentous hyphae and fruiting bodies (molds) further delineates these two large groups. Depending on the fungus, identification to the level of genus and species usually requires more detailed morphologic characterization supplemented by specific biochemical and physiologic tests (49) (Table 7). Increasingly, definitive identification of fungi is accomplished by immunologic and molecular characterization (50,51).

Yeasts are usually characterized morphologically as single cells that reproduce by simple budding; however, under certain conditions some yeasts may form true hyphae, pseudohyphae, capsules, arthroconidia, and other reproductive structures (49). Colonies form on most agar media within a few (2–5) days and are usually round, opaque, moist or mucoid, and white or cream colored. Because *C. albicans* constitutes the vast majority of yeasts recovered from clinical specimens, several rapid and simple tests have been devised to distinguish it from other yeasts (52). The most widely used test for the identification of *C. albicans* is the germ tube test. *Candida albicans* forms germ tubes in 3 hr when incubated in serum or plasma at 35°C. Other *Candida* species are capable of germ-tube formation but require extended incubation. *Candida dubliniensis* and *C. stellatoidea* are capable of forming germ tubes within 3 hr and may be difficult or impossible to differentiate from *C. albicans* without performing additional physiologic, immunologic, or nucleic acid-based testing (53–55). More recently, a rapid colorimetric test based on the detection of *C. albicans-specific* enzymes (L-proline aminopeptidase and β-galactosaminidase) or the use of agar medium containing chromogenic substrates (CHROMagar Candida, Hardy Diagnostics, Santa Maria, California, U.S.A.) has proven to be useful in the rapid presumptive identification of yeasts (41,42,56,57). Although a single presumptive identification test is not sufficient for identifying most yeasts, a positive germ tube, colorimetric test, characteristic green colony on CHROMagar medium is generally considered to be acceptable for the identification of *C. albicans*

(52). Importantly, although the appearance of small hyphal projections or "feet" from the edge of a colony has been cited as characteristic of *C. albicans* (52,58,59), further investigation has shown that both *C. tropicalis* and *C. krusei* are also capable of producing this phenotype (60).

Although more than 100 species of *Candida* have been identified, 95–98% of invasive candidal infections are caused by only five species: *C. albicans* (56%), *C. glabrata* (16%), *C. parapsilosis* (13%), *C. tropicalis* (10%), and *C. krusei* (3%) (3,61,62). Recent reports suggest that shifts have occurred in the distribution of non-*albicans* species with the emergence of *C. glabrata*, *C. krusei*, *C. lusitaniae*, and other less common species (16,61,63). Infections with these various species may require different therapeutic considerations (64,65a), and so further identification of all germ tube-negative or colorimetric test-negative yeasts is mandatory for isolates obtained from blood and other normally sterile body fluids (64,65a). Due to the pathogenic potential of *C. neoformans*, all encapsulated yeasts from any body site should also be identified. There are several rapid screening tests that may be used for the presumptive identification of *C. neoformans* including the urease test (positive), nitrate test (negative), and production of phenol oxidase (positive) (49).

Further identification of germ tube-negative yeasts to species requires the determination of biochemical and physiologic profiles and an assessment of their morphology when grown on a medium such as cornmeal agar or yeast morphology agar (49). In addition to the identification of *C. albicans*, colony morphology on CHROMagar allows the presumptive identification of *C. tropicalis* and *C. krusei* (41,42). Likewise, *C. glabrata* may be identified by a rapid trehalose test (49) or by differential growth on blood (no growth or slow growth) vs. eosin methylene blue (rapid growth) agar (66). Carbohydrate assimilation tests provide definitive identification of most of these species and may be performed by using one of the several commercial identification systems (55). Differentiation of yeasts with similar biochemical profiles can be accomplished by observing their microscopic characteristics on cornmeal agar (Table 7).

In contrast to yeasts, the identification of molds is largely based upon morphologic features such as gross colony appearance and microscopic morphology (Table 7). Visible growth on agar media may be obtained within 1–5 days for the Zygomycetes, most hyaline (light colored hyphae and conidia) hyphomycetes, and some, but not all, dematiaceous (dark pigmented hyphae and conidia) fungi. In contrast, the dimorphic fungi (*H. capsulatum*, *B. dermatitidis*, *C. immitis*, *Sporothrix schenckii*, and *Paracoccidioides brasiliensis*) grow much more slowly and may require 2–4 weeks of incubation. Furthermore, the dimorphic fungi are not inhibited by cycloheximide, an agent that inhibits the growth of most of the more rapidly growing molds that may represent either clinically unimportant "contaminants" or opportunistic pathogens causing infections in immunocompromised hosts.

The macroscopic appearance of many filamentous fungi when growing on solid media may provide clues as to the identification of the fungus. Variations in colonial morphology that may be medium- or strain-specific preclude the use of this feature as the sole criterion for identification. Surface texture, topography, color, reverse pigmentation, growth at 37°C, and requirements for specific vitamins are all useful characteristics. Potato glucose agar and cornmeal agar are considered two of the more reliable media for assessment of gross colonial morphology. Color development may be dependent on exposure to light.

Definitive identification of most molds is dependent upon visualization of the microscopic morphology of the fungus. Key morphologic features include the size, the shape, the method of production, and the arrangement of the conidia or spores, as well as the size and appearance of the hyphal structures. Material must be prepared for microscopic examination in such a way as to minimize any disruption of the relationship of the conidia or spores to their respective reproductive structures. This is usually best accomplished by the use of slide cultures whereby a cover slip is placed on the agar in such a way that the fungus spreads over the glass surface. The cover slip is then removed and placed on a slide for examination under the microscope. Determination of melanin and temperature-regulated dimorphism are also important characteristics. The dimorphic pathogens may also be characterized by immunologic- or nucleic acid probe–based methods in addition to morphology and thermal dimorphism. The typical features of selected filamentous and dimorphic pathogens are listed in Table 7.

F. Role of Surveillance Cultures

Fungal surveillance cultures of immunocompromised patients have been studied as potential predictors of invasive or disseminated mycoses (67–71). Although active surveillance of high-risk patients may enhance case detection of invasive candidiasis and aspergillosis, the data are quite variable (11,69,70,72–80). In the light of this problem, guidelines for the development of microbiologic surveillance protocols have been published and include (67,71,81) consideration of (i) the probability and severity of a specific infection in the patient population; (ii) the time period in which the risk of infection exists relative to the onset of immunosuppression; (iii) the accuracy, timeliness, and the cost of the tests used for surveillance; (iv) the sensitivity, specificity, positive (PPVs) and negative predictive values of a test result in an asymptomatic patient; (v) the efficacy of prophylactic therapy and the risk of development of resistance; and (vi) the expected impact on the clinical outcome.

It is generally acknowledged that the primary reservoir for hematogenously disseminated candidiasis is the GI tract and, to a lesser extent, the GU system (82). As such, one might expect that those immunocompromised patients with demonstrated colonization of several anatomic sites by *Candida* spp. to be at increased risk of invasive candidiasis compared with similar patients without colonization (69,78,83–85). Although several studies have shown this to be the case, it is clear that colonization without infection is very common, with the result that the PPV of a positive surveillance culture for *Candida* is quite low (11,69,71,75). Conversely, negative surveillance cultures may be helpful because individuals without colonization by *Candida* spp. rarely develop candidiasis (11,69,70,75).

The PPV of surveillance cultures for *Candida* may improve when species such as *C. tropicalis*, *C. glabrata*, or *C. krusei* are found colonizing high-risk patients (69,70,86). Detection of *C. glabrata* and *C. krusei* as colonizing agents may be of additional importance given that these species are typically less susceptible to azoles and other systemically active antifungal agents than *C. albicans* (3,63,86), thus prompting a change in empirical antifungal coverage for patients colonized by those species (64).

The poor sensitivity of routine nasal and respiratory cultures for *Aspergillus* spp. limits the usefulness of surveillance cultures for early detection of IA (25,67). The isolation of *Aspergillus* from respiratory specimens is often considered to represent contamination or colonization (67); however, it is now well established that a positive respiratory culture for *Aspergillus* in a host at high risk for IA is very suggestive of invasive disease and is an indication for more aggressive attempts at diagnosis and early empiric antifungal therapy (25,73,74,76,80).

The performance of surveillance cultures for *Candida* and *Aspergillus* may have some value in highly selected patient groups. However, the use of *routine* surveillance cultures of asymptomatic immunocompromised patients remains of questionable value and generally should be discouraged (71).

Environmental surveillance for *Aspergillus* and other molds is another controversial area (71). Clearly, environmental monitoring should be performed in an outbreak setting in an effort to detect and eliminate the source of infection (68,71,87,88). Beyond that specific situation, there are only a few additional indications for environmental surveillance (68,87). Specifically, air-quality monitoring to detect *Aspergillus* spores in air should be performed: (i) when clinical surveillance demonstrates a possible increase in mold infections; (ii) during periods of construction or renovation that take place near high-risk areas; (iii) before patients enter a new protected area or after renovation of the protected area; and (iv) when there is suspicion of dysfunction in the quality of air systems (68,87). Many centers also perform routine periodic air cultures (in addition to particulate counts) in protected environments to monitor the effectiveness of high-efficiency particulate air filters.

Unfortunately, specific standards for air-quality monitoring have not been established. A variety of air-sampling techniques exist. Although each may have its own specific merits, the preferred method for use in the hospital setting is based on filtration and the impacting of particles (spores) from an air stream onto an agar surface. Once the air has been sampled, the number of colony forming units (CFUs) per cubic millimeter can be determined; however, interpretation of this number is also problematic because of a lack of agreement over the specific threshold of CFU per cubic millimeter above which the risk of IA is increased (89). Counts of $<0.1\text{--}1$ CFU/mm^3 are desirable; however, most experts recommend counts of <5 CFU/mm^3 in protected isolation units and selected operating rooms (68). It should be emphasized that such air sampling is just an aspect of a more comprehensive program of prevention (87). Routine air sampling in the absence of a specific problem generally should be discouraged (71).

V. ANTIFUNGAL SUSCEPTIBILITY TESTING

The field of antifungal susceptibility testing has progressed and matured over the past 15–20 years. In vitro susceptibility tests with antifungal agents are performed for the same reasons that tests with antibacterial agents are performed (65a,90–92): (i) to provide a reliable estimate of the relative activities of two or more agents; (ii) to correlate with in vivo activity and predict the likely outcome of therapy; (iii) to provide means by which to monitor the development of resistance among a normally susceptible population of organisms; and (iv) to predict the therapeutic potential of newly discovered investigational agents.

At the present time, the state of the art for susceptibility testing of yeasts is comparable to that of bacteria (65a,90–92). Standardized methods for performing antifungal susceptibility testing are reproducible, accurate, and available for use in clinical laboratories (93–95). The establishment of quality-control guidelines and interpretative criteria for a limited number of antifungal agents (Table 9) provides the basis for the application of this testing in the clinical laboratory (65a,90–92).

Table 9 Antifungal Susceptibility Testing: Interpretive Breakpoints Using NCCLS Methods[a]

Antifungal Agent	Interpretive breakpoints (µg/ml)			Comments (ref.)
	S	S-DD	R	
Fluconazole	≤8	16–32	≥64	NCCLS M27-A2, follows 90-60 rule of clinical response (65a)[b]
Itraconazole	≤0.12	0.25–.05	≥1	NCCLS M27-A2, follows 90-60 rule of 90-60 rule of clinical response (65a)
Flucytosine	≤4	8–16[c]	≥32	NCCLS M 27-A2 follows 90–60 rule of clinical response (65a)
Amphotericin B	≤1		>1	Use Etest or antibiotic medium 3
Caspofungin	NA	NA	NA	96% ≤ 2 µg/ml by NCCLS M27-A2(65b)
Voriconazole	≤1	2	≥4	98% ≤ 1 µg/ml by NCCLS M27-A2 (62)

[a]Pertains to *Candida* spp. only.
[b]90–60 rule: infections caused by susceptible isolates respond to appropriate therapy 90% of the time, whereas infections caused by resistant isolates (or infections treated with inappropriate antimicrobials) respond 60% of the time.

Establishing a clinical correlation between in vitro susceptibility tests and clinical outcome has been difficult; however, it is now clear that antifungal susceptibility testing can predict outcome in several situations including candidemia and mucosal infections (Table 10)(65a,91). The National Committee for Clinical Laboratory Standards (NCCLS) Sub-Committee on Antifungal Susceptibility Tests has

Table 10 Correlations of Susceptibility Testing with Outcome for Fungal and Bacterial Infections[ab]

Organism group	Number of studies	Number of patients	Cases with successful outcome % (no. of cases/total) by susceptibility class[c]		
			S	R	p Value
Fungi[d]	13	1,197	91 (828/923)	48 (131/274)	<0.001
Bacteria[e]	12	5,447	89 (4,521/5,081)	59 (215/366)	<0.001

[a]Antifungal testing performed according to NCCLS M27-A2.
[b]Susceptibility to antibacterial agents determined by MIC, zone diameter, AUC/MIC ratio, or peak/MIC ratio.
[c]Outcome measurement varied from clinical and/or microbiologic response to therapy.
[d]Includes mucosal, fungemia, meningitis, and disseminated infections treated with fluconazole, itraconazole, or ketoconazole.
[e]Includes bacteremia, otitis, and severe infections treated with various agents including cephalosporins, β-lactamase inhibitor combinations, aminoglycosides, and fluoroquinolones.
Source: Adapted from Ref. 65a.

Table 11 Recommendations for Studies of Fungal Isolates in the Clinical Laboratory

Clinical setting	Recommendation
Routine	Species level identification of all *Candida* isolates from deep sites
	Genus level identification of molds (species level preferred for *Aspergillus*)
	Routine antifungal testing of fluconazole and flucytosine against *Candida* isolated from blood and normally sterile body fluids and tissue
Oropharyngeal candidiasis	Determination of susceptibility to fluconazole and itraconazole may be helpful but not routinely necessary
	Susceptibility testing may be useful for patients unresponsive to azole therapy
Invasive disease with clinical failure of initial therapy	Consider susceptibility testing as an adjunct
	Candida species and amphotericin B
	Cryptococcus neoformans and fluconazole, flucytosine, or amphotericin B
	Histoplasma capsulatum and fluconazole
	Consultation with an experienced microbiologist recommended
Infection with species with high rates of intrinsic or acquired resistance	Susceptibility testing not necessary when intrinsic resistance is known (e.g., *C. krusei* vs. fluconazole; *A. terreus* vs. amphotericin B)
	Select therapy based on literature. When high rates of acquired resistance (e.g., *C. glabrata* and fluconazole) monitor closely for signs of failure and perform susceptibility testing
New treatment options (e.g., caspofungin, voriconazole) or unusual organisms	Select therapy based on published consensus guidelines and review of survey data on the organism–drug combination in question
Patients who respond to therapy despite being infected with an isolate later found to be resistant	Best approach not clear
	Take into account severity of infection, patient immune status, consequences of recurrence of infection, etc.
	Consider alternative therapy for infections with isolates that appear to be highly resistant to therapy selected
Mold infections	Susceptibility testing not recommended as a routine. Interpretive criteria have not been established
Selection of susceptibility testing method	Standardized methods
	NCCLS broth-based methods
	Yeasts; M27-A2
	Molds; M38-A
	Agar-based methods
	Etest, numerous agents, yeast, and molds
	Disk (fluconazole, voriconazole), NCCLS M44-P method for yeasts

Source: Adapted from Ref. 65a.

developed and published approved reference methods for broth dilution testing of yeasts (93) and filamentous fungi (94) and has proposed a standard method for disk diffusion testing of yeasts against fluconazole (62,95,96). Studies are now ongoing to further refine these methods and to examine the in vivo correlation with the in vitro data for molds (97).

Despite this progress, it remains to be seen how useful antifungal susceptibility testing will be in guiding therapeutic decision making. Guidelines for the use of laboratory studies, including antifungal testing have been developed (Table 11) (65a). Selective application of in vitro susceptibility testing, coupled with broader identification of fungi to the species level, should prove to be useful, especially in difficult to manage fungal infections (64,65a). Future efforts will be directed toward further validation of interpretive breakpoints for established antifungal agents and developing them for newly introduced systemically active agents. In addition, procedures must be optimized for testing non-*Candida* yeasts (e.g., *C. neoformans*, *Trichosporon*) and molds (90).

VI. SUMMARY AND CONCLUSIONS

The infectious fungi now constitute one of the most important threats to the survival of immunocompromised hosts. There is little doubt that in addition to *C. albicans* and *A. fumigatus*, a vast array of fungi, previously considered to be non-pathogens, have now emerged as significant human pathogens. Recognition of these emerging fungal pathogens has resulted in a better understanding of their clinical presentation and response to the available therapeutic measures. Conventional laboratory-based methods for diagnosis of fungal infections remain useful but are often slow and lack sensitivity. Clearly, there is a need for improved diagnosis and management of these difficult infections. Newer broad-spectrum antifungal agents should prove useful but may require more sensitive methods for diagnosing the infections, as well as for estimating the extent of disease to significantly impact disease outcome. Broad application of both new and established antifungal agents may also select more resistant organisms from the vast pool of environmental opportunistic fungi. Such "emerging" fungal pathogens will pose yet another set of diagnostic and therapeutic challenges and will require that they are both visualized in tissue and identified in culture to truly define their pathogenesis and response to treatment.

REFERENCES

1. Chiller TM, Galgiani JN, Stevens DA. Coccidioidomycosis. Infect Dis Clin North Am 2003; 17:41–57.
2. Patterson TF, Kirkpatrick WR, White M. Invasive aspergillosis: disease spectrum, treatment practices, and outcomes. Medicine 2000; 79:250–260.
3. Pfaller MA, Diekema DJ. 12 Years of fluconazole in clinical practice: Global trends in species distribution and fluconazole susceptibility of bloodstream isolates of *Candida*. Clin Microbiol Infect 2003; Suppl 1: 11–23.
4. Rees JR, Pinner RW, Hajjeh RA, Brandt MR, Reingold AL. The epidemiologic features of invasive mycotic infection in the San Francisco Bay Area 1992–1993: results of a population-based laboratory active surveillance. Clin Infect Dis 1998; 27:1138–1147.
5. Trick WE, Fridkin SK, Edwards JR, Hajjeh RA, Gaynes RA. The National Nosocomial Infections Surveillance System Hospitals. Secular trends of hospital acquired candidemia

among intensive care unit patents in the United States during 1998–1999. Clin Infect Dis 2002; 35:627–630.

6. Walsh TJ, Groll AH. Emerging fungal pathogens: evolving challenges to immuno-compromised patients for the twenty-first century. Transpl Infect Dis 1999; 1:247–261.

7. Wheat LJ, Kauffman CA. Histoplasmosis. Infect Dis Clin North Am 2003; 17:1–19.

8. Gudlaugsson O, Gilespie S, Lee K, Vande Berg J, Messer S, Herwaldt L, Pfaller M, Diekema D. Nosocomial candidemia: attributable mortality and excess length of stay revisited. Clin Infect Dis 2003; 37:1172–1177.

9. Lin S, Schranz J, Teutsch S. Aspergillosis case-fatality rate: systematic review of the literature. Clin Infect Dis 2001; 32:358–366.

10. McNeil MM, Nash SL, Hajjeh RA, Phelan MA, Conn LA, Pilkaytis BD, Warnock DW. Trends in mortality due to invasive mycotic diseases in the United States, 1980–1997. Clin Infect Dis 2001; 33:641–647.

11. Blumberg HM, Jarvis WR, Soucie JM, Edwards JE, Patterson JE, Pfaller MA, Rangel-Frausto MS, Rinaldi MG, Saiman L, Wiblin RT, Wenzel RP. The NEMIS study group. Risk factors for candidal bloodstream infection in surgical intensive care unit patients: The NEMIS perspective multicenter study. Clin Infect Dis 2001; 33:177–186.

12. Saiman L, Ludington E, Pfaller M, Rangel-Frausto S, Wiblin RT, Dawson J, Blumberg HM, Patterson JE, Rinaldi M, Edwards JE, Wenzel RP, Jarvis W. Risk factors for candidemia in neonatal intensive care unit patients. The National Epidemiology of Mycosis Study Group. Pediatr Infect Dis 2000; 19:319–324.

13. Singh N. Fungal infections in recipients of solid organ transplantation. Infect Dis Clin North Am 2003; 17:113–134.

14. Mirza SA, Phelan M, Rimland D, Graviss E, Hamill R, Brandt ME, Gardner T, Sattah M, Ponce de Leon G, Baughman W, Hajjeh RA. The changing epidemiology of crypto-coccosis: an update from population-based active surveillance in 2 large metropolitan areas, 1992–2000. Clin Infect Dis 2003; 36:789–794.

15. Pfaller MA. The fungal pathogen shift in the United States. J Crit Illness 2001; 16(suppl): S35–S42.

16. Pfaller MA, McGinnis MR. The laboratory and clinical mycology. In: Anaissie EJ, McGinnis MR, Pfaller MA, eds. Clinical Mycology. New York: Churchill Livingstone, 2003:67–79.

17. Nesky MA, McDougal EC, Peacock JE Jr. *Pseudallescheria boydii* brain abscess successfully treated with voriconazole and surgical drainage: case report and literature review of central nervous system pseudallescheriasis. Clin Infect Dis 2000; 31:673–677.

18. Richter S, Cormican MG, Pfaller MA, Lee CK, Gingrich R, Rinaldi MG, Sutton DA. Fatal disseminated *Trichoderma longibrachiatum* infection in an adult bone marrow transplant patient: species identification and review of the literature. J Clin Microbiol 1999; 37:1154–1160.

19. Torres HA, Rivero GA, Lewis RE, Hachem R, Raad II, Kontoyiannis DP. Aspergillosis caused by non-*fumigatus Aspergillus* species: risk factors and in vitro susceptibility compared with *Aspergillus fumigatus*. Diagn Microbiol Infect Dis 2003; 46:25–28.

20. Perfect JR, Marr KA, Walsh TJ, Greenberg RN, DuPont B, de la Torre-Cisneros J, Just- Nübling G, Schlaman HT, Lutsar I, Espinel-Ingroff A, Johnson E. Voriconazole treatment for less-common, emerging, or refractory fungal infections. Clin Infect Dis 2003; 36:1122–1131.

21. Schell WA. New aspects of emerging fungal pathogens: a multifaceted challenge. Clin Lab Med 1995; 15:365–386.

22. Koneman EW, Roberts GD. The appearance of fungi in tissues. Lab Med 2002; 33: 927–933.

23. O'Shaughnessy EM, Shea YM, Witebsky FG. Laboratory diagnosis of invasive mycoses. Infect Dis Clin North Am 2003; 17:135–158.

24. Merz WG, Roberts GD. Algorithms for detection and identification of fungi. In: Murray PR, Baron EJ, Jorgensen JH, Pfaller MA, Yolken RH, eds. Manual of Clinical Microbiology. Washington DC: American Society for Microbiology, 2003:1668–1685.

25. Perfect JR, Cox GM, Lee JY, Kauffman CA, de Repentigny L, Chapman SW, Morrison VA, Pappas P, Hiemenz JW, Stevens DA. The Mycoses Study Group. The impact of culture isolation of *Aspergillus* species: a hospital-based survey of aspergillosis. Clin Infect Dis 2001; 33:1824–1833.

26. Pfaller MA. Laboratory aids in the diagnosis of invasive candidiasis. Mycopathologia 1992; 120:65–72.

27. Woods GH, Schnadig VJ. Histopathology of fungal infections. In: Anaissie EJ, McGinnis MR, Pfaller MA, eds. Clinical Mycology. New York: Churchill Livingstone, 2003:80–95.

28. Fleming RV, Walsh TJ, Anaissie EJ. Emerging and less common fungal pathogens. Infect Dis Clin North Am 2002; 16:915–934.

29. Diekema DJ, Messer SA, Hollis RJ, Jones RN, Pfaller MA. Activity of caspofungin and the new trizoles compared with itraconazole and amphotericin B against 462 recent clinical isolates of filamentous fungi. J Clin Microbiol 2003; 41:3623–3626.

30. Dictar MO, Maiolo E, Alexander B, Jacob N, Veron MT. Mycoses in the transplanted patient. Med Mycol 2000; 38(suppl 1):251–258.

31. Kao AS, Brandt ME, Pruitt WR, Conn LA, Perkins BA, Stephens DS, Baughman WS, Reingold AL, Rothrock GA, Pfaller MA, Pinner RW, Hajjeh RA. The epidemiology of candidemia in two United States cities: results of a population-based active surveillance. Clin Infect Dis 1999; 29:1164–1170.

32. Marr KA, Carter RA, Crippa F, Wald A, Corey L. Epidemiology and outcome of mould infections in hematopoietic stem cell transplant recipients. Clin Infect Dis 2002; 34:909–917.

33. Miller JM, Holmes HT, Krisher K. General principles of specimen collection and handling. In: Murray PR, Baron EJ, Jorgensen JH, Pfaller MA, Yolken RH, eds. Manual of Clinical Microbiology. Washington DC: American Society for Microbiology, 2003:55–66.

34. Sutton DA. Specimen collection, transport, and processing: mycology. In: Murray PR, Baron EJ, Jorgensen JH, Pfaller MA, Yolken RH, eds. Manual of Clinical Microbiology. Washington, DC: American Society for Microbiology, 2003:1712–1725.

35. Cushion MT. Pneumocystis. In: Murray PR, Baron EJ, Jorgensen JH, Pfaller MA, Yolken RH, eds. Manual of Clinical Microbiology. Washington, DC: American Society for Microbiology, 2003:1712–1725.

36. Powers CN. Diagnosis of infectious diseases: a cytopathologists' perspective. Clin Microbiol Rev 1998; 11:341–365.

37. Procop GW, Wilson M. Infectious disease pathology. Clin Infect Dis 2001; 32:1589–1601.

38. Woods GL, Walker DH. Detection of infection or infectious agents by use of cytologic and histologic stains. Clin Microbiol Rev 1996; 9:382–404.

39. Kaufman L, Standard PG, Jalberl M, Kraft DE. Immunohistologic identification of *Aspergillus* spp. and other hyaline fungi by using polyclonal fluorescent antibodies. J Clin Microbiol 1997; 35:2206–2209.

40. Hayden RT, Qian X, Roberts GD. In situ hybridization for the identification of yeast-like organisms in tissue section. Diagn Mol Pathol 2001; 10:15–23.

41. Odds FC, Bernaerts R. CHROMagar *Candida*, a new differential isolation medium for presumptive identification of clinically important *Candida* species. J Clin Microbiol 1994; 32:1923–1929.

42. Pfaller MA, Houston A, Coffman S. Application of CHROMagar *Candida* for rapid screening of clinical specimens for *Candida albicans, Candida tropicalis, Candida krusei* and *Candida (Torulopsis) glabrata*. J Clin Microbiol 1996; 34:58–61.

43. Magadia R, Weinstein MP. Laboratory diagnosis of bacteremia and fungemia. Infect Dis Clin North Am 2001; 15:1009–1024.

44. Reimer LG, Wilson ML, Weinstein MP. Update on bacteremia and fungemia. Clin Microbiol Rev 1997; 10:444–465.

45. Lyon R, Woods G. Comparison of the BacT/Alert and isolator blood culture systems for recovery of fungi. Am J Clin Pathol 1995; 103:660–662.

46. Duthie R, Denning DW. *Aspergillus fungemia*: report of 2 cases review. Clin Infect Dis 1995; 20:598–605.

47. Groll AH, Gea-Banacloche JC, Glasmacher A, Just-Nüebling G, Maschmeyer G, Walsh TJ. Clinical pharmacology of antifungal compounds. Infect Dis Clin North Am 2003; 17:159–191.

48. Roilides E, Lyman CA, Panagopoulou P, Chanock S. Immunomodulation of invasive fungal infections. Infect Dis Clin North Am 2003; 17:193–219.

49. Larone DH. Medically important fungi: a guide to identification. 4th ed.Washington, DC: American Society for Microbiology, 2002.

50. Guarro J, Genē J, Stchigel AM. Developments in fungal taxonomy. Clin Microbiol Rev 1999; 12:454–500.

51. Kurtzman CP, Fell JW. The yeasts, A Taxonomic Study. 4th ed. Elsevier Science B.V.Amsterdam. 1998.

52. National Committee for Clinical Laboratory Standards. Abbreviated Identification of Bacteria and Yeast; Approved Guideline. NCCLS document M35-A. Wayne, PA: NCCLS, 2002.

53. Gales AC, Pfaller MA, Houston AK, Joly S, Sullivan DJ, Coleman DC, Soll DR. Identification of *Candida dubliniensis* based on temperature and utilization of xylose and α-methyl-D-glucoside as determined with the API 20C AUX and Vitek YBC systems. J Clin Microbiol 1999; 37:3804–3808.

54. Pinjon E, Sullivan D, Salkin I, Shanley D, Coleman D. Simple, inexpensive, reliable method for differentiation f *CAndida dubliniensis* from *Candida albicans*. J Clin Microbiol 1998; 36:2093–2095.

55. Hazen KC, Howell SA. *Candida, Cryptococcus; and other ueasts of medical importance.* In: Murray PR, Baron EJ, Jorgensen JH, Pfaller MA, Yolken RH, eds. Manual of Clinical Microbiology. 8th ed. Washington, DC: American Society for Microbiology, 2003: 1693–1711.

56. Hazen KC. New and emerging yeast pathogens. Clin Microbiol Rev 1995; 8:462–478.

57. Koehler AP, Chu KC, Houang ETS, Cheng AFB. Simple, reliable, and cost-effective yeast identification scheme for the clinical laboratory. J Clin Microbiol 1999; 37:422–426.

58. Nagashi K, Baron EJ. Identification of *Candida albicans* by colony morphology. Clin Microbiol Newsletter 1997; 19:112.

59. Calvin C, Freeman C, Masterson R, Miles D, Straedey V, Vineyard M. Identification of *Candida albicans* by colony morphology. Clin Microbiol Newsletter 1998; 20:16.

60. Buschelman B, Jones RN, Pfaller MA, Koontz FP, Doern GV. Colony morphology of *Candida* spp. as a guide to species identification. Diagn Microbiol Infect Dis 1999; 35: 89–91.

61. Pfaller MA, Diekema DJ. Role of sentinel surveillance of candidemia: trends in species distribution and antifungal susceptibility. J Clin Microbiol 2002; 40:3551–3557.

62. Pfaller MA, Diekema DJ, Messer SA, Boyken L, Hollis RJ. Activities of fluconazole and voriconazole against 1,586 recent clinical isolates of *Candida* species determined by broth microdilution, disk diffusion, and Etest methods: report from the ARTEMIS Global Antifungal Susceptibility Program, 2001. J Clin Microbiol 2003; 41:1440–1446.

63. Pfaller MA, Diekema DJ, Messer SA, Boyken L, Hollis RJ, Jones RN. The International Fungal Surveillance Participant Group. In vitro activities of voriconazole, posaconazole, and four licensed systemic antifungal agents against *Candida* species infrequently isolated from blood. J Clin Microbiol 2003; 41:78–83.

64. Rex JH, Walsh TJ, Sobel JC, Filler SG, Pappas PG, Dismukes WE, Edwards JE. Practice guidelines for the treatment of candidiasis. Clin Infect Dis 2000; 30:662–678.

65a. Rex JH, Pfaller MA. Has antifungal susceptibility testing come of age? Clin Infect Dis 2002; 35:982–989;

65b. Pfaller MA, Diekema DJ, Messer SA, Hollis RJ, Jones RN. In vitro activities of caspofungin compared with those of fluconazole and itraconazole against 3,959 clinical isolates of *Candida* spp., including 157 fluconazole-resistant isolates. Antimicrob Agents Chemother 2003; 47:1068–1071.

66. Bale MJ, Yang C, Pfaller MA. Evaluation of growth characteristics on blook agar and eosin methylene blue agar for the identification of *Candida* (Torulopsis) glabrata. Diagn Microbiol Infect Dis 1997; 29:65–67.

67. La Rocco MT, Burgert SJ. Infection in the bone marrow transplant recipient and role of the microbiology laboratory in clinical transplantation. Clin Microbiol Rev 1997; 10: 277–297.

68. Muñoz P, Burillo A, Bouza E. Environmental surveillance and other control measures in the prevention of nosocomial fungal infections. Clin Microbiol Infect 2001; 7(suppl 2): 38–45.

69. Pfaller M, Cabezudo I, Koontz F, Bale M, Gingrich R. Predictive value of surveillance cultures for systemic infection due to *Candida* species. Eur J Clin Microbiol 1987; 6:628–633.

70. Sanford GR, Merz WG, Wingard JR, Charache P, Saral R. The value of fungal surveillance cultures as predictors of systemic fungal infections. J Infect Dis 1980; 142:503–509.

71. Snydman DR. Posttransplant microbiological surveillance. Clin Infect Dis 2001; 33(suppl 1):S22–S25.

72. Collins LA, Samore MH, Roberts MS, Luzzati R, Jenkins RL, Lewis WD, Karchmer AW. Risk factors for invasive fungal infections complicating orthotopic liver transplantation. J Infect Dis 1994; 170:644–652.

73. Kusne S, Torre-Cisneros J, Manez R, Rish W, Martin M, Fung J, Simmons RL, Starzl TE. Factors associated with invasive lung aspergillosis and the significance of positive *Aspergillus* culture after liver transplantation. J Infect Dis 1992; 66:1379–1383.

74. Nalesnk MA, Myerowitz RL, Jenkins R, Lenkey J, Herbert D. Significance of *Aspergillus* species isolated from respiratory secretions in the diagnosis of invasive pulmonary aspergillosis. J Clin Microbiol 1980; 11:370–376.

75. Riley DK, Pavia AT, Beatty PG, Denton D, Carroll KC. Surveillance cultures inbone marrow recipients: worthwhile or wasteful? Bone Marrow Transplant 1995; 15:469–473.

76. Rogers TR, Visscher DW, Bartlett MS, Smith JW. Diagnosis of pulmonary infection caused by *Aspergillus*: Usefulness of respiratory cultures. J Infect Dis 1985; 152:572–576.

77. Saiman L, Ludington E, Dawson JD, Patterson JE, Rangel-Frausto S, Wiblin RT, Blumberg HM, Pfaller M, Rinaldi M, Edwards JE, Wenzel RP, Jarvis W. The National Epidemiology of Mycoses Study Group. Risk factors for *Candida* species colonization of neonatal intensive care unit patients. Pediatr Infect Dis J 2002; 20:1119–1124.

78. Tollemar J, Holmberg K, Ringden O, Lonnqvist B. Surveillance tests for the diagnosis of invasive fungal infections in bone marrow transplant recipients. Scand J Infect Dis 1989; 21:205–212.

79. Tollemar J, Ericzon BG, Holmberg K, Andersson J. The incidence and diagnosis of invasive fungal infections in liver transplant recipients. Transplant Proc 1990; 22:242–244.

80. Yu VL, Muder RR, Poorsattar A. Significance of isolation of *Aspergillus* from the respiratory tract in diagnosis of invasive pulmonary aspergillosis. Results from a three-year prospective study. Am J Med 1986; 81:249–254.

81. Walker RC. The role of the clinical microbiology laboratory in transplantation. Arch Pathol Lab Med 1991; 115:299–305.

82. Pfaller MA. Nosocomial candidiasis: emerging species, reservoirs and modes of transmission. Clin Infect Dis 1996; 22(suppl 2):S89–S94.

83. Rossetti F, Brawner DL, Bowden R, Meyer WG, Schoch HG, Fisher L, Myerson D, Hackman RC, Shulman HM, Sale GE, Meyers JD, McDonald GB. Fungal liver infection in marrow transplant recipients: prevalence at autopsy, predisposing factors, and clinical features. Clin Infect Dis 1995; 20:801–811.

84. Vervaillei C, Weisdorf D, Haake R, Hostetter RM, Ramsay NK, McGlave P. *Candida* infections in bone marrow transplant recipients. Bone Marow Transplant 1991; 8:177–184.

85. Wey SB, Mori M, Pfaller MA, Woolson RF, Wenzel RP. Risk factors for hospital-acquired candidemia. Arch Intern Med 1989; 149:2349–2353.

86. Wingard JR, Merz WG, Rinaldi MG, Johnson TR, Karp JE, Saral R. Increase in *Candida krusei* infection among patients with bone marrow transplantation and neutropenia treated prophylactically with fluconazole. N Engl J Med 1991; 325:1274–1277.

87. Centers for Disease Control and Prevention. Guideline for preventing opportunistic infections among hematopoietic stem cell transplant recipients. Recommendations of CDC, the Infectious Disease Society of America, and the American Society of Blood and Marrow Transplantation. MMWR 2000; 49(RR-10): 1–125.

88. Richardson M, Rennie S, Marshall I. Fungal surveillance of an open haematology ward. J Hospital Infect 2000; 45:288–292.

89. Latge J. *Aspergillus fumigatus* and aspergillosis. Clin Microbiol Rev 1999; 12:310–350.

90. Pfaller MA, Yu WL. Antifungal susceptibility testing: new technology and clinical applications. Infect Dis Clin North Am 2001; 15:1222–1261.

91. Rex JH, Pfaller MA, Galgiani JN, Bartlett MS, Espinel-Ingroff A, Ghannoum MA, Lancaster M, Rinaldi MG, Walsh TJ, Barry AL. Development of interpretive breakpoints for antifungal susceptibility testing: conceptual framework and analysis of in vitro–in vivo correlation data for fluconazole, itraconazole and *Candida* infections. Clin Infect Dis 1997; 24:235–247.

92. Rex JH, Pfaller MA, Walsh TJ, Chaturvedi V, Espinel-Ingroff A, Ghannoum MA, Gosey LL, Odds FC, Rinaldi MG, Sheehan DJ, Warnock DW. Antifungal susceptibility testing: practical aspects and current challenges. Clin Microbiol Rev 2001; 14:643–658.

93. National Committee for Clinical Laboratory Standards. Reference Method for Broth Dilution Antifungal Susceptibility Testing of Yeasts; Approved Standard. National Committee for Clinical Laboratory Standards, Wayne, PA: 2nd ed. M27-A2. 2002.

94. National Committee for Clinical Laboratory Standards. Reference Method for Broth Dilution Antifungal Susceptibility Testing of Filamentous Fungi; Approved Standard M38- A. Wayne, PA: National Committee for Clinical Laboratory Standards, 2002.

95. National Committee for Clinical Laboratory Standards. Method for Antifungal Disk Diffusion Susceptibility Testing of Yeasts; Proposed Guideline M44-P. Wayne, PA: National Committee for Clinical Laboratory Standards, 2002.

96. Barry AL, Pfaller MA, Rennie RP, Fuchs PC, Brown SD. Precision and accuracy of fluconazole susceptibility testing by broth microdilution, Etest, and disk diffusion methods. Antimicrob Agents Chemother 2002; 46:1781–1784.

97. Odds FC, Von Ferven F, Espinel-Ingroff A, Bartlett MS, Ghannoum MA, Lancaster MV, Pfaller MA, Rex JH, Rinaldi MG, Walsh TJ. Evaluation of possible correlations between antifungal susceptibilities of filamentous fungi in vitro and antifungal treatment outcomes in animal infection models. Antimicrob Agents Chemother 1998; 42:282–288.

14

Serological and Molecular Approaches to the Diagnosis of Invasive Fungal Infections in Immunocompromised Patients

José L. López-Ribot and Thomas F. Patterson
Department of Medicine/Division of Infectious Diseases, The University of Texas, Health Science Center at San Antonio, San Antonio, Texas, U.S.A.

I. INTRODUCTION

Fungal infections have become increasingly important in the last few decades as advances in modern medicine prolong the lives of severely debilitated patients. A wide variety of hosts with compromised host defenses are at risk for these infections. These include HIV-infected, cancer, transplant, surgical and Intensive Care Unit (ICU) patients, and also newborn infants. Neutropenia, use of broad spectrum antibiotics, indwelling catheters, immunosuppression and disruption of mucosal barriers due to chemotherapy and radiotherapy constitute some of the main predisposing factors for these opportunistic infections.

Formulating effective strategies to improve the outcome for patients with invasive fungal infections represents a formidable challenge. Making the diagnosis of invasive fungal infections early and accurately enough to allow institution of timely and effective antifungal therapy is critical, and better diagnostic tools are urgently needed to identify infected patients. However, the diagnosis of invasive fungal infections remains difficult; the lack of sensitive and specific noninvasive diagnostic tests constitutes a major impediment for therapeutic advance. The most important issue remains the need for tests or procedures that allow early detection of disease or, equally important, to provide reliable evidence for the absence of fungal infection. The diagnosis of invasive fungal infections is usually difficult to establish by clinical criteria. Moreover, noninvasive diagnostic techniques have been limited in most opportunistic fungal pathogens. Thus, conventional diagnostic tests (histology, microscopy, and culture)—reviewed in the previous chapters of this book—remain the cornerstone of proving the presence or absence of fungal disease; however, their sensitivity is low and isolation of fungi from clinical specimens take valuable time, ranging from days to weeks; therefore, their impact on clinical decisions to treat patients is often limited. Many times, microbiological cultures become positive at a late stage of infection, and delayed therapy is clearly associated with a poor outcome. Development of methods for the detection of fungal antigens and antibodies, as well as molecular (PCR-based) methods represent promising noninvasive tools for the diagnosis of fungal infections. Because *Candida* and *Aspergiilus* account for a significant number of these infections, this review focuses mainly on noninvasive diagnostic advances for invasive candidiasis and aspergillosis, and reviews the current status for nonculture based methods for other more common pathogenic and endemic mycoses.

II. SERODIAGNOSIS OF INVASIVE CANDIDIASIS

Candidiasis represents now the fourth most frequent nosocomial infection in hospitals in the US and worldwide (1–4). These infections are caused by yeast-like fungi of the genus *Candida*. These are normally commensal organisms found colonizing human mucous membranes. *C. albicans* remains the most frequent causative agent of candidiasis but other species have been increasingly associated with infections in an expanding population of immunocompromised patients (2,3).

Morbidity and mortality rates associated with invasive candidiasis remain unacceptably high (5), the main reasons being the difficulties encountered in the diagnosis and treatment of this type of infection. Development of nonculture based laboratory methods for invasive candidiasis faces the difficult challenge of differentiating normal commensalism/colonization from tissue invasion and from candidemia requiring antifungal treatment. Blood cultures for *Candida* species generally exhibit low sensitivity, with less than 50% of cultures from patients with disseminated disease being positive, even when lysis of centrifugation tubes is performed that reportedly increases sensitivity of the technique (6–8). To date, most of the nonculture based diagnostic techniques can be considered investigational, limited to research laboratories, with several commercial tests having ended in only limited success due to the intrinsic problems associated with the diagnosis of these infections.

A. Antibody Detection

Standard serological tests to detect *anti-Candida* antibodies usually have failed to discriminate between colonization and invasive candidiasis, since anti-*Candida* antibodies are ubiquitous in human sera, leading to poor specificity values (false positives) (9). Additionally, the tests may present a low sensitivity (false negatives) in severely immunosuppressed patients in whom the antibody response may be delayed, reduced, or altogether absent (9). Thus, despite more than 50 years of experience in this field, to date the development of useful tests based on antibody detections remains a formidable unconquered challenge.

Early studies on antibody detection for diagnosis suffered from the fact that they used mostly whole cells or crude antigenic preparations that were difficult to standardize. Additionally, most of these antigenic preparations contained cell wall mannan, and antimannan antibodies are almost ubiquitous in human sera (8,10). These early assays for antibody detection used techniques such as latex agglutination, complement fixation, immunodiffusion, counter-immonoelectrophoresis and indirect immunofluorescence. In general, the resulting tests lacked sensitivity and specificity and were found to be of limited diagnostic value (11,12).

More recent studies have attempted to improve on previous results by using purified antigens (or alternatively defined antigenic preparations) and more sensitive techniques such as immunoblotting, radioimmunoassay, and most importantly enzyme-linked immuno sorbent assay (ELISA). Initially, there was a differentiation between antibodies against cell wall and cytoplasmic antigens; however, this differentiation is difficult because it has become evident that some "cytoplasmic" antigens can also be found as bona fide components of the cell wall (13).

Mannan is one of the main cell wall components of *Candida*. Most of the mannan in the wall structure is found in covalent association with proteins (mannoproteins) (10,13). As mentioned before, antimannan antibodies have been shown to be ubiquitous in human sera, presumably because the immune system can be stimulated as a result of colonization by *C. albicans* in the absence of disease (7–10). In any defined population, levels of antimannan antibodies are usually distributed about a mean; sera having the highest levels give positive precipitin tests when tested against cell wall mannan (14). When antimannan antibodies were measured in serially drawn sera from neutropenic patients, a frequency distribution plot showed that antibodies from patients with invasive candidiasis were elevated and tended to skew the normal distribution curve to the right. However, a clear bimodal distribution of these antibody values was not observed; thus, after establishing a cut-off value for anticell wall mannan antibodies, the best sensitivity value was about 65% (15). Sensitivities of 23–100% and specificities of 92–100% have been reported in ELISA assays for mannan detection (16). Most of these analyses considered mannan to be a single molecule, but failed to take into consideration its chemical and immunological complexity. More recently, several groups have reconsidered the diagnostic value of antimannan antibody detection. Several oligomannosidic epitopes were identified that react with antibodies in human sera (17–20). Based on these, the newer Platelia *Candida* antibody test (Bio-Rad, Redmond, WA) uses a standardized mannan preparation to coat ELISA plates to capture circulating antimannan antibodies in sera from patients, with reported specificity and sensitivity values of 94% and 53%, respectively (21). When performed simultaneously in combination with a mannan antigen detection test, the technique gave a specificity of 93% and a sensitivity of 80% (21,22). Similarly, van Deventer et al. (23) reported that a test measuring the antimannan antibodies was 64% sensitive and 89% specific in determining invasive candidiasis. In this report, antimannan antibody titers determined longitudinally in a group of immunocompromised patients with invasive candidiasis increased during the course of infection, as opposed to those who were only colonized.

Identification of antigens specific to the filamentous form of C. *albicans* could offer certain advantages, since filamentation is associated with invasive disease (24). By using an ELISA to detect antibodies against a defined cell wall extract from C. *albicans* germ tubes in sera previously depleted of antimannan antibodies, Navarro et al. (25) described a sensitivity of 89.2% and a specificity of 98.6% for the diagnosis of systemic candidiasis in a population of patients, including bone marrow transplant patients. Also, an indirect immunofluorescence test was developed that detected antibodies in patients' sera directed against germ-tube specific antigens (26–28). This test was useful in the diagnosis of invasive candidiasis in different patient populations, and showed an overall sensitivity of 77–89% and a specificity of 91–100% (27,29,30). The test was also valuable for the therapeutic monitoring of patients with invasive disease.

MacDonald and Odds (31) compared the titers of antibodies to candidal secreted aspartyl proteinase (SAP) and to cytoplasmic antigens in the sera of healthy individuals, patients with candidiasis, and other hospitalized patients without candidiasis. Levels of anti-SAP antibodies in human sera were higher in patients with candidiasis than in healthy individuals, while the antibody titer against candidal cytoplasmic antigens was similar in the two groups. Thus SAP could be a specific antigen for the serological diagnosis of candidiasis (31,32). Detection of anti-SAP antibodies for serodiagnosis has been attempted (33). Elevated levels of IgG antibodies to SAP were also observed in patients with invasive or disseminated candidiasis (34,35). However, it was reported that monitoring of anti-SAP antibodies alone was not useful for the diagnosis of invasive candidiasis (34).

Immunoblotting experiments with sera from patients suffering from systemic candidiasis showed the presence of a 47-kDa immunodominant antigen present in whole cell extracts of the fungus (36–38). This 47-kDa antigen was further identified as a heat-stable breakdown product of hsp90 with a cell wall location (39). Antibody to the 47-kDa antigen is present in serum samples from a high proportion of patients with chronic mucocutaneous candidiasis (CMC) and AIDS (36,40). Patients who recover from systemic candidiasis produce a major antibody response to the 47-kDa component, whereas fatal cases have little antibody or falling titers (36,38,41,42). In another report, Zoller et al. (43) used purified somatic antigens of *C. albicans,* including a 47-kDa component, in enzyme immunoassays for antibody detection in sera from patients with confirmed disseminated candidiasis. The assay had a sensitivity of 81.5% and a specificity of 97%. However, the identity of this 47-kDa antigen remains to be resolved, since it could actually be enolase (see below).

Despite the complex antigenic make-up and considerable heterogeneity of the antibody responses to candidal antigens in humans (9,13), several immunodominant antigens have been identified. Perhaps, the most prominent of these is the cytosolic glycolytic enzyme enolase (although it has to be noted that it has been demonstrated that enolase is also present in the cell wall of *C. albicans* (44)). Strockbine et al. (45) characterized the antigenic components in cytoplasmic extracts of *C. albicans* recognized by sera from patients with disseminated candidiasis. They found that these patients had circulating antibodies directed against a 48-kDa protein antigen, which was subsequently identified as enolase (46,47). Circulating antienolase antibodies may have potential value for the diagnosis of candidiasis (48,49). Thus, an ELISA using purified *C. albicans* enolase as target was devised to detect antibodies in sera from patients with proven candidiasis. Statistical analysis of the results obtained indicated that the assay was able to discriminate between invasive infection and simple colonization (48). However, the test suffered from low sensitivity. Using purified candidal enolase as antigen in immunoblotting experiments, another group detected antienolase IgG antibodies in serial samples drawn from 92.5% of the patients with systemic candidiasis examined with a specificity of 95% (49).

Greenfield and Jones (50,51) described a major *C. albicans* cytoplasmic antigen of a molecular mass of 54.3 kDa that was also present in *C. tropicalis* and *C. guillerrmondii.* An ELISA test was developed to detect antibodies against this antigen in serum samples from patients with acute leukemia. Despite its excellent specificity (100%) unfortunately, the authors reported only a sensitivity of 21.4%, possibly indicating that patients with candidiasis often failed to produce antibodies against antigen.

B. Antigen Detection

To overcome problems (mainly specificity problems) with the detection of anti-*Candida* antibodies, many investigators have focused their effort in the detection of circulating *Candida* antigens (8,9,12,42). However, from experience to date, it is clear that tests for determination of *Candida* antigens as markers for invasive disease need further fine-tuning to improve their sensitivity and specificity, so that they will be valuable in guiding clinical treatment decisions. Many times, the use of crude preparations of candidal antigens cannot be standardized enough to allow good test reproducibility among laboratories, which complicates development of such tests. Therefore, identification, characterization, and detection of defined fungal antigens may provide a suitable procedure for diagnosis of invasive-candidiasis (9,12).

Mannan is the major circulating antigen in patients with invasive candidiasis. Because antimannan antibodies are ubiquitous, mannan frequently circulates in the form of immunocomplexes, a dissociation of antigen–antibody complexes is required for optimal detection of circulating mannan (9,10,12,16). Sensitivities of 23–100% and specificities of 92–100% have been reported in ELISA assays for mannan detection (16). A commercial system to detect *Candida* mannan in serum, the Pastorex Candida test (Sanofi Diagnostics Pasteur, Mames-la-Coquette, France), appeared promising (11); however, Gutierrez et al. (52), who conducted a prospective clinical trial, found 0% sensitivity for this test. Lack of sensitivity is due to the rapid clearance of the antigen from patients' sera and the test format (latex agglutination). Of note, the sensitivity of the Pastorex system was improved when serial assays using multiple consecutive serum samples were used (53). More recently, a double-sandwich ELISA using the same monoclonal antibody (EBCA1) used in the Pastorex *Candida* has been developed, which improved the detection limit up to 0.1 ng of mannan/mL and resulted in increased sensitivity. This test now constitutes the basis for the Platelia *Candida* antigen test (Bio Rad) with reported sensitivity and specificity values of 40% and 98%, respectively (21,22). As mentioned before, the utility of this assay is maximized when used in combination with the antibody detection test, but further evaluation and validation are needed to confirm its utility.

An extracellular proteinase activity from *C. albicans,* first reported by Staib (54), has been characterized as secreted aspartyl proteinases (SAPs). SAPs are important virulence factors in candidiasis (55); hence, the usefulness of SAP as a diagnostic antigen emanates from the idea that these enzymes are only produced during active tissue invasion during infection. Morrison et al. (56) purified this enzyme and removed contaminating mannan by column chromatography with sequential anion-exchange, gel permeation, and linear gradient anion-exchange steps. The polyclonal antibodies prepared against this purified SAP were used in a competitive binding enzyme immunoassay in an immunosuppressed rabbit model of disseminated candidiasis. This assay was able to detect SAP antigenuria within 24 h of IV challenge and could discriminate between gastrointestinal *C. albicans* colonization and disseminated candidiasis (57). Ruchel et al. (34) examined serum samples from patients with candidiasis for the presence of circulating SAP using a polyclonal anti-SAP antibody in a ELISA format. Proteinase antigen was detected in approximately 50% of suspected plus confirmed cases, indicating that detection of SAP has only limited diagnostic utility. However, a confounding factor could be the fact that SAP forms complexes in circulation.

C. albicans hsp90 circulates in body fluids of patients with disseminated candidiasis and its 47-kDa antigenic fragment was isolated from patients' sera by affinity chromatography (37). An enzyme-linked immunodot assay using affinity-purified antibody against the 47-kDa moiety was capable of detecting circulating antigen in the serum of patients (36). With this assay, systemic candidiasis was detected in 77% of neutropenic patients, and in 87% of non-neutropenic patients. The sensitivity and specificity of detection was improved over that of other commercially available products (36).

Antigenemia with the 48-kDa antigen (later found to be enolase) as detected by ELISA was observed in a murine model of disseminated candidiasis in the absence of fungemia and correlated with deep tissue infection (58). An assay was commercialized as a double sandwich assay using antienolase monoclonal antibody immobilized on nitrocellulose membrane for antigen capture, and subsequent detection with an anti-enolase polyclonal antibody (Directigen; Becton Dickinson) (58). To investigate the expression of this candidal cytoplasmic antigen in the serum of patients with cancer who are at high risk for deep invasive candidiasis, Walsh et al. (58) conducted a prospective clinical trial among patients from four medical oncology centers over a two-year period. They concluded that *C. albicans* enolase antigenemia is a marker for deep tissue invasion even in the absence of fungemia. The serum enolase immunoassay complemented rather than replaced blood cultures for the diagnosis of such infections (7,58). The assay was very specific (96%), but the sensitivity was low (only 54% in patients with proven deep tissue invasion). Testing of multiple samples improved the sensitivity for antigen detection to 85% for patients with proven deep tissue infection and to 64% in proven cases of candidemia (58). Gutierrez et al. (52) described similar values of specificity and sensitivity using the Directigen test. Unfortunately, this test is no longer commercially available. Mitsutake et al. (59) used an in-house developed dot-immunobloting assay for the detection of enolase in serum samples from candidiasis and reported a sensitivity of 71.8% and a specificity of 100%.

Gentry et al. (60) developed a reverse passive latex agglutination assay for the detection of a structurally uncharacterized 56°C heat-labile antigen of *C. albicans* (60). The test was commercialized as the Cand-Tec test (Ramco Laboratories, Houston, Texas). It used latex particles that were sensitized with polyclonal sera from rabbits immunized with heat-killed *C. albicans* blastoconidia. The antigen seems to be a glycoprotein and may represent a neoantigen after processing by human cells. The test did not need the dissociation of immune complexes. Although early studies showed good sensitivity and specificity of this latex-agglutination tests (61), later studies were less favorable (62,63), particularly in patients with malignancies (64). Overall, although easy to perform, the test suffered from both poor sensitivity and specificity, and its usefulness for the reliable diagnosis of invasive candidiasis is limited.

III. SERODIAGNOSIS OF INVASIVE ASPERGILLOSIS

Over the past two decades, *Aspergillus fumigatus* has become the most prevalent airborne fungal pathogen, causing severe and usually fatal invasive infections in immunosuppressed patients (65–67). Invasive aspergillosis is now a major cause of death at leukemia treatment centers, and bone marrow and solid organ transplantation units (65–67). Other spp. of *Aspergillus,* such as *A. terreus, A. flavus,* and *A. niger* can also cause invasive aspergillosis (66). This severe opportunistic fungal infection is characterized by a high mortality rate in these at-risk patients (68) (the crude mortality rate of invasive aspergillosis approaches 100%). The diagnosis of these infections at an early stage of the disease remains a significant clinical problem, which is compounded by the fact that antifungal agents must be begun promptly in these highly immunosuppressed patients if therapy is likely to be successful (69,70).

However, the diagnosis of invasive aspergillosis is difficult; the lack of sensitive and specific noninvasive diagnostic tests remains a major obstacle. Conventional diagnostic tests (histology, microscopy, and culture) remain the cornerstone of proving the presence or absence of fungal disease; however, their sensitivity is low and, therefore, their impact on clinical decisions to treat patients limited. Cultures become positive at a late stage of infection and delayed institution of adequate antifungal therapy is clearly associated with a poor outcome. Performance of biopsy is often precluded by profound cytopenias or by the critical condition of the patient. More recently, the use of high-resolution computed tomography (CT), with the halo-sign as early indicator of fungal infection evolving into the air-crescent sign later in the course of infection, has become an important diagnostic tool (71,72). Unfortunately, although the halo sign is frequently seen in neutropenic patients, it is neither specific for aspergillosis nor is it commonly seen in solid-organ transplant recipients with aspergillosis (73,74). Consequently, in daily clinical practice, physicians combine clinical, radiological, and/or microbiological criteria to define the level of probability of invasive aspergillosis.

A. Antibody Detection

Sera from most healthy individuals contain anti-*Aspergillus* antibodies due to continuous environmental exposure. In contrast to immunocompetent hosts, growth of *A. fumigatus* in the tissues of an immunocompromised host, who either lack a sufficient antibody response or who mount variable antibody response, is not correlated with an increase in *anti-Aspergillus* antibody titers. Indeed, presence of antibodies against *Aspergillus* in immunosuppressed individuals is more likely to represent circulating antibodies prior to the onset of immunosuppressive therapy, rather than antibodies formed during invasive infection (75). Increasing antibody titers at the end of immunosuppression are normally indicative of recovery from invasive aspergillosis, whereas declining antibody levels are normally associated with poor prognosis. These tests are further complicated by the use of uncharacterized antigenic preparations (75). Even if antigen-specific antibodies could be identified, because of the rapid progression of infection, a test is needed to detect very low levels of antibodies at a very early stage during infection. These facts and considerations highlight the difficulties of using antibody detection for the serodiagnosis of invasive aspergillosis in this patient population. In a rather comprehensive evaluation of eight *Aspergillus* antibody detection assays (three indirect hemagglutination tests, three enzyme immunoassays, and two complement fixation tests), sensitivity ranged from 14% to 36% and specificity from 72% to 99% (76). The authors concluded that commercially available antibody detection assays for the serodiagnosis of invasive aspergillosis are inadequate. It is clear that further evaluation is needed in order to clearly establish the diagnostic value of antibody detection in different types of patients with invasive aspergillosis.

B. Antigen Detection

Because of the problems with the detection of antibodies for the serodiagnosis of invasive aspergillosis in immunocompromised patients, much attention has been paid to the detection of circulating antigens in biological fluids (serum, urine, and broncheoalveolar lavage fluid), obtained from patients (77). As in candidiasis, an essential step in the detection of antigen in body fluids is the dissociation of immune complexes that result from the ubiquitous presence of *anti-Aspergillus* antibodies because of continuous environmental exposure in most individuals (75). Although several immunoreactive proteins have been detected that circulate in the blood of patients with invasive aspergillosis, this review focuses on the detection of galacto-mannan, which represents the most promising serologic tool for the diagnosis of these infections.

Galactomannan (GM), a component of the *Aspergillus* cell wall, was the first antigen detected in experimentally infected animals and in patients with invasive aspergillosis (78–80). Recently, Stynen et al. (81) have introduced a sandwich ELISA that is currently the most sensitive method developed for the diagnosis of invasive infection. Several studies performed in Europe have shown that this method shows promise for the early diagnosis of invasive aspergillosis, and the inter- and intra-laboratory reproducibility of the method is reasonably good (82–91). The FDA cleared the test—Platelia *Aspergillus* EIA (Bio Rad)—in May 2003 (92). This is a rapid (approximately 3 h) one-stage immunoenzymatic sandwich microplate assay method that employs the rat monoclonal antibody EB-A2, which recognizes the $(1\rightarrow5)$-β-D-galactofuranoside side chain of the GM molecule. Since each GM mole-cule harbors several epitopes, the same monoclonal antibody can function as capture and detector antibody (75,81). This sandwich technique results in a significantly lower limit of detection of GM of 0.5–1.0 ng/mL of serum, whereas, the previous latex agglutination test using the same antibody—Pastorex *Aspergillus* latex aggluti-nation test—had a 15 ng/mL threshold (81,93–95). Detection of circulating GM at a lower threshold should allow earlier diagnosis of invasive aspergillosis, which is of paramount importance in determining outcome. The galactomannan ELISA results are reported as a ratio between the optical density of the patient's sample and that of a control with a low but detectable amount of galactomannan, and data are expressed as a serum galactomannan index (GMI). Most published studies used a cut-off GMI of less than 1.0 as a negative value, a value greater than 1.5 positive, and those between 1.0 and 1.5 were indeterminate, as recommended by the manufac-turer. Those recommendations for a positive result required 2 or more samples to be tested positive. However, some studies have indicated that this cut-off may be low-ered (90). Based on these studies, the approval by the Food and Drug Administra-tion (FDA) is based on a cut-off of 0.5 (92). Importantly, positive results, as approved in the United States, are based on a single sample being tested positive more than once—rather than multiple samples testing positive. Data presented to the FDA showed a sensitivity of 80.7% in 31 patients with invasive aspergillosis and a specificis of 89.2% (92).The impact of this lowered threshold for positivity should increase sensitivity of the test, but its impact on specificity, particularly in patients at lower risk for invasive aspergillosis remain to be determined.

In addition to variable sensitivity, false-positive results have been a significant issue in interpreting the results of this test with false-positive results occurring in 1–8% of patients in most series (81,93,95–98). Importantly, false positive results have been reported more frequently in certain settings, including, children—in whom absorption of galactomannan from food seems higher (99), and also with some other fungi, like *Penicillium*, which has related antigens (96). More recently, false-positive results have been reported in patients receiving the semi-synthetic penicillin antibio-tic pipercillin-tazobactam, which is derived from a fermentation product of *Penicil-lium*, although the specific cause of the apparent false-positive results remains under investigation (100,101).

Importantly, in addition to the chosen cut-off, the gradual increase in the index in consecutive samples is a very strong indication of infection and should be considered when interpreting the results. The reported results with this test can be influenced by the extent of invasive aspergillosis at time of diagnosis, the prevalence of aspergillosis among the patients studied, the cut-off ratio used, and whether multiple consecutive positive tests were or not required for significance. In a patient population with a high incidence of aspergillosis the test had a sensitivity of almost 93% and specificity of 95% (91). However, in a study of both adult and pediatric patients with hematological malignancies who had a lower prevalence of aspergillosis, sensitivity was 28% and specificity was 99% (90).

Thus, performance and utility of this test seems to depend to a great extent on the patient population under study and the cut-offs used to consider positive results (102). Circulating galactomannan was detected in the serum from approximately 65% of patients before diagnosis was made by clinical examination and radiology, and at the same time as conventional diagnosis in 10% of patients. However, in approximately 25% of patients circulating antigen was detected after diagnosis was made. Also important is the fact that course of the antigen titer seems to correlate well with clinical outcome in patients; hence, this test could be important for monitoring therapeutic responses (102).

Studies of combining galactomannan with other diagnostic modalities such as CT scans of the chest suggest that this test can be a useful adjunct to establish a likely diagnosis of invasive aspergillosis (103,104). For example, in the study by Becker et al. (103), galactomannan was detected in both CT-directed BAL fluid and in serial serum samples. Although not approved for use in nonserum samples, this study showed that the sensitivity of serial serum samples was only 47%, which increased to 85% when combined with CT-directed BAL fluid galactomannan testing, with a specificity of 100% using that approach.

Galactomannan detection in CSF has also been used to diagnose *Aspergillus* meningitis and in a limited number of patients to follow the course of infection in those patients, although the use of the EIA for body fluids other than serum remains investigational (105).

IV. DETECTION OF FUNGAL METABOLITES AND OTHER NONANTIGENIC COMPONENTS

Detection of different nonantigenic components released by fungal cells during infections can also be employed in the diagnosis of invasive candidiasis. Among these, arabinitol (for the diagnosis of candidiasis) and glucan (for a nonspecific fungal diagnosis) are perhaps the most promising and have received most attention of late.

D-arabinitol is a metabolite of many pathogenic *Candida* species and can be determined by gas chromatography or enzymatic analysis (7,106,107). However, *C. krusei* and *C. glabrata*, two species of increasing clinical importance, do not produce this metabolite (108). Most frequently, to correct for human-produced arabinitol and differences in kidney metabolism, the normalized D-arabinitol/L-arabinitol or the D-arabinitol/creatinine ratios are used. In a limited number of prospective clinical studies, elevated ratios in serum or urine from patients with invasive candidiasis were detected, which occurred before positive blood cultures. In addition, these ratios have been correlated with therapeutic response. Overall assay sensitivity seems to be in the proximity of only 50% (7,12). Further investigation of various patient groups in well-designed studies is needed to establish the applicability of this method for the diagnosis of invasive candidiasis.

Glucan (β-1-3-glucan), which is another component of the cell wall of *Candida, Aspergillus,* and many other pathogenic fungi, can also be used diagnostically and possibly as surrogate marker of infection, even though it is not an immunogenic molecule. Human cells lack this polysaccharide, and thus it has been proposed as a good indicator of systemic fungal infection, if detectable in blood or other normally sterile body fluids. The Fungitec G test MK (Seikagaku/Tokyo, Japan; Glucatell, Associates of Cape Cod, Inc., Falmouth, MA), is a commercially available—and recently approved for diagnostic purposes in the United States—colorimetric assay that can indirectly determine the concentration of 1-3-β-glucan in serum samples (109). In this case, the detection system is based on the activation of a proteolytic coagulation cascade, whose components are purified from the horseshoe crab (110). The components of the assay include factor G, which triggers the β-1-3-glucan glucan-sensitive hemolymph-clotting pathway specifically, and a chromogenic Leu-Gly-Arg-pNA tripeptide, which is cleaved by the last component of this proteolytic cascade. The assay can measure picogram amounts of β-1-3-glucan and has been used to demonstrate the presence of this polysaccharide during a variety of systemic fungal infections, including candidiasis and aspergillosis, but not cryptococcosis nor infections caused by Zygomycetes which lack this component (59,109,111). The small quantities of β-1-3-glucan found in serum can be explained by the fact that β-1-3-glucan is an integral component of the cell wall skeleton and, in contrast to other cell wall carbohydrate components, is not normally released from the fungal cell. The high degree of specificity and sensitivity of this test suggest that it may be useful for the early and rapid diagnosis of deep-seated fungal infections. A sensitivity of 90% and a specificity of 100% were reported in a study of over 200 febrile episodes in patients who underwent treatment for hematological malignancies (111), Most experience to date has been obtained in Japan and results of further evaluation in other countries are awaited; however, standardization of this method may prove problematic.

V. PCR-BASED DIAGNOSIS

The detection of microbial DNA by PCR is without question one of the most powerful tools for the early diagnosis and identification of different types of micro-organisms pathogenic to humans (112). Amplification of gene sequences unique to fungi may allow for early diagnosis of invasive fungal infections and subsequent treatment (113–115). Since fungal DNA sequences have been studied for the last few decades, and particularly now with the availability of data from genomic sequencing projects for different fungi, probes for both highly conserved regions as well as genus- and species-specific variable regions are available (113,116). This offers potential for sensitive panfungal markers for detection of invasive fungal infection, followed by identification at the species level of the causative agent. It is normally advisable to target a region of the fungal genome where repeated sequences are present, i.e., ribosomal or mitochondrial regions, to ensure good sensitivity of amplification (113,116). Important procedural considerations need to be taken for removing contaminating nonfungal DNA, breaking fungal cells for DNA extraction, and preventing destruction of fungal DNA. Irrespective of the technology used, most reports from different laboratories seem to indicate that the sensitivity of PCR-base diagnosis is often better than other currently used diagnostic technologies (113,116). Additionally, PCR might be useful for monitoring the response to antifungal therapy. Contamination has been the main obstacle to the clinical application of PCR; it can occur by airborne spore inoculation during the extraction process, by product carry-over, and by the presence of nonviable fungal spores found in reusable equipment, even after autoclaving (116,117). One additional caveat is that these are all in-house protocols developed by different groups of investigators; they use different samples, e.g. serum vs. plasma vs. whole-blood, different protocols for sample preparation, and different genes. Hence, comparisons and standardization between different assays are virtually impossible (113,114).

Early protocols for the detection of fungal DNA in human specimens focused on the DNA detection of single species or genus. Different studies in animals demonstrated that PCR with blood is more sensitive than culture for detecting candidemia (118). A higher sensitivity was also found for clinical samples obtained from patients with candidemia and those with histologically confirmed invasive candidiasis (119). Different types of clinical samples were analyzed including blood, serum, and blood culture bottles (114). An important observation was that *Candida* PCR of blood was negative in most patients and animals with gastrointestinal colonization with *Candida* species (118,120,121). During the past decade, PCR assays for the diagnosis of candidiasis have been reported using a variety of genes, such as *ERG11,* hsp90, secreted aspartyl proteinase, chitin synthase, actin, tubulin, mitochondrial DNA, a number of rRNA gene fragments derived from internal transcribed regions (ITS), and 5S, 18S and 28S rRNA [reviewed in Ref. (113)].

PCR has also been successfully used for early detection of *Aspergillus* DNA in peripheral blood (122,123). Moreover, PCR monitoring of high-risk patients allowed early diagnosis of invasive aspergillosis with good sensitivity and specificity, both in BMT recipients and in allogeneic stem cell transplant recipients indicating that in patients with a negative PCR result the probability of an invasive fungal infection was extremely low (122,123). A potential problem complicating the use of diagnostic PCR to detect *Aspergillus* DNA in respiratory specimens is the potential false positives because of contamination or colonization. Despite this fact, a number of reports have successfully used PCR-based methods for the diagnosis of invasive aspergillosis in different types of patients and clinical samples (124–136). Overall, results from these tests yielded similar levels of sensitivity and specificity (most often superior to other diagnostic tests), but comparative trials are still lacking (114,115).

Because of the changing epidemiology of fungal infections and the increasing recognition of the pathogenic potential of a number of fungal species in these patients, the ability to detect a wide range of medically important fungi is important. Different PCR-based protocols have been developed to such objective. The method developed by Hopfer et al. (137) targeted a multicopy rDNA highly conserved throughout the fungal kingdom, obtaining positive PCR results for all genera and species of fungi tested (137). By performing restriction fragment length polymorphism (RFLP) analysis of the resulting amplicons, they could subsequently differentiate between different groups of medically important fungi. Similarly, a test was developed that could detect a rDNA fragment present in all pathogenic fungi except *Mucor* spp. (138). Sandhu et al. first sequenced the 28S rDNA from 50 medically important fungi and designed universal primers and species-specific probes (139). Their results indicated a high level of specificity. Van Burik et al. (140) developed a novel panfungal PCR assay for the detection of fungal infections in blood from patients. The panfungal primers, which targeted the small-subunit rRNA gene were optimized separately for *Candida albicans* and *Aspergillus fumigatus*. Another method uses a combination of seven digoxigenin labeled probes following amplification of a 482–503-bp fragment of 18S rRNA genes and could detect DNA from seven *Candida* spp and six *Aspergillus* spp (122,123) with excellent sensitivity.

The methods mentioned above use conventional PCR for the diagnosis of invasive fungal infections. The majority of these procedures include time consuming in-house DNA extraction protocols and require the use of gel-electrophoresis or other slow detection steps. The use of standardized DNA extraction protocols and real-time PCR may address many of the limitations of conventional PCR (141). Recently, a quantitative real-time PCR assay using the LightCycler instrument (Roche Molecular Diagnostics) has been reported to show great potential for the rapid diagnosis of candidiasis and aspergillosis (142). The LightCycler technology combines the fast in vitro amplification of DNA with immediate fluorescence detection of the amplicon. This allows the real-time quantification of the amount of DNA. A proven method for the highly specific detection of the PCR products uses the fluorescence resonance energy transfer (FRET) system with sequence-specific hybridization probes. A recent report by Pryce et al. (143) describes the use of a new real-time PCR assay with FRET and melting curve analysis to detect *C. albicans* and *A. fumigatus* DNA in whole blood and its preliminary evaluation in a number of high-risk patients. In this report, the real-time assay demonstrated an analytical sensitivity of 10 fg of purified fungal DNA, was highly reproducible, and detected *C. albicans* and *A. fumigatus* DNA in two patients with proven and in one patient with possible invasive fungal infection. Similarly, other investigators have used the TaqMan assay (Applied Biosystems) for the automated detection of fungal DNA in clinical isolates and in experimentally infected animal tissues (130,144–146). Loeffler et al. (130) compared the results of quantitative culture, PCR-ELISA, and a quantitative Light-Cycler assay of blood and organ specimens of experimentally infected mice and rabbits. The PCR assay was almost 20-fold more sensitive than culture from both blood and organ cultures. None of the 68 blood cultures from mice and rabbits were positive for *Aspergillus fumigatus,* whereas, PCR detected Aspergillus DNA in 17 out of 68 blood samples. Quantitative PCR analysis of blood samples showed a fungus load of 10–100 cfu/mL of blood.

Other groups of investigators are implementing simitar technologies, mostly for *Candida* and *Aspergillus* infections, but other pathogenic fungi can readily be accommodated in these assays (147–153). It is anticipated that the use of quantitative real-time PCR could be readily introduced into the routine clinical microbiology laboratory and may result in drastically reduced turnaround times for results.

The potential clinical utility of PCR for the early diagnosis of invasive aspergillosis was evaluated by Hebart et al. (127) who evaluated 84 patients undergoing allogeneic stem cell transplantation. Of 1193 blood samples analyzed, 169 (14.2%) were positive by PCR. In 7 patients with newly diagnosed invasive aspergillosis, PCR positivity preceded the first clinical signs by a median of 2 days (range, 1–23 days) and preceded clinical diagnosis of IA by a median of 9 days (range, 2–34 days). The PCR assay revealed a sensitivity of 100% and a specificity of 65%, and none of the PCR-negative patients developed invasive aspergillosis during the study period, suggesting that prospective PCR screening may allow for early identification of patients at high risk for subsequent onset of invasive aspergillosis. Those same investigators showed that PCR-based techniques was sensitive in detecting early invasive aspergillosis in patients with febrile neutropenia (123).

VI. NONCULTURE BASED DIAGNOSIS OF PATHOGENIC AND ENDEMIC MYCOSES

The occurrence of true pathogenic, and endemic mycoses, including cryptococcosis, histoplasmosis, blastomycosis, and coccidioidomycosis in immunosuppressed hematological patients are less common than infections caused by *Candida, Aspergillus,* and opportunistic moulds (154,155). Nevertheless, the diagnosis of these infections through classical culture-based methods is often difficult. This is because their sensitivity, like with the opportunistic pathogens described above, is low and the time required for a positive culture result of these is often slow as the growth of these organisms may delay diagnosis and treatment significantly. Consequently, interest has been high in developing nonculture-based methods for these infections as well.

A. Cryptococcosis

The most useful nonculture-based method in systemic mycoses is the one developed for detecting the capsular polysaccharide antigen of *Cryptococcus.* While direct visualization of the organism in cerebrospinal fluid or other body fluids is sufficient to establish a presumptive diagnosis of cryptococcosis (156), cultures of the organisms may take several days to detect and identify the organism. Detection of cryptococcal antigen by latex agglutination based on latex particles coated with antibody raised against cryptococcal capsule has been widely used to diagnose this infection (112). False-positive results can occur with some other fungi—particularly *Trichosporon* species which shares a common antigenic component (157). More recently, the PREMIER Cryptococcal antigen assay (Meridian Diagnostics, Inc.) is an EIA that has become widely used for the diagnosis of cryptococcosis, because of its lack of reactivity with rheumatoid factor, fewer false positives, excellent sensitivity, and being easy to run on a large number of samples (158). The sensitivity of the assay in serum is greater than that in cerebrospinal fluid, even in patients with meningitis, although the sensitivity of the newer assays approaches is more than 95% and false-negative results can occur particularly in capsule-deficient strains (159). Higher titers clearly predict poorer outcomes, although the value of serial measurement is limited, with only serial CSF values correlating with response (160). Development of antibody to *Cryptococcus* is common following infection and may indicate a more favorable long-term prognosis, although it has limited value as a clinical tool and is seldom measured (159,161).

B. Histoplasmosis

While isolation of *Histoplasma capsulatum* from tissues remains the standard for establishing a diagnosis of histoplasmosis, cultures for the organism may take as long as 2–4 weeks to grow and be identified. Thus, nonculture-based methods, including both antibody and antigen detection, may significantly reduce the time required to diagnose this endemic organism. Antibody detection may give a clue to the diagnosis of this infection, even in immunosuppressed hosts. Antibodies to the H antigen of histoplasmin develop during active histoplasmosis, while those to M antigen are indicative of prior infection and is the first to rise with seroconversion (162). Nevertheless, limitations of serological detection of histoplasmosis include lack of humoral response in those patients with more severe immunosuppression, and because of the lack of sensitivity or specificity of that response (162). More useful, particularly in immunosuppressed hosts, is the detection of histoplasma poly-saccharide, which is detectable in disseminated infection and correlates with response to therapy (163–165). This assay system developed by Wheat et al. (165), originally a radioimmunoassay (RIA) is now performed as an EIA, and detects antigen in urine as well as serum, with higher sensitivity in the urine. In addition, antigen can be detected in the CSF as a means to establish the presence of histoplasmosis in the central nervous system (166).

C. Blastomycosis

The diagnosis of blastomycosis is usually made either by isolating the organism in culture or by identifying the typical broad-based budding yeast in pathological mate-rial or lesion scrapings. Serological approaches can occasionally be helpful in estab-lishing the diagnosis as antibodies to *Blastomyces dermatiditis* are produced in response to the infection. Early tests detected antibodies to *Blastomyces* A antigen, a yeast antigen (167), but recent efforts by Klein et al. (168) have focused on WI-1 antigen. Antibodies to this 120-kDa cell surface protein are detected earlier than A antigen and decline by 6 months after illness in patients who respond to therapy. A major problem complicating interpretation of serological tests for blastomycosis is cross-reactivity with other mycoses, including histoplasmosis, coccidioidomycosis, paracoccioidomycosis, and even nonfungal infections (167,169).

D. Coccidioidomycosis

The diagnosis of coccidioidomycosis can be established by demonstration of the characteristic spherule in infected tissues, which is relatively insensitive, or by isolat-ing the organism in tissues—that can be associated with risk of infectivity to labora-tory personnel for unsuspected infections and requires the use of biological safety hoods. Thus, serological techniques for this mycosis are important in establishing a diagnosis. Serologic studies using crude antigens prepared from filtrates, or lysates of mycelial, or spherule-endospore phases are useful in establishing a diagnosis of coccidioidomycosis and in determining prognosis (170). Currently used qualitative tests include EIA, immunodiffusion (ID) and tube precipitin (TP) for the detection of IgM (IDTP) and EIA, ID and CF for the detection of IgG (IDCF) (171). IgM antibody may be detected within the first few weeks while IgG is detected after a few weeks of infection and usually disappears in several months if the infection resolves. A positive IDCF is highly suggestive of infection, and titers of 1:16 or greater typically indicate disseminated, extrapulmonary disease. Serum IDCF titers can be negative with single-site extrapulmonary infection. A positive CSF IDCF is useful in the diagnosis of the disease because cultures of CSF are uncommonly posi-tive and serum IgG levels may not be elevated. Serial serum titers can be used to assess efficacy of therapy: rising titers are a poor prognostic sign, while falling titers are associated with a favorable clinical response (172).

VII. SUMMARY

The diagnosis of invasive fungal infection remains a significant challenge in the management of hematological patients. Since traditional culture based diagnosis is often not sensitive and invasive procedures are reluctantly undertaken in these compromised hosts, nonculture-based methods offer substantial opportunities to establish an early diagnosis of these often lethal infections. Much attention has been focused on nonculture-based methods not only to establish an early diagnosis of systemic candidiasis or invasive aspergillosis because of the frequency of these infections in immunosuppressed hosts, but are also available for true pathogenic fungi and endemic mycoses. Nonculture-based methods for diagnosing serious *Candida* infection remain limited, with significant challenges of distinguishing invasive infection from colonization. Recent advances in aspergillosis have improved early diagnosis, including both detection of the antigen galactomannan and PCR-based techniques, but significant limitations to these methods remain, which significantly reduce their clinical utility. Ongoing research efforts hope to capitalize on data derived from the sequencing of the *Aspergillus* genome, which is aimed at identifying new targets and new methods for diagnosing this often lethal infection.

ACKNOWLEDGMENTS

The authors gratefully acknowledge the support of the National Institutes of Health through grants R03 AI 054447 and R21 DE 15079 (to JLL-R) and contract N01-AI-30041 (to TFP). JLL-R is the recipient of a New Investigator Award in Molecular Pathogenic Mycology from the Burroughs Wellcome Fund.

REFERENCES

1. Banerjee SN, Emori TG, Culver DH, et al. Secular trends in nosocomial primary bloodstream infections in the United States, 1980–1989. National Nosocomial Infections Surveillance System. Am J Med 1991; 91:86S–89S.
2. Pfaller MA, Jones RN, Doern GV, Sader HS, Hollis RJ, Messer SA. International surveillance of bloodstream infections due to Candida species: frequency of occurrence and antifungal susceptibilities of isolates collected in 1997 in the United States, Canada, and South America for the SENTRY Program. The SENTRY Participant Group. J Clin Microbiol 1998; 36:1886–1889.
3. Pfaller MA, Jones RN, Doern GV, et al. International surveillance of blood stream infections due to Candida species in the European SENTRY Program: species distribution and antifungal susceptibility including the investigational triazole and echinocandin agents. SENTRY Participant Group (Europe). Diagn Microbiol Infect Dis 1999; 35: 19–25.
4. Viudes A, Peman J, Canton E, Ubeda P, Lopez-Ribot JL, Gobernado M. Candidemia at a tertiary-care hospital: epidemiology, treatment, clinical outcome and risk factors for death. Eur J Clin Microbiol Infect Dis 2002; 21:767–774.
5. Wey SB, Mori M, Pfaller MA, Wooison RF, Wenzel RP. Hospital-acquired candidemia. The attributable mortality and excess length of stay. Arch Intern Med 1988; 148:2642–2645.
6. De Repentigny L, Kaufman L, Cole GT, Kruse D, Latge JP, Matthews RC. Immunodiagnosis of invasive fungal infections. J Med Vet Mycol 1994; 32(suppl 1):239–252.
7. Reiss E, Morrison CJ. Nonculture methods for diagnosis of disseminated candidiasis. Clin Microbiol Rev 1993; 6:311–323.
8. Jones JM. Laboratory diagnosis of invasive candidiasis. Clin Microbiol Rev 1990; 3: 32–45.
9. Martinez JP, Gil ML, Lopez-Ribot JL, Chaffin WL. Serologic response to cell wall mannoproteins and proteins of *Candida albicans*. Clin Microbiol Rev 1998; 11:121–141.

10. Domer JE. Candida cell wall mannan: a polysaccharide with diverse immunologic properties. Crit Rev Microbiol 1989; 17:33–51.
11. Herent P, Stynen D, Hernando F, Fruit J, Poulain D. Retrospective evaluation of two latex agglutination tests for detection of circulating antigens during invasive candidosis. J Clin Microbiol 1992; 30:2158–2164.
12. Ponton J, Moragues MD, Quindos G. Non-culture based diagnostics. In: Calderone RA, ed. Candida and Candidiasis. Washington, DC: ASM Press, 2002:395–425.
13. Chaffin WL, Lopez-Ribot JL, Casanova M, Gozalbo D, Martinez JP. Cell wall and secreted proteins of *Candida albicans*: identification, function, and expression. Microbiol Mol Biol Rev 1998; 62:130–180.
14. Jones JM. Quantitation of antibody against cell wall mannan and a major cytoplasmic antigen of Candida in rabbits, mice, and humans. Infect Immun 1980; 30:78–89.
15. Greenfield RA, Stephens JL, Bussey MJ, Jones JM. Quantitation of antibody to Candida mannan by enzyme-linked immunosorbent assay. J Lab Clin Med 1983; 101: 758–771.
16. de Repentigny L, Reiss E. Current trends in immunodiagnosis of candidiasis and aspergillosis. Rev Infect Dis 1984; 6:301–312.
17. Faille C, Wieruszeski JM, Michalski JC, Poulain D, Strecker G. Complete 1H- and 13C-resonance assignments for D-mannooligosaccharides of the beta-D-(1–>2)-linked series released from the phosphopeptidomannan of *Candida albicans* VW.32 (serotype A). Carbohydr Res 1992; 236:17–27.
18. Trinel PA, Faille C, Jacquinot PM, Cailliez JC, Poulain D. Mapping of *Candida albicans* oligomannosidic epitopes by using monoclonal antibodies. Infect Immun 1992; 60:3845–3851.
19. Faille C, Mackenzie DW, Michalski JC, Poulain D. Evaluation of an enzyme immunoassay using neoglycolipids constructed from *Candida albicans* oligomannosides to define the specificity of anti-mannan antibodies. Eur J Clin Microbiol Infect Dis 1992; 11:438–446.
20. Faille C, Michalski JC, Strecker G, Mackenzie DW, Camus D, Poulain D. Immunoreactivity of neoglycolipids constructed from oligomannosidic residues of the *Candida albicans* cell wall. Infect Immun 1990; 58:3537–3544.
21. Sendid B, Tabouret M, Poirot JL, Mathieu D, Fruit J, Poulain D. New enzyme immunoassays for sensitive detection of circulating *Candida albicans* mannan and antimannan antibodies: useful combined test for diagnosis of systemic candidiasis. J Clin Microbiol 1999; 37:1510–1517.
22. Sendid B, Poirot JL, Tabouret M, et al. Combined detection of mannanaemia and antimannan antibodies as a strategy for the diagnosis of systemic infection caused by pathogenic Candida species. J Med Microbiol 2002; 51:433–442.
23. van Deventer AJ, Goessens WH, van Zeijl JH, Mouton JW, Michel MF, Verbrugh HA. Kinetics of anti-mannan antibodies useful in confirming invasive candidiasis in immunocompromised patients. Microbiol Immunol 1996; 40:125–131.
24. Saville SP, Lazzell AL, Monteagudo C, Lopez-Ribot JL. Engineered control of cell morphology in vivo reveals distinct roles for yeast and filamentous ferms of *Candida albicans* during infection. Eukaryot Cell 2003; 2:1053–1060.
25. Navarro D, Monzonis E, Lopez-Ribot JL, et al. Diagnosis of systemic candidiasis by enzyme immunoassay detection of specific antibodies to mycelial phase cell wall and cytoplasmic candidal antigens. Eur J Clin Microbiol Infect Dis 1993; 12: 839–846.
26. Garcia-Ruiz JC, del Carmen Arilla M, Regulez P, Quindos G, Alvarez A, Ponton J. Detection of antibodies to *Candida albicans* germ tubes for diagnosis and therapeutic monitoring of invasive candidiasis in patients with hematologic malignancies. J Clin Microbiol 1997; 35:3284–3287.
27. Quindos G, Ponton J, Cisterna R. Detection of antibodies to *Candida albicans* germ tube in the diagnosis of systemic candidiasis. Eur J Clin Microbiol 1987; 6:142–146.

28. Bikandi J, San Millan R, Regulez P, Moragues MD, Quindos G, Ponton J. Detection of antibodies to *Candida albicans* germ tubes during experimental infections by different Candida species. Clin Diagn Lab Immunol 1998; 5:369–374.

29. Ponton J, Quindos G, Arilla MC, Mackenzie DW. Simplified adsorption method for detection of antibodies to *Candida albicans* germ tubes. J Clin Microbiol 1994; 32: 217–219.

30. Quindos G, Ponton J, Cisterna R, Mackenzie DW. Value of detection of antibodies to *Candida albicans* germ tube in the diagnosis of systemic candidosis. Eur J Clin Microbiol Infect Dis 1990; 9:178–183.

31. MacDonald F, Odds FC. Inducible proteinase of *Candida albicans* in diagnostic serology and in the pathogenesis of systemic candidosis. J Med Microbiol 1980; 13:423–435.

32. MacDonald F, Odds FC. Purified *Candida albicans* proteinase in the serologicai diagnosis of systemic candidosis. JAMA 1980; 243:2409–2411.

33. Odds FC. *Candida albicans* proteinase as a virulence factor in the pathogenesis of Candida infections. Zentralbl Bakteriol Mikrobiol Hyg [A] 1985; 260:539–542.

34. Ruchel R, Boning-Stutzer B, Mari A. A synoptical approach to the diagnosis of candidosis, relying on serological antigen and antibody tests, on culture, and on evaluation of clinical data. Mycoses 1988; 31:87–106.

35. Ray TL, Payne CD. Detection of *Candida* acid proteinase (CAP) antibodies in systemic candidiasis by enzyme immunoassay. Clin Res 1987; 35:711A.

36. Matthews R, Burnie J. Diagnosis of systemic candidiasis by an enzyme-linked dot immunobinding assay for a circulating immunodominant 47-kilodalton antigen. J Clin Microbiol 1988; 26:459–463.

37. Matthews RC, Burnie JP, Tabaqchali S. Isolation of immunodominant antigens from sera of patients with systemic candidiasis and characterization of serological response to *Candida albicans*. J Clin Microbiol 1987; 25:230–237.

38. Matthews RC, Burnie JP, Tabaqchali S. Immunoblot analysis of the serological response in systemic candidosis. Lancet 1984; 2:1415–1418.

39. Matthews R, Burnie J. Cloning of a DNA sequence encoding a major fragment of the 47 kilodalton stress protein homologue of *Candida albicans*. FEMS Microbiol Lett 1989; 51:25–30.

40. Burford-Mason AP, Matthews RC, Williams JR. Transient abrogation of immunosuppression in a patient with chronic mucocutaneous candidiasis following vaccination with *Candida albicans*. J Infect 1987; 14:147–157.

41. Matthews R, Burnie J, Smith D, et al. Candida and AIDS: evidence for protective antibody. Lancet 1988; 2:263–266.

42. Burnie JP, Matthews RC, Tabaqchali S. Developments in the serological diagnosis of opportunistic fungal infections Isolation of immunodominant antigens from sera of patients with systemic candidiasis and characterization of seroiogical response to *Candida albicans*. J Antimicrob Chemother 1991; 28(suppl A):23–33.

43. Zoller L, Kramer I, Kappe R, Sonntag HG. Enzyme immunoassays for invasive Candida infections: reactivity of somatic antigens of *Candida albicans*. J Clin Microbiol 1991; 29:1860–1867.

44. Angiolella L, Facchin M, Stringaro A, Maras B, Simonetti N, Cassone A. Identification of a glucan-associated enolase as a main cell wall protein of *Candida albicans* and an indirect target of lipopeptide antimycotics. J Infect Dis 1996; 173:684–690.

45. Strockbine NA, Largen MT, Zweibel SM, Buckley HR. Identification and molecular weight characterization of antigens from *Candida albicans* that are recognized by human sera. Infect Immun 1984; 43:715–721.

46. Mason AB, Brandt ME, Buckley HR. Enolase activity associated with a C. albicans cytoplasmic antigen. Yeast 1989; 5 Spec No:S231–S239.

47. Franklyn KM, Warmington JR, Ott AK, Ashman RB. An immunodominant antigen of *Candida albicans* shows homoiogy to the enzyme enolase. Immunol Cell Biol 1990; 68:173–178.

48. van Deventer AJ, van Vliet HJ, Hop WC, Goessens WH. Diagnostic value of anti-Candida enolase antibodies. J Clin Microbiol 1994; 32:17–23.

49. Mitsutake K, Kohno S, Miyazaki T, Miyazaki H, Maesaki S, Koga H. Detection of Candida enolase antibody in patients with candidiasis. J Clin Lab Anal 1994; 8: 207–210.

50. Greenfield RA, Jones JM. Comparison of cytoplasmic extracts of eight Candida species and Saccharomyces cerevisiae. Infect Immun 1982; 35:1157–1161.

51. Greenfield RA, Jones JM. Purification and characterization of a major cytoplasmic antigen of *Candida albicans*. Infect Immun 1981; 34:469–477.

52. Gutierrez J, Maroto C, Piedrola G, Martin E, Perez JA. Circulating Candida antigens and antibodies: useful markers of candidemia. J Clin Microbiol 1993; 31:2550–2552.

53. Gutierrez J, Liebana J. Immunological methods for the detection of structural components and metabolites of bacteria and fungi in blood. Ann Biol Clin (Paris) 1993; 51: 83–90.

54. Staib F. Serum-proteins as nitrogen source for yeastlike fungi. Sabouraudia 1965; 4:187–193.

55. Naglik JR, Challacombe SJ, Hube B. *Candida albicans* secreted aspartyl proteinases in virulence and pathogenesis. Microbiol Mol Biol Rev 2003; 67:400–428, table of contents.

56. Morrison CJ, Hurst SF, Bragg SL, et al. Purification and characterization of the extracellular aspartyl proteinase of *Candida albicans*: removal of extraneous proteins and cell wall mannoprotein and evidence for lack of glycosylation. J Gen Microbiol 1993; 139:1177–1186.

57. Morrison CJ, Hurst SF, Reiss E. Competitive binding inhibition enzyme-linked immunosorbent assay that uses the secreted aspartyl proteinase of *Candida albicans* as an antigenic marker for diagnosis of disseminated candidiasis. Clin Diagn Lab Immunol 2003; 10:835–848.

58. Walsh TJ, Hathorn JW, Sobel JD, et al. Detection of circulating Candida enolase by immunoassay in patients with cancer and invasive candidiasis. N Engl J Med 1991; 324:1026–1031.

59. Mitsutake K, Miyazaki T, Tashiro T, et al. Enolase antigen, mannan antigen, Cand-Tec antigen, and beta-glucan in patients with candidemia. J Clin Microbiol 1996; 34: 1918–1921.

60. Gentry LO, Wilkinson ID, Lea AS, Price MF. Latex agglutination test for detection of Candida antigen in patients with disseminated disease. Eur J Clin Microbiol 1983; 2:122–128.

61. Fung JC, Donta ST, Tilton RC. Candida detection system (CAND-TEC) to differentiate between *Candida albicans* colonization and disease. J Clin Microbiol 1986; 24: 542–547.

62. Lemieux C, St-Germain G, Vincelette J, Kaufman L, de Repentigny L. Collaborative evaluation of antigen detection by a commercial latex agglutination test and enzyme immunoassay in the diagnosis of invasive candidiasis. J Clin Microbiol 1990; 28: 249–253.

63. Cabezudo I, Pfaller M, Gerarden T, et al. Value of the Cand-Tec Candida antigen assay in the diagnosis and therapy of systemic candidiasis in high-risk patients. Eur J Clin Microbiol Infect Dis 1989; 8:770–777.

64. Escuro RS, Jacobs M, Gerson SL, Machicao AR, Lazarus HM. Prospective evaluation of a Candida antigen detection test for invasive candidiasis in immunocompromised adult patients with cancer. Am J Med 1989; 87:621–627.

65. Patel R, Paya CV. Infections in solid-organ transplant recipients. Clin Microbiol Rev 1997; 10:86–124.

66. Marr KA, Patterson T, Denning D. Aspergillosis. Pathogenesis, clinical manifestations, and therapy. Infect Dis Clin North Am 2002; 16:875–894, vi.

67. Denning DW. Invasive aspergillosis. Clin Infect Dis 1998; 26:781–803; quiz 804–805.

68. Lin SJ, Schranz J, Teutsch SM. Aspergillosis case-fatality rate: systematic review of the literature. Clin Infect Dis 2001; 32:358–366.

69. Patterson TF. Early use of antifungai therapy in high-risk patients. Curr Opin Infect Dis 2002; 15:561–563.

70. Patterson TF. Approaches to fungal diagnosis in transplantation. Transpl Infect Dis 1999; 1:262–272.

71. Caillot D, Casasnovas O, Bernard A, et al. Improved management of invasive pulmonary aspergillosis in neutropenic patients using early thoracic computed tomographic scan and surgery. J Clin Oncol 1997; 15:139–147.

72. Caillot D, Couaillier JF, Bernard A, et al. Increasing volume and changing characteristics of invasive pulmonary aspergillosis on sequential thoracic computed tomography scans in patients with neutropenia. J Clin Oncol 2001; 19:253–259.

73. Singh N. Fungal infections in the recipients of solid organ transplantation. Infect Dis Clin North Am 2003; 17:113–134, viii.

74. Diederich S, Scadeng M, Dennis C, Stewart S, Flower CD. Aspergillus infection of the respiratory tract after lung transplantation: chest radiographic and CT findings. Eur Radiol 1998; 8:306–312.

75. Latge JP. Aspergillus fumigatus and aspergillosis. Clin Microbiol Rev 1999; 12:310–350.

76. Kappe R, Schulze-Berge A, Sonntag HG. Evaluation of eight antibody tests and one antigen test for the diagnosis of invasive aspergillosis. Mycoses 1996; 39:13–23.

77. Latge JP. Tools and trends in the detection of Aspergillus fumigatus. Curr Top Med Mycol 1995; 6:245–281.

78. Patterson T, Miniter P, Ryan J, Andriole V. Effect of Immunosuppression and amphotericin B on aspergillus antigenemia in an experimental model. J Infec Dis 1938; 158:415–422.

79. Reiss E, Lehmann PF. Galactomannan antigenemia in invasive aspergillosis. Infect Immun 1979; 25:357–365.

80. Dupont B, Huber M, Kim SJ, Bennett JE. Galactomannan antigenemia and antigenuria in aspergillosis: Studies in patients and experimentally infected rabbits. J Infect Dis 1987; 155:1–11.

81. Stynen D, Goris A, Sarfati J, Latge JP. A new sensitive sandwich enzyme-linked immunosorbent assay to detect galactofuran in patients with invasive aspergillosis. J Clin Microbiol 1995; 33:497–500.

82. Pinel C, Fricker-Hidalgo H, Lebeau B, et al. Detection of circulating *Aspergillus fumigatus* galactomannan: value and limits of the Platelia test for diagnosing invasive aspergillosis. J Clin Microbiol 2003; 41:2184–2186.

83. Lombardi G, Farina C, Andreoni S, et al. Multicenter evaluation of an enzyme immunoassay (Platelia Aspergillus) for the detection of Aspergillus antigen in serum. Mycopathologia 2002; 155:129–133.

84. Centeno-Lima S, de Lacerda JM, do Carmo JA, Abecasis M, Casimiro C, Exposto F. Follow-up of anti-Aspergillus IgG and IgA antibodies in bone marrow transplanted patients with invasive aspergillosis. J Clin Lab Anal 2002; 16:156–162.

85. Siemann M, Koch-Dorfler M. The Platelia Aspergillus ELISA in diagnosis of invasive pulmonary aspergilosis (IPA). Mycoses 2001; 44:266–272.

86. Fortun J, Martin-Davila P, Alvarez ME, et al. Aspergillus antigenemia sandwich-enzyme immunoassay test as a serodiagnostic method for invasive aspergillosis in liver transplant recipients. Transplantation 2001; 71:145–149.

87. Sulahian A, Boutboul F, Ribaud P, Leblanc T, Lacroix C, Derouin F. Value of antigen detection using an enzyme immunoassay in the diagnosis and prediction of invasive aspergillosis in two adult and pediatric hematology units during a 4-year prospective study. Cancer 2001; 91:311–318.

88. Salonen J, Lehtonen OP, Terasjarvi MR, Nikoskelainen J. Aspergillus antigen in serum, urine and bronchoalveolar lavage specimens of neutropenic patients in relation to clinical outcome. Scand J Infect Dis 2000; 32:485–490.

89. Verweij PE, Erjavec Z, Sluiters W, et al. Detection of antigen in sera of patients with invasive aspergillosis: intra- and interlaboratory reproducibility. The Dutch Interuniversity Working Party for Invasive Mycoses. J Clin Microbiol 1998; 36:1612–1616.

90. Herbrecht R, Letscher-Bru V, Oprea C, et al. Aspergillus galactomannan detection in the diagnosis of invasive aspergillosis in cancer patients. J Clin Oncol 2002; 20:1898–1906.

91. Maertens J, Verhaegen J, Demuynck H, et al. Autopsy-controlled prospective evaluation of serial screening for circulating galactomannan by a sandwich enzyme-linked immunosorbent assay for hematological patients at risk for invasive Aspergillosis. J Clin Microbiol 1999; 37:3223–3228.

92. Anonymous. FDA clears rapid test for *Aspergillus* infection. http://www.fda.gov/bbs/topics/NEWS/2003/NEW00907.html U.S. Food and Drug Administration, 2003.

93. Machetti M, Feasi M, Mordini N, et al. Comparison of an enzyme immunoassay and a latex agglutination system for the diagnosis of invasive aspergillosis in bone marrow transplant recipients. Bone Marrow Transplant 1998; 21:917–921.

94. Verweij PE, Rijs AJ, De Pauw BE, Horrevorts AM, Hoogkamp-Korstanje JA, Meis JF. Clinical evaluation and reproducibility of the Pastorex Aspergillus antigen latex agglutination test for diagnosing invasive aspergillosis. J Clin Pathol 1995; 48:474–476.

95. Verweij PE, Stynen D, Rijs AJ, de Pauw BE, Hoogkamp-Korstanje JA, Meis JF. Sandwich enzyme-linked immunosorbent assay compared with Pastorex latex agglutination test for diagnosing invasive aspergiilosis in immunocompromised patients. J Clin Microbiol 1995; 33:1912–1914.

96. Verweij PE, Poulain D, Obayashi T, Patterson TF, Denning DW, Ponton J. Current trends in the detection of antigenaemia, metabolites and cell wall markers for the diagnosis and therapeutic monitoring of fungal infections. Med Mycol 1998; 36:146–155.

97. Sulahian A, Tabouret M, Ribaud P, et al. Comparison of an enzyme immunoassay and latex agglutination test for detection of galactomannan in the diagnosis of aspergillosis. Eur J Clin Microbiol Infect D 1996; 15:139–145.

98. Swanink CMA, Meis JFGM, Rijs AJMM, Donnelly JP, Verweij PE. Specificity of a sandwich enzyme-linked immunosorbent assay for detecting *Aspergillus* galactomannan. J Clin Microbiol 1997; 35:257–260.

99. Letscher-Bru V, Cavalier A, Pernot-Marino E, et al. Aspergillus galactomannan antigen detection with Platelia (R) Aspergillus: multiple positive antigenemia without Aspergillus infection. J Mycologie Medicale 1998; 8:112–113.

100. Viscoli C, Machetti M, Cappellano P, Bucci B, Bruzzi P, Bacigalupo A. False-positive platelia *Aspergillus* (PA) test in patients (pts) receiving piperacillin-tazobactam (P/T) (abstract M-2062b). In: Abstracts of the 43rd Interscience Conference on Antimicrobial Agents and Chemotherapy, Chicago, IL, September, 14–17. Washington, DC: Am Soc Microb, 2003.

101. Sulahian A, Touratier S, Ribaud P. False positive test for aspergillus antigenemia related to concomitant administration of piperacillin and tazobactam. N Engl J Med 2003; 349:2366–2367.

102. Bennett JE, Kauffman C, Walsh T, et al. Forum report: issues in the evaluation of diagnostic tests, use of historical controls, and merits of the current multicenter collaborative groups. Clin Infect Dis 2003; 36:S123–S127.

103. Becker MJ, Lugtenburg EJ, Cornelissen JJ, Van Der Schee C, Hoogsteden HC, De Marie S. Galactomannan detection in computerized tomography-based bronchoalveolar lavage fluid and serum in haematological patients at risk for invasive pulmonary aspergillosis. Br J Haematol 2003; 121:448–457.

104. Severens JL, Donnelly JP, Meis JFGM, De Vries Robbe PF, De Pauw BE, Verweij PE. Two strategies for managing invasive aspergillosis: A decision analysis. Clinical Infectious Diseases 1997; 25:1148–1154.

105. Verweij PE, Brinkman K, Kremer HPH, Kullberg BJ, Meis J. *Aspergillus* meningitis: Diagnosis by non-culture-based microbiological methods management. J Clin Microbiol 1999; 37:1186–1189.

106. Christensson B, Wiebe T, Pehrson C, Larsson L. Diagnosis of invasive candidiasis in neutropenic children with cancer by determination of D-arabinitol/L-arabinitol ratios in urine. J Clin Microbiol 1997; 35:636–640.

107. Christensson B, Sigmundsdottir G, Larsson L. D-arabinitol–a marker for invasive candidiasis. Med Mycol 1999; 37:391–396.

108. Tokunaga S, Ohkawa M, Takashima M, Hisazumi H. Clinical significance of measurement of serum D-arabinitol levels in candiduria patients. Urol Int 1992; 48:195–199.

109. Miyazaki T, Kohno S, Mitsutake K, et al. Plasma $(1\rightarrow3)$-beta-D-glucan and fungal antigenemia in patients with candidemia, aspergillosis, and cryptococcosis. J Clin Microbiol 1995; 33:3115–3118.

110. Tamura H, Tanaka S, Ikeda T, Obayashi T, Hashimoto Y. Plasma $(1\rightarrow3)$- beta-D-glucan assay and immunohistochemical staining of $(1\rightarrow3)$-beta-D- glucan in the fungal cell walls using a novel horseshoe crab protein (T-GBP) that specifically binds to $(1\rightarrow3)$-beta-D-glucan. J Clin Lab Anal 1997; 11:104–109.

111. Obayashi T, Yoshida M, Mori T, et al. Plasma $(1\rightarrow3)$-beta-D-glucan measurement in diagnosis of invasive deep mycosis and fungal febrile episodes. Lancet 1995; 345:17–20.

112. Yeo SF, Wong B. Current status of nonculture methods for diagnosis of invasive fungal infections. Clin Microbiol Rev 2002; 15:465–484.

113. Hopfer RL, Amjadi D. Molecular diagnosis of fungal infections. In: Calderone RA, Cihlar RL, eds. Fungal Pathogenesis. New York: Marcel Dekker, Inc., 2002:649–665.

114. Verweij PE, Meis JF. Microbiological diagnosis of invasive fungal infections in transplant recipients. Transpl Infect Dis 2000; 2:80–87.

115. Erjavec Z, Verweij PE. Recent progress in the diagnosis of fungal infections in the immunocompromised host. Drug Resist Updat 2002; 5:3–10.

116. Hopfer RL. Use of molecular biological techniques in the diagnostic laboratory for detecting and differentiating fungi. Arch Med Res 1995; 26:287–292.

117. Loeffler J, Hebart H, Bialek R, et al. Contaminations occurring in fungal PCR assays. J Clin Microbiol 1999; 37:1200–1202.

118. van Deventer AJ, Goessens WH, van Belkum A, van Vliet HJ, van Etten EW, Verbrugh HA. Improved detection of *Candida albicans* by PCR in blood of neutropenic mice with systemic candidiasis. J Clin Microbiol 1995; 33:625–628.

119. Flahaut M, Sanglard D, Monod M, Bille J, Rossier M. Rapid detection of *Candida albicans* in clinical samples by DNA amplification of common regions from C. albicans-secreted aspartic proteinase genes. J Clin Microbiol 1998; 36:395–401.

120. Chryssanthou E, Klingspor L, Tollemar J, et al. PCR and other non-culture methods for diagnosis of invasive Candida infections in allogeneic bone marrow and solid organ transplant recipients. Mycoses 1999; 42:239–247.

121. Burnie JP, Golbang N, Matthews RC. Semiquantitative polymerase chain reaction enzyme immunoassay for diagnosis of disseminated candidiasis. Eur J Clin Microbiol Infect Dis 1997; 16:346–350.

122. Einsele H, Hebart H, Roller G, et al. Detection and identification of fungal pathogens in blood by using molecular probes. J Clin Microbiol 1997; 35:1353–1360.

123. Hebart H, Loffler J, Reitze H, et al. Prospective screening by a panfungal polymerase chain reaction assay in patients at risk for fungal infections: implications for the management of febrile neutropenia. Br J Haematol 2000; 111:635–640.

124. Buchheidt D, Baust C, Skladny H, et al. Detection of Aspergillus species in blood and bronchoalveolar lavage samples from immunocompromised patients by means of 2-step polymerase chain reaction: clinical results. Clin Infect Dis 2001; 33:428–435.

125. Buchheidt D, Baust C, Skladny H, Baldus M, Brauninger S, Hehlmann R. Clinical evaluation of a polymerase chain reaction assay to detect Aspergillus species in bronchoalveolar lavage samples of neutropenic patients. Br J Haematol 2002; 116:803–811.

126. Hayette MP, Vaira D, Susin F, et al. Detection of Aspergillus species DNA by PCR in bronchoalveolar lavage fluid. J Clin Microbiol 2001; 39:2338–2340.
127. Hebart H, Loffler J, Meisner C, et al. Early detection of aspergillus infection after allogeneic stem cell transplantation by polymerase chain reaction screening. J Infect Dis 2000; 181:1713–1729.
128. Jones ME, Fox AJ, Barnes AJ, et al. PCR-ELISA for the early diagnosis of invasive pulmonary aspergillus infection in neutropenic patients. J Clin Pathol 1998; 51:652–656.
129. Lass-Florl C, Aigner J, Gunsilius E, et al. Screening for Aspergillus spp. using polymerase chain reaction of whole blood samples from patients with haematological malignancies. Br J Haematol 2001; 113:180–184.
130. Loeffler J, Kloepfer K, Hebart H, et al. Polymerase chain reaction detection of aspergillus DNA in experimental models of invasive aspergillosis. J Infect Dis 2002; 185:1203–1206.
131. Raad I, Hanna H, Huaringa A, Sumoza D, Hachem R, Albitar M. Diagnosis of invasive pulmonary aspergillosis using polymerase chain reaction-based detection of aspergillus in BAL. Chest 2002; 121:1171–1176.
132. Raad I, Hanna H, Sumoza D, Albitar M. Polymerase chain reaction on blood for the diagnosis of invasive pulmonary aspergillosis in cancer patients. Cancer 2002; 94:1032–1036.
133. Skladny H, Buchheidt D, Baust C, et al. Specific detection of Aspergillus species in blood and bronchoalveolar lavage samples of immunocompromised patients by two-step PCR. J Clin Microbiol 1999; 37:3865–3871.
134. Spreadbury C, Holden D, Aufauvre-Brown A, Bainbridge B, Cohen J. Detection of *Aspergillus fumigatus* by polymerase chain reaction. J Clin Microbiol 1993; 31:615–821.
135. Tang CM, Holden DW, Aufauvre-Brown A, Cohen J. The detection of Aspergillus spp by the polymerase chain reaction and its evaluation in bronchoalveolar lavage fluid. Am Rev Respir Dis 1993; 148:1313–1317.
136. Williamson EC, Leeming JP, Palmer HM, et al. Diagnosis of invasive aspergillosis in bone marrow transplant recipients by polymerase chain reaction. Br J Haematol 2000; 108:132–139.
137. Hopfer RL, Walden P, Setterquist S, Highsmith WE. Detection and differentiation of fungi in clinical specimens using polymerase chain reaction (PCR) amplification and restriction enzyme analysis. J Med Vet Mycol 1993; 31:65–75.
138. Makimura K, Murayama SY, Yamaguchi H. Detection of a wide range of medically important fungi by the polymerase chain reaction. J Med Microbiol 1994; 40:358–364.
139. Sandhu GS, Kline BC, Stockman L, Roberts GD. Molecular probes for diagnosis of fungal infections. J Clin Microbiol 1995; 33:2913–2919.
140. Van Burik JA, Myerson D, Schreckhise RW, Bowden RA. Panfungal PCR assay for detection of fungal infection in human blood specimens. J Clin Microbiol 1998; 36:1169–1175.
141. Loeffler J, Schmidt K, Hebart H, Schumacher U, Einsele H. Automated extraction of genomic DNA from medically important yeast species and filamentous fungi by using the MagNA Pure LC system. J Clin Microbiol 2002; 40:2240–2243.
142. Loeffler J, Henke N, Hebart H, et al. Quantification of fungal DNA by using fluorescence resonance energy transfer and the light cycler system. J Clin Microbiol 2000; 38:586–590.
143. Pryce TM, Kay ID, Palladino S, Heath CH. Real-time automated polymerase chain reaction (PCR) to detect *Candida albicans* and *Aspergillus fumigatus* DNA in whole blood from high-risk patients. Diagn Microbiol Infect Dis 2003; 47:487–496.
144. Guiver M, Levi K, Oppenheim BA. Rapid identification of Candida species by TaqMan PCR. J Clin Pathol 2001; 54:362–366.
145. Bowman JC, Abruzzo GK, Anderson JW, et al. Quantitative PCR assay to measure *Aspergillus fumigatus* burden in a murine model of disseminated aspergillosis:

demonstration of efficacy of caspofungin acetate. Antimicrob Agents Chemother 2001; 45:3474–3481.

146. Maaroufi Y, Heymans C, De Bruyne JM, et al. Rapid detection of *Candida albicans* in clinical blood samples by using a TaqMan-based PCR assay. J Clin Microbiol 2003; 41:3293–3298.

147. Imhof A, Schaer C, Schoedon G, et al. Rapid detection of pathogenic fungi from clinical specimens using LightCycler real-time fluorescence PCR. Eur J Clin Microbiol Infect Dis 2003; 22:558–560.

148. Sanguinetti M, Posteraro B, Pagano L, et al. Comparison of real-time PCR, conventional PCR, and galactomannan antigen detection by enzyme-linked immunosorbent assay using bronchoalveolar lavage fluid samples from hematology patients for diagnosis of invasive pulmonary aspergillosis. J Clin Microbiol 2003; 41:3922–3925.

149. Spiess B, Buchheidt D, Baust C, et al. Development of a LightCycler PCR assay for detection and quantification of *Aspergillus fumigatus* DNA in clinical samples from neutropenic patients. J Clin Microbiol 2003; 41:1811–1818.

150. White PL, Shetty A, Barnes RA. Detection of seven Candida species using the Light-Cycler system. J Med Microbiol 2003; 52:229–238.

151. Pham AS, Tarrand JJ, May GS, Lee MS, Kontoyiannis DP, Han XY. Diagnosis of invasive mold infection by real-time quantitative PCR. Am J Clin Pathol 2003; 119:38–44.

152. Kami M, Fukui T, Ogawa S, et al. Use of real-time PCR on blood samples for diagnosis of invasive aspergillosis. Clin Infect Dis 2001; 33:1504–1512.

153. Costa C, Vidaud D, Olivi M, Bart-Delabesse E, Vidaud M, Bretagne S. Development of two real-time quantitative TaqMan PCR assays to detect circulating Aspergillus fumigatus DNA in serum. J Microbiol Methods 2001; 44:263–269.

154. Morrison VA, Haake RJ, Weisdorf DJ. The spectrum of non-Candida fungal infections following bone marrow transplantation. Medicine (Baltimore) 1993; 72:78–89.

155. Kaplan MH, Rosen PP, Armstrong D. Cryptococcosis in a cancer hospital: clinical and pathological correlates in forty-six patients. Cancer 1977; 39:2265–2274.

156. Asciogiu S, Rex JH, de Pauw B, et al. Defining opportunistic invasive fungal infections in immunocompromised patients with cancer and hematopoietic stem cell transplants: An international consensus. Clin Infect Dis 2002; 34:7–14.

157. McManus EJ, Jones JM. Detection of a *Trichosporon beigelii* antigen cross-reactive with *Cryptococcus neoformans* capsular polysaccharide in serum from a patient with disseminated Trichosporon infection. J Clin Microbiol 1985; 21:681–685.

158. Gade W, Hinnefeld SW, Babcock P, et al. Comparison of the PREMIER cryptococcal antigen enzyme immunoassay and the latex agglutination assay for detection of cryptococcal antigens. J Clin Microbiol 1991; 29:1616–1629.

159. Patterson TF, Andriole VT. Current concepts in cryptococcosis. Eur J Clin Micro 1989; 8:457–465.

160. Powderly WG, Cloud GA, Dismukes WE, Saag MS. Measurement of cryptococcal antigen in serum and cerebrospinal fluid: Value in the management of AIDS-associated cryptococcal meningitis. Clin Infect Dis 1994; 18:789–792.

161. Chen LC, Goldman DL, Doering TL, Pirofski LA, Casadevall A. Antibody response to Cryptococcus neoformans proteins in rodents and humans. Infec Immunity 1999; 67:2218–2224.

162. Wheat LJ, Kohler RB, French ML, et al. Immunoglobulin M and G histoplasmal antibody response in histoplasmosis. Amer Rev Resp Dis 1983; 128:65–70.

163. Wheat LJ, Cloud G, Johnson PC, et al. Clearance of fungal burden during treatment of disseminated histoplasmosis with liposomal amphotericin B versus itraconazole. Antimicrob Agents Chemother 2001; 45:2354–2357.

164. Wheat LJ, Connolly P, Haddad N, Le Monte A, Brizendine E, Hafner R. Antigen clearance during treatment of disseminated histoplasmosis with itraconazole versus fluconazole in patients with AIDS. Antimicrob Agents Chemother 2002; 46:248–250.

165. Wheat LJ, Connolly-Stringfield P, Kohler RB, Frame PT, Gupta MR. *Histoplasma capsulatum* polysaccharide antigen detection in diagnosis and management of disseminated histoplasmosis in patients with acquired immunodeficiency syndrome. Amer J Med 1989; 87:396–400.

166. Wheat LJ, Kohler RB, Tewari RP, Garten M, French MLV. Significance of *Histoplasma* antigen in the cerebrospinai fluid of patients with meningitis. Archives of Internal Medicine 1989; 149:302–304.

167. Klein BS, Kuritsky JN, Chappell WA, et al. Comparison of the enzyme immunoassay, immunodiffusion, and complement fixation tests in detecting antibody in human serum to the A antigen of *Blastomyces dermatitidis.* Am Rev Resp Dis 1986; 133:144–148.

168. Klein BS, Jones JM. Purification and characterization of the major antigen WI-1 from *Blastomyces dermatitidis* yeasts and immunological comparison with A antigen. Infec Immunity 1994; 62:3890–3900.

169. Klein BS, Vergeront JM, Kaufman L, et al. Serological tests for blastomycosis: Assessments during a large point-source outbreak in Wisconsin. J Infec Dis 1987; 155: 262–268.

170. Pappagianis D, Zimmer BL. Serology of coccidiodomycosis. Clin Microbiol Rev 1990; 3:247–268.

171. Gade W, Ledman DW, Wethington R, Yi A. Serological responses to various Coccidoides antigen preparation in a new enzyme immunoassay. J Clin Microbiol 1992; 30:1907–1912.

172. Stevens DA. Coccidioidomycosis. N Engl J Med 1995; 332:1077–1082.

15

Radiology of Fungal Infections in the Immunocompromised Patient

Reginald Greene
Massachusetts General Hospital, Boston, Massachusetts, U.S.A.

I. OVERVIEW

Imaging is increasingly important in the management of the immunocompromised patient with suspected invasive fungal infection, largely because early-targeted treatment is the key to improved outcome. Modern cross-sectional imaging provides a powerful means of detecting occult disease and of narrowing the differential diagnosis when invasive fungal diseases might otherwise go undetected. For patients whose condition permits, imaging also serves as a guide for tissue sampling and as an essential tool for longitudinal assessment of treatment response.

Although etiologic diagnosis usually depends on culture, direct visualization of a specific fungus in clinical specimens, or on certain serologic tests, initial imaging findings are of great utility in identifying further diagnostic and treatment strategies when an etiologic diagnosis is not made. The probability that a particular imaging finding will be associated with a specific infection depends mostly on the prior probability of that infection, i.e., on the entire clinical context in which imaging abnormalities is identified. The prior probability of infection depends on the underlying condition, the type and severity of immunosuppression, the past medical history, coexisting conditions, the duration of infection, the pathogenesis of the infectious process, and clinical tests and findings (1). The unique contribution of imaging to the differential diagnosis depends mainly on the type, extent, and distribution of lesions detected with cross-sectional imaging, i.e., CT, MRI, and US.

A few clinical circumstances may be associated with very distinctive imaging findings that can provide highly suggestive diagnoses of invasive fungal infection. In the HSCT recipient, and in the patient with a hematological condition associated with neutropenia, the CT "halo sign" or the "air crescent sign" are highly suggestive of invasive pulmonary aspergillosis. Similarly, in the AIDS patient with a low CD4 count, diffuse "miliary" nodules are highly likely to indicate a disseminated endemic fungal infection.

II. CLINICAL–ETIOLOGIC CONSTELLATIONS

The lung is an important portal of entry for fungal infection, so chest imaging is of central importance in the early detection of disease. Initial imaging findings of invasive fungal infection are in general, nonspecific, but when taken in clinical context, they may greatly narrow the differential diagnostic possibilities. From an imaging point of view, the vast majority of invasive mycoses affecting the immune-deficient patient fall into one of four clinical–etiological constellations that have varied but prototypical imaging findings.

The first constellation is caused by ubiquitous opportunistic fungi that rarely cause invasive infection in the immune-competent host, but often cause life-threatening primary fungal pneumonia in the immune-deficient patient, particularly in the HSCT recipient, and in the patient with a hematologic condition associated with severe neutropenia. The angio-invasive fungus *Aspergillus* is by far the most common example, and the angio-invasive *Mucorales* fungus is a rare example. The most prototypical initial CT finding in this constellation is the pulmonary macronodule (≥ 1 cm diameter); less commonly, consolidation and the consolidative infarct. With prompt CT imaging, these findings are often discoverable prior to systemic fungal dissemination.

The second constellation is caused by ubiquitous opportunistic fungi that rarely cause primary invasive pneumonia even in the immune-deficient patient. These infections are usually widely disseminated at the time of first detection. A variety of portals of entry are utilized. These fungi rarely cause primary pneumonia, but they can cause secondary pneumonias from hematogenous dissemination to the lungs from an extra-pulmonary site of infection, and from super-infection of lung, damaged by prior infection from other microbes or by noninfectious processes (2,3).

Candida sp., are by far the most common example, and *Sporothrix schenckii*, the soil fungus for which the lung is an uncommon portal of entry is a very rare example. CT imaging of extra-pulmonary candidiasis tends to produce characteristic disseminated 5–15 mm diameter nodules. Secondary pneumonias associated with candidiasis are highly variable and unpredictable in appearance, often demonstrating diffuse or multifocal infection that is often multimicrobial.

The third constellation is caused by ubiquitous pathogenic fungi that use the lung as the primary portal of entry, but uncommonly cause clinically obvious or progressive infection in the immune-competent patient, but commonly cause life-threatening disseminated fungal infection in the immune-deficient patient, especially in the host with severe T-cell immune-deficiency. *Cryptococcus neoformans* is the main example. The most common imaging findings in this constellation include focal or disseminated lesions in the brain and meninges. Lung lesions include focal nodules or focal consolidations, or diffuse miliary nodules. The vast majority of patients first discovered with pulmonary cryptococcosis already have disseminated CNS infection.

The fourth constellation is caused by geographically endemic fungi that produce only trivial or subclinical pneumonia in immune-competent hosts, but cause disseminated infection and progressive pulmonary infection in patients with marked T-cell immune-deficiency. In the United States, endemic fungi include, *Histoplasma capsulatum, Coccidioides immitis,* and *Blastomyces dermatitidis.* On initial CT studies, chest findings often consist of residue of previously dormant primary infection, or widespread lesions such as miliary or larger-sized nodules consistent with systemic dissemination to the lungs. Abnormalities are also commonly found in solid viscera and lymph nodes.

   Identifying one of these constellations can be useful in narrowing the differential diagnosis, planning further etiologic diagnostic testing, and deciding on presumptive treatment. Identifying a constellation, however, can be complicated by variations from the prototypical imaging findings described above, and by synchronous or metachronous fungal infections, nonfungal infections, or noninfectious complications (4).

   Seriously immunocompromised patients who are at risk of invasive fungal infection are also at increased risk of a wide range of other potentially serious infectious and noninfectious conditions. These include bacterial and viral pneumonias, aspiration, septic or bland pulmonary emboli and infarcts, pulmonary hemorrhage, drug toxicities, lymphoproliferative disorders, vasculitis, and localized and disseminated malignancy.

   This chapter includes discussions on the use of imaging techniques pertinent to the diagnosis of suspected fungal infection in the immunocompromised patient, and imaging findings of infections caused by fungi in the four clinical–etiologic constellations described above.

III. IMAGING TECHNIQUES

The chest, sinuses, CNS, abdominal organs, and bones are the main affected anatomic regions that require imaging assessment for invasive fungal infection. Efficient use of imaging can expedite and simplify patient management, and can help avoid errors. The chest is the central focus for imaging suspected invasive fungal infection because the lung is the most common portal of entry.

A. Chest Imaging

1. Computed Tomography

Many studies have confirmed that CT is both much more sensitive (5,6) and more specific (7) than radiography in the detection and diagnosis of pulmonary lesions. Modern CT provides high-resolution tomographic anatomic detail that has become the gold standard for lung imaging, and reduced respiratory artifacts in the tachypneic patient with pneumonia. There is growing availability of state-of-the-art scanners that provide improved speed, image quality, and radiation dose reduction. As a result, there is justifiably growing reliance on CT for both screening detection as well as for differential diagnosis. CT is the most dependable means of detecting chest lesions associated with clinically occult invasive fungal infection, and the most accurate means of determining the location, extent, distribution, and type of lung lesions; the imaging parameters most necessary in narrowing the differential diagnosis. CT also serves as the modality of choice for guiding percutaneous lung biopsy, a procedure that in the immunocompromised patient can be expected to identify etiologic organisms about 80% of the time (8). Because many patients are not suitable candidates for expeditious biopsy, specific etiologic diagnosis is often not known. Thus, early treatment is often based on the most likely diagnosis based on clinical background, imaging, and other tests (9,10). Today, few important clinical management decisions in the immunocompromised patient with suspected fungal infection are made without reference to chest CT studies.

2. Radiography

Despite the now dominant position of CT in chest imaging, radiography continues to be a practical day-to-day management tool in the evaluation of chest infection.

Standard, state-of-the-art, high-quality, erect, full inspiration, posteroanterior digital chest radiographs obtained in a modern radiology department provide a reasonably dependable gross survey of chest anatomy. Unfortunately, even these high-quality studies frequently produce false-negative results in the immunosuppressed patient with fungal infection. Low-quality, anteroposterior, supine, shallow inspiration bedside chest radiography that has even lower sensitivity and specificity than high-quality-studies cannot be relied upon to exclude chest disease; or when positive, be relied upon to accurately portray the type and extent of lung abnormality.

Thus, in a patient at high risk of fungal infection, a CT study is almost always needed to confirm the type, severity, extent, and distribution of disease when radiography is positive, and is often necessary to exclude lung disease in the symptomatic patient even when radiography is negative.

B. Extrapulmonary Imaging

Magnetic resonance imaging (MRI) and CT are the main modalities used to image the sinuses, bones and joints, and CNS. Contrast-enhanced CT is the main modality used for imaging the abdominopelvic compartment in patients with suspected invasive fungal infection. As compared with either ultrasound or MRI, CT provides the best means of global assessment of the entire abdominopelvic compartment. Sonography has the advantage of being suitable for bedside studies when necessary, and not requiring iodinated intravenous contrast. Like sonography, MRI, is best suited for focused problem-solving examinations of specific organs or regions, rather than for overall assessment of the abdominopelvic compartment. Whole body scintigraphic screening for infection with F-18 fluorodeoxyglucose positron emission tomography (PET) is rapidly replacing Gallium-67-labeled radiopharmaceuticals, but it has not been much used to detect invasive fungal infection because there are cross-over positive results with malignant tumors (11), and other noninfectious inflammations, e.g., drug-induced pulmonary toxicity (12).

IV. IMAGING IN SPECIFIC INVASIVE MYCOSES

A. Aspergillosis

Aspergillus is the main example of the clinical–etiological constellation caused by ubiquitous opportunistic fungi that rarely cause invasive infection in the immune-competent host, but often cause life-threatening primary fungal pneumonia in the immune-deficient patient. The HSCT recipient and the patient with a hematologic condition associated with severe neutropenia are at particularly high risk of infection. Two peak periods of especially high infection risk for the HSCT recipient occur during the first 30 days following engraftment when neutropenia may be severe, and later after the first 90 days when chronic graft versus host disease (GVHD) may require prolonged high levels of immunosuppression. Thus, slightly more than half of *Aspergillus* infections in HSCT recipients occur after hospital discharge (13). Sporadic invasive aspergillosis also occurs in patients with other underlying causes of immune-suppression but at a lower incidence than in the above high risk groups, such as in solid organ transplant recipients, high-dose corticosteroid recipients, and in patients with AIDS.

The lung is the main portal of entry, and the most common primary site of invasive infection (~90%) (14). *Aspergillus* is the most common cause of primary opportunistic invasive pulmonary fungal pneumonia in the immune-deficient patient (14).

Angio-invasion is the dominant pathogenetic method of disease progression, and responsible for the most important imaging findings. Immune mechanisms that normally prevent the tiny inhaled ubiquitous *Aspergillus* spores, which are regularly inhaled into the peripheral airspaces, from germinating into invasive hyphae allow the development of a core of infection. Vascular invasion by *Aspergillus* hyphae produces a tangle of small infected necrotic vessels that become incorporated into the core of infection (15). The resulting vascular thrombosis and infarction are responsible for a perimeter of hemorrhage and infection surrounding the core of infection (16). This pathogenetic sequence is responsible for the development of the pulmonary nodule and the perimeter of ground-glass opacity due to infection and hemorrhage, i.e., the "halo sign" (17). Occasionally, hyphal elements invade adjacent large vessels to cause thrombosis, pseudoaneurysm, and the risk of rupture and exsanguination. In a small fraction of patients (~10%), *aspergillosis* infection progresses via airway invasion, i.e., via the radial airway route resulting in centrilobular infection, which includes the bronchi, bronchioli, and peripheral airspaces (18).

1. Similarities to Mucormycosis

Mucormycosis is a much rarer cause of this constellation. Invasive aspergillosis and mucormycosis have indistinguishable clinical presentations, pathogenetic mechanisms, pathology, and imaging findings (19–21). For this reason, the vast majority of the discussion of imaging findings in invasive aspergillosis can be extrapolated to mucormycosis. Angio-invasive mucormycosis differs angio-invasive aspergillosis primarily in its rarity (22), even in the at-risk groups described above, and in its resistance to standard anti-*Aspergillus* therapy with amphotericin B. Mucormycosis is frequently treated with surgical resection. Thus, lesions attributed to *Aspergillus* without confirmatory mycology should always be regarded as potential signs of mucormycosis, especially when standard treatment with standard anti-Aspergillus drugs is not effective.

2. Pulmonary Aspergillosis

Initial CT imaging findings in invasive aspergillosis are dominated by the nodule and associated "halo sign." Cavities and the "air crescent sign" are primarily features of late invasive aspergillosis. Consolidations and consolidative infarcts are much less common than nodules as initial CT features. Subcentimeter lung nodules, singly or in clusters, and the bronchiolitis–bronchopneumonia pattern are uncommonly detected on initial CT studies. Ancillary pleural or pericardial effusions, and hilar or mediastinal adenopathy are each found in a very small fraction of patients (~10%).

  a. Macronodule. The main finding in invasive aspergillosis is a pulmonary nodule ≥1 cm in maximum diameter, i.e., the macronodule. It is defined as a localized space-occupying, ovoid soft tissue opacity that displaces rather than conforms to the shape of the pre-existing aerated lung. The soft tissue nodule completely obscures the background bronchovasculature. The macronodule is the imaging analog of the angio-invasive core of infection in the peripheral airspaces (16), and the most common initial CT finding in patients with mycologically proven invasive aspergillosis. More than 90% of patients with mycologically proven invasive aspergillosis have at least one pulmonary nodule (10). The macronodule is such a common feature on initial CT that its absence argues against the likelihood of invasive aspergillosis (10,16).

The "roughly nodular infarct" is a subcategory of the macronodule that has a characteristic hump-shape and subpleural location; sometimes referred to as a "Hampton's hump" (23).

Macronodules can be caused by any invasive fungal infection, as well as by many other infectious processes including nocardiosis, tuberculosis, and lung abscess. Common noninfectious causes include bland pulmonary infarcts, lung cancer, lung metastases, lymphoproliferative disorders, and vasculitis.

b. Halo Sign.   The halo sign is a modifier of the macronodule. It is defined as a perimeter of CT ground-glass lung opacity that surrounds a pulmonary nodule (10,15–17,24) (Fig. 1). The ground glass perimeter should be substantial enough to permit clear visualization of background vasculature through it (10). The nodule with a halo sign is differentiated from the nodule with unsharp margination because of irregularity of outline or partial volume effect caused by thick CT sections or respiratory motion.

On initial CT study of patients with mycologically proven invasive aspergillosis, about one-third of patients have one or more macronoduies with a halo sign (14).

In the patient with a compatible illness who is at particularly high risk of invasive aspergillosis, i.e., the HSCT recipient, and the patient with a hematologic condition associated with neutropenia, the halo sign is considered a specific indicator of the fungal infection (14–17,25,26).

The halo sign is also an important imaging sign because it tends to identify patients with invasive aspergillosis who are most likely to respond to aggressive specific anti*Aspergillus* therapy (10,25).

There is relatively little experience with MRI in early invasive aspergillosis. Nodular and segmental non-nodular lung lesions have demonstrated target,like

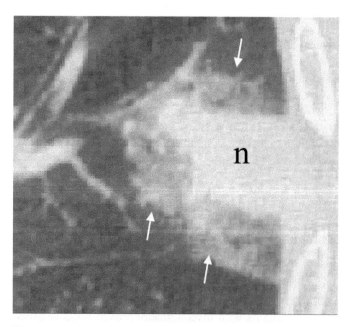

Figure 1 Halo Sign.

Tl-weighted central hyperintensities, and rim-enhancement after intravenous gadolinium injection (27). Hyperintensity on T-l weighted imaging correlates with subacute hemorrhage permeated by *Aspergillus* organisms (27). A comparative study found that the CT halo sign was much more specific than the analogous MRI halo sign in identifying patients with invasive aspergillosis (28).

The differential diagnosis of the halo sign is broad. The halo sign is not unique only to infection by angio-invasive *Aspergillus.* Other causes include the rare angio-invasive Mucorales sp., and other even rarer normally saprophytic angio-invasive fungi, such as *Trichosporon* sp., (29), *Penicillium* sp., (30) and *Fusarium* sp., (31). The pathogenetic mechanism responsible for the halo sign can also be found in angio-invasive bacterial infections, most notably those caused by *Pseudomonas aeruginosa* (32). The CT halo sign has also been reported in lung infections due to endemic fungi, e.g., *Coccidioides immitis,* as well as due to infections caused by *Nocardia* sp., *Mycobacterium tuberculosis, cytomegalovirus,* and *herpes simplex* virus. Noninfectious conditions reported to cause the halo sign include bronchoalveolar cell carcinoma, lymphoproliferative disorders, metastatic angiosarcoma, Kaposi sarcoma, Wegener granulomatosis, eosinophilic lung disease, and organizing pneumonia (24,33,34).

    c. Air Crescent Signs and Cavities. The air crescent sign on CT is defined as a CT nodule containing a semilunar pocket of gas surmounting a partially detached sequestrum of devitalized lung (16,35) (Fig. 2).

In the patient with a compatible illness who is at particularly high risk of invasive aspergillosis, i.e., the HSCT recipient, and the patient with a hematologic condition associated with neutropenia, the air crescent sign is considered a specific indicator of the fungal infection (14–17,25,26). The air crescent sign is attributed to a crescentic cap of air between a devitalized sequestrum pulmonary aspergillosis that has separated from the remaining viable lung.

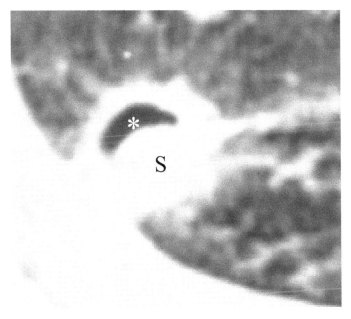

Figure 2 Air Crescent Sign.

Over time, necrosis tends to develop in nodular foci of *Aspergillus* infection often leading to cavitation. Sometimes an air crescent sign will develop. The air crescent sign is detected in only 5–10% of patients on initial CT studies (10). In a week to 10 days following an initial chest CT, macronodules with halo signs will become progressively less frequent (28,36), while macronodules with cavitation and air crescent signs will become more frequent.

The air-crescent sign tends to develop after recovery from neutropenia. Like the halo sign, the air crescent sign is an indicator of likely invasive aspergillosis when it is detected in a patient at high risk of the infection (16,37,38).

Thick-walled and thin-walled cavities without air crescents can be found in about 10% of initial CT studies of patients with invasive aspergillosis, but these findings do not seem to have the same diagnostic predictive value as the air crescent sign, from which they should be differentiated (39).

In limited experience with invasive aspergillosis, MRI studies have demonstrated necrotic target lesions with a rim with T-2 weighted hyperintensity, and gadolinium rim enhancement (28).

The differential diagnosis of the air crescent sign is broad, but like the halo sign, invasive aspergillosis is the most common cause when it is found in the HSCT recipient or the patient with hematologic malignancy with neutropenia who has a compatible illness. The sign is also found in many conditions other than invasive aspergillosis, e.g., nocardiosis, tuberculosis, bacterial lung abscess, cavitary hematoma, and cavitary lung cancer (40,41). The sequestrum of the air crescent sign needs to be differentiated from the often free-floating fungus ball of saprophytic aspergillosis. The sign also needs to be differentiated from thin and thick-walled cavities that lack air crescents.

d. Consolidation and Consolidative Infarct. Consolidation is defined as a nonspace-occupying lung opacification of the peripheral airspaces, such that the background of underlying bronchovascular structures is totally obscured, except where bronchi contain residual gas, i.e., air bronchograms (42). Consolidations usually maintain the general shape of the pre-existing aerated lung anatomy. The consolidative infarct is a subcategory of consolidation that is wedge-shaped and pleural-based (16,17). In angio-invasive aspergillosis, the consolidative infarct is attributed to a segment- or larger-sized lung infarct (16).

On initial CT studies, about one-third of patients with invasive aspergillosis demonstrate one or more consolidations, or consolidative infarcts (10).

The differential diagnosis of localized lung consolidation includes any invasive fungal infection, as well as a wide range of pneumonias due to bacteria, *Legionella*, and viruses. Common noninfectious causes include aspiration, infarction, hemorrhage, partial atelectasis, lymphoproliferative disorders, and radiation injury.

e. Centrilobular, Tree-in-Bud, and Peri-bronchial Opacities. Centrilobular opacities are discrete subcentimeter nodular opacities located in the center of secondary lobules, and are often found in conjunction with opacified segments of small branching bronchi and bronchioli, i.e., tree-in-bud opacities, and/or patches of peribronchial consolidation. They form what is called the bronchiolitis–bronchopneumonia pattern.

These findings, identified either separately or in combination, are taken as general indicators of bronchiolitis or bronchopneumonia that result from spread of infection along the airways (18). In the specific clinical context of the patient at high risk of opportunistic or endemic fungal infection, such findings may be because of airway invasive progression of fungal infection, such as because of *Aspergillus* or *Cryptococcus*.

These findings have been noted in about 10% of patients with invasive pulmonary aspergillosis, and attributed to airway invasion (10,18,43,44).

A chronic form of airway invasive aspergillosis, i.e., chronic tracheobronchial aspergillosis infection spreads along the airways, resulting in bronchial wall thickening and nodularity, bronchostenosis, and bronchiectasis that can lead to peribronchial consolidation and atelectasis, especially in HSCT and lung transplant recipients, and in AIDS patients (18,45).

The differential diagnosis of the bronchiolitis–bronchopneumonia pattern is broad, and not specific for invasive aspergillosis. It may be found in a wide variety of other conditions, including atypical mycobacterial infection, tuberculosis, and bronchopneumonia of any cause (18).

Direct intrathoracic invasion into extra-pulmonary tissues such as the pleura and pericardium (~10%), and hila and mediastinum (~1%) is very low on initial CT studies (10). Blood-borne dissemination into the lungs may result in disseminated lung nodules, or diffuse consolidation.

f. Treatment Response. Follow-up imaging of initial pulmonary findings shows that the halo and air crescent signs vary inversely with each other over time, i.e., the frequency of the halo sign falls, and the frequency of the air crescent sign rises. In one longitudinal CT study, 72% of patients had halo signs early in the course of disease, but only 22% of patients had halo signs after the first 10 days (28). In another study, the frequency of the halo sign rapidly decreased to about one fifth of its initial frequency 7–10 days following an initial CT scan (36). Some data suggest that there may even be a significant fall off in the frequency of the halo sign during the first three days following the initial CT scan (36).

Over the first seven days following discovery, a three to four-fold increase in the volume of CT lung opacities has been observed in patients who do not seem to show other signs of unsatisfactory response to treatment (36). This phenomenon may be because of increased host responsiveness to infection and not because of treatment failure.

3. Extrapulmonary Aspergillosis

Cerebral aspergillosis occurs by direct extension from sino-nasal aspergillosis, or from systemic hematogenous dissemination (Fig. 3). Sino-nasal aspergillosis may demonstrate soft tissue masses or abscesses in the nasal cavities or paranasal sinuses. Extension to the brain or orbit may be seen through the cribriform plate, sometimes associated with bone destruction or cavernous sinus thrombosis (46). Initial brain lesions are similar in appearance to those in the lung; usually well-defined macronodular hypodensities or large vessel infarcts surrounded by edema on CT. On MRI, cerebral lesions are T2W hyperintensities surrounded by edema that enhance after intravenous gadolinium (47). In later stages, central necrosis and rim enhancement are the primary findings (48).

Visceral dissemination is associated with solid nodular masses, abscesses or infarcts in the liver, spleen, and kidneys.

B. Candidiasis

Candida is the main example of the clinical–etiological constellation caused by ubiquitous opportunistic fungi that rarely result in primary invasive pneumonia, but commonly cause solid organ and/or lung dissemination that is often identifiable

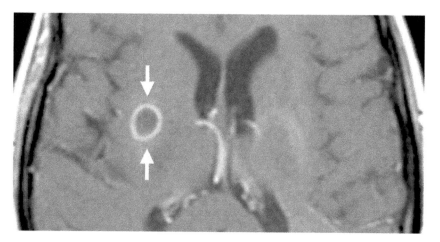

Figure 3 Cerebral IPA.

on an initial imaging study. Candidiasis is commonly associated with synchronous infection by other pathogenic and opportunistic microbes. Those at high risk are usually severely immunosuppressed patients, especially those with leukemia and those who are neutropenic.

1. Pulmonary Candidiasis

Candida pneumonia may be due to hematogenous dissemination or to super-infection of lung that has been damaged by prior or contemporaneous infection, by other microbes or by some other noninfectious processes.

In pulmonary candidiasis, imaging findings defy meaningful categorization because the fungus is often found in lung tissue without convincing evidence of significant lung damage (49). It is usually found in severely immunocompromised patients who have disseminated candidiasis that often coexists with invasive infection because of other opportunistic and pathogenic microbes (50).

The pulmonary imaging findings that have been attributed to invasive Candidiasis are often bilateral and diffuse as a result of systemic dissemination. Focal findings may also occur in areas of damaged lung that has become infected. On CT, a wide variety of both focal or diffuse lesions have been identified, including nodules (50), lesions of the bronchiolitis-bronchopneumonia pattern (51), and diffuse miliary nodules (1–3mm discrete nodules too numerous to count). Focal nodules detected in pulmonary candidiasis do not seem to have the same clinical relevance as early nodular lesions found in invasive aspergillosis, where early detection and treatment may have an impact on outcome (52). The lack of correlation between the detection of localized and diffuse imaging findings on improved outcome holds whether candidiasis is considered "primary," i.e., due to airway aspiration, or "secondary," i.e., due to hematogenous dissemination. Contemporaneous initial abdominal CT studies may also demonstrate disseminated nodular lesions in the liver, spleen, or kidneys.

The differential diagnosis of diffuse lung opacification in the immunosuppressed patient is broad and mainly dependent on the particular type of lung lesions that make up the diffuse opacification. The detailed differential diagnosis based on the type and distribution of particular lung lesions is beyond the scope of this chapter.

In general, in the immune-deficient patient, diffused lung opacification may be found in candidiasis, PCP, viral pneumonia, toxoplasmosis, and disseminated endemic or opportunistic mycoses. It can also be found in pulmonary edema, Kaposi sarcoma, ARDS, capillary leak syndromes, pulmonary hemorrhage, alveolar proteinosis, transfusion reactions, drug toxicity, idiopathic interstitial pneumonias, and metastatic cancer.

2. Extra-pulmonary Candidiasis

The portal of entry is variable, e.g., because of transcutaneous infusion lines or aspiration. The infection is usually disseminated in multiple organs at the time of the initial CT study. CT studies may demonstrate pulmonary lesions alone or in combination with extrapulmonary infection.

    a. Hepatosplenic Candidiasis. Chronic hepatosplenic candidiasis is a condition often of patients recovering from prolonged neutropenia, usually after remission induction chemotherapy for acute leukemia (53). The recovered neutrophil function in chronic candidiasis allows for focal granuloma formation (54).

    In chronic hepatosplenic candidiasis, studies of the abdomen with CT, MRI or US characteristically demonstrate multiple, 5–15 mm, well-defined, solid nodules in the liver, spleen, and/or kidneys. In acute hepatosplenic candidiasis before neutrophil function has recovered, these same nodules consist of liquefied or partially liquefied abscesses, rather than solid focal lesions.

    Patients suspected of chronic disseminated candidiasis are best studied with contrast-enhanced CT. Upper abdominal US may also be useful because lesions that are not visible on CT may be apparent with US (55). The converse is also true. On CT, multiple, well-defined, low-attenuation nodules of 5–15 mm are detected in the liver, spleen, and/or kidneys (56) (Fig. 4). Disseminated granulomatous infection can be found most often in the liver, spleen, or kidneys (56) when chest radiographic studies are usually normal.

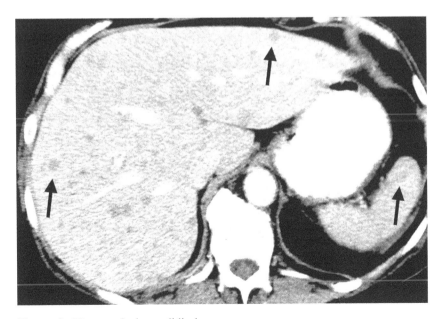

Figure 4 Hepatosplenic candidiasis.

In US, the nodules are well defined and hypoechoic, often with a "wheels within wheels" appearance consisting of a hypoechoic outer rim, hyperechoic inner rim, and hypoechoic infectious-necrotic core. Sometimes the hypoechoic nodules have hyperechoic cores called "Bull's eye" lesions (55,57). In MRI, deep visceral candidiasis appears as well-defined, T-2 hyperintense nodules (58).

Similar appearing, multiple subacute or chronic macroscopic hepatosplenic nodules (hypoechoic on US and hypoattenuating on CT) can be found in immunosuppressed patients with other disseminated fungal infections, such as disseminated aspergillosis and fusariosis, miliary tuberculosis and disseminated mycobacterial infection, and multiple bacterial abscesses.

b. Treatment Response. Even after satisfactory clinical response to treatment, hepatosplenic nodules tend to persist for long periods (55,57,59).

C. Cryptococcosis

Cryptococcus neoformans is the main example of the clinical–etiological constellation caused by ubiquitous pathogenic fungi, which use the lung as the primary portal of entry that uncommonly cause clinically obvious or progressive infection in immune-competent patients, but also commonly cause life-threatening disseminated fungal infection in immune-deficient patients. The main high-risk groups have severe T-cell immune-deficiency, especially those with AIDS and very low CD4 counts. The pathogenesis sequence includes inhalation of fungi, pneumonia, and prompt blood-borne dissemination in the immune-deficient patient. The pulmonary infection is the result of either a new primary pulmonary infection, or an activated dormant focus of infection.

1. Pulmonary Cryptococcosis

In the immune-competent patient, cryptococcosis can produce a wide variety of initial pulmonary imaging findings, most often of the focal type. In dormant infection, there may be no imaging residue, or a silent subpleural soft tissue nodule or mass. Other positive chest findings may include hilar lymphadenopathy and pleural effusion.

In the immune-deficient patient, cryptococcosis is the most common cause of fungal pneumonia in the severely immune-deficient AIDS patient, usually associated with concomitant CNS infection (86%) that may be clinically silent (60). Conversely, about one-fourth of AIDS patients who present with CNS cryptococcosis have clinically silent pulmonary lesions (Fig. 5). Other common sites of disseminated mycosis include skin, bone, or genitourinary tract.

In the immune-deficient patient, a subpleural pulmonary nodule is a characteristic localized finding (61), and may be observed to progress into a peribronchial, segmental, or Iobar opacity or into a fulminant, widespread ARDS-like picture (61). Hematogenous dissemination to the lung often takes on a pattern of miliary nodules (1–3 mm diameter discrete nodules too numerous to count) identical to the appearance of hematogenous spread of endemic mycoses (61).

The differential diagnosis of diffuse miliary nodules includes other hematogenously disseminated mycoses, such as endemic mycoses and other nonfungal infectious etiologies. The other infections that are likely to cause diffuse miliary nodules in the immunocompromised patient include disseminated tuberculosis, disseminated nontuberculous mycobacterial infection, and viral pneumonia. Other

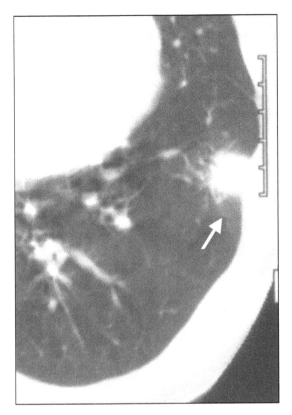

Figure 5 Pulmonary Cryptococcosis.

causes of diffuse miliary nodules include noninfectious granulomatous disease, such as sarcoidosis and pneumoconiosis, and hematogenous metastases to the lung. See Sec.IV.B.1 for a discussion of the more general differential diagnosis of diffuse lung opacification in the immunosuppressed patient.

2. Extra-pulmonary Cryptococcosis

a. Cerebral Cryptococcosis. Cerebral cryptococcosis is the most common invasive fungal infection of the CNS. On CT and MRI, it presents in approximately equal frequencies as (a) one or more nonenhancing solid lesions, hypodense pseudo-cysts, or space-occupying lesions in the basal ganglia, as (b) meningitis/meningoencephalitis with gyral enhancement, or as (c) normal studies (62). Commonly, there are signs of hydrocephalus (62). Imaging can identify the most useful site for biopsy when necessary (63). MRI studies show meningeal enhancement. Other signs include a solid parenchymal mass without hemorrhage (granuloma), atrophy, cerebral edema, or hydrocephalus. Basal ganglia lesions are hypointense on Tl-weighted images, hyperintense on T2-weighted images, and usually hyperintense on Tl-weighted images after intervention gadolinium.

b. Abdominal Cryptococcosis. Abdominal cryptococcosis can affect the solid abdominal viscera such as the liver, and may be seen as multiple, small, and low attenuation nodules similar to other those found with disseminated infections by opportunistic or other endemic fungi.

In the AIDS patient with a very low CD4 count and diffuse nodular CT lung opacities, diagnostic considerations for small miliary nodules should include disseminated endemic fungal infection, disseminated mycobacterial infection, *pneumocystis carinii* pneumonia, viral pneumonia, pulmonary edema, diffuse lung damage (ARDS), treatment-induced lung reactions, bronchiolitis obliterans-organized pneumonia, lymphoproliferative disorders, Kaposi sarcoma, hematogenous metastases, and allergic pneumopathy. Up to one-third of pulmonary nodules have been diagnosed with halo signs (64), or cavitation (61). The differential diagnosis of a cavitary pulmonary nodule in the AIDS patient must include PCP (61). Hilar and/or mediastinal adenopathy, and pleural effusions can also be found (60,61).

In the AIDS patient with neurologic findings and a very low CD4 count at-risk, the differential diagnosis must include toxoplasmosis, a cause of parenchymal lesions with ring enhancement, solid enhancement, and nonenhancing focal edema.

D. Endemic Mycoses

Histoplasma capsulatum, Coccidioides immitis, and *Blastomyces dermatididis* are the main causes of a clinical–etiological constellation resulting from geographically endemic fungi encountered in the United States. Infection in immune-competent hosts usually produces trivial or subclinical pneumonia that spontaneously resolves, but in immunosuppressed patients it can cause disseminated life-threatening infection. Dissemination has usually already occurred at the time of initial detection. The main risk factor is severe impairment in T-cell immunity, such as in the AIDS patient with very low CD4 count. (61,65).

The lung is the main portal of entry of endemic mycoses. Infection in immune-deficient patients usually arises from one of two pathogenetic sequences. In the first, deficiency of T-cell immunity results in failure to maintain inactivity of a dormant focus of a previous primary infection. In the second, deficiency of T-cell immunity results in failure to prevent new primary pulmonary infection, in an endemic area. In each case, there is rapid hematologic dissemination to extra-pulmonary sites and the lungs. Nonpulmonary sites of initial infection include the paranasal sinuses and skin. Sites of extra-pulmonary dissemination that have significant imaging implications include the brain and meninges, and the solid abdominal viscera, gastrointestinal tract, and bones.

Initial chest radiographs are negative as often as half the time even when the disease is disseminated. Positive initial chest findings are varied (66), but tend to occur in three types of presentations. In one presentation, initial studies show focal or multifocal lung lesions such as nodules or consolidations because of a reactivated dormant focus, or a progressive primary infection.

In a second presentation, there are diffuse lung lesions because of hematogenous dissemination from a progressive primary pulmonary infection or from secondary sites of extra-pulmonary infection. The diffuse lung lesions may be composed of discrete miliary nodules (1–3 mm diameter), larger nodules, or consolidation. In radiography, the discrete miliary lesions seen on CT may appear as vague, nonspecific reticulonodular opacities. When the miliary nodules of hematogenous dissemination are present, larger nodules or consolidation of the focus of previously dormant primary lung infection, or the main new site of progressive primary infection may be visible.

In the third presentation, the initial imaging finding is due to extra-pulmonary dissemination to the CNS, intra-abdominal organs, or lymph nodes.

For a discussion on the differential diagnosis of the macronodule and consolidation in the immunocompromised patient, see Sec. IV.A.2. For a discussion on the differential diagnosis of diffuse lung opacification in general, see Sec. IV.B.1. For a discussion on the differential diagnosis of diffuse miliary nodules, see Sec. IV.C.1.

The same underlying conditions and immunodeficiency that make these patients susceptible to endemic mycoses also put them at increased risk of infection caused by other organisms such as other fungi, bacteria, viruses, and protozoa, including especially mycobacteria, *Nocardia asteroides,* and *Legionella* sp., varicella-zoster virus, herpes simplex virus, cytomegalovirus, Epstein-Barr virus, *P. carinii,* and *T. gondii.* Each of these alternative infections, and a variety of noninfectious conditions must be kept in mind when arriving at a differential diagnosis of imaging findings (67,44). Hilar, mediastinal, and intra-abdominal lymphadenopathy are common features of endemic mycoses, and need to be differentiated from similar findings in disseminated tuberculosis, atypical mycobacteria, metastatic tumor, and lymphoma.

1. Histoplasmosis

a. Pulmonary Histoplasmosis. *Histoplasma capsulation* causes endemic infection in central United States. Like other endemic fungi, it generally produces a mild, self-limited infection of the lungs, and only rarely causes progressive or disseminated infection (<0.05 %) (68). The immune-competent patient with histoplasmosis is capable of reacting to infection with well-developed ruberculoid granulomas that usually become dormant and calcify.

In the immunocompromised patient, histoplasmosis is uncommon even in endemic areas (3). When it occurs, infection is often disseminated on first discovery. Dissemination is the result of activation of a dormant focus, or progressive primary infection. Impaired T-cell immunity limits the ability to produce well-developed granulomas.

In the lung, a diffuse radiographic abnormality reflecting hematogenous dissemination is identified in about half of the patients (69). The diffuse lung lesions consist of miliary nodules, macronodules, vague reticulonodular opacities or consolidations (Fig. 6). See Sec. On IV.A.2 and IV.C.1 for differential diagnosis. Almost half the time, chest radiographs are interpreted as normal even in disseminated disease (69,70). Focal radiographic lung opacities are identified in only about 10% of patients (69). Enlarged hilar and mediastinal lymph nodes, calcified granulomas, and cavitation are uncommonly identified (<5% each) (69). Increased focal opacity and/or cavitation within the diffuse lung disease may indicate a site of an activated dormant focus. Even when imaging does identify findings consistent with disseminated histoplasmosis, concurrent tuberculosis must be considered, especially in the AIDS patient with a low CD4 count.

b. Extra-pulmonary Histoplasmosis. Extra-pulmonary findings include hepatosplenomegaly, lymphadenopathy, and solid organ enlargement. The specific diagnosis is based on *H. capsulatum* in a tissue specimen or grown in culture or the presence of *Histoplasma* antigen in blood or urine. At the onset of infection, histoplasmosis is often widely disseminated, and can be rapidly diagnosed with antigen levels in urine or serum, or by blood cultures or pathologic specimens. Disseminated extra-pulmonary histoplasmosis is an important diagnostic consideration in the immunocompromised patient from an endemic area who develops a febrile illness associated with pneumonic consolidation, paratracheal mediastinal and intra-abdominal lymphadenopathy, superior vena cava syndrome, and in the patient with

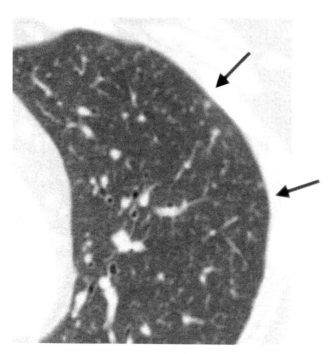

Figure 6 Miliary Histoplasmosis.

miliary lesions in the lung, spleen, or adrenal glands. These lesions may or may not be calcified.

2. Coccidioidomycosis

a. Pulmonary Coccidioidomycosis. The lung is the primary portal of entry of *Coccidioides immitis,* a cause of endemic mycosis in southwestern United States. In the immunocompetent person, an intact T-cell immunity helps confine coccidioido-mycosis to the lungs and intrathoracic lymph nodes during which the disease is usually self-limited, and flu-like. Only a small fraction of symptomatic immunocompetent patients exhibits imaging evidence of pneumonia (about 5%). When they do, the findings are most often segmental or lobar airspace opacities, sometimes associated with hilar adenopathy and/or pleural effusion. Any residue of these infections are usually one or more soft tissue nodules or cavities that gradually resolve, or evolve into thin-walled cysts in a matter of several months (71).

In the immunocompromised patient with defective T-cell immunity, a dormant focus of coccidioidomycosis may activate, or in an endemic region a new primary pulmonary infection may become progressive and/or promptly disseminate to involve the skin, bones, joints, kidneys, and meninges. Dissemination carries a high risk of mortality (about 70%). CNS involvement is usually fatal.

Blood-borne pulmonary dissemination results in diffuse micro nodular (miliary) abnormality (72) or diffuse reticulonodular opacities, sometimes with hilar lymphadenopathy and pleural effusions (73). In about one-fourth of patients with disseminated disease, localized lung disease will be found. CT and radiographic images often demonstrate diffuse miliary or reticulonodular opacities in patients with hematogenous dissemination to the lungs (74). Hilar and mediastinal adenopathy are frequent findings in disseminated coccidioidomycosis. Pericardial involvement may lead to pericardial effusion, cardiac tamponade, or constrictive pericarditis.

See the following sections for discussions on differential diagnosis: nodules and consolidations in Sec.IV.A.2., diffuse lung opacification in Sec.IV.B.1, diffuse miliary nodules in.

b. Extra-pulmonary Coccidioidomycosis. In a CT and/or an MRI, dissemination to the brain may show meningitis, i.e., marked thickening of basal meninges and intense contrast enhancement. Other CNS findings include communicating hydrocephalus in the cervical subarachnoid space and cisterns (basilar, sylvian, and inter-hemispheric) (46,75). Focal parenchymal MRI abnormalities may suggest ischemia or infarction, brain abscess, or granulomas (76). Extra-pulmonary dissemination can also produce bone abscesses, synovitis, abscesses, or granulomas in the liver and other infra-abdominal organs in CT or MRI.

3. Blastomycosis

a. Pulmonary Blastomycosis. *Blastomyces dermatitidis,* is a soil fungus coendemic with *H. capsulatum* in south-central and mid-western United States. It is an uncommon cause of invasive mycoses in severely immunocompromised HIV patients. The two main portals of entry are the lung and the skin. Etiologic diagnoses depend solely on culture or direct visualization of the fungus in clinical specimens because there are no reliable serological tests. Cell-mediated immunity appears to be less important for protection against blastomycosis than it is for protection against other endemic mycoses.

In immunocompetent patients with acute blastomycosis, imaging findings usually consist of airspace opacification most of which also have air bronchograms (86%) (77). Mass lesions usually indicate chronic disease (78). CT studies demonstrate airspace disease, and mass-like opacities in more than half of patients (78,79). Other presentations, such as nodules, cavities, and interstitial lung findings are uncommon (~10%). Miliary lesions and diffuse alveolar damage are rare in the immunocompetent patient (less than 10% of patients) (78).

In the immunosuppressed patient, imaging findings consist of consolidations and mass lesions that are often extensive and progressive (80), and may be complicated by the superimposition of disseminated miliary lung lesions or an ARDS-like pattern (about a quarter of patients (81) (Fig. 7). Cavitation and pleural abnormalities occur in a minority of patients.

Microbial confirmation and/or histopathology is required to document an etiologic diagnosis. See the discussions on differential diagnosis: nodules and consolidations in the sections on Pulmonary Aspergillosis, diffuse lung opacification in Pulmonary Candidiasis, diffuse miliary nodules in Pulmonary Cryptococcosis.

b. Extra-pulmonary Blastomycosis. Dissemination to liver, spleen, bone marrow, pancreas, brain, meninges, and endocrine glands are commonly seen in AIDS patients. CNS involvement typically demonstrates evidence of meningitis or cerebral abscess. The highest rate of CNS dissemination and the most severe disease are found in patients with advanced HIV disease.

E. Other Rare Invasive Mycoses

Scedosporium apiospermum is an asexual anamorph of the fungus *Pseudallescheria boydii,* an emerging cause of disseminated infection in immunocompromised patients

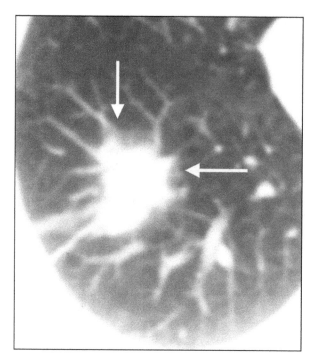

Figure 7 Pulmonary Blastomycosis.

that may rarely simulate the imaging findings of invasive aspergillosis, but is resistant to amphotericin B (82).

Sporotrichosis is a dimorphic soil fungus that usually gains access to the body through the skin, a rare cause of a chronic re-infection tuberculosis-like pattern with apical cavities in immunocompetent patients after heavy soil exposure (83). In the immunocompromised patient with a deficiency of cell-mediated immunity, the fungus rarely causes disseminated lesions in the lungs, brain, and bones similar to those found in disseminated endemic fungal infections (84).

Rare angio-invasive fungi include three normally saprophytic fungi, i.e., *Trichosporon* sp., (29) *Penicillium* sp., (30), and *Fusarium* sp., (31). These fungi rarely cause angio-invasive infection with imaging features similar to invasive aspergillosis and mucormycosis. They may also cause disseminated disease.

V. SUMMARY

This chapter provides an overview of the role of imaging in the management of invasive fungal infection in the immunocompromised patient.

It stresses the importance of cross-sectional imaging in the detection and differential diagnosis of infection, and the importance of prior probability in interpreting imaging findings.

It identifies a few coherent prototypical patterns out of a wide variety of imaging findings in the patient with a compatible illness. Four such clinical–etiological imaging constellations include:

1. One or more pulmonary nodules with halo signs or air crescent signs due to lung infection by a ubiquitous angio-invasive opportunistic fungus typified by *Aspergillus* in an HSCT recipient or in a patient with a hematologic condition with neutropenia.
2. Multiple chronic 5–15 mm nodules in the liver and/or spleen due to a hematogenously disseminated infection by a ubiquitous opportunistic fungus typified by *Candida* in an HSCT recipient or in a patient with a hematologic condition recovering from neutropenia.
3. One or more enhancing cerebral gyri, cerebral nodules, and/or diffuse miliary or focal lung opacities due to a disseminated ubiquitous fungus typified by *Cryptococcus* in a patient with severe T-cell immunodeficiency.
4. Diffuse miliary lung nodules and/or intra-abdominal abnormalities due to a hematogenously disseminated geographically endemic fungus in the United States typified by *Histoplasma capsulatum, Coccidioides immitis,* and *Blastomyces dermatitidis* in a patient with marked T-cell immunodeficiency.

REFERENCES

1. Rubin RH, Greene R. Etiology and management of the compromised patient with fever and pulmonary infiltrates. In: Rubin RH, Young LS, eds. Clinical Approach to Infection in the Compromised Host. 4 ed. NY: Plenum, 2002:111–163.
2. Wilson WR, Cockerill FR III, Rosenow EC III. Pulmonary disease in the immunocompromised host (2). Mayo Clin Proc 1985; 60:610–631.
3. Williams DM, Krick JA, Remington JS. Pulmonary infection in the compromised host. Part II. AM Rev Respir Dis 1976; 114:593–627.
4. Ramirez-Ortiz R, Rodriguez J, Soto Z, Rivas M, Rodriguez-Cintron W. Synchronous pulmonary cryptococcosis and histoplasmosis. South Med J 1997; 90:729–732.
5. Warner GC, Cox GJ. Evaluation of chest radiography versus chest computed tomography in screening for pulmonary malignancy in advanced head and neck cancer. J Otolaryngol 2003; 32:107–109.
6. Henschke CI, McCauley DI, Yankelevitz DF, et al. Early lung cancer action project: overall design and findings from baseline screening. Lancet 1999; 354:99–105.
7. Grenier P, Valeyre D, Cluzel P, et al. Chronic diffuse interstitial lung disease: diagnostic value of chest radiography and high-resolution CT. Radiology 1991; 179:123–132.
8. Hwang SS, Kim HH, Park SH, Jung JI, Jang HS. The value of CT-guided percutaneous needle aspiration in immunocompromised patients with suspected pulmonary infection. AJR Am J Roentgenol 2000; 175:235–238.
9. Ascioglu S, Rex JH, de Pauw B, et al. Defining opportunistic invasive fungal infections in immunocompromised patients with cancer and hematopoietic stem cell transplants: an international consensus. Clin Infect Dis 2002; 34:7–14.
10. Greene RE, Oestmann JW, Schlamm HT, et al. Early imaging findings in acute invasive pulmonary aspergillosis: utility of the halo sign for early diagnosis and treatment in severely immunocompromised patients. Under review. Submitted.
11. Filmont JE, Czernin J, Yap C, et al. Value of F-18 fluorodeoxyglucose positron emission tomography for predicting the clinical outcome of patients with aggressive lymphoma prior to and after autologous stem-cell transplantation. Chest 2003; 124:608–613.
12. Stumpe KD, Dazzi H, Schaffner A, von Schulthess GK. Infection imaging using whole-body FDG-PET. Eur J Nucl Med 2000; 27:822–832.
13. Patterson JE, Zidouh A, Miniter P, Andriole VT, Patterson TF. Hospital epidemiologic surveillance for invasive aspergillosis: patient demographics and the utility of antigen detection. Infect Control Hosp Epidemiol 1997; 18:104–108.

14. Herbrecht R, Denning DW, Patterson TF, et al. Voriconazole versus amphotericin B for primary therapy of invasive aspergillosis. N Engl J Med 2002; 347:408–415.

15. Hruban RH, Meziane MA, Zerhouni EA, et al. Radiologic-pathologic correlation of the CT halo sign in invasive pulmonary aspergillosis. J Comput Assist Tomogr 1987; 11: 534–536.

16. Orr DP, Myerowitz RL, Dubois PJ. Patho-radiologic correlation of invasive pulmonary aspergillosis in the compromised host. Cancer 1978; 41:2028–2039.

17. Kuhlman JE, Fishman EK, Siegelman SS. Invasive pulmonary aspergillosis in acute leukemia: characteristic findings on CT, the CT halo sign, and the role of CT in early diagnosis. Radiology 1985; 157:611–614.

18. Logan PM, Primack SL, Miller RR, Muller NL. Invasive aspergillosis of the airways: radiographic, CT, and pathologic findings. Radiology 1994; 193:383–388.

19. Funada H, Misawa T, Nakao S, Saga T, Hattori KI. The air crescent sign of invasive pulmonary mucormycosis in acute leukemia. Cancer 1984; 53:2721–2723.

20. Vogl TJ, Hinrichs T, Jacobi V, Bohme A, Hoelzer D. Computed tomographic appearance of pulmonary mucormycosis. Rofo Fortschr Geb Rontgenstr Neuen Bildgeb Verfahr 2000; 172:604–608.

21. Jamadar DA, Kazerooni EA, Daly BD, White CS, Gross BH. Pulmonary zygomycosis: CT appearance. J Comput Assist Tomogr 1995; 19:733–738.

22. Wheat LJ. Fungal infections in the immunocompromised host. In: Rubin RH, Young LS, eds. Clinical Approach to Infection in the Compromised Host.: Plenum, 1981:211–237.

23. Worsley DF, Alavi A, Aronchick JM, et al. Chest radiographic findings in patients with acute pulmonary embolism: observations from the PIOPED Study. Radiology 1993; 189:133–136.

24. Primack SL, Hartman TE, Lee KS, Muller NL. Pulmonary nodules and the CT halo sign. Radiology 1994; 190:513–515.

25. Caillot D, Casasnovas O, Bernard A, et al. Improved management of invasive pulmonary aspergillosis in neutropenic patients using early thoracic computed tomographic scan and surgery. J Clin Oncol 1997; 15:139–147.

26. Denning DW. Invasive aspergillosis. Clin Infect Dis 1998; 26:781–803.

27. Herold CJ, Kramer J, Sertl K, et al. Invasive pulmonary aspergillosis—Evaluation with MR Imaging. Radiology 1989; 173:717–721.

28. Blum U, Windfuhr M, Buitrago-Tellez C, et al. Invasive pulmonary aspergillosis. MRI, CT, and plain radiographic findings and their contribution for early diagnosis. Chest 1994; 106:1156–1161.

29. Saul SH, Khachatoorian T, Poorsattar A, et al. Opportunistic Trichosporon pneumonia. Association with invasive aspergillosis. Arch Pathol Lab Med 1981; 105:456–459.

30. Huang SN, Harris LS. Acute disseminated penicilliosis: report of a case and review of pertinent literature. Am J Clin Pathol 1963; 39:167–174.

31. Young NA, Kwon-Chung KJ, Kubota TT, Jennings AE, Fisher RI. Disseminated infection by *Fusarium moniliforme* during treatment for malignant lymphoma. J Clin Microbiol 1978; 7:589–594.

32. Armstrong D, Young LS, Meyer RD, Blevins AH. Infectious complications of neoplastic disease. Med Clin North Am 1971; 55:729–745.

33. Kim Y, Lee KS, Jung KJ, et al. Halo sign on high resolution CT: findings in spectrum of pulmonary diseases with pathologic correlation. J Comput Assist Tomogr 1999; 23:622–626.

34. Gaeta M, Blandino A, Scribano E, et al. Computed tomography halo sign in pulmonary nodules: frequency and diagnostic value. J Thorac Imaging 1999; 14:109–113.

35. Curtis AM, Smith GJ, Ravin CE. Air crescent sign of invasive aspergillosis. Radiology 1979; 133:17–21.

36. Caillot D, Couaillier JF, Bernard A, et al. Increasing volume and changing characteristics of invasive pulmonary aspergillosis on sequential thoracic computed tomography scans in patients with neutropenia. J Clin Oncol 2001; 19:253–259.

37. Gefter WB, Albelda SM, Talbot GH, et al. Invasive pulmonary aspergillosis and acute leukemia. Limitations in the diagnostic utility of the air crescent sign. Radiology 1985; 157:605–610.

38. Aquino SL, Kee ST, Warnock ML, Gamsu G. Pulmonary aspergillosis: imaging findings with pathologic correlation. AJR Am J Roentgenol 1994; 163:811–815.

39. Godwin JD, Webb WR, Savoca CJ, Gamsu G, Goodman PC. Multiple, thin-walled cystic lesions of the lung. AJR Am J Roentgenol 1980; 135:593–604.

40. Ryu JH, Swensen SJ. Cystic and cavitary lung diseases: focal and diffuse. Mayo Clin Proc 2003; 78:744–752.

41. Tuncel E. Pulmonary air meniscus sign. Respiration 1984; 46:139–144.

42. Austin JH, Muller NL, Friedman PJ, Hansell DM, Naidich DP, Remy-Jardin M, et al. Glossary of terms for CT of the lungs: recommendations of the Nomenclature Committee of the Fleischner Society. Radiology. 1996; 200:327–331.

43. Won HJ, Lee KS, Cheon JE, et al. Invasive pulmonary aspergillosis: prediction at thin-section CT in patients with neutropenia—a prospective study. Radiology 1998; 208:777–782.

44. Oh YW, Effmann EL, Godwin JD. Pulmonary infections in irnrnunocompromised hosts: the importance of correlating the conventional radiologic appearance with the clinical setting. Radiology 2000; 217:647–656.

45. Kramer MR, Denning DW, Marshall SE, et al. Ulcerative tracheobronchitis after lung transplantation. A new form of invasive aspergillosis. Am Rev Respir Dis 1991; 144:552–556.

46. Bowen BC, Post MJD. Intracranial infection. In: Atlas SW, ed. Magnetic Resonance Imaging of the Brain and Spine. New York: Raven Press, 1991:501–538.

47. Cox J, Murtagh FR, Wilfong A, Brenner J. Cerebral aspergillosis: MR imaging and histopathologic correlation. AJNR Am J Neuroradiol 1992; 13:1489–1492.

48. Osborn AG. Diagnostic Neuroradiology. St. Louis: Mosby, 1994:706–709.

49. Masur H, Rosen PP, Armstrong D. Pulmonary disease caused by *Candida* species. Am J Med 1977; 63:914–925.

50. Dubois PJ, Myerowitz RL, Allen CM. Pathoradiologic correlation of pulmonary candidiasis in immunosuppressed patients. Cancer 1977; 40:1026–1036.

51. Buff SJ, McLelland R, Gallis HA, Matthay R, Putman CE. *Candida albicans* pneumonia: radiographic appearance. AJR Am J Roentgenol 1982; 138:645–648.

52. Cairns MRI, Durack DT. Fungal pneumonia in the immunocompromised host. Semin Respir Infect 1986; 1:166–185.

53. Haron E, Feld R, Tuffnell P, et al. Hepatic candidiasis: an increasing problem in immunocompromised patients. Am J Med 1987; 83:17–26.

54. Haron E, Vartivarian S, Anaissie E, Dekmezian R, Bodey GP. Primary *Candida* pneumonia. Experience at a large cancer center and review of the literature. Medicine (Baltimore) 1993; 72:137–142.

55. Pastakia B, Shawker TH, Thaler M, O'Leary T, Pizzo PA. Hepatosplenic candidiasis: wheels within wheels. Radiology 1988; 166:417–421.

56. Thaler M, Pastakia B, Shawker TH, O'Leary T, Pizzo PA. Hepatic candidiasis in cancer patients: the evolving picture of the syndrome. Ann Intern Med 1988; 108:88–100.

57. Shirkhoda A. CT findings in hepatosplenic and renal candidiasis. J Comput Assist Tomogr 1987; 11:795–798.

58. Mudad R, Vredenburgh J, Paulson EK, et al. A radiologic syndrome after high dose chemotherapy and autologous bone marrow transplantation, with clinical and pathologic features of systemic candidiasis. Cancer 1994; 74:1360–1366.

59. Shirkhoda A, Lopez-Berestein G, Holbert JM, Luna MA. Hepatosplenic fungal infection: CT and pathologic evaluation after treatment with liposomal amphotericin B. Radiology 1986; 159:349–353.

60. McGuinness G. Changing trends in the pulmonary manifestations of AIDS. Radiol Clin North Am 1997; 35:1029–1082.

61. Woodring JH, Ciporkin G, Lee C, Worm B, Woolley S. Pulmonary cryptococcosis. Semin Roentgenol 1996; 31:67–75.
62. Cornell SH, Jacoby CG. The varied computed tomographic appearance of intracranial cryptococcosis. Radiology 1982; 143:703–707.
63. Whelan MA, Kricheff II, Handler M, et al. Acquired immunodeficiency syndrome: cerebral computed tomographic manifestations. Radiology 1983; 149:477–484.
64. Zinck SE, Leung AN, Frost M, Berry GJ, Muller NL. Pulmonary cryptococcosis: CT and pathologic findings. J Comput Assist Tomogr 2002; 26:330–334.
65. Connolly JE Jr, McAdams HP, Erasmus JJ, Rosado-de-Christenson ML. Opportunistic fungal pneumonia. J Thorac Imaging 1999; 14:51–62.
66. Conces DJ Jr. Endemic fungal pneumonia in immunocompromised patients. J Thorac Imaging 1999; 14:1–8.
67. Greene R. Opportunistic pneumonias. Semin Roentgenol 1980; 15:50–72.
68. Wheat J. Histoplasmosis Experience during outbreaks in Indianapolis and review of the literature. Medicine (Baltimore) 1997; 76:339–354.
69. Vathesatogkit P, Goldenberg R, Parsey M. A 27-year-old HIV-infected woman with severe sepsis and pulmonary infiltrates Disseminated histoplasmosis with severe sepsis and acute respiratory failure. Chest 2003; 123:272–276.
70. Conces DJ Jr, Stockberger SM, Tarver RD, Wheat LJ. Disseminated histoplasmosis in AIDS: findings on chest radiographs. AJR Am J Roentgenol 1993; 160:15–19.
71. Dublin AB, Phillips HE. Computed tomography of disseminated coccidiodomycosis. Radiology 1980; 135:361–368.
72. Goldstein E. Miliary and disseminated coccidioidomycosis. Ann Intern Med 1978; 89:365–366.
73. Batra P, Batra RS. Thoracic coccidioidomycosis. Semin Roentgenol 1996; 31:28–44.
74. Ampel NM, Dols CL, Galgiani JN. Coccidioidomycosis during human immunodeficiency virus infection: results of a prospective study in a coccidioidal endemic area. Am J Med 1993; 94:235–240.
75. Wrobel CJ, Meyer S, Johnson RH, Hesselink JR. MR findings in acute and chronic coccidioidomycosis meningitis. AJNR Am J Neuroradiol 1992; 13:1241–1245.
76. Erly WK, Bellon RJ, Seeger JF, Carmody RF. MR imaging of acute coccidioidal meningitis. AJNR Am J Neuroradiol 1999; 20:509–514.
77. Winer-Muram HT, Beals DH, Cole FH Jr. Blastomycosis of the lung: CT features. Radiology 1992; 182:829–832.
78. Brown LR, Swensen SJ, Van Scoy RE, et al. Roentgenologic features of pulmonary blastomycosis. Mayo Clin Proc 1991;66:29–38.
79. Halvorsen RA, Duncan JD, Merten DF, Gallis HA, Putman CE. Pulmonary blastomycosis: radiologic manifestations. Radiology 1984; 150:1–5.
80. Pappas PG, Pottage JC, Powderly WG, et al. Blastomycosis in patients with the acquired immunodeficiency syndrome. Ann Intern Med 1992; 116:847–853.
81. Evans ME, Haynes JB, Atkinson JB, Delvaux TC Jr, Kaiser AB. *Blastomyces dermatitidis* and the adult respiratory distress syndrome. Case reports and review of the literature. Am Rev Respir Dis 1982; 126:1099–1102.
82. Raj R, Frost AE. *Scedosporium apiospermum* fungemia in a lung transplant recipient. Chest 2002; 121:1714–1716.
83. Shaffer K, Smith D. Sporotrichosis. FIRE (File of Images for Radiology Education), Harvard Medical Center 2001.
84. Ware AJ, Cockerell CJ, Skiest DJ, Kussman HM. Disseminated sporotrichosis with extensive cutaneous involvement in a patient with AIDS. J Am Acad Dermatol 1999; 40:350–355.

16
Polyenes

John Hiemenz

Sections of Hematology, Oncology and Infectious Diseases, Medical College of Georgia, Augusta, Georgia, U.S.A.

Thomas J. Walsh

National Institutes of Health, National Cancer Institute/Pediatric Oncology Branch, Bethesda, Maryland, U.S.A.

I. INTRODUCTION

The polyenes are a family of several hundred naturally derived macrolide antibiotics. Those most well studied to date possess an internal cyclic ester, with 4–7 conjugated double bonds. They exhibit a broad spectrum of antifungal activity and have a common mechanism of action (1). The polyenes bind to sterols in all eukaryotic cells, but some have greater affinity for ergosterol found in fungal cell membranes, as opposed to cholesterol found in mammalian cell membranes. This difference in affinity between fungal and mammalian sterols has allowed for human use, a select few of the polyenes that have been studied. Amphotericin B, nystatin, and pimaricin are the most commonly used polyenes in clinical practice. This chapter will focus exclusively on amphotericin B and its lipid formulations.

Amphotericin B is a lipophilic, rod-like macrolide, first isolated by Gold and colleagues (2) from an aerobic actinomycete (*Streptomyces nodosus*), found in the Orinico Valley of Venezuela in 1955. Because of its broad spectrum of antifungal activity, the increasing importance of invasive mycosis in clinical medicine, and the lack of effective alternative therapy, amphotericin B soon became the treatment of choice for invasive fungal infections, particularly in the immunocompromised host (3,4). Like other polyenes studied, amphotericin B binds to sterols, primarily ergosterol, in the fungal cell membrane. The binding of amphotericin B to the sterols of susceptible fungi allows for the development of pores, which increase cytoplasmic membrane permeability leading to loss of intracellular potassium and other small intracellular molecules and eventual fungal cell death (Fig. 1). Antifungal activity does not require metabolism of amphotericin B and is rapid in onset. Oxidative damage to fungal cells caused by amphotericin B has also been suggested as an additional mechanism of antifungal action (1,5).

Amphotericin B has a broad range of activity against most pathogenic fungi in vitro. Standards for susceptibility testing of amphotericin B against isolates of yeasts and molds have been developed by the national committee for clinical laboratory

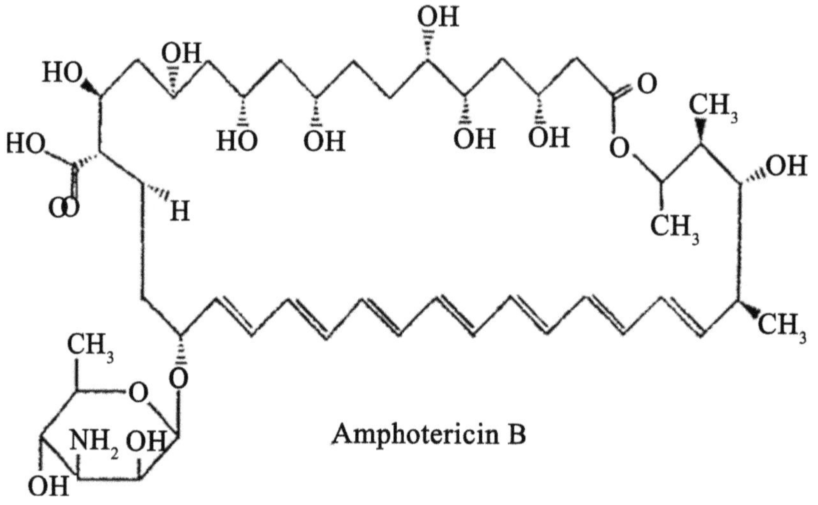

Figure 1 Molecular structure of amphotericin B.

standards (6,7) (NCCLS). Although susceptibility testing does not always clearly separate sensitive from resistant organisms, a number of investigators have reported a relative correlation between outcome and results they obtained from in vitro testing of amphotericin B, against clinical isolates utilizing modifications of the NCCLS methodology (8,9). Emergence of previously less common fungi as causes of life-threatening invasive infections (10,15), however, make it important to mention fungi, which have poor susceptibility to amphotericin B. These include the moulds *Pseudallescheria boydii* (*Scedosporium apiospermum*) (12), *Aspergillus terreus* (13), *Fusarium* spp. (14), and the yeasts *Trichosporon* spp. (15,16), and *Blastoshizomyces capitatus* (17).

II. AMPHOTERICIN B DEOXYCHOLATE

Amphotericin B is a lipophilic molecule that is poorly absorbed from the gastrointestinal tract and is insoluble in water at physiologic pH. In order to allow for intravenous use, amphotericin B is dispersed as a colloid formation in sodium deoxycholate with sodium phosphate buffer. Amphotericin B will aggregate in electrolyte solutions and must be reconstituted in 5% dextrose solutions. The use of inline filters with pore size of 0.22 μm or less may remove significant amounts of drug from solution and is not recommended (18). All of the lipid formulations of amphotericin B also require reconstitution in 5% dextrose water and inline filters are not recommended.

Amphotericin B deoxycholate is usually infused over 2–4 hr with doses of 0.5–1.0 mg/kg/day. A maximum of approximately 1.5 mg/kg/day of conventional amphotericin B deoxycholate has been utilized for more serious infections; however, toxicity at this dosage usually limits length of therapy. The drug is best administered through a central venous catheter due to associated phlebitis. Although the pharmacokinetics of amphotericin B are not well understood, concentrations of the drug in biological fluids have been measured by a variety of methods including high pressure liquid chromatography (19), immunoassay (20), and bioassay (21). Amphotericin B separates from deoxycholate in serum with greater than 95% binding to serum proteins. The drug rapidly leaves the circulation, distributing throughout tissues presumably by combining with cholesterol containing membranes. Amphotericin B then re-enters the circulation slowly with only a small percentage being excreted in the urine or bile acid (22). Blood levels of amphotericin B are not affected by hepatic or renal dysfunction and the drug is not cleared by hemodialysis. The drug concentrates in the reticulo-endothelial system with higher concentrations in the liver and spleen. Amphotericin B penetrates poorly into brain, meninges, pancreas, muscle, and bone. Peak blood levels of amphotericin B after infusion of standard doses amphotericin B deoxycholate are approximately 0.5–2.0 µg/mL. The initial half-life is 24 hr with a β phase of approximately 15 days. Amphotericin B can be detected in blood even 7 weeks after end of treatment, suggesting continued release from tissues (21).

Unfortunately, a number of acute and chronic toxicities have made treatment with amphotericin B deoxycholate difficult for patients to tolerate. Infusion-related reactions occurred such as fever, rigors, and chills occur in as approximately 50% of patients (23,24), but were usually treated symptomatically without discontinuation of the drug in the setting of life-threatening infection. When severe, however, rigors can be accompanied by bronchospasm with wheezing and hypoxia. These less common infusion-related reactions to amphotericin B deoxycholate, which also include hypertension, hypotension, and hypoxemia, may adversely affect antifungal drug therapy. Although infusion-related toxicities frequently diminish after several days, a variety of medications including acetaminophen, nonsteroidal anti-inflammatory drugs (NSAIDs), diphenhydramine, and hydrocortisone have been utilized as premedications in an attempt to ameliorate the discomfort of therapy with amphotericin B deoxycholate (25). Merperidine at doses of 25–50 mg has been utilized successfully to blunt serious rigors, but may lead to seizures after accumulation of the neurotoxic metabolite normeperidine in patients with serum creatinine >2 mg/dL. Few controlled studies have been done to show benefit of premedication and the use of these drugs is not without risk. Use of NSAIDs in the thrombocytopenic patient is not recommended, and long-term use of steroids may worsen the immune suppression that lead to development of invasive mycosis in the compromised host initially.

Reduction in dosage or discontinuation of therapy with amphotericin B deoxycholate is more commonly because of the adverse effects of this polyene on renal function. Amphotericin B deoxycholate treatment causes constriction of the afferent renal arterioles leading to reduced blood flow to glomeruli and renal tubules (26). Continued use of amphotericin B deoxycholate frequently leads to azotemia, renal tubular acidosis, and impaired urinary concentrating ability with subsequent electrolyte imbalance. Factors that have been identified for increased risk of nephrotoxicity with amphotericin B deoxycholate treatment include underlying chronic renal disease, concurrent use of other nephrotoxic agents (e.g., aminoglycosides and cyclosporine), duration of therapy, and a mean daily dose of ≥35 mg/day (27,28). Amphotericin B deoxycholate-related nephrotoxicity has been shown to increase the duration of hospital stay and cost (27,29,30). Moreover, although nephrotoxicity associated with amphotericin B, deoxycholate has long been considered reversible after drug discontinuation; treatment leading to the need for hemodialysis has been shown to increase the risk of death (27,28).

A number of strategies have been utilized in an attempt to reduce the risk of nephrotoxicity related to treatment with amphotericin B deoxycholate. These include reduced dosage, alternate day therapy, the use of mannitol, saline loading, low-dose dopamine, and prolonging the infusion time (31–35). The use of low-dose dopamine has been common in many centers; however, a study by Camp et al shows no benefit in a group of high risk leukemia and BMT patients. In addition, there were signifi-

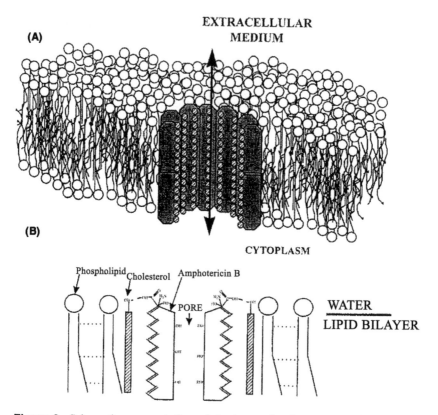

Figure 2 Schematic representation of the interaction between amphotericin B and cholesterol in a phospholipid bilayer. **(A)** The conducting pore is formed by the end-to-end union
of two wells or half pores, and **(B)** Molecular orientation in an amphotericin B-cholesterol
pore. The dotted lines between the hydrocarbon chains of phospholipids represent short-range
London-van der Waals forces. The dashed lines represent hydrogen bonds formed between
amphotericin B and cholesterol molecules.

cantly more adverse events including cardiac arrhythmias in the dopamine treated
patients (33). Reducing the dose of drug or giving the same dose on alternate days
risks reduced efficacy, Mannitol has not been found to be particularly effective
(31), but saline loading has been found to be beneficial (32). Eriksson et al. (34)
found that they could reduce the risk of nephrotoxicity associated with amphotericin
B deoxycholate by prolonging the infusion time to 24 hr. This reduced risk extended
to slightly higher daily doses of the amphotericin B deoxycholate up to 2 mg/kg day
in a follow-up study by Imhof et al. (35). The daily doses given in the second study
did not equal the daily doses routinely achieved when amphotericin B is given as
lipid formulation. Moreover, because of its incompatibility with electrolyte containing solutions, dedicating one intravenous line to amphotericin B deoxycholate over
24 hr each day may become problematic in complicated patients requiring multiple
drug infusions (11).

Along with reduced glomerular filtration rate with resulting increase in serum
creatinine, electrolyte losses are an important result of amphotericin B deoxycholate-
related nephrotoxicity. Magnesium loss is a commonly overlooked occurrence and
needs to be considered when amphotericin B-related hypokalemia appears to be
refractory to replacement therapy.

Other toxicities that may occur with amphotericin B deoxycholate treatment include fatigue, anorexia, nausea, vomiting, and weight loss. Anemia due to hemolysis and/or renal insufficiency with suppression of erythropoiesis may also be seen. Leukoencephalopathy has been reported in patients receiving systemic chemotherapy, intrathecal chemotherapy, or whole brain radiation (36). Wright et al. (37) reported the development of severe pulmonary reactions leading to acute respiratory distress syndrome when granulocyte transfusions were given to a group of patients who simultaneously received treatment with amphotericin B deoxycholate. Other investigators have not been able to document the same pulmonary reaction when white cell transfusions and amphotericin B are given together, and therefore, the interaction between the two has been questioned (38–40). In the study by Wright et al. (37), all patients receiving white cell transfusions had concurrent Gram-negative sepsis. It has been speculated that if the relationship between white cell transfusions and the use of amphotericin B exists, the presence of Gram-negative endotoxin may be required as a cofactor, leading to excess trafficking of the infused white cells to the microvasculature in the lungs and subsequent respiratory distress. Regardless, when given together in the same patient, it has been suggested that the antifungal and white cells be given at least 4–12 hr apart.

Even in the setting of maximally tolerated doses of drug, treatment with amphotericin B deoxycholate frequently fails to control invasive fungal infections in the immunocompromised host. Mortality rates for invasive aspergillosis remain high for neutropenic patients with the majority of these severely immunocompromised patients dying of infection despite therapy (41–43).

III. LIPID FORMULATIONS OF AMPHOTERICIN B

Incorporation of the highly lipophilic drug amphotericin B into liposomes to improve its therapeutic index, was recognized almost two decades ago. New et al. (44) reported reduced amphotericin B-related toxicity associated with the use of liposomal-associated drug in an animal model of leshmaniasis. This was followed by reports from Graybill et al. (45) and Taylor et al. (46) that liposomal-associated amphotericin B could significantly reduce the toxicities associated with free drug, without compromising efficacy in animal models of cryptococcosis and histoplasmosis. Lopez-Berestein and Juliano developed a lipid formulation of this polyene by combining a mixture of the two phospholipids dimyristoyl phosphatidylcholine (DMPC) and dimyristoyl phosphatidylglycerol (DMPG) in a 7:3 molar ratio containing 5–10% mole ratio of amphotericin B and showed a significant improvement in therapeutic index, as compared to conventional drug in a neutropenic mouse model of disseminated candidiasis (47). They subsequently reported the preliminary compassionate use experience with this lipid formulation in patients treated at the MD Anderson Cancer Center (Houston, Texas). They suggested that life-threatening invasive fungal infections could be controlled even in patients who had failed to respond to treatment with conventional doses of amphotericin B deoxycholate. Moreover, the liposomal product they had created had significantly less nephrotoxicity than conventional amphotericin B even at higher doses (48,49). Similar findings were observed at the Institute Jules Bordet (Brussels, Belgium), in a group of cancer patients treated there with a small unilamellar liposomal formulation of amphotericin B (50). Although these initial products were not further developed, the use of lipid-based biotechnology by the pharmaceutical industry has led to the development

Table 1 Structure, Biochemical Composition, and Pharmacokinetics of Amphotericin B and Its Lipid Formulations

Compound	Brand name	Lipid configuration	Size (n.m)	Lipids	Mean C in g/mL (dose)	Mean Vdss in l/kg (dosage)*	Mean CL in mL/[min kg] (dosage)	Mean AUC in g h/mL (dosage)	Human plasm pharmacokins References
Amphotericin B	Fungizone	NA	NA	Deoxycholate	0.98 (0.25 mg/kg) 2.9 (0.68 mg/kg)	4 (1.0 mg/kg) 0.76 (0.68 mg/kg)	0.43 (1.0 mg/kg) 0.76 (0.68 mg/kg)	8.6 (0.25 mg/kg)	(48–50)
L-AMB	AmBisome	Small unilamellar vesicle (liposome)	80	Hydrogenated soy phosphatidylcholine, distearoyl-phosphatidylglycerol	7.3 (1.0 mg/kg) 17.2 (2.5 mg/kg) 57.6 (5.0 mg/kg) Increased	0.58 (1.0 mg/kg) 0.69 (2.5 mg/kg) 0.22 (5.0 mg/kg) Decreased	0.27 (1.0 mg/kg) 0.33 (2.5 mg/kg) 0.17 (5.0 mg/kg) Decreased	69 (1.0 mg/kg) 206 (2.5 mg/kg) 713 (5.0 mg/kg) Increased	(51–53) (51)
ABCD	Amphocil	Disklike	120–140	Cholesteryl sulfate	0.84 (0.5 mg/kg) Decreased	5.7 (0.5 mg/kg) 7.2 (1.0 mg/kg) 7.9 (1.5 mg/kg) Increased	0.42 (0.5 mg/kg) 0.36 (1.0 mg/kg) 0.47 (1.5 mg/kg) Similar	21 (0.5 mg/kg) 46 (1.0 mg/kg) 57 (1.5 mg/kg) Decreased	(49,52)
ABLC	ABELCET	Ribbonlike	1,600 – 11,000	Dimyristoyl phosphatidylcholine, dimyristoyl phosphatidylglycerol	0.27 (0.5 mg/kg) 1.1 (2.5 mg/kg) Decreased	3.9 (0.5 mg/kg) Not determined Similar	1.3 (0.5 mg/kg) 3.6 (2.5 mg/kg) Increased	2.8 (0.5 mg/kg) 8.9(2.5 mg/kg) Decreased	(52,53,55,56)

Note. "Decreased," "increased," and "similar" are in reference to values for amphotericin B.
ABCD = amphotericin B colloidal dispersion; ABLC amphotericin B lipid complex; AUC = area under the curve; C pharmacokinetics in children; Cmax = maximum drug concentration; Cl = clearance; L-AMB liposomal amphotericin B; NA = not applicable; VdSS = volume of distribution.
*Model dependent.

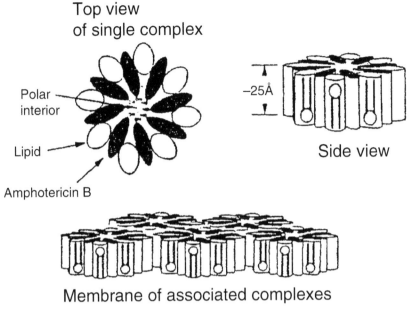

Top view
of single complex

Polar interior

Lipid

Amphotericin B

~25Å

Side view

Membrane of associated complexes

Figure 3 The putative structure of amphotericin B lipid complex (ABLC). Amphotericin B and lipid are arranged in a 1:1 interdigitated complex. *Source:* From Ref. 137.

of three commercially available lipid formulations of amphotericin B (amphotericin B lipid complex (ABLC), amphotericin B colloidal dispersion (ABCD), and liposomal amphotericin- [L-AMB]) that have been available for clinical use worldwide for the last several years (Table 1) (51–56). The lipid formulations of amphotericin B have the same antifungal spectrum as, but are significantly less nephrotoxic than, amphotericin B deoxycholate at doses up to 4–6 mg/kg day (24,57–63). With increased availability and experience in the use of the lipid formulations of amphotericin B, along with the newer broad spectrum azoles and the echinocandins, amphotericin B deoxycholate's role as the "gold standard" has recently come in to question (64).

A. Amphotericin B Lipid Complex

ABLC, manufactured by Enzon Pharmaceuticals, Bridgewater, New Jersey, is similar to the original formulation of Berestein and Juliano in that it contains amphotericin B complexed with the two phospholipids DMPC and DMPG in a 7:3 molar ratio. ABLC, however, is a ribbon-like structure measuring 1600–11,000 nm in diameter and is not made up of liposomes. Studying a mixture of phospholipids and amphotericin B similar to the Berestein/Juliano product, Janoff et al. (65) at The Liposome Company discovered that it contained a variety of liposomal and nonliposomal structures of lipid bilayers. It appeared that the nonliposomal structures in the formulation that they called "ribbons" were responsible for the reduction in toxicity. A varying concentration of amphotericin B was mixed with the combination of phospholipids DMPC and DMPG in a fixed molar concentration of 7:3 Freeze-etch electron microscopy of formulations made with 0,5,25, and 50 mol% of amphotericin B showed significant differences in the structures formed (Fig. 2) (66,67). Amphotericin B in a 5 mole%

concentration resulted in a product similar to the original Berestein/Juliano mixture with both liposomes and ribbon-like structures. With increased concentration of amphotericin B, liposomes disappeared, leaving tightly packed ribbon-like structures. At concentrations > 50 mol% amphotericin B, the formulation appeared as ribbon structures; however, the lipids and total amphotericin B were no longer closely complexed, with the appearance of free amphotericin. ABLC was the name given to the formulation of ribbon-like structures created by complexing DMPC and DMPG in a 7:3 molar ratio with a 1:1 molar concentration of amphotericin B.

Hemolytic activity at low concentrations (<3 mole% of amphotericin B) was similar to conventional amphotericin B. As the concentration of amphotericin B was increased and the ribbon structures formed, there was a marked reduction in toxicity. As the ribbon structures formed, the amount of free amphotericin in solution decreased, presumably accounting for the reduced toxicity.

ABLC has been compared to amphotericin B in a number of animal models including mice, rats, rabbits, and dog. Amphotericin B concentrations in the liver, spleen, and lungs of mice and rats appear to be much higher after a single dose of ABLC than after a single dose of amphotericin B deoxycholate. Amphotericin B levels in the kidney of mice after injection of 1 mg/kg of ABLC appeared similar to levels achieved with conventional amphotericin B. However, plasma levels of amphotericin were significantly lower after dosing with ABLC as compared to amphotericin B deoxycholate. Moreover, when increasing the dose of the lipid complex, the levels of drug in the liver, spleen, and lung tissue rise dramatically with little change in the level of amphotericin found in the kidney and with essentially no rise in plasma levels (68–70). The LD_{50} after a single i.v. dose for ABLC was found to be 40 mg/kg whereas for conventional amphotericin B it was 3 mg/kg. Multiple dose studies of ABLC continued to show reduced toxicity even at 10 times the standard dose of conventional amphotericin B in mice (69) and four times the standard dose in rabbits (71). The efficacy of ABLC was found to be comparable to conventional amphotericin B in a number of animal models of fungal infection. Moreover, in a number of cases, the lipid complex was found to be effective when conventional amphotericin B was found ineffective in controlling the fungal infection (68,69,72,73). As an example, in a model of experimental murine disseminated candidiasis, Mitsutake et al. (71) found that ABLC was as effective as conventional amphotericin B at doses of 0.5 and 1.0 mg/kg but more efficacious at 10 mg/kg. The ability to deliver much higher doses of amphotericin B in the form of lipid complex without reaching the maximum tolerated dose may account for the improved therapeutic index (68).

Bhamra et al. (74) reported results of pharmacokinetic studies comparing the behavior of ABLC relative to amphotericin B deoxycholate in plasma in vitro and in circulation in rats. Rat blood or plasma spiked with ABLC was assayed for amphotericin B released from the complex after centrifugation. At 0–15 min approximately 90% of amphotericin B remained complexed in the phospholipid formulation. The amphotericin B released from the complex was found to be associated with plasma lipoprotein and nonlipoprotein proteins. The area under the curve ($AUC_{0-24\,hr}$) for total amphotericin B in whole blood of rats given a single i.v. dose of 1 mg ABLC per kg of body weight was four-fold lower than that in rats given 1 mg of amphotericin B deoxycholate per kg. Complexed amphotericin B was rapidly removed from the circulation and was distributed to the tissues. Further study looked at rats treated intravenously with 10 mg/kg/day of ABLC compared to 0.5 mg/kg/day of amphotericin B deoxycholate for 15 days. Blood samples taken at 15 and 180 min after the last dose of drug, showed total levels of amphotericin B in rats administered ABLC to be 3–5 times greater than those given amphotericin B deoxycholate. The concentration of uncomplexed, protein bound amphotericin B in plasma of ABLC treated rats was only 1–2 times that of those treated with amphotericin B deoxycholate, despite a 20-fold difference in dose given. The rapid uptake of amphotericin B by tissues in the form of the lipid complex and the very low levels of circulating protein-bound amphotericin B in plasma was suggested to possibly account in part for the improved therapeutic index of this lipid formulation.

Pharmacokinetics of ABLC in humans resembles those in animals. Circulating blood levels of amphotericin B were much lower in male volunteers after single-dose infusion of ABLC than after conventional amphotericin B deoxycholate (55). The lipid complex is believed to be rapidly taken up by the reticulo-endothelial system and concentrated in the liver, spleen, lungs, and other tissues of the body. Tissue levels of amphotericin B were measured at autopsy of a heart transplant patient after 3 days of treatment with ABLC. Relatively high concentrations of amphotericin were detected in the spleen (290 g/g), liver (196 g/g), and lungs (222 g/g). Lower concentrations were detected in kidney (6.9 g/g), lymph nodes (7.6 g/g), brain (1.6 g/g), and heart (4.9 g/g) (75).

The safety, tolerance, and pharmacokinetics of ABLC were studied in a cohort of pediatric patients enrolled in a phase I/II trial (54). Six children received ABLC at 2.5 mg/kg/day for 6 weeks for a total dose of 105 mg/kg for the treatment of hepatosplenic candidiasis. Mean baseline serum creatinine of 0.85 ± 0.12 mg/dL was stable at the end of therapy at 0.85 ± 0.18 mg/dL and at 1-month follow-up at 0.72 ± 0.12 mg/dL. There was no increase in transaminases. Mean plasma concentrations over the dosing interval and $AUC_{0-24 \, hr}$ increased between doses 1 and 7 but were similar between doses 7 and 42, suggesting that a steady state was achieved by day 7 of therapy. After the final dose of ABLC therapy (42nd), mean $AUC_{0-24 \, hr}$ was 11.9 ± 2.6 g/mL/hr, mean plasma concentration over the dosing interval was 0.50 ± 0.11 g/mL, maximum concentration of drug was 1.69 ± 0.75 g/mL, and clearance was 3.64 ± 0.78 (mL/kg/min). Response of hepatic and splenic lesions was monitored by serial computed tomographic and magnetic resonance imaging scans. Five patients evaluated for response to ABLC showed complete or partial resolutions of physical findings and radiographic lesions of infection. During the treatment course, there was no evidence of progression of infection, breakthrough fungemia, or recurrence of hepatosplenic candidiasis post-therapy. Hepatic lesions continued to resolve even after completion of treatment with ABLC. This study suggests that ABLC administered in multiple doses was safe and effective in the treatment of children with hepatosplenic candidiasis.

ABLC has been given in substantially larger doses than conventional amphotericin B. When given over several months, these large doses of amphotericin B appear to be relatively less toxic than those of conventional amphotericin B. Six patients with invasive fungal infection were reported by Kline et al. (76) to have received large cumulative doses (23.3–73.6 g) of ABLC over 21–121 weeks. These patients were reported to tolerate the therapy well. Although the mean serum creatinine level for this group of patients rose from 1 mg/dL (range, 0.4–1.9 mg/dL) at the start of ABLC to 1.5 mg/dL (range, 1.0–2.0 mg/dL) at the end of therapy, none had dose-limiting toxicity necessitating discontinuation of treatment.

ABLC has been compared to conventional amphotericin B in a number of small phase II and III clincal trials of patients with coccidiodomycosis and cryptococcosis. In a study by Sharkey et al. (77), ABLC was studied in a sequential dose escalation for the treatment of cryptococcosis in HIV-infected patients. Fifty-five patients were randomly assigned to 6 weeks of therapy with ABLC (1.2–5.0 mg/kg/day, with ascending doses for three sequential cohorts) or conventional amphotericin B (0.7–1.2 mg/kg/day). Forty-six patients received 12 or more doses. Transfusion requirements, mean decreases in blood hemoglobin, and mean increases in serum creatinine were significantly greater in patients treated with conventional amphotericin B when compared to ABLC. The total number of adverse events, infusion-related events, and occurrences of hypomagnesemia and hypokalemia were similar in the two groups of patients. Among patients treated with ABLC at a dose of 5 mg/kg (daily for 2 weeks and then three times per week for 4 weeks), symptoms and signs of infection resolved in 18 patients (86%). This study suggests that ABLC is effective in the treatment of HIV-related cryptococcal meningitis and is associated with less hematologic and renal toxicity when compared to conventional amphotericin B.

ABLC was compared to amphotericin B deoxycholate in a randomized, controlled trial of the treatment of invasive candidasis (57). Two hundred and thirty-one patients from 27 centers were randomized (2:1) to receive ABLC 5 mg/kg/day vs. amphotericin B 0.6–1.0 mg/kg/day for hematogenous and invasive candidiasis. One hundred and fifty-three patients were assigned to treatment with ABLC and 78 to amphotericin B. Response rates (68% for ABLC vs. 68% for amphotericin) were not significantly different ($P > 0.5$). Nephrotoxicity; however, was less significant with ABLC. In patients treated with ABLC, serum creatinine doubled by the end of therapy in 28%, when compared to 47% of patients treated with conventional amphotericin B ($P = 0.007$).

There is extensive experience with the use of ABLC in emergency-use protocols for patients with invasive fungal infections, who were felt to be refractory or intolerant to treatment with amphotericin B desoxycholate. Walsh et al. (78) reviewed the safety and antifungal efficacy of ABLC in 556 cases of invasive fungal infection treated on single patient emergency use protocols for patients refractory or intolerant of conventional antifungal therapy. In order to be eligible to receive therapy with ABLC, patients had to have met one of the following criteria: (1) patients must have failed treatment with previous systemic antifungal therapy, including amphotericin B at a cumulative dose of at least 500 mg; (2) developed nephrotoxicity defined as a serum creatinine of 2.5 mg/dL in adult or 1.5 mg/dL in children while undergoing antifungal therapy with amphotericin B or other drugs; (3) had severe acute toxicity secondary to amphotericin B or (4) had pretreatment renal insufficiency defined as a serum creatinine of 2.5 mg/dL or creatinine clearance rate of <25 mL/min precluding treatment with amphotericin B. In this open-labeled study, serum creatinine levels decreased significantly from baseline ($P < 0.02$) during the course of ABLC treatment. Moreover, in the 162 patients who began therapy with a baseline serum creatinine 2.5 mg/dL, the mean serum creatinine value decreased significantly from the first to the sixth week of treatment ($P < 0.0003$). There was either complete or partial response to treatment with ABLC in 57% (167/291) of cases of mycologically confirmed invasive fungal infection, which were evaluable for therapeutic response. This included 55/130 (42%) cases of aspergillosis, 28/42 (67%) cases of disseminated candidiasis, 17/24 (71%) cases of zygomycosis, and 9/11 (82%) cases of fusariosis.

Wingard (79) reported the results of efficacy and toxicity from a subgroup of 95 bone marrow transplant recipients with presumed or documented invasive fungal infection treated with ABLC on this open-label emergency use clinical trial. Seventy one (75%) had undergone allogeneic bone marrow transplantation and 24 (25%)

had received an autologous transplant. The most common underlying diagnosis before transplant was leukemia (59 patients). Forty-one patients were neutropenic ($< 500/mm^3$) at baseline. Fifty-nine patients undergoing bone marrow transplantation were felt to be clinically evaluable for response. Thirty-one patients (53%) responded to treatment: 23 patients (39%) were designated as cured, and eight patients (14%) were designated as improved. All 95 patients were evaluable for nephrotoxicity. Overall, only two patients discontinued therapy due to renal toxicity. Moreover, for 30 patients who began ABLC treatment with a serum creatinine of > 221 mol/L, significant improvement in renal function was observed at weeks 1–3 ($P < 0.01$) and 6 ($P<0.001$). Trends in serum creatinine during ABLC therapy between autologous and allogeneic transplant recipients were similar.

In a preliminary report of the treatment of invasive aspergillosis (80), 151 patients treated with ABLC on the emergency-use protocols were compared to medical records of 122 control patients treated with conventional amphotericin B deoxycholate. Complete and partial responses were seen in 43% of patients treated with ABLC vs. 23% of patients treated with amphotericin B deoxycholate. Moreover, in patients with a baseline serum creatinine of 2.5 mg/dL at the beginning of treatment with ABLC, significant decreases in serum creatinine were observed at 2 and 5 weeks ($P < 0.004$) despite continued therapy at 5 mg/kg/day. Although historical control trials are difficult to interpret, these data suggest that ABLC is effective in the treatment of invasive aspergillosis, and less nephrotoxic than treatment with amphotericin B deoxycholate. These include infections due to *Fusarium* species and Zygomycetes (81), in which conventional amphotericin B rarely controls disease and the value of ABLC for individual patients was particularly apparent.

Sundar and Murray (82) reported the use of ABLC in 21 Indian patients with visceral leishmaniasis, who did not respond to or relapsed after 28–60 days of pentavalent antimony therapy. Five infusions (3 mg/kg each), given every second day over 9 days (total dose, 15 mg/kg), resulted in a curative response in all patients treated with this regimen. In four other patients who had not responded to antimony, an apparent cure was also induced by ABLC, given 3 mg/kg/day for 5 consecutive days (total dose, 15 mg/kg). Fever and chills developed routinely during the initial 2-hr infusions; however, these reactions were tolerated and diminished with successive infusions. Six months after treatment, all 25 patients were healthy, had parasite-free bone marrow aspirates, and were considered cured.

Based upon current data, ABLC is considered to be active against a variety of invasive mycoses in immunocompromised hosts even in the setting of prior failure of amphotericin B deoxycholate. ABLC is also less nephrotoxic than conventional therapy, which may account for its improved therapeutic index. This drug is currently approved for clinical use in the United States, as well as numerous countries worldwide, for patients with invasive fungal infections who are refractory or intolerant to treatment with amphotericin B deoxycholate. Additional clinical study of ABLC is in progress to further define its role in the treatment of life-threatening fungal infections.

B. Amphotericin B Colloidal Dispersion

Amphotericin B colloidal dispersion (InterMune, Brisbane, California) is a combination of amphotericin B and cholesteryl sulfate in a 1:1 ratio. This formulation of amphotericin B forms disk-like structures approximately 115 nm in diameter when combined with the cholesteryl sulfate (83). The discs are made up of aggregates of

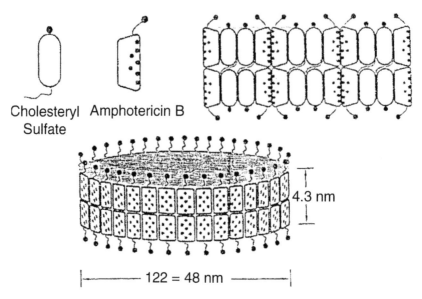

Cholesteryl Amphotericin B
Sulfate

Figure 4 The putative structure of amphotericin B colloidal dispersion (ABCD). *Source:*
From Ref. 137.

tetramers of amphotericin B and cholesteryl sulfate coalesced into spiral arms. Each
tretramer consists of two molecules of amphotericin B with two molecules of cholesteryl sulfate with a hydrophobic core and hydrophilic regions exposed to water
(Fig. 3). Hanson and Stevens (84) documented in vitro activity of ABCD against
41 isolates of 15 pathogenic species of fungus. Mean inhibitory concentrations and
mean fungicidal concentrations of ABCD appeared similar to those of conventional
amphotericin B.

Plasma levels of amphotericin B after a single intravenous bolus injection in the
rat are significantly less at 1 hr when ABCD is compared with amphotericin B deoxycholate. The half-life of the lipid formulation, however, is much longer, and its
volume of distribution is much greater. Tissue concentrations of amphotericin B
in the liver are 2–3 times higher after injection of ABCD vs. amphotericin B deoxycholate. At the same time, amphotericin B concentrations in the kidney are significantly reduced even after 5 mg/kg of the colloidal dispersion (85). Similar findings of
lower plasma concentrations, increased liver deposition, and decreased kidney concentration of amphotericin B have been reported in the dog model (86). Dosages of
as much as 5 mg/kg/day could be given to dogs before ABCD produced adverse
effects similar to those of 0.6 mg/kg/day of amphotericin B deoxycholate.

The efficacy of ABCD compared with amphotericin B deoxycholate has been
studied in animal models of coccidioidomycosis, cryptococcosis, and aspergillosis
(73,87,88). Despite lower doses of amphotericin B deoxycholate (1–3 mg/kg)
required to clear organs of fungus in a murine model of coccidiodomycosis compared with ABCD (5.0 mg/kg), conventional amphotericin B was found to be 5–8
times more toxic resulting in an improved therapeutic index for the lipid formulation
(73).

In a murine model of cryptococcosis, ABCD was found to have equal efficacy,
compared to amphotericin B on a milligram per kilogram basis. ABCD was also
found to be less toxic, again resulting in an improvement in therapeutic index for

the lipid formulation when compared to amphotericin B deoxycholate. ABCD treatment of persistently granulocytopenic rabbits in a model of pulmonary aspergillosis resulted in improved survival when comparing 5 mg/kg/day of ABCD and 1 mg/kg/day of amphotericin B deoxycholate (88). The improved therapeutic index may be because of an enhanced rate of tissue clearance, decreased pulmonary injury, and reduced nephrotoxicity in the rabbits treated with 5 mg/kg/day of ABCD. These findings were further confirmed in a study of the evolution of pulmonary infarcts in experimental pulmonary aspergillosis. Through ultrafast computed tomographic scanning and an image-analysis algorithm, a dose-dependent clearance of pulmonary infiltrates in rabbits treated with ABCD was found (89). In an immunocompromised rabbit model of experimental disseminated aspergillosis, Patterson et al. (90) again demonstrated a dose-dependent response of ABCD. Animal models of both disseminated and pulmonary invasive aspergillosis suggested that ABCD was less effective than amphotericin B deoxycholate in tissue clearance of fungus at equal doses of 1 mg/kg (88–90).

Bowden et al. (91) reported results of a phase I sequential dose-escalation study of ABCD in 75 bone marrow transplant recipients with invasive fungal infections (primarily *Aspergillus* or *Candida* species). This study was designed to evaluate the toxicity profile, maximum tolerated dose, and clinical response to ABCD. Dosages were escalated from 0.5–8.0 mg/kg/day in 0.5 mg/kg per patient increments with an upper limit of 6 weeks of treatment duration. No infusion-related toxicity was observed in 32% of the patients; 52% had grade 2 toxicity, and 5% had grade 3 toxicity. Significant renal toxicity was not observed at any dose level. Maximum tolerated dose was considered to be 7.5 mg/kg, based upon rigors, chills, and hypotension in three of five patients at 8.0 mg/kg. The overall complete or partial response rate across dose levels and infection types was 52%. 53% of patients with fungemia had complete responses, and 52% of patients with fungal pneumonia had complete or partial responses. ABCD was considered to be safe at doses up to 7.5 mg/kg, with tolerable infusion-related toxicity and documented antifungal activity in this patient population.

The safety of ABCD in five open-label phase I and II clinical trials was recently reviewed by Herbrecht (92). In a total of 572 selected patients treated ABCD for invasive fungal infections, ABCD was administered to 442 patients after therapy with amphotericin B. In 192 patients, conventional amphotericin B had been withdrawn because of toxicity. One hundred and forty patients had pre-existing nephrotoxicity. No alterations in serum creatinine were seen with dosages of ABCD as high as 6 mg/kg/day even in those patients with pre-existing renal failure. ABCD therapy also resulted in no significant changes in liver function from baseline as measured by serum levels of aspartate aminotransferase, alkaline phosphatase, and total bilirubin in comparison. Apart from thrombocytopenia, there was no significant alteration in hematologic parameters. Adverse events attributable to ABCD requiring discontinuation of therapy occurred in 70 patients (12.2%). The most toxicity resulting in discontinuation of ABCD in this group of patients was infusion-related adverse events, occurring in 5.4% of patients.

White et al. (93), retrospectively, compared the records of 82 patients with proven or probable aspergillosis who were treated in clinical trials with ABCD with 261 patients with aspergillosis who were treated with amphotericin B, at six cancer or transplantation centers, between January 1990 and June 1994. Although the groups were balanced in terms of underlying disease, ABCD recipients were younger and more likely to have pre-existing renal insufficiency than amphotericin B recipients

(40.7% vs. 8.7%) Amphotericin B recipients were more likely to be neutropenic at baseline than ABCD recipients (42.5% vs. 15.9%). Patients in the ABCD treated group had higher response rates (48.8%) and survival rates (50%) than those patients treated only with conventional amphotericin B deoxycholate (23.4% and 28.4%, respectively) ($P < 0.001$ for both comparisons). ABCD recipients were less likely to develop renal impairment when compared to amphotericin B deoxycholate recipients (8.2% vs. 43.1%, respectively; $P < 0.001$). ABCD was considered to be less nephrotoxic and similarly efficacious as amphotericin B deoxycholate in this study of the treatment of invasive aspergillosis. A prospective double-blind, randomized, and controlled multicenter trial comparing conventional amphotericin B and ABCD (at a dose of 6 mg/kg/day) in patients with invasive aspergillosis was recently reported by Bowden et al. (59). Although no significant difference in overall efficacy was noted, ABCD was significantly less nephrotoxic than amphotericin B deoxycholate. Another phase III trial compared ABCD and conventional amphotericin B for empiric treatment of the persistently febrile neutropenic patient (58). Although this study again showed that ABCD was less nephrotoxic, this lipid formulation had increased infusion related toxicity when compared to amphotericin B deoxycholate.

C. Liposomal Amphotericin B, L-AMB (AmBisome™)

L-AMB (Gilead Sciences, Inc., San Dimas, CA) is the third lipid formulation of amphotericin B to be approved by the Food and Drug Administration for clinical use in the United States. It has been used for the treatment of proven or suspected invasive fungal infections in numerous countries worldwide. This formulation of amphotericin B differs from ABLC and ABCD in that the lipids involved form small unilamellar lipid vesicles (true "liposomes") that are uniform and spherical in size, averaging 60–70 nm. The lipid bilayer is made up of hydrogenated soy phosphatidylcholine and distearoyl phosphatidylglycerol, stabilized by cholesterol, and combined with lipophilic amphotericin B in a 2:0.8:1:0.4 molar ratio (94) (Fig. 4). Antifungal activity of L-AMB in vitro was found to be comparable to that of amphotericin B when a number of clinical isolates from a large cancer center were tested (95).

A number of animal models have been used to study the pharmacokinetics, toxicity, and efficacy of L-AMB (96–104). Pharmacokinetic evaluation of liposomal amphotericin B in mice, rats, and rabbits revealed similar peak plasma levels. Similar to the other lipid formulations of amphotericin B, L-AMB is preferentially concentrated in the liver and spleen of animals. The rate of uptake by the reticulo-endothelial system; however, appears to be much slower than that of ABLC or ABCD. It is hypothesized that the larger lipid complexes and dispersions may be more readily phagocytosed by the macrophages of the reticulo-endothelial system when compared with the smaller unilamellar vesicles. The negative charge on the L-AMB particle also may delay uptake by the reticulo-endothelial system. These mechanisms may account for the much higher peak plasma levels and prolonged circulation time of the liposomal form of amphotericin B as opposed to its larger counterparts.

L-AMB has been found to be less nephrotoxic than conventional amphotericin B in mice, rats, and rabbits. There does however, appear to be a slight rise in liver transaminases with repeated infusions of liposomal amphotericin B at high dosages in rodents (101). The LD_{50} after a single injection of liposomal amphotericin B was >175 mg/kg in mice and 50 mg/kg in rats. This LD_{50} was 30–60 times greater than that of a single injection of conventional amphotericin B (96). Boswell et al. (101)

recently reported on the pharmacokinetics and toxicity profile of L-AMB in a rat model. Single and multiple dose pharmacokinetics were evaluated for doses of 1, 3, 9, and 20 mg/kg/day. Mean plasma amphotericin B concentrations reached 500 and 380 g/mL (males and females respectively) following 30 days of L-AMB at 20 mg/kg. The overall apparent half-life was 11.2 ± 4.5 hr (males) or 8.7 ± 2.2 hr (females). The overall clearance was 9.4 ± 5.5 mL/hr/kg (males) and 10.2 ± 4.1 mL/hr/kg (females). L-AMB appeared to have a saturable disposition. This resulted in a nondose proportional AUC for amphotericin B and a lower clearance at higher doses. Histopathological evaluation revealed transitional cell hyperplasia of the epithelium of the urinary tract that was dose dependent. Moderate hepatocellular necrosis was seen at the highest dose (20 mg/kg/day). However, the toxicities seen in this animal model were considered to be considerably less than that expected with amphotericin B at much lower doses.

Murine models of disseminated candidiasis, cryptococcosis, and blastomycosis have been used to study the efficacy of L-AMB. Gondal et al. (102) showed survival benefit in mice infected with *Candida albicans*, if treated early with all doses of liposomal amphotericin B studied except for 1 mg/kg. Delay in treatment until 3 days after inoculation, required 5 mg/kg of the drug to achieve optimal benefit. The maximum dose of conventional amphotericin B given to mice by single injection was 2 mg/kg, with 1.5 mg/kg /day the maximum tolerated dose with multiple injections. Although Phals and Schaffner (104) found L-AMB to be significantly less toxic in their mouse model of candidiasis, these investigators suggested that liposomal amphotericin B was 4–8 times less active in clearing the infection. L-AMB was given in divided daily doses in this study, and may have altered the pharmacodynamics of the compound.

A study by Francis et al. (103) reported the results of a comparison of amphotericin B deoxycholate with the small unilamellar liposomal form of amphotericin B in a neutropenic rabbit model of pulmonary aspergillosis. Rabbits were evaluated for survival, lung tissue infection, and hemorrhagic pulmonary lesions by the use of ultrafast CT scans. Treatment with the liposomal form of amphotericin was studied at 1, 5, and 10 mg/kg, compared with 1 mg/kg of amphotericin B deoxycholate. Although all doses of L-AMB showed survival benefit compared with amphotericin B, the rate of reduction of pulmonary injury was greatest above 5 mg/kg/day. Although the 10 mg/kg/day dosage was capable of irradicating tissue infection, it was found to be more nephrotoxic. Based on these findings, 5 mg/kg/day was proposed as the optimal dosage between safety and efficacy in this model of pulmonary aspergillosis.

The pharmacokinetics, safety, and tolerance of L-AMB were studied in 24 persistently febrile neutropenic patients receiving this liposomal formulation of amphotericin B as empiric antifungal therapy in a sequential dose-escalation study of 1.0, 2.5, and 5.0 mg/kg (105). Serial measurements of serum creatinine, potassium, and magnesium were not significantly changed from baseline, and there was no net increase in hepatic transaminases during the duration of therapy. There were, however, increases in serum bilirubin and alkaline phosphatase levels in patients from all dosage groups. L-AMB followed a nonlinear dosage relationship that was consistent with reticuloendothelial uptake and redistribution. This study demonstrates that L-AMB was safe and well tolerated when administered as empirical antifungal therapy in febrile neutropenic patients receiving cytotoxic chemotherapy. This study is not designed to assess efficacy; however, no breakthrough fungal infections developed during the course of empiric antifungal treatment with L-AMB.

Pharmacokinetics of L-AMB in 10 patients treated with dosages of 2.8–3.0 mg/kg/day were compared with the pharmacokinetics observed in six patients treated with amphotericin B deoxycholate at a dosage of 1.0 mg/kg/day by Heinemann et al. (106). When administered approximately three-fold greater doses of amphotericin B as L-AMB formulation, patients were found to have a median maximal concentration of drug 8.4-fold higher (14.4) than that in patients treated with amphotericin B deoxycholate (1.7 g/mL). The median AUCs in the L-AMB treated patients also exceeded the AUCs in patients treated with amphotericin B deoxycholate by nine-fold. This was partly explained by a 5.7-fold lower volume of distribution (0.42 L/kg) in L-AMB treated patients ($P = 0.001$). Elimination of amphotericin from the serum was biphasic for both liposomal and deoxycholate amphotericin B. Compared to amphotericin B deoxycholate; however, the plasma half-life of L-AMB was twice as short ($P = 0.003$). L-AMB was less nephrotoxic than conventional amphotericin B, despite being given at higher dosages in this study.

European investigators have had extensive experience with the use of L-AMB in immunocompromised patients with proven or suspected invasive fungal infections. Much of this experience has been published as the results of a number of phase II clinical trials (106–110). Similar to the initial clinical experience with ABLC and ABCD in the United States, patients in Europe were eligible to receive therapy with liposomal amphotericin B if they failed to respond to or could not tolerate treatment with amphotericin B deoxycholate. Additionally, they could also receive the lipid formulation if they had significant underlying renal insufficiency before antifungal therapy was started. The most common fungal pathogen isolated was *Candida* species and *Aspergillus* species. Patients with underlying malignancies, AIDs, and bone marrow and solid organ transplant recipients were the most commonly treated. Even in patients with documented invasive fungal infections who had previously failed treatment with amphotericin B deoxycholate, clinical responses were noted. Neutropenic patients also appeared to respond to therapy, although recovery from neutropenia, remission from underlying malignancy, and continued therapy with the liposomal form of amphotericin B appeared to be necessary for resolution of the fungal infection. Pediatric experience with the use of L-AMB in immunocompromised children has also been published (111–115), suggesting efficacy and safety in this patient population.

Prentice et al. (60) conducted a randomized phase III clinical trial in Europe comparing the empirical use of conventional amphotericin B deoxycholate vs. L-AMB for patients with persistent fever and neutropenia unresponsive to antibacterial therapy. 134 adults and 204 children were randomized in two separate, but parallel prospective, multi-institutional trials. Patients were eligible for study if they were neutropenic ($< 500/mm^3$) and had fever of unknown origin ($> 38°$ centigrade) for more than 96 hr not responding to antibacterial antibiotics. They were randomized to receive 1 mg/kg/day amphotericin B deoxycholate, 1 mg/kg/day liposomal amphotericin B, or 3 mg/kg/day of liposomal amphotericin B. In patients not receiving concurrent nephrotoxic agents, no one treated with 1 mg/kg/day was observed to have a doubling of serum creatinine from baseline. 3% of patients treated with 3 mg/kg/day were found to double their serum creatinine from baseline as opposed to 23% of patients treated with amphotericin B deoxycholate. Analysis of breakthrough fungal infections and time to resolution of fever revealed no overall difference between the study arms. The authors concluded that L-AMB was significantly less toxic than conventional amphotericin B deoxycholate.

Walsh et al. (24) reported the results of a multicenter trial comparing empirical antifungal therapy with L-AMB vs. amphotericin B deoxycholate in a similar patient population in North Amercia. Unlike the European trial, this study was double-blind and was designed to have improved statistical power to assess antifungal efficacy. A total of 687 patients were randomized to receive empirical antifungal therapy with either conventional amphotericin B (CAB) or liposomal amphotericin B (L-AMB). The two arms of the study were assessed for both antifungal efficacy as well as safety. Overall survival rates (93% for L-AMB vs. 90% for CAB) and fever resolution during neutropenia (58% for L-AMB vs. 58% for CAB) were similar in on both arms of the study. However, there was a significant reduction in the development of breakthrough fungal infections in patients treated with L-AMB as compared to amphotericin B deoxycholate (5% L-AMB vs. 9% CAB) ($P = 0.021$). Treatment with L-AMB was associated with significantly less infusion related fever, including increases in temperature of 1° Centigrade ($P \leq 0.01$), chills and rigor ($P \leq 0.01$), and cardiorespiratory events such as dyspnea, hypotension, hypertension, tachycardia and hypoxia ($P = 0.01$) when compared with conventional amphotericin B. All patients in the North American study were assessed for nephrotoxicity regardless of concurrent treatment with other nephrotoxic agents. Only 19% of patients treated with L-AMB vs. 34% of patients treated with CAB developed a significant rise in serum creatinine from baseline defined as, in children a rise >2 times baseline, and in adults a rise >2 times baseline, along with a rise >1.2 mg/dL. This double-blind, randomized controlled trial confirmed the superior safety profile of liposomal amphotericin B previously seen in European trials. Moreover, the larger number of patients included in the North American study allowed improved assessment of efficacy. Although there was no overall difference in outcome, there was a statistically significant decrease in the number of breakthrough fungal infections in patients treated with L-AMB.

There are only a few published reports of prophylactic studies of lipid formulations of amphotericin B to date. Tollemar et al. (116) has reported the results of a double-blind, randomized trial comparing L-AMB at 1 mg/kg/day with placebo for antifungal prophylaxis in a group of patients undergoing bone marrow transplantation in Sweden. 84 allogeneic and 15 autologous bone marrow transplant recipients were entered on this phase III study. There was no significant difference in the incidence of documented invasive fungal infection in patients receiving prophylactic L-AMB as compared to patients receiving placebo (3% vs. 8%, respectively). All documented fungal infections were in allogeneic transplant recipients. There was no survival advantage seen in the group of bone marrow transplant patients treated prophylactically with liposomal amphotericin B even in the subset of allogeneic transplant recipients. The authors suggest that the low incidence of invasive fungal infection and the small number of bone marrow transplant patients entered in the study made it difficult to show benefit from antifungal prophylaxis with L-AMB. Further study of antifungal prophylaxis with lipid formulations of amphotericin B in patients at higher risk for invasive fungal infection, such as recipients of unrelated donor marrow or those who develop graft vs. host disease post-transplant, are in progress.

Tollemar et al. (117) also reported the results of a trial of liposomal amphotericin B in liver transplant recipients. A reduction in invasive fungal infections was found, but the benefit was mostly because of a decrease in *Candida* infections, a result that one surmises could be achieved with fluconazole, at less expense and toxicity. Liver transplant patients with certain risk features are at high risk for invasive fungal infections. The utility of lipid amphotericin B formulations was evaluated in an historical control study recently (118). In this very high-risk subset of patients, there were suggestions of benefit, especially seen in patients receiving hemodialysis.

Lung transplant recipients are particularly susceptible for invasive aspergillosis. These appear to invade tissue via the airway, especially at the anastomosis site. Perfect and colleagues have conducted several trials of delivery of amphotericin directly to the site of infection by aerosolization of amphotericin B or amphotericin B in lipid complex. Early results appears promising and the lipid formulation is better tolerated and appears more easily delivered to the lower respiratory tract (119).

Patients with undergoing induction therapy for acute myelogenous leukemia are especially susceptible for *Candida* and *Aspergillus* infections. In a randomized trial of liposomal amphotericin B, given at a dose of 3 mg/kg three times weekly compared with the combination of fluconazole plus itraconazole, both groups had very low rates of invasive fungal infections and the rates of infection were not different (120). However, there was significantly more nephrotoxicity and elevated levels of bilirubin with liposomal amphotericin B. Leukemic patients who have had invasive *aspergillus* infections, which have been treated but require additional antineoplastic therapy, are at very high risk for recurrence. "Secondary" prophylaxis with amphotericin B has beeen shown to be associated with a reduced rate of reactivation; similarly, several case series show that lipid amphotericin B has a similar protective benefit (121).

Cryptococcal meningitis is one of the AIDS-defining illnesses in patients infected with HIV. Initial therapy with intravenous amphotericin B deoxycholate followed by oral fluconazole has been considered standard therapy for this fungal infection for the last several years. A phase III randomized trial of L-AMB at a dose of 4 mg/kg/day or conventional amphotericin B deoxycholate at 0.7 mg/kg/day for 3 weeks followed by oral fluconazole 400 mg/day for 7 weeks in 28 evaluable patients with AIDS- related cryptococcol meningitis was conducted by Leenders et al. (61) in the Netherlands. Patients treated with L-AMB and amphotericin B deoxycholate were found to have similar rates of clinical response; however, treatment with liposomal amphotericin B showed a more rapid conversion of CSF fungal culture to negative ($P < 0.05$; median time between 7 and 14 days for L-AMB vs. >21 days for amphotericin B deoxycholate by Kaplan–Meier estimate).

Similar to ABLC, liposomal amphotericin B has been studied for the treatment of cutaneous and visceral leishmaniasis in both experimental and clinical settings (122,123).

D. Lipid Emulsion Mixtures of Amphotericin B Deoxycholate

The development of each of the lipid formulations of amphotericin B previously described has taken as much as a decade before they were approved for routine clinical use. The processes involved in their preparation and quality control are complex and expensive. For these reasons, a number of investigators have studied the use of an admixture of commercially available lipid emulsion in a 20% with conventional amphotericin B.

Kirsh et al. (124) reported reduced amphotericin B toxicity without loss of antifungal activity in a murine model of murine candidiasis when amphotericin B was mixed with lipid emulsion; Chavanet et al. (125) recently reported improved efficacy and reduced toxicity in a neutropenic rabbit model of candidiasis. Randall et al. (126), however, found no difference in the degree of nephrotoxicity between amphotericin B deoxycholate prepared in 5% dextrose vs. 20% fat emulsion in a canine model of adult male Beagles.

Limited pharmacokinetic studies suggest that the combination of conventional amphotericin B with lipid emulsion has a similar profile to ABLC or ABCD, with lower peak concentrations and AUC values in serum than conventional amphotericin B, corresponding to faster deposition of the lipid emulsion amphotericin B mixture in tissues (106,127). There have been several reports describing the clinical use of this mixture for HIV-infected patients with candidiasis or cryptocococcol meningitis, as well as in patients with fever and neutropenia (125,128–132). Although Lopez et al. (133) found that amphotericin B at concentrations of 1 and 2 mg/mL were stable in 20% fat emulsion for four days at 20–25° C exposed to fluorescent light, studies by Trissel (134) as well as Ranchere et al. (135) have found this mixture to be quite unstable. Even when amphotericin B was first diluted in 5% dextrose, the amphotericin B/intralipid combination was found to be unstable with the development of a yellow precipitate. Despite the suggestion by Shadkhan et al. (136) that the mixture can be stabilized by extended agitation, methods of drug preparation have not been standardized. The admixture of this amphotericin B with fat emulsion in the pharmacy has not been approved by the U.S. Food and Drug Administration, and exposure of patients to parenteral lipid formulations may carry the risk of infections, coagulopathy, and hepatic disease. Further study of standardized preparations of this mixture are required to define the safety and efficacy of this combination before it can be recommended for routine clinical use.

E. Comparisons of the Lipid Formulations of Amphotericin B

Although there is general agreement that all of the lipid formulations are less nephrotoxic than amphotericin B deoxycholate, a number of questions still remain unanswered. Although there are clear differences in the structure and pharmacokinetics of the lipid formulations of amphotericin B (137,138), what clinical significance does this have, if any (139,140)? Two small controlled trials showed liposomal amphotericin B to be less nephrotoxic than ABLC, however, severe nephrotoxicity leading to the need for hemodialysis was rare with both products (141,142). Although infusion-related reactions are least common with liposomal amphotericin B (24,58,141), reactions such as chest, back, or flank pain have been seen in up to 5% of patients treated with this formulation (143). Does dosage make a difference? Although neutropenic animal models of candidiasis have not shown superior efficacy, models of disseminated aspergillosis have suggested an advantage to the higher daily doses of amphotericin B that can be achieved by administering the drug in a lipid formulation. Unfortunately, despite dose-excalation studies showing safety at doses as high as 15 mg/kg/day (144), clinical trials have not shown superior efficacy with higher doses of lipid formulation (59,145). Studies of empirical therapy have also used doses of 1–3 mg/kg/day. Although there appeared to be no difference in efficacy between 3 and 5 mg/kg/day in one study (141), 1 mg/kg/day appeared less effective in terms of defervescence as compared to 3 mg/kg/day in another study. Current recommendations at this point suggest that higher dosages in the range of 4–6 mg/kg/day be utilized in the setting of documented infections, particularly with invasive aspergillosis and other filamentous fungal infections. Lower doses in the range of 1–3 mg/kg/day may be reasonable for empirical therapy (146).

REFERENCES

1. Bennett JE. Antifungal Agents. 9th ed. In: Hardman JG, Limbird LE, Molinoff PB, Ruddon RW, Gilman AG, eds. Goodman & Gilman's The Pharmacological Basis of Therapeutics. New York: McGraw-Hill, 1996:1176–1179.
2. Donovick R, Gold W, Pagano JF, Stout HA. Amphotericins A and B, antifungal antibiotics produced by a *streptomycete*. I. In vitro studies. Antibiot Annu 1955; 3: 579–586.
3. Sarosi GA. Amphotericin B. Still the 'gold standard' for antifungal therapy. Postgrad Med 1990; 88(1):151–152, 155–161,165–166.
4. Gallis HA, Drew RH, Pickard WW. Amphotericin B: 30 years of clinical experience. Rev Infect Dis 1990; 12(2):308–329.
5. Stevens DA, Bennett JE. Antifungal Agents. In: Mandell GL, Bennett JE, Dolin R, eds. Mandell, Douglas, and Bennett's Principles and Practice of Infectious Diseases. 5th ed. Churchill Livingstone: Philadelphia, 2000:452–454.
6. National Committee for Clinical Laboratory Standards. Reference Method for Broth Dilution Antifungal Susceptibility Testing for Yeasts: Approved Standard. Document 27-A. Wayne, PA, 1997.
7. National Committee for Clinical Laboratory Standards. Reference Method for Broth Dilution Antifungal Susceptibility Testing of Conidium-Forming Filamentous Fungi: Proposed Standard M38-P. Wayne, PA, 1998.
8. Clancy CJ, Nguyen MH. Correlation between in vitro susceptibility determined by E test and response to therapy with amphotericin B: results from a multicenter prospective study of candidemia. Antimicrob Agents Chemother 1999; 43(5):1289–1290.
9. Nguyen MH, Clancy CJ, Yu VL, Yu YC, Morris AJ, Snydman DR, Sutton DA, Rinaldi MG. Do in vitro susceptibility data predict the microbiologic response to amphotericin B? Results of a prospective study of patients with *Candida fungemia*. J Infect Dis 1998; 177(2):425–430.
10. Groll AH, Walsh TJ. Uncommon opportunistic fungi: new nosocomial threats. Clin Microbiol Infect 2001; 7(suppl 2):8–24.
11. Hiemenz JW. Amphotericin B deoxycholate administered by continuous infusion: does the dosage make a difference? Clin Infect Dis 2003; 36(8):952–953.
12. Walsh TJ, Peter J, McGough DA, Fothergill AW, Rinaldi MG, Pizzo PA. Activities of amphotericin B and antifungal azoles alone and in combination against *Pseudallescheria boydii*. Antimicrob Agents Chemother 1995; 39(6):1361–1364.
13. Sutton DA, Sanche SE, Revankar SG, Fothergill AW, Rinaldi MG. In vitro amphotericin B resistance in clinical isolates of *Aspergillus terreus*, with a head-to-head comparison to voriconazole. J Clin Microbiol 1999; 37(7):2343–2345.
14. Arikan S, Lozano-Chiu M, Paetznick V, Nangia S, Rex JH. Microdilution susceptibility testing of amphotericin B, itraconazole, and voriconazole against clinical isolates of *Aspergillus* and *Fusarium* species. J Clin Microbiol 1999; 37(12):3946–3951.
15. Walsh TJ, Melcher G, Rinaldi M, Lecciones J, McGough D, Lee J, Callender D, Rubin M, Pizzo PA. Trichosporon beigelii: an emerging pathogen resistant to amphotericin B. J Clin Microbiol 1990; 28:1616–1622.
16. Walsh TJ, Lee JW, Melcher GP, Navarro E, Bacher J, Callender D, Reed KD, Wu T, Lopez-Berestein G, Pizzo PA. Experimental disseminated trichosporonosis in persistently granulocytopenic rabbits: implications for pathogenesis, diagnosis, and treatment of an emerging opportunistic infection. J Infect Dis 1992; 166:121–133.
17. Sanz MA, Lopez F, Martinez ML, Sanz GF, Martinez JA, Martin G, Gobernado M. Disseminated *Blastoschizomyces capitatus* infection in acute myeloblastic leukaemia. Report of three cases. Support Care Cancer 1996; 4(4):291–293.
18. Tipple M, Shadomy S, Espinelingroff A. Availability of active amphotericin-B after filtration through membrane filters. Am Rev Respir Dis 1977; 115(5):879–881.

19. Mayhew JW, Fiore C, Murray T, Barza M. An internally-standardized assay for amphotericin B in tissues and plasma. J Chromatogr 1983; 274:271–279.

20. Cleary JD, Chapman SW, Hardin TC, Rinaldi MG, Spencer JL, Deng J, Pennick GJ, Lobb CJ. Amphotericin B enzyme-linked immunoassay for clinical use: comparison with bioassay and HPLC. Ann Pharmacother 1997; 31(1):39–44.

21. Bindschadler DD, Bennett JE. A pharmacologic guide to the clinical use of amphotericin B. J Infect Dis 1969; 120(4):427–436.

22. Adamson PC, Rinaldi MG, Pizzo PA, Walsh TJ. Amphotericin B in treatment of Candida cholecystitis. Pediatr Infect Dis 1989; 8:408–411.

23. Stamm AM, Diasio RB, Dismukes WE, Shadomy S, Cloud GA, Bowles CA, Karam GH, Espinel-Ingroff A. Toxicity of amphotericin B plus flucytosine in 194 patients with cryptococcal meningitis. Am J Med 1987; 83(2):236–242.

24. Walsh TJ, Finberg RW, Arndt C, Hiemenz J, Schwartz C, Bodensteiner D, Pappas P, Seibel N, Greenberg RN, Dummer S, Schuster M, Holcenberg JS. Liposomal amphotericin B for empirical therapy in patients with persistent fever and neutropenia. National Institute of Allergy and Infectious Diseases Mycoses Study Group. N Engl J Med 1999; 340(10):764–771.

25. Goodwin SD, Cleary JD, Walawander CA, Taylor JW, Grasela TH Jr. Pretreatment regimens for adverse events related to infusion of amphotericin B. Clin Infect Dis 1995; 20(4):755–761.

26. Sawaya BP, Weihprecht H, Campbell WR, Lorenz JN, Webb RC, Briggs JP, Schnermann J. Direct vasoconstriction as a possible cause for amphotericin B-induced nephrotoxicity in rats. J Clin Invest 1991; 87(6):2097–2107.

27. Bates DW, Su L, Yu DT, Chertow GM, Seger DL, Gomes DR, Dasbach EJ, Platt R. Mortality and costs of acute renal failure associated with amphotericin B therapy. Clin Infect Dis 2001; 32(5):686–693.

28. Wingard JR, Kubilis P, Lee L, Yee G, White M, Walshe L, Bowden R, Anaissie E, Hiemenz J, Lister J. Clinical significance of nephrotoxicity in patients treated with amphotericin B for suspected or proven aspergillosis. Clin Infect Dis 1999; 29(6): 1402–1407.

29. Harbarth S, Pestotnik SL, Lloyd JF, Burke JP, Samore MH. The epidemiology of nephrotoxicity associated with conventional amphotericin B therapy. Am J Med 2001; 111(7):528–534.

30. Cagnoni PJ, Walsh TJ, Prendergast MM, Bodensteiner D, Hiemenz S, Greenberg RN, Arndt CA, Schuster M, Seibel N, Yeldandi V, Tong KB. Pharmacoeconomic analysis of liposomal amphotericin B versus conventional amphotericin B in the empirical treatment of persistently febrile neutropenic patients. J Clin Oncol 2000; 18(12):2476–2483.

31. Bullock WE, Luke RG, Nuttall CE, Bhathena D. Can mannitol reduce amphotericin B nephrotixicity? Double-blind study and description of a new vascular lesion in kidneys Antimicrob Agents Chemother 1976; 10(3):555–563.

32. Llanos A, Cieza J, Bernardo J, Echevarria J, Biaggioni I, Sabra R, Branch RA. Effect of salt supplementation on amphotericin B nephrotoxicity. Kidney Int 1991; 40(2): 302–308.

33. Camp MJ, Wingard JR, Gilmore CE, Lin LS, Dix SP, Davidson TG, Geller RB. Efficacy of low-dose dopamine in preventing amphotericin B nephrotoxicity in bone marrow transplant patients and leukemia patients. Antimicrob Agents Chemother 1998; 42(12):3103–3106.

34. Eriksson U, Seifert B, Schaffner A. Comparison of effects of amphotericin B deoxycholate infused over 4 or 24 hours: randomized controlled trial. BMJ 2001; 322(7286): 579–582.

35. Imhof A, Walter RB, Schaffner A. Continuous infusion of escalated doses of amphotericin B deoxycholate: an open-label observational study. Clin Infect Dis 2003; 36(8): 943–951.

36. Walker RW, Rosenblum MK. Amphotericin B-associated leukoencephalopathy. Neurology 1992; 42(10):2005–2010.

37. Wright DG, Robichaud KJ, Pizzo PA, Deisseroth AB. Lethal pulmonary reactions associated with the combined use of amphotericin B and leukocyte transfusions. N Engl J Med 1981; 304(20):1185–1189.

38. Dana BW, Durie BG, White RF, Huestis DW. Concomitant administration of granulocyte transfusions and amphotericin B in neutropenic patients: absence of significant pulmonary toxicity. Blood 1981; 57:90–94.

39. Bow EJ, Schroeder ML, Louie TJ. Pulmonary complications in patients receiving granulocyte transfusions and amphotericin B. Can Med Assoc J 1984; 130:593–597.

40. Dutcher JP, Kendall J, Norris D, Schiffer C, Aisner J, Wiernik PH. Granulocyte transfusion therapy and amphotericin B: adverse reactions? Am J Hematol 1989; 31:102–108

41. Walsh TJ, Dixon DM. Nosocomial aspergillosis: environmental microbiology, hospital epidemiology, diagnosis and treatment. Eur J Epidemiol 1989; 5(2):131–142.

42. Denning DW, Stevens DA. Antifungal and surgical treatment of invasive aspergillosis: review of 2,121 published cases. Rev Infect Dis 1990; 12(6):1147–1201.

43. Patterson TF, Kirkpatrick WR, White M, Hiemenz JW, Wingard JR, Dupont B, Rinaldi MG, Stevens DA, Graybill JR. Invasive aspergillosis. Disease spectrum, treatment practices, and outcomes: I3 Aspergillus Study Group. Medicine (Baltimore) 2000; 79(4):250–260.

44. New RR, Chance ML, Heath S. Antileishmanial activity of amphotericin and other antifungal agents entrapped in liposomes. J Antimicrob Chemother 1981; 8(5):371–381.

45. Graybill JR, Craven PC, Taylor RL, Williams DM, Magee WE. Treatment of murine cryptococcosis with liposome-associated amphotericin B. J Infect Dis 1982; 145(5):748–752.

46. Taylor RL, Williams DM, Craven PC, Graybill JR, Drutz DJ, Magee WE. Amphotericin B in liposomes: a novel therapy for histoplasmosis. Am Rev Respir Dis 1982; 125(5):610–611.

47. Lopez-Berestein G, Rosenblum MG, Mehta R. Altered tissue distribution of amphotericin B by liposomal encapsulation: comparison of normal mice to mice infected with *Candida albicans*. Cancer Drug Deliv 1984; 1(3):199–205.

48. Lopez-Berestein G, Fainstein V, Hopfer R, Mehta K, Sullivan MP, Keating M, Rosenblum MG, Mehta R, Luna M, Hersh EM. Liposomal amphotericin B for the treatment of systemic fungal infections in patients with cancer: a preliminary study. J Infect Dis 1985; 151(4):704–710.

49. Lopez-Berestein G, Bodey GP, Frankel LS, Mehta K. Treatment of hepatosplenic candidiasis with liposomal-amphotericin B. J Clin Oncol 1987; 5(2):310–317.

50. Sculier JP, Coune A, Meunier F, Brassinne C, Laduron C, Hollaert C, Collette N, Heymans C, Klastersky J. Pilot study of amphotericin B entrapped in sonicated liposomes in cancer patients with fungal infections. Eur J Cancer Clin Oncol 1988; 24(3):527–538.

51. Atkinson AJ Jr, Bennett JE. Amphotericin B pharmacokinetics in humans. Antimicrob Agents Chemother 1978; 13(2):271–276.

52. Sanders SW, Buchi KN, Goddard MS, Lang JK, Tolman KG. Single-dose pharmacokinetics and tolerance of a cholesteryl sulfate complex of amphotericin B administered to healthy volunteers. Antimicrob Agents Chemother 1991; 35(6):1029–1034.

53. Benson JM, Nahata MC. Pharmacokinetics of amphotericin B in children. Antimicrob Agents Chemother 1989; 33(11):1989–1993.

54. Walsh TJ, Yeldandi V, McEvoy M, Gonzalez C, Chanock S, Freifeld A, Seibel NI Whitcomb PO, Jarosinski P, Boswell G, Bekersky I, Alak A, Buell D, Barret J, Wilson W. Safety, tolerance, and pharmacokinetics of a small unilamellar liposomal formulation of amphotericin B (AmBisome) in neutropenic patients. Antimicrob Agents Chemother 1998; 42(9):2391–2398.

55. Kan VL, Bennett JE, Amantea MA, Smolskis MC, McManus E, Grasela DM, Sherman JW. Comparative safety, tolerance, and pharmacokinetics of amphotericin B lipid complex and amphotericin B deoxycholate in healthy male volunteers. J Infect Dis 1991; 164(2):418–421.

56. Walsh TJ, Whitcomb P, Piscitelli S, Figg WD, Hill S, Chanock SJ, Jarosinski P, Gupta R, Pizzo PA. Safety, tolerance, and pharmacokinetics of amphotericin B lipid complex in children with hepatosplenic candidiasis. Antimicrob Agents Chemother 1997; 41(9): 1944–1948.

57. Anaissie EJ, White M, Ozun O, et.al. Amphotericin B lipid complex versus amphotericin B for treatment of invasive candidasis: a prospective, randomized, multicenter trail [Poster session; Abstract LM21]. In: Programs and Abstracts of the 35th Interscience Conference on Antimicrobial Agents and Chemotherapy. ASM Press, Washington, DC, 330:1995.

58. White MH, Bowden RA, Sandler ES, Graham ML, Noskin GA, Wingard JR, Goldman M, Van Burik JA, McCabe A, Lin JS, Gurwith M, Miller CB. Randomized, double-blind clinical trial of amphotericin B colloidal dispersion vs. amphotericin B in the empirical treatment of fever and neutropenia. Clin Infect Dis 1998; 27(2):296–302.

59. Bowden R, Chandrasekar P, White MH, Li X, Pietrelli L, Gurwith M, Van Burik JA, Laverdiere M, Safrin S, Wingard JR. A double-blind, randomized, controlled trial of amphotericin B colloidal dispersion versus amphotericin B for treatment of invasive aspergillosis in immunocompromised patients. Clin Infect Dis 2002; 35(4):359–366.

60. Prentice HG, Hann IM, Herbrecht R, Aoun M, Kvaloy S, Catovsky D, Pinkerton CR, Schey SA, Jacobs F, Oakhill A, Stevens RF, Darbyshire PJ, Gibson BE. A randomized comparison of liposomal versus conventional amphotericin B for the treatment of pyrexia of unknown origin in neutropenic patients. Br J Haematol 1997; 98(3):711–718.

61. Leenders AC, Reiss P, Portegies P, Clezy K, Hop WC, Hoy J, Borleffs JC, Allworth T, Kauffmann RH, Jones P, Kroon FP, Verbrugh HA, de Marie S. Liposomal amphotericin B (AmBisome) compared with amphotericin B both followed by oral fluconazole in the treatment of AIDS-associated cryptococcal meningitis. AIDS 1997; 11(12): 1463–1471.

62. Hamill RJ, Sobel J, El-Sadr W, et al. Randomized double-blind trial of AmBisome (liposomal amphotericin B) and amphotericin B in acute cryptococcal meningitis in AIDS patients [abstract 1161]. In: Programs and abstracts of the 39th Interscience Conference on Antimicrobial Agents and Chemotherapy. ASM Press, Washington, DC, 1999; 489.

63. Johnson PC, Wheat LJ, Cloud GA, Goldman M, Lancaster D, Bamberger DM, Powderly WG, Hafner R, Kauffman CA, Dismukes WE. Safety efficacy of liposomal amphotericin B compared with conventional amphotericin B for induction therapy of histoplasmosis in patients with AIDS. Ann Intern Med 2002; 137(2):105–109.

64. Ostrosky-Zeichner L, Marr KA, Rex JH, Cohen SH. Amphotericin B: time for a new "gold standard." Clin Infect Dis 2003; 37(3):415–425

65. Janoff AS, Boni LT, Popescu MC, Minchey SR, Cullis PR, Madden TD, Taraschi T, Gruner SM, Shyamsunder E, Tate MW. Unusual lipid structures selectively reduce the toxicity of amphotericin B. Proc Natl Acad Sci USA 1988; 85(16):6122–6126.

66. Defever KS, Whelan WL, Rogers AL, Beneke ES, Veselenak JM, Soil DR. *Candida albicans* resistance to 5-fluorocytosine: frequency of partially resistant strains among clinical isolates. Antimicrob Agents Chemother 1982; 22(5):810–815.

67. Ghannoum MA, Rice LB. Antifungal agents: mode of action, mechanisms of resistance, and correlation of these mechanisms with bacterial resistance. Clin Microbiol Rev 1999; 12(4):501–517.

68. Janoff AS, Perkins WR, Saletan SL, Swenson CE. Amphotericin B Lipid Complex (ABLC): a molecular rationale for the attenuation of amphotericin B related toxicities. J Liposome Res 1993; 3:451–471.

69. Clark JM, Whitney RR, Olsen SJ, George RJ, Swerdel MR, Kunselman L, Bonner DP. Amphotericin B lipid complex therapy of experimental fungal infections in mice. Antimicrob Agents Chemother 1991; 35(4):615–621.

70. Olsen SJ, Swerdel MR, Blue B, Clark JM, Bonner DP. Tissue distribution of amphotericin B lipid complex in laboratory animals. J Pharm Pharmacol 1991; 43(12):831–835.

71. Mitsutake K, Kohno S, Miyazaki Y, Noda T, Miyazaki H, Miyazaki T, Kaku M, Koga H, Hara K. In-vitro and In-vivo Antifungal Activities of liposomal amphotericin-B, and amphotericin-B lipid complex. Mycopathologia 1994; 128(1):13–17.

72. Perfect JR, Wright KA. Amphotericin B lipid complex in the treatment of experimental cryptococcal meningitis and disseminated candidosis. J Antimicrob Chemother 1994; 33(1):73–81.

73. Clemons KV, Stevens DA. Comparative efficacy of amphotericin B colloidal dispersion and amphotericin B deoxycholate suspension in treatment of murine coccidioidomycosis. Antimicrob Agents Chemother 1991; 35(9):1829–1833.

74. Bhamra R, Sa'ad A, Bolcsak LE, Janoff AS, Swenson CE. Behavior of amphotericin B lipid complex in plasma in vitro and in the circulation of rats. Antimicrob Agents Chemother 1997; 41(5):886–892.

75. Williams P, Waskin H, Bolcsak L, Swenson C. Amphotericin B concentrations in autopsy tissues of organ transplant patients administered amphotericin B lipid complex infection. [Abstr no. 348] 18th Annual Meeting. Chicago, IL: American Society of Transplantation, 1999.

76. Kline S, Larsen TA, Fieber L, Fishbach R, Greenwood M, Harris R, Kline MW, Tennican PO, Janoff EN. Limited toxicity of prolonged therapy with high doses of amphotericin B lipid complex. Clin Infect Dis 1995; 21(5):1154–1158.

77. Sharkey PK, Graybill JR, Johnson ES, Hausrath SG, Pollard RB, Kolokathis A, Mildvan D, Fan-Havard P, Eng RH, Patterson TF, Pottage JC Jr, Simberkoff MS, Wolf J, Meyer RD, Gupta R, Lee LW, Gordon DS. Amphotericin B lipid complex compared with amphotericin B in the treatment of cryptococcal meningitis in patients with AIDS. Clin Infect Dis 1996; 22(2):315–321.

78. Walsh TJ, Hiemenz JW, Seibel NL, Perfect JR, Horwith G, Lee L, Silber JL, DiNubile MJ, Reboli A, Bow E, Lister J, Anaissie EJ. Amphotericin B lipid complex for invasive fungal infections: analysis of safety and efficacy in 556 cases. Clin Infect Dis 1998; 26(6):1383–1396.

79. Wingard JR. Efficacy of amphotericin B lipid complex injection (ABLC) in bone marrow transplant recipients with life-threatening systemic mycoses. Bone Marrow Transplant 1997; 19(4):343–347.

80. Hiemenz JW, Lister J, Anaissie EJ, White MH, Dinubile M, Silber J, Horwith G, Lee LW. Emergency-use amphotericin B lipid complex (ABLC) in the treatment of patients with aspergillosis: historical-control comparison with amphotericin B, [Abstr 3383]. Blood 1995; 86(10):849a.

81. Larkin JA, Montero JA. Efficacy and safety of amphotericin B lipid complex for zygomycosis. Infect Med 2003; 20(4):201–206.

82. Sundar S, Murray HW. Cure of antimony-unresponsive Indian visceral leishmaniasis with amphotericin B lipid complex. J Infect Dis 1996; 173(3):762–765.

83. Luke S, Guo S, Fielding RM, Lasic DD, Hamilton RL, Mufson D. Novel antifungal drug delivery: stable amphotericin B-cholesteryl sulfate discs. Int J Pharm 1991; 75(1):45–54.

84. Hanson LH, Stevens DA. Comparison of antifungal activity of amphotericin B deoxycholate suspension with that of amphotericin B cholesteryl sulfate colloidal dispersion. Antimicrob Agents Chemother 1992; 36(2):486–488.

85. Wang LH, Fielding RM, Smith PC, Guo LS. Comparative tissue distribution and elimination of amphotericin B colloidal dispersion (Amphocil) and Fungizone after repeated dosing in rats. Pharm Res 1995; 12(2):275–283.

86. Fielding RM, Singer AW, Wang LH, Babbar S, Guo LS. Relationship of pharmacokinetics and drug distribution in tissue to increased safety of amphotericin B colloidal dispersion in dogs. Antimicrob Agents Chemother 1992; 36(2):299–307.

87. Hostetler JS, Clemons KV, Hanson LH, Stevens DA. Efficacy and safety of amphotericin B colloidal dispersion compared with those of amphotericin B deoxycholate suspension for treatment of disseminated murine cryptococcosis. Antimicrob Agents Chemother 1992; 36(12):2656–2660.

88. Allende MC, Lee JW, Francis P, Garrett K, Dollenberg H, Berenguer J, Lyman CA, Pizzo PA, Walsh TJ. Dose-dependent antifungal activity and nephrotoxicity of amphotericin B colloidal dispersion in experimental pulmonary aspergillosis. Antimicrob Agents Chemother 1994; 38(3):518–522.

89. Walsh TJ, Garrett K, Feurerstein E, Girton M, Allende M, Bacher J, Francesconi A, Schaufele R, Pizzo PA. Therapeutic monitoring of experimental invasive pulmonary aspergillosis by ultrafast computerized tomography, a novel, noninvasive method for measuring responses to antifungal therapy. Antimicrob Agents Chemother 1995; 39(5): 1065–1069.

90. Patterson TF, Miniter P, Dijkstra J, Szoka FC Jr, Ryan JL, Andriole VT. Treatment of experimental invasive aspergillosis with novel amphotericin B/cholesterol-sulfate complexes. J Infect Dis 1989; 159(4):717–724.

91. Bowden RA, Cays M, Gooley T, Mamelok RD, van Burik JA. Phase I study of amphotericin B colloidal dispersion for the treatment of invasive fungal infections after marrow transplant. J Infect Dis 1996; 173(5):1208–1215.

92. Herbrecht R. Safety of amphotericin B colloidal dispersion. Eur J Clin Microbiol Infect Dis 1997; 16(1):74–80.

93. White MH, Anaissie EJ, Kusne S, Wingard JR, Hiemenz JW, Cantor A, Gurwith M, Du MC, Mamelok RD, Bowden RA. Amphotericin B colloidal dispersion vs. amphotericin B as therapy for invasive aspergillosis. Clin Infect Dis 1997; 24(4):635–642.

94. Adler-Moore JP, Proffitt T. Development, characterization, efficacy and mode of action of AmBisome, a unilarnellar liposomal formulation of amphotericin B. J Liposomal Res 1993; 3:429–450.

95. Anaissie E, Paetznick V, Proffitt R, Adler-Moore J, Bodey GP. Comparison of the in vitro antifungal activity of free and liposome-encapsulated amphotericin B. Eur J Clin Microbiol Infect Dis 1991; 10(8):665–668.

96. Proffitt RT, Satorius A, Chiang SM, Sullivan L, Adler-Moore JP. Pharmacology and toxicology of a liposomal formulation of amphotericin B (AmBisome) in rodents. J Antimicrob Chemother 1991; 28(suppl B):49–61.

97. Graybill JR, Bocanegra R. Liposomal amphotericin B therapy of murine histoplasmosis. Antimicrob Agents Chemother 1995; 39(8):1885–1887.

98. Albert MM, Adams K, Luther MJ, Sun SH, Graybill JR. Efficacy of AmBisome in murine coccidioidomycosis. J Med Vet Mycol 1994; 32(6):467–471.

99. Allen SD, Sorensen KN, Nejdl MJ, Durrant C, Proffit RT. Prophylactic efficacy of aerosolized liposomal (AmBisome) and non-liposomal (Fungizone) amphotericin B in murine pulmonary aspergillosis. J Antimicrob Chemother 1994; 34(6):1001–1013.

100. Lee JW, Amantea MA, Francis PA, Navarro EE, Bacher J, Pizzo PA, Walsh TJ. Pharmacokinetics and safety of a unilamellar liposomal formulation of amphotericin B (AmBisome) in rabbits. Antimicrob Agents Chemother 1994; 38(4):713–718.

101. Boswell GW, Bekersky I, Buell D, Hiles R, Walsh TJ. Toxicological profile and pharmacokinetics of a unilamellar liposomal vesicle formulation of amphotericin B in rats. Antimicrob Agents Chemother 1998; 42(2):263–268.

102. Gondal JA, Swartz RP, Rahman A. Therapeutic evaluation of free and liposome-encapsulated amphotericin B in the treatment of systemic candidiasis in mice. Antimicrob Agents Chemother 1989; 33(9):1544–1548.

103. Francis P, Lee JW, Hoffman A, Peter J, Francesconi A, Bacher J, Shelhamer J, Pizzo PA, Walsh TJ. Efficacy of unilamellar liposomal amphotericin B in treatment of pulmonary

aspergillosis in persistently granulocytopenic rabbits: the potential role of bronchoalveo-lar D-mannitol and serum galactomannan as markers of infection. J Infect Dis 1994; 169(2):356–368.

104. Pahls S, Schaffner A. Comparison of the activity of free and liposomal amphotericin B in vitro and in a model of systemic and localized murine candidiasis. J Infect Dis 1994; 169(5):1057–1061.

105. Walsh TJ, Yeldandi V, McEvoy M, Gonzalez C, Chanock SJ, Freifeld A, Seibel NI, Jar-osinski P, Boswell G, Bekersky I, Alak A, Buell D, Barret J, Wilson W. Safety, toler-ance, and pharmacokinetics of a small unilamellar liposomal formulation of amphotericin B (AmBisome) in neutropenic patients. Antimicrob Agents Chemother 1998; 42:2391–2398.

106. Heinemann V, Bosse D, Jehn U, Kahny B, Wachholz K, Debus A, Scholz P, Kolb HJ, Wilmanns W. Pharmacokinetics of liposomal amphotericin B (Ambisome) in critically ill patients. Antimicrob Agents Chemother 1997; 41(6):1275–1280.

107. Meunier F, Prentice HG, Ringden O. Liposomal amphotericin B (AmBisome): safety data from a phase II/III clinical trial. J Antimicrob Chemother 1991; 28(suppl B):83–91.

108. Ringden O, Meunier F, Tollemar J, Ricci P, Tura S, Kuse E, Viviani MA, Gorin NC, Klastersky J, Fenaux P. Efficacy of amphotericin B encapsulated in liposomes (AmBi-some) in the treatment of invasive fungal infections in immunocompromised patients. J Antimicrob Chemother 1991; 28(suppl B):73–82.

109. Mills W, Chopra R, Linch DC, Goldstone AH. Liposomal amphotericin B in the treatment of fungal infections in neutropenic patients: a single-centre experience of 133 episodes in 116 patients. Br J Haematol 1994; 86(4):754–760.

110. Ng TT, Denning DW. Liposomal amphotericin B (AmBisome) therapy in invasive fun-gal infections. Evaluation of United Kingdom compassionate use data. Arch Intern Med 1995; 155(10):1093–1098.

111. Ringden O, Tollemar J. Liposomal amphotericin B (AmBisome) treatment of invasive fungal infections in immunocompromised children. Mycoses 1993; 36(5–6):187–192.

112. Tollemar J, Duraj F, Ericzon BG. Liposomal amphotericin B treatment in a 9-month-old liver recipient. Mycoses 1990; 33(5):251–252.

113. Pasic S, Flannagan L, Cant AJ. Liposomal amphotericin (AmBisome) is safe in bone marrow transplantation for primary immunodeficiency. Bone Marrow Transplant 1997; 19(12):1229–1232.

114. Jarlov JO, Born P, Bruun B. *Candida albicans* meningitis in a 27 weeks premature infant treated with liposomal amphotericin-B (AmBisome). Scand J Infect Dis 1995; 27(4):419–420.

115. Dornbusch HJ, Urban CE, Pinter H, Ginter G, Fotter R, Becker H, Miorini T, Berghold C. Treatment of invasive pulmonary aspergillosis in severely neutropenic children with malignant disorders using liposomal amphotericin B (AmBisome), granu-locyte colony-stimulating factor, and surgery: report of five cases. Pediatr Hematol Oncol 1995; 12(6):577–586.

116. Tollemar J, Ringden O, Andersson S, Sundberg B, Ljungman P, Tyden G. Randomized double-blind study of liposomal amphotericin B (Ambisome) prophylaxis of invasive fungal infections in bone marrow transplant recipients. Bone Marrow Transplant 1993; 12(6):577–582.

117. Tollemar J, Hockerstedt K, Ericzon BG, Jalanko H, Ringden O. Liposomal amphoter-icin B prevents invasive fungal infections in liver transplant recipients: a randomized, placebo-controlled study. Transplantation 1995; 59:45–50.

118. Fortun J, Martin-Davila P, Moreno S et al. Prevention of invasive fungal infections in liver transplant recipients: the role of prophylaxis with lipid formulations of amphoter-icin B in high-risk patients. J Antimicrob Chemother 2003; 52:813–819.

119. Drew RH, Dodds AE, Benjamin DK Jr, Duane DR Palmer SM, Perfect JR. Com-parative safety of amphotericin B lipid complex and amphotericin B deoxycholate as

aerosolized antifungal prophylaxis in lung-transplant recipients. Transplantation 2004; 77:232–237.

120. Mattiuzzi GN, Estey E, Raad I, et al. Liposomal amphotericin B versus the combination of fluconazole and itraconazole as prophylaxis for invasive fungal infections during induction chemotherapy for patients with acute myelogenous leukemia and myelodysplastic syndrome. Cancer 2003; 97:450–456.

121. Mele L, Pagano L, Equitani F, Leone G. Case reports. Secondary prophylaxis with liposomal amphotericin B after invasive aspergillosis following treatment for haematological malignancy. Mycoses 2001; 44:201–203.

122. Yardley V, Croft SL. Activity of liposomal amphotericin B against experimental cutaneous leishmaniasis. Antimicrob Agents Chemother 1997; 41(4):752–756.

123. Davidson RN, di Martino L, Gradoni L, Giacchino R, Gaeta GB, Pempinello R, Scotti S, Cascio A, Castagnola E, Maisto A, Gramiccia M, di Caprio D, Wilkinson RJ, Bryceson AD. Short-course treatment of visceral leishmaniasis with liposomal amphotericin B (AmBisome). Clin Infect Dis 1996; 22(6):938–943.

124. Kirsh R, Goldstein R, Tarloff J, Parris D, Hook J, Hanna N, Bugelski P, Poste G. An emulsion formulation of amphotericin B improves the therapeutic index when treating systemic murine candidiasis. J Infect Dis 1988; 158(5):1065–1070.

125. Chavanet PY, Garry I, Charlier N, Caillot D, Kisterman JP, D'Athis M, Portier H. Trial of glucose versus fat emulsion in preparation of amphotericin for use in HIV infected patients with candidiasis. BMJ 1992; 305(6859):921–925.

126. Randall SR, Adams LG, White MR, DeNicola DB. Nephrotoxicity of amphotericin B administered to dogs in a fat emulsion versus five percent dextrose solution. Am J Vet Res 1996; 57(7):1054–1058.

127. Ayestaran A, Lopez RM, Montoro JB, Estibalez A, Pou L, Julia A, Lopez A, Pascual B. Pharmacokinetics of conventional formulation versus fat emulsion formulation of amphotericin B in a group of patients with neutropenia. Antimicrob Agents Chemother 1996; 40(3):609–612.

128. Caillot D, Casasnovas O, Solary E, Chavanet P, Bonnotte B, Reny G, Entezam F, Lopez J, Bonnin A, Guy H. Efficacy and tolerance of an amphotericin B lipid (Intralipid) emulsion in the treatment of candidaemia in neutropenic patients. J Antimicrob Chemother 1993; 31(1):161–169.

129. Moreau P, Milpied N, Fayette N, Ramee JF, Harousseau JL. Reduced renal toxicity and improved clinical tolerance of amphotericin B mixed with intralipid compared with conventional amphotericin B in neutropenic patients. J Antimicrob Chemother 1992; 30(4):535–541.

130. Pascual B, Ayestaran A, Montoro JB, Oliveras J, Estibalez A, Julia A, Lopez A. Administration of lipid-emulsion versus conventional amphotericin B in patients with neutropenia. Ann Pharmacother 1995; 29(12):1197–1201.

131. Joly V, Geoffray C, Reynes J, Goujard C, Mechali D, Maslo C, Raffi F, Yeni P. Amphotericin B in a lipid emulsion for the treatment of cryptococcal meningitis in AIDS patients. J Antimicrob Chemother 1996; 38(1):117–126.

132. Sorkine P, Nagar H, Weinbroum A, Setton A, Israitel E, Scarlatt A, Silbiger A, Rudick V, Kluger Y, Halpern P. Administration of amphotericin B in lipid emulsion decreases nephrotoxicity: results of a prospective, randomized, controlled study in critically ill patients. Crit Care Med 1996; 24(8):1311–1315.

133. Lopez RM, Ayestaran A, Pou L, Montoro JB, Hernandez M, Caragol I. Stability of amphotericin B in an extemporaneously prepared i.v. fat emulsion. Am J Health Syst Pharm 1996; 53(22):2724–2727.

134. Trissel LA. Amphotericin B does not mix with fat emulsion. Am J Health Syst Pharm 1995; 52(13):1463–1464.

135. Ranchere JY, Latour JF, Fuhrmann C, Lagallarde C, Loreuil F. Amphotericin B intralipid formulation: stability and particle size. J Antimicrob Chemother 1996; 37(6): 1165–1169.

136. Shadkhan Y, Segal E, Bor A, Gov Y, Rubin M, Lichtenberg D. The use of commercially available lipid emulsions for the preparation of amphotericin B-lipid admixtures. J Antimicrob Chemother 1997; 39(5):655–658.

137. Hiemenz JW, Walsh TJ. Lipid formulations of amphotericin B: recent progress and future directions. Clin Infect Dis 1996; 22(suppl 2):133–144.

138. Wong-Beringer A, Jacobs RA, Guglielmo BJ. Lipid formulations of amphotericin B: clinical efficacy and toxicities. Clin Infect Dis 1998; 27(3):603–618.

139. Wingard JR. Lipid formulations of amphotericins: are you a lumper or a splitter? Clin Infect Dis 2002; 35(7):891–895

140. Bellmann R, Egger P, Wiedermann CJ. Differences in pharmacokinetics of amphotericin B lipid formulations despite clinical equivalence. Clin Infect Dis 2003; 36(11):1500–1501.

141. Wingard JR, White MH, Anaissie E, Raffalli J, Goodman J, Arrieta A. A randomized, double-blind comparative trial evaluating the safety of liposomal amphotericin B versus amphotericin B lipid complex in the empirical treatment of febrile neutropenia. L Amph/ABLC Collaborative Study Group. Clin Infect Dis 2000; 31(5):1155–1163.

142. Fleming RV, Kantarjian HM, Husni R, Rolston K, Lim J, Raad I, Pierce S, Cortes J, Estey E. Comparison of amphotericin B lipid complex (ABLC) Vs. AmBisome in the treatment of suspected or documented fungal infections in patients with leukemia. Leuk Lymphoma 2001; 40(5–6):511–520.

143. Roden MM, Nelson LD, Knudsen TA, Jarosinski PF, Starling JM, Shiflett SE, Calis K, DeChristoforo R, Donowitz GR, Buell D, Walsh TJ. Triad of acute infusion-related reactions associated with liposomal amphotericin B: analysis of clinical and epidemiological characteristics. Clin Infect Dis 2003; 36(10):1213–1220.

144. Walsh TJ, Goodman JL, Pappas P, Bekersky I, Buell DN, Roden M, Barrett J, Anaissie EJ. Safety, tolerance, and pharmacokinetics of high-dose liposomal amphotericin B (AmBisome) in 46 patients infected with Aspergillus species and other filamentous fungi: maximum tolerated dose study. Antimicrob Agents Chemother 2001; 45(12): 3487–3496.

145. Ellis M, Spence D, de Pauw B, Meunier F, Marinus A, Collette L, Sylvester R, Meis J, Boogaerts M, Selleslag D, Krcmery V, von Sinner W, MacDonald P, Doyen C, Vandercam B. An EORTC international multicenter randomized trial (EORTC number 19923) comparing two dosages of liposomal amphotericin B for treatment of invasive aspergillosis. Clin Infect Dis 1998; 27(6):1406–1412.

146. Wingard JR, Leather H. A new era of antifungal therapy. Biol Blood Marrow Transplant 2004; 10(2):73–90.

147. Gotzsche PC, Johansen HK. Meta-analysis of prophylactic or empirical antifungal treatment versus placebo or no treatment in patients with cancer complicated by neutropenia. BMJ 1997; 314:1238–1244.

148. Bow EJ, Laverdiere M, Lussier N, Rotstein C, Cheang MS, Ioannou S. Antifungal prophylaxis for severely neutropenic chemotherapy recipients: a meta analysis of randomized-controlled clinical trials. Cancer 2002; 94:3230–3246.

17

The Systemically Acting Azoles

Paul O. Gubbins
Department of Pharmacy Practice, College of Pharmacy, University of Arkansas for Medical Sciences, Little Rock, Arkansas, U.S.A.

I. INTRODUCTION

Ketoconazole, the first oral systemically acting azole, was introduced in 1981 and at the time it represented an advance in antifungal therapy. Prior to this, choices of systemic antifungal therapy were limited to intravenous (IV) amphotericin B or miconazole, oral flucytosine. All these agents were associated with significant toxicity, and flucytosine had a narrow spectrum of activity. The use of ketoconazole was limited over time as a result of the subsequent introductions of fluconazole in 1990, and itraconazole in 1992, These azoles were designed to be more specific for fungal cells, and to be associated with less human toxicity. Consequently ketoconazole is now relegated to second-line status for the treatment of many systemic mycoses. Voriconazole, the most recent addition to this class, possesses a broad spectrum of activity and thus, it represents yet another advance in this growing class of antimycotics. The safety and efficacy of fluconazole, itraconazole, and voriconazole, make them significant additions to the antifungal arsenal. These azoles represent relatively safe and effective alternatives to other systemically acting antifungal agents. This chapter will review the pharmacology of the azole class of antifungal agents.

A. Chemistry

The systemic azoles are synthetic compounds and are divided into the imidazole and triazole classes based on their chemical structure (Fig. 1). Ketoconazole, the remaining systemically acting imidazole, contains two nitrogen atoms on the five-membered azole ring, whereas the triazoles, fluconazole, itraconazole, and voriconazole, contain three nitrogens in the five-membered azole ring. The chemical structure and properties of ketoconazole and itraconazole are somewhat similar. Ketoconazole is a lipophilic, weak dibasic compound with low-water solubility at pH greater than 3 (1). Itraconazole is a weak base that is extremely lipophilic, essentially water-insoluble ($<5\,\mu g/mL$) and ionized at only low pH (2). Both ketoconazole and itraconazole undergo optimal dissolution at pH less than 3 (1,2). The poor aqueous solubility made the development of IV formulations of these compounds challenging, thus ketoconazole is available only as a solid oral dosage form.

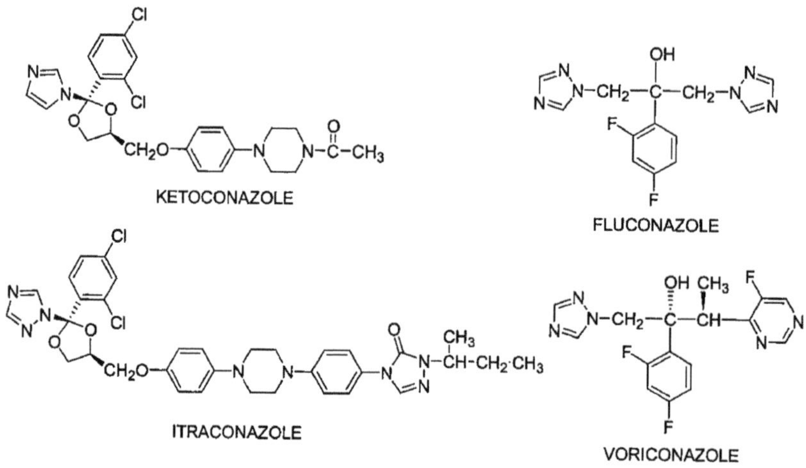

Figure 1 The chemical structures of the systemically acting azoles.

Fluconazole is also a weak base, but it is only slightly lipophilic, and thus more polar than either ketoconazole or itraconazole. As a result, it circumvents much of the hepatic metabolism required by the other azoles, achieves high-serum concentrations, and exhibits low-protein binding (3). In addition, since fluconazole is water soluble, it is readily formulated as an IV dosage form.

Voriconazole is a derivative of fluconazole (Fig. 1). Chemically, voriconazole differs from fluconazole in that a fluropyrimidine group replaced one triazole moiety and a methyl group was added to the propanol backbone of the molecule (4). These alterations enhance the potency and expand the spectrum of activity to include filamentous fungi, especially *Aspergillus* sp. (4).

II. MECHANISM OF ACTION

A. Effects on 14α-Demethylase

The sterol ergosterol is a key component of the fungal cell membrane that is not present in mammalian cells. Therefore, this sterol is an ideal target for antifungal activity. Ergosterol is critical to the integrity of the fungal cell membrane and functions in regulating membrane fluidity and asymmetry (5). Sterols that are incorporated into the cell membrane must lack C-4 methyl groups in order for membrane integrity to be maintained (5). This is accomplished in the sterol biosynthesis pathway by cytochrome P450 (CYP) – dependent 14α-demethylase. Inhibition of the enzyme 14α-demethylase leads to depletion of the essential cell membrane sterol, ergosterol, and accumulation of sterol precursors, including 14α-methylated sterols (lanosterol, 14-dimethyl lanosterol, and 24-methylenedihydrolanosterol) (Fig. 2). The net result of this inhibition is the formation of a plasma membrane with altered structure and function (5).

The systemic azoles are generally believed to exert a fungistatic effect by inhibiting this step via binding of the azole ring to the heme iron of the enzyme, which catalyzes the CYP-dependent 14α-demethylation of lanosterol (7). However, ketoconazole may have a secondary mechanism of action. Ketoconazole also inhibits several membrane-bound enzymes and may interact directly with membrane lipid

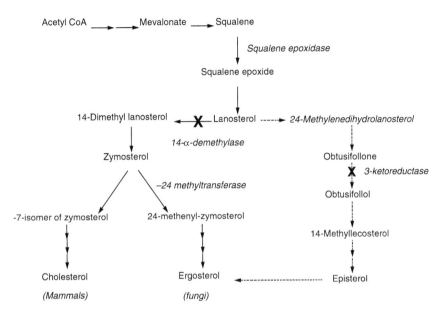

Figure 2 Probable biosynthesis pathway of ergosterol (fungi) and cholesterol (mammals). selected enzymes (*italicized*) shown, alternative pathway shown with dashed lines, primary path shown with solid lines. Azole site of inhibition marked with "X". *Source*: Adapted from Refs. 5,6 and 10.

biosynthesis (5). Likewise, in addition to inhibiting 14α-demethylation of lanosterol, voriconazole may also affect chitin synthesis (8). However, studies show that the triazoles act primarily on the enzyme 14α-demethylase (5,9).

The 14α-demethylase inhibitory activity of the triazoles may vary with genus. For example, in addition to inhibiting 14α-demethylase in *Cryptococcus neoformans*, itraconazole and fluconazole inhibit the reduction of the 3-ketosteroid obtusifolone to obtusifoliol, presumably by inhibiting 3-ketoreductase (Fig. 2) (5). The resultant accumulation of the 3-ketosteroid obtusifolone and other methylated sterol precursors increases the fragility of the membrane. In *Histoplasma capsulatum* var. *capsulatum*, investigators have hypothesized that 3-ketoreductase may be more sensitive to inhibition by itraconazole than by fluconazole (10). This may explain why itraconazole is more active than fluconazole against this pathogen.

The 14α-demethylase inhibitory activity of the triazoles also varies with species, in fluconazole susceptible *Candida albicans* voriconazole completely blocks ergosterol and obtusifoliol synthesis, whereas fluconazole only partially inhibits ergosterol and completely blocks obtusifoliol synthesis (9). Similarly, in *Candida krusei*, both voriconazole and fluconazole completely blocked obtusifoliol synthesis, but voriconazole inhibited ergosterol synthesis more than fluconazole (9). Variability in the 14α-demethylase inhibitory potencies among the azoles likely explains the differences in their activity.

B. Pharmacokinetics

The triazoles differ subtly in chemical properties, which form the basis of the pharmacokinetic differences between the agents and the propensity of this class to interact with other medications. These properties can limit the use of these agents,

Table 1 Summary of Pharmacological and Pharmacokinetic Characteristics of Systemic Azoles

Parameter	KTZ	ITZ Cap	ITZ Soln	FCZ	VCZ
pH-dependent dissolution	Yes	Yes	No	No	No
Rate of absorption	Rapid	Slow	Rapid	Rapid	Rapid
Extent of absorption	Variable	Variable	Less variable	Nearly complete	Nearly complete
Bioavailability (%)	80	<50	60–70	>93	90–96
Steady state conc. (mg/L)					
After IV dosing	n/a	n/a	1.3–1.6	4–6	3–6
After oral dosing	1–4	0.5–2	1.2–2	2–3	2–3
Usual daily dosage (mg)					
IV	n/a	n/a	200–400	6 mg/kg	3–6 mg/kg
Oral	200–400	200–400	200–400	200–400	200–400
Intestinal metabolism	Significant	Significant	Minimal	None	None
Half-life (hr)	2–10	24–33		30	6
Non-linear PK	Yes	Yes		No	Yes
Protein binding	Extensive	Extensive		Minimal	Moderate
Metabolism	Extensive	Extensive		Minimal	Extensive
CYP enzyme inhibited	3A4	3A4		2C9/19 > 3A4	2C9/19 > 3A4
Metabolites (active)	Many (none)	Many (one)		Few (none)	Several (none)
P-gp substrate	Yes	Yes		No	No
CSF conc. (%serum)	<10	<1		>70	30–70
Urinary Elimination	<5%	<5%		89%	<5%

particularly ketoconazole or itraconazole. The pharmacokinetic properties of the commonly used systemic acting azoles are provided in Table 1.

1. Ketoconazole

For systemic use ketoconazole is available only as 200 mg tablets. Due to its chemistry and low water solubility, ketoconazole undergoes optimal dissolution at pH less than 3. Food does not consistently alter the absorption and systemic availability of ketoconazole (11). The absorption of ketoconazole is rapid and somewhat complete. The relative bioavailability of the ketoconazole tablet is approximately 80% (11). Ketoconazole is highly lipophilic, therefore in the serum it is highly protein bound (99%) and widely distributed in the body (11). As a result of high-protein binding, the unbound concentrations of ketoconazole in body fluids [i.e., urine, cerebral spinal fluid (CSF), etc.] are low (11). Ketoconazole is hepatically metabolized to inactive metabolites by CYP3A4, and exhibits non-linear (i.e., dose-dependent) elimination. Less than 5% of an administered dose of ketoconazole is eliminated unchanged in the urine (11). Ketoconazole also interacts extensively with the heme moiety of CYP3A resulting in non-competitive inhibition of oxidative metabolism of many CYP3A substrates (12). To a lesser extent ketoconazole also inhibits other CYP enzymes involved in drug metabolism (13). Ketoconazole also interacts somewhat with the transport P-glycoprotein (P-gp) (14).

P-gp is a transmembrane efflux pump/transport protein that is expressed in a variety of tissues, where it interacts with a diverse array of substrates, including itraconazole and ketoconazole, but not fluconazole (14). Although it has not been characterized, the interaction between voriconazole and P-gp is likely negligible. The P-gp is extensively expressed in the GI tract, liver, cells of the blood–brain barrier, and in the renal epithelia of the proximal tubule (15). In these tissues P-gp acts to limit systemic exposure of its substrate. In the GI tract P-gp reduces drug absorption, whereas in the liver and proximal tubules of the kidney it enhances drug elimination. In the blood–brain barrier, P-gp limits distribution to central nervous system (CNS) tissues (12). This protein is the basis of several azole drug–drug interactions.

2. Itraconazole

Itraconazole is available as 100 mg capsules containing itraconazole-coated pellets, and solubilized in a 40% hydroxpropyl-β-cyclodextrin (HP-βCD) 10 mg/mL solution for oral and IV use. The absorption of itraconazole from the capsule form is slow and incomplete, consequently the drug is subjected to significant metabolism in the intestine and liver before reaching the systemic circulation. As a result, absorption from the capsule is variable and optimal under acidic gastric conditions or in the fed state (16). In contrast, HP-βCD significantly enhances the solubility of itraconazole. Therefore, the oral solution form requires no dissolution so its absorption is not influenced by gastric pH and is rapid. As a result, itraconazole is delivered to the intestinal epithelium in high concentrations, which may cause transient saturation of intestinal CYP3A4 (i.e., a component of first pass metabolism) (17,18). With less first pass metabolism, higher and more consistent serum concentrations can be achieved. The absorption of itraconazole from the oral solution is optimal in the absence of food (17). Consequently, with an empty stomach peak plasma concentrations of both itraconazole and its primary metabolite, hydroxyitraconazole, are higher and are achieved earlier, compared to non-fasting conditions (17,18). Absorption of the oral solution on an empty stomach is more rapid and less variable than the absorption of the capsule under fed conditions. This results in a pharmacokinetic profile with less inter- and intrapatient variability (19). However, even in the presence of food, higher serum concentrations are achieved with the oral solution than with the capsule. The absolute bioavailability of the oral solution is 55% and approximately 30% higher than that of the capsule formulation, nonetheless the two formulations are considered bioequivalent in many pharmacokinetic parameters (16,19).

The HP-βCD is a carrier molecule modified from natural breakdown products of starch, and when given orally it is poorly absorbed from the intestine, stimulates gastrointestinal secretion and propulsion, and causes diarrhea. While, this compound improves the pharmacokinetics of the oral dosage form of itraconazole, it hinders the IV form of itraconazole. Following IV administration, the amount of itraconazole that is cleared by the kidney is negligible, but HP-βCD is primarily eliminated by the kidneys (80–90%) (20,21). With severe renal impairment (creatinine clearance (CrCl) $\leq 19\,\text{mL/min}$) renal elimination of this compound decreases sixfold (22). Currently the use of IV itraconazole is contraindicated in patients with $\text{CrCl} \leq 30\,\text{mL/min}$ due to concern that the renal accumulation of HP-βCD may cause histological damage to the kidney (22). These changes have been observed in animals, but there is no human data describing this toxicity.

Itraconazole is highly lipophilic, therefore in the serum it is highly bound (99.8%) to albumin and widely distributed in the body (2). As a result of high protein binding, the unbound concentrations of itraconazole in body fluids (i.e., CSF, saliva, and urine) are very low (2). Itraconazole has high affinity for tissues (i.e., vaginal mucosa, horny layer of nails, etc.), and concentrations in these tissues can persist well after the serum concentrations are undetectable (2). Like ketoconazole, itraconazole also exhibits non-linear elimination. However, itraconazole is extensively metabolized to many metabolites by CYP3A4. The principle metabolite, hydroxyitraconazole is formed primarily during gut wall metabolism and is bioactive (16). The complete metabolic pathway of itraconazole is not fully understood and it may interact with additional CYP enzymes. Itraconazole primarily inhibits the CYP3A4 enzyme (13,23). In addition, it is a substrate and inhibitor of P-gp, and its interaction with this protein is the basis for several notable drug interactions involving itraconazole (i.e., vinca alkaloids, digoxin, etc.) (13,23).

3. Fluconazole

Fluconazole is available as 50, 100, 150, and 200 mg tablets as well as a 2 mg/mL solution for IV administration, and in a powder form for reconstitution as a 10 or 40 mg/mL oral suspension. The oral formulations of fluconazole are rapidly and nearly completely absorbed, with a bioavailability in excess of 93% (24). Consequently, serum concentrations after oral dosing are similar to those obtained with IV dosing. Therefore, the IV formulation should be used only in patients who cannot take oral medications, or in whom oral absorption cannot be assured. The administration of fluconazole in through enteral feeding tubes has been studied and most data seem to indicate that the systemic availability of fluconazole is relatively unaffected by this mode of administration. However, one large study demonstrated that serum concentrations obtained with standard doses administered via an enteral feeding tube may not be adequate to treat *Candida glabrata* infections (25). Absorption of fluconazole is not dependent on acidic gastric conditions or the presence of food (24). Fluconazole binds minimally to plasma proteins (11%), and circulates mostly as free drug, thus it distributes extensively into a variety of body fluids including the CSF, urine, as well as hepatic, renal, and CNS tissues (24).

The chemical properties of fluconazole also allow it to circumvent much of the intestinal and hepatic metabolism required by ketoconazole or itraconazole for elimination. Fluconazole exhibits linear pharmacokinetics, that is, increases in dosage produce proportional changes in serum concentration and systemic exposure. Fluconazole is unique among systemic azoles, in that approximately 91% of an orally administered dose is excreted in the urine, mostly (80%) as unchanged drug, two inactive metabolites account for the remaining 11%(26). Although fluconazole undergoes minimal CYP-mediated metabolism, like the other azoles, in vitro it inhibits CYP3A4, albeit much more weakly than other agents in this class (27). However, in vitro fluconazole also inhibits several other CYP enzymes (27). When evaluating in vitro studies of the CYP inhibitory potential it is important to note fluconazole binds non-competitively to CYP, and in vivo it circulates largely as free drug. Therefore, determination of the ability of fluconazole to inhibit CYP in vitro may not accurately predict its potential to inhibit CYP in vivo.

4. Voriconazole

Voriconazole is available in both IV and oral formulations. The IV formulation is formulated as a powder for reconstitution containing 200 mg voriconazole solubilized with sulfobutyl ether β-cyclodextrin. When reconstituted the final solution contains 10 mg/mL. The oral tablets contain either 50 or 200 mg of voriconazole. Like fluconazole, dissolution of voriconazole is not affected by increases in gastric pH. Voriconazole absorption is rapid and nearly complete following oral dosing, with a relative bioavailability of approximately 90% (28). Peak serum concentrations are achieved within 2 hr of oral dosing. Voriconazole is moderately bound to plasma proteins, and is widely distributed throughout the body. In case reports, CSF concentrations achieved with standard dosing have been approximately 30–60% of plasma concentrations (28,29). Voriconazole concentrations in brain tissue concentrations are higher than those in the CSF (30).

In adults, increases in voriconazole dosage produce disproportional changes in drug levels (i.e., non-linear pharmacokinetics). In contrast, in children, increases in voriconazole dosage produce proportional changes in drug levels (i.e., linear pharmacokinetics). Moreover, higher doses are required in children (28). These age related differences are probably due to the saturation of CYP enzymes in adults or age related differences in CYP expression.

Voriconazole undergoes extensive hepatic metabolism by CYP enzymes. However, the metabolism of voriconazole is more complex than other azoles and involves several different CYP enzymes, namely, CYP2C9, CYP2C19, and CYP3A4 (28,30). Voriconazole is primarily metabolized by CYP2C19, which exhibits genetic polymorphism. To date there have been eight variant alleles identified with this polymorphism. All variants are associated with reduced enzyme activity that manifests as a poor metabolizing phenotype (PM). The PM phenotype is an inherited autosomal recessive trait, and is present in 3–5% of Caucasians, 12–23% of Asian populations, and 38–79% of Polynesians and Micronesians (31). Populations that exhibit the homozygous PM phenotype will have approximately a four fold increase in drug exposure compared to those who exhibit the homozygous efficient metabolizer (EM) phenotype. Populations that are heterozygous for the EM phenotype will have nearly a two fold increase in drug exposure compared to the homozygous EM phenotype (28).

Voriconazole is also metabolized by CYP2C9, which also exhibits polymorphisms. To date six variant alleles have been identified with this polymorphism, and a two are associated with reduced enzyme activity. Therefore, clearance of a substrate, such as voriconazole will be reduced when these variants are present. The variant alleles are expressed among Caucasians, and less frequently among African-Americans. They are not expressed in Asian populations (31,32). Lastly, CYP3A4 is also involved in voriconazole metabolism, however, to date significant polymorphisms have not been identified with this enzyme. Genotyping is not clinically indicated, but nonetheless clinicians should be aware of the complexities of voriconazole metabolism. In addition to being a substrate of these three CYP enzymes, voriconazole inhibits them as well. Therefore, it has the potential to interact with a wide array of other medicines. As a consequence of its complex CYP-mediated metabolism, less than 5% of voriconazole is eliminated by the kidneys unchanged (28). The affinity of voriconazole for P-gp has not been fully evaluated. However, since it is a derivative of fluconazole, and has activity in CNS infections, it is likely not a P-gp substrate.

C. Adverse Effects

In general the azoles are associated with few serious adverse effects and are considered a relatively safe class of drugs. Table 2 summarizes common and serious adverse

Table 2 Common and Serious Adverse Effects of the Azoles

Organ System	KTZ	FCZ	ITZ	VCZ
GI tract				
Nausea	+	+	++	+
Vomiting	+	+	++	+
Diarrhea	+	+	++	+
Dermatological				
Itching	+	+	+	+
Rash	+	++	+	++
Photosensitivity	–	–	–	+
Stevens–Johnson	+	++	+	+
Hepatic				
Increased transaminases	++	+	+	++
Hepatitis	++	+	+	++
Bone marrow				
	–	–	–	–
Renal				
	–	–	–	–
Endocrine				
Adrenal insufficiency	++	–	–	–
Mineralocorticoid excess	++	–	++	–
Other				
Headache	+	+	+	+
Visual disturbances	–	–	–	++

Abbreviations: KTZ, ketoconazole; FCZ, fluconazole; ITZ, itraconazole; VCZ, voriconazole; (–), uncommon; (+), common; (++), most common within class.

effects of the azoles. The advent of the triazoles greatly improved the safety of this class. As a class, dose related GI symptoms are the most common side effects, particularly with the oral itraconazole solution (11). These effects are typically seen at the upper ends of the recommended dosage ranges of these compounds, and rarely are the symptoms severe enough to warrant discontinuation of therapy. Transient increases in serum aminotransferase concentrations are also commonly observed with all agents in this class. In general, patients who experience azole-associated increases in serum aminotransferases are asymptomatic, but these increases can, on rare occasion, evolve into fatal drug-induced hepatitis (11). Consequently, baseline liver function tests should be performed prior to initiating azole therapy, and the patient should be monitored periodically for evidence of drug-induced hepatitis (11). The azoles can also produce allergic skin rashes that are generally mild, and subside with discontinuation of the drug. The azoles produce teratogenic effects in mice and therefore their use should be avoided in pregnancy (category C).

1. Ketoconazole

The biosynthesis pathways of fungal and mammalian sterols have several CYP-mediated steps in common. For example the azoles can block synthesis mammalian sterols, specifically cholesterol, at the 14α-demethylation step. However, the triazoles have reduced affinity for the mammalian enzymes, and thus supra-pharmacologic doses would be required to produce the degree of inhibition observed in fungal cells (5). However, ketoconazole is non-specific in its inhibition of sterol biosynthesis, which is the primary difference between the imidazole, and the triazoles. Consequently, inhibition of human sterol biosynthesis is most commonly observed with use of ketoconazole, than with the triazoles.

Ketoconazole reversibly inhibits the synthesis of several mammalian sterols including testosterone, estradiol, and cortisol, especially when given in daily doses in excess of 400 mg (33). Consequently, a variety of endocrine disturbances can be observed in patients receiving ketoconazole. Within 6 months of starting therapy up to 20% of men can experience a dose-dependent inhibition of testosterone that causes symptoms such as gynecomastia, or diminished libido (33). In addition, oligospermia, or impotence can also occur. Women also can experience endocrine abnormalities associated with ketoconazole therapy. Menstrual irregularities can occur in up to 16%, and reversible alopecia can be seen in 8% (33). These endocrine abnormalities subside with drug discontinuation. In rare cases ketoconazole can cause adrenal insufficiency as a consequence of its ability to inhibit steroidogenesis (11). Limiting the dose to no more than 400 mg/day lowers the risk of endocrine or GI adverse effects associated with ketoconazole (34).

2. Itraconazole

Itraconazole in dosages of 400 mg/day or less generally produces little toxicity. Reports of adverse effects increase with prolonged courses of at least 400 mg/day. Nonetheless this toxicity rarely necessitates discontinuation of the drug (34). The primary adverse effects associated with itraconazole administration are GI symptoms, particularly nausea, abdominal pain, and diarrhea (34). These symptoms are generally described as mild by patients receiving the capsule or IV formulations of itraconazole. However, the symptoms are most frequently reported with the use of the oral solution and are generally more severe (35). In clinical trials of the oral solution in patients with AIDS, the frequency of GI adverse events were severe enough to necessitate withdrawal of therapy in 8–10%, which is a higher discontinuation rate than seen other populations (35). The propensity of the oral solution to cause diarrhea is likely due to the cyclodextrin, HP-βCD that helps to solubilize itraconazole. When given orally, HP-βCD is converted its basic glucose molecules by cyclodextrin transglycolase, which is produced by intestinal microflora (35). The glucose breakdown products are then absorbed and metabolized in the liver (22). The diarrhea associated with the oral solution is generally attributed to an osmotic effect of the HP-βCD in the GI tract (35).

Adverse effects with the IV formulation are generally mild and rare. The most common reactions reported with this formulation are phlebitis and other injection site reactions (35). As mentioned previously, use of the IV solution in patients with significant renal impairment is contraindicated. The concern stems from the fact that when administered IV, HP-βCD is primarily eliminated rapidly by glomerular filtration, and animal data suggesting high concentrations of cyclodextrins can damage renal tissue (20,21,36). Whether these animal data are applicable to HP-βCD, is unknown. Cyclodextrins are classified as "α," "β," or "γ" by the number of α-1, 4-linked glucose units in their molecular structure (36). β-Cyclodextrin has limited aqueous solubility due to intramolecular hydrogen bonding (36). The low aqueous solubility of β-cyclodextrin carries toxicological consequences. In mice and rats the parenteral administration of β-cyclodextrin leads to increases in blood urea nitrogen (BUN), a reduction in the rate of weight gain, decreases in liver mass (36). In addition, kidney mass is increased and the activity of numerous enzymes in the kidney are diminished (36). β-Cyclodextrin undergoes tubular reabsorption and concentrates in vacuoles, where, it precipitates due to its low aqueous solubility, (36). Histologically the resultant damage manifests as nephrosis (36). Clinicians should understand that HP-βCD, the cyclodextrin used in the IV and oral itraconazole solutions, is a hydroxylated β-cyclodextrin. The non-selective hydroxylation of β-cyclodextrin increases its water solubility and therefore may decrease its potential to cause renal toxicity (36). Rare life-threatening reactions (liver failure and CHF) can also occur with itraconazole therapy. Clinicians should keep this in mind when using itraconazole to treat non–life-threatening infections of the skin and nailbeds. Lastly, in contrast to ketoconazole, when given in standard doses, itraconazole has little or no inhibitory effect on human steroidogenesis. However, occasionally with doses in excess of 400 mg/day or with protracted courses, patients may experience a mineralocorticoid excess syndrome manifested by hypokalemia, hypertension, and edema (36).

3. Fluconazole

Fluconazole is considered the safest azole, and doses 4–5 times in excess of the recommended daily dose have been well tolerated. Similar to ketoconazole and itraconazole GI symptoms are the most commonly reported adverse effects, but with fluconazole they occur in less than 2% of patients and are frequently considered mild. As previously mentioned, transient elevations in serum transaminase levels occur, but progression to severe drug-induced hepatitis is exceedingly rare. Like itraconazole, fluconazole does not interfere with human steroidogenesis. Nonetheless, reversible alopecia has been reported in up to 20% of patients receiving at least 400 mg/day for more than 2 months (37). This adverse effect resolves within 6 months of stopping therapy or reducing the dose by 50% (37).

4. Voriconazole

In general like other azoles voriconazole is well tolerated. However, voriconazole is commonly associated with a unique adverse effect. Approximately 30% of patients experience reversible visual disturbances (30). Although noxious, these disturbances rarely lead to discontinuation of therapy. The reported visual disturbances include changes in color discrimination, blurred vision, increased sensitivity to light, and the appearance of bright spots. These disturbances are acute and diminish shortly into a course of therapy, and apparently there is no lasting damage to the retina (30). The underlying mechanism for this adverse effect is unknown.

Other common adverse effects include skin rash and elevations in serum transaminase levels. Like the other azoles, the elevations in serum transaminase levels are generally benign, however, life-threatening hepatitis associated with voriconazole use has been described (38). The risk of hepatitis associated with voriconazole use, appears to correlate with elevated serum drug concentrations (38). More rigorous monitoring of liver function tests is recommended for patients who will be treated with voriconazole (30).

III. IN VITRO ACTIVITY

A. Susceptibilty Testing

1. Susceptibility Testing and Interpretive Breakpoints

For many years clinically relevant antifungal susceptibility testing was non-existent. Consequently antifungal therapy was largely empiric and not guided by susceptibility data. Clinically relevant antifungal susceptibility testing has developed over the past two decades. Currently the National Committee for Clinical Laboratory Standards (NCCLS) has published an approved reference method for yeasts (M27-A). This method is fairly established for interpreting susceptibility data for azole antifungal agents. The NCCLS has also published a proposed reference method for molds (M38-P). However, the development of this method is still in its infancy. A comprehensive discussion of the specific methods used to test the susceptibility of fungal pathogens against the azoles is beyond the scope of this chapter. The reader is referred to two excellent comprehensive reviews that were recently published on the subject (5,39). Breakpoints exist for *Candida* sp. tested against

Table 3 NCCLS Breakpoints for the Azole Antifungals Agents Against *Candida* sp.

Agent	Susceptible (S) (μg/mL)	Susceptible-Dose Dependent (S-DD) (μg/mL)	Resistant (R) (μg/mL)
Ketoconazole	n/a	n/a	n/a
Fluconazole	≤8	16–32	≥64
Itraconazole	≤0.125	0.25–0.5[a]	≥1
Voriconazole	unk	unk	unk

[a]For isolates classified S-DD, plasma concentrations should be maintained in excess of 0.5 μg/mL.
Abbreviations: n/a, No specific breakpoints proposed, data suggest MIC > 0.125 μg/mL associated with diminished response (5).unk, Not yet determined.

the azoles (Table 3). There were no specific breakpoints proposed for ketoconazole against yeasts or molds. However, aggregate data suggest that *Candida* sp. with an MIC of >125 µg/mL as determined by the reference M27-A method will have reduced susceptibility (39). Breakpoints for fluconazole were established based on data from mucosal and invasive disease. The breakpoints contain a unique category known as "susceptibility is dose-dependent" (S-DD). This breakpoint considers the pharmacokinetics of fluconazole and emphasizes the importance of optimizing fluconazole blood and tissue concentrations for isolates with elevated MICs (39).

For itraconazole breakpoints against *Candida* sp. exist only for mucosal infections (39). Like fluconazole, there is an S-DD breakpoint that suggests the susceptibility depends upon drug delivery to the infection site (39). Depending on the formulation, itraconazole absorption is unpredictable and somewhat erratic. Therefore, lack of drug delivery to the infection site may be the true cause of the apparent reduced susceptibility. The correlation between itraconazole serum concentrations or MICs and outcome are unclear (39).

The NCCLS has yet to establish breakpoints for voriconazole against clinically relevant fungal pathogens, and the relationship between clinical outcome and in vitro susceptibility has yet to be determined (28). Interpretive breakpoints for *C. neoformans* and other molds against the azoles have yet to be established.

B. In Vitro Spectrum of Activity

1. Ketoconazole

Based upon in vitro observations, ketoconazole is considered to be fungistatic. Ketoconazole is very active in vitro against many yeasts including *C. neoformans* and *C. albicans.* Ketoconazole is active, but has less potency than other agents against non-albicans *Candida* sp., such as *C. glabrata, C. krusei,* and *C. parapsilosis.* In addition, ketoconazole also is active against common dimorphic or endemic fungi such as *Coccidioides immitis, H. capsulatum, B. dermatitidis, Paracoccidioides brasiliensis, Sporothrix schenckii* (11). The activity of ketoconazole against *Aspergillus* sp. is variable, and it is not active against *Aspergillus fumigatis.* Despite a fairly broad spectrum of activity, clinically ketoconazole has been relegated to a second-line drug by the more potent and safer triazoles.

2. Fluconazole

The in vitro activity of fluconazole is generally considered to be fungistatic (40). In addition, its activity is essentially limited to yeasts. Fluconazole is highly active against *C. neoformans* and *C. albicans.* Moreover, fluconazole is also active against certain *non-albicans Candida* sp., such as *C. parapsilosis, C. tropicalis,* and *C. lusitaniae* (41,42). However, the activity of fluconazole against other *albicans Candida* sp. is poor. *C. krusei* is inherently resistant, and *C. glabrata* is often resistant to fluconazole. Fluconazole has activity against *C. immitis,* but it has poor activity against other dimorphic fungi such as *H. capsulatum* and *B. dermatitidis.* Fluconazole is devoid of activity against *Aspergillus* sp., *Fusarium* sp., and the agents of Zygomycetes.

3. Itraconazole

The activity of itraconazole is species- and strain-dependent. In vitro itraconazole exerts fungicidal activity against filamentous fungi, and some strains *of C. neoformans* (40). However, against yeasts itraconazole is generally fungistatic. Itraconazole has a very broad spectrum of in vitro activity and is very active against dermatophytes and many yeasts including *C. neoformans, C. albicans.* Moreover, itraconazole is also active in vitro against certain *non-albicans Candida* sp., such as *C. parapsilosis, C. tropicalis,* and *C. lusitaniae* (42). In addition, itraconazole has varying in vitro activity against other non-*albicans Candida* sp., such as *C. glabrata, C. krusei* (42). Itraconazole has excellent in vitro activity against common dimorphic or endemic fungi including *B. dermatitidis,* C. immitis, *H. capsulatum, H. duboisii,* and *P. brasiliensis* (11,43). Itraconazole also possesses good activity against *S. schenckii* (11). Prior to the development of voriconazole, itraconazole was the only azole with clinically significant activity against *Aspergillus* sp. Like other early azoles, itraconazole is devoid of activity against *Fusarium* sp., and the agents of Zygomycetes. In addition, itraconazole is unique in that hydroxyitraconazole, its primary metabolite in humans, is bioactive (16).

There are few data assessing the activity of hydroxyitraconazole against fungal pathogens. The antifungal activity of hydroxyitraconazole was tested in a study of quantitative differences between biologic and chemical analytical methods used to measure itraconazole concentrations in body fluids. Accordingly, the antifungal activity of hydroxyitraconazole was found to be nearly identical to that of itraconazole. Hydroxyitraconazole was twice as active against *C. pseudotropicalis,* which was the isolate used in the bioassay (44). Because the bioassay measures total activity and does not distinguish the contribution of hydroxyitraconazole from itraconazole, these data explain why, compared to chemical analytical methods, bioassays overestimate itraconazole concentrations in body fluids (44). Of more interest, the activity of hydroxyitraconazole *A. fumigatus, A. terreus, C. neoformans, and C. immitis* was the same as that of itraconazole (44). In drug interaction studies, the two compounds were additive against *A. fumigatus,* and slight synergy was observed against *C. pseudotropicalis* and C. neoformans (44). Interestingly, more pronounced synergy were observed against *C. immitis* (44). Whether this additive or synergistic activity occurs in vivo or how much hydroxyitraconazole contributes to the clinical activity of itraconazole is unknown. However, in the body, it circulates at 1–2 times the concentration of the parent compound after IV or oral administration, respectively (16).

4. Voriconazole

Similar to itraconazole, voriconazole exerts fungicidal activity against select opportunistic fungi (40). In addition, fungicidal activity against certain *non-albicans Candida* isolates and C. *neoformans* has been observed (40). However, against most yeasts, voriconazole exerts fungistatic activity (40). Voriconazole is the most potent azole available, and it possesses as very broad spectrum of activity against dermatophytes, yeasts, and molds. Voriconazole is active against all *Candida* sp., including those with acquired (i.e., *C. albicans)* or inherent (i.e., C. *glabrata* and C. *krusei)* resistance to fluconazole (30). Voriconazole is very active against other yeasts including *C. neoformans,* and *Trichosporon beigelii,* which is typically resistant to the other azoles and polyenes (30).

Voriconazole is also highly active against filamentous fungi such as *Aspergillus* sp., and its activity against *A. fumigatis* and *A. flavus* is comparable to that of itraconazole (28). Most notably it possesses activity against resistant *Aspergillus* sp., including *A. terreus*, which is often resistant to amphotericin B, and a clinical isolate of *A. fumigatus* resistant to itraconazole (30,45). Voriconazole is very active against the dimorphic fungi including *B. dermatitidisp, C. immitis,* and *H. capsulatum.* However, against *S. schenckii* it is less active. Voriconazole is active against many amphotericin resistant molds, including certain strains of *Pseudoallescheria boydii, Fusarium* sp., and other less common opportunistic pathogens (30). Similar to the other azoles, voriconazole is devoid of activity against the agents of Zygomycetes (30).

C. Pharmacodynamic Properties

The study of pharmacodynamics examines relationships among drug concentrations, time, and pharmacological effects (46). These relationships can be elucidated in vivo through the use of infected animal models, which incorporate pharmacokinetic measurements and antibiotic effect. In-vitro, these relationships are characterized by the use of classic time-kill assays, the study of persistent and subinhibitory effects, and in vitro models or cell cultures (40). While these methods have been employed in the study of antibacterials for many years, they have only recently been applied to antifungal agents, specifically the azoles. Consequently, the pharmacodynamic behavior of ketoconazole has not been well characterized.

The pharmacodynamic characteristics of an antimicrobial are defined by two important relationships. The first relationship is the effect of drug concentration on the rate and extent of organism killing (46). When increasing drug concentrations enhance the rate and extent of killing, the relationship is referred to as "concentration dependent" killing. In this case optimal killing is achieved by maximizing the peak drug concentration in relation to the MIC of the organism. Thus, this relationship is defined by the pharmacodynamic parameter known as the "peak-to-MIC ratio" (peak/MIC). When the rate and extent of killing is enhanced by the time course of drug exposure rather than by increasing drug concentration, the relationship is referred to as "concentration independent" killing. In this case optimal killing is achieved by maximizing the time the drug concentration remains above the MIC by some factor over the course of the dosing interval. Thus, this relationship is defined by the two pharmacodynamic parameters known as the "percentage of time that serum drug concentration exceeds the MIC" (T > MIC), and "the area under the serum concentration–time curve in relation to the MIC" (AUC/MIC). The second relationship that defines the pharmacodynamic characteristics of an antimicrobial is the ability of the organism to grow after drug exposure. In terms of antifungals, the key parameter describing this relationship is the so-called "postantifungal effect" (PAE). This parameter is a measure of time during which there is continued suppression of growth at concentrations below the MIC.

1. Fluconazole

Pharmacodynamic behavior of fluconazole is well characterized. Classic in vitro time-kill studies and an in vitro dynamic bloodstream infection model reveal that against *C. albicans* fluconazole exhibits concentration-independent fungistatic activity (47–49). Similarly, in vitro time-kill assays revealed that against *C. neoformans,* fluconazole exhibits concentration-independent fungistatic activity (50,51). Studies using incubation periods longer than 72 hr and non-proliferating growth conditions have suggested fluconazole may also exert a direct fungicidal effect on *C. albicans*

(52). In vivo animal infection models have confirmed that the pharmacodynamic value of fluconazole that best predicts outcome is the AUC:MIC ratio, which indicates concentration-independent behavior (40). Moreover, the infection models revealed that fungal burdens were similarly reduced regardless of the frequency of administration of a given total dose, and the optimal AUC:MIC was similar regardless of strain susceptibility (40). Fluconazole pharmacodynamic relationships have not been examined in infected patients. The in vitro persistent effects of fluconazole are apparently dependent upon the presence of human serum. In serum-free growth media there was no measurable PAE against C. albicans and C. neoformans (53,54). However, in the presence of fresh serum a short PAE was observed against C. albicans (53).

2. Itraconazole

The pharmacodynamic behavior of itraconazole is genus dependent. Classic in vitro time-kill experiments in conventional media reveal that against Candida sp. and C. neoformans, itraconazole exhibits concentration-independent fungistatic activity (49,51,55). In these studies maximum effectiveness occurred when concentrations were maintained at two times the MIC for Candida species, and 4–8 times above the MIC of C. neoformans (51,55). Similar pharmacodynamic behavior of itraconazole against Candida species was observed in time-kill assays in the presence of 80% human serum (56). In contrast to the yeasts, the pharmacodynamic behavior of itraconazole against Aspergillus sp., demonstrated both concentration- and time-dependent cidal activity (57).

The relationship between itraconazole serum concentration and efficacy has been assessed in a model of invasive pulmonary aspergillosis in immunocompromised rabbits. Like humans, peak serum concentrations were highly variable, however, a pharmacodynamic relationship between itraconazole serum concentrations, and efficacy as a function of fungal burden in lung tissue was observed. Higher plasma concentrations were associated with decreases in tissue burden of A. fumigatus (58). This study suggested that a threshold value of serum-drug concentration maybe required for optimal effectiveness. However, whether the results of this study can be extrapolated to humans is questionable. The study used an extemporaneous prepared suspension using the capsules, and a recent study has found that the rabbit is not an ideal animal model in predicting the oral absorption of itraconazole in humans (59).

Given the above animal data, the erratic pharmacokinetics and the differential pharmacodynamic behavior of itraconazole several studies have tried to establish a threshold concentration in humans that is predicative of response. The results of these studies vary, but in general, for optimal effectiveness, investigators advocate itraconazole plasma trough concentration of at least $0.25\,\mu g/mL$ (measured by HPLC) (2). However, recent preliminary work suggests that $0.5\,\mu g/mL$ is the minimal desirable target concentration for the prevention and treatment of invasive fungal infections, especially in neutropenic hosts (60).

3. Voriconazole

Pharmacodynamic relationships for voriconazole not been fully characterized, and have only been studied in vitro using time-kill assays. These methods indicate that voriconazole exhibits concentration-independent fungistatic activity C. albicans, C. glabrata, C. tropicalis, and C. neoformans (57,61). In contrast, voriconazole displayed concentration-independent fungicidal activity against *A.fumigatus,* further suggesting that the fungicidal activity of the azoles may be organisms specific (57). Similar to fluconazole, the in vitro persistent effects of voriconazole are apparently dependent upon the presence of human serum. In serum-free growth media there was no measurable PAE against *C. albicans,* but in the presence of fresh serum a relatively short PAE was observed (62).

IV. MECHANISMS OF RESISTANCE TO AZOLES

A comprehensive discussion of the specific mechanisms of resistance employed by fungal pathogens against the azoles is beyond the scope of this chapter. The reader is referred to two excellent comprehensive reviews that were recently published on the subject (5,63).

In general microbes resist the effects of antimicrobials by producing enzymes to modify the antibiotic; by qualitative or quantitative modifications in the cellular target; or reducing access to the cellular target. Fungi resist the effects of the azoles by modifying the target or reducing the access to the target or a combination of both (5). The underlying mechanism of fluconazole resistance has been examined by comparing sterol composition, fluconazole accumulation, and inhibition of 14α-demethylase in clinical isolates of *Candida* sp., that express intrinsic fluconazole resistance (*C. krusei*), and a fluconazole-susceptible *C. albicans* isolate (64). Sterol content did not differ between the species, but the affinity of 14α-demethylase for fluconazole was greater in *C. albicans* (64). Moreover, over-time fluconazole accumulation in *C. krusei* was less than that in *C. albicans* (64). Thus, in this study, qualitative modifications and active efflux were implicated as coexisting resistance mechanisms in the strains of *C. krusei*. Yet, other studies examining clinical isolates have implicated only a single mechanism, (i.e., qualitative alterations in the target enzyme) (5).

Over expression of 14α-demethylase represents a quantitative modification of the target and it has also been identified as a mechanism of resistance to the azoles in a strain of *C. glabrata*. In this strain an increase in the ergosterol content led to a corresponding decrease in susceptibility to fluconazole, itraconazole, and amphotericin B (65). The increased ergosterol content was attributed to over expression of 14α-demethylase, but the strain also had evidence of active efflux of fluconazole (65). Interestingly, there was no evidence of itraconazole efflux in this strain, indicating that the azole cross-resistance was likely due to over expression of 14α-demethylase. The importance of over expression of 14α-demethylase as a mechanism of resistance is difficult to ascertain since it has only been observed in *C. glabrata*, and at least for fluconazole, other mechanisms may contribute to the resistance phenotype.

Active efflux is likely a primary method by which fungi resist the effects of the azoles. Fungi possess two types of efflux pumps. These transporters belong to either the "major facilitator" (MF) or "ATP-binding cassette" (ABC) superfamilies of proteins. Both superfamilies transport a diverse array of substrates and are involved in transport of a variety of toxic compounds out of the cell (5). Resistance to azoles is rare, and the understanding of the mechanisms involved and how they manifest clinically are evolving. Although the primary mechanism of resistance to the azoles is active efflux, high-level resistance is in fact due to multiple mechanisms acting in concert. In contrast over-expression of a target enzyme may result in cross-resistance to other azoles.

Most clinical reports of azole resistance, specifically fluconazole, involve *Candida* sp. Azole resistance is commonly observed in HIV infected patients. Estimates suggest overall, approximately one third of patients with advanced HIV will develop an azole-resistant infection (66). Azole resistant *C. albicans* are commonly isolated in AIDS patients with oropharyngeal candidasis (67). However, azole resistance to non-*albicans Candida* has also been observed in this population (67). In these cases the same strain is repeatedly isolated and over time, its MIC increases with subsequent azole therapy. As the MIC climbs, clinicians often increase the dose of fluconazole. This is approach is generally successful up to an MIC of $64\,\mu g/mL$ (67), at higher MIC values even high dose fluconazole therapy ($>800\,mg/day$) frequently fails, but other azoles maybe effective. Risk factors for the development of azole resistance in this population includes patients with $CD4^+$ cell counts of $<50/mm^3$, prior exposure to azoles and a cumulative azole dose $\geq 10\,g$ (68).

Azole resistant infections among non-HIV infected patients are most often due to non-*albicans Candida* sp., particularly *C. krusei* and *C. glabrata* (67), and occur in patients with malignancies. Risk factors for the development of azole resistance include leukemia, lymphoma, solid tumor, BMT, neutropenia, diabetes, and high-dose steroid therapy. Although azole resistance, if observed, occurs most often in *Candida* sp., it has also been observed in a variety of clinical isolates, including fluconazole resistant *C. neoformans,* and *H. capsulatum* and itraconazole resistant *A. fumigatus* and with more use it will likely surface with voriconazole (10,68–70).

V. IN VIVO EXPERIMENTAL ACTIVITY

A number of animal models, both immunosuppressed and non-immuosuppressed have been developed and used in the study of the pathogenesis of invasive mycoses, antifungal pharmacodynamics, and toxicities. These models have provided invaluable information on the activity and dose–response relationship of a drug or drug combination against a pathogen, In addition, in contrast to the clinical setting, these models allow for control of confounding variables, and thus provide for more specific outcome measures. A comprehensive review of the many infection models for a number of life-threatening systemic mycoses is beyond the scope of this chapter. Since most work has been directed at studying the effectiveness of an azole in the treatment of disseminated candidiasis, or invasive aspergillosis, models of these infections are discussed below.

A. *Candida* Species

The effectiveness of the azoles in the treatment of disseminated candidiasis and other serious candidal infections has been evaluated in a variety of neutropenic and non-neutropenic animal models including mice, rats, guinea pigs, and rabbits. When evaluating the results of these studies clinicians should be cognizant of interspecies differences in azole pharmacokinetics, and the route of drug administration as both may affect the performance of the model. This consideration is particularly germane when evaluating the experimental efficacy of itraconazole in fungal infection models. Itraconazole efficacy in an infection model may vary with dose, administration route, formulation, diet, and fungal species. In addition, the results will vary among animal models.

The effective itraconazole dose for the treatment of experimental disseminated candidiasis in murine models is quite variable (71). Some investigators even noted no effect with oral itraconazole despite administration of doses up to 80 mg/kg (72). Consequently, itraconazole has been associated with poor activity in mice. This lack of activity likely reflects differences in murine pharmacokinetics, or is related to the difficulty of formulating an oral-dosage itraconazole form for animal consumption. Significantly higher itraconazole plasma concentrations are achieved in DBA/2 mice than in BALB/c mice, regardless of whether the drug is administered intraperitoneally (i.p.) or orally (73). Additionally, prior to the advent of the oral HP-βCD solution form of itraconazole, non-standardized preparations were studied, and bioavailability data for these products in animals were often lacking. Such formulations have been studied in humans and they are poorly absorbed (74).

In contrast, to murine models, oral or parenterally administered itraconazole in guinea pigs has good activity and significantly enhances survival in candidiasis and several other fungal pathogen models (75,76). Whether this is due to differences in pharmacokinetics or the itraconazole formulation used is unclear. Itraconazole plasma concentrations are lower in guinea pigs than in mice, but the oral HP-βCD solution form of itraconazole, rather than non-standardized preparations have been used in the guinea pig models (73). Itraconazole efficacy in a given animal model may ultimately depend upon the formulation employed. In contrast to oral administration, IV itraconazole prolonged the survival of mice, but had little effect on reducing fungal burden in the end organs (71). Moreover, diet may influence efficacy by altering the pharmacokinetics of specific azoles in certain animals. Substituting grapefruit juice for water in the animal's diet has been shown to enhance serum voriconazole concentrations in mice (77). However, the effect varies across animals and between animals. Grapefruit juice had no effect on serum itraconazole concentrations in DBA/2 or BALB/c mice regardless of whether the drug was administered orally or parenterally, yet in the same study it increased plasma itraconazole concentrations following oral administration in guinea pigs (73). Collectively, the experimental efficacy data for itraconazole in the treatment of candidiasis are consistent with the experience in humans. That is, because of its unpredictable pharmacokinetics, oral itraconazole is not appropriate for the treatment of disseminated candidiasis. Rather, if itraconazole is to be used for the treatment of disseminated candidiasis, then it should be administered parenterally so that adequate serum concentrations are achieved.

Fluconazole for the treatment of disseminated candidiasis has been extensively studied in a variety of animal models. In general, fluconazole is significantly more active in the prevention (i.e., prophylaxis) and early (i.e., empirical) treatment of disseminated candidiasis than in the treatment of established (i.e., chronic) infection (78). In comparisons using granulocytopenic rabbit models of disseminated candidiasis, fluconazole was as effective as amphotericin B with or without flucytosine when used for preventative or early treatment. However, in a chronic disseminated candidiasis model, fluconazole was less active than amphotericin B plus flucytosine (78).

Similar to itraconazole, there are unique interspecies differences in voriconazole that affect its activity in certain animal models. In early experimental infection models it was noted that serum voriconazole concentrations are negligible in mice, consequently other models, namely the guinea pig, were used for the study of this azole (77). In a model of disseminated candidiasis in non-neutropenic and neutropenic guinea pigs, voriconazole produced efficacy similar to that of fluconazole or itraconazole, and was more active than amphotericin B (79). Voriconazole produced good activity in animals infected with fluconazole resistant strains of *C. glabrata*, *C. krusei*, and *C. albicans* (79). In a neutropenic guinea-pig model of hematogenously disseminated *C. krusei* infection voriconazole was significantly more effective than either amphotericin B or fluconazole in eradicating *C. krusei* from brain, liver, and kidney tissue (80).

B. Invasive Aspergillosis

Similar to disseminated candidiasis models, studies of oral itraconazole in murine aspergillosis models usually demonstrate little activity. In contrast, in an immuno-suppressed, temporarily leukopenic rabbit model of invasive aspergillosis the oral HP-βCD solution form of itraconazole improved animal survival. At high doses (40 mg/kg/day) it also significantly reduced antigen levels, significantly eradicated *A. fumigatus* from tissues and was as effective as amphotericin B (81). Oral itracona-zole is highly effective as prophylaxis or treatment of established invasive aspergillo-sis in guinea-pig infection models (82,83). In addition, IV itraconazole has produced significant activity in a invasive aspergillosis guinea-pig model (76).

Voriconazole has been studied extensively in a variety of experimental infection models of invasive aspergillosis. Compared to control, and to itraconazole oral voriconazole significantly improved survival in a rat model of invasive pulmonary aspergillosis (84). Similar data were observed in a model of disseminated aspergillosis due to *A.fumigatus*, in an immunosuppressed, leukopenic rabbit and guinea pig (75,85). Because of their fungistatic activity, azoles have not had good activity in experimental models of fungal endocarditis. However, voriconazole has demon-strated unique activity in the prevention and treatment of experimental *A. fumigatus* endocarditis in guinea pigs (86).

VI. CLINICAL EFFICACY OF THE AZOLES

The azoles have been evaluated in large prospective randomized trials, key clinical trials, focused primarily in neutropenic hosts. The studies that demonstrate the effi-cacy of the azoles in the treatment or prevention of systemic infections due to oppor-tunistic fungal pathogens are summarized below. Ketoconazole has been supplanted by the newer azoles and is primarily considered only as an alternative agent, and therefore will not be discussed further.

A. Fluconazole

Currently fluconazole is the most widely used azole for the treatment of infections due to *Candida* sp., Fluconazole is devoid of activity against *Aspergillus* sp., there-fore, it is studied in clinical trials for its use in the treatment of invasive or dissemi-nated candidiasis. The results of two large prospective studies indicate that fluconazole 400 mg/day as effective as amphotericin B 0.5–0.6 mg/kg/day in the treatment of invasive candidiasis in non-neutropenic hosts. In these studies response rates for fluconazole and amphotericin B were similar, (57–70% vs. 62–79%, respec-tively), (87,88). In both studies the incidence of non-*albicans Candida* sp., was low. Moreover, observed mortality rates were consistent with that associated with candi-demia and there was no difference in mortality rates between the treatments. When the source of the infection is related to a vascular catheter, removal and replacement of the catheter was an important therapeutic modality (89).

There are no large prospective studies comparing the efficacy of fluconazole to amphotericin B in neutropenic hosts, but data from observational studies suggest the two treatments may be similarly effective (42). Based upon these data in non-neutropenic patients who are medically stable, or in whom the infecting pathogen is known fluconazole is a safe and effective alternative to amphotericin B in the treatment of candidemia.

Several large clinical trials have evaluated fluconazole as prophylactic therapy in the immunocompromised hosts (i.e., neutropenic cancer patients, BMT, etc.). Administering antifungal therapy to persistently febrile neutropenic patients several days after the initiation of antibacterial therapy has become standard practice. Although this practice stems from the results of two classic prospective trials performed nearly two decades ago, some have suggested that this practice has evolved largely based on theoretical priniciples rather than clinical science (90). The first randomized trial of fluconazole in this setting demonstrated that it as effective as amphotericin B in patients at low risk for invasive aspergillosis (91). Subsequently a larger trial also demonstrated that fluconazole was not inferior to amphotericin B in this setting (90). In patients who are at high risk for amphotericin B nephrotoxicity, these studies indicate that fluconazole is a reasonable alternative.

Two large-randomized, placebo-controlled trials established that fluconazole 400 mg administered as prophylaxis decreased the risk of superficial and invasive fungal infections after allogeneic and autologous blood and marrow transplantation (91,92). In one study, fluconazole was administered to primarily autologous graft recipients and only during neutropenia, while in the other it was used primarily in allogeneic graft recipients and administered for 75 days. Only one trial demonstrated a decrease in overall mortality (92). Whether fluconazole prophylaxis needs to be continued for 75 days in all blood and marrow transplant recipients or only allogeneic graft recipients has been debated. Data from an 8-year long-term follow up study demonstrate that the survival benefit of prophylactic fluconazole administered for 75-days is realized only by allogeneic graft recipients. Furthermore the study demonstrated that the survival benefit is a result of a reduction in candidiasis related deaths, which frequently occur during acute graft-versus-host disease (93).

B. Itraconazole

Although itraconazole is active against *Candida* sp., there are no prospective data from large clinical trials describing the efficacy of itraconazole for the treatment of candidemia. In addition, there have been no large, randomized clinical trials comparing the efficacy of itraconazole to other agents with activity against *Aspergillus* sp., However, because of its activity against *Aspergillus* sp., itraconazole has been evaluated in large clinical trials for antifungal therapy in persistently febrile neutropenic patients, and as long-term antifungal prophylaxis in allogeneic hematopoietic stem-cell transplant recipients.

In a randomized controlled trial IV and oral itraconazole was compared to amphotericin B deoxycholate as empiric antifungal therapy in persistently febrile neutropenic patients, who had not responded to antibacterial therapy. Patients were randomized to receive amphotericin B deoxycholate 0.7–1.0 mg/kg/day, or IV itraconazole 200 mg/day for 1–2 weeks, at which time they were switched to itraconazole oral solution 400 mg/day (94). The intent-to-treat analysis revealed that overall 47%

of patients randomized to itraconazole responded, in contrast to only 38% of the patients who received amphotericin B. Most of the patients had received prior recent antifungal prophylaxis, and when this was considered the difference in response rate was maintained (94). Significantly fewer drug-related toxicities were seen in patients receiving itraconazole. Consequently, significantly fewer patients receiving itraconazole were withdrawn from the study due to toxicities (94). The study suggests that itraconazole is safer than, and at least as effective as amphotericin B as empirical antifungal therapy in persistently febrile neutropenic patients (94). However, this study was unblinded, which may have introduced bias into the study, particularly in the decision to discontinue the investigational drug due to toxicity (90).

As described above, fluconazole prophylaxis in allogeneic blood and marrow transplant recipients has been shown to reduce the incidence of invasive infections and in allogeneic graft recipients its long-term use is associated with a demonstrable survival benefit (92,93). Infections due to *Aspergillus* sp., are a significant concern throughout the transplant process. Given the safety profile of itraconazole, and its activity against *Aspergillus* sp., it is an attractive alternative to amphotericin B deoxycholate and fluconazole in this setting. IV and oral itraconazole were compared to IV and oral fluconazole as long-term prophylaxis in allogeneic hematopoietic stem-cell transplant recipients. Patients were randomized to receive itraconazole 200 mg/day or fluconazole 400 mg/day IV and then orally for 100 days after transplantation (95). Proven invasive fungal infections were significantly less common among patients receiving itraconazole (9%), compared to those receiving fluconazole (25%) (95). Infections due to *C. albicans* occurred in both groups, but patients receiving itraconazole had fewer invasive fungal infections due to *C. glabrata*, *C. krusei*, and *Aspergillus* sp., (95). Adverse events were less common with fluconazole (95). Based upon the data it was concluded that itraconazole is more effective than fluconazole for long-term prophylaxis in allogeneic hematopoietic stem-cell transplant recipients. However, this study was unblinded, which may have introduced bias into the analysis of the study. In centers with a high incidence of fungal isolates with reduced susceptibility towards fluconazole, itraconazole administered as the IV and oral solution may be a reasonable alternative to fluconazole. However, clinicians must balance its potential benefits with the uncertainty of using the IV formulation in patients with reduced renal function, and the drugs' inherent potential to interact with other medications.

C. Voriconazole

Voriconazole was compared to liposomal amphotericin B as empiric antifungal therapy in persistently febrile neutropenic patients in a large, randomized trial (96). This study was unblinded, which may have introduced bias into the study, particularly in the decision to discontinue the investigational drug (90). The study was also designed to demonstrate non-inferiority of voriconazole by a difference in success rate not in excess of 10% for the composite endpoint. A modified intent-to-treat analysis revealed the overall success rate for voriconazole was 26% compared to 30.6% for liposomal amphotericin B. However, the lower bounds of the 95% CI for the differences in treatment groups slightly exceeded the 10% bounds set in the non-inferiority definition. A secondary analysis of the individual components of the composite endpoint revealed that there were significantly fewer proven or probable breakthrough fungal infections with voriconazole (96). The authors concluded that voriconazole is a suitable alternative to amphotericin B preparations for empiric antifungal therapy in persistently febrile neutropenic patients (96).

However, in light of the study design the analysis was questioned and the subsequent conclusion was somewhat disputed (97). The analysis presented was unstratified, yet a stratified analysis was initially planned and given the design of the study, it was deemed the more appropriate primary analysis (97). Second, voriconazole did not fulfill that criterion for non-inferiority to liposomal amphotericin B. In addition, even voriconazole treatment was associated with breakthrough fungal infections, the analyses of the other four components of the composite end point favored liposomal amphotericin B (97). Therefore, whether voriconazole is not as good as liposomal amphotericin B as empiric therapy in persistently febrile neutropenic hosts is still a matter of debate. Clinicians should interpret the results of the study in terms of their own clinical experience and determine what difference in success rate is acceptable to them.

VII. DRUG INTERACTIONS

Drug interactions involving the azoles are discussed in Chapter 17. In general, drug interactions occur primarily in the GI tract, liver, and kidneys by a variety of mechanisms. In the GI tract azole drug interactions result from alterations in pH, complexation with ions, or interference with transport and enzymatic processes involved in gut wall (i.e., presystemic) drug metabolism. In the liver they occur as a result of interference with phase I or II drug metabolism, or interactions with transport proteins. In the kidney–drug interactions can occur through interference with glomerular filtration, active tubular excretion, or interactions with transport proteins. The azoles are one of the few drug classes that can cause or be involved in drug interactions at all of these sites, by one or more of the above mechanisms. Many of the drug–drug interactions involving the azoles occur class-wide. Therefore, when using the azoles, the clinician must be aware of the many drug–drug interactions, both real and potential, associated with this class. For a comprehensive review of drug interactions specifically involving the azoles, the reader is referred to Chapter 17 and two recent reviews on this topic (4,13).

VIII. CONCLUSION

The systemically acting azoles are one of the largest classes of systemically acting antifungals. The chemical properties of these drugs influence their pharmacokinetics, and are the basis of the many drug interactions associated with these agents. They act at a key step in ergosterol synthesis. Unlike other classes of antifungals they are available as oral and IV dosage forms. Each agent has a unique pharmacokinetic profile and among existing antifungals as a class they among the safest agents. Additionally they are broad spectrum in activity, and they typically exhibit concentration-independent, static pharmacodynamic effects. As a class these agents possess potent yet diverse spectrum of activity. Fluconazole possesses perhaps the narrowest spectrum of activity and is primarily active against *Candida* and *Cryptococcus* sp., In contrast itraconazole, and voriconazole possesses activity against yeasts and molds including *Candida* and *Aspergillus* species, and other opportunistic pathogens. Although antifungal susceptibility testing is still in its infancy, the susceptibility testing methods and breakpoints for *Candida* species are well defined. Resistance to the azoles is relatively uncommon, but when it occurs it is most likely due to either alterations in the target enzyme, or active efflux or a combination of both. Clinically, resistance is most often observed in the setting of HIV infection and AIDS.

The azoles have demonstrated potency in against many pathogens in a variety of experimental animal models of infection. However, in order to interpret the results obtained in these models clinicians should be cognizant of the complex pharmacokinetics displayed by itraconazole and voriconazole, and the impact the dosage form may have on the function of the model. Lastly, in large clinical trials in immunocompromised hosts the azoles have demonstrated efficacy as prophylactic and empirical therapy. Thus, they are alternative treatments to amphotericin B for a variety of systemic mycoses. As the azoles continue to grow as a class, so too will the options available to clinicians in selecting therapy for life-threatening mycoses in immunocompromised hosts. Future agents will likely continue to expand the spectrum of activity and offer improved pharmacokinetics.

REFERENCES

1. Daneshmend TK, Warnock DW. Clinical phamacokinetics of systemic antifungal drugs. Clin pharmacokinet 1983; 8:17–42.
2. Poirier JM, Cheymol G. Optimization of itraconazole therapy using target drug concentrations. Clin Pharmacokinet 1998; 35:461–473.
3. Richardson K, Cooper K, Marriott MS, Tarbit MH, Troke PF, Whittle PJ. Discovery of fluconazole, a novel antifungal agent. Rev Infect Dis 1990; 12(suppl 3):S267–S271.
4. Chiou CC, Groll AH, Walsh TJ. New drugs and novel targets for the treatment of invasive fungal infections in patients with cancer. Oncologist 2000; 5:120–135.
5. Ghannoum MA, Rice LB. Antifungal agents: mode of action, mechanisms of resistance, and correlation of these mechanisms with bacterial resistance. Clin Microbiol Rev 1999; 12:501–517.
6. Zacchino SA, Yunes RA, Filho VC, Enriz RD, Kouznetsov V, Ribas JC. The need for new antifungal drugs; screening for antifungal compounds with a selective mode of action with emphasis on inhibitors of the fungal cell wall. In: Rai M, Mares D, eds. Plant-derived Antimycotics, Current Trends and Future Prospects. New York: Haworth Press Inc., 2003:1–48.
7. Hitchcock CK, Dickinson K, Brown SB, Evans EG, Adams DJ. Interaction of azole antifungal antibiotics with cytochrome P450-dependent 14α-sterol demethylase purified from *Candida albicans*. J Biochem 1990; 266:475–480.
8. Bellanger P, Nast CC, Fratti R, Sanati H, Ghannoum M. Voriconazole (UK-109,496) inhibits the growth and alters the morphology of fluconazole-susceptible and -resistant *Candida* species. Antimicrob Agents Chemother 1997; 41:1840–1842.
9. Sanati H, Belanger P, Rutilio F, Ghannoum M. A new triazole, voriconazole (UK-109,496), blocks sterol biosynthesis in *Candida albicans* and *Candida krusei*. Antimicrob Agents Chemother 1997; 41:2492–2496.
10. Wheat J, Marichal P, Vanden Bossche H, Le Monte A, Connolly P. Hypothesis on the mechanism of resistance to fluconazole in *Histoplasma capsulatum*. Antimicrob Agents Chemother 1997; 41:410–414.
11. Como JA, Dismukes WE. Oral azole drugs as systemic antifungal therapy. N Engl J Med 1994; 330:263–272.
12. Thummel KE, Wilkinson GR. In vitro and in vivo drug interactions involving human CYP3A. Annu Rev Pharmacol Toxicol 1998; 38:389–430.

13. Venkatakrishnan K, von Moltke LL, Greenblatt DJ. Effects of the antifungal agents on oxidative drug metabolism: clinical relevance. Clin Pharmacokinet 2000; 38:111–180.

14. Wang E, Lew K, Casciano CN, Clement RP, Johnson WW. Interaction of common azole antifungals with P-glycoprotein. Antimicrob Agents Chemother 2002; 46:160–165.

15. Wacher VJ, Wu CJ, Benet LZ. Overlapping substrate specificities and tissue distribution of cytochrome P450 3A and P-glycoprotein: implications for drug delivery and activity in cancer chemotherapy. Mol Carcinog 1995; 13:129–134.

16. Heykants J, Van Peer A, Van de Velde V, Van Rooy P, Meuldermans W, Lavrijsen K, Woestenborghs R, Van Cutsem J, Cauwenbergh G. The clinical pharmacokinetics of itraconazole: an overview. Mycoses 1989; 32 (suppl 1):67–87.

17. Van de Velde VJS, Van Peer A, Heykants JJP, Woestenborghs RJH, Eng C, Van Rooy P, DeBeule KL, Cauwenbergh GFMJ. Effect of food on the pharmacokinetics of a new hydroxypropyl-β-cyclodextrin formulation of itraconazole. Pharmacotherapy 1996; 16:424–428.

18. Barone JA, Moskovitz BL, Guarnieri J, Hassell AE, Colaizzi JL, Bierman RH, Jessen L. Food interaction and steady-state pharmacokinetics of itraconazole oral solution in healthy volunteers. Pharmacotherapy 1998; 18:295–301.

19. Barone JA, Moskovitz BL, Guarnieri J, Hassell AE, Colaizzi JL, Bierman RH, Jessen L. Enhanced bioavailability of itraconazole in hydroxypropyl-β-cyclodextrin solution versus capsules in healthy volunteers. Antimicrob Agents Chemother 1998; 42:1862–1865.

20. Zhou H, Goldman M, Wu J, Woestenborghs R, Hassell AE, Lee P, Baruch A, Pesco-Koplowitz L, Borum J, Wheat LJ. A pharmacokinetic study of intravenous itraconazole followed by oral administration of itraconazole oral capsules in patients with human immunodeficiency virus infection. J Clin Pharmacol 1998; 38:593–602.

21. Zhao Q, Zhou H, Pesco-Koplowitz L. Pharmacokinetics of intravenous itraconazole followed by itraconazole oral solution in patients with human immunodeficiency virus infection. J Clin Pharmacol 2001; 41:1319–1328.

22. Stevens DA. Itraconazole in cyclodextrin solution. Pharmacotherapy 1999; 19:603–611.

23. Gubbins PO, McConnell SA, Penzak SR. Drug interactions associated with antifungal agents. In: Piscitelli SC, Rodvold KA, eds. Drug Interactions in Infectious Diseases. Totowa, New Jersey: Humana Press, 2001:185–217.

24. Debruyne D, Ryckelynk JP. Clinical pharmacokinetics of fluconazole. Clin Pharmacokinet 1993; 24:10–27.

25. Pelz RK, Lipsett PA, Swoboda MS, Merz W, Rinaldi MG, Hendrix CW. Enteral fluconazole is well absorbed in critically ill surgical patients. Surgery 2002; 131:534–540.

26. Brammer KW, Coakley AJ, Jezequel SG, Tarbit MH. The disposition and metabolism of [^{14}C] fluconazole in humans. Drug Metab Dispos 1991; 19:764–767.

27. Black DJ, Kunze KL, Wienkers LC, Gidal BE, Seaton TL, McDonnell ND, Evans JS, Bauwers JE, Trager WF. Warfarin-fluconazole II A metabolically based drug interaction: in vivo studies. Drug Metab Dispos 1996; 24:422–428.

28. Pearson MM, Rogers PD, Cleary JD, Chapman SW. Voriconazole: a new triazole antifungal. Ann Pharmacother 2003; 37:420–432.

29. Schwartz S, Milatovic D, Thiel E. Successful treatment of cerebral aspergillosis with a novel triazole (voriconazole) in a patient with acute leukemia. Br J Haematol 1997; 97:663–665.

30. Johnson LB, Kauffman CA. Voriconazole: a new triazole antifungal agent. Clin Infect Dis 2003; 36:630–637.

31. Goldstein JA. Clinical relevance of genetic polymorphisms in the human CYP2C subfamily. Br J Clin Pharmacol 2001; 52:349–355.

32. Lee CR, Goldstein JA, Pieper JA. Cytochrome P450 2C9 polymorphisms: a comprehensive review of the in-vitro and human data. Pharmacogenetics 2002; 12:251–263.

33. Sugar AM, Alsip SG, Galgiani JN, Graybill JR, Dismukes WE, Cloud GA, Craven PC, Stevens DA. Pharmacology and toxicology of high dose ketoconazole. Antimicrob Agents Chemother 1987; 31:(12)1874–1878.

34. Terrell CL. Antifungal agents. Part II. The azoles. Mayo Clin Proc 1999; 74:78–100.
35. Willems L, van der Geest R, de Beule K. Itraconazole oral solution and intravenous formulations: a review of pharmacokinetics and pharmacodynamics. J Clin Pharm Ther 2001; 26:159–169.
36. Brewster ME, Simpkins JW, Hora MS, Stern WC, Bodor N. The potential use of cyclodextrins in parenteral formulations. J Parenter Sci Tech 1989; 43:231–240.
37. Pappas PG, Kauffman CA, Perfect J, Johnson PC, McKinsey DS, Bamberger DM, Hamill R, Sharkey PK, Chapman SW, Sobel JD. Alopecia associated with fluconazole therapy. Ann Intern Med 1995; 123:354–357.
38. Tan KKC, Brayshaw N, Oakes M. Investigation into the relationship between plasma voriconazole concentrations and liver function test abnormalities in therapeutic trials. 41st Interscience Conference on Antimicrobial Agents and Chemotherapy, Chicago, IL, Dec 2001.
39. Rex JH, Pfaller MA, Walsh TJ, Chaturvedi V, Espinel-Ingroff A, Ghannoum MA, Gosey LL, Odds FC, Rinaldi MG, Sheehan DJ, Warnock DW. Antifungal susceptibility testing: practical aspects and current challenges. Clin Microbiol Rev 2001; 14:643–658.
40. Groll AH, Piscitelli SC, Walsh TJ. Antifungal pharmacodynamics: concentration–effect relationships in vitro and in vivo. Pharmacotherapy 2001; 21(8 (Pt 2)):133S–148S.
41. Grant SM, Clissold SP. Fluconazole: a review of its pharmacodynamic and pharmacokinetic properties, and therapeutic potential in superficial and systemic mycoses. Drugs 1990; 39:877–916.
42. Rex JH, Walsh TJ, Sobel JD, Filler SG, Pappas PG, Dismukes WE, Edwards JE. Practice guidelines for the treatment of candidiasis. Clin Infect Dis 2000; 30:662–678.
43. Slain D, Rogers PD, Cleary JD, Chapman SW. Intravenous itraconazole. Ann Pharmacother 2001; 35:720–729.
44. Hostetler JS, Heykants J, Clemons KV, Woestenborghs R, Hanson LH, Stevens DA. Discrepancies in bioassay and chromatography determinations explained by metabolism of itraconazole to hydroxyitraconazole: studies of interpatient variations in concentrations. Antimicrob Agents Chemother 1993; 37:2224–2227.
45. Johnston D, Cannom RRM, Filler SG. Amino acid substitutions in the *Aspergillus ERG11* gene product renders it resistant to itraconazole, yet susceptibility to voriconazole is maintained. 40th Interscience Conference on Antimicrobial Agents and Chemotherapy, Toronto, Sep 19, 2000.
46. Andes D. In vivo pharmacodynamics of antifungal drugs in the treatment of candidiasis. Antimicrob Agents Chemother 2003; 47:1179–1186.
47. Klepser ME, Wolfe EJ, Jones RN, Nightingale CH, Pfaller MA. Antifungal pharmacodynamic characteristics of fluconazole and amphotericin B tested against *Candida albicans*. Antimicrob Agents Chemother 1997; 41:1392–1395.
48. Lewis RE, Lund BC, Klepser ME, Ernst EJ, Pfaller MA. Assessment of antifungal activities of fluconazole and amphotericin B administered alone and in combination against *Candida albicans* by using a dynamic in vitro mycotic infection model. Antimicrob Agents Chemother 1998; 42:1382–1386.
49. Burgess DS, Hastings RW, Summers KK, Hardin TC, Rinaldi MG. Pharmacodynamics of fluconazole, itraconazole, and amphotericin B against *Candida albicans*. Diagn Microbiol Infect Dis 2000; 36:13–18.
50. Klepser ME, Wolfe EJ, Pfaller MA. Antifungal pharmacodynamic characteristics of fluconazole and amphotericin B against *Cryptococcus neoformans*. J Antimicrob Chemother 1998; 41:397–401.
51. Burgess DS, Hastings RW. A comparison of dynamic characteristics of fluconazole, itraconazole, and amphotericin B against *Cryptococcus neoformans* using time-kill methodology. Diagn Microbiol Infect Dis 2000; 38:87–93.
52. Sohnle PG, Hahn BL, Erdmann MD. Effect of fluconazole on viability of *Candida albicans* over extended periods of time. Antimicrob Agents Chemother 1996; 40:2622–2625.

53. Minguez F, Chiu ML, Lima JE, Nique R, Prieto J. Activity of fluconazole:postantifungal effect, effects of low concentrations and pretreatment on susceptibility of *Candida albicans* to leukocytes. J Antimicrob Chemother 1994; 34:93–100.

54. Ernst E, Klepser ME, Pfaller MA. Postantifungal effects of echinocandin, azole, and polyene antifungal agents against *Candida albicans* and *Cryptococcus neoformans*. Antimicrob Agents Chemother 2000; 44:1108–1111.

55. Fung-Tomc JC, White TC, Minassian B, Huczko E, Bonner DP. In vitro antifungal activity of BMS 207147 and itraconazole against yeast strains that are non-susceptible to fluconazole. Diagn Microbiol Infect Dis 1999; 35:163–167.

56. Zhanel GG, Saunders DG, Hoban DJ, Karlowsky JA. Influence of human serum on antifungal pharmacodynamics with *Candida albicans*. Antimicrob Agents Chemother 2001; 45:2018–2022.

57. Manavuathu EK, Cutright JL, Chandrasekar PH. Organism dependent fungicidal activity of azoles. Antimicrob Agents Chemother 1998; 42:3018–3021.

58. Berenguer J, Ali NM, Allende MC, Lee J, Garrett K, Battaglia S, Piscitelli SC, Rinaldi MG, Pizzo PA, Walsh TJ. Itraconazole for experimental pulmonary aspergillosis: comparison with amphotericin B, interaction with cyclosporine A and correlation between therapeutic response and itraconazole concentration in plasma. Antimicrob Agents Chemother 1994; 38:1303–1308.

59. Yoo SD, Kang E, Shin BS, Jun H, Lee SH, Lee KC, Lee KH. Interspecies comparison of the oral absorption of itraconazole in laboratory animals. Arch Pharm Res 2002; 25: 387–391.

60. Glasmacher A, Hahn C, Molitor E, Sauerbruch T, Marklein G, Schmidt-Wolf IGH. Definition of a minimal effective trough concentration of itraconazole for antifungal prophylaxis in severely neutropenic patients with hematologic malignancies. 39th Interscience Conference on Antimicrobial Agents and Chemotherapy, San Francisco, CA, Sep 26–29, 1999.

61. Klepser ME, Malone D, Lewis RE, Ernst EJ, Pfaller MA. Evaluation of voriconazole pharmacodynamics using time-kill methodology. Antimicrob Agents Chemother 2000; 44:1917–1920.

62. Garcia MT, Llorente MT, Lima JE, Minguez F, Del Moral F, Prieto J. Activity of voriconazole: post-antifungal effect, effects of low concentrations and of pretreatment on susceptibility of *Candida albicans* to leucocytes. Scand J Infect Dis 1999; 31:501–504.

63. Klepser ME. Antifungal resistance among *Candida* species. Pharmacotherapy 2001; 21 (8 Pt 2):124S–132S.

64. Orozco A, Higginbotham L, Hitchcock T, Parkinson D, Falconer A, Ibrahim M, Ghannoum M, Filler SG. Mechanisms of fluconazole resistance in *Candida krusei*. Antimicrob Agents Chemother 1998; 42:2645–2649.

65. Vanden Bossche H, Marichal HP, Odds F, LeJeune L, Coene MC. Characterization of azole-resistant *Candida glabrata* isolate. Antimicrob Agents Chemother 1992; 36:2602–2610.

66. Maenza JR, Merz WG, Romagnoli MJ, Keruly JC, Moore RD, Gallant JE. Infection due to fluconazole resistant *Candida* in patients with AIDS: prevalence and microbiology. Clin Infect Dis 1997; 24:28–34.

67. Sheenhan DJ, Hitchcock CA, Sibley CM. Current and emerging azole antifungal agents. Clin Microbiol Rev 1999; 12:40–79.

68. Penzak SR, Gubbins PO. Preventing and treating azole-resistant oropharyngeal candidiasis in HIV-infected patients. Am J Health Syst Pharm 1998; 55:279–283.

69. Venkateswarlu K, Taylor M, Manning NJ, Rinaldi MG, Kelly SL. Fluconazole tolerance in clinical isolates of *Cryptococcus neoformans*. Antimicrob Agents Chemother 1997; 41: 748–751.

70. Denning DW, Venkateswarlu K, Oakley KL, Anderson MJ, Manning NJ, Stevens DA, Warnock DW, Kelly SL. Itraconazole resistance in *Aspergillus fumigatus*. Antimicrob Agents Chemother 1997; 41:1364–1368.

71. MacCallum DM, Odds FC. Efficacy of parenteral itraconazole against disseminated *Candida albicans* infection in two mouse strains. J Antimicrob Chemother 2002; 50:225–229.

72. Abbruzzo GK, Flattery AM, Gill CJ, Kong L, Smith JG, Krupa D, Picounis B, Kropp H, Bartizal K. Evaluation of water-soluble pneumocandin analogs L-733560, L-705589, and L731373 with mouse models of disseminated aspergillosis, candidiasis, and cryptococcosis. Antimicrob Agents Chemother 1995; 39:1077–1081.

73. MacCallum DM, Odds FC. Influence of grapefruit juice on itraconazole plasma levels in mice and guinea pigs. J Antimicrob Chemother 2002; 50:219–224.

74. Christensen K, Gubbins PO, Gurley BJ, Bowman JL, Buice RG. A study to determine single-dose absorption and relative bioavailability of an extemporaneous oral suspension preparation of itraconazole. Am J Health Syst Pharm 1998; 55:261–265.

75. Kirkpatrick WR, McAtee RK, Fothergill AW, Rinaldi MG, Patterson TF. Efficacy of voriconazole in a guinea pig model of disseminated invasive aspergillosis. Antimicrob Agents Chemother 2000; 44:2865–2868.

76. Odds FC, Oris M, Van Dorsselaer P, Van Gervan F. Activities of an intravenous formulation of itraconazole in experimental disseminated *Aspergillus, Candida,* and *Cryptococcus* infections. Antimicrob Agents Chemother 2000; 44:3180–3183.

77. Sugar AM, Liu XP. Effect of grapefruit juice on serum voriconazole concentrations in the mouse. Med Mycol 2000; 38:209–212.

78. Walsh TJ, Lee JW, Roilides E, Francis P, Bacher J, Lyman CA, Pizzo PA. Experimental antifungal chemotherapy in granulocytopenic animal models of disseminated candidiasis: approaches to understanding investigational antifungal compounds for patients with neoplastic diseases. Clin Infect Dis 1992; 14(suppl 1):S139–S147.

79. Troke PF, Brammer KW, Hitchcock CA, Youren S, Sarantis N. UK-109,496, A novel, wide-spectrum triazole derivative for the treatment of fungal infections: activity in systemic candidiasis models and early clinical efficacy in oropharyngeal candidiasis (OPC). 35th Interscience Conference on Antimicrobial Agents and Chemotherapy, San Francisco, CA, Sep 17–20, 1995.

80. Ghannoum MA, Okogbule-Wonodi I, Bhat N, Sanati H. Antifungal activity of voriconazole (UK-109,496), fluconazole and amphotericin B against hematogenous *Candida krusei* infection in neutropenic guinea pig model. J Chemother 1999; 11:34–39.

81. Patterson TF, Fothergill AW, Rinaldi MG. Efficacy of itraconazole solution in a rabbit model of invasive aspergillosis. Antimicrob Agents Chemother 1993; 37:2307–2310.

82. Arrese JE, Delvenne P, Van Cutsem J, Pierard-Franchimont C, Pierard GE. Experimental aspergillosis in guinea pigs: influence of itraconazole on fungaemia and invasive fungal growth. Mycoses 1994; 37:117–112.

83. Van Cutsem J. Prophylaxis of *Candida* and *Aspergillus* infections with oral administration of itraconazole. Mycoses 1994; 37:243–248.

84. Murphy M, Bernard EM, Ishimaru T, Armstrong D. Activity of voriconazole (UK-109,496) against clinical isolates of *Aspergillus* species and its effectiveness in an experimental model of invasive pulmonary aspergillosis. Antimicrob Agents Chemother 1997; 41:696–698.

85. George D, Miniter P, Andriole VT. Efficacy of UK-109496, a new azole antifungal agent, in an experimental model of invasive aspergillosis. Antimicrob Agents Chemother 1996; 40:86–91.

86. Martin MV, Yates J, Hitchcock CA. Comparison of voriconazole (UK-109,496) and itraconazole in prevention and treatment of *Aspergillus fumigatus* endocarditis in guinea pigs. Antimicrob Agents Chemother 1997; 41:13–16.

87. Rex JH, Bennett JE, Sugar AM, Pappas PG, van der Horst CM, Edwards JE, Washburn RG, Scheld WM, Karchmer AW, Dine AP, Levenstein MJ, Webb CD. The Candidemia Study Group the National Institute of Allergy and Infectious Diseases Mycoses Study Group. A randomized trial comparing fluconazole with amphoteric in

B for the treatment of candidemia in patients without neutropenia. N Engl J Med 1994; 331:1325–1330.

88. Phillips P, Shafran S, Garber G, Rotstein C, Smaill F, Fong I, Salit I, Miller M, Williams K, Conly JM, Singer J, Ioannou S. Multicenter randomized trial of fluconazole versus amphotericin B for treatment of candidemia in non-neutropenic patients. Canadian Candidemia Study Group. Eur J Clin Microbiol Infect Dis 1997; 16:337–345.

89. Rex JH, Bennett JE, Sugar AM, Pappas PG, Serody J, Edwards JE, Washburn RG. Intravascular catheter exchange and duration of candidemia. NIAID Mycoses Study Group and the Candidemia Study Group. Clin Infect Dis 1995; 21:994–996.

90. Bennett JE, Powers J, Walsh T, Viscoli C, de Pauw B, Dismukes W, Galgiani J, Glauser M, Herbrecht R, Kauffman C, Lee J, Pappas P, Rex J, Verweij P. Forum Report: issues in Clinical trials of empirical antifungal therapy in treating febrile neutropenic patients. Clin Infect Dis 2003; 36(suppl 3):S117–S122.

91. Goodman JL, Winston DJ, Greenfield RA, Chandrasekar PH, Fox B, Kaizer H, Shadduck RK, Shea TC, Stiff P, Friedman DJ, Powderly WG, Silber JL, Horowitz H, Lichtin A, Wolff SN, Mangan KF, Silver SM, Weisdorf D, Ho WG, Gilbert G, Buell D. A controlled trial of fluconazole to prevent fungal infections in patients undergoing bone marrow transplantation. N Engl J Med 1992; 326:845–851.

92. Slavin MA, Osborne B, Adams R, Levenstein MJ, Schoch HG, Feldman AR, Meyers JD, Bowden RA. Efficacy and safety of fluconazole prophylaxis for fungal infections after marrow transplantation—a prospective, randomized, double-blind study. J Infect Dis 1995; 171:1545–1552.

93. Marr KA, Seidel K, Slavin MA, Bowden RA, Schoch G, Flowers ME, Corey L, Boeckh M. Prolonged fluconazole prophylaxis is associated with persistent protection against candidiasis-related death in allogeneic marrow transplant recipients: long-term follow-up of randomized, placebo-controlled trial. Blood 2000; 96:2055–2061.

94. Boogaerts M, Winston DJ, Bow EJ, Garber G, Reboli AC, Schwarer AP, Novitzky N, Boehme A, Chwetzoff E, De Beule K. Intravenous and oral itraconazole versus intravenous amphotericin B deoxycholate as empirical antifungal therapy for persistent fever in neutropenic patients with cancer who are receiving broad-spectrum antibacterial therapy. A randomized, controlled trial. Ann Intern Med 2001; 135:412–422.

95. Winston DJ, Maziarz RT, Chandrasekar PH, Lazarus HM, Goldman M, Blumer JL, Leitz GJ, Territo MC. Intravenous and oral itraconazole versus intravenous and oral fluconazole for long-term antifungal prophylaxis in allogeneic hematopoietic stem-cell transplant recipients. A multicenter, randomized trial. Ann Intern Med 2003; 138: 705–713.

96. Walsh TJ, Pappas P, Wiston DJ, Lazarus HM, Petersen F, Rafalli J, Yanovich S, Stiff P, Greenberg R, Donowitz G, Lee J. National Institute of Allergy and Infectious Disease Mycoses Study Group. Voriconazole compared with liposomal amphotericin B for empirical antifungal therapy in patients with neutropenia and persistent fever. N Engl J Med 2002; 346:225–234.

97. Powers JH, Dixon CA, Goldberger MJ. Voriconazole versus liposomal amphotericin B in patients with neutropenia and persistent fever. N Engl J Med 2002; 346:289–290.

18
Echinocandin Antifungal Drugs

John R Graybill
Department of Medicine, Division of Infectious Diseases, University of Texas Health Science Center, San Antonio, Texas, U.S.A.

Gregory M. Anstead
Department of Medicine, South Texas Veterans Healthcare System, San Antonio, Texas, U.S.A.

I. A NEW ANTIFUNGAL TARGET

The fungal cell wall is composed largely of chitins, mannoproteins, and glucans. The cell wall fulfills a number of critical functions for the fungal cell, including defining its shape, providing docking sites for fungal enzymes, filtering the passage of multiple ions and compounds into the cell, and functioning as the site for adherence of fungi to the vascular endothelium and other structures (1). The fungal cell wall is a highly desirable target for drug design because there is no equivalent in mammalian cells; thus, there may be less drug toxicity.

Disruption of the fungal cell wall was attempted some years ago by inhibiting chitin synthase with Nikkomycin Z. Although this drug was effective in vitro and in vivo against *Coccidioides immitis,* and to lesser degree *Candida, Histoplasma capsulatum,* and *Aspergillus*, and reached Phase I clinical trials, it was not further developed, in part because of bankruptcy of the parent company, Shaman (2–6). Efforts were also directed at attack on the fungal mannoproteins, primarily with development of pradimycin. This compound was highly effective in animals (7,8). However, in phase I clinical trials there was hepatotoxicity and the drug was withdrawn.

The third class of cell wall constituents, the glucans, was more amenable to antifungal drug development. Aculaecin A and other related cyclic lipopeptides were initially tested against fungi. They showed some activity, but were not suitable for further development (1). The first compound of significant medical interest was cilofungin, developed by Lilly (Fig. 1) (9,10). However, cilofungin as a first start was quickly aborted in phase I trials. The drug was poorly soluble in water, and the vehicle used in the initial clinical trials was nephrotoxic. Nevertheless, before it was abandoned, cilofungin provided some very useful information. First, the drug acts against FKS1 synthase, an enzyme responsible for synthesis of beta-1,3-D-glucans (11). Second, it is highly effective in vitro against *Candida albicans* (12). Third, while

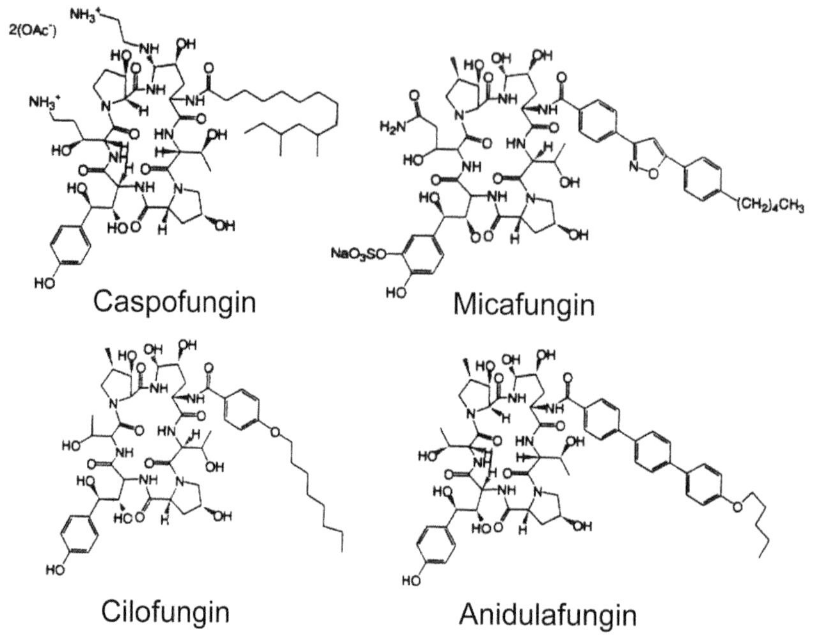

Figure 1 Structures of echinocandins.

ineffective in vitro against *Aspergillus fumigatus* (using NCCLS methods), the drug was highly effective in vivo in murine aspergillosis (13,14). Fourth, its non-linear kinetics and the saturable clearance of the drug in animals suggested hepatic metabolism of this class of drugs (15,16). Fifth, cilofungin was active against *C. immitis,* an organism very rich in glucans (17). Sixth, in a series of studies which may predict clinical use of this class, cilofungin was additive or synergistic with amphotericin B against several fungal pathogens (18–21).

Despite the limitations of cilofungin, by the 1990s interest in the echinocandins had broadened considerably. Lilly continued development of drugs, and eventually produced what is now anidulafungin (Versicor). Fujisawa independently developed micafungin, and Merck developed caspofungin. At the time of this writing, caspofungin is licensed, micafungin is on the verge of licensure, and anidulafungin is well into clinical trials. Drugs focused on this new antifungal target had reached the clinic.

II. MECHANISM OF ACTION

Although the cell wall has multiple components, beta-1,3-D-glucans are critical components for many (but not all) fungal species. Double deletion mutants of FKS1 (glucan synthase) are non-viable (11). Echinocandin-induced inhibition of glucan synthesis causes *Candida* cells to lose their rigidity, become deformed, and ultimately form a protoplast-like mass (Fig. 2) (22). Echinocandin binding may occur within moments, and an exposure of just minutes is sufficient to reduce cell viability sharply (Fig. 3) (23).

One advantage of the echinocandins is that they act independently of the fungal cell membrane. Thus, as expected, triazole-resistant *Candida* are susceptible

(A) **Control**

(B) **MIC$_{80}$**

Wounded

(C) **16x MIC**

Dead

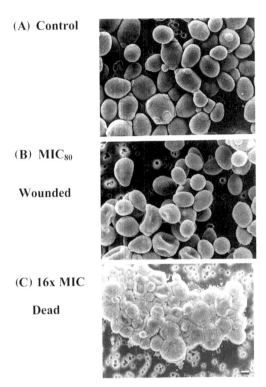

Figure 2 Scanning electron micrographs showing viable *C. albicans* control cells, damaged cells at 80% of the minimum inhibitory concentration (MIC) for anidulafungin, and non-viable cells at 16 times the MIC (22).

in vitro to echinocandins (24–27). The echinocandins have a long postantifungal effect, and are considered fungicidal to *Candida* (28,29). Unfortunately, this broad susceptibility does not apply to all fungi. *Cryptococcus neoformans*, also a yeast, does not contain high quantities of beta-1,3-D-glucans, and thus is resistant both in vitro and in animal models (30). Other investigators have found that overexpression of a gene coding for synthesis of a Golgi protein also confers resistance to caspofungin in *Saccharromyces cerevesiae* (31).

Another potential advantage of echinocandins is that they, and lipid preparations of amphotericin B, appear unusually potent in reducing *Candida* in biofilms (32). This is of potential importance, as *Candida* are particularly difficult to treat when associated with prosthetic devices such as catheters and artificial heart valves (33,34). Whether this in vitro phenomenon can be translated into the clinical arena is unclear.

Further, glucan synthesis occurs relatively evenly in yeast cell walls, but occurs primarily at new growth tips of hyphae in mycelial fungi (35,36). Thus, we see a different picture in *A. fumigatus* exposed to echinocandins. The growing tips of fungi are damaged by the drug, and killed, but older more sessile mycelial structures remain viable (Fig. 4) (37). If susceptibilities are performed by NCCLS methods for hyphae, the resulting MIC is extremely high, (above 64 μg/mL) as fungal colonies are blunted in growth but there are few clear end points (36,38). However, if the fungal colonies are examined using a change from diffuse hyphal growth to a clumped pattern, with little new hyphal extension, then end points fall within the range of ≤2 μg/mL or less. This

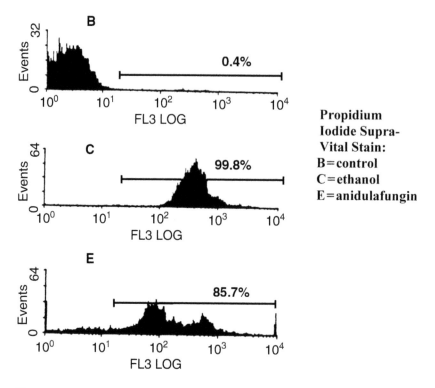

Figure 3 Flow cytometric evaluation of *C. albicans* treated with anidulafungin. The uptake of propidium iodide corresponds to fungicidal activity. B is the control; only a small amount of autofluorescence is observed. In panel C, treatment of yeast cells with 70% ethanol results in >100%-fold increase in PI fluorescence intensity, with death of almost 100% of cells. In panel E, treatment of *C. albicans* with anidulafungin at the minimal fungicidal concentration for 5-mins results in 85.7% of the yeast cells taking up propidium iodide. *Source*: Modified from Ref. 23.

end point, based on the "minimum effective concentration (MEC)" may accurately predict the efficacy of echinocandins against mycelial pathogens. The MEC may be generalizable to other moulds as well, with the mycelial phase of *C. immitis* showing the same pattern (39). Although *Aspergillus* fares well with the MEC method, other mycelial pathogens such as *Fusarium* appear resistant using even this optimized method (40,41). There is some variability in results with other mycelial fungi. Interpretation is difficult, as "resistance" may have been measured as an artifact of turbidimetric methods rather than the change in morphology which is a preferable end point (41,42). Disc diffusion has also been utilized to measure antifungal efficacy (Table 1) (9). If the antifungal drugs are removed, *Aspergillus* begin to grow rather quickly, showing very little postantifungal effect. The echinocandins are thus only considered fungistatic to mycelial pathogens (43).

III. CORRELATING IN VITRO AND IN VIVO ACTIVITY

As with other antifungal drugs, in vitro activity of the echinocandins must be proven in vivo using animal models, before the drug is taken to clinical evaluation. Here the

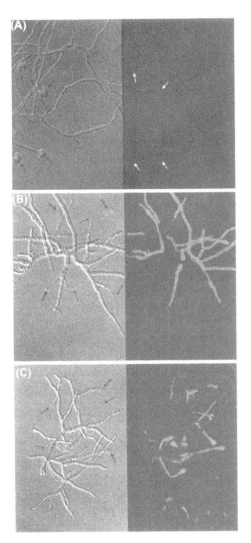

Figure 4 Effect of extended drug treatment on *A. fumigatus* fluorescent dye staining. **(A)** Untreated, DiBAC-stained germlings harvested 24-hour after vehicle addition. Magnification 400×. Arrows indicate conidiophores. Caspofungin treated germlings (0.3 µg/mL) harvested 72 hr after drug addition were stained with CFDA**(B)** or DiBAC**(C)** (magnification 800×). In panels B and C, arrows with single tails indicate lysed apical cells and arrows with double tails indicate lysed conidophores. The fluorescent micrographs in panel A required a 20-sec exposure. Left panels, Normarski optics; right panels, epifluorescence with an FITC filter set (35).

echinocandins gave some surprising results. As expected, in an animal model studied with fluconazole-susceptible and -resistant *C. albicans* and non-*albicans* species, the echinocandins showed high efficacy, down to as low as <0.1 µg/kg/dose. *C. neoformans* is predictably resistant in vitro and in vivo (27,30,45–47). However, in vitro surveys showed up a number of isolates of *Candida parapsilosis* with relatively high in vitro MIC values, up to 8 µg/mL or more. Because there were no good animal models for this low virulence species, correlation of in vitro and in vivo results had to await clinical experience.

Table 1 Minimum Effective Concentration of Caspofungin by the Method of Kurtz (MEC) (44) Vs. Zone of Inhibition (IZ, Expressed in mm Diameter Inhibition) for *Aspergillus* and *Fusarium* (41)

Species (*N*)	IZ Range in mm (Mean)	MEC Range in Conc'n (Mean)
A. flavus (27)	16–25 (21.2)	0.125–0.5 (0.26)
A. fumigatus (26)	12–23 (16)	0.25–0.5 (0.31)
A. niger (16)	15–24 (18)	0.125–0.25 (0.2)
A. terreus (9)	12–26 (19.6)	0.25 (0.25)
F. solani (18)	No zone	>16
F. oxysporum (4)	No zone	>16

No activity is observed against *Fusarium*.

More impressive surprises awaited those working with mycelial fungi. The early model was aspergillosis. In mice and rats, echinocandins prolonged the survival of treated mice, though the effects on tissue counts were variable (30,46,48,49). Further, micafungin appears highly effective in murine aspergillosis caused by amphotericin B-resistant *A. fumigatus* (50). In this model, survival was prolonged and lung tissue burden was reduced sharply. However, when chronically immuno-suppressed rabbits were infected with *A. fumigatus* and treated with echinocandins, survival was prolonged, size of pulmonary infarct lesions was reduced, and yet there was no reduction of colony counts of infected pulmonary tissues (Fig. 5) (51).

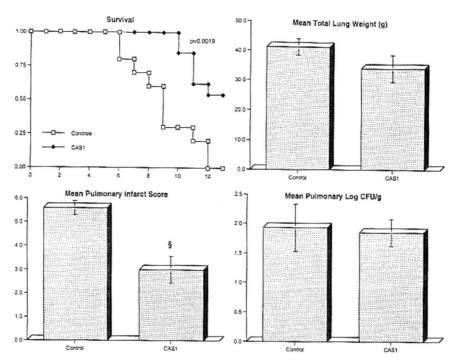

Figure 5 Effects of caspofungin treatment on survival, infarct size, and tissue burden of rabbits infected with *A. fumigatus* (52).

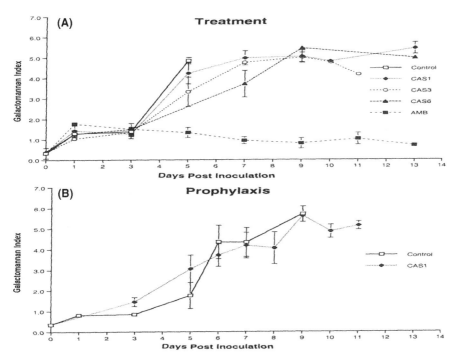

Figure 6 Effects of caspofungin treatment or preinfection prophylaxis on galactomannan antigen (52).

Furthermore, this happened not only with micafungin, but also with anidulafungin. This indicates that the effect is class specific, not drug specific (51).

The lack of effect on colony counts raises the question as to whether echino- candins actually reduce the fungal burden or somehow just hold the organism in check, with benefit in survival only. Petraitis et al. indicate that not only do fungal colony counts remain unchanged with caspofungin therapy, but galactomannan antigen, a measure of fungal biomass, also remains stable, or increases (51). The lack of effect of echinocandins on tissue burden stands in distinction from amphotericin B, where the galactomannan titer drops (Fig. 6). There is not uniform agreement on this, however, as Bowman et al. have found, with different molecular methods, that *Aspergillus* burden does decline on caspofungin therapy (Fig. 7) (37,53). The infer- ence here is that the fungi are broken up into smaller particles, each of which can form a colony, though the total burden is reduced. Resolution of this difference awaits future studies.

Other mycelial and dimorphic pathogens might behave in similar ways. At pre- sent our information is incomplete. There is animal evidence of good efficacy in cocci- dioidomycosis, and conflicting data in histoplasmosis (39,54,55). In vitro data on other moulds need follow-up with animal studies before clinical trials are launched (56).

IV. CLINICAL EVALUATION: HOW ARE THESE DRUGS HANDLED?

Of the three echinocandins in clinical use, none are absorbed very well when admi- nistered orally. All drugs must be given intravenously. One advantage of these drugs

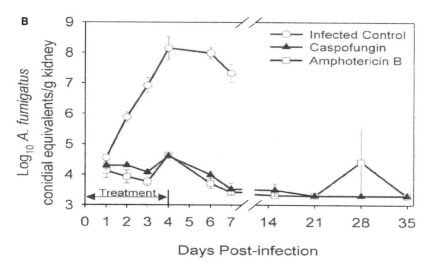

Figure 7 Effect of caspofungin therapy on kidney burden of *Aspergillus* in mice, as determined by quantitative polymerase chain reaction (Taqman) (53).

is that they are sufficiently water soluble that special vehicles, such as the cyclodextrins used for triazoles, are not required. Plasma protein binding is well over 90% for caspofungin, and approximately 85% for anidulafungin. However, the drugs are sufficiently potent that high plasma protein binding does not impair activity. Animal studies have shown that echinocandins are distributed well to most tissues. However, for micafungin, penetration of the brain was reduced compared to the lung, liver, and plasma (57). The caspofungin plasma concentration 1 hr after infusion of 10 mg was 1.6 µg/mL, and after 100 mg was 14.03 µg/mL (58). Clearance occurred slowly and was similar over a broad range of doses. The caspofungin plasma half-life is 9–10 hr, and is linear from 5 to 100 mg doses. The micafungin half-life is 10–16 hr, and the anidulafungin half-life is as long as 50 hr (59,60). This allows for once daily dosing for all three drugs. Chemical hydrolysis in plasma to inactive metabolites may be the primary route of clearance (61). With anidulafungin, this occurs at the same rate in saline as in serum, with a half-life at body temperature and pH 7.4 of approximately 24 hr. These drugs may be further cleared hepatically, but not via the cytochrome oxidase system used by the triazoles (61). A third advantage of the echinocandins is that there are virtually none of the complex drug interactions which plague the triazoles (62,63). One unresolved question is whether the combination of caspofungin and cyclosporine A causes liver toxicity (elevated liver enzymes were noted in a small number of healthy volunteers). Studies with anidulafungin in vitro showed that up to 30 µg/mL did not affect hepatic microsomal degradation of cylosporin (64). Tacrolimus and mycophenolate do not affect any of these drugs. Despite secondary hepatic metabolism of some components, clearance is almost linear over the dose ranges explored thus far. Liver failure significantly impedes clearance (Table 2) (65–67). Peak serum concentrations after a single 50-mg dose in normal patients were 2.07 µg/mL vs. 2.24 µg/mL in those on dialysis. Peaks of 1.57 µg/mL vs. 2.87 µg/mL were observed in those with severe hepatic impairment. Anidulafungin is not dialyzable. A fourth advantage of the echinocandins is that all three drugs appear to have a very broad therapeutic index, and significant dose-dependent toxicity has not been a problem for any of these drugs (Table 3). In effect,

Table 2 Clearance of Anidulafungin in Patients with Severe Liver or Renal Failure (65,67)

	N	C_{max} (µg/mL)	Clearance (L/hr)
Hepatic Failure			
Control	6	1.57 ± 0.4	1.23 ± 0.3
Severe	5	2.87 ± 0.7	0.74 ± 0.2
Renal Failure			
Control	8	2.07 ± 0.2	0.99 ± 0.1
Hemodialysis	3	2.24 ± 0.7	1.00 ± 0.2

The daily dose was 50 mg/day for 7 days.
The half-life is increased by hepatic failure.

Table 3 Selected Clinical and Laboratory Adverse Reactions

	Caspofungin				Micafungin (69)		Anidulafungin[a]	
	Systemic (63)		Mucosal (68)					
	Patients (N)	%	Patients (N)	%	Patients (N)	%	Patients (N)	%
Total	114	100	83	100	67	100	300	100
Fever/chills	8	7	3	4	1	1	26	8.7
Abdominal Pain	NS		3	4	NS		NS	
Phlebitis	4	3.5	13	16	2	3	16	5.3
Nausea	2	1.8	5	6	NS		19	6.3
Vomiting	4	3.5	NS		NS		20	6.7
Diarrhea	NS		3	4	2	3	23	7.7
Headache	NS		5	6	1	1	25	8.3
Rash	1	0.9	2	2	2	3	NS	
Dizziness	NS		NS		NS		5	2.0
Cough	NS		NS		NS		11	3.7
Increased SGOT	4	24.3	4	5	1	1	10[b]	3.3
Increased SGPT	2	1.9	7	9	2	3	NS	
Increased bilirubin	3	2.8	0	0	NS		NS	
Increased alkaline Phosphatase	9	8.3	7	9	3	4	NS	
Decreased hemoglobin	1	0.9	11	4	NS		10	3.3
Leukopenia and/or neutropenia	NS		7	13	1	1	11	3.7
Decreased albumin	NS		5	9	NS		NS	
Increased creatinine or Urea nitrogen	4	3.7			3	4		
Polyarthritis	NS		NS		NS		1	1

[a]J. Schranz, personal communication, Versicor.
[b]sum of patients with any liver function test abnormal.
Abbreviation: NS, not specified.

the maximum tolerated dose for none of these drugs has been determined. Courses of >1 week in adults have been used with caspofungin at 140 mg/day, micafungin up to 8 mg/kg/day, and anidulafungin at up to 130 mg/day (60). However, at the 100 mg anidulafungin/day dose, three of 10 healthy subjects had >2x normal elevations of the alanine or aspartate aminotransferase.

There are fewer data available for children. Micafungin has been administered at 4 mg/kg/day. Pharmacokinetics in children aged 2–17-year old were evaluated by Walsh et al. (70). The geometric mean ratios of AUC and 1-hour serum concentrations in children/adults were 0.62 and 0.87 on day-1 of treatment, and 0.52 and 0.80 on day-4 of treatment. The β-phase half-life was reduced 32–43% in children vs. adults.

With such a broad safety range and so few signs of intolerance, how are these drugs administered clinically? At this relatively early phase of experience, it appears that the potency of each echinocandin appears to be quite similar to the other, and one might almost interchange recommendations. In the initial studies of caspofungin, mouse studies were used to estimate human doses. The desired goal was a plasma concentration which consistently exceeded the MIC for *C. albicans* at a 24-hour postdose trough, and was effective in mice. Because of the long half-life, an initial loading dose of caspofungin was used at 70 mg. Maintenance doses in initial clinical studies of *Candida* esophagitis bracketed 50 mg/day (71).

Another advantage for use in the intensive care unit is the striking absence of severe adverse reactions (Table 3). The echinocandins have virtually no effect on the kidneys, the liver, or the myelopoietic system. Initial concerns about potential anaphylaxis have proven unfounded. Indeed, in the phase III trial in candidemia, there were 16 cases of anaphylaxis with amphotericin B and only one with caspofungin.

All of the above considerations, plus the ease of administration, suggest that the echinocandins will be excellent alternatives in patients with liver or renal failure, and in patients with known or suspected fluconazole resistance. Indeed, the cost of these new drugs may be the only reason they do not replace amphotericin B completely in hospitalized patients.

V. CLINICAL EFFICACY

A. *Candida*

Although animal studies suggest that efficacy may be broader, at present our clinical data are limited to experience with *Candida* and *Aspergillus* species. Uniformity of in vitro resistance and animal study failures in cryptococcal disease suggests that we should proceed cautiously in expanding clinical experience beyond *Candida* and *Aspergillus* (72).

For all three echinocandins in clinical use, the first studies were conducted in mucosal candidiasis, particularly in patients with HIV infection and *Candida* esophagitis. Initial open dose ranging studies were followed by randomized clinical trials. It is remarkably how similarly the three echinocandins behaved. Using a modified intent-to-treat analysis, the endoscopic response rates were 85% for 81 recipients of caspofungin at 50 mg/day, and 86% for 94 recipients of fluconazole at 200 mg/day (68). A large randomized trial comparing anidulafungin at 50 mg/day (249 patients evaluable with endoscopy) with fluconazole at 100 mg/day (255 patients evaluable with endoscopy) and using 1 grade reduction of endoscopy score, showed 97% success for anidulafungin and 99% for fluconazole (J Schranz, personal

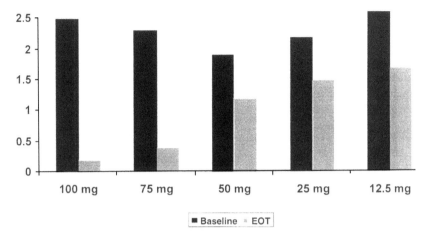

Figure 8 Response of esophagitis to micafungin (51,75,76). Esophagoscopy scale Y axis, Grade 0–3, none to severe. Daily dose in mg indicated on X axis.

communication, Versicor). A dose finding study of micafungin for esophageal candidiasis had 120 patients divided into cohorts treated with 12.5, 25, 50, 75, or 100 mg/day (Protocol 97-7-003, Monograph Echinocandins in the Management of Invasive Fungal Infections, 2001, C. Brown, Project Coordinator Marketing, Fujisawa Healthcare Inc., Deerfield, IL). The clinical responses at end of therapy were above 80% at $\geq$50 mg/day, and <80% at lower doses. However, the endoscopic responses showed a dose-response all the way up to 100 mg/day (mean reduction of endoscopy score from 2.5 to 0.2 at the highest dose, vs. reduction from 1.8 to 1.1 at 50 mg/day dose) (Fig. 8). This study, while having an average of only 20 patients in each treatment group, suggested a dose-dependent response all the way from 12.5 to 100 mg/day. The study with micafungin in humans is reminiscent of a trial in rabbits, in which micafungin responses were clearly dose-dependent in fluconazole-resistant esophageal candidiasis (73). In a follow-up open label study, 97 patients were treated with at least five doses of micafungin, 50 mg/day, for esophageal candidiasis (74). Of those with end-of-treatment esophagoscopy, 91% were cured or improved compared to the baseline.

As shown in Table 4, responses of patients with thrush (complete clearing required and resolution of symptoms) and esophagitis (two grades of improvement

Table 4 Efficacy of Caspofungin in Oropharyngeal and Esophageal Candidiasis

		Caspofungin			Amphotericin B	Fluconazole
	N	35 mg	50 mg	70 mg	0.5 mg/kg	200 mg
Thrush (71)	128	ND	(74)/46	(89)/28	(63)/54	ND
Mucosal (62)						
Thrush	52	(85)/13	(93)/14	(92)/13	(67)/12	ND
Esophagitis	86	(67)/21	(90)/20	(77)/22	(61)/23	ND
Esophagitis (43)	175	ND	(81)/82	ND	ND	(85)/94

Responses given as (%)/N in group.
Source: Modified from Ref. 78.

required on endoscopy, and resolution of symptoms) were as effective with caspofungin at 50 mg/day as with amphotericin B (62). Because there was slightly lower response at 35 mg/day, the 50 mg/day maintenance dose was accepted for caspofungin for further study in systemic candidiasis. In another study of patients with fluconazole-resistant mucosal disease, caspofungin was found to be no less effective than with fluconazole for susceptible disease (77).

The reason initial trials were conducted with mucosal candidiasis was that a failure of therapy simply meant persistent esophagitis, while failure of therapy for disseminated disease could be lethal. Armed with the initial data from mucosal disease, Merck and Fujisawa proceeded in different directions. Caspofungin was evaluated in a large phase III blinded randomized trial for documented systemic disease (63). The trial was sufficiently powered to give results for an overall group with systemic disease and also for the subgroup with candidemia. Patients were stratified for presence or absence of neutropenia, APACHE II score over or under 20, and randomized to caspofungin at 70 mg load then 50 mg/day vs. amphotericin B at 0.6–1 mg/kg/day. In the modified intent-to-treat analysis (MITT—each patient was randomized and received at least one dose of study drug), the caspofungin response rate in 109 patients was 73.4%, while the amphotericin B response rate in 115 patients with 61.7% (Table 5). This was not quite statistically significant ($p = 0.09$). Of 185 patients who could be evaluated clinically for cure, the response to caspofungin was 80.7% vs. 64.9%. The comparison in this group significantly favored caspofungin over amphotericin B for efficacy ($p = 0.03$). Overall mortality was 34% in the caspofungin recipients, and 30% in the amphotericin B recipients (not statistically significant).

Also of interest, there were no dramatic differences between caspofungin and amphotericin B for treatment of patients with *C. parapsilosis* infection (high MIC to caspofungin, >4 μg/mL) or *Candida glabrata or C. krusei* infection (traditionally resistant to fluconazole), or in patients with neutropenia (<500 or 100 neutrophils/mm^3) or high APACHE scores (over 20) (Table 6). However, it must be emphasized that none of these subgroups is large enough for statistical comparison.

Micafungin was subjected to a phase III trial of prevention rather than the treatment of systemic candidiasis in hematopoietic stem cell transplant recipients (80).

Table 5 Response to Treatment of Disseminated Candidiasis; Caspofundin Vs. Amphotericin B

| Analysis | Overall response at end of IV therapy (test of cure) number with a favorable response/total number (%) | | Estimated difference adjusted for strata (%) (95.6 CI) |
	Caspofungin 70 mg induction 50 mg maintainence	Amphotericin B 0.6–1.0 mg/kg	
MITT[a] ($n = 224$)	80/109 (73.4)	71/115 (61.7)	12.7 (-0.7, 26.0)[*]
Evaluable patients ($n = 185$)	71/88 (80.7)	63/97 (64.9)	15.4 (1.1, 29.7)[**]

[a]Modified Intent-to-Treat (each patient was randomized and received at least one dose of study drug).
[*]$p = 0.09$.
[**]$p = 0.03$.
Source: Modified from Ref. 63.

Table 6 Response by Organism; Caspofungin Vs. Amphotericin B

Pathogen	Overall response at end of IV therapy (test of cure) number with a favorable response/total number (%)	
	Caspofungin 70 mg induction 50 mg maintainence	Amphotericin B 0.6–1.0 mg/kg
C. albicans	23/36 (63.9)	34/59 (57.6)
C. parasiolopsis	14/20 (70.0)	13/20 (65.5)
C. tropicalis	17/20 (85.0)	10/14 (71.4)
C. glabrata	10/13 (76.9)	8/10 (80.0)
C. guilliermondii	3/3 (100.0)	1/1 (100.0)
C. krusei	4/4 (100.0)	0/1 (0.0)
Mixed Infection	3/3 (100.0)	2/4 (100.0)
Neutropenia (<500 cells/mm^3)	7/14 (50.0)	4/10 (40.0)
Apache II Score >20	12/21 (957.1)	10/23 (43.5)

Source: Modified from Refs. 63 and 79.

In a large study of 882 patients, van Burik et al. found similar efficacy of micafungin and fluconazole in prevention of systemic fungal infections in both adults and children. They used 50 mg/day for adults and 1 mg/kg/day for children. Fewer micafungin recipients (15%) than fluconazole recipients (21%, $p = 0.018$) required systemic antifungal therapy. Seven breakthrough infections with *Aspergillus* occurred in patients receiving fluconazole, vs. one in a patient receiving micafungin. The difference was almost significant ($p = 0.07$). Thus, micafungin was at least as effective as fluconazole in prevention of overall deep and superficial mycoses.

From the above information one can make some tentative recommendations for the use of echinocandins for treatment of *Candida* infection. For mucosal candidiasis, and for prophylaxis of *Candida* deep infection in predisposed patients, it is clear that echinocandins are as effective as fluconazole. Most of these patients are infected with *C. albicans* susceptible to fluconazole. However, because fluconazole is effective, it is hard to justify the markedly increased cost and IV delivery of echinocandins. However, in a small group of patients with fluconazole-resistant *C. albicans* esophagitis, the echinocandins clearly are successful, and reasonable, non-toxic alternatives to amphotericin B. A daily dose of 50–100 mg/day would seem sufficient. In a study of four patients with mucosal candidiasis refractory to fluconazole, itraconazole, and amphotericin B, all four had dramatic improvements with caspofungin, with no evidence of candidiasis within 7–10 days (44). Nevertheless, treatment needs to be done daily to prevent relapse, and this is a limitation. A recent presentation found that four patients relapsed when caspofungin was reduced to 3–5 times weekly after an initial successful course (81).

For deep candidiasis, caspofungin is clearly effective, better tolerated than amphotericin B, and likely more effective than amphotericin B (63). However, the current drug of choice is fluconazole, and there is no evidence that caspofungin, as initial therapy, would be sufficiently superior to fluconazole to merit its much higher costs (82). However, there are several circumstances which would warrant the use of caspofungin. One of these is nephrotoxicity and another similar reason is concurrent administration of nephrotoxic drugs (tacrolimus, gentamicin, etc.). In these cases, echinocandins would be preferred over amphotericin B desoxycholate or lipid formulations, but not fluconazole. Another circumstance is intolerance of fluconazole or other triazoles, either from toxicity (usually hepatic) or drug interactions. The latter are usually more problematic in the broad-spectrum triazoles itraconazole, voriconazole, and potentially posaconazole (83,84). Yet another circumstance is the suspicion or documentation of a *Candida* species (usually *C. glabrata*) resistant to fluconazole. *C. glabrata* may have up to 20% high-level resistance to fluconazole, and tends to emerge in oncology populations, where the use of fluconazole as a prophylactic agent is common (85,86). A similar circumstance would be in the patient who has developed candidemia while receiving or shortly after receiving fluconazole or another triazole. While the above are supported by evidence, there is one more circumstance in which I would instinctively utilize echinocandins as first line drugs. This would be in the intensive care unit patient who has fungemia and who is critically ill and hypotensive. In such a patient it is reasonable to prefer a fungicidal agent with very little toxicity and great potency and echinocandins seem to best fit those characteristics.

Taken together, these data support the contention that echinocandins are highly efficacious against both mucocutaneous (vs. fluconazole) and disseminated (vs. amphotericin B) *Candida* infection, that they are similarly effective against fluconazole-susceptible and -resistant organisms, and that are at least as effective as fluconazole in prevention of mycotic infections in patients undergoing allogeneic stem cell transplantation. There is also the suggestion that they may not be antagonistic to AmBisome when used in combinations. However, because of poor penetration into the urine as the active drug, the echinocandins are not likely to be useful for the treatment of *Candida* urinary tract infection. Finally, efficacy in severely ill patients, and the requirement for intravenous administration, suggest that these agents may find their optimal use in the intensive care unit.

B. *Aspergillus* and Other Moulds

Invasive mould infections are generally acquired by inhalation of conidia, and development of fungal pneumonia or sinusitis. A major problem has been in defining which pneumonias are likely to be fungal and which are not. This has led to problems comparing present results of recent results with prior experience. Prior experience used varied definitions of invasive filamentous fungal infections. More recently, a consensus on redefinition of invasive mould infection has been reached by investigators in the United States and Europe. They have established criteria for "documented" and "probable" mycelial invasive disease, but have considered "possible" mycelial infection (essentially pneumonia in a predisposed person, with no specific indicators for filamentous fungal pathogens) as too nonspecific (87). Recent studies of *Aspergillus* galactomannan detection have suggested that "possible" mycoses are likely not mycoses at all (88,89). Using the EORTC/MSG definitions for documented and probable invasive aspergillosis, response rates have been in the order of 10–20% in bone marrow transplant recipients, and 40–60% in lung transplant recipients (87,90). Most of these patients had received amphotericin B in its various forms. Amphotericin B lipid formulations appear similar in efficacy to the desoxycholate preparation (91). In this discouraging setting, the recent publication of a multi-center trial found voriconazole is markedly superior to amphotericin B for treatment of documented invasive aspergillosis (84). The data significantly favored voriconazole in terms of drug tolerance, complete and partial responses, and survival. Voriconazole is now clearly the drug of choice for acute invasive aspergillosis.

Nevertheless, many patients still fail primary therapy with voriconazole or amphotericin B preparations. For these patients, physicians have often had salvage therapy success rates of 40–50% at best. Given the limited efficacy of the polyenes and itraconazole, and the efficacy of echinocandins in animal models, all three echinocandins are undergoing clinical evaluation in invasive aspergillosis. Preliminary data are available for caspofungin. At present there are no phase III comparative trials with echinocandins, as there are for voriconazole. The clearest data come from Merck's open study of caspofungin in acute invasive aspergillosis. This study, which was the basis for FDA approval for caspofungin, involved salvage therapy with caspofungin for patients with either progressive disease after a week on primary therapy with another drug, or with intolerance of other therapy. This was primarily renal failure from amphotericin B. The initial experience with 56 patients was enlarged to 83 patients (79,92). Caspofungin was given at 70 mg initial loading dose, then 50 mg/day. Patients had severe predisposing diseases, including 48% with hematologic malignancy and 25% with allogeneic bone marrow transplant. The complete and partial response rates were 50% of 32 patients with pulmonary disease, 23% of 13 patients with disseminated disease, and 33% of six patients with single organ extra-pulmonary disease. Unlike candidiasis, in which neutropenia did not affect outcome, only 26% of 19 neutropenic patients had a complete or partial response. The overall response rate was 45%.

Of interest, in the initial series, 34% of 44 patients responded to caspofungin, vs. 70% of 10 patients treated because of intolerance to other antifungal drugs (79). This suggests that primary therapy of invasive aspergillosis, undertaken at an earlier time in the course of disease, might show a more favorable response than one sees in those given salvage for progressive disease.

There is a small unreported experience collected with micafungin therapy of aspergillosis. Micafungin was administered to some patients alone, and to some patients combined with liposomal amphotericin B. There are no data yet available in the public arena. The prophylaxis study by van Burik et al. found nearly significant (7 vs. 1) protection by micafungin against invasive aspergillosis (80). This suggests a role for micafungin against aspergillosis. Similarly, information on anidulafungin for invasive aspergillosis are not yet available. Although animal experience supports activity in coccidioidomycosis, there are no clinical data available. A single patient treated by us for refractory disease received caspofungin for less than 2 weeks before the drug supply was exhausted. We were unable to ascertain a change in her course.

VI. COMBINATION THERAPY OF MYCOSES

Combinations of echinocandins and other antifungals have been evaluated in numerous in vitro and some animal studies. The strongest data supporting combination therapy have come from in vitro studies. Perhaps the strongest interaction effects occur between two cell wall active agents, micafungin and anidulafungin, which inhibit glucan synthesis, and Nikkomycin Z, which inhibits chitin synthesis (93,94). While the interaction was additive to indifferent against *Fusarium solanae* and *Rhizopus oryzae*, against *A. fumigatus* there was marked synergistic activity. The hyphae showed extensive damage over a wide range of drug concentrations. Unfortunately, Nikkomycin Z is not under active development at present.

Other studies have shown a favorable interaction of triazoles and echinocandins against *C. neoformans* (95). However, Roling et al. found only indifference of caspofungin or anidulafungin and fluconazole against *C. albicans, C. tropicalis, C. glabrata, C. krusei,* and *C. neoformans* (96). Against *Aspergillus* and *Fusarium,* Arikan et al. found synergistic activity in a few and additive activity in more isolates (97). Bartizal et al. have also found additive activity of echinocandin combinations (98).

Likewise, animal studies have been mixed. Early studies with cilofungin (not in clinical use) and amphotericin B showed additive effects in mice with candidiasis (20,21). Another study showed antagonism of cilofungin and amphotericin B in murine aspergillosis (19). In contrast, Nakajima et al. found additive effects of micafungin and amphotericin B in murine aspergillosis (99). Perhaps of greatest interest, Kirkpatrick et al. found "additive" effects of voriconazole and caspofungin in a guinea-pig model of aspergillosis (100). In the same laboratory, synergistic effects were found in vitro. However, there is some controversy on whether the effects of the combination were truly superior to voriconazole alone.

Given the limited successes of single drug therapy, and the in vitro/animal studies which show mixed results, clinicians have interpreted these data in the best positive terms possible, and are beginning to use caspofungin plus either amphotericin B or voriconazole clinically. Patients are treated usually for progressing disease, and in general the salvage rate for alternative antifungals has been in the 30–40% range (101,102). The combinations used seem to have responses also in this range, and it is very unclear what, if anything, these costly regimens add to improvement of the clinical outcome. In one "positive" study, 20 of 30 patients treated with caspofungin and liposomal amphotericin B had "possible" rather than "probable" or "documented" infection (103). Thus, the authors of the recent study of mainly "possible" mycoses, in which the patients may not really have had fungal infection, attribute good responses to caspofungin and voriconazole combined. In another study, 28 patients with documented invasive aspergillosis and 22 patients with possible invasive aspergillosis were treated with caspofungin added to liposomal amphotericin B, as salvage therapy (104). The response rates were 21% in documented disease and 77% in possible disease, or similar to prior response rates of 16% in documented invasive aspergillosis. The investigators at MD Anderson were not impressed that caspofungin addition improved outcome of patients on liposomal amphotericin B. In yet another study, combined liposomal amphotericin B and caspofungin or voriconazole and caspofungin were given to six patients with definite or probable invasive aspergillosis "refractory" to lipid formulations of amphotericin B (105). All patients improved, and none of the three deaths were attributed to aspergillosis. Finally, Thebaut et al. treated nine refractory patients with caspofungin and amphotericin B, four patients with caspofungin and voriconazole, and one patient with all three drugs (103). Overall, five patients (36%) had a favorable response.

From the above studies, there does not appear to emerge a clear and dramatic message that the echinocandins add significantly to either amphotericin B or to triazoles. Although there appears to be no added toxicity, these regimens are very costly. Accordingly, in the absence of Phase III studies, the anecdotes reported may be of interest but should not be taken as conclusive evidence of improved outcome in seriously ill patients. More deliberate comparative studies should be done before aggressive practitioners utilize these combinations as standard therapy.

In summary, we can glean that caspofungin (and likely micafungin and possibly anidulafungin as well) have activity against *Aspergillus* species. Data are fewer than for *Candida*, only apply to secondary or salvage therapy, and do not give us any indication of relative potency vs. other antifungals. Merck has recommended that caspofungin daily doses be raised to 70 mg in patients with aspergillosis. There are no clinical data on dose dependency of clinical responses. However, the absence of a maximal tolerable dose suggests that higher doses may be explored. Clinical data on other mycoses await presentation/publication of further information.

VII. A FOOTNOTE ON *PNEUMOCYSTIS*

In addition to classic fungi, *Pneumocystis carinii* also includes ß-1,3-glucans in the walls of its cysts, though not in the trophozoites (106,107). When rats with *P. carinii* infection were treated with anidulafungin, the cyst walls were deformed and lacked cyst wall ß-1,3-glucans. Echinocandins have been effective against *P. carinii* in infected rats and mice (108). Micafungin has been found effective for prophylaxis of *P. carinii* in mice (109). Although the cysts are rapidly eliminated in mice, trophozoites, which do not contain glucans, persist after caspofungin treatment (110). For this reason, and despite the success of animal treatment regimens for infected animals, the echinocandins have not been developed clinically for use in *P. carinii* pneumonia.

REFERENCES

1. Hector RF. Compounds active against cell walls of medically important fungi. Clin Microbiol Rev 1993; 6:1–21.
2. Chapman T, Kinsman O, Houston J. Chitin biosynthesis in *Candida albicans* grown *in vitro* and *in vivo* and its inhibitin by nikkomycin Z. Antimicrob Agents Chemother 1992; 36(9):1909–1914.
3. Debono M, Gordee RS. Antibiotics that inhibit fungal cell wall development. Ann Rev Microbiol 1994; 48:471–497.
4. DeLucca A, Walsh TJ. Antifungal agents: novel therapeutic compounds against emerging pathogens. Antimicrob Agents Chemother 1999; 43:1–11.
5. Graybill JR, Najvar LK, Bocanegra R, Hector RF, Luther MF. Efficacy of Nikkomycin Z in the treatment of murine histoplasmosis. Antimicrob Agents Chemother 1998; 42:2371–2374.
6. Hector RF, Schaller K. Positive interaction of nikkomycins and azoles against *Candida albicans* in vitro and in vivo. Antimicrob Agents Chemother 1992; 36(6):1284–1289.
7. Kakushima M, Masuyoshi S, Hirano M, Shinoda M, Ohta A, Kamei H, Oki T. In vitro and in vivo antifungal activities of BMY-28864, a water-soluble pradimycin derivative. Antimicrob Agents Chemother 1991; 35:2185–2190.
8. Oki TM, Konishi M, Tomatsu K, Tomita K, Saitoh M, Tsunakawa M, Nishio M, Miyaki T, Kawaguchi H. Pradimycin, a novel class of potent antifungal antibiotics. J Antibiot (Tokyo) 1988; 41:1701–1704.
9. Angiolella L, Simonetti N, Cassone A. The lipopeptide antimycotic, cilofungin modulates the incorporation of glucan-associated proteins into the cell wall of *Candida albicans*. J Antimicrob Chemother 1994; 33:1137–1146.
10. Taft CS, Stark T, Selitrennikoff CP. Cilofungin (LY12109) inhibits Candida albicans (1-3)-beta-D-glucan synthase activity. Antimicrob Agents Chemother 1988; 32:1901–1903.

11. Douglas CM, D'ippolito JA, Shei GJ, Meinz M, Onishi J, Marrinan JA, Li W, Abruzzo GK, Flattery A, Bartizal K, Mitchell A, Kurtz MB. Identification of the FKS1 gene of Candida albicans as the essential target of 1,3-beta,D-glucan synthase inhibitors. Antimicrob Agents Chemother 1997; 41:2471–2479.

12. Perfect JR, Hobbs MM, Wright KA, Durack DT. Treatment of experimental disseminated candidiasis with cilofungin. Antimicrob Agents Chemother 1989; 33(10): 1811–1812.

13. Beaulieu D, Tang J, Yan B, Vessels JM, Radding JA, Parr TR. Characterization and cilofungin inhibition of solubilized *Aspergillus fumigatus* (1,3)-beta-D-glucan synthase. Antimicrob Agents Chemother 1994; 38:937–944.

14. Beaulieu D, Tang J, Zeckner DJ, Parr TR Jr. Correlation of cilofungin in vivo efficacy with its activity against *Aspergillus fumigatus* (1,3)-β-D-glucan synthase. FEMS Microbiol Lett 1993; 108:133–138.

15. Rouse MS, Tallan BM, Steckelberg JM, Henry NK, Wilson WR. Efficacy of cilofungin therapy administered by continuous intravenous infusion for experimental disseminated candidiasis in rabbits. Antimicrob Agents Chemother 1992; 36(1):56–58.

16. Walsh TJ, Lee JW, Bacher J, Lecciones J, Thomas V, Lyman C, Coleman D, Gordee R, Pizzo PA. Antifungal effects of the nonlinear pharmacokinetis of cilofungin, a 1,3-beta-D-glucan synthase inhibitor, during continuous and intermittent infusions in treatment of experimental disseminated candidiasis. Antimicrob Agents Chemother 1991; 35:1321–1328.

17. Galgiani JN, Sun SH, Clemons KV, Stevens DA. Activity of cilofungin against *Coccidioides immitis*: differential in vitro effects in mycelia and spherules correlated with in vivo studies. J Infect Dis 1990; 162:944–948.

18. Bulo AN, Bradley SF, Kauffman CA. The effect of cilofungin (LY 121019) in combination with amphotericin B or flucytosine against *Candida* species. Mycoses 1989; 32(3): 151–157.

19. Denning DW, Stevens DA. Efficacy of cilofungin alone and in combination with amphotericin B in a murine model of disseminated aspergillosis. Antimicrob Agents Chemother 1991; 35(7):1329–1333.

20. Hanson LH, Perlman AM, Clemons KD, Stevens DA. Synergy between cilofungin and amphotericin B in a murine model of candidiasis. Antimicrob Agents Chemother 1991; 35(7):1334–1337.

21. Sugar AM, Goldani LZ, Picard M. Treatment of murine invasive candidiasis with amphotericin B and cilofungin: evidence of enhanced activity with combination therapy. Antimicrob Agents Chemother 1991; 35(10):2128–2130.

22. Klepser ME, Ernst EJ, Ernst ME, Messer SA, Pfaller MA. Evaluation of endpoints for antifungal susceptibility determinations with LY303366. Antimicrob Agents Chemother 1998; 42:1387–1391.

23. Green LJ, Marder P, Mann LL, Chio LC, Current WL. LY303366 exhibits rapid and potent fungicidal activity in flow cytometric assays of yeast viability. Antimicrob Agents Chemother 1999; 43:830–835.

24. Nelson PW, Lozano-Chiu M, Rex JH. In vitro activity of L-743872 against putatively amphotericin B (AmB) and fluconazole (Flu)-resistant Candida isolates. 36th Interscience Conference on Antimicrobial Agents and Chemotherapy 1996; [Abstr F28], 104.

25. Pfaller MA, Messer SA, Coffman S. In vitro susceptibilities of clinical yeast isolates to a new echinocandin derivative, LY303366, and other antifungal agents. Antimicrob Agents Chemother 1997; 41:763–766.

26. Pfaller MA, Messer SA, Mills K, Bolmström A, Jones RN. Evaluation of E-test method for determining caspofungin (MK-0991) susceptibilities of 726 clinical isolates of *Candida* species. J Clin Microbiol 2001; 39:4387–4389.

27. Barchiesi F, Schimizzi AM, Fothergill AW, Scalise G, Rinaldi MG. In vitro activity of the new echinocandin antifungal, MK-0991, against common and uncommon clinical isolates of *Candida* species. Eur J Clin Microbiol Infect Dis 1999; 18:302–304.

28. Ernst EJ, Klepser ME, Pfaller M. Postantifungal effects of echinocandin, azole, and polyene antifungal agents against *Candida albicans* and *Cryptococcus neoformans.* Antimicrob Agents Chemother 2000; 44:1108–1111.

29. Gunderson SM, Hoffman H, Ernst EJ, Pfaller MA, Klepser ME. In vitro pharmaco-dynamic characteristics of nystatin including time-kill and postantifungal effect. Antimicrob Agents Chemother 2000; 44:2887–2890.

30. Bartizal KF, Abruzzo G, Trainor C, Krupa D, Nollstadt K, Schmatz D, Schwartz R, Hammond M, Balkovec J, Vanmiddlesworth F. *In vitro* antifungal activities and *in vivo* efficacies of 1,3-β-D-Glucan synthesis inhibitors L-671,329, L-646,991, tetrahydroechinocandin B, and L-687,781, a papulacandin. Antimicrob Agents Chemother 1992; 36(8):1648–1657.

31. Osherov N, May G, Albert MD, Kontoyiannis DP. Overexpression of Sbe2p, a Golgi protein, results in resistance to caspofungin in *Saccharromyces cerevesiae.* Antimicrob Agents Chemother. 2002; 46:2462–2469.

32. Kuhn DM, George T, Chandra J, Mukherjee PK, Ghannoum MA. Antifungal suscept-ibility of *Candida* biofilms: Unique efficacy of amphotericin B lipid formulations and echinocandins. Antimicrob Agents Chemother 2002; 46:1773–1780.

33. Rex JH. Catheters and candidemia - editorial response. Clin Infect Dis 1996; 22:467–470.

34. Rex JH, Bennett JE, Sugar AM, Pappas PG, Serody J, Edwards JE, Washburn RG. Intravascular catheter exchange and duration of candidemia. Clin Infect Dis 1995; 21:994–996.

35. Bowman JC, Hicks PS, Kurtz MB, Rosen H, Schmatz DM, Liberator PA, Douglas CM. The antifungal echinocandin caspofungin acetate kills growing cells of *Aspergillus fumigatus* in vitro. Antimicrob Agents Chemother 2002; 46:3001–3012.

36. Kurtz MB, Heath IB, Marrinan J, Dreikorn S, Onishi J, Douglas C. Morphological effects of lipopeptides against *Aspergillus fumigatus* correlate with activities against (1,3)-β-D-glucan synthase. Antimicrob Agents Chemother 1994; 38:1480–1489.

37. Douglas CM, Bowman JC, Abruzzo GK, Flattery AM, Gill CJ, Long K, Leighton C, Smith JG, Pikounis VB, Bartizal K, Kurtz MB, Rosen H. The glucan synthesis inhibitor caspofungin acetate kills *Aspergillus fumigatus* hyphal tips in vitro and is effecive against disseminated aspergillosis in cyclophosphamide induced chronically leukopenic mice. Fortieth Interscience Conference on Antimicrobial Agents and Chemotherapy 2000; 40:387.

38. National Committee for Clinical Laboratory Standards. Unpublished data. 1998.

39. Gonzalez G, Tijerina R, Najvar L, Bocanegra R, Luther M, Rinaldi M, Graybill J. Correlation between antifungal susceptibilities of *Coccidioides immitis* (CI) in vitro and antifungal treatment with caspofungin in a mouse model. Antimicrob Agents Chemother 2001; 45:1854–1859.

40. Arikan S, Lozano-Chiu M, Paetznick V, Rex JH. In vitro susceptibility testing methods for caspofungin against *Aspergillus* and *Fusarium* isolates. Antimicrob Agents Chemother 2001; 45:327–330.

41. Arikan S, Paetznick V, Rex JH. Comparative evaluation of disk diffusion with micro-dilution assay in susceptibility testing of caspofungin against *Aspergillus* and *Fusarium* isolates. Antimicrob Agents Chemother 2002; 46:3084–3087.

42. Del Poeta M, Schell WA, Perfect J. In vitro antifungal activity of pneumocandin L-743,872 against a variety of clinically important molds. Antimicrob Agents Chemother 1997; 41:1835–1836.

43. Vitale RG, Mouton JW, Afeltra J, Meis JFGM, Verweij PE. Method for measuring postantifungal effect in *Aspergillus* species. Antimicrob Agents Chemother 2002; 46:1960–1965.

44. Kutler C, Koll B, Raucher B, Saltznab B. Treatment of resistant oral and esopageal candidiasis with caspofungin in patients with AIDS. Fortieth Annual Meeting of IDSA 2002 [Abstr 350].

45. Maesaki S, Hossain MA, Miyazaki Y, Tomono K, Tashiro T, Kohno S. Efficacy of FK4634, a 1,3-beta-D-glucan synthase inhibitor, in dissemianted azole-resistant *Candida albicans* infection in mice. Antimicrob Agents Chemother 2000; 44:1728–1730.

46. Abruzzo GK, Flattery AM, Gill CJ, Kong L, Smith JG, Pikounis VB, Balkovec JM, Bouffard AF, Dropinksi JF, Rosen H, Kropp H, Bartizal K. Evaluation of the echinocandin antifungal MK-0991 (L-743,872) efficacies in mouse models of disseminated aspergillosis, candidiasis, and cryptococcosis. Antimicrob Agents Chemother 1997; 41:2333–2338.

47. Graybill J, Bocanegra R, Luther M, Fothergill A, Rinaldi MG. Treatment of murine *Candida krusei* or *Candida glabrata* infection with L-743,872. Antimicrob Agents Chemother 1997; 41:1937–1939.

48. Abruzzo GK, Gill CJ, Flattery AM, Kong L, Leighton C, Smith JG, Pikounis VB, Bartizal K, Rosen H. Efficacy of the echinocandin caspofungin against disseminated aspergillosis and candidiasis in cyclophosphamide-induced immunosuppressed mice. Antimicrob Agents Chemother 2000; 44:2310–2318.

49. Bernard EM, Ishimaru T, Armstrong D. Low doses of pneumocandin L-743872, are effective in prevention and treatment in an animal model of pulmonary aspergillosis. 36th Interscience Conference on Antimicrobial Agents and Chemotherapy [Abstr F38], 1996; 106.

50. Verweij PE, Oakley KL, Morrissey J, Morrissey G, Denning DW. Efficacy of LY303366 against amphotericin B susceptible and resistant *Aspergillus fumigatus* in a murine model of invasive aspergillosis. Antimicrob Agents Chemother 1998; 42:873–878.

51. Petraitis V, Petraitiene R, Groll A, Roussillon K, Hemmings M, Lyman CA, Sein T, Bacher J, Bekersky I, Walsh TJ. Comparative antifungal activities and plasma pharmacokinetics of micafungin (FK463) against disseminated candidiasis and invasive pulmonary aspergillosis in persistently neutropenic rabbits. Antimicrob Agents Chemother 2002; 46:1857–1869.

52. Petraitiene R, Petrikkou E, Groll AH, Sein T, Schaufele R, Francesconi A, Avila NA, Walsh TJ. Anitifungal efficacy of caspofungin (MK-0991) in experimental pulmonary aspergillosis in persistently neutropenic rabbits: pharmacokinetics, drug disposition, and relationship to galactomannan antigenemia. Antimicrob Agents Chemother 2002; 46:12–23.

53. Bowman JC, Abruzzo GK, Anderson JW, Flattery AM, Gill CJ, Pikounis VB, Schmatz DM, Liberator PA, Douglas CM. Quantitative PCR assay to measure *Aspergillus fumigatus* burden in a murine model of disseminated aspergillosis: Demonstration of efficacy of caspofungin acetate. Antimicrob Agents Chemother 2001; 45:3474–3481.

54. Graybill JR, Najvar LC, Montalbo EM, Barchiesi FJ, Luther MF, Rinaldi MG. Treatment of histoplasmosis with MK-991 (L-743,872). Antimicrob Agents Chemother 1998; 42:151–153.

55. Kohler S, Wheat J, Connoly P, Schnizlein-Bick C, Durkin C, Smedema M, Goldberg J, Brizendine E. Comparison of the echinocandin caspofungin with amphotericin B for treatment of histoplasmosis following pulmonary challenge in the murine model. Antimicrob Agents Chemother 2000; 44:1850–1854.

56. Del Poeta M, Schell WA, Perfect JR. In vitro antifungal activity of L-743872 against a variety of moulds. 36th Interscience Conference on Antimicrobial Agents and Chemotherapy [Abstr F33], 1996; 105.

57. Groll AH, Mickiene D, Werner K, Petratiene R, Petraitis V, Calendario M, Field-Ridley A, Crisp J, Piscitelli SC, Walsh TJ. Compartmental pharmacokinetics and tissue distribution of multilamellar liposomal nystatin in rabbits. Antimicrob Agents Chemother 2000; 44:950–957.

58. Stone JA, Hollana SD, Wickersham PJ, Sterrett A, Schwartz M, Bonfiglio C, Hesney M, Winchell GA, Deutsch PJ, Greenberg H, Hunt TL, Waldman SA. Single- and multiple-dose pharmacokinetics of caspofungin in healthy men. Antimicrob Agents Chemother 2002; 46:739–745.

59. Hiemenz J, Cagnoni P, Simpson D, Devine S, Chao M. Maximum tolerated dose and pharmacokinetics of FK463 in combination with fluconazole for the prophylaxis of fungal infections in adult bone marrow or peripheral stem cell transplant recipients. 39th Interscience Conference on Antimicrobial Agents and Chemotherapy 1999; 39:576 [Abstr 1648].

60. Thye D, Shepherd B, White RJ, Weston IE, Henkel T. Anidulafungin: a phase I study to determine the maximum tolerated daily dose in healthy volunteers. Abstracts of the 41st Interscience Conference on Antimicrobial Agents and Chemotherapy 2002; 42:[Abstr 36].

61. Balani SK, Xu X, Arison BH, Silva MV, Gries A, DeLuna FA, Cui DH, Kari PH, Ly T, Hop CECA, Singh R, Wallace MA, Dean DC, Lin JH, Pearson PG, Baillie TA. Metabolites of caspofungin acetate, a potent antifungal agent, in human plasma and urine. Drug Metab Dispos 2000; 28:1274–1278.

62. Arathoon EG, Gotuzzo E, Noriega LM, Berman RS, DiNubile MJ, Sable CA. Randomized, double-blind, multicenter study of caspofungin versus amphotericin B for treatment of oropharyngeal and esophageal candidiases. Antimicrob Agents Chemother 2002; 46:451–457.

63. Mora-Duarte J, Betts R, Rotstein C, Colombo A, Thompson-Moya L, Smietana J, Lupinacci R, Sable C, Kartsonis N, Perfect J. Comparison of caspofungin and amphotericin B for invasive candidiasis. N Engl J Med 2002; 347:2020–2029.

64. White RJ, Thye D. Anidulafungin does not affect metabolism of cyclosporine by human hepatic microsomes. Abstracts of the 41st Interscience Conference on Antimicrobial Agents and Chemotherapy 2001; 41[Abstr 36].

65. Thye D, Kilfoil T, Kilfoil G, Henkel T. Anidulafungin: pharmacokinetics (PK) in subjects with severe liver failure. Abstracts of the 42nd Interscience Conference on Antimicrobial Agents and Chemotherapy 2002; 42:19[A-1392].

66. Thye D, Kilfoil T, White RJ, Lasseter K. Anidulafungin: pharmacokinetics in subjects with mild and moderate hepatic dysfunction. Abstracts of the 41st Interscience Conference on Antimicrobial Agents and Chemotherapy 2001; 41[Abstr 34].

67. Thye D, Marbury T, Kilfoil T, Kilfoil G, Henkel T. Anidulafungin: pharmacokinetics in subjects receiving hemodialysis. Abstracts of the 42nd Interscience Conference on Antimicrobial Agents and Chemotherapy 2002; 42:19[Abstr A-1390].

68. Villanueva A, Gotuzzo E, Arathoon EG, Noriega LM, Kartsonis NA, Lupinacci RJ, Smietana JM, DiNubile MJ, Sable CA. A randomized double-blind study of caspofungin versus fluconazole for the treatment of esophageal candidiasis. Am J Med 2002; 113:294–299.

69. Kohno S, Masoka T, Yamaguchi H. A multi-center, open-label clinical study of FK463 in patients with deep mycosis in Japan. Abstracts of the 41st Interscience Conference on Antimicrobial Agents and Chemotherapy 2001; 41:384[Abstr J-834].

70. Walsh TJ, Adamson PC, Seibel NL, Flynn PM, Neely MN, Miller A, Sable CA. Pharmacokinetics of caspofungin (CAS) in pediatric patients. Abstracts of the 42nd Interscience Conference on Antimicrobial Agents and Chemotherapy 2002; 42:395 [Abstr M-896].

71. Villanueva A, Arathoon EG, Gotuzzo E, Berman RS, DiNubile MJ, Sable CA. A randomized double-blind study of caspofungin versus amphotericin for the treatment of candidal esophagitis. Clin Infect Dis 2001; 33:1529–1535.

72. Abruzzo GK, Flattery AM, Gill CJ, Kong L, Smith JG, Krupa D, Pikounis VB, Kropp H, Bartizal K. Evaluation of water-soluble pneumocandin analogs L-733560, L-705589, and L-731373 with mouse models of disseminated aspergillosis, candidiasis, and cryptococcosis. Antimicrob Agents Chemother 1995; 39:1077–1081.

73. Petraitis V, Petraitiene R, Groll AH, Sein T, Schaufele RL, Lyman CA, Francesconi A, Bacher J, Piscitelli SC, Walsh TJ. Dosage-dependent antifungal efficacy of V-echinocandin (LY303366) against experimental fluconazole-resistant oropharyngeal and esophageal candidiasis. Antimicrob Agents Chemother 2001; 45:471–479.

74. Suleiman J, Della Negra M, LLanos-Cuentra A, Ticona E, Rex JH, Buell D. Open label study of micafungin in the treatment of esophageal candidiasis (EC). Abstracts of the 42nd Interscience Conference on Antimicrobial Agents and Chemotherapy 2002; 42:394 [Abstr M-893].

75. Pettengell K, Mynhardt J, Kluyts T, Soni P. A multicenter study to determine the minimal effective dose of FK463 for the treatment of esophageal candidiasis in HIV-positive patients. 39th Interscience Conference on Antimicrobial Agents and Chemotherapy 1999; 39:567 [Abstr 1421].

76. Stadler P, Ito T, Brown C. Unpublished data. 2001.

77. Kartsonis N, DiNubile MJ, Bartizal K, Hicks PS, Sable CA. Efficacy of caspofungin in the treatment of esophageal candidiasis resistant to fluconazole. JAIDS 2003; 31: 183–187.

78. Letscher-Bru V, Herbrecht R. Caspofungin: the first representative of a new antifungal class. J Antimicrob Chemother 2003; 51:513–521.

79. Maertens J, Raad I, Sable CA, Ngai A, Berman R, Patterson TF, Denning D, Walsh T. Multicenter, noncomparative study to evaluate the safety and efficacy of caspofungin (CAS) in adults with invasive aspergillosis (IA) refractory (R) or intolerant (I) to standard therapy (ST). Fortieth Interscience Conference on Antimicrobial Agents and Chemotherapy 2000; 40:371.

80. Van Burik JA, Ratanatharathorn V, Lipton JM, Miller C, Bunin N, Walsh TJ. Randomized double-blind trial of micafungin (MI) versus fluconazole (FLU) for prophylaxis of invasive fungal infections in patients (pts) undergoing hematopoietic stem cell transplant (HSCT), NIAID/BAMSG Protocol 46. Abstracts of the 42nd Interscience Conference on Antimicrobial Agents and Chemotherapy 2002; 42: 401 [Abstr M-1238].

81. Waldrop TW, Keiser P, Ware A, Race E, Rossi D, Moore T, Garrison L, Zetka E, Pickle P, Sinclair G. Failure of intermittent caspofungin therapy to treat fluconazole-resistant mucocutaneous *Candida* despite apparent in vitro susceptibility. Abstracts of the 42nd Interscience Conference on Antimicrobial Agents and Chemotherapy 2002; 42:393 [Abstr M-891].

82. Rex JH, Walsh TJ, Sobel JD, Filler SG, Pappas PG, Dismukes WE, Edwards JE. Practice guidelines for the treatment of candidiasis. Clin Infect Dis 2000; 30:662–678.

83. Como JA, Dismukes WE. Oral azole drugs as systemic antifungal therapy. N Engl J Med 1994; 330:263–272.

84. Herbrecht R, Denning DW, Patterson TF, Bennett JE, Greene RE, Oestman J-W, Kern WV, Marr KA, Ribaud P, Lortholary J, Sylvester R, Rubin RH, Wingard J, Stark P, Durand C, Caillot D, Thiel E, Chandrasekar PH, Hodges M, Schlamm H, Troke PF, DePauw BE. Voriconazole versus amphotericin B for primary therapy of invasive aspergillosis. N Engl J Med 2002; 347:408–415.

85. Pfaller MA, Jones RN, Doern GV, Sader HS, Messer SA, Houston A, Coffman S, Hollis RJ, Sentry PG. Bloodstream infections due to *Candida* species: SENTRY Antimicrobial Surveillance Program in North America and Latin America, 1997–1998. Antimicrob Agents Chemother 2000; 44:747–751.

86. Wingard JR, Merz WG, Rinaldi MG, Miller CB, Karp JE, Saral R. Association of *Torulopsis glabrata* infections with fluconazole prophylaxis in neutropenic bone marrow transplant patients. Antimicrob Agents Chemother 1993; 37:1847–1849.

87. Ascioglu S, Rex JH, De Pauw B, Bennett JE, Bille J, Crokaert F, Denning DW, Donnelly JP, Edwards JE, Erjavec Z, Fiere D, Lortholary O, Maertens J, Meis JF, Patterson TF, Ritter J, Selleslag D, Shah PM, Stevens DA, Walsh TJ, Invasive F. Defining opportunistic invasive fungal infections in immunocompromised patients with cancer and hematopoietic stem cell transplants: an international consensus. Clin Infect Dis 2002; 34:7–14.

88. Herbrecht R, Letscher-Bru V, Oprea C, Lioure B, Waller J, Campos F, Villard O, Liu KL, Natarajan-Amé S, Lutz P, Dufour P, Bergerat JP, Candolfi E. *Aspergillus*

galactomannan detection in the diagnosis of invasive aspergillosis in cancer patients. J Clin Oncol 2002; 20:1898–1906.

89. Maertens J, Verhaegen J, Lagrou K, Van Eldere J, Boogaerts M. Screening for circulating galactomannan as a noninvasive diagnostic tool for invasive aspergillosis in prolonged neutropenic patients and stem cell transplantation recipients: a prospective validation. Blood 2001; 97:1604–1610.

90. Lin SJ, Schranz J, Teutsch SM. Aspergillosis case - Fatality rate: Systematic review of the literature. Clin Infect Dis 2001; 32:358–366.

91. White MH, Anaissie EJ, Kisne S, Wingard JR, Hiemenz JW, Cantor A, Gurwith M, DuMond C, Mamelok RD, Bowden RA. Amphotericin B colloidal dispersion vs. amphotericin B as therapy for invasive aspergillosis. Clin Infect Dis 1997; 24:635–642.

92. Maertens J, Raad I, Petrikkous G, Selleslag D, Petersen F, Sable C, Kartsonis N, Ngai A, Taylor A, Patterson T, Denning D, Walsh T. Update of the multicenter noncomparative styudy of caspofungin (CAS) in adults with invasive aspergillosis (IA) refractory (R) or intolerant (I) to other antifungal agents: analysis of 90 patients. Abstracts of the 42nd Interscience Conference on Antimicrobial Agents and Chemotherapy 2002; 42:388 [Abstr M-868].

93. Chiou CC, Mavrogiorgos N, Tillem E, Hector R, Walsh TJ. Synergy, pharmacodynamics, and time-sequenced ultrastructural changes of the interaction between nikkomycin Z and the echinocandin FK463 against *Aspergillus fumigatus*. Antimicrob Agents Chemother 2001; 45:3310–3321.

94. Stevens DA. Drug interaction studies of a glucan synthase inhibitor (LY 303366) and a chitin synthase inhibitor (nikkomycin Z) for inhibition and killing of fungal pathogens. Antimicrob Agents Chemother 2000; 44:2547–2548.

95. Franzot SP, Casadevall A. Pneumocandin L-743,872 enhances the activities of amphotericin B and fluconazole against *Cryptococcus neoformans* in vitro. Antimicrob Agents Chemother 1997; 41:331–336.

96. Roling EE, Klepser ME, Lewis WA, Ernst EJ, Pfaller MA. Antifungal activities of fluconazole, caspofungin (MK0991), and anidulafungin (LY303366) alone and in combination against *Candida* spp. and *Cryptococcus neoformans via time-kill methods. Diagn Microbiol Infect Dis 2002; 43:13–27.*

97. Arikan S, Lozano-Chiu M, Paetznick V, Rex JH. In vitro synergy of caspofungin and amphotericin B against *Aspergillus* and *Fusarium* isolates. Antimicrob Agents Chemother 2002; 46:245–247.

98. Bartizal K, Gill CJ, Abruzzo G, Flattery A, Kong LI, Scott PM, Smith JG, Bouffard AF, Dropinksi JF, Balkovec J. In vitro preclinical evaluation studies with the echinocandin antifungal MK-0991 (L-743,872). Antimicrob Agents Chemother 1997; 41:2326–2332.

99. Nakajima M, Tamada S, Yoshida K, Wakai Y, Nakai T, Ikeda F, Goto T, Niki Y, Mathushima T. Pathological findings in a murine pulmonary aspergillosis model: treatment with FK463, amphotericin B, and a combination of FK463 and amphoericin B. Fortieth Interscience Conference on Antimicrobial Agents and Chemotherapy 2000; 40:387.

100. Kirkpatrick WR, Perea S, Coco BJ, Patterson TF. Efficacy of caspofungin alone and in combination with voriconazole in a guinea pig model of invasive aspergillosis. Antimicrob Agents Chemother 2002; 46:2564–2568.

101. De Pauw BE, Meunier F. The challenge of invasive fungal infection. Chemotherapy 1999; 45:1–14.

102. Rex JH, Walsh TJ, Nettleman M, Anaissie EJ, Bennett JE, Bow EJ, Carillo-Munoz AJ, Chavanet P, Cloud GA, Denning DW, De Pauw BE, Edwards JE Jr, Hiemenz JW, Kauffman CA, Lopez-Berestein G, Martino P, Sobel JD, Stevens DA, Sylvester R, Tollemar J, Viscoli C, Viviani MA, Wu T. Need for alternative trial designs and evaluation strategies for therapeutic studies of invasive mycoses. Clin Infect Dis 2001; 33:95–106.

103. Aliff TB, Maslak PG, Jurcic JG, Heaney ML, Cathcart KN, Sepkowitz KA, Weiss MA. Refractory aspergillus pneumonia in patients with acute leukemia - Successful therapy with combination caspofungin and liposomal amphotericin. Cancer 2003; 97: 1025–1032.

104. Kontoyiannis DP, Hachem R, Lewis RE, Rivero G, Kantarjian H, Raad II. Efficacy and toxicity of the caspofungin/liposomal amphotericin B (CAS/Lipo AMB) combination in documented or possible invasive aspergillosis (IA) in patients (Pts) with hematologic malignancies. Abstracts of the 42nd Interscience Conference on Antimicrobial Agents and Chemotherapy 2002; 42:416 [Abstr M-1820].

105. Gentina T, deBotton S, Alfandari S, de Lomez J, Jaillard S, Lerow O, Marquette C, Beaucaire G, Bauters F, Fenaux P. Combination antifungals for treatment of pulmonary invasive aspergillosis (IA) refractory to amphotericin B (AmB) in leukemia patients. Abstracts of the 42nd Interscience Conference on Antimicrobial Agents and Chemotherapy 2002; 42:386 [Abstr M-860].

106. Bartlett MS, Current WL, Goheen MP, Boylan CJ, Lee CH, Shaw MM, Queener SF, Smith JW. Semisynthetic echinocandins affect cell wall deposition of *Pneumocystis carinii* in vitro and in vivo. Antimicrob Agents Chemother 1996; 40:1811–1816.

107. Nollstadt K, Powles MA, Fujioka H, Aikawa M, Schmatz D. Use of B-1,3,glucan-specific antibody to study the cyst wall of *Pneumocystis carinii* and effects of pneumocandin Bo analogue L-733,560. Antimicrob Agents Chemother 1994; 38:2258–2265.

108. Schmatz D, Powles MA, McFadden D, Nollstadt K, Bouffard AA, Dropinksi JF, Liberator P, Andersen J. New semisynthetic pneumocandins with improved efficacies agaisnt *Pneumocystis carinii* in the rat. Antimicrob Agents Chemother 1995; 39: 1320–1323.

109. Ito M, Nozu R, Kuramochi T, Eguchi N, Suzuki S, Hioki K, Itoh T, Ikeda F. Prophylactic effect of FK463, a novel antifungal lipopeptide, against *Pneumocystis carinii* infection in mice. Antimicrob Agents Chemother 2000; 44:2259–2262.

110. Powles MA, Liberator P, Anderson J, Karkhanis Y, Dropinksi JF, Bouffard FA, Balkovec JM, Fujioka H, Aikawa M, McFadden D, Schmatz D. Efficacy of MK-991 (L743–872), a semisynthetic pneumocandin, in murine models of *Pneumocystis carinii*. Antimicrob Agents Chemother 1998; 42:1985–1989.

19

Antifungal Agents: Other Classes and Compounds

Andreas H. Groll
Infectious Disease Research Program, Center for Bone Marrow Transplantation, Department of Pediatric Hematology/Oncology, University Children's Hospital, Münster, Germany

Thomas J. Walsh
National Institutes of Health, National Cancer Institute/Pediatric Oncology Branch, Bethesda, Maryland, U.S.A.

I. AGENTS FOR SYSTEMIC TREATMENT OF INVASIVE MYCOSES

A. Inhibitors of Protein Synthesis

1. *Flucytosine*

Flucytosine (5-fluorocytosine; 5-FC) is low-molecular weight water-soluble synthetic fluorinated pyrimidine-analogue (Fig. 1). It is taken up into the fungal cell by the fungus-specific enzyme cytosine permease and converted in the cytoplasm by cytosine deaminase to 5-fluorouracil which causes RNA miscoding and inhibits DNA-synthesis (1). The 5-FC is relatively non-toxic to mammalian cells because of the absence or very low level of activity of cytosine deaminase. In the United States, 5-FC is available only as oral formulation; outside the United States, an IV formulation is available in select countries.

   a. **Antifungal Activity.**   The antifungal spectrum of 5-FC in vitro includes *Candida* spp., *Cryptococcus neoformans*, *Saccharomyces cerevisiae*, and selected dematiaceous molds. The 5-FC has no or weak activity against *Aspergillus* spp., and other hyaline molds (1–3). Synergistic or additive effects in combination with amphotericin B (AmB) have been observed against *Candida* spp., and in combination with AmB or fluconazole against *C. neoformans* (4). Resistance to 5-FC in susceptible species may involve either mutations in enzymes necessary for cellular uptake, transport, or metabolism, or competitive upregulation of pyrimidine synthesis (1). While the exact prevalence is unclear, primary resistance has been reported in up to 8% and 22% of clinical *Candida albicans* and non-*albicans Candida* spp., respectively, and in ≤ 2% of *C. neoformans* isolates (5). Secondary resistance, predominantly by selection of resistant clones, can evolve rapidly, at least in *C. albicans*

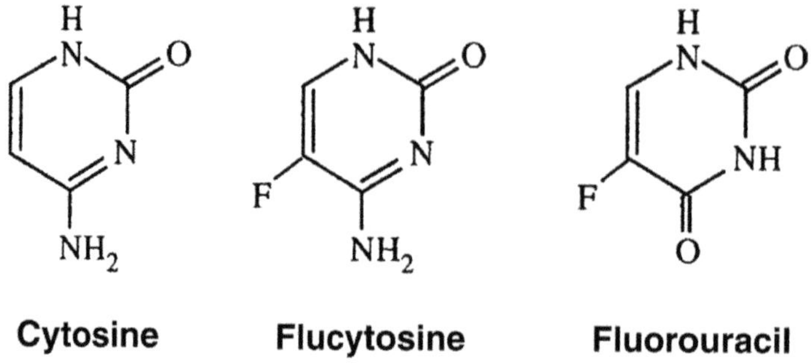

Figure 1 Chemical structures of cytosine, flucytosine, and fluorouracil.

(3). As a consequence, 5-FC is rarely given alone but in combination with AmB, or more recently, fluconazole.

b. Pharmacodynamics. The 5-FC has demonstrated predominantly concentration-independent fungistatic activity against *Candida* species and *C. neoformans* in time-kill assays and prolonged concentration- and exposure-dependent postantifungal effects of up to 10 hr; pharmacodynamic studies in mice with experimental disseminated candidiasis revealed that both the time above the MIC and AUC/MIC were important in predicting efficacy. Maximum efficacy was observed when levels exceeded the MIC for only 20–25% of the 24-hour dosing interval (6). Thus, lower dosages or less-frequent dosing may yield identical antifungal efficacy while further reducing potential toxicities, which are mostly dose-dependent (3).

c. Pharmacokinetics. The 5-FC is readily absorbed from the gastrointestinal tract, has negligible protein binding and distributes evenly into tissues and body fluids, including the CSF, peritoneal fluid, inflamed joints, and the eye. At usual dosages, the drug undergoes negligible hepatic metabolism and is eliminated predominantly in active form by glomerular filtration into the urine with a half-life in plasma of 3–6 hr. Individual dosage adjustment is necessary in patients with impaired renal function and those undergoing hemofiltration. In patients undergoing hemodialysis, a dose of 37.5 mg/kg is recommended following dialysis; in peritoneal dialysis, the compound can be administered systemically or intraperitoneally. Although the data are limited, impaired liver function does not appear to alter the disposition of 5-FC (2,4). The pharmacokinetics of 5-FC in pediatric patients has not been systematically characterized, and uniform dosing recommendations in this population cannot be made (7).

d. Adverse Effects. Common adverse effects of 5-FC that occur in 5–6% of patients include gastrointestinal intolerance and reversible elevations of hepatic transaminases and alkaline phosphatase. More rare side effects are skin rashes, blood eosinophilia, and crystalluria (4). Hematological adverse effects have been reported in overall 6% of patients receiving oral 5-FC, and may include neutropenia, thrombocytopenia, or pancytopenia. While they are usually reversible following discontinuation of the drug or dosage reduction, fatal outcomes have been reported (3). Some of the adverse effects of 5-FC may be due to the compound's conversion to 5-fluorouracil by the gastrointestinal bacterial flora (8) or toxic effects of endogenous metabolites. Hematological adverse effects are less frequent if plasma levels of 5-FC do not exceed 100 μg/mL (3,9).

e. Drug Interactions. Orally administered, non-resorbable antibiotics and aluminum/magnesium hydroxide-based antacids may delay absorption of 5-FC from the gastrointestinal tract (4). The 5-FC is not known to interfere with CYP450 enzyme system. However, any drug that can cause a reduction in the glomerular filtration rate may lead to increased 5-FC serum levels and thereby has the potential to enhance 5-FC-associated toxicity. This includes AmB as well as number of antimicrobial agents, anticancer drugs, and cyclosporin (2). Cytosine arabinoside (ARA-C) competitively inhibits 5-FC and both drugs should not be given concomitantly.

f. Indications and Dosing. Due to the propensity for secondary resistance (10), 5-FC is generally not administered as a single agent. An established indication for its use in combination with amphotericin B deoxycholate (DAMB) is that for induction therapy of cryptococcal meningitis (11,12). The combination of DAMB with 5-FC can also be recommended for the treatment of *Candida* infections involving deep tissues, particularly in critically ill patients and when non-*albicans Candida* species are involved (3). This includes *Candida* meningitis, endophthalmitis, endocarditis, vasculitis, and peritonitis, as well as osteoarticular, renal, and chronic disseminated candidiasis (4). The combination of 5-FC with fluconazole may be used for cryptococcal meningitis, when treatment with AmB is not feasible. In addition, this combination may also be useful as second-line therapy for individual patients with invasive *Candida* infections involving aqueous body compartments. Currently, we recommend a starting dosage for both adults and children of 100 mg/kg daily divided in three or four doses.

g. Therapeutic Monitoring. Monitoring of plasma concentrations is essential to adjust dosage to changing renal function and to avoid toxicity. Following oral administration, near peak levels 2 hr postdosing overlap with trough levels as patients reach steady state and are thus sufficient for therapeutic monitoring (3). Peak plasma levels between 40 and 60 μg/mL correlate with antifungal efficacy and are seldom associated with hematological adverse effects (3,9).

2. Sordarins

The sordarins (Fig. 2) are a distinct class of investigational semisynthetic antifungal agents that selectively inhibit fungal protein synthesis by an interaction with translation elongation factor 2 and the large ribosomal subunit stalk rpP0 (13,14). More

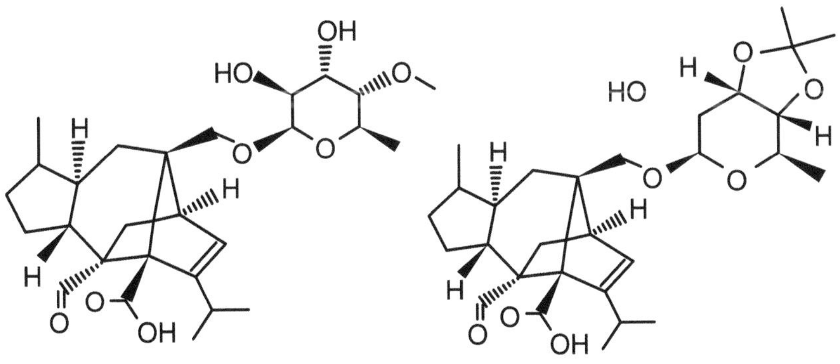

Sordarin   **GM 193663**

Figure 2 Sordarin and the semisynthetic sordarin derivative GM193663. The sordarins are composed of a pyranose sugar and a variable ring structure attached to C3'-C4'. The parent sordarin is a natural product of the fungus *Sordaria oraneosa*.

recently, several novel derivatives (GM-193663, GM-211676, GM-222712, and GM-327354) have undergone preclinical investigation and have demonstrated the potential of this class for clinical development (15).

a. **Spectrum and Pharmacodynamics in Vitro.** The sordarins have potent antifungal activity in vitro against *C. albicans* and non-*albicans Candida* spp., (*C. krusei* exempted), *C. neoformans*, other yeast-like fungi and endemic molds. With few exceptions, they appear to have lesser or no activity against opportunistic filamentous fungi and dermatophytes (16). In time-kill assays, consistent with their mechanism of action, the sordarins exhibited time-dependent fungicidal dynamics against *C. albicans* (17). Using an in vitro one compartment pharmacodynamic model, unbound plasma concentrations of the lead compound GM 237354 were simulated and antifungal activity in vitro compared to antifungal efficacy in an in vivo murine model of systemic candidiasis. The compound displayed concordant fungicidal activity in vitro and in vivo; the in vitro model predicted accurately the in vivo antifungal efficacy of GM 237354 and might thus be useful to forecast in vivo outcome in conjunction with clinical trials (18).

b. **Pharmacokinetics.** The plasma pharmacokinetics of GM-237354 have been investigated in rodents and *Cynomolgus* monkeys. GM-237354 achieved considerable exposure as measured by the plasma AUC and a half-life ranging from 0.45 hr in mice to 1.75 hr in monkeys. The compound exhibited high ($>95\%$) protein binding and exhibited linear pharmacokinetics. No information is available on metabolism, routes of excretion as well as safety and pharmacokinetics in humans. Based on interspecies-scaling, the half-life in humans was estimated to be around 9 hr (19,20).

c. **Antifungal Efficacy and Pharmacodynamics in Vivo.** Promising therapeutic efficacy of sordarins has been demonstrated in non-immunocompromised murine models of disseminated and mucosal candidiasis (21,22), histoplasmosis (23) and coccidioidomycosis (24). Efficacy in non-immunocompromised murine models of disseminated aspergillosis was limited (21,25). Sordarins have shown strong inhibitory activity on protein synthesis and replication of *Pneumocystis carinii* in vitro that translated into promising in vivo efficacy in murine models of pneumocystosis (21,26). Relationship between pharmacokinetic parameters of GM-237354 and outcome were investigated in a lethal murine kidney target model of systemic *C. albicans* candidiasis (27). Across all dosing regimens, the AUC correlated best with survival and clearance of the organism from the kidney, while C_{max} and the Ttau $>$ MIC were not predictive. Using pharmacodynamic modeling and E_{max} functions, the predicted AUC for an efficacy target of 90% survival was 67 µg/hr/mL.

d. **State of Development.** The example of the sordarins clearly reflects the progress in antifungal drug development with pharmacodynamic studies being incorporated in early steps of the preclinical drug development process. Although preclinical safety data were favorable, sordarin compounds have not yet entered the stages of clinical development.

3. Cispentacin Derivatives: PLD-118 (BAY 10–8888)

PLD-118[(-) (1R,2S)-2-amino-4-methylene-cyclopentane carboxylic acid] is a novel synthetic, water-soluble orally bio-available antifungal agent of the beta-amino acid class that is structurally related to the naturally occurring beta-amino acid cispentacin and that is currently undergoing phase II clinical trials for oral treatment of mucocutaneous *Candida*-infections. The PLD acts by a dual mode of action (Fig. 3): first, it is accumulated in yeast cells by active transport via permeases specific for branched amino acids. Inside the cell, PLD-118 specifically inhibits

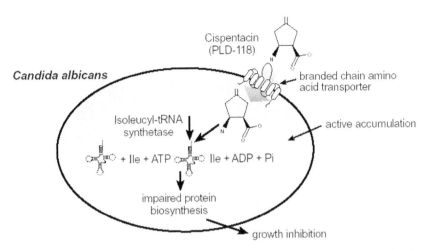

Figure 3 Chemical structure and mechanism of action of the cispentacin derivative, PLD-118.

isoleucyl t-RNA synthetase, resulting in inhibition of protein synthesis and cell growth (28,29). Of note, efflux of PLD-118 from the cell occurs by diffusion and is not carrier mediated (28). *C. albicans* and *C. tropicalis* isolates resistant to PLD-118 showed either decreased accumulation or increased isoleucyl-tRNA synthetase activity (30).

   a.   **Antifungal Spectrum and In Vivo Efficacy.**   The in vitro activity of PLD-118 depends strongly on assay conditions, mainly due to the expression of the transporter for active transport (31,32). Using a microtiter plate dilution assay and YPG medium, PLD-118 showed antifungal activity against *C. albicans* (32), including azole-resistant isolates (31), *C. glabrata, C. krusei*, and to a lesser extent, *C. tropicalis* and *C. parapsilosis* (33). Time-kill assays against fluconazole-resistant *C. albicans* showed concentration-dependent pharmacodynamics in vitro (34). In vivo, oral PLD achieved complete survival in lethal models of disseminated azole-susceptible and azole-resistant *C. albicans* infections in mice and rats at dosages of 10 and 4 mg/kg BID, respectively (35,31). Against experimental esophageal candidiasis caused by fluconazole-resistant *C. albicans* in corticosteroid-immunosuppressed rabbits, PLD-118 demonstrated significant dose-dependent antifungal efficacy (34).

   b.   **Preclinical Pharmacokinetics and Safety.**   Plasma pharmacokinetics in rats, rabbits, and dogs revealed linear pharmacokinetics following single oral dosing over a concentration range of 1–100 mg/kg. The half-life increased from 3 hr in mice to 10 hr in dogs. Plasma protein binding was less than 1%, and studies with radiolabeled compound showed a homogeneous distribution within all tissues. Almost complete renal elimination of unchanged compound was observed in rats and dogs, and no major metabolites were detected. Using pooled liver microsomes and specific probe substrates, PLD did not inhibit the most prevalent human liver cytochrome P450 isoenzymes. The PLD was well tolerated in experimental animals with an LD50 exceeding 2000 mg/kg in mice and rats and a no effect level of 30 mg/kg in rats and dogs after 4 weeks of administration (36,37).

   c.   **Clinical Trials.**   In healthy volunteers, tolerance, safety, and pharmacokinetics of oral PLD-118 were investigated in a double-blind, randomized, and placebo-controlled cross-over study at dosages ranging from 17.5 to 280 mg. The PLD exhibited linear plasma pharmacokinetics. Peak plasma concentrations ranged from 0.5 to 8.5 µg/mL and were achieved at approximately 1 hr after dosing. Elimination half-life was 6–7 hr and 70–90% of unchanged compound was recovered in urine within 72 hr after dosing. The PLD appeared to be well tolerated without significant acute adverse events (38). Following multiple dosing at 50–200 mg q8h and 150 or 300 mg q12h for 7 days, steady-state plasma levels were dose-proportional and achieved within 2–3 days of multiple dosing. Similar to single dosing, half-life was around 7 hr, and more than 80% of compound were recovered in urine in unchanged form. The PLD was well tolerated. The most common adverse event was a dry mouth, occurring in six subjects receiving PLD (39).

    d. Perspectives. Based on its unique mechanism of action, promising activity against *Candida* spp., in vitro and in vivo, favorable pharmacokinetic and safety profiles, and the potential for oral and IV administration of PLD-118 warrants further preclinical and clinical investigation as therapeutic agent against superficial and perhaps, invasive *Candida* infections.

II. CELL WALL ACTIVE AGENTS

A. Nikkomycin Z

The nikkomycins and the structurally closely related polyoxins are antifungal antibiotics produced by Streptomycetes and were discovered in the 1970s through programs searching for new fungicides and insecticides for agricultural use (40). The nikkomycins and polyoxins are pyrimidine nucleosides that are linked to a di- or tripeptide moiety (Fig. 4). They are structurally similar to UDP-*N*-acetyl-glucosamine, the precursor substrate for chitin, a linear polymer of b-(1-4)-linked *N*-acetylglucosamine residues.

    The nikkomycins and polyoxins act as competitive inhibitors of chitin synthesis, leading to inhibition of septation, chaining, and osmotic swelling of the fungal cell (40,41). In *C. albicans*, three different membrane-bound isoenzymes of chitin synthase have been described. Although the absence of all three isoenzymes is uniformly lethal, no single one is essential, and each may be inhibited to different degrees by different compounds. Of note, the chitin-synthase inhibitors are required

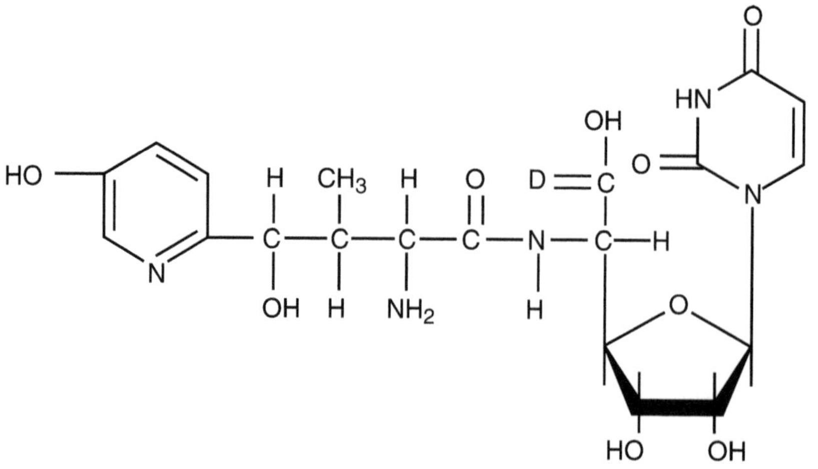

Figure 4 Chemical structure of nikkomycin Z.

to be transported into the cell via one or more permeases. This transport system, however, is subject to antagonism by extracellular peptides. In addition, various proteases can inactivate the nucleoside-peptide compounds. This results in a wide range of susceptibility of intact fungi, even though their isolated enzyme preparations are uniformly sensitive (4,40,41).

1. Antifungal Spectrum and In Vivo Efficacy

Among the nucleoside-peptide chitin-synthase inhibitors, only nikkomycin Z has been investigated to a greater extent. Nikkomycin Z has been shown to have particularly good activity against the chitinous dimorphic fungi *Coccidioides immitis* and *Blastomyces dermatitidis*, both in vitro and in vivo (42,43). Its in vitro activity against *Histoplasma capsulatum, C. albicans*, and *C. neoformans* was only moderate, and non-*albicans Candida* spp., and filamentous fungi appear essentially resistant (44). However, the compound had inhibitory activity in murine models of systemic candidiasis and histoplasmosis, respectively (45–47).

Notably, synergy between nikkomycin Z and antifungal triazoles against *C. albicans, C. neoformans*, and *Aspergillus fumigatus* has been observed in vitro (45,48,49), and synergy with fluconazole could be demonstrated in a mouse model of systemic candidiasis (45). Whereas synergy with glucan synthesis inhibitors against *C. albicans* in vitro has been described early on (50,51), more recent in vitro studies also provided strong evidence for additive or synergistic cooperation against *A. fumigatus* and, more variably, against other filamentous fungi (52–54).

2. State of Clinical Development

Apart from a phase I study of safety and pharmacokinetics of single oral doses of 0.25–2.0 mg/kg in human volunteers, nikkomycin Z is being evaluated for treatment of coccidioidomycosis. The compound may be useful for other mycoses as well, particularly in combination with other antifungals such as triazoles and echinocandins and remains a candidate for clinical development as well as natural peptidyl nucleoside lead compounds that continue to be investigated.

III. CELL MEMBRANE ACTIVE AGENTS

A. Pradimicins

The pradimicins and the structurally similar benanomycins constitute a unique class of antifungal antibiotics derived from *Actinomycetes* with broad-spectrum fungicidal activity (55,56). The chemical structure of these compounds is characterized by a benzonaphthacene quinone skeleton substituted by a D-amino acid and a disaccharide side chain (Fig. 5). Since their discovery in the late 1980s, numerous natural and semisynthetic congeners have been developed, which differ from one another by virtue of substitutents and type of D-amino acid and hexose sugar (57). The pradimicins and benanomycins possess a novel mechanism of action, consisting of a calcium-dependent complexing with the saccharide portion of cell surface mannoproteins, leading to perturbation of the cell membrane, leakage of intracellular contents, disintegration of intracellular organelles, and ultimately, cell death (58).

1. Antifungal Spectrum and In Vivo Efficacy

Both pradimicins and benanomicins possess broad-spectrum antifungal activity in vitro and in vivo, including *Candida* spp., *C. neoformans, Aspergillus* spp.,

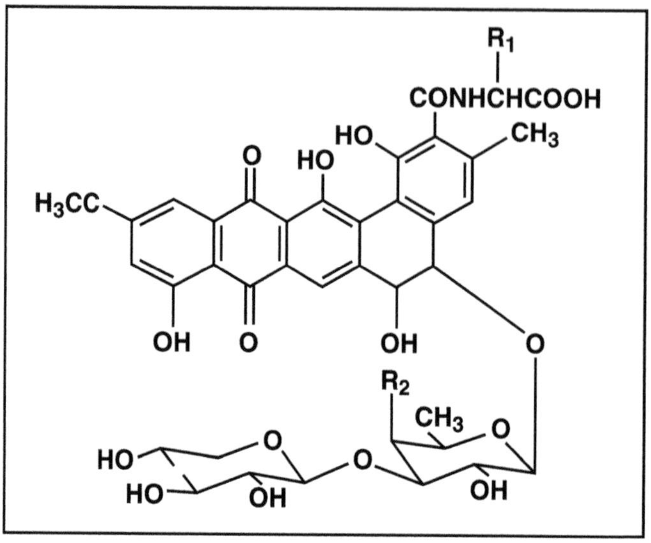

	R_1	R_2
Benanomycin A	CH_3	OH
BMS 181184	CH_2OH	OH

Figure 5 Chemical structures of the pradimicin antibiotics, BMS 181184 and benanomycin A.

dematiaceous molds and dermatophytic fungi without cross-resistance to cross-resistance to polyenes, antifungal azoles and 5-FC (57,59–61). Pradimicins also have antiviral activity, possibly due to an interaction with mannose-containing glycoproteins on the surface of those viruses (57).

The pradimicins have demonstrated potent efficacy in murine models of systemic candidiasis, cryptococcosis and aspergillosis, both in immunocompetent and immunosuppressed animals (57). BMS 181184, a 4'hydroxy analog of the earlier BMY 28864 with excellent water solubility, was the first pradimicin targeted for clinical development. The compound had promising antifungal efficacy in rabbit models of subacute disseminated candidiasis, disseminated aspergillosis, and invasive pulmonary aspergillosis in profoundly neutropenic rabbits (62–64). Among the benanomycins, benanomycin A exhibited the best activity. Apart from therapeutic efficacy against disseminated candidiasis, cryptococcosis, and aspergillosis in non-immunocompromised mice (65) the compound also demonstrated activity in a murine model of *P. carinii* pneumonia (66).

2. State of Development

A high-therapeutic index permitted the administration of large doses of BMS 181184 to animals with minimal toxicity. Significant findings in unpublished preclinical toxicity studies were red discoloration of body fluids and numerous tissues associated with reversible granulomatous inflammation in these tissues; renal tubular degeneration at high dosages and dose-dependent, species specific hemolysis in *Cynomolgus* monkeys. Unexpected hepatic toxicity in early phase I studies led to the stop of further development of this compound; no new pradimicin or benenomycin lead compounds have been reported in the interim.

B. Antimicrobial Peptides

Potentially promising approaches to antifungal therapy are naturally occuring cationic peptides or their synthetic derivatives. These molecules are part of the mammalian oxygen independent microbial host defense mechanisms [histatins, indolicidin, bactericidal/permeability increasing (BPI) factor, lactoferrin, and defensins] or belong to the antimicrobial response of insects (cecropins), bees, amphibes, plants, and various other species. Cationic peptides may bind to the lipid bilayer of biological membranes, form pores and ultimately produce cell death; others may traverse the membrane and interact with intracellular molecules. They may possess broad-spectrum, non-crossresistant antifungal activity, and probably do not induce resistance at measurable frequencies. While some of these peptides are quite toxic, others have only weak activity against mammalian cells (67–69).

Naturally occurring, cationic peptides with potentially exploitable antifungal activity in vitro include, among others, the defensins, the protegrins, gallinacin I, cecropin A, thanatin, and the dermaseptins. Cecropin, an antimicrobial lytic peptide not lethal to mammalian cells, is derived from the silk moth and appears to bind to fungal ergosterol. Its antifungal properties are genus and species-dependent, and include prevention of spore germination, reduced hyphal viability, and potential lethality to hyphae (70). In vivo, a liposomal formulation of indolicin was effective against experimental systemic aspergillosis (71). Similarly, synthetic derivatives of the BPI protein demonstrated dose-dependent effects on survival and fungal burden in mouse models of systemic candidiasis and disseminated aspergillosis (72); in the latter study, combination with AmB significantly increased survival when compared with either agent alone. Finally, genes encoding cationic peptides with antifungal activity have been successfully transferred to the salivary glands of laboratory animals, thus allowing the investigation of their effect on mucosal candidiasis in permanently imunosuppressed subjects (73).

First clinical trials involving antimicrobial therapy with cationic peptides are under way (68,69). However, the potential usefulness of these peptides in treating human diseases of infectious origin remains to be determined.

IV. AGENTS FOR SYSTEMIC TREATMENT OF MYCOSES OF THE SKIN AND ITS APPENDAGES

A. Griseofulvin

Griseofulvin (Fig. 6) was originally isolated in 1939 as a natural product of *Penicillium griseofulvum*. Griseofulvin interferes with fungal microtubule formation, disrupting the cell's mitotic spindle formation and arresting the metaphase of cell division. Griseofulvin is a fungistatic compound. It is active against *Trichophyton, Microsporon,* and *Epidermophyton* species. The drug has no activity against yeast-like organisms, opportunistic hyaline and dematiaceous molds, and the dimorphic (endemic) molds. Of note, in-vitro resistance of dermatophytes to griseofulvin has been reported and may be the cause for therapeutic failure (74,75).

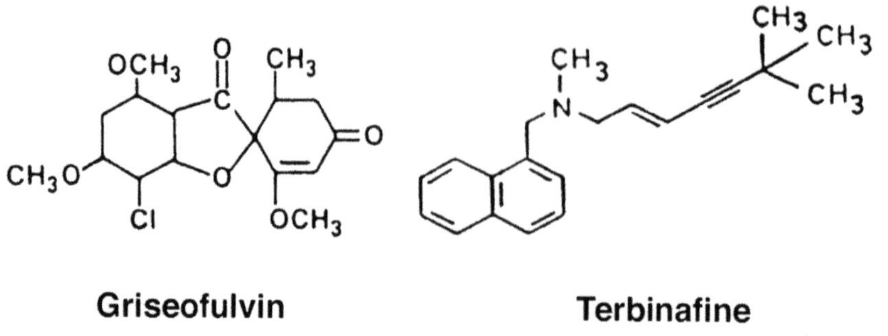

Griseofulvin   **Terbinafine**

Figure 6 Chemical structures of griseofulvin and terbinafine.

1. Pharmacokinetics

Griseofulvin is commercially available for oral administration only as griseofulvin microsize (4 μm particle size) and griseofulvin ultramicrosize (1 μm particle size). Oral bioavailability of the micronized formulation is variable and ranges from 25% to 70%; ultramicronized griseofulvin, in contrast, is almost completely absorbed (76). Peak plasma concentrations occur approximately 4 hr after dosing. Griseoful-vin distributes to keratin precursor cells and is concentrated in skin, hair, nails, liver, adipose tissue, and skeletal muscles. In skin, over time, a concentration gradient is established, with the highest concentrations in the outermost stratum corneum. However, within 48–72 hr after discontinuation, plasma concentrations of griseoful-vin are markedly reduced and the compound is no longer detectable in the stratum corneum (75,76). The elimination of griseofulvin from plasma is bi-exponential with a terminal elimination half-life of 9–21 hr (77). The compound is oxidatively demethylated and conjugated with glucuronic acid primarily in the liver; its major metabolite, 6-desmethylgriseofulvin, is microbiologically inactive; within 5 days, approximately one third of a single dose of micronized griseofulvin is excreted in feces, and 50% in urine, predominantly as glucuronized 6-desmethylgriseofulvin (78).

2. Adverse Effects and Drug Interactions

Griseofulvin is generally well tolerated. More common adverse effects include headaches and a variety of gastrointestinal symptoms. Griseofulvin can cause photo-sensitivity and exacerbate lupus and porphyria. Cases of erythema multiforme-like reactions, toxic epidermal necrolysis, and a reaction resembling serum sickness have been reported. Proteinuria, nephrosis, hapatotoxicity, leukopenia, menstrual irregu-larities, estrogen-like effects, and reversible diminuition of hearing have been reported rarely in association with griseofulvin therapy (75,76). The compound has been shown to be teratogenic in animals. Griseofulvin also has mutagenic and carcinogenic potential; the significance of these observations for humans, however, is unclear. Griseofulvin has been noted to enhance the clearance of oral contracep-tives, cyclosporine, theophylline, aspirin, and warfarin. Concurrent use of phenobar-bital may lead to decreased griseofulvin levels. Finally, concurrent alcohol ingestion may lead to a disulfiram-like reaction (74).

3. Clinical Indications and Dosing

Griseofulvin remains an important agent for the treatment of tinea capitis and refractory tinea corporis caused by dermatophytes. For tinea capitis, 6–8 weeks of treatment are usually required; the usual duration of therapy for refractory tinea corporis is 4 weeks (75,79). Nail infections usually fail to respond to therapy with griseofulvin and are better treated with itraconazole or terbinafine. The recommended dosage in adults ranges from 500 to 1000 mg (microsize) and 330 to 750 mg (ultramicrossize) as a single daily dose or in 2–4 equally divided doses. The compound is approved for children older than 2 years of age. The recommended pediatric dosage of microsize griseofulvin is 10–20 mg/kg/day (maximum 1 g), and that of ultramicronized griseofulvin is 5–10 mg/kg/day (maximum 750 mg), respectively, administered in two equally divided doses (7).

B. Terbinafine

The synthetic allylamine terbinafine (Fig. 6) is a newer antifungal agent that is useful for topical and systemic (oral) treatment of superficial infections of the skin and its appendages by dermatophytes and yeasts, and possibly, for cutaneous sporotrichosis. It acts by inhibiting the biosynthesis of fungal ergosterol at the level of squalene epoxidase (Fig. 2), leading to depletion of ergosterol and accumulation of toxic squalenes in the fungal cell membrane (80). Terbinafine has potent, fungicidal in vitro activity against dermatophytes. It is also highly active against *Aspergillus* species, *Fusarium* spp. dematiaceous and dimorphic fungi and *P. carinii*. Its in vitro activity against yeasts appears more variable (4,81). Of note, synergy with triazoles, and more variable, with AmB, has been reported against yeasts and filamentous fungi in vitro (82–84).

1. Pharmacokinetics

Terbinafine displays linear plasma pharmacokinetics over the current dosage range. Independent of food, oral bioavailability is 70–80%, and peak plasma concentrations of are measured within 2 hr (85). Steady-state in plasma is reached after 10–14 days after only twofold accumulation. As a lipophilic drug, terbinafine is strongly bound to plasma proteins. The compound is extensively distributed to tissues, accumulating throughout adipose tissues, dermis, epidermis, and nail. It exhibits a triphasic distribution pattern in plasma with a terminal half-life of up to 3 weeks; microbiologically active concentrations can be measured in plasma for weeks to months after the last dose, which is consistent with a slow redistribution from peripheral tissue and adipose tissue sites (85,86). Terbinafine undergoes extensive and complex hepatic biotransformation that involves at least seven CYP450 enzymes (87); none of its metabolites has been shown to be mycologically active (86). Urinary excretion accounts for more than 70% and fecal elimination for 10% of total excretion; the extent of enterohepatic recycling is yet unknown. Due to the compound's extensive hepatic metabolization and urinary excretion, caution is warranted in patients with severe hepatic and renal impairment (80). The plasma pharmacokinetics of terbinafine in pediatric patients have been comparatively well investigated (88). Whereas no apparent differences in metabolization were observed, on a mg/kg and mg/m^2 basis, children had a shorter B half-life, a lower mean AUC, and a higher volume of distribution, reflecting the higher proportion of lipophilic tissues in pediatric age groups.

2. Adverse Effects

At dosages of up to 500 mg/day, terbinafine is usually well tolerated. The most common adverse effects include gastrointestinal upsets and skin reactions in 2–7%

of patients. Terbinafine can cause hepatitis and liver failure; potentially severe hepatotoxicity is estimated to occur in 1:120,000 patients, and asymptomatic rises in liver enzyme activities are likely to occur at a frequency of 1:200. The drug should not be administered in patients with an underlying liver problem, and liver function tests should be obtained prior to the prescription of terbinafine. Less common significant adverse effects have included reversible loss of taste, severe skin eruptions, Stevens–Johnson syndrome, and blood dyscrasias (4).

3. Drug Interactions

With the possible exception of CYP2D6 substrates, in vitro studies revealed little or no effect of terbinafine on the metabolism of many characteristic CYP substrates (87). Inhibition of CYP2D6-mediated metabolism may be relevant with the concomitant use of tricyclic antidepressants, beta-blockers, selective serotonine reuptake inhibitors, and type-B monoaminooxidase inhibitors. Terbinafine can reduce the clearance of theophylline, increase levels of nortryptiline, increase or reduce warfarin exposure, and can reduce the trough cyclosporine concentration in transplant patients. The metabolism of terbinafine may be decreased by cimetidine and increased by rifampin (4).

4. Clinical Indications and Dosing

Terbinafine is indicated for treatment of superficial infections of the skin and its appendages by dermatophytes (80), and possibly, for cutaneous sporotrichosis (89). The recommended dosage range in adults is 250–500 mg once daily, and the recommended durations of treatment for tinea capitis, tinea corporis and pedis, fingernail onychomycosis, and toenail onychomycosis are 4, 2, 6, and 12 weeks, respectively (80,90). Several clinical studies have documented the safety of terbinafine in pediatric patients aged 2–17 years (90); based on the experience with dosages of 10 mg/kg and less in adults and the described pharmacokinetic profile of the compound in children, a dose of 250 mg/day has been proposed for children weighing >40 kg, a dose of 125 mg/day for children weighing 20–40 kg, and 62.5 mg/day for children weighing less than 20 kg (90).

The broad-spectrum, fungicidal in vitro activity, systemic availability, and the lack of significant side effects suggested potential against selected deep-seated fungal infections. Unfortunately, terbinafine was ineffective in rodent models of pulmonary aspergillosis (91), systemic sporotrichosis (92), cerebral phaeohyphomycosis (93), systemic Candida infection, and pulmonary cryptococcosis (94). This ineffectiveness is likely due to the compound's non-saturable protein binding in serum (91). Of note, terbinafine was as effective as TMP/SMZ in a rat model of pulmonary pneumocystosis, as rated by survival, lung weight, infection rate, and microbial tissue burden (95,96), indicating potential usefulness for treatment of selected compartments.

V. TOPICAL ANTIFUNGAL AGENTS

Apart from fungal keratitis, the use of topical agents is confined to superficial infections of the skin and mucosal surfaces. The decision to use a topical or a systemic agent depends mainly on the site and extent of the infection. Immunocompromised patients, however, usually require systemic therapies as do patients with tinea capitis and onychomycosis (97).

A. Superficial Skin Infections

Dermatophytosis is caused by the filamentous fungi *Microsporon* spp., *Trichophyton* spp., and *Epidermophyton floccosum*. A large variety of agents and formulations are available for topical treatment of dermatophytic skin infections (tinea corporis, facialis, or pedis), including allylamines, benzylamines, thiocarbamates, morpholines, and azoles. Agents for treatment of *Candida* dermatitis and Tinea (pityriasis) versicolor (caused by *Malassezia furfur* or *M. pachydermatidis*) include various topical azoles and topical polyenes. Most topical agents are usually applied twice daily well beyond the clinical resolution of the infection. A detailed review of the treatment of cutaneous mycoses is beyond the scope of this chapter and can be found elsewhere (75,76,79).

B. Mucosal Candidiasis

Agents for the topical treatment of vulvovaginal candidiasis include a large variety of antifungal azoles and the polyene nystatin. Of note, azole agents maybe absorbed to a minor extent and can potentially interfere with the metabolism of concomitant drugs. For example, potentiation of the anticoagulatory effects of acenocoumarol has been noted after vaginal administration of miconazole capsules and after oral administration of miconazole gel (7).

Antifungal azoles such as clotrimazole and miconazole and antifungal polyenes such as AmB and nystatin are effective in the treatment of oropharyngeal candidiasis. Many clinical trials have evaluated the usefulness of these agents for prevention of fungal infections in immunocompromised cancer or hematopoietic stem-cell transplant patients. While most agents have documented efficacy in the prevention of oropharyngeal candidiasis, they are not effective in preventing invasive mycoses and improving infection related and overall mortality in this setting (98–100).

REFERENCES

1. Vermes A, Guchelaar HJ, Dankert J. Flucytosine: a review of its pharmacology, clinical indications, pharmacokinetics, toxicity and drug interactions. J Antimicrob Chemother 2000; 46:171–179.
2. Daneshmend TK, Warnock DW. Clinical pharmacokinetics of systemic antifungal drugs. Clin Pharmacokinet 1983; 8:17–42.
3. Francis P, Walsh TJ. Evolving role of flucytosine in immunocompromised patients: new insights into safety, pharmacokinetics, and antifungal therapy. Clin Infect Dis 1992; 15:1003–1018.
4. Groll AH, Piscitelli SC, Walsh TJ. Clinical pharmacology of systemic antifungal agents: a comprehensive review of agents in clinical use, current investigational compounds, and putative targets for antifungal drug development. Adv Pharmacol 1998; 44: 343–500.
5. Medoff G, Kobayashi GS. Strategies in the treatment of systemic fungal infections. N Engl J Med N 1980; 302:1451–1455.
6. Groll AH, Piscitelli SC, Walsh TJ. Antifungal pharmacodynamics: concentration-effect relationships in vitro and in vivo. Pharmacotherapy 2001; 21(8 Pt 2):133S–148S.
7. Groll AH, Walsh TJ. Antifungal agents. In: Feigin RD, Cherry JD, Demmler GJ, Kaplan SL, eds. Textbook of Pediatric Infectious Diseases, 5th ed. Philadelphia: Harcourt Health Sciences, Chapter 239, 2004; 3075–3107.

8.   Harris BE, Manning BW, Federle TW. Conversion of 5-fluorocytosine to 5-fluorouracil by human intestinal microflora. Antimicrob Agents Chemother 1986; 29:44–48.

9.   Vermes A, van Der Sijs H, Guchelaar HJ. Flucytosine: correlation between toxicity and pharmacokinetic parameters. Chemotherapy 2000; 46:86–94.

10. Polak A. Mode of action studies. In: Ryley JF, ed. Handbook of Experimental Pharmacology. Vol. 96. Berlin: Springer-Verlag, 1990:153–182.

11. Bennett JE, Dismukes WE, Haywood M, et al. A comparison of amphotericin B alone and in combination with flucytosine in the treatment of cryptococcal meningitis. N Engl J Med 1979; 301:126–131.

12. Van der Horst CM, Saag MS, Cloud GA, et al. Treatment of cryptococcal meningitis associated with the Acquired Immunodeficiency Syndrome. N Engl J Med 1997; 337: 15–21.

13. Dominguez JM, Martin JJ. Identification of elongation factor 2 as the essential protein targeted by sordarins in *Candida albicans*. Antimicrob Agents Chemother 1998; 42: 2279–2283.

14. Dominguez JM, Kelly VA, Kinsman OS, Marriott MS, Gomez de las Heras F, Martin JJ. Sordarins: a new class of antifungals with selective inhibition of the protein synthesis elongation cycle in yeasts. Antimicrob Agents Chemother 1998; 42:2274–2278.

15. Gargallo-Viola D. Sordarins as antifungal compounds. Curr Opin Anti-infect Invest Drugs 1999; 1:297–305.

16. Herreros E, Martinez CM, Almela MJ, Marriott MS, De Las Heras FG, Gargallo-Viola D. Sordarins: in vitro activities of new antifungal derivatives against pathogenic yeasts, *Pneumocystis carinii*, and filamentous fungi. Antimicrob Agents Chemother 1998; 42: 2863–2869.

17. Herreros E, Martinez CM, Almela MJ, Lozano S, Gomez de las Heras F, Gargallo-Viola G. Fungicidal activity of sordarins against *Candida albicans* determined by time-kill methods. Abstracts of the 38th Interscience Conference on Antimicrobial Agents and Chemotherapy [abstr J-13], American Society for Microbiology, Washington, DC, 1998.

18. Aviles P, Falcoz C, Guillen MJ, San Roman R, Gargallo-Viola D. Correlation between in vitro and in vivo activity of sordarin derivatives against *C. albicans* by using an in vitro pharmacodynamic model. Abstracts of the 39th Interscience Conference on Antimicrobial Agents and Chemotherapy [abstr 2000], American Society for Microbiology, Washington, DC, 1999.

19. Aviles P, Pateman A, San Roman R, Gargallo D. Single-dose pharmacokinetic studies in rodents with GM237354, a new systemic antifungal agent. Abstracts of the 37th Interscience Conference on Antimicrobial Agents and Chemotherapy [abstr F-66], American Society for Microbiology, Washington, DC, 1997.

20. Aviles P, Pateman A, San Roman R, Gomez de las Heras F, Gargallo-Viola G. Interspecies pharmacokinetic scaling of sordarin derivatives: a new class of antifungal agents. Abstracts of the 38th Interscience Conference on Antimicrobial Agents and Chemotherapy [abstr J-71], American Society for Microbiology, Washington, DC, 1998.

21. Martinez A, Aviles P, Jimenez E, Caballero J, Gargallo-Viola D. Activities of sordarins in experimental models of candidiasis, aspergillosis, and pneumocystosis. Antimicrob Agents Chemother 2000; 44:3389–3394.

22. Martinez A, Ferrer S, Jimenez E, Sparrowe J, Gomez de las Heras F, Gargallo-Viola G. Antifungal activity of sordarin derivatives against nonlethal models of candidiasis in rats. Abstracts of the 39th Interscience Conference on Antimicrobial Agents and Chemotherapy [abstr 1999], American Society for Microbiology, Washington, DC, 1999.

23. Najvar LK, Bocanegra RA, Fothergil AW, Luther MF, Graybill JR. New sordarin antifungal drugs active in murine histoplasmosis. Abstracts of the 37th Interscience Conference on Antimicrobial Agents and Chemotherapy [abstr F-63], American Society for Microbiology, Washington, DC, 1997.

24. Clemons KV, Stevens DA. Efficacies of sordarin derivatives GM193663, GM211676 or GM237354 in a murine model of systemic coccidioidomycosis. Abstracts of the 37th Interscience Conference on Antimicrobial Agents and Chemotherapy [abstr F-62], American Society for Microbiology, Washington, DC, 1997.

25. Oakley KL, Verweij PW, Morrissey G, Denning DW. In vivo activity of GM237354 in a neutropenic murine model of aspergillosis. Abstracts of the 37th Interscience Conference on Antimicrobial Agents and Chemotherapy [abstr F-61], American Society for Microbiology, Washington, DC, 1997.

26. Aviles P, Aliouat EM, Martinez A, Dei-Cas E, Herreros E, Dujardin L, Gargallo-Viola D. In vitro pharmacodynamic parameters of sordarin derivatives in comparison with those of marketed compounds against *Pneumocystis carinii* isolated from rats. Antimicrob Agents Chemother 2000; 44:1284–1290.

27. Aviles P, Falcoz C, San Roman R, Gargallo-Viola D. Pharmacokinetics–pharmacodynamics of a sordarin derivative (GM 237354) in a murine model of lethal candidiasis. Antimicrob Agents Chemother 2000; 44:2333–2340.

28. Ziegelbauer K. Decreased accumulation or increased isoleucyl-tRNA synthtase activity confers resistance to the cyclic b-amino acid BAY 10–8888 in *Candida albicans* and *Candida* tropicalis. Antimicrob Agents Chemother 1998; 42:1581–1586.

29. Schoenfeld W. Discovery, synthesis and SAR of the b-amino acid BAY 10–8888/PLD-1 18, a novel antifungal for treatment of yeast infections. Abstracts of the 42nd Interscience Conference on Antimicrobial Agents and Chemotherapy [abstr F-811], American Society for Microbiology, Washington, DC, 2002.

30. Ziegelbauer K, Babczinski P, Schoenfeld W. Molecular mode of action of the antifungal b-amino acid BAY 10–8888. Antimicrob Agents Chemother 1998; 42:2197–2205.

31. Schoenfeld W. PLD-118: a cyclopentane amino acid with antifungal activity. Abstracts of the 41st Interscience Conference on Antimicrobial Agents and Chemotherapy [abstr 11], American Society for Microbiology, Washington, DC, 2001.

32. Hasenoehrl A, Skerlev M, Marsic N, Schoenfeld W. PLD-118: a novel antifungal for treatment of yeast infections: in vitro activity against clinical isolates of *Candida albicans*. Abstracts of the 41st Interscience Conference on Antimicrobial Agents and Chemotherapy [abstr F-2143], American Society for Microbiology, Washington, DC, 2001.

33. Schoenfeld W. PLD-118: In vitro activity on *Candida* non-*albicans* species by MIC and time-kill. Abstracts of the 42nd Interscience Conference on Antimicrobial Agents and Chemotherapy [abstr F-812], American Society for Microbiology, Washington, DC, 2002.

34. Petraitis V, Petraitine R, Kelaher A, Sarafandi A, Lyman CA, Sein T, Schaufele RL, Bacher J, Walsh TJ. Efficacy of PLD-118, a novel inhibitor of *Candida* isoleucyl-tRNA synthase, against experimental fluconazole-resistant esophageal candidiasis. Abstracts of the 42nd Interscience Conference on Antimicrobial Agents and Chemotherapy [abstr F-813], American Society for Microbiology, Washington, DC, 2002.

35. Schoenfeld W, Mittendorf J, Schmidt A, Geschke U. PLD-118, a novel antifungal for treatment of yeast infections: in vivo efficacy in *Candida albicans* infection in mice and rats. Abstracts of the 41st Interscience Conference on Antimicrobial Agents and Chemotherapy [abstr F-2144], American Society for Microbiology, Washington, DC, 2001.

36. Schoenfeld W, Parnham M. PLD-118: a novel antifungal for treatment of yeast infections: animal pharmacokinetics. Abstracts of the 41st Interscience Conference on Antimicrobial Agents and Chemotherapy [abstr F-2145], American Society for Microbiology, Washington, DC, 2001.

37. Bogaards JJP, Schut MW, Mildner B, Parnham MJ. The novel antifungal PLD-118 does not inhibit cytochrome P450 enzymes in vitro. Abstracts of the 42nd Interscience Conference on Antimicrobial Agents and Chemotherapy [abstr F-814], American Society for Microbiology, Washington, DC, 2002.

38. Oreskovic K, Bischoff A, Pavicic-Stedul H, Avdagic A, Dumic M, Kralj Z, Schoenfeld W, Schroedter A, Knoeller J. PLD-118: tolerability, safety and pharmacokinetics following single oral dose in healthy volunteers. Abstracts of the 41st Interscience Conference on Antimicrobial Agents and Chemotherapy [abstr F-2146], American Society for Microbiology, Washington, DC, 2001.

39. Schroedter A, Bischoff A, Oreskovic K, Knoeler J, Radosevic S, Schoenfeld W, Peterson J. A phase I multiple dose study of a novel oral antifungal PLD-118. Abstracts of the 42nd Interscience Conference on Antimicrobial Agents and Chemotherapy [abstr F-815], American Society for Microbiology, Washington, DC, 2002.

40. Hector RF. Compounds active against cell walls of medically important fungi. Clin Microbiol Rev 1993; 6:1–21.

41. Debono M, Gordee RS. Antibiotics that inhibit fungal cell wall development. Annu Rev Microbiol 1994; 48:471–497.

42. Hector RF, Zimmer BL, Pappagianis D. Evaluation of nikkomycin X and Z in murine models of coccidiodomycosis, histoplasmosis, and blastomycosis. Antimicrob Agents Chemother 1990; 34:587–593.

43. Clemons KV, Stevens DA. Efficacy of nikkomycin Z against experimental pulmonary blastomycosis. Antimicrob Agents Chemother 1997; 41:2026–2028.

44. Hector RF, Yee E. Evaluation of Bay R 3783 in rodent models of superficial and systemic candidiasis, meningeal cryptococcosis, and pulmonary aspergillosis. Antimicrob Agents Chemother 1990; 34:448–454.

45. Hector RF, Schaller K. Positive interaction of nikkomycins and azoles against *Candida albicans* in vitro and in vivo. Antimicrob Agents Chemother 1992; 36:1284–1289.

46. Graybill JR, Najvar LK, Montalbo EM, Barchiesi FJ, Luther MF, Rinaldi MG. Treatment of histoplasmosis with MK-991 (L-743,872). Antimicrob Agents Chemother 1998; 42:151–153.

47. Goldberg J, Connolly P, Schnizlein-Bick C, Durkin M, Kohler S, Smedema M, Brizendine E, Hector R, Wheat J. Comparison of nikkomycin Z with amphotericin B and itraconazole for treatment of histoplasmosis in a murine model. Antimicrob Agents Chemother 2000; 44:1624–1629.

48. Milewski S, Mignini F, Borowski E. Synergistic action of nikkomycin X/Z with azole antifungals on *Candida albicans*. J Gen Microbiol 1991; 137:2155–2161.

49. Li RK, Rinaldi MG. In vitro antifungal activity of nikkomycin Z in combination with fluconazole or itraconazole. Antimicrob Agents Chemother 1999; 43:1401–1405.

50. Hector RF, Braun PC. Synergistic action of nikkomycin X and Z with papulacandin B on whole cells and regenerating protoplasts of *Candida albicans*. Antimicrob Agents Chemother 1986; 29:389–394.

51. Pfaller MA, Wey S, Gerarden T, Houston A, Wenzel RP. Susceptibility of nosocomial isolates of *Candida* species to LY121019 and other antifungal agents. Diagn Microbiol Infect Dis 1989; 12:1–4.

52. Stevens DA. Drug interaction studies of a glucan synthase inhibitor (LY 303366) and a chitin synthase inhibitor (Nikkomycin Z) for inhibition and killing of fungal pathogens. Antimicrob Agents Chemother 2000; 44:2547–2548.

53. Capilla-Luque J, Clemons KV, Stevens DA. Efficacy of FK-463 alone and in combination against systemic murine aspergillosis. Abstracts of the 41st Interscience Conference on Antimicrobial Agents and Chemotherapy [abstr J-1834], American Society for Microbiology, Washington, DC, 2001.

54. Chiou CC, Mavrogiorgos N, Tillem E, Hector R, Walsh TJ. Synergy, pharmacodynamics, and time-sequenced ultrastructural changes of the interaction between nikkomycin Z and the echinocandin FK463 against *Aspergillus fumigatus*. Antimicrob Agents Chemother 2001; 45:3310–3321.

55. Oki K, Konishi M, Tomatsu K, Tomita K, Saitoh K. Pradimicin, a novel class of potent antifungal antibiotics. J Antibiot 1988; 41:1701–1704.

56. Takeuchi T, Hara T, Naganawa H, Okada M, Hamada M, Umezawa H, Gomi S, Sezaki M, Kondo S. New antifungal antibiotics, benanomicins A and B from an Actinomycete. J Antibiot 1988; 41:807–811.
57. Walsh TJ, Giri N. Pradimicins: a novel class of broad-spectrum antifungal compounds. Eur J Clin Microbiol Infect Dis 1997; 16:93–97.
58. Sawada Y, Numata K, Murakami T, Tanimichi H, Yamamoto S, Oki T. Calcium-dependent anti*Candida*1 action of pradimicin A. J Antibiot (Tokyo) 1990; 43:715–721.
59. Fung-Tomc JC, Minassian B, Huczko E, Kolek B, Bonner DP, Kessler RE. In vitro antifungal and fungicidal spectra of a new pradimicin derivative, BMS-181184. Antimicrob Agents Chemother 1995; 39:295–300.
60. Wardle HM, Law D, Denning DW. In vitro activity of BMS-181184 compared with those of fluconzole and amphotericin B against various *Candida* spp., Antimicrob Agents Chemother 1996; 40:2229–2231.
61. Watanabe M, Hiratani T, Uchida K, Ohtsuka K, Watabe H, Inouye S, Kondo S, Takeuchi T, Yamaguchi H. The in vitro activity of an antifungal antibiotic benanomicin A in comparison with amphotericin B. J Antimicrob Chemother 1996; 38:1073–1077.
62. Gonzales CE, Shetty D, Giri N, Love W, Klygis K, Lyman C, Bacher J, Walsh TJ. Efficacy of pradimicin against disseminated candidiasis. Abstracts of the 36th Interscience Conference on Antimicrobial Agents and Chemotherapy [abstr 131], American Society for Microbiology, Washington, DC, 1996.
63. Gonzalez CE, Groll AH, Giri N, Shetty D, Al-Mohsen I, Sein T, Feuerstein E, Bacher J, Piscitelli S, Walsh TJ. Antifungal activity of the pradimicin derivative BMS 181184 in the treatment of experimental pulmonary aspergillosis in persistently neutropenic rabbits. Antimicrob Agents Chemother 1998; 42:2399–2404.
64. Patterson TF, Kirkpatrick WR, Mcatee RK. The activity of pradimicin (BMS-181184) in experimental invasive aspergillosis. Abstracts of the 36th Interscience Conference on Antimicrobial Agents and Chemotherapy [abstr 31], American Society for Microbiology, Washington, DC, 1996.
65. Ohtsuka K, Watanabe M, Orikasa Y, Inouye S, Uchida K, Yamaguchi H, Kondo S, Takeuchi T. The in vivo activity of an antifungal antibiotic, benanomicin A, in comparison with amphotericin B and fluconazole. J Antimicrob Chemother 1997; 39:71–77.
66. Yasuoka A, Oka S, Komuro K. Successful treatment of *pneumocystis carinii* pneumonia in mice with benanomicin A (ME1451). Antimicrob Agents Chemother 1995; 39:720–724.
67. Hancock RE, Falla T, Brown M. Cationic bactericidal peptides. Adv Microb Physiol 1995; 37:135–175.
68. Hancock RE. Peptide antibiotics. Lancet 1979; 349:418–422.
69. Muller FM, Lyman CA, Walsh TJ. Antimicrobial peptides as potential new antifungals. Mycoses 1999; 42(suppl 2):77–82.
70. DeLucca AJ, Bland JM, Jacks TJ, Grimm C, Cleveland TE, Walsh TJ. Fungicidal activity of Cecropin A. Antimicrob Agents Chemother 1997; 41:481–483.
71. Ahmad I, Perkins WR, Lupan DM, Selsted ME, Janoff AS. Liposomal entrapment of the neutrophil-derived peptide indolicidin endows it with in vivo antifungal activity. Biochim Biophys Acta 1995; 1237:109–114.
72. Appenzeller L, Lim E, Wong P, Fadem M, Motchnik P, Bakalinsky M, Little R. In vivo fungicidal activity of optimized domain III peptides derived from bactericidal/permeability increasing protein (BPI). Abstracts of the 36th Interscience Conference on Antimicrobial Agents and Chemotherapy [abstr F187], American Society for Microbiology, Washington, DC, 1996.
73. O'Connell BC, Xu T, Walsh TJ, Sein T, Mastrangeli A, Crystal RG, Oppenheim FG, Baum BJ. Transfer of a gene encoding the anticandidal protein histatin 3 to salivary glands. Hum Gene Ther 1996; 7:2255–2261.
74. Friedlander SF, Suarez S. Pediatric antifungal therapy. Dermatol Clin 1998; 16:527–537.

75. Gupta AK, Sauder DN, Shear NH. Antifungal agents: an overview. J Am Acad Dermatol 1994; 30:677–698 and 911–933.
76. Blumer JL. Pharmacologic basis for the treatment of tinea capitis. Pediatr Infect Dis J 1999; 18:191–199.
77. Rowland M, Riegelman S, Epstein WL. Absorption kinetics of griseofulvin in man. J Pharm Sci 1968; 57:984–989.
78. Lin C, Symchowicz S. Absorption, distribution, metabolism, and excretion of griseofulvin in man and animals. Drug Metab Rev 1975; 4:75–95.
79. Howard RM, Frieden IJ. Dermatophyte infections in children. Adv Pediatr Infect Dis 1999; 14:73–107.
80. Balfour JA, Faulds D. Terbinafine. A review of its pharmacodynamic and pharmacokinetic properties, and therapeutic potential in superficial mycoses. Drugs 1992; 43:259–284.
81. Jessup CJ, Ryder NS, Ghannoum MA. An evaluation of the in vitro activity of terbinafine. Med Mycol 2000; 38:155–159.
82. Meletiadis J, Mouton JW, Rodriguez-Tudela JL, Meis JF, Verweij PE. In vitro interaction of terbinafine with itraconazole against clinical isolates of *Scedosporium prolificans*. Antimicrob Agents Chemother 2000; 44:470–472.
83. Ryder NS, Leitner I. Synergistic interaction of terbinafine with triazoles or amphotericin B against *Aspergillus* species. Med Mycol 2001; 39:91–95.
84. Weig M, Muller FM. Synergism of voriconazole and terbinafine against *Candida albicans* isolates from human immunodeficiency virus-infected patients with oropharyngeal candidiasis. Antimicrob Agents Chemother 2001; 45:966–968.
85. Kovarik JM, Kirkesseli S, Humbert H, Grass P, Kutz K. Dose-proportional pharmacokinetics of terbinafine and its *N*-demethylated metabolite in healthy volunteers. Br J Dermatol 1992; 126(suppl 39):8–13.
86. Kovarik JM, Mueller EA, Zehender H, Denouel J, Caplain H, Millerioux L. Multiple-dose pharmacokinetics and distribution in tissue of terbinafine and metabolites. Antimicrob Agents Chemother 1995; 39:2738–2741.
87. Vickers AE, Sinclair JR, Zollinger M, et al. Multiple cytochrome P-450s involved in the metabolism of terbinafine suggest a limited potential for drug–drug interactions. Drug Metab Dispos 1999; 27:1029–1038.
88. Humbert H, Denouel J, Cabiac MD, Lakhdar H, Sioufi A. Pharmacokinetics of terbinafine and five known metabolites in children, after oral administration. Biopharm Drug Dispos 1998; 19:417–423.
89. Hull PR, Vismer HF. Treatment of cutaneous sporotrichosis with terbinafine. J Dermatol 1992; 126(suppl 39):51–55.
90. Jones TC. Overview of the use of terbinafine (Lamisil) in children. Br J Dermatol 1995; 132:683–689.
91. Schmitt HJ, Andrade J, Edwards F, Niki Y, Bernard E, Armstrong D. Inactivity of terbinafine in a rat model of pulmonary aspergillosis. Eur J Clin Microbiol Infect Dis 1990; 9:832–835.
92. Kan VL, Bennett JE. Efficacies of four antifungal agents in experimental murine sporotrichosis. Antimicrob Agent Chemother 1988; 32:1619–1623.
93. Dixon DM, Polak A. In vitro and in vivo drug studies with three agents of central nervous system phaeohyphomycosis. Chemotherapy 1987; 33:129–140.
94. Ryley JF, McGregor S, Wilson RG. Activity of ICI 195,739—a novel, orally active bistriazole—in rodent models of fungal and protozoal infections. Ann NY Acad Sci 1988; 544:310–328.
95. Contini C, Manganaro M, Romani R, Tzantzoglou S, Poggesi I, Vullo V, Delia S, De Simone C. Activity of terbinafine against *Pneumocystis carinii* in vitro and its efficacy in the treatment of experimental pneumonia. J Antimicrob Chemother 1994; 34:727–735.

96. Contini C, Colombo D, Cultrera R, Prini E, Sechi T, Angelici E, Canipari R. Employment of terbinafine against *Pneumocystis carinii* infection in rat models. Br J Dermatol 1996; 134(suppl 46):30–32.

97. Groll AH, Walsh TJ. Uncommon opportunistic fungi: new nosocomial threats. Clin Microbiol Infect 2001; 7(suppl 2):8–24.

98. Lortholary O, Dupont B. Antifungal prophylaxis during neutropenia and immunodeficiency. Clin Microbiol Rev 1997; 10:477–504.

99. Uzun O, Anaissie EJ. Antifungal prophylaxis in patients with hematologic malignancies: a reappraisal. Blood 1995; 86:2063–2072.

100. Groll AH, Ritter J, Muller FM. Prevention of fungal infections in children and adolescents with cancer. Klin Padiatr 2001; 213(suppl 1):A50–A68.

20

Clinically Relevant Drug Interactions with Systemic Antifungal Therapy

Helen L. Leather
BMT/Leukemia, Shands at the University of Florida, Gainesville, Florida, U.S.A.

I. INTRODUCTION

A drug interaction is best defined as "the possibility that one drug may alter the intensity of pharmacological effects of another drug that is given concurrently." This results in either enhanced activity of the affected drug, which may lead to toxicity, or reduced activity of the affected drug, leading to therapeutic failure. It is also possible that there may be the appearance of a new effect that is not seen with either drug alone, such as caspofungin and cyclosporine coadministration leading to elevated liver function tests. Drug interactions can be divided into either pharmacokinetic (PK) or pharmacodynamic (PD) interactions.

A. Pharmacokinetic Drug Interactions

Pharmacokinetic drug interactions influence the disposition of the drug in the body. When drugs are ingested, they undergo several processes to produce an end-effect, including absorption, distribution, metabolism, and excretion. Interactions between two or more drugs may affect any of these phases, including modulation of hepatic drug biotransformation, renal clearance, altered distribution, or changes in plasma protein binding.

The most clinically relevant mechanisms of PK drug interactions relate to metabolism and elimination of drugs from the body, and involve the cytochrome P450 (CYP) enzymes and the transporter P-glycoprotein at the hepatic and intestinal levels, and glomerular filtration and tubular secretion at the renal level. The CYP microsomal enzyme system is a family of hemoproteins that is responsible for the oxidative biotransformation of endogenous substrates and xenobiotics. CYP's are expressed in several tissues, with the main drug metabolizing CYP's concentrated in the smooth endoplasmic reticulum in the liver, with lower expression in the lungs, kidneys, intestines, and brain (1). Of the several different CYP isoforms identified, CYP1A2, CYP2C9, CYP2C19, CYP2D6, and CYP3A4 have the greatest involvement in drug metabolism. An extensive list of drugs metabolized by the various isoenzymes is outlined in Table 1 (2). CYP1A2 accounts for approximately 15% of

Table 1 Cytochrome P450 Isoenzymes Involved in Drug Metabolism (2)

Cytochrome P450 isoenzyme	Substrates	Inhibitors	Inducers
CYP 1A2	Amitriptyline, caffeine, haloperidol, ondansetron, propranolol, theophylline verapamil, (R) warfarin	Amiodarone, cimetidine, fluoroquinolones, ticlopidine	Broccoli, brussel sprouts, chargrilled meat, insulin, tobacco
CYP 2C9	Oral hypoglycemics, celecoxib, fluoxetine, fluvastatin, NSAID's, phenytoin, tamoxifen, S-warfarin, voriconazole	Fluconazole, fluvastatin, isoniazid, lovastatin, paroxetine, sertraline, teniposide, trrmethoprim, voriconazole	Rifampin
CYP 2C19	Cyclophosphamide, diazepam, nelfinavir, phenobarbitone, phenytoin, primidone, proton pump inhibitors, teniposide, voriconazole	Cimetidine, fluconazole, fluoxetine, ketoconazole, omeprazole, voriconazole	Carbamazepine, prednisone, rifampin
CYP 2D6	Fluoxetine, haloperidol, paroxetine, methadone, metoclopramide, morphine, ondansetron, propranolol, risperidone, tamoxifen, tricyclic antidepressants	Celecoxib, doxorubicin, fluoxetine, lopinavir, metoclopramide, paroxetine, ritonavir, sertraline	Dexamethasone? Rifampin
CYP 3A4/5	Antifungals: itraconazole Antihistamines (astemizole, terfenadine) Benzodiazepines (alprazolam, diazepam, midazolam, triazolam) Calcium channel antagonists (amlodipine, diltiazem, nifedipine, felodipine, verapamil) HIV antivirals (indinavir, nelfinavir, ritonavir, saquinavir) HMG Co A reductase inhibitors (atorvastatin, lovastatin, simvastatin) Immunosuppressants (cyclosporine, sirolimus, tacrolimus) Macrolides (clarithromycin, erythromycin) Others (cisapride, dapsone, irinotecan, ondansetron, tamoxifen, thiotepa, vincristine voriconazole)	Amprenavir, cimetidine, ciprofloxacin, clarithromycin, delaviridine, diltiazem, efavirenz, erythromycin, fluconazole, grapefruit juice, indinavir, itraconazole, ketoconazole, lopinavir, nelfinavir, posaconazole, ritonavir, saquinavir, voriconazole	Amprenavir, barbiturates, carbamazepine, efavirenz, glucocorticoids, lopinavirnevirapine, phenobarbital, phenytoin, rifampin, rifabutin, ritonavir, St John's wort, troglitazone

hepatic CYP and CYP2D6 represents 1.5% of total hepatic CYP. The CYP2C isoforms are abundant in the liver, second only to CYP3A4. There are two isoforms of CYP2C, namely 2C9 and 2C19, which share 91% identity in amino acid sequences, therefore, most substrates of CYP2C9 are metabolized by CYP2C19 as well (1). The majority of oxidatively biotransformed drugs are metabolized, at least in part, by the CYP3A4 isoenzyme, which is responsible for drug metabolism both in the liver and the small intestine.

CYP-mediated drug interactions can occur by two separate mechanisms, enzyme inhibition and enzyme induction. Inhibition is the process whereby there is either enzyme inactivation or mutual competition of substrates at a catalytic site. The net response is inhibition of drug metabolism leading to increased serum concentrations, increased trough concentrations, and a prolongation of half-life. This causes potentiation of the pharmacodynamic effect, and often leads to enhanced toxicity, particularly among those agents with a very narrow therapeutic index, such as cyclosporine and tacrolimus. Examples of substrates whose bioavailability is increased by inhibition includes benzodiazepines (midazolam, triazolam), immunosuppressants (cyclosporine, tacrolimus, sirolimus), nonsedating antihistamines (astemizole, terfenadine), calcium channel blockers (amlodipine, diltiazem, nifedipine, verapamil), HMG CoA-reductase inhibitors (atorvastatin, lovastatin, simvastatin), and many of the antineoplastic agents (etoposide, ifosfamide, cyclophosphamide, vinca alkaloids). Examples of inhibitors include the azole antifungals (fluconazole, itraconazole, ketoconazole, voriconazole), and the macrolide antibiotics (clarithromycin, erythromycin). Grapefruit juice, a commonly ingested "health" drink, is also a potent inhibitor of CYP enzymes and must be considered when reviewing drug interactions.

Induction is a process whereby there is increased synthesis or decreased degradation of CYP enzymes, resulting in decreased plasma levels of the substrate, and a decrease in its pharmacodynamic effects. Examples of enzyme inducers are rifampin, rifabutin, phenytoin, carbamazepine, phenobarbital, and St John's wort.

Drugs that require metabolism by the same CYP enzyme compete for binding to, and metabolism by CYP (3). Therefore, in theory, any two drugs metabolized by identical CYP enzymes have a potential for interaction, although the clinical significance of the interaction will rely on the drug's relative affinities for binding to these enzymes, concentrations achieved in the endoplasmic reticulum after therapeutic doses, dependence on CYP for elimination, and therapeutic ratios (3).

A second potential mechanism of pharmacokinetic drug interactions is thought to occur by modulation of P-glycoprotein. P-glycoprotein, the product of the multidrug resistance gene (MDR1), is an ATP-dependent plasma membrane transporter. It is present in the proximal tubular cells of the kidneys, the bile cannalicular membrane of hepatocytes, endothelial cells of the blood–brain barrier and blood–testis barriers. P-glyoprotein is best known for its role in resistance of cancer cells to antineoplastic agents, namely paclitaxel, vinca alkaloids, the epipodophyllotoxins, and the anthracycline antibiotics. P-glycoprotein also promotes the excretion of many other drugs, including digoxin, HIV protease inhibitors, and cyclosporine from renal tubule and intestinal cells (4). Administration of an agent that inhibits or induces P-glycoprotein activity can increase or decrease the clearance of P-glycoprotein substrates at the renal level, and increase or decrease bioavailability at the intestinal level (4).

B. Pharmacodynamic Drug Interactions

In addition to PK mediated drug-interactions, there are also pharmacodynamic inter-actions. These occur when a medication induces a change in the patient's response to a drug without altering the pharmacokinetics of the object drug, e.g., amphotericin B-induced hypokalemia in a patient on digoxin, leading to enhanced digoxin toxicity. Pharmacodynamic interactions are primarily seen with the polyene antifungal agents, e.g., amphotericin B. Examples of pharmacodynamic interactions are listed in Table 2

II. DRUG–DRUG INTERACTIONS

With the large number of pharmaceuticals available today, it is not surprising that drug interactions occur commonly, particularly, in diseases that require polyphar-macy, Immunocompromised patients, including recipients of solid organ transplant (SOT), hematopoietic stem cell transplantation (HSCT), neonates, surgical candi-dates, and patients infected with the human immunodeficiency virus (HIV), frequently receive complex medication regimens, with the potential for numerous drug interactions. Due to the vast number of potential drug interactions that can occur in a patient, only PK and PD drug interactions involving antifungal therapy is discussed in detail in this chapter.

A. Polyenes

1. *Amphotericin B*

Amphotericin B is a potent nephrotoxin, causing toxicity by arteriolar vasoconstric-tion, which leads to renal ischemia and a decreased glomerular filtration rate. Nephrotoxicity is one of the main mechanisms by which pharmacodynamic drug

Table 2 Pharmacodynamic Drug Interactions with Amphotericin B

Drug A	DrugB	Clinical Effect
Amphotericin B	Aminoglycosides	Additive or synergistic nephrotoxicity
	Antineoplastic agents (e.g., cisplatin, bleomycin)	Additive or synergistic nephrotoxicity (i.e., cisplatin) Delayed clearance of other renally excreted drugs leading to enhanced toxicity (i.e., bleomycin)
	Cidofovir	Additive or synergistic nephrotoxicity
	Cyclosporine	Additive or synergistic nephrotoxicity
	Digoxin	Hypokalemia induced by amphotericin B promotes inhibition of Na^+, K^+ATPase by digoxin
	Flucytosine [5-FC]	Enhanced bone marrow suppression due to delayed clearance of 5-FC in the presence of renal dysfunction induced by amphotericin B
	Foscarnet	Additive or synergistic nephrotoxicity Additive or synergistic electrolyte abnormalities
	Ganciclovir	Hematological toxicity due to delayed clearance; dose reduce ganciclovir
	Tacrolimus	Additive or synergistic nephrotoxicity
	Zidovudine	Hematological toxicity
5-Flucytosine	Zidovudine	Hematological toxicity
	Ganciclovir	Potentially greater hematological toxicity

interactions occur with amphotericin B (and its analogues). Pharmacodynamic inter-actions of importance are listed in Table 2, along with the likely clinical effects. Another type of pharmacodynamic interaction that can occur is via the electrolyte imbalances that result from amphotericin B administration. The third type of pharmacodynamic interaction that may occur results from additive myelotoxic inter-actions, e.g., enhanced myelosuppressive toxicity in patients who are coadministered zidovudine and amphotericin B products.

The main interaction of concern with the polyene products arises when combi-nation antifungal therapy with amphotericin B and an azole is considered. Theore-tically these two classes of drug may interact negatively. Amphotericin B exerts its effects by binding to ergosterol whereas azole antifungals block the enzyme 14-α demethylase, a necessary enzyme to convert lanosterol to ergosterol. By depleting ergosterol, the target of amphotericin B, clinical efficacy of amphotericin B may be diminished, potentially leading to higher mortality rates when combination ther-apy is used. Based on the potential for theoretical antagonism, several in vitro and animal studies have been conducted to address this issue. In vitro and animal models suggest an attenuation of response in animals with prior exposure to an azole before receiving a polyene (5–13). Increasing the dose of amphotericin B does not overcome the noted antagonism. There does appear to be some sequence dependence to the interaction. Pretreatment with an azole, as would be a common practice in immuno-compromised patients that were receiving fungal prophylaxis decreases the ability of amphotericin B to prolong survival. Similarly, the same effect is seen when a polyene and an azole are administered simultaneously. The interaction is not noted when a polyene is administered first, followed by an azole. There are limited clinical data supporting these animal and in vitro models. The only available clinical data is in the setting of candidemia, in a trial conducted by the National Institute of Allergy and Infectious Diseases Mycoses Study Group (14). This trial compared high-dose fluconazole (800 mg/day) in combination with either placebo or amphotericin B deoxycholate (0.7 mg/kg/day, with the placebo/amphotericin B component given only for the first 5–6 days). Overall success rates were 56% and 69%, respectively ($p = 0.043$), with failure to clear the bloodstream occurring in 17% and 6% of patients, respectively ($p = 0.02$) (14). Based on these results, one can conclude that the combination of fluconazole and amphotericin B was not antagonistic when compared to fluconazole monotherapy, and that the combination trended towards improved success and more rapid bloodstream clearance. Whether there are differences in outcome, based on the underlying fungal pathogen, remains to be determined.

B. Azoles

When one agent within a class of drugs is reported to interact with a medication, a frequent assumption is that it is a "class effect." This assumption must not be made when considering clinically relevant drug interactions with azole antifungals. Drugs within the class have distinct differences, some with very different metabolic path-ways. As a consequence, the presence of a drug interaction with one agent cannot be extrapolated to others within the class, nor can be the magnitude of the interac-tion, as the azoles have different affinities for the CYP isoenzymes.

1. Ketoconazole

In 1981, ketoconazole was the first azole to be introduced into clinical practice, and was used widely for a variety of fungal infections. Its use is now relegated to second-line therapy, behind the newer azoles that possess more favorable side effect profiles and a broader spectrum of activity. Ketoconazole is metabolized primarily by the CYP3A4 isoenzyme system, with other CYP enzymes involved to a lesser extent. Ketoconazole has also been reported to interact with the transport protein P-glycoprotein, another mechanism by which drug–drug interactions can occur.

Drug interactions of most concern in immunocompromised patients include the calcineurin inhibitors cyclosporine, tacrolimus and sirolimus, and the antiretrovirals and antineoplastic agents. Ketoconazole was first noticed to reduce the daily cyclosporine requirements in renal transplant patients in 1982 (15). Since that time it has been widely accepted as a method to reduce costs associated with organ transplantation. Concomitant administration of ketoconazole and cyclosporine leads to a reduction in the cyclosporine dose of 70–80% (16–18). This then reduces the overall cost of the transplant immunosuppression by this percentage. Initially, many centers were concerned about introducing another drug that had a known side-effect profile to reduce the dose of another agent purely for financial reasons. Long-term follow-up of patients treated with combination ketoconazole and cyclosporine have not shown any detrimental effects, with a similar number of acute rejection episodes and chronic graft dysfunction (17), a similar rate of hepatotoxicity to those not receiving ketoconazole, and had better metabolic profiles in the ketoconazole/cyclosporine recipients. The dose of ketoconazole required to induce the cyclosporine sparing effect is 87 mg. A similar interaction has been observed among recipients of tacrolimus (19,20), although it has not been studied formally. Similar dose reductions should be made to tacrolimus when initiating ketoconazole therapy.

Patients infected with HIV are immunocompromised and may develop either topical or systemic fungal infections requiring antifungal therapy. Ketoconazole is known to alter the metabolism of several of the protease inhibitors (PI) and the non-nucleoside reverse transcriptase inhibitors (NNRTI's), and many drugs within these classes in turn affect the PK of ketoconazole. Importantly, the drug interactions between ketoconazole and each of the agents within these classes are not the same. For example, within the PI class of drugs, only indinavir requires a dosage adjustment whereas no dosage modifications are necessary for amprenavir and nelfinavir. The lopinavir/ritonavir combination, ritonavir, and saquinavir have all been shown to increase the exposure of ketoconazole several fold, and as a consequence, a maximum dose of 200 mg/day of ketoconazole is recommended. Clinically significant interactions between ketoconazole and the PI's and the NNRTI's are summarized in Table 3 (21–35).

Lastly, interactions between ketoconazole and antineoplastic chemotherapy must be considered. These interactions are poorly characterized with the majority of data arising from animal models or the use of test systems in vitro. As a consequence limited data is available. Ketoconazole is a model CYP3A4 inhibitor, and has been studied in combination with irinotecan, a commonly used agent in colorectal cancer. It is also a partial substrate of CYP3A4 isoenzymes (25). Patients were initially exposed to irinotecan monotherapy, at a standard dose of 350 mg/m^2, and then 3 weeks later were exposed to a lower dose of irinotecan (100 mg/m^2) in combination with ketoconazole 200 mg/day. Irinotecan is metabolized to several metabolites, including the pharmacologically active metabolite SN-38. Following concomitant

Table 3 Clinically Relevant Pharmacokinetic Drug Interactions with Ketoconazole (21–35)

Drug	Data type	Proposed Mechanism of Interaction by Ketoconazole (K) or Drug (D)	Clinical Effect (Potential or Actual)	Recommended Action
Antiarrhythmics Dofetilide (21)	Case reports	CYP3A4 inhibition Inhibition of tubular secretion via the cation transport system	↑ Dofetilide [ ] by 53% males; ↑ Dofetilide [ ] by 97% females	Stop dofetilide 2 days prior to starting ketoconazole
Antihistamines (astemizole, terfenadine) (22)	Case reports	CYP3A4 inhibition by K	↑ Astemizole and Terfenadine [ ] → QTc prolongation	Contraindicated. Avoid
Benzodiazepines (midazolam, triazolam) (22)	Case reports	CYP3A4 inhibition by K	↑ Midazolam/Triazolarm [ ]	Prolonged sedative and hypnotic effects
Bosentan (23)	PK study	CYP3A4 inhibition by K	↑ C_{max} Bosentan 2.1-fold; ↑ AUC Bosentan 2.3-fold	
Calcineurin Inhibitors Cyclosporine (16–18,24)	Case reports PK studies	CYP3A4 inhibition by K	↑ C_{min}, ↑ AUC cyclosporine	Reduce the dose of cyclosporine or tacrolimus by 75–80% when starting ketoconazole
Tacrolimus (19,20)	Case reports	CYP3A4 inhibition by K	↑ C_{min}, AUC tacrolimus	
Cisparide (22)	Case reports	CYP3A4 inhibition by K	↑ cisparide AUC 8-fold	Contraindicated. Avoid
Cytotoxic chemotherapy Irinotecan (25)	PK study	CYP3A4 inhibition by K	↑ AUC SN-38 (pharmacologically active metabolite of irinotecan) 109%	↓ Dose irinotecan by 75% Monitor for hematological toxicity
HMG-CoA reductase inhibitors (26)	Case reports	CYP3A4 inhibition by K	↑ Simvastatin [ ] - > toxicity	Monitor for signs of rhabdo-myolysis

(Continued)

Table 3 Clinically Relevant Pharmacokinetic Drug Interactions with Ketoconazole (21–35) (*Continued*)

Drug	Data type	Proposed Mechanism of Interaction by Ketoconazole (K) or Drug (D)	Clinical Effect (Potential or Actual)	Recommended Action
NNRTI's Nevirapine (27)	PK study	CYP3A4 induction by D	↓ Ketoconazole AUC 72% ↓ Ketoconazole C_{max} 44%	Avoid
Protease inhibitors Amprenavir (28)	PK study	CYP3A4 inhibition by D	↑ Ketoconazole AUC 44%	No dose modification
Indinavir (29)	PK study	CYP3A4 inhibition by K	↑ Ketoconazole C_{max} 19% ↑ Indinavir AUC by 68%[a]	↓ Indinavir dose to 600 mg TTD
Lopinavir/Ritonavir (30)	PK study	CYP3A4 inhibition by D	↑ Ketoconazole AUC 3-fold	Do not exceed 200 mg/day ketoconazole
Nelfinavir (31)	PK study	CYP3A4 inhibition by K	↑ Nelfinavir AUC 35%; C_{max} 25%	No dose adjustments necessary. Monitor for PI toxicity
Ritonavir (32)	PK study	CYP3A4 inhibition by D	↑ Ketoconazole AUC 3.4-fold ↑ Ketoconazole C_{max} 55%	Use with caution. Do not exceed ketoconazole 200 mg/day
Saquinavir (33)	PK study	CYP3A4 inhibition by K	↑ Saquinavir AUC_{0-8} by 190%	If ketoconazole dose is > 200 mg monitor for saquinavir toxicity
Rifampin (22)	PK study	CYP3A4 induction by D	↓ AUC Ketoconazole	Avoid concomitant use where possible. If essential, increase dose
Telithromycin (34)	PK study	CYP3A4 inhibition by K	↑ Telithromycin C_{max} and AUC by 51.3% and 94.5%	Unknown
Warfarin (35)	PK study	CYP2C9 inhibition by D	↑ INR → bleeding	Monitor INR

[], concentration, ↑, increased; →, leads to; ↓, decreased; AUC, area under the curve; C_{min}, trough concentration; C_{max}, peak concentration; PK, pharmacokinetic; CYP3A4, cytochrome P450 3A4 isoenzyme; NNRTI's, non-nucleoside reverse transcriptase inhibitors.

[a]Single dose study. In multiple dosing study, 18% decrease in AUC of indinavir seen.

administration of ketoconazole, circulating SN-38 concentrations are increased by approximately 109%. Similarly, the principal oxidative metabolite, 7-ethyl-10-[4-N-(5-aminopentanoic acid)-l-piperidinol-carbonyloxycamptothecin (APC), was reduced by 87%. A paired analysis of hematologic toxicity demonstrated a similar degree of myelosuppression, despite a 3.5-fold reduction in irinotecan dose, when administered in combination with ketoconazole compared to irinotecan monotherapy. This study highlights the importance of understanding metabolic pathways prior to administering medications. Irinotecan is not the only antineoplastic that is likely to be subject to such an interaction; potentially docetaxel, etoposide, cyclophosphamide, and ifosfamide may interact similarly.

2. Fluconazole

Fluconazole, a bis-triazole antifungal, is widely used in high-risk population (neonates, surgical candidates, HIV, HSCT, and SOT patients) to prevent superficial and systemic fungal infections. Recent studies have shown that fluconazole can reduce systemic and superficial fungal infections, reduce fungal colonization, and reduce the use of empiric amphotericin B in high-risk populations (36–45). Fluconazole is metabolized by CYP3A4 isoenzymes, and is also a potent inhibitor of CYP2C9 isoenzymes, leading to several potential drug interactions (see Table 4) (46–87). One of the interactions of most concern, related to the transplantation community, is that of fluconazole and the calcineurin inhibitors, cyclosporine, and tacrolimus. Many centers have reported a clinically significant drug interaction between these two agents, although the magnitude of the interaction is smaller than seen with itraconazole, ketoconazole, and voriconazole. Two issues warrant consideration: first, does the interaction occur when the agents are administered intravenously as well as orally, and second, does the interaction occur at all doses of fluconazole, or is it a dose-dependent phenomenon?

Several case reports in the literature document a drug interaction between fluconazole and the calcineurin inhibitors (52–69), although these are retrospective and uncontrolled observations. Osowski and colleagues performed a controlled PK study of the interaction between intravenous cyclosporine/tacrolimus and intravenous fluconazole 400 mg daily in HSCT recipients (52). They observed no statistically or clinically significant differences in steady-state concentration or clearance of tacrolimus, and a statistically but not clinically significant difference in the clearance.of cyclosporine A. These results did not reflect the experience seen with oral administration of both agents in many of the earlier case reports.

CYP3A4 isoenzymes are the most abundant isoforms of CYP, accounting for nearly 30% of the total P450 content in the human liver, and as much as 70% in the gut wall (88). It has been postulated that tacrolimus and cyclosporine are also metabolized in the intestine by gut CYP3A4 isoenzymes. If this does occur, it would explain why a drug interaction is seen between azole antifungals and tacrolimus/cyclosporine when administered orally, and not when administered intravenously. In addition to tacrolimus and cyclosporine being metabolized in this manner, there is also evidence that fluconazole inhibits CYP3A4 substrate, which could result in increased serum tacrolimus or cyclosporine concentrations, with resultant toxicities. These differing observations lead to the conclusion that the interaction between tacrolimus and fluconazole is because of the inhibition of gut metabolism of tacrolimus by fluconazole, resulting in increased absorption, an increased AUC, and increased trough concentrations when these agents are administered orally.

Table 4 Clinically Relevant Pharmacokinetic Drug Interactions with Fluconazole (FLU) (46–87)

Drug (D)	Data type	Proposed mechanism of interaction by FLU (F) or (D)	Clinical effect (potential or actual)	Recommended Action
All-trans retinoic acid (ATRA) (46,47)	Case reports	CYP3A4 inhibition by F	↑ ATRA [] → ↑ CNS toxicity	Monitor closely for toxicities associated with ATRA
Antihistamines (astemizole, terfenadine) (48)	Case reports	CYP3A4 inhibition by F	↑ Astemizole/Terfenadine [] → prolonged QTc interval	Avoid. Contraindicated
Benzodiazepines				
Midazolam (49,50)	PK study	CYP3A4 inhibition by F	↑ Midazolam [] 0–4 fold → ↑ sedation	Monitor sedation; ↓ Midazolam dose; > interaction with oral Rx and high dose/continuous infusion ↑ Sedation; monitor
Triazolam (51)	PK study	CYP3A4 inhibition by F	↑ Triazolam AUC and $t_{1/2}$ (fluconazole dose dependent increases)	
Calcineurin inhibitors				
Tacrolimus (52–54)	Case reports, PK Studies	CYP3A4 inhibition by F	↑ Tacrolimus C_{min} → ↑ toxicity[a]	Monitor levels, ↓ Tacrolimus dose[a]
Cyclosporine (55–68)	Case reports	CYP3A4 inhibition by F	↑ Cyclosporine C_{min} → ↑ toxicity	Monitor levels; ↓ Cyclosporine dose[a]
Sirolimus (69)	Case report	CYP3A4 inhibition by F	↑ Sirolimus C_{min} → ↑ toxicity	Monitor levels; ↓ Sirolimus dose
Carbamazepine (70,71)	Case reports	CYP3A4 inhibition by F	↑ Carbamazepine [] → ↑ toxicity	Monitor levels; ↓ Carbamazepine dose
HMGCoA reductase inhibitor (simvastatin) (72)	Case report	CYP3A4 inhibition by F	↑ Simvastatin [] → ↑ musculo skeletal toxicity	Monitor patient closely for symptoms of rhabdomyolysis
Opioids				
Alfentanil (73)	PK study	CYP3A4 inhibition by F	↓ Alfentanil CL 55%; ↓ respiratory rate	Monitor sedation and respiratory rate
Phenytoin (74–77)	Case reports	CYP2C9/CYP3A4 inhibition by F	↑ Phenytoin []	Monitor phenytoin []
Rifamycins		CYP3A4 induction by D	↓ Fluconazole []	Monitor clinically for antifungal response
Rifabutin (78)	PK study	CYP3A4 inhibition by F	↑ Rifabutin exposure	Treatment failure of antifungal; monitor for response
Rifampin (79,80)	Case reports	CYP3A4 induction by D	↓ Fluconazole AUC; $t_{1/2}$; ↑ CL	
Sulfonylureas				
Glimepiride (81)	Case report	CYP2C9 inhibition by F	↑ Glimepiride AUC; $t_{1/2}$	Monitor blood sugar; ↓ glimepiride dose
Warfarin (82–87)	Case reports	CYP2C9 and CYP3A4 inhibition by F	↑ Warfarin [] → ↑ bleeding	Monitor INR; ↓ Warfarin dose

[], concentration; ↑, increased; →, leads to; ↓, decreased; AUC, area under the curve; C_{min}, trough concentration; F, bioavailability; $t_{1/2}$, half-life; CL, clearance; GVHD, graft vs. host disease; PK, pharmacokinetic; CYP3A4, cytochrome P450 3A4, isoenzyme; CYP2C9, cytochrome P450 2C9 isoenzyme.
[a]Drug interaction occurs when both agents administered orally and where fluconazole dose is >200 mg/day.

Therefore, appropriate dose reductions in cyclosporine and tacrolimus should be made when administered orally, but are unnecessary when given intravenously.

At the University of Florida HSCT program, lower doses of fluconazole (100 mg for autologous HSCT recipients were used; 200 mg for allogeneic HSCT recipients) as part of our antifungal prophylaxis strategy. When the calcineurin inhibitors are concomitantly administered with fluconazole at these doses, appreciable increases in cyclosporine or tacrolimus serum concentrations are not noted. This suggests that the drug interaction is dose-dependent, and that at doses of fluconazole of greater than 200 mg per day the interaction is much more likely to occur, requiring reductions in cyclosporine/tacrolimus doses (60,62,66). Fluconazole doses < 200 mg daily typically do not require a dose adjustment of the calcineurin inhibitor. Other investigators have made similar observations (60,62,64,68).

The other drugs with which fluconazole has been reported to interact include rifampin, phenytoin, and warfarin. Rifampin, a potent CYP3A4, CYP2C9, and CYP2C19 isoenzyme inducer, was shown to significantly lower the AUC of fluconazole by 52%, increase clearance by 93%, and shorten the half-life of fluconazole when concomitantly prescribed (79). In this case series, the dose of rifampin was higher than the doses used for HSCT antibiotic prophylaxis (1200 mg daily vs. 600 mg daily), and may account for the differences seen in this trial compared to earlier healthy volunteer studies, where the mean decrease in exposure was 23% (80). Relapse or failure of fluconazole therapy in cryptococcal meningitis has been reported due to this enzyme induction.

Phenytoin, a known potent inducer of CYP3A4 enzymes, is itself metabolized by CYP2C9 and CYP2C19. Fluconazole is a potent inhibitor of these isoenzymes, leading to increased serum concentrations of phenytoin and clinical toxicity. Several case reports have indicated clinical phenytoin toxicity when phenytoin is administered with fluconazole at doses of 200 mg or greater per day (74–77). In healthy volunteers, fluconazole administration increases phenytoin trough concentrations and AUC by 128% and 75%, respectively. The onset of the interaction is relatively quick, within 2–6 days of concomitant administration. Phenytoin dosage should be reduced, and serum concentrations closely monitored. Warfarin also requires close monitoring and potential dosage adjustment when prescribed with fluconazole. Fluconazole inhibits the metabolism of warfarin by CYP2C9, thus potentiating the hypoprothrombinemic response of warfarin, usually in the first few days of concomitant administration. Frequent monitoring of the INR should occur in this population. In healthy volunteer studies, the mean change in the INR was 38% (range 16–64%) (84–87).

3. Itraconazole

Itraconazole, a triazole compound with activity against yeasts and molds, has been used as prophylaxis against fungal infections in immunocompromised patients (89,90), in the empiric setting for fever unresponsive to broad-spectrum antibiotics (91), and in the treatment of documented fungal infections (92–94), Like other members of the azole family, it undergoes extensive metabolism via the CYP3A4 enzyme system, and is subject to drug interactions with agents metabolized by a similar pathway (95–134).

Itraconazole differs from fluconazole in that there is a relationship between drug dose, serum drug concentration, and efficacy. Serum concentrations of itraconazole greater than 500 ng/mL are required to prevent invasive fungal infection

(120). If enzyme inducers are coadministered, there is potential for increased metabolism of itraconazole leading to reduced serum concentrations and potential drug failure. Drugs that decrease plasma concentrations of itraconazole include carbamazepine (106,107), phenobarbital, phenytoin (116), isoniazid, rifampin (117,118), and rifabutin (119). Whenever possible, these should not be prescribed concomitantly with itraconazole, although if no suitable alternative exists, routine drug monitoring of itraconazole levels is recommended to ensure that therapeutic levels are achieved (i.e., >500 ng/mL).

Itraconazole also has the ability to increase concentrations of many other medications (see Table 5) (95–134). Numerous case reports in the literature document an interaction between oral itraconazole and oral tacrolimus (122,125–129), and oral itraconazole and oral cyclosporine (122–124). These cases demonstrate that the addition of itraconazole to calcineurin inhibitor therapy increases the trough concentrations of the calcineurin inhibitors by two-to three-fold. In each of these case reports, additional factors could affect outcome, so the frequency of occurrence and the magnitude of the drug interaction is not clear. Despite these uncertainties, the dose of cyclosporine and tacrolimus must be reduced, and based on available data, the reduction should be at least 50% at the time itraconazole is added to therapy. Evaluation of the pharmacokinetic drug interaction between intravenous itraconazole and intravenous calcineurin inhibitors has also been conducted (122). In a controlled environment, allogeneic HSCT recipients were stabilized on intravenous calcineurin inhibitors. Once steady state was reached, intravenous itraconazole was added to therapy. Among the 16 patients studied, the mean steady-state tough concentration of cyclosporine and tacrolimus increased by 123–249% and 126–207%, respectively. This is accompanied by a corresponding mean decrease in clearance of 46.4% and 44%, respectively. The increase in serum cyclosporine and tacrolimus concentrations is evident at the completion of the intravenous loading dose, when steady state is achieved. A 50% reduction in dose of cyclosporine and tacrolimus doses should occur when starting intravenous itraconazole therapy.

Many critically ill patients require narcotic analgesics for pain relief. Phenylpiperidine opiates, which include fentanyl, sufentanil, and alfentanil, are extensively metabolized by CYP3A4 isoenzymes. There is potential for elevated serum concentrations of these opioids if coadministered with medications that inhibit CYP3A4 isoenzymes. When administration of both agents is essential, patients should be monitored closely for excessive sedation and for low respiratory rates.

The other major class of drugs that requires consideration when prescribing itraconazole is the antineoplastic agents. Numerous case reports exist in the literature documenting greater neurotoxicity when itraconazole is prescribed during vinca alkaloid administration (98–102). Cyclophosphamide, a cytotoxic agent used in many chemotherapy regimens, is a prodrug that must undergo metabolism by CYP enzymes to produce the alkylator species required for its antineoplastic effect. The CYP's most involved in this process are CYP3A4 and CP2C9 (135). Coadministration of inhibitors of these isoenzymes may lead to increased exposure of cyclophosphamide, and increased toxicity. It has been suggested that concomitant administration of itraconazole with cyclophosphamide preparative regimens may lead to greater toxicity. Itraconazole has also been reported to reduce the clearance of busulfan when concomitantly prescribed with itraconazole. Clearance was reduced by 20%, and was accompanied by increased toxicity (136). Similarly, other antineoplastic agents that are metabolized by the CYP enzymes may have their serum concentrations enhanced leading to greater toxicity. Metabolic pathways of

Table 5 Clinically Relevant Pharmacokinetic Drug Interactions with Itraconazole (96–134)

Drug (D)	Data type	Proposed mechanism of interaction by Itraconazole (I) or drug (D)	Clinical effect (potential or actual)	Recommended action
Antiarrhythmics Dofetilide (121)	Case report	CYP3A4 inhibition by I; inhibition of tubular secretion via the cation transport system	↑ Dofetilide [ ]	Contraindicated together. Stop dofetilide 2 days prior to starting at interacting drugs
Antihistamines Terfenadine (96,97) Antemizole	PK study PK study	CYP3A4 inhibition by I	↑ [ ] unmetabolized terfenadine; ↑ C_{max}, $t_{1/2}$ → prolonged QTc	Contraindicated—Avoid
Antineoplastics e.g., vinca alkaloids, busulfan, ifosfamide, cyclophosphamide, docetaxel; epipodophyllotoxins (98–102)	Case reports/ Theoretical	CYP3A4 inhibition by I	↑ Antineoplastic [ ] due to ↓ metabolism → ↑ toxicity e.g., neurotoxicity with vinca alkaloids	Avoid concomitant therapy. Use alternative nonazole antifungal during chemotherapy administration and until antineoplastic elimination complete
Benzodiazepines (BZD) (alprazolam, midazolam—oral, triazolam) (103,104)	Case reports	CYP3A4 inhibition by I	↑ BZD C_{max}, ↑ AUC, $t_{\frac{1}{2}}$ → prolonged hypnotic and sedative effects; prolonged psychomotor impairment	Avoid where possible. Use alternative BZD e.g., lorazepam, temazepam
Calcineurin Inhibitors Cyclosporine (CyA) IV (122)	PK study	CYP3A4 inhibition by I	↑ CyA C_{min} 1.23–2.49-fold → nephrotoxicity	Decrease dose of CyA by 50% when starting intravenous itraconazole
Cyclosporine (oral) (123,124)	Case reports	CYP3A4 inhibition by I	↑ CyA C_{min} by 33–85% → potential nephrotoxicity	Decrease dose of CyA by 50% when starting itraconazole (Kramer).

(Continued)

Table 5 Clinically Relevant Pharmacokinetic Drug Interactions with Itraconazole (96–134) (*Continued*)

Drug (D)	Data type	Proposed mechanism of interaction by Itraconazole (I) or drug (D)	Clinical effect (potential or actual)	Recommended action
Tacrolimus(IV) (122)	PK study	CYP3 A4 inhibition	↑ Tacrolimus C_{min},1.26–2.07-fold → ↑ toxicity	Reduce tacrolimus dose by 50% at the time of initiating itraconazole therapy
Tacrolimus (oral) (125–129)	Case reports	CYP3A4 inhibition	↑ Tacrolimus C_{min}	Reduce the dose of tacrolimus by 50–67% when initiating itraconazole therapy
			↓ Tacrolimus CL → ↑ toxicity	
Cisapride (121)	Case reports	CYP3A4 inhibition by I	↑ Cisparide [ ] → *Torsades de points*/QTc prolongation	Contraindicated—Avoid
Corticosteroids				
Intravenous MP (130)	PK studies	CYP3A4 inhibition by I	↓ CL MP;t½	Enhanced steroid side effects
Inhaled (131,132)	PK studies	CYP3A4 inhibition by I		Enhanced steroid side effects
Oral	PK studies	CYP3A4 inhibition by I	↑ AUC Methylprednisolone (no effect on prednisone); ↑ t½	Enhanced suppression of exogenous cortisol secretion
Digoxin (108–111)	Case reports	↓ renal CL due to inhibition of digoxin p-glycoprotein pump	↑ Digoxin [ ] 2–4 fold → toxicity ↓ CL	Decrease dose of digoxin 60–75%. Monitor digoxin levels closely. Note: interaction occurs 7–13 days after starting itraconazole
HMG Co-A reductase inhibitors (lovastatin (112), atorvastatin (113), Simvastatin (114,115)	Case reports	CYP3A4 inhibition by I	L: ↑ C_{max} 22-fold; ↑ AUC 13-fold; 97% ↓ clearance S: ↑ C_{max} > 10-fold; ↑ AUC 19-fold; > 90% ↓ clearance A: ↑ AUC 4-fold; 70% ↓ clearance → ↑ risk of rhabdomyolysis	Avoid atorvastatin, lovastatin, and simvastatin = contraindicated Fluvastatin and pravastatin are suitable alternatives, as they do not interact with itraconazole.

Opioids				
Fentanyl (133)	Case report	CYP3A4 inhibition by I	↑ Fentanyl []	MOnitro for CNS depression
Phenytoin (116)	Case reports	CYP3A4 induction by D	↓ Itraconazole C_{max} 95% ↓ Itraconazole AUC 93% ↓ Itraconazole $t_{\frac{1}{2}}$ 83%	Switch to alternative antiepileptic agent
Protease inhibitors				
Amprenavir	Theoretical	CYP3 A4 inhibition by D	↑ Itraconazole [], AUC	Increased itraconazole levels
Indinavir	PK study	CYP3A4 inhibition by D	↑ Itraconazole [], AUC	↓ Indinavir to 600 mg PO Q8H
Lopinavir/ritonavir (134)		CYP3A4 inhibition by D	↑ Itraconazole [], AUC	
Rifampin (117,118)	Case reports	CYP3A4 induction by D	Itraconazole [] → treatment failure	Avoid
Rifabutin (119)	Case report	CYP3A4 induction by D	↑ Itraconazole [] → treatment failure	Avoid
Sirolimus[a]	Hypothesis	CYP3A4 inhibition; ?P-gp inhibition by I	↑ Sirolimus AUC, C_{max}, and t to C_{max} → ↑ toxicity	Monitor sirolimus levels. Decrease sirolimus dose
Warfarin (95)	Case report	CYP2C9 inhibition by I	Prolonged INR, ↑ PT → ↑ bleeding risk	Close monitoring of INR/PT (every 2 days) and dose reduction of warfarin

CYP, cytochrome P450; CYP3A4, cytochrome P450 3A4, isoenzyme; CYP2C9, cytochrome P450 2C9 isoenzyme ↑, increase; ↓, decrease; [], concentration; →, leads to; INR, international normalized ratio; PK, pharmacokinetic; BP, blood pressure; HR, heart rate; CL, clearance; C_{min}, trough concentration; C_{max}, maximum concentration; AUC, area under the curve; $t_{\frac{1}{2}}$, half-life; P-gp, P-glycoprotein; MP, methyprednisolone; INR, international normalized ratio; PT, prothrombin time; QTc, QTc interval on an EKG; F, bioavailability.

[a]There are literature reports of an interaction between voriconazole/sirolimus, and ketoconazole/sirolimus. Significant ↑ in AUC, C_{max} seen.

the antineoplastic agent should be verified prior to coadministering with itraconazole. Patient's receiving antineoplastic agents metabolized by the CYP3A4 isoenzyme system should have the itraconazole therapy held during the chemotherapy administration. One must be mindful of the long half-life of itraconazole (64 hr with oral dosing when at steady state), and stop the drug early enough to permit complete excretion of itraconazole and its metabolites.

4. *Voriconazole*

Voriconazole, the most recent commercially available azole, offers new challenges to the prescribing clinician. It is similar to other members of the azole family in that it is subject to several drug interactions (137–146). Voriconazole, however, is metabolized by three separate cytochrome P450 enzyme systems, namely CYP2C9, CYP2C19, and CYP3A4. This differs from the other azoles (fluconazole, itraconazole, ketoconazole, posaconazole, and ravuconazole), which are metabolized primarily by CYP3 A4. In vitro metabolism studies show that voriconazole is both a substrate and an inhibitor of these three enzymes. Due to extensive hepatic microsomal metabolism, caution is needed when prescribing voriconazole to immunocompromised patients receiving multiple medications. Prior to starting any new drug, a screen of potential interactions should always be performed, and if there are no data, evaluate the metabolic pathways of the new agent to evaluate the hypothetical risk of a drug interaction occurring.

Based on data from in vitro drug metabolism studies, voriconazole was subject to extensive clinical PK drug interaction studies prior to marketing. These PK interaction studies were designed around target drugs that were likely to be coadministered to target patient populations and/or when an interaction might be expected on mechanistic grounds. The main clinically significant drug interactions that are known to occur when coprescribed with voriconazole are summarized in Table 6 (137,139,140,142–146), and the effect of other drugs on voriconazole metabolism are summarized in Table 7 (137,139,141–143). There are several agents that are contraindicated in patients receiving voriconazole, including sirolimus, ergot alkaloids, terfenadine, astemizole, cisapride, pimozide, quinidine, rifampin, and rifabutin. Coadministration of sirolimus with voriconazole results in an increased maximal concentration (C_{max}) by 556%, and an increased exposure, or "area-under-the curve" of sirolimus by 1014%, prohibiting dose reduction to a safe level (137). The interaction with astemizole, cisapride, pimozide, quinidine, and ergot derivatives is due to potential prolongation of the QTc interval leading to *Torsades de pointes*. A similar reaction is noted to occur when these agents are administered with several other members of the azole family (itraconazole, ketoconazole). Rifampin, however, induces the metabolism of voriconazole to such an extent that there is no dose of voriconazole that could be safely administered to a patient to overcome this inhibition. It should be noted that increasing the dose of voriconazole when coadministered with rifabutin can overcome the enzyme induction, although this approach should be avoided.

Again, the one therapeutic class of drugs where there is a lack of available information regarding drug interactions with voriconazole, is antineoplastic therapy. This is an area that should be addressed because immunocompromised patients will often require antifungal therapy with ongoing chemotherapy. Several antineoplastic agents are metabolized by the CYP3A4 enzyme system. The ramifications of the potential drug interaction include elevated concentrations of the antineoplastic

Table 6 Clinically Relevant Pharmacokinetic Drug Interactions with Voriconazole (VORI): Effect of Voriconazole on the Pharmacokinetics of Other Drugs (137,139,140,142–146)

Target drug	Population	Proposed mechanism of interaction	Clinical effect on target drug	Recommended action
Antihistamines Astemizole, terfenadine (137)	Theoretical	CYP3A4 inhibition	↑ Astemizole and terfenadine [ ] → QTc prolongation	Contraindicated. Potential for QT prolongation and *Torsades de pointes*
Benzodiazepines (BZD) (137)	In vitro studies	CYP3 A4 inhibition	Potential for inhibition of metabolism of BZD → ↑ sedation	Frequent monitoring for adverse events and toxicity Dose reduce BZD if symptomatic
Calcineurin inhibitors Cyclosporine (144)	PK study Stable renal transplant patients Stable renal transplant patients	CYP3A4 inhibition	↑ CyA AUC 70% ↑ CyA C_{min} 2.5-fold → ↑ toxicity	When initiating VORI in patients already on CyA, ↑ CyA dose by 50% and closely monitor blood levels Interaction evident on day 4 of coadministration ↑CyA dose when VORI discontinued
Tacrolimus (FK) (145,146)	PK study Healthy volunteers	CYP3A4 inhibition	↑ Tacrolimus AUC 321% ↑C_{max} 217% → ↑ toxicity	When initiating VORI in patients on FK, ↓ dose of FK by 67–90%, ↑ FK dose when VORI is discontinued
Sirolimus (solution) (137)	PK study Healthy volunteers	CYP3A4 inhibition	↑ Sirolimus AUC 1014% ↑ Sirolimus C_{max} 556% → toxicity	Contraindicated
Calcium channel blockers (CCB) (dihydropyridine class) (137)	In vitro studies	CYP3A4 inhibition	Potential for inhibition of metabolism of CCB → hypotension	Monitor blood pressure and pulse. Dose reduction of CCB may be needed if symptomatic
Chemotherapy/ cytotoxics (metabolized by CYP 3A4, 2C19, or 2C9)	Hypothesized interaction	CYP3A4, 2C9, 2C19 inhibition	Potentially ↑ exposure to chemotherapeutic agent and enhanced toxicity	Avoid coadministration with cytotoxic agents metabolized by the CYP 3A4, 2C9, 2C19 pathways. If fungal coverage necessary, change to alternative nonazole antifungal with similar spectrum

(Continued)

Table 6 Clinically Relevant Pharmacokinetic Drug Interactions with Voriconazole (VORI): Effect of Voriconazole on the Pharmacokinetics of Other Drugs (137,139,140,142–146) (*Continued*)

Target drug	Population	Proposed mechanism of interaction	Clinical effect on target drug	Recommended action
Ergot alkaloids (137)	Hypothesized interaction	CYP3A4 inhibition	↑ Ergot alkaloid [ ]	Contraindicated. Potential for QT prolongation and *Torsades de pointes*
HMG-CoA reductase inhibitors (Statins) (137)	In vitro studies	CYP3A4 inhibition	↑ Plasma exposure of the statins, → ↑ toxicity	Monitor for increased muscle pain/weakness and rhabdomyolysis
NNRTI's (137)	In vitro studies	CYP3A4 inhibition	↑ Plasma exposure of NNRTI's	Monitor frequently for adverse events
Phenytoin (143)	PK study Healthy volunteers	CYP2C9 inhibition	↑ AUC 81% ↑ C_{max} 67%	Monitor phenytoin concentrations and adjust the dose accordingly
Prednisolone (138)	Healthy volunteers	CYP3A4 inhibition	↑ AUC 34% prednisolone	None recommended
HIV protease inhibitors (137)	In vitro studies	CYP3A4 inhibition	↑ Plasma exposure HIV protease inhibitors	Monitor frequently for adverse events
Proton pump inhibitors Omeprazole (142)	Healthy volunteers	CYP3A4 inhibition	↑ AUC 280% ↑ C_{max} 116%	Doses > 40 mg omeprazole per day may be reduced by 50%
Quinidine (137)	Theoretical	CYP3A4 inhibition	↑ Quinidine [ ]	Contraindicated. Potential for QT prolongation and *Torsades depointes*
Rifabutin (139)	Healthy volunteers	CYP3A4 inhibition	↑ Rifabutin AUC 331% ↑ Rifabutin C_{max} 195%	Contraindicated
Rifampin (139)	Healthy volunteers	CYP3A4 induction		Contraindicated
Sulfonylurea oral hypoglycemics (137)	Theoretical	CYP2C9 inhibition	↑ Plasma exposure to sulfonylurea → ↑ BSL	Frequent BSL monitoring → ↓dose of sulfonylurea
Vinca alkaloids (also see chemotherapy)	Hypothesis	CYP3A4 inhibition	↑ Exposure to vinca's → ↑ neurotoxicity	Avoid coadministration with vinca alkaloids
Warfarin (140)	Healthy volunteers	CYP2C9 inhibition	↑ PT, INR → bleeding	Monitor INR/PT closely ↓ Warfarin dose

CYP 3A4, Cytochrome P450 3A4 isoenzyme; CYP2C9, cytochrome P450 2C9 isoenzyme; CYP2C19, cytochrome P450 2C19 isoenzyme; AUC, area under the curve; ↑, increase; ↓, decrease; →, leads to; NNRTI's, non-nucleoside reverse transcriptase inhibitors.

Table 7 Clinically Relevant Pharmacokinetic Drug Interactions with Voriconazole (VORI): Effect of Other Drugs on the Pharmacokinetics of Voriconazole (137,139,141–143).

Drug	Population	Proposed mechanism of interaction	Clinical effect	Recommended Action
Barbiturates (long acting) (137)	Hypothesized interaction	CYP3A4 induction	Likely to result in ↓ VORI exposure	Contraindicated
Carbamazepine (137)	Hypothesized interaction	CYP3A4 induction	Enzyme induction → enhanced VORI metabolism → potential VORI treatment failure	Contraindicated
NNRTI's (137)	In vitro	CYP3A4 inhibition or induction	↑ and ↓ VORI []	Monitor for VORI-associated toxicity and lack of response
Omeprazole (141,142)	PK study	CYP2C19 inhibition Healthy volunteers	↑ VORI AUC 41%	None ↑ VORI C_{max} 15%
Phenytoin (143)	PK study Healthy volunteers	CYP3A4 induction	↓ VORI AUC 69% ↓ VORI C_{max} 49%	Increase VORI maintenance to 5 mg/kg IV BID (from 4 mg/kg); or from 200 mg to 400 mg PO BID (100–200 mg PO BID in patients <40 kg)
Protease inhibitors (PI's) (137)	In vitro studies	CYP3A4 inhibition	↑ VORI []	Monitor for VORI-associated toxicity. NO adjustment required when coadministered with indinavir. Frequent monitoring for ADR's when prescribed with other PI's
Rifabutin (139)	PK study Healthy volunteers	CYP3A4 induction	↓ VORI AUC 78% ↓ VORI C_{max} 69% → treatment failure	Contraindicated
Rifampin (139)	PK study Healthy volunteers	CYP3A4 induction	↓ AUC 96%; ↓ C_{max} 93% → treatment failure	Contraindicated

CYP 3A4, cytochrome P450 3A4 isoenzyme; CYP2C9, cytochrome P450 2C9 isoenzyme; CYP2C19, cytochrome P450 2C19 isoenzyme; AUC, area under the curve; ↑, increase; ↓, decrease; →, leads to; VORI, voriconazole; C_{max}, maximum "peak" concentration; ADR's, adverse drug reactions.

agent, leading to greater chemotherapy or preparative regimen associated toxicity. Increased toxicity has been noted both with itraconazole and ketoconazole when administered at the same time as antineoplastic therapy as discussed previously. These case reports and studies clearly highlight the potential the azole antifungal agents have to increase concentrations of antineoplastic agents metabolized by CYP 3A4, leading to greater toxicity if dose reductions are not made. If a patient is receiving voriconazole for a pre-existing fungal infection, and is scheduled to undergo chemotherapy metabolized by CYP2C9, CYP2C19, or CYP3A4 (whether that be a HSCT preparative regimen or conventional chemotherapy), the best course of action would be to stop the voriconazole at least 30 hr prior to the chemotherapy/ preparative regimen, and continue to hold during chemotherapy. Once the antineoplastic agent has been eliminated (approximately 5 half-lives of the antineoplastic agent), voriconazole can be restarted. Other suitable nonazole antifungals can be instituted during the preparative regimen.

In some of the clinical trials, adverse events including visual hallucinations and confusion were reported. When evaluated more closely, there appeared to be a relationship between these side effects and the use of benzodiazepines and/or opioid analgesic consumption in conjunction with voriconazole. Many of the benzodiazepines are metabolized by the CYP3A4 isoenzymes, including midazolam, triazolam, and alprazolam. Diazepam is metabolized by CYP2C19 in addition to CYP3A4. If the BZD's are coadministered with a drug that is a potent inhibitor of CYP3A4, there will be an increase in serum concentrations of the BZD, with potential for increased sedation. Lorazepam, a commonly used component of antiemetic regimens, is eliminated by conjugation, and therefore, does not undergo a PK drug interaction with CYP3A4 modulators, and can be safely used. Similarly, oxazepam and temazepam are safe to use in combination with CYP3A4 agents.

In addition to these listed interactions, it is important to note that several drug interaction studies did not demonstrate an increase in either voriconazole or the concomitant medication when coadministered. Agents studied that are safe to coadminister with voriconazole include erythromycin, azithromycin, indinavir, prednisolone, ranitidine, digoxin, and mycophenolate mofetil. It is clear that there are many other mediations that may theoretically interact with voriconazole, yet have not been studied. Whenever prescribing voriconazole, it is prudent to monitor the patient very closely in the early phase of concomitant administration, looking for both toxicities as well as a lack of effect of the concomitant medication as well as voriconazole. Despite the numerous known drug interactions with voriconazole, if appropriate caution is used and modifications to target drugs are made, it is relatively safe to use voriconazole in the majority of patients.

5. *Posaconazole*

Posaconazole is an investigational "extended spectrum triazole" with clinical activity demonstrated in *Candida* spp. (147–149), *Coccidiomycosis* spp. (150), *Aspergillus* spp. (147), *Fusarium* spp. (147), and *Mucor* spp. (147) infections. Posaconazole is an inhibitor of CYP3A4, and has not been shown to affect the activity of CYP1A2, CYP 2C8/9, CYP2D6, and CYP2E1 (151). Therefore, interactions are likely to occur with drugs that are metabolized via the CYP3A4 isoenzyme system. Because of the investigational status of posaconazole, there are limited data on drug interactions with this agent (Table 8) (152–157). It appears that there is an interaction with cyclosporine, although the magnitude of this interaction is not as great as that seen with

Table 8 Clinically Relevant Pharmacokmetic Drug Interactions with Posaconazole (POS) (152–157)

Drug (D)	Data type	Proposed mechanism of interaction by Posaconazole (P) or (D)	Clinical effect (potential or actual)	Recommended action
Calcineurin inhibitors				
Cyclosporine (152)	PK study	CYP3A4 inhibition by P	↑ CyA C_{min} → ↑ toxicity	Monitor levels. ↓ CyA dose (0–29%)
Tacrolimus (153)	PK study	CYP3A4 inhibition by P	↑ AUC, 469% → toxicity	Monitor levels, ↓ tacrolimus dose (at least 50%)
			↑ C_{max} 221%;↓ CL5-fold, ↑ $t\frac{1}{2}$ 7.5 hr	
Cimetidine (154)	PK study	CYP3A4 induction by D	↓ Posaconazole C_{max}, AUC	Increase posaconazole dose
Glipizide (155)	PK study	CYP3A4 inhibition by P	↓ 15% mean plasma glucose	Monitor blood glucose closely
Phenytoin (156)	PK study	CYP3A4 induction by D	↑ Posaconazole CL by 90%	Avoid
Rifabutin (157)	PK study	CYP3A4 induction by D	↓ Posaconazole C_{max}, AUC	Avoid
	PK study	CYP3A4 inhibition by P	↑ Rifabutin C_{max}, AUC	

[], concentration; ↑ increased; →, leads to; ↓, decreased; AUC, area under the curve; C_{min}, trough concentration; C_{max}, peak concentration; CL, clearance; $t\frac{1}{2}$, half-life; PK, pharmacokinetic; CYP3A4, cytochrome P4503A4 isoenzyme.

voriconazole and itraconazole. In a limited number of cardiac transplant candidates, the dose reductions of cyclosporine ranged from 0% to 29% (152). Like the other azoles, the magnitude of the drug interaction with the various calcineurin inhibitors is not consistent within the class. Posaconazole has been shown to interact with tacrolimus, and the magnitude of this interaction is greater than the interaction with cyclosporine. In a healthy volunteer study, the concomitant administration of posaconazole and tacrolimus resulted in a 469% increase in the AUC1 and a 221% increase in the C_{max} concentration (153). Clearance of tacrolimus decreased 5-fold, and there was an extension in the half-life of tacrolimus to 7.5 hr (153). While no specific dosage recommendations have been made, and since we do not have the relative C_{min} concentrations, it is clear that a dose reduction of tacrolimus will be necessary, most likely in the vicinity of 50%.

The hepatic microsomal enzyme inducer, rifabutin, has been shown to increase the clearance of posaconazole two-fold, resulting in a 57% reduction in the C_{max}, and a 51% reduction in exposure (AUC) (157). When rifabutin and posaconazole are coadministered there is also an increase in the PK parameters of rifabutin. Plasma rifabutin C_{max} and AUC are increased 31% and 72%, respectively (157). Phenytoin also reduces the bioavailability of posaconazole 2–3-fold, however, there is no effect of posaconazole on serum phenytoin concentration (156). Both phenytoin and rifabutin should be avoided in patients receiving posaconazole.

Other drugs that have been studied in combination with posaconazole include the H_2-antagonist cimetidine, as well as the antiretroviral agents zidovudine/lamivudine and indinavir. Concomitant administration of posaconazole and cimetidine results in a 40% reduction in the C_{max} and AUC of posaconazole compared to posaconazole alone (154). The mechanism by which this interaction takes place is not clear. A similar study evaluating the effect of antacids on the PK of posaconazole did not demonstrate an effect of antacid on C_{max} or AUC of posaconazole thus, suggesting that the cause of the interaction is not pH mediated (158). Similarly, administration of posaconazole with zidovudine/lamivudine and indinavir in HIV infected patients does not lead to any significant interaction and no dosage modification is required.

6. Ravuconazole

Ravuconazole is also a broad-spectrum triazole, currently under investigation, and as a consequence there are limited data on the drug interaction profile of this agent. Pharmacokinetic data are available evaluating the interaction between ravuconazole and nelfinavir (159). There were no significant changes in the C_{max} and AUC of nelfinavir when both drugs were administered together compared to one drug alone, thus, it is safe for these to be coadministered. There are also data evaluating the drug interaction between ravuconazole and simvastatin in healthy subjects. Concomitant administration of these agents lead to an initial doubling of the AUC and C_{max}, and over repeated dosing (14 days) the C_{max} increased 4-fold and the AUC increased 4-fold (160). While an interaction does occur, it does not appear to be as great as the interaction seen with other azoles and the HMG CoA reductase inhibitors. As this drug moves further along the investigational pipeline, we can anticipate more PK data.

C. Echinocandins

1. Caspofungin

Caspofungin, the first echinocandin approved by the Food and Drug Administration (FDA), is used widely in the treatment of *Aspergillus* fungal infections in immunocompromised patients (161,162). The echinocandin class of agents is unique in that they are subject to few drug interactions. Caspofungin is neither a substrate nor an inhibitor of the cytochrome P450 enzyme system. PK studies demonstrate that caspofungin is not affected by the administration of itraconazole (163), amphotericin B (164), or mycophenolate mofetil (164), nor does it affect the pharmacokinetics of these target drugs. Caspofungin has been shown to decrease the peak plasma concentration, the 12-hr trough concentration, and AUC of tacrolimus when these two agents are concomitantly administered (165), and a corresponding increase in the dose of tacrolimus may be required. Close monitoring of tacrolimus concentrations should occur.

The interaction noted with tacrolimus is not a calcineurin inhibitor class effect, as a completely different interaction occurs when cyclosporine and caspofungin are administered concomitantly. Cyclosporine increases the AUC of caspofungin by 35% whereas cyclosporine concentrations are unaffected by caspofungin (164). In a healthy volunteer study, concomitant administration of cyclosporine and caspofungin resulted in significant elevations in liver function tests. In the first cohort of this study, healthy volunteers received caspofungin 70 mg intravenously once daily from day one to ten. Cyclosporine 3 mg/kg per dose was administered twice on day 10, each dose 12 hr apart. On day 11, transiently elevated alanine aminotransferase (ALT), approximately 2–3 times the upper limit of normal was noted in three out of four (75%) patients (164). A separate group of patients on the same study received caspofungin at a lower dose of 35 mg intravenously daily on day 1–3. Cyclosporine was administered at the same dose as the first cohort on day 1. On day 2, two out of eight patients (25%) had small increases in ALT, only slightly above the upper limit of normal (164). Based on these results, concomitant administration of caspofungin with cyclosporine is not recommended unless the potential benefit outweighs the risks. Until further information is available, the alternative is to change cyclosporine to tacrolimus.

Concomitant administration of caspofungin with inducers of drug clearance or mixed inducers/inhibitors may result in clinically meaningful reductions in serum caspofungin concentrations. Based on regression analyses of PK data, consideration should be given to increasing the daily dose of caspofungin to 70 mg when coadministering efavirenz, nelfinavir, nevirapine, phenytoin, rifampin, dexamethasone, or carbamazepine (164).

2. Micafungin

Micafungin, formerly known as FK463, is a new echinocandin antifungal that is pending final FDA approval. Micafungin differs from caspofungin in that it is not subject to the same drug interaction with cyclosporine. In the recently completed trial comparing fluconazole to micafungin in the prophylaxis of fungal infection in HSCT recipient's (166), approximately half of the 882 patients enrolled received concomitant micafungin and cyclosporine. No elevations in cyclosporine levels were seen. Similarly, no increases in liver function tests occurred, including AST, ALT, and bilirubin over time, which included baseline assessments, evaluation at week 1, 2, 3, and 4, as well as end of therapy assessments. These data have been confirmed in a formal PK study where healthy volunteers received a single dose of cyclosporine (5 mg/kg) on study days 1, 5, and 9, and a single infusion of micafungin on days 11–15. PK data demonstrated no significant interaction effects of single or multiple doses of micafungin on cyclosporine, and similarly no PK interaction effect of single dose cyclosporine on micafungin (167). Based on these data, micafungin would be the preferred echinocandin in patients requiring concomitant cyclosporine, once final FDA approval is granted. The effect of micafungin on the PK of tacrolimus, and the effects of tacrolimus on the PK of micafungin have also been evaluated in healthy volunteers. A similar result was seen with no drug–drug interaction effects on single-dose tacrolimus PK, and single dose tacrolimus exposure did not alter the PK of micafungin (168).

3.   Anidulafungin (LY303366, V-echinocandin, VER-002)

Anidulafungin is an experimental echinocandin being evaluated for its activity against *Candida* and *Aspergillus* spp., infections. Because of the investigational nature of the drug, there is limited information on drug interactions. In preclinical murine models, coadminisration of anidulafungin with glucocorticoids resulted in lethal toxicity. Deaths occurred in the DBA/2 mice treated with cortisone acetate prior to intranasal innoculation with *Aspergillus,* as well as the mice treated as above but with anidulafungin. Studies were also conducted with other corticosteroids, including hydrocortisone and triamcinolone, with similar outcomes. The use of dexamethasone did not result in the death of any mice. The rationale for the lethal effects of anidulafungin and corticosteroids remains unknown (169).

The effect of cyclosporine on the PK profile of anidulafungin has been evaluated. Healthy volunteers were administered anidulafungin 200 mg IV on day 1, followed by 100 mg/day on days 2–8. Oral cyclosporine solution was administered on days 5–8, at a dose of 1.25 mg/kg twice a day. The PK profile of cyclosporine A was characterized on day 4 (absence of cyclosporine) and on day 8 (presence of anidulafungin). The changes in the C_{max} and AUC of anidulafungin, both in the presence and absence of cyclosporine, were clinically insignificant (170). To assess the effect of anidulafungin on cyclosporine metabolism, a small in vitro study assessed different doses of anidulafungin in combination with cyclosporine in human hepatic protein in vitro. This study concluded that anidulafungin at concentrations of up to 30 µg/mL does not affect the in vitro metabolism of cyclosporine (171). Further clinical data is necessary before conclusive recommendations can be made.

D.   Miscellaneous

1.   Terbinafine

Terbinafine, an allylamine derivative, is structurally unrelated to other available antifungal agents. It is a potent competitive inhibitor of CYP2D6, but at least six other CYP450 enzymes are involved in its metabolism, including CYP1A2, CYP2C9, and CYP3A4 (172). Terbinafine is weakly bound to hepatic cytochromes with its metabolism involving only 5% of the metabolizing capacity of hepatic CYP450 enzymes (173). In recent years, attention has been paid to the inhibition of CYP2D6, the isoenzyme system responsible for the metabolism of a wide variety of medications including anti depressants, neuroleptics, antihypertensives, opioids, and antiarrhythmics (174). When prescribing warfarin (175), theophylline, nortriptyline (176), desipramine (177), cimetidine, or rifampin concomitantly with terbinafine, the prescriber must consider the potential for toxicity or lack of effect to occur. Unlike the azole antifungal agents, terbinafine can be coadministered with cyclosporine without any significant changes in cyclosporine concentrations (178).

2. 5-Flucytosine (5-FC)

5-Flucytosine, first synthesized in 1957, is an antimetabolite antifungal agent whose spectrum of activity includes *Candida* spp., and *Cryptococcus neoformans.* 5-FC is not subject to the same interactions as the azoles and interacts with relatively few agents. When administered with cytosine arabinoside, there is a reduction in its anti-mycotic activity, most likely due to competitive inhibition. Inhibition is thought to result from 5-FC being taken up by susceptible cells by the same transport system as cytarabine (179), Administration of 5-FC in close proximity to antacids containing aluminum hydroxide or magnesium hydroxide results in delayed absorption, although this is clinically insignificant.

Pharmacodynamically, there is a concern that 5-FC may enhance the marrow suppressive effects of other medications that are marrow suppressive. As a consequence, caution should be exercised when prescribing this agents with medications such as zidovudine, ganciclovir, etc.

3. Griseofulvin

Griseofulvin is primarily restricted to the treatment of topical fungal infections. There are a couple of noteworthy drug interactions that occur, and patients should be monitored closely when concomitantly prescribing warfarin, oral contraceptives, and phenobarbital. Concomitant administration of griseofulvin and warfarin leads to a diminished anticoagulant effect (180–182). Repeated administration of griseofulvin induces the enzymes that metabolize warfarin, whereas a single dose of griseofulvin has been reported to increase the international normalized ratio and increase serum warfarin concentration (183). With prolonged treatment, the dose of warfarin required for therapeutic anticoagulation is likely to increase, and similarly, close monitoring of the INR on withdrawal of griseofulvin should occur.

The other notable drug interaction is between griseofulvin and oral contraceptive medications (184). Griseofulvin induces the metabolism of estrogens, both endogenous and exogenous, thus, leading to loss of oral contraceptive efficacy. Patients should be informed of the interaction and counseled to use alternative contraceptive measures while receiving griseofulvin.

Finally, griseofulvin has been shown to have its concentrations affected by phenobarbital. Whether this occurs by decreased absorption, or by enzyme induction is not clear, but concomitant griseofulvin and phenobarbital leads to a reduction in griseofulvin concentrations and may lead to antifungal failure.

E. Antifungal Combinations

The recent approval of caspofungin, an echinocandin whose target is β 1,3 glucan, and voriconazole, a second-generation triazole with an extended spectrum of action, has encouraged the infectious disease community caring for immunocompromised patients to assess the efficacy of combination antifungal therapy. This approach is similar to that of antineoplastic therapy, where using two drugs with different mechanisms of action to improve outcomes. Historically, this has not been possible mostly due to the limited antifungal armamenatrium. Up until 2001, we only had the polyenes, first-generation azoles, terbinafine, and flucytosine available. Many institutions used combinations of itraconazole and amphotericin B in patients with *Aspergillus* infections who were not responding to monotherapy. The fear with this approach was that there could be antagonism between the drugs based on their mechanisms of action, leading to a worse outcome (see azole section in this chapter). In a candidiasis model, this has not occurred (14). Whether this is an agent specific interaction requires clarification. With the availability of new classes of antifungal agents, there seems little reason to pursue the azoles in combination with a polyene with this controversy, and combinations of azoles and echinocandins, or polyenes and echinocandins make greater theoretical sense.

Researchers involved in mycology and the treatment of high-risk patients with invasive fungal infections are now evaluating several antifungal combinations for synergy, indifference, and antagonism both in vitro and in animal models (185–194). The clinical relevance of these combinations remains untested in large prospective randomized trials, although observational data in limited patients does exist (195,196). Hopefully, the most promising laboratory combination identified will be pursued in a large clinical trial to definitively conclude that this is an effective strategy. At least from a pharmacokinetic standpoint, there does not appear to be any interaction, and preliminary "observational" clinical data do not suggest any negative effects.

III. CONCLUSION

Drug interactions are common among critical care, HIV, and transplant patients due to the large number of medications and the complexity of prescribed regimens. It is important that the medical teams caring for these populations are aware of the potential for drug interactions, and screen all new medications against a full history to attempt the decrease of the probability of interaction occurring. With the availability of new medications each year, it is clear that we must ensure and understand the metabolic routes of these drugs, and in the absence of any substantive data, make out "best guess" as to the possibility of a potential drug interaction. Knowledge of the dominant CYPs involved in the metabolism of a drug makes it possible to anticipate from a list of inducers and inhibitors which drugs might cause significant interactions.

REFERENCES

1. Venkatakrishnan K, von Moltke LL, Greenblatt DJ. Effects of the antifungal agents on oxidative drug metabolism clinical relevance. Clin Pharmacokinet 2000; 38:111–180.
2. Flockhart DA. Cytochrome P450 drug interaction table (online). Available from URL: http://medicine.iupui.edu/flockhart/ [accessed August 14, 2003].
3. Watkins PB. Role of cytochromes P450 in drug metabolism and hepatotoxicity. Semin Liver Dis 1990; 10:235–250.
4. Pea F, Farlanut M. Pharmacokinetic aspects of treating infections in the intensive care unit: focus on drug interactions. Clin Pharmacokinet 2001; 40:833–868.
5. Lewis RE, Prince RA, Chi J, Kontoyiannis DP. Itraconazole pre-exposure attenuates the efficacy of subsequent amphotericin B therapy in a murine model of acute invasive pulmonary aspergillosis. Antimicrob Agents Chemother 2003; 46:3208–3214.
6. Lewis RE, Klepser ME, Pfaller MA. Combination systemic antifungal therapy for cryptococcosis, candidiasis, and aspergillosis. J Infect Dis Pharmacother 1999; 3:61–83.
7. Sugar AM. Use of amphotericin B with azole antifungal drugs: what are we doing? Antimicrob Agents Chemother 1995; 39:1907–1912

8. Sanati H, Ramos CF, Bayer AS, Ghannoum MA. Combination therapy with amphotericin B and fluconazole against invasive candidiasis in neutropenic-mouse and infective-endocarditis rabbit models. Antimicrob Agents Chemother 1997; 41:1345–1348.

9. Schacter LP, Owellen RJ, Rathbun HK, Buchanan B. Antagonism between miconazole and amphotericin B. Lancet 1976; 2:318.

10. Schaffner A, Bohler A. Amphotericin B refractory aspergillosis after itraconazole: evidence for significant antagonism. Mycoses 1993; 36:421–424.

11. Scheven M, Scheven ML. Interaction between azoles and amphotericin B in the treatment of candidiasis. Clin Infect Dis 1995; 20:1079.

12. Scheven M, Schwegler F. Antagonistic interactions between azoles and amphotericin B with yeast depend on azole lipophilia for special test conditions in vitro. Antimicrob Agents Chemother 1995; 39:1779–1783.

13. Van Etten EW, Van De Rhee NE, Van Kampen KM, et al. Effects of amphotericin B and fluconazole on the extracellular and intracellular growth of *Candida albicans*. Antimicrob Agents Chemother 1991; 35:2275–2281.

14. Rex JH, Pappas PG, Karchmer AW, Sobel J, Edwards JE, Hadley S, Brass C, Vazquez JA, Chapman SW, Horowitz HW, Zervos M, McKinsey D, Lee J, Babinchak T, Bradshewr RW, Cleary JD, Cohen DM, Danzingert L, Goldman M, Goodman J, Hilton E, Hyslop NE, Kett DH, Lutz J, Rubin RH, Scheld M, Schuster M, Simmons B, Stein DK, Washburn RG, Mautner L, Chu T-C, Panzer H, Rosenstein RB, Booth J for the National Institute of Allergy and Infectious Diseases Mycoses Study Group. A randomized and blinded multicenter trial of high-dose fluconazole plus placebo versus fluconazole plus amphotericin B as therapy for Candidemia and its consequences in nonneutropenic subjects. Clin Infect Dis 2003; 36:1221–1228.

15. Ferguson RM, Sutherland DE, Simmons RL, Najarian JS. Ketoconazole, cyclosporin metabolism, and renal transplantation. Lancet 1982; 2(8304):882–883.

16. Abraham MA, Thomas PP, John GT, Job V, Shankar V, Jacob CK. Efficacy and safety of low-dose ketoconazole (50 mg) to reduce the cost of cyclosporine in renal allograft recipients. Transplant Proc 2003; 35:215–216.

17. Sobh MA, Hamdy AF, El Agroudy AE, El Sayed K, El-Diasty T, Bakr MA, Ghoneim MA. Coadministration of ketoconazole and cyclosporine for kidney transplant recipients: long-term follow-up and study of metabolic consequences. Am J Kidney Dis 2001; 37: 510–517.

18. Keogh A, Spratt P, McCosker C, Macdonald P, Mundy J, Kaan A. Ketoconazole to reduce the need for cyclosporine after cardiac transplantation. N Engl J Med 1995; 333:628–633.

19. Soltero L, Carbajal H, Rodriguez-Montalvo C, Valdes A. Soltero L, Carbajal H, Rodriguez-Montalvo C, Valdes A. Coadministration of tacrolimus and ketoconazole in renal transplant recipients: cost analysis and review of metabolic effects. Transplant Proc 2003; 35:1319–1321.

20. Moreno M, Latorre A, Manzanares C, Morales E, Herrero JC, Dominguez-Gil B, Carreno A, Cubas A, Delgado M, Andres A, Morales JM. Clinical management of tacrolimus drug interactions in renal transplant patients. Transplant Proc 1999; 31: 2252–2253.

21. Pfizer Pharmaceuticals. Tikosyn (dofetilide) Package Insert. New York, NY, 1999.

22. Janssen Pharmaceutica. Nizoral (ketoconazole) Package Insert. Titusville, NJ, 1998.

23. Van Giersbergen PL, Halabi A, Dingemanse J. Single- and multiple-dose pharmacokinetics of bosentan and its interaction with ketoconazole. Br J Clin Pharmacol 2002; 53:589–595.

24. First MR, Schroeder TJ, Weiskittel P, Myre SA, Alexander JW, Pesce AJ. Concomitant administration of cyclosporin and ketoconazole in renal transplant recipients. Lancet 1989; 2:1198–1201.

25. Kehrer DF, Mathijssen RH, Verweij J, de Bruijn P, Sparreboom A. Modulation of irinotecan metabolism by ketoconazole. J Clin Oncol 2002; 20:3122–3129.

26. Itakura H, Vaughn D, Haller DG, O'Dwyer PJ. Rhabdomyolysis from cytochrome p-450 interaction of ketoconazole and simvastatin in prostate cancer. Urolosy 2003; 169:613.

27. Roxane Laboratories. Viramune (nevirapine) Package Insert. Columbus, OH, 2003.

28. GlaxoWellcome. Agenerase (amprenavir) Package Insert. Research Triangle Park, NC, 1999.

29. Merck and Co, Inc. Crixivan (indinavir) Package Insert. West Point, PA, 2003.

30. Abbott Laboratories. Kaletra (lopinavir/ritonavir) Package Insert. Abbott Park, IL, 2000.

31. Agouron Pharmaceuticals. Viracept (nelfinavir) Package Insert. La Jolla, CA, 2002.

32. Abbott Laboratories. Norvir (ritonavir) Package Insert. Abbott Park, IL, 2001.

33. Grub S, Bryson H, Goggin T, Ludin E, Jorga K. The interaction of saquinavir (soft gelatin capsule) with ketoconazole, erythromycin and rifampicin: comparison of the effect in healthy volunteers and in HIV-infected patients. Eur J Clin Pharmacol 2001; 57:115–121.

34. Shi J, Montay G, Leroy B, Bhargava V. Effects of ketoconazole and itraconazole on the pharmacokinetics of telithromycin, a new ketolide antibiotic. In: Program and Abstracts of the 42nd Interscience Conference on Antimicrobial Agents and Chemotherapy. [abst A-1833]. San Diego, California, USA, September 27–30 2002, Washington, DC, American Society of Microbiology, 2002.

35. Smith AG. Potentiation of oral anticoagulants by ketoconazole. Br Med J 1984; 288:188–189.

36. Havir DV, Dube MP, McCutchan JA, Forthal DN, Kemper CA, Dunne MW, Parenti DM, Kumar PN, White AC, Witt MD, Nightingale SD, Sepkowitz KA, MacGregor RR, Cheeseman SH, Torriani FJ, Zelasky MT, Sattler FR, Bozzette SA. Prophylaxis with weekly versus daily fluconazole for fungal infections in patients with AIDS. Clin Infect Dis 1998; 27:1369–1375.

37. MacMillan ML, Goodman JL, DeFor TE, Weisdorf DJ. Fluconazole to prevent yeast infections in bone marrow transplantation patients: a randomized trial of high versus reduced dose, and determination of the value of maintenance therapy. Am J Med 2002; 11:369–379.

38. Chariyalertsak S, Supparatpinyo K, Sirisanthana T, Nelson KE. A controlled trial of itraconazole as primary prophylaxis for systemic fungal infections in patients with advanced human immunodeficiency virus infection in Thailand. Clin Infect Dis 2002; 34:277–284.

39. Kaufman D, Boyle R, Hazen K, Patrie JT, Robinson M, Donowitz LG. Fluconazole prophylaxis against fungal colonization and infection in preterm infants. N Engl J Med 2001; 345:1660–1666.

40. Garbino J, Lew DP, Romand JA, Hugonnet S, Auckenthaler R, Pittet D. Prevention of severe Candida infections in non-neutropenic, high-risk, critically ill patients: a randomized, double-blind, placebo-controlled trial in patients treated by selective digestive contamination. Intensive Care Med 2002; 28:1708–1717.

41. Pelz RK, Hendrix CW, Swoboda SM, Diener-West M, Merz WG, Hammond J, Lipsett PA. Double-blind placebo-controlled trial of fluconazole to prevent candidal infections in critically ill surgical patients. Ann Surg 2001; 233:542–548.

42. Winston DJ, Busuttil RW. Randomized controlled trial of oral itraconazole solution versus intravenous/oral fluconazole for prevention of fungal infections in liver transplant recipients. Transplantation 2002; 74:688–695.

43. Dykewicz CA, Jaffe HW, Kaplan JE, in collaboration with The Guidelines Working Group Members from the CDC, the Infectious Diseases Society of America, and the American Society of Blood and Marrow Transplantation. Guidelines for preventing opportunistic infections among hematopoietic stem cell transplant recipients. Biol Blood Marrow Transplant 2000; 6:659–737.

44. Marr KA, Seidel K, Slavin MA, Bowden RA, Schoch HG, Flowers ME, Corey L, Boeckh M. Prolonged fluconazole prophylaxis is associated with persistent protection against candidiasis-related death in allogeneic marrow transplant recipients: long-term follow-up of a randomized, placebo- controlled trial. Blood 2000; 96:2055–2061.

45. Slavin MA, Osborne B, Adams R, Levenstein MJ, Feldman AR, Myers JD, Bowden RA. Efficacy and safety of fluconazole prophylaxis for fungal infections after marrow transplantation—a prospective, randomized, double-blind study. J Infect Dis 1995; 171: 1545–1552.

46. Vanier KL, Mattiussi AJ, Johnston DL. Interaction of all-trans-retinoic acid with fluconazole in acute promyelocytic leukemia. J Pediatr Hematol Oncol 2003; 25: 403–404.

47. Schwartz EL, Hallam S, Gallagher RE, Wiernik PH. Inhibition of all-trans-retinoic acid metabolism by fluconazole in vitro and in patients with acute promyelocytic leukemia. Biochem Pharmacol 1995; 50:923–928.

48. Pfizer. Diflucan (fluconazole) Package Insert. New York, NY, 1998.

49. Ahonen J, Olkkola KT, Takala A, Neuvonen PJ. Interaction between fluconazole and midazolam in intensive care patients. Acta Anaesthesiol Scand 1999; 43:509–514.

50. Olkkola KT, Ahonen J, Neuvonen PJ, The effects of the systemic antimycotics, itraconazole and fluconazole, on the pharmacokinetics and pharmacodynamics of intravenous and oral midazolam. Anesth Analg 1996; 82:511–516.

51. Varhe A, Olkkola KT, Neuvonen PJ. Effect of fluconazole dose on the extent of fluconazole- triazolam interaction. Br J Clin Pharmacol 1996; 42:465–470.

52. Osowski CL, Dix SP, Lin L, Mullins RE, Geller RB, Wingard JR. Evaluation of the drug interaction between high dose fluconazole and cyclosporine or tacrolimus in bone marrow transplant patients. Transplantation 1996; 61:1268–1272.

53. Manez R, Martin M, Raman D, Silverman D, Jain A, Warty V, Gonzalez-Pintol, Kusne S, Starzl TE. Fluconazole therapy in transplant recipients receiving FK506. Transplantation 1994; 57:1521–1523.

54. Toda F, Tanabe K, Ito S, Shinmura H, Tokumoto T, Ishida H, Toma H. Tacrolimus trough level adjustment after administration of fluconazole to kidney recipients. Transplant Proc 2002; 34:1733–1735.

55. Hebert MF, Fisher RM, Marsh CL, Dressler D, Bekersky I. Effects of rifampin on tacrolimus pharmacokinetics in healthy volunteers. J Clin Pharmacol 1999; 339:91–96.

56. Chenhsu RY, Loong CC, Chou MH, Lin MF, Yang WC. Renal allograft dysfunction associated with rifampin–tacrolimus interaction. Ann Pharmacother 2000; 34:27–31.

57. Furlan V, Perello L, Jacquemin E, Debray D, Taburet AM. Interaction between FK506 and rifampicin or erythromycin in pediatric liver recipients. Transplantation 1995; 59:1217–1218.

58. Bolley R, Zulke C, Kammerl M, Fischereder M, Kramer BK. Tacrolimus-induced nephrotoxicity unmasked by induction of the CYP3A4 system with St John's wort. Transplantation 2002; 73:1009–1010.

59. Boubenider S, Vincent I, Lambotte O, Roy S, Hiesse C, Taburet AM, Charpentier B. Interaction between theophylline and tacrolimus in a renal transplant patient. Nephrol Dial Transplant 2000; 15:1066–1068.

60. Collignon P, Hurley B, Mitchell D. Interaction of fluconazole with cyclosporin. Lancet 1989; 1:1262.

61. Tett S, Carey D, Lee HS. Drug interactions with fluconazole. Med J Aust 1992; 156:365.

62. Sugar AM, Saunders C, Idelson BA, Bernard DB. Interaction of fluconazole and cyclosporine. Ann Intern Med 1989; 110:844.

63. Graves NM, Matas AJ, Hilligoss DM, et al. Fluconazole/cyclosporine interaction. Clin Pharmacol Ther 1990; 47:208.

64. Ehninger G, Jaschonek K, Schuler U, Kruger HU. Interaction of fluconazole with cyclosporin. Lancet 1989; 2:104–105.

65. Lucey MR, Kolars JC, Merion RM, Campbell DA, Aldrich M, Watkins PB. Cyclosporin toxicity at therapeutic blood levels and cytochrome P-450 IIIA. Lancet 1990; 335:11–15.
66. Lopez-Gill JA. Fluconazole–cylosporine interaction: a dose-dependent effect? Ann Pharmacother 1993; 27:427–430
67. Canafax DM, Graves NM, Hilligoss DM, Carleton BC, Gardner MJ, Matas AJ. Interaction between cyclosporin and fluconazole in renal allograft recipients. Transplantation 1991; 51:1014–1018.
68. Kruger HU, Schuler U, Zimmermann R, Ehninger G. Absence of significant interaction of fluconazole with cyclosporin. J Antimicrob Chemother 1989; 24:781–786.
69. Cervelli MJ. Fluconazole–sirolimus drug interaction. Transplantation 2002; 74:1477–1478.
70. Finch CK, Green CA, Self TH. Fluconazole–carbamazepine interaction. South Med J 2002; 95:1099–1100.
71. Nair DR, Morris HH. Potential fluconazole-induced carbamazepine toxicity. Ann Pharmacother 1999; 33:790–792.
72. Haukat A, Benekli M, Vladutiu GD, Slack JL, Wetzler M, Baer MR. Simvastatin–fluconazole causing rhabdomyolysis. Ann Pharmacother 2003; 37:1032–1035.
73. Palkama VJ, Isohanni MH, Neuvonen PJ, Olkkola KT. The effect of intravenous and oral fluconazole on the pharmacokinetics and pharmacodynamics of intravenous alfentanil. Anesth Analg. 1998; 87:190–194.
74. Blum RA, Wilton JH, Hilligoss DM, Gardner MJ, Henry EB, Harrison NJ, Schentag JJ. Effect of fluconazole on the disposition of phenytoin. Clin Pharmacol Ther 1991; 49:420–425.
75. Cadle RM, Zenon GJ, Rodriguez-Barradas MC, et al. Fluconazole-induced symptomatic phenytoin toxicity. Ann Pharmacother 1994; 28:191–195.
76. Mitchell AS, Holland JT. Fluconazole and phenytoin: a predictable interaction. BMJ 1989; 298:1315.
77. Howitt KM, Oziemski MA. Phenytoin toxicity induced by fluconazole. Med J Aust 1989; 151:603–604.
78. Trapnell CB, Narang PK, Li R, Lavelle JP. Increased plasma rifabutin levels with concomitant fluconazole therapy in HIV-infected patients. Ann Intern Med 1996; 124:573–576.
79. Nicolau DP, Crowe HM, Nightingale CH, et al. Rifampin-fluconazole interaction in critically ill patients. Ann Pharmacother 1995; 29:994–996.
80. Apseloff G, Hilligoss DM, Gardner MJ, et al. Induction of fluconazole metabolism by rifampin: in vivo study in humans. J Clin Pharmacol 1991; 31:358–361.
81. Niemi M, Backman JT, Neuvonen M, et al. Effects of fluconazole and fluvoxamine on the pharmacokinetics and pharmacodynamics of glimepiride. Clin Pharmacol Ther 2001; 69:194–200.
82. Mootha VV, Schluter ML, Das A. Intraocular hemorrhages due to warfarin fluconazole drug interaction in a patient with presumed Candida endophthalmitis. Arch Ophthalmol 2002; 120:94–95.
83. Black DJ, Kunze KL, Wienkers LC, Gidal BE, Seaton TL, McDonnell ND, Evans JS, Bauwens JE, Trager WF. Warfarin-fluconazole. II. A metabolically based drug interaction: in vivo studies. . Drug Metab Dispos 1996; 24:422–428.
84. Crussell-Porter LL, Rindone JP, Ford MA, Jaskar DW. Low-dose fluconazole therapy potentiates the hypoprothrombinemic response of warfarin sodium. Arch Intern Med 1993; 153:102–104.
85. Back DJ, Tjia JF. Comparative effects of the antimycotic drugs ketoconazole, fluconazole, itraconazole and terbinafine on the metabolism of cyclosporin by human liver microsomes. Br J Clin Pharmacol 1991; 32:624–626.
86. Baciewicz AM, Menke JJ, Bokar JA, Baud EB. Fluconazole–warfarin interaction. Ann Pharmacother 1994; 28:1111.

87. Gericke KR. Possible interaction between warfarin and fluconazole. Pharmacotherapy 1993; 13:508–509.
88. Slaughter RL, Edwards DJ. Recent advances: the cytochrome P450 enzymes. Ann Pharmacother 1995; 29:619–624.
89. Winston DJ, Maziarz RT, Chandrasekar PH, et al. Long-term antifungal prophylaxis in allogeneic bone marrow transplant patients: a multicenter, randomized trial of intravenous/oral itraconazole versus intravenous/oral fluconazole. [abstr 2002]. Blood 2001; 98:489a.
90. Nucci M, Biasoli I, Akiti T, Silveira F, Solza C, Barrieros G, Spector N, Derossi A, Pulcheri W. A double-blind, randomized, placebo-controlled trial of itraconazole capsules as antifungal prophylaxis for neutropenic patients. Clin Infect Dis 2000; 30: 300–305.
91. Boogaerts M, Winston DJ, Bow EJ, Garber G, Reboli AC, Schwarer AP, Novitsky N, Boehme A, Chwetzoff E, De Buele K for the Itraconazole Neutropenia Study Group. Intravenous and oral itraconazole versus intravenous amphotericin B deoxycholate as empirical antifungal therapy for persistent fever in neutropenic patients with cancer who are receiving broad-spectrum antibacterial therapy. A randomized, controlled trial. Ann Intern Med 2001; 135:412–422.
92. Denning DW, Lee JY, Hostetler JS, Pappas P, Kauffman CA, Dewsnup DH, Galgiani JK Graybill JR, Sugar AM. NIAID Mycoses Study Group Multicenter Trial of oral itraconazole therapy for invasive aspergillosis. Am J Med 1994; 97:135–144.
93. Denning DW, Tucker RM, Hanson LH, Stevens DA. Treatment of invasive aspergilliosis with itraconazole. Am J Med 1989; 86:791–800.
94. Stevens DA, Lee JY. Analysis of compassionate use itraconazole therapy for invasive aspergillosis by the NIAID mycoses study group criteria. Arch Intern Med 1997; 157:1857–1862.
95. Yeh J, Soo SC, Summerton C, Richardson C. Potentiation of action of warfarin by itraconazole. BMJ 1990; 301:669.
96. Crane JK, Shih HT. Syncope and cardiac arrhythmia due to an interaction between itraconazole and terfenadine. Am J Med 1993; 95:445–446.
97. Pohjola-Sintonen S, Viitasalo M, Toivonene L, Neuvonen P. Torsades de pointes after terfenadine–itraconazole interaction. BMJ 1993; 306:186.
98. Kamaluddin M, McNally P, Breatnach F, O'Marcaig A, Webb D, O'Dell E, Scanlon P, Butler K, O'Meara A. Potentiation of vincristine toxicity by itraconazole in children with lymphoid malignancies. Aeta Paediatr 2001; 90:1204–1207.
99. Jeng MR, Feusner J. Itraconazole-enhanced vincristine neurotoxicity in a child with acute lymphoblastic leukemia. Pediatr Hematol Oncol 2001; 18:137–142.
100. Sathiapalan RK, El-Solh H. Enhanced vincristine neurotoxicity from drug interactions: case report and review of the literature. Pediatr Hematol Oncol 2001; 18:543–546.
101. Bohme A, Ganser A, Hoelzer D. Aggravation of vincristine-induced neurotoxicity by itraconazole in the treatment of adult ALL. Ann Hematol 1995; 71:311–312.
102. Murphy JA, Ross LM, Gibson BE. Vincristine toxicity in five children with acute lymphoblastic leukaemia. Lancet 1995; 346:443.
103. Olkkola KT, Backman JT, Neuvonen PJ. Midazolam should be avoided in patients receiving systemic antimycotics ketoconazole or itraconazole. Clin Pharmacol Ther 1994; 55:481–485.
104. Varhe A, Olkkola KT, Neuvonen PJ. Oral triazolam is potentially hazardous to patients receiving systemic antimycotics ketoconazole or itraconazole. Clin Pharmacol Ther 1994; 56:601–607.
105. Jalalava KM, Olkkola KT, Neuvonen PJ. Itraconazole greatly increases plasma concentrations and effects of felodipine. Clin Pharmacol Ther 1997; 61:410–415.
106. Tucker RM, Denning DW, Hanson LH, et al. Interaction of azoles with rifampin, phenytoin, and carbamazepine: in vitro and clinical observations. Clin Infect Dis 1992; 14:165–174.

107. Bonay M, Jonville-Bera AP, Diot P, et al. Possible interaction between phenobarbital, carbamazepine and itraconazole. Drug Saf 1993; 9:309–311.

108. Alderman CP, Allcroft PD. Digoxin–itraconazole interaction: possible mechanisms. Ann Pharmacother 1997; 31:438–440.

109. Sachs MK, Blanchard LM, Green PJ. Interaction of itraconazole and digoxin. Clin Infect Dis 1993; 16:400–403.

110. Rex J. Itraconazole–digoxin interaction. Ann Intern Med 1992; 116:525.

111. Kauffman CA, Bagnasco FA. Digoxin toxicity associated with itraconazole therapy. Clin Infect Dis 1992; 15:886–887.

112. Neuvonen PJ, Jalava KM. Itraconazole drastically increases plasma concentrations of lovastatin and lovastatin acid. Clin Pharmacol Ther 1996; 60:54–61.

113. Kantola T, Kivisto KT, Neuvonen PJ. Effect of itraconazole on the pharmacokinetics of atorvastatin. Clin Pharmacol Ther 1998; 64:58–65.

114. Neuvonen PJ, Kantola T, Kivisto KJ. Simvastatin but not pravastatin is very susceptible to interactions with the CYP3A4 inhibitor itraconazole. Clin Pharmacol Ther 1998; 63:332–341.

115. Vlahakos DV, Manginas A, Chilidou D, Zamanika C, Alivizatos PA. Itraconazole-induced rhabdomyolysis and acute renal failure in a heart transplant recipient treated with simvastatin and cyclosporine. Transplantation 2002; 73:1962–1964.

116. Ducharme MP, Slaughter RL, Warbasse LH, Chandrasekar PH, Van de Velde V, Mannens G, Edwards DJ. Itraconazole and hydroxyitraconazole serum concentrations are reduced more than tenfold by phenytoin. Clin Pharmacol Ther 1995; 58:617–624.

117. Jaruratanasirikul S, Sriwiriyajan S. Effect of rifampicin on the pharmacokinetics of itraconazole in normal volunteers and AIDS patients. Eur J Clin Pharmacol 1998; 54:155–158.

118. Drayton J, Dickinson G, Rinaldi MG. Coadministration of rifampin and itraconazole leads to undetectable levels of serum itraconazole. Clin Infect Dis 1994; 18:266–267.

119. Smith JA, Hardin TC, Patterson TF, et al. Rifabutin decreases itraconazole plasma levels in patients with HIV-infection [abstr]. 2nd National Conference on Human Retro viruses and Related Infections, Washington DC, January 1995.

120. Glasmacher A, Hahn C, Molitor E, et al. Definition of an itraconazole target concentration for antifungal prophylaxis. Program and Abstracts of the 40th Interscience Conference on Antimicrobial Agents and Chemotherapy. [abstr 700]. Toronto, Ont September 17–20, 2000, Washington, DC: American Society of Microbiology, 2000.

121. Ortho Biotech, Inc. Sporanox (itraconazole) Package Insert. Raritan, NJ, 2002.

122. Leather HL, Wingard JR. Characterizing the pharmacokinetic (PK) drug interaction between intravenous (IV) itraconazole (ITRA) and IV tacrolimus (FK506) or IV cyclosporine (CyA) in allogeneic bone marrow transplant (alloBMT) patients. Program and Abstracts of the 41st Interscience Conference on Antimicrobial Agents and Chemotherapy. Chicago, IL, 16–19.

123. Kramer MR, Marshall SE, Denning DW, Keogh AM, Tucker RM, Galgiani JN, Lewiston NJ, Stevens DA, Theodore J. Cyclosporine and itraconazole interaction in heart and lung transplant recipients. Ann Intern Med 1990; 113:327–329.

124. Kwan JT, Foxall PJ, Davidson DG, Bending MR, Eisinger AJ. Interaction of cyclosporin and itraconazole. Lancet 1987; 2:282.

125. Banerjee R, Leaver N, Lyster H, Banner NR. Coadministration of itraconazole and tacrolimus after thoracic organ transplantation. Transplant Proc 2001; 33:1600–1602.

126. Billaud EM, Guillemain R, Tacco F, Chevalier P. Evidence for a pharmacokinetic interaction between itraconazoie and tacrolimus in organ transplant patients. Br J Clin Pharmacol 1998; 46:271–272.

127. Capone D, Gentile A, Imperatore P, Palmiero G, Basile V. Effects of itraconazole on tacrolimus blood concentrations in a renal transplant recipient. Ann Pharmacother 1999; 33:1124–1125.

128. Furlan V, Parquin F, Penaud JF, Cerrina J, Ladurie FL, Dartevelle P, Taburet AM. Interaction between tacrolimus and itraconazole in a heart–lung transplant recipient. Transplant Proc 1998; 30:187–188.

129. Outeda Macias M, Salvador P, Hurtado JL, Martin I. Tacrolimus–itraconazole interaction in a kidney transplant patient. Ann Pharmacother 2000; 34:536.

130. Varis T, Kivisto KT, Backman JT, Neuvonen PJ. Itraconazole decreases the clearance and enhances the effects of intravenously administered methylprednisolone in healthy volunteers. Pharmacol Toxicol 1999; 85:29–32.

131. Skov M, Main KM, Sillesen IB, Muller J, Kock C, Lanng S. Iatrogenic adrenal insufficiency as a side-effect of combined treatment of itraconazole and budesonide. Eur Respir J 2002; 20:127–133.

132. Raaska K, Niemi M, Neuvonen M, Neuvonen PJ, Kivisto KT. Plasma concentrations of inhaled budesonide and its effects on plasma cortisol are increased by the cytochrome P4503A4 inhibitor itraconazole. Clin Pharmacol Ther 2002; 72:362–369.

133. Mercadante S, Villari P, Ferrera P. Itraconazole–fentanyl interactions in a cancer patient. Pain Symptom Manage 2002; 24:284–286.

134. Bertz R, Hsu A, Lam W, et al. Pharmacokinetic interactions between Kaletra. (lopinavir/ritonavir or ABT- 378/r) and other non-HIV drugs [poster no. 438]. 5th International Congress on Drug Therapy in HIV Infection, Glasgow, Oct 22–26, 2000.

135. Yule SM, Walker D, Cole M, McSorley L, Cholerton S, Daly AK, Pearson AD, Boddy AV. The effect of fluconazole on cyclophosphamide metabolism in children. Drug Metab Dispos 1999; 27:417–421.

136. Buggia I, Zecca M, Alessandrino EP, Locatelli F, Rosti G, Bosi A, Pession A, Rotoli B, Majolino I, Dallorso A, Regazzi MB. Itraconazole can increase systemic exposure to busulfan in patients given bone marrow transplantation. GITMO (Gruppo Italiano Trapianto di Midollo Osseo). Anticancer Res 1996; 16:2083–2088.

137. Pfizer. Vfend (vorinconazole) Package Insert. New York, NY, 2003.

138. Ghahramani P, Purkins L, Kleinermans D, et al. The pharmacokinetics of voriconazole and its effect on prednisolone disposition. Program and Abstracts of the 40th Interscience Conference on Antimicrobial Agents and Chemotherapy [abstr 842]. Toronto, Ont September 17–20 2000, Washington, DC: American Society of Microbiology, 2000.

139. Ghahramani P, Purkins L, Kleinermans D, et al. Effects of rifampicin and rifabutin on the pharmacokinetics of voriconazole. Program and Abstracts of the 40th Interscience Conference on Antimicrobial Agents and Chemotherapy [abstr 844]. Toronto, Ont September 17–20 2000, Washington, DC: American Society of Microbiology, 2000.

140. Ghahramani P, Purkins L, Kleinermans D, et al. Voriconazole potentiates warfarin-induced prolongation of prothrombin time. Program and Abstracts of the 40th Interscience Conference on Antimicrobial Agents and Chemotherapy [abstr 846]. Toronto, Ont September 17–20 2000, Washington, DC: American Society of Microbiology, 2000.

141. Ghahramani P, Purkins L, Kleinermans DJ, et al. Effect of omeprazole on the pharmacokinetics of voriconazole. Program and Abstracts of the 40th Interscience Conference on Antimicrobial Agents and Chemotherapy [abstr 843]. Toronto, Ont September 17–20 2000, Washington, DC: American Society of Microbiology, 2000.

142. Wood N, Tan K, Allan R, et al. Effect of voriconazole on the pharmacokinetics of omeprazole. Program and Abstracts of the 41st Interscience Conference on Antimicrobial Agents and Chemotherapy [abstr A-19]. Chicago, IL, December 16–19 2001, Washington, DC: American Society of Microbiology, 2001.

143. Ghahramani P, Purkins L, Love ER, et al. Drug interactions between voriconazole and phenytoin. Program and Abstracts of the 40th Interscience Conference on Antimicrobial Agents and Chemotherapy [abstr 847]. Toronto, Ont September 17–20 2000, Washington, DC: American Society of Microbiology, 2000.

144. Romero AJ, Pogamp PL, Nilsson LG, Wood N. Effect of voriconazole on the pharmacokinetics of cyclosporine in renal transplant patients. Clin Pharmacol Ther 2002; 71:226–234.

145. Wood N, Tan K, Allan R, et al. Effect of voriconazole on the pharmacokinetics of tacrolimus. Program and Abstracts of the 41st Interscience Conference on Antimicrobial Agents and Chemotherapy [abstr A-20]. Chicago, IL, December 16–19 2001, Washington, DC: American Society of Microbiology, 2001.

146. Pai MP, Allen S. Voriconazole inhibition of tacrolimus metabolism. Clin Infect Dis 2003; 36:1089–1091.

147. Hachem RY, Raad II, Afif CM, et al. An open, non-comparative multicenter study to evaluate efficacy and safety of posaconazole (SCH56592) in the treatment of invasive fungal infections (IFI) refractory (R) or intolerant (I) to standard therapy (ST). Program and Abstracts of the 40th Interscience Conference on Antimicrobial Agents and Chemotherapy [abstr 1109]. Toronto, Ont, Canada, September 17–20 2000, Washington, DC: American Society of Microbiology, 2000.

148. Nieto L, Northland R, Pittisuttithum P, et al. Posaconazole equivalent to fluconazole in the treatment of oropharyngeal candidiasis. Program and Abstracts of the 40th Interscience Conference on Antimicrobial Agents and Chemotherapy [abstr 1109]. Toronto, Ont, Canada, September 17–20 2000, Washington, DC: American Society of Microbiology, 2000.

149. Vasquez JA, Northland R, Miller S, et al. Posaconazole compared to fluconazole for oropharyngeal candidiasis in HIV-positive patients. Program and Abstracts of the 40th Interscience Conference on Antimicrobial Agents and Chemotherapy [abstr 1107]. Toronto, Ont, Canada, September 17–20 2000, Washington, DC: American Society of Microbiology, 2000.

150. Catanzaro A, Cloud G, Stevens D, et al. Safety and tolerability of posaconazole (SCH56592) in patients with nonmeningeal disseminated coccidiomycosis. Program and Abstracts of the 40th Interscience Conference on Antimicrobial Agents and Chemotherapy [abstr 1417]. Toronto, Ont, Canada, September 17–20 2000, Washington, DC: American Society of Microbiology, 2000.

151. Wexler D, Laughlin M, Courtney R, et al. Effects of posaconazole on drug metabolizing enzymes. Program and Abstracts of the 42nd Interscience Conference on Antimicrobial Agents and Chemotherapy [Abstr A-1839]. San Diego, California, USA, September 27–30 2002, Washington, DC: American Society of Microbiology, 2002.

152. Courtney RD, Statkevich P, Laughlin M, Lim J, Clement RP, Batra VK. Effect of posaconazole on the pharmacokinetics of cyclosporine. Program and Abstracts of the 41st Interscience Conference on Antimicrobial Agents and Chemotherapy [abstr A-27]. Chicago, IL, December 16–19 2001. Washington, DC: American Society of Microbiology, 2001.

153. Belle D, Snsone A, Statkevich P, Joseph D, Kantesaria B, Laughlin M, Courtney R. Effect of posaconazole on the pharmacokinetics of tacrolimus in healthy volunteers. Program and Abstracts of the 43rd Interscience Conference on Antimicrobial Agents and Chemotherapy [abstr number pending]. Chicago, Illinois, USA, September 13–17 2000, Washington, DC: American Society of Microbiology, 2003.

154. Courtney R, Wexler D, Statkevich P, Lim J, Batra V, Laughlin M. Effect of cimetidine on the pharmacokinetics of posaconazole in healthy volunteers. Program and Abstracts of the 42nd Interscience Conference on Antimicrobial Agents and Chemotherapy [abstr A-1838]. San Diego, California, USA, September 27–30 2002, Washington, DC: American Society of Microbiology, 2002.

155. Courtney R, Sansone A, Statkevich P, Martinho M, Laughlin M. Assessment of the pharmacokinetic (PK), and pharmacodynamic (PD) interaction potential between posaconazole and glipizide in healthy volunteers. Presented at ***** 2003.

156. Courtney RD, Statkevich P, Laughlin M, Pai S, Lim J, Clement RP, Batra VK. Potential for a drug interaction between posaconazole and phenytoin. Program and Abstracts of the 41st Interscience Conference on Antimicrobial Agents and Chemotherapy [abstr A-28]. Chicago, Illinois, USA, December 16–19 2001, Washington, DC: American Society of Microbiology, 2001.

157. Courtney RD, Statkevich P, Laughlin M, Radwanski E, Lim J, Clement RP, Batra VK. Potential for a drug interaction between posaconazole and rifabutin. Program and Abstracts of the 41st Interscience Conference on Antimicrobial Agents and Chemotherapy [abstr A-29]. Chicago, Illinois, USA, December 16–19 2001, Washington, DC: American Society of Microbiology, 2001.

158. Courtney R, Statkevich P, Lim J, Laughlin M, Batra V. Effect of food and antacid on the pharmacokinetics of posaconazole in healthy volunteers. Program and Abstracts of the 42nd Interscience Conference on Antimicrobial Agents and Chemotherapy [abstr A-1837]. San Diego, California, USA, September 27–30 2002, Washington, DC: American Society of Microbiology, 2002.

159. Mummaneni V, Hadjilambris OW, Nichola P, et al. Ravuconazole does not affect the pharmacokinetics of nelfinavir. Program and Abstracts of the 41st Interscience Conference on Antimicrobial Agents and Chemotherapy [abstr A-25]. Chicago, Illinois, USA, December 16–19 2001, Washington, DC: American Society of Microbiology, 2001.

160. Mummaneni V, Geraldes M, Hadjilambris OW, Ouyang Z. Effect of ravuconazole on the pharmacokinetics of simvastatin in healthy subjects. Program and Abstracts of the 40th Interscience Conference on Antimicrobial Agents and Chemotherapy [abstr 841]. Toronto, Ont, Canada, September 17–20 2000, Washington, DC: American Society of Microbiology, 2000.

161. Maertens J, Raad I, Petrikkos G, et al. Update of the multicenter noncomparative study of caspofungin (CAS) in adults with invasive aspergillosis (IA) refractory (R) or intolerant (I) to other antifungal agents: analysis of 90 patients. Program and Abstracts of the 42nd Interscience Conference on Antimicrobial Agents and Chemotherapy [abstr M-868]. San Diego, California, September 27–30 2002, Washington, DC: American Society of Microbiology, 2002.

162. Maertens J, Raad I, Sable CA, et al. Multicenter, noncomparative study to evaluate safety and efficacy of caspofungin (CAS) in adults with invasive aspergillosis (IA) refractory (R) to or intolerant (I) to amphotericin B (AMB), AMB lipid formulations (lipid AMB) or azoles. Program and Abstracts of the 40th Interscience Conference on Antimicrobial Agents and Chemotherapy [Abstr 1103]. Toronto, Ont, September 17–20 2000, Washington, DC: American Society of Microbiology, 2000.

163. Stone JA, McCrea JB, Wickersham PJ, et al. A Phase I study of caspofungin evaluating the potential for drug interactions with itraconazole, the effect of gender and the use of a loading dose regimen. Program and Abstracts of the 40th Interscience Conference on Antimicrobial Agents and Chemotherapy [abstr 854]. Toronto, Ont, September 17–20. 2000, Washington, DC: American Society of Microbiology, 2000.

164. Merck & Co. Inc. Cancidas (caspofungin) Package Insert. West Point, PA, 2003.

165. Stone J, Holland S, Wickersham P, et al. Drug interactions between caspofungin and tacrolimus. Program and Abstracts of the 41st Interscience Conference on Antimicrobial Agents and Chemotherapy [abstr A-13]. Chicago, Illinois, December 16–19 2001, Washington, DC: American Society of Microbiology, 2001.

166. Van Burik J, Ratanatharathorn V, Lipton J, et al. Randomized, double-blind trial of micafungin (MI) versus fluconazole (FL) for prophylaxis of invasive fungal infections in patients (pts) undergoing hematopoietic stem cell transplant (HSCT), NIAID/ BAMSG Protocol 46. Program and Abstracts of the 42nd Interscience Conference on Antimicrobial Agents and Chemotherapy [Abstr M-1238]. San Diego, California, September 27–30 2002, Washington, DC: American Society of Microbiology, 2002.

167. Townsend R, Hebert M, Wisemandle W, Bekersky I. Concomitant pharmacokinetics (PK) of micafungin, and echinocandin antifungal, and cyclosporine in healthy volunteers [abstr 15]. J Clin Pharmacol 2002; 42:1054.

168. Townsend R, Hebert M, Wisemandle W, Bekersky I. Concomitant pharmacokinetics (PK) of micafungin, and echinocandin antifungal, and tacrolimus in healthy volunteers [abstr 18]. J Clin Pharmacol 2002; 42:1055.

169. Clemons KV, Sobel RA, Stevens DA. Toxicity of LY303366, and echinocandin antifungal, in mice pretreated with glucocorticoids. Antimicrob Agents Chemother 2000; 44:378–381.

170. Thye D, Kilfoil T, Kilfoil G, Henkel T. Anidulafungin: safety and pharmacokinetics in subjects receiving concomitant cyclosporine. Program and Abstracts of the 42nd Interscience Conference on Antimicrobial Agents and Chemotherapy [abstr A-1836]. San Diego, California, USA, September 27–30 2002, Washington, DC: American Society of Microbiology, 2002.

171. White RJ, Thye D. Anidulafungin does not affect the metabolism of cyclosporin by human hepatic microsomes. Program and Abstracts of the 41st Interscience Conference on Antimicrobial Agents and Chemotherapy [abstr A-35]. Chicago, Illinois, USA, December 16–19 2001, Washington, DC: American Society of Microbiology, 2001.

172. Vickers AE, Sinclair JR, Zollinger M, et al. Multiple cytochrome P-450s involved in the metabolism of terbinafine suggests a limited potential for drug–drug interactions. Drug Metab Dispos 1999; 27:1029–1038.

173. Albengres E, Le Louet H, Tillement JP. Systemic antifungal agents. Drug interactions of clinical significance. Drug Saf 1998; 18:83–87.

174. Shear N, Drake L, Gupta AK, Lambert J, Yaniv R. The implications and management of drug interactions with itraconazole, fluconazole, and terbinafine. Dermatology 2000; 201:196–203.

175. Gupta AK, Ross GS. Interaction between terbinafine and warfarin. Dermatology 1998; 196:266–267.

176. Van Der Kuy PH, Van Den Heuvel HA, Kempen RW, Vanmolkot LM. Pharmacokinetic interaction between nortriptyline and terbinafine. Ann Pharmacother 2002; 36: 1712–1714.

177. Madani MS, Barilla D, Cramer J, Wang Y, Paul C. Effect of terbinafine on the pharmacokinetics and pharmacodynamics of desipramine in healthy volunteers identified as cytochrome P450 2D6 (CYP2D6) extensive metabolizers. J Clin Pharmacol 2002; 42: 1211–1218.

178. Long CC, Hill SA, Thomas RC, Johnston A, Smith SG, Kendall F, Finlay AY. Effect of terbinafine on the pharmacokinetics of cyclosporin in humans. J Invest Dermatol 1994; 102:740–743.

179. Polak A, Grenson M. Evidence for a common transport system for cytosine, adenine and hypoxanthine in Saccharomyces cerevisiae and Candida albicans. Eur J Biochem 1973; 32:276–282.

180. Okino K, Weibert RT. Warfarin–griseofulvin interaction. Drug Intell Clin Pharm 1986; 20:291–293.

181. Wells PS, Holbrook AM, Crowther NR, Hirsh J. Interactions of warfarin with drugs and food. Ann Intern Med 1994; 121:676–683.

182. Cropp JS, Bussey HI. A review of enzyme induction of warfarin metabolism with recommendations for patient management. Pharmacotherapy 1997; 17:917–928.

183. Matsumura Y, Yokota M, Yoshioka H, Shibata S, Ida S, Takiguchi Y. Acute effects of griseofulvin on the pharmacokinetics and pharmacodynamics of warfarin in rats. J Int Med Res 1999; 27:167–175.

184. Weisberg E. Interactions between oral contraceptives and antifungals/antibacterials. Is contraceptive failure the result? Clin Pharmacokinet 1999; 36:309–313

185. Petraitis V, Petraitiene R, Sarafandi AA, Kelaher AM, Lyman CA, Casler HE, Sein T, Groll AH, Bacher J, Avila NA, Walsh TJ. Combination therapy in treatment of experimental pulmonary aspergillosis: synergistic interaction between an antifungal triazole and an echinocandin. Clin Infect Dis 2003; 187:1834–1843.

186. Manavathu EK, Alangaden GJ, Chandresakar PH. Differential activity of triazoles in two-drug combinations with the echinocandin caspofungin against Aspergillus fumigatus. J Antimicrob Chemother 2003; Advance access published April 25, 2003: 1–3.

187. Hossain MA, Reyes GH, Long LA, Mukherjee PK, Ghannoum MA. Efficacy of caspofungin combined with amphotericin B against azole-resistant Candida albicans. J Antimicrob Chemother 2003; Advance access published April 25, 2003:1–3.
188. Luque JC, Clemons KV, Stevens DA. Efficacy of micafungin alone or in combination against systemic murine aspergillosis. Antimicrob Agents Chemother 2003; 47: 1452–1455.
189. Gomez-Lopez A, Cuenca-Estrella M, Mellado E, Rodriguez-Tudela JL. In vitro evaluation of combination of terbinafine with itraconazole or amphotericin B against Zygomycota. Diagn Microbiol Infect Dis 2003; 45:199–202.
190. Weig M, Muller FM. Synergism of voriconazole and terbinafine against Candida albicans isolates from human immunodeficiency virus-infected patients with oropharyngeal candidiasis. Antimicrob Agents Chemother 2001; 45:966–968.
191. Meletiadis J, Mouton JW, Meis JF, Verweij PE. In vitro drug interaction modeling of combinations of azoles with terbinafine against clinical Scedosporium prolificans isolates. Antimicrob Agents Chemother 2003; 47:106–117.
192. Kirkpatrick WR, Perea S, Coco BJ, Patterson TF. Efficacy of caspofungin alone and in combination with voriconazole in a guinea pig model of invasive aspergillosis. Antimicrob Agents Chemother 2002; 46:2564–2568.
193. Perea S, Gonzalez G, Fothergill AW, Kirkpatrick WR, Rinaldi MG, Patterson TF. In vitro interaction of caspofungin acetate with voriconazole against clinical isolates of Aspergillus spp. Antimicrob Agents Chemother 2002; 46:3039–3041.
194. Arikan S, Lozano-Chiu M, Paetznick V, Rex JH. In vitro synergy of caspofungin and amphotericin B against Aspergillus and Fusarium spp. Antimicrob Agents Chemother 2002; 46:245–247.
195. Kontoyiannis DP, Hachem R, Lewis RE, Rivera GA, Torres HA, Thornby J, Champlin D, Kantarjian H, Bodey GP, Raad II. Efficacy and toxicity of caspofungin in combination with liposomal amphotericin B as primary or salvage treatment of invasive aspergillosis in patients with hematologic malignancies. Cancer 2003; 98:292–299.
196. Aliff TB, Maslak PG, Jurcic JG, Heaney ML, Cathcart KN, Sepkowitz KA, Weiss MA. Refractory Aspergillus pneumonia in patients with acute leukemia. Successful therapy with combination caspofungin and liposomal amphotericin. Cancer 2003; 97:1025–1032.

21
Adjunctive Immunotherapy Against Opportunistic Fungal Infections

Emmanuel Roilides and John Dotis
Third Department of Pediatrics, Hippokration Hospital, Thessaloniki, Greece

Thomas J. Walsh
National Institutes of Health, National Cancer Institute/Pediatric Oncology Branch, Bethesda, Maryland, U.S.A.

I. INTRODUCTION

A. Invasive Fungal Infections in Immunocompromised Patients

During the last two decades invasive fungal infections (IFIs) have emerged as important medical problems, particularly among immunocompromised patients. This trend is alarming problems, IFIs are associated with significant morbidity and high mortality, which in some cases may exceed 90% (1,2). While endemic fungi may also cause infections in immunocompromised patients in certain areas of the world, opportunistic fungi are by far the most important causes of IFIs in these patients worldwide. While infections due to *Candida* spp. remain an important problem in immunocompromised patients, infections due to filamentous fungi have become progressively more frequent and retain their extremely high mortality in susceptible patients (2,3). It is especially against these refractory infections that host defenses and immune reconstitution are very important in order to improve their dismal outcome.

B. Settings of IFIs

The underlying immunological status is the major contributor to host defense against opportunistic fungal infections. These infections occur when host defense mechanisms are absent or dysfunctional. Since innate host defense against fungi is primarily based on the antifungal activity of phagocytes, patients with deficient number or function of phagocytes are at increased risk of IFIs. Such deficiencies occur in a variety of patients (Table 1) including those with cancer and chemotherapy-related neutropenia, transplant recipients with neutropenia or receiving corticosteroids or other immunosuppressants (3–5), and other functional deficiencies of phagocytes, most importantly chronic granulomatous disease (CGD) (6). Therefore, immunotherapy aimed at augmenting host defense mechanisms may improve outcome in these patients (7).

Table 1 Diseases and Conditions Predisposing to Development of IFIs

High-dose chemotherapy-associated neutropenia

High-dose corticosteroid therapy

Hematological disorders (main risk factors: persistent and profound neutropenia, use of broad-spectrum antibacterial agents, indwelling central venous catheters, and damage of normal host barriers following intensive cytotoxic chemotherapy)

Hospitalization in surgical, neonatal, and intensive care units: extensive burn injury and extensive surgery operations (main risk factors: use of broad-spectrum antibacterial agents, prematurity, indwelling central venous catheters, and damage of normal host barriers)

Transplantation [bone marrow transplantation (BMT), peripheral blood stem cell transplantation (PBSCT), and solid organ transplantation]

Acquired immunodeficiency syndrome (AIDS) (main risk factors: neutropenia and high-dose corticosteroid therapy)

Chronic granulomatous disease (CGD)

II. OVERVIEW OF ANTIFUNGAL HOST DEFENSES

A. Innate Host Defense

The human host defense against opportunistic fungi is divided into innate and adaptive immunity. The innate immunity is served mainly by phagocytes, such as tissue macrophages, circulating monocytes (MNCs), and neutrophils (PMNs) and does not involve T-cell memory (Table 2). Its great importance in the defense against IFIs due to opportunistic pathogens is demonstrated by their high incidence in patients with deficient macrophage (i.e., corticosteroids) or PMN (i.e., neutropenia) host defense systems. Adaptive immunity appears to be less important against opportunistic fungi in immunocompromised patients.

Table 2 Innate Immune Response to Specific Groups of Fungi

Fungi	Innate Immune Response
Skin and gut fungi (mainly *Candida albicans* and other *Candida* spp.)	Macrophages (peritoneal, Kupffer cells, spleen adherent cells, etc.) phagocytose and kill blastoconidia intracellularly by oxidative and non-oxidative mechanisms, produce monokines (i.e., TNF-α)
	Neutrophils (bloodstream circulating and in tissues) ingest and kill blastoconidia intracellularly, damage pseudohyphae and hyphae extracellularly by oxidative burst, and non-oxidative mechanisms
	T lymphocytes produce lymphokines (i.e., IL-18, IFN-γ)
Airborne fungi (i.e., *Aspergillus* spp., Zygomycetes, *Fusarium* spp., *Scedosporium* spp.)	Pulmonary alveolar macrophages ingest and kill conidia intracellularly by oxidative and non-oxidative mechanisms, produce monokines (i.e., TNF-α)
	Neutrophils damage escaping hyphae extracellularly by oxidative burst and non-oxidative mechanisms
	T lymphocytes produce lymphokines (i.e., IL-18, IFN-γ)
Cryptococcus neoformans (and *Trichosporon* spp.)	Polysaccharide-specific antibody mediated response, phagocytosis by macrophages and neutrophils, and inhibition of immune functions

Source: Modified from Ref. 8.

B. Phagocytes

Depending on the fungus and the route of acquisition, specific macrophage-type phagocytes recognize particular ligands on the surface of fungi, ingest them, become activated, and destroy the intracellular forms of fungi. The roles of oxygen-dependent intermediates as well as antimicrobial peptides and other non-oxygen dependent metabolites are very important for intracellular killing (9–12). When the fungal conidia escape and germinate to hyphae, macrophages cannot handle them. Circulating PMNs and MNCs are attracted by the action of a number of cytokines and chemokines that are released at the site of infection, attach to the surface of the hyphae and inflict damage by mainly oxygen-dependent antifungal intermediates (reviewed in Refs. 9 and 13).

C. Hematopoietic Growth Factors (HGFs) and Other Cytokines

A number of hematopoietic growth factors (HGFs) and other cytokines are capable to act on immature or end-stage phagocytes and either increase their number (HGFs) or modulate their antifungal function (HGFs and cytokines). The most clinically relevant HGFs acting on phagocytes are granulocyte colony-stimulating factor (G-CSF), granulocyte-macrophage colony-stimulating factor (GM-CSF), and macrophage colony-stimulating factor (M-CSF) (Table 3). Cytokines that affect the function of phagocytes against fungi include Thl cytokines, such as interferon-γ (IFN-γ), interleukin (IL) -12, IL-15, and tumor necrosis factor-α (TNF-α). Additionally, cytokines of Th2 pattern, such as IL-4 and IL-10, exert an overall suppressive effect on antifungal function of phagocytes (14).

III. RATIONALE OF ADJUNCTIVE IMMUNOTHERAPY

Despite the development of new potent and less toxic antifungal agents such as lipid formulations of amphotericin B, second generation of triazoles, and echinocandins, the mortality of IFIs in immunocompromised patients is still unacceptable reaching the frequency of 90% in some fungal syndromes (1,15). A critical factor for the increased frequency of IFIs and their resistance to therapy nowadays is the profound compromise of the immune system that is created by potent immunosuppressive therapies and the prolonged survival of patients in such profound immunocompromised state. Therefore, alternative or adjunctive therapeutic approaches have been investigated for the management of IFIs that are still a challenge for clinicians.

Table 3 Clinically Relevant Hematopoietic Growth Factors and Cytokines with Potential Utility as Adjunctive Antifungal Therapy

Hematopoietic Growth Factors	Cytokines	
Granulocyte colony-stimulating factor (G-CSF)	Interferon-γ (IFN-γ)	Interleukin (IL)-4
Granulocyte-macrophage colony-stimulating factor (GM-CSF)	Tumor necrosis factor-α (TNF-α)	Interleukin (IL)-10
Macrophage colony-stimulating factor (M-CSF)	Interleukin (IL)-12	
	Interleukin (IL)-15	

Because of the importance of intact innate immune response to the fight against IFIs, and thanks to advances in understanding pathogenesis of IFIs as well as the availability of recombinant cytokines, immunotherapeutic approaches have become very appealing. These can be either reconstitution of effector cells numerically and/or functionally with cytokines and/or white blood cell transfusions (WBCTx), or manipulation of cytokine dysbalance (16).

IV. PRECLINICAL BASIS OF IMMUNOTHERAPY

A. In Vitro and In Vivo Laboratory Investigations

Many preclinical studies have shown that certain HGFs and cytokines augment the antifungal host defense by increasing the number and/or enhancing the function of phagocytes. The most important results of these studies have extensively been reviewed elsewhere (17) and are briefly summarized in this chapter. Data from experimental animal models have suggested the utility of cytokines prophylactically or as adjunctive therapy in combination with conventional antifungal chemotherapy in the setting of certain IFIs (18–22) (Table 4).

The G-CSF acts upon PMNs promoting their maturation and increasing their number in peripheral blood (43,44). The G-CSF enhances the antimicrobial activity of PMNs against a wide variety of bacteria (45). It also regulates the function of intact PMNs against fungi including C. albicans and A. fumigatus hyphae, mainly by enhancement of PMN oxidative burst (46–48). This enhancement occurs even in cases of corticosteroid-suppressed PMNs (49). In various animal models of infection, therapeutic administration of G-CSF has been shown to enhance pathogen eradication and to decrease morbidity and/or mortality (50). The G-CSF enhances host resistance to disseminated candidiasis in non-neutropenic mice through activation of PMNs and their recruitment to the site of infection (23) and also has a protective effect on bacterial and fungal infections in neutropenic mice (51). In addition, it can induce dendritic cells with a Th2 response profile (52) and, accordingly, may down-regulate the proinflammatory response having a more favorable benefit-to-toxicity ratio against infections for which PMNs are the predominant effector cells. The antifungal effects of G-CSF in vitro and in animal models of IFIs are reviewed in an excellent recent paper (50).

The PMNs from patients treated with G-CSF have been found to possess enhanced activity not only against A. fumigatus but also against Rhizopus arrhizus, C. albicans (48), and Candida neoformans (53). The last two fungi were killed even by PMNs from HIV-infected patients who had received G-CSF (5 μg/kg), a finding suggesting that this cytokine restores the suppressed function (53).

The effect of G-CSF also has been studied in vitro in combination with fluconazole and voriconazole where an additive effect has been found against C. albicans and A. fumigatus, respectively (54,55). A similar effect has been demonstrated in a neutropenic murine model of invasive aspergillosis with G-CSF and posaconazole (20). When G-CSF and posaconazole were given to corticosteroid-immunosuppressed mice, however, the antifungal effect was either antagonistic or indifferent (20), indicating that the type of immune deficit is important in enhancing in vivo host response.

The GM-CSF promotes the differentiation and proliferation of mononuclear cells as well as PMNs (50,56). Although it is biologically similar to G-CSF, GM-CSF acts on progenitor cells capable of differentiating into both granulocytic and monocytic lineages. Consequently, it can increase the numbers of PMNs,

Table 4 Effects of Cytokines in Animal Models of Candidiasis and Aspergillosis

Cytokines	Animal Model	Organism	Antifungal Rx	Outcome
G-CSF	Immuncompetent mice	C. albicans		↓ Mortality and fungal growth of organs (23)
	Immunocompetent and neutropenic mice	C. albicans	Fluconazole	Additive effect, ↑ survival, and renal clearance (24)
	Neutropenic mice	C. albicans		Protective (19) or no effect (23)
	Neutropenic mice	C. albicans	Alone	↑ Survival, ↓ the number of Candida in kidneys
			± Amphotericin B	↑↑ Survival (25)
	Neutropenic mice	C. albicans		Protective effect ↓ Candida growth of kidney (26)
	Neutropenic mice	Aspergillus fumigatus		Protective effect (26)
	Neutropenic mice	A. fumigatus	Posaconazole	Additive effect (20)
GM-CSF	Neutropenic mice	C. albicans		↑ Resistance, ↓ Candida recovery from the organs (27)
M-CSF	Immunocompetent mice	C. albicans		↑ Survival ↓ Candida recovery (28)
	Immunocompetent rats	C. albicans	Fluconazole	Improved survival (29)
	Neutropenic mice	C. albicans	+ Fluconazole	↑ Survival
			+ Amphotericin B	↑↑ Survival (30)
	Neutropenic rabbits	A. fumigatus		↑ Survival ↑ PAM activation (31)
IFN-γ	Immunocompetent and corticosteroid-treated mice	C. albicans		↓ Candida growth (32)
	Neutropenic mice	Paracoccidioides brasiliensis		Protective effect major mediator of resistance against paracoccidioidomycosis (33)
IFN-γ, TNF-α	Corticosteroid-treated mice	A. fumigatus		↓ Mortality and organ clearance (34)
TNF-α	Immunocompetent mice	C. albicans		Protective effect ↑ Resistance (34)
TNF-α, GM-CSF	Immunocompetent mice	A. fumigatus		Role in recruitment of neutrophils (↑ fungal clearance) (35)

(Continued)

Table 4 Effects of Cytokines in Animal Models of Candidiasis and Aspergillosis (*Continued*)

Cytokines	Animal Model	Organism	Antifungal Rx	Outcome
TNF-α agonist	Neutropenic mice	*A. fumigatus*		↑ Survival (22)
IL-1	Neutropenic mice	*C. albicans*		↑ survival (36)
	Neutropenic mice	*C. albicans*	Fluconazole	↓↓ The number of *Candida* in organs (37)
IL-4	Immunocompetent mice	*C. albicans*		↓ Survival (38)
		A. fumigatus		↓ Survival IL-4-deficiency protected (39)
IL-10	Immunocompetent mice	*C. albicans*		↓ Survival IL-10-neutralization protected (40) IL-10-deficiency protected (41)
		A. fumigatus		↓ Survival IL-10-deficiency protected (41)
IL-12	Neutropenic mice	*P. brasiliensis*		Protects against disseminated infection but enhances pulmonary inflammation (42)

eosinophils, and MNCs. The GM-CSF enhances antifungal activities of intact PMNs and/or MNCs against *C. albicans* (57), *A. fumigatus* (58), and other less frequently isolated fungi (59). Its effect has been tested in vitro in combination with voriconazole and PMNs and an additive effect, similar with G-CSF, has been found against *A. fumigatus* (55). Such an effect has not, however, been seen with GM-CSF, voriconazole, and MNCs suggesting that there are differences in the way that phagocytes interact with antifungal drugs under cytokine-induced activation.

The GM-CSF also primes macrophages to release mediators of inflammation such as IL-1 and TNF-α (56) that can overcome dexamethasone-mediated suppression of antifungal monocytic activity against *Aspergillus* (60). Some forms of GM-CSF, particularly non-glycosylated preparations, have been associated with toxicity that may reflect its ability to increase proinflammatory mediators and there has also been a theoretical concern that GM-CSF therapy could hinder PMNs migration to sites of infection (16). Indeed, a deleterious GM-CSF-mediated proinflammatory response may have resulted in worsened outcome in an animal model of disseminated trichosporonosis (61).

The M-CSF promotes the differentiation, proliferation, and activation of MNCs and macrophages. It enhances the antifungal activity of MNCs and macrophages against *Candida* spp. (62), *A. fumigatus* (63), and other fungi (59). Animal studies have revealed complex effects with regard to the immunomodulatory activity of M-CSF (29,64). In a rabbit model of invasive aspergillosis, administration of

M-CSF augmented pulmonary host defense against *A. fumigatus* suggesting potential role for this cytokine as adjunctive therapy in the treatment of pulmonary aspergillosis in the setting of profound neutropenia (31). In a murine model of candidiasis, M-CSF synergized with amphotericin B but not with fluconazole for an improved outcome of infection as this was documented by decreased mortality in the animals (30).

The IFN-γ is a potent activator of both PMN and macrophage function (65) that can enhance the phagocytic activity against a number of fungal pathogens. Depending on the experimental conditions, IFN-γ has been shown to have an enhancing effect (66) or no effect (67) on fungicidal activities of human or murine PMNs against *C. albicans* blastoconidia. While dexamethasone suppresses the fungicidal activity of human MNCs against *A. fumigatus* evidenced as oxidative burst in response to hyphae and as hyphal damage, IFN-γ is able to restore these activities (60). An up-regulatory role of IFN-γ on both PMNs and MNCs against *Aspergillus* hyphae has been shown as well as an additive effect of the combination of IFN-γ and G-CSF at high concentrations (46,58). Compared to G-CSF and GM-CSF, IFN-γ has been shown to be a very potent activator of phagocytes against opportunistic fungal pathogens (68). Synergy between IFN-γ and antifungal agents against *Candida* spp., *A. fumigatus*, *C. neoformans*, *P. brasiliensis*, and *Blastomyces dermatiditis* has been demonstrated in vitro by use of macrophages (56) and in vivo for experimental cryptococcosis (69).

The IL-12 plays a key role in promoting Th1 responses and subsequent cell mediated immunity (70). It is produced primarily by antigen presenting cells. Its major biologic function is to enhance proliferation and cytolytic activity of natural killer (NK) and T cells, and stimulate their IFN-γ production (71). Th1 type cellular responses are essential for protection against fungal pathogens, including *Candida* spp., *Aspergillus* spp., and *C. neoformans* (72). The IL-12 has activity in experimental murine cryptococcosis (73), histoplasmosis (74), coccidioidomycosis (75), and early in the course of aspergillosis (76). In addition, it can enhance fluconazole's efficacy against *Candida* infections in mice with neurropenia (77). Thus, IL-12 may be useful adjunctive therapy against various IFIs in the setting of neutropenia. However, IL-12 may be detrimental in hosts that are not neutropenic because it can induce an excessive inflammatory response (78). Adjustment of dosage of IL-12 may ameliorate these adverse effects.

The IL-15 has similar biologic properties in vitro with IL-2, consistent with their shared receptor signaling components (IL-2/15Rc). However, specificity for IL-15 vs. IL-2 also exists (79). Both IL-15 and IL-15R transcripts have a much broader tissue distribution than IL-2/IL-2R. Studies to date examining the biology of IL-15 have identified several key roles, such as IL-15's importance during NK and T-cell development and function. The IL-15 has important activity in host defense against fungi. It has been shown to enhance oxidative burst and antifungal activities of PMNs and MNCs including the abilities to ingest and inhibit growth of *C. albicans* (80,81). Similarly, it enhances PMN-induced hyphal damage in a number of filamentous fungi including *A. fumigatus, Scedosporium prolificans,* and *Fusarium* spp., but not *Aspergillus flavus* or *Scedosporium apiospermum* (*Pseudallescheria bodyii*) (82). Similar to IFN-γ, IL-15 may be a candidate for adjunctive immunotherapy in cases of Th1/Th2 dysregulation.

The TNF-α is a potent immunoenhancing cytokine augmenting the production of other cytokines, such as GM-CSF as well as enhancing several PMN functions, mainly by increasing O_2^- and H_2O_2 release (83). This cytokine has a protective role on systemic infections by *C. albicans* (84). The TNF-α stimulates PMNs to damage hyphae, enhances pulmonary alveolar macrophage (PAM) phagocytosis of conidia, augments PMN oxidative respiratory burst, and the degranulation induced by opsonized fungi (83). Fungicidal activity of PMNs against blastoconidia of C. albicans and Candida glabrata also has been shown to be enhanced (66,85), whereas the results with pseudohyphae of C. albicans have been equivocal (86). Underscoring its critical role in host response to pathogenic fungi, suppression of TNF-α by infliximab (anti-TNF-α antibody) may result in invasive aspergillosis (87,88).

The IL-4 has anti-inflammatory properties and primarily exerts a suppressive effect on immune cells. It has been shown to suppress the oxidative burst of MNCs and the killing of C. albicans blastoconidia (89). In the case of A. fumigatus, IL-4 significantly suppresses MNC-induced damage of hyphae, but it does not alter phagocytic activity or inhibition of conidial germination. In murine models of candidiasis and aspergillosis, IL-4 had detrimental effects (39,90) and its inhibition improved outcome. Its administration to patients with renal carcinoma, however, did not induce serious infections (91).

The IL-10 affects MNCs by suppressing oxidative burst and antifungal activity against A. fumigatus hyphae. The IFN-γ and GM-CSF may counteract suppressive effects of IL-10 (92). The IL-10 also affects PMN function against C. albicans by suppressing phagocytosis of blastoconidia and by reducing PMN-induced damage of C. albicans pseudohyphae (93). In murine models of candidiasis and aspergillosis, IL-10 had detrimental effects (40) and its inhibition improved outcome. Administration of IL-10 to patients with psoriasis or Crohn's disease, however, did not result in serious infections probably because of production of IFN-γ that high doses of IL-10 may induce (94,95).

B. Combined Activity of Antifungal Drugs, Phagocytes, and Cytokines

Antifungal drugs such as conventional and lipid formulations of amphotericin B, triazoles, and echinocandins have been studied in combination with PMNs or other phagocytes against fungal pathogens (55,96). These studies aimed first to exclude any adverse effect of the antifungal drugs on the antifungal activity of phagocytes, and second to find whether a synergistic effect exists between the two components. In these studies, no adverse effects were documented with any of the antifungal drug classes studied. Amphotericin B formulations have been shown to exert overall additive antifungal effects (conidiocidal activity and hyphal damage) in combination with PAMs and PMNs against A. fumigatus (97). Similar combinational effects have been found with caspofungin and phagocytes against the same organism (98). Triazoles and PMNs are synergistic to cause increased hyphal damage to S. prolificans and S. apiospermum, two therapy-refractory fungi (99). Further, amphotericin B lipid complex (ABLC) exerts additive antifungal activity in combination with PMNs against the two Scedosporium spp. (100). The ABLC exerts additive antifungal activity in combination with PAMs against Fusarium solani (unpublished authors' results). Taken all these data together, it appears that certain antifungal drugs, e.g., ABLC, have the capacity to be synergistic with the antifungal host response to an improved defense against the infection.

Beside the direct effects of cytokines on effector cells in inhibiting fungal growth, cytokines may collaborate with antifungal drugs in producing larger antifungal effects. As an example, when voriconazole was combined with GM-CSF or G-CSF treatment of PMNs against A. fumigatus hyphae, growth inhibition was

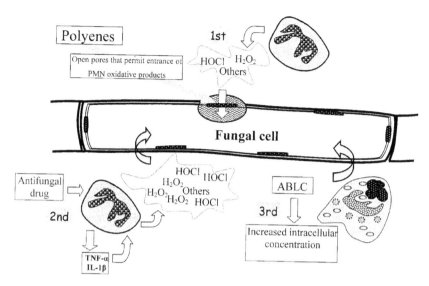

Figure 1 Hypothetical mechanisms of additive or synergistic activity of antifungal drugs and phagocytes against fungal pathogens.

significantly increased compared to growth inhibition due to unstimulated PMNs (101). Similar phenomena were observed when voriconazole was combined with IFN-γ treated PMNs (102). However, such collaboration between GM-CSF and voriconazole in inhibiting *A. fumigatus* hyphal growth was not observed when MNCs were used.

This antifungal–cytokine collaboration may occur through the fungi, through the effector cells, or through both of them (Fig. 1). Antifungal drugs such as polyenes and azoles, which alter the fungal membrane, or echinocandins, which damage the cell wall, may render fungi more susceptible to oxidative and non-oxidative products. Furthermore, antifungal drugs may have direct immunomodulatory activity on phagocytes as it was found for amphotericin B and voriconazole, which enhanced the conidiocidal and antihyphal activity of PAMs and PMNs against *A. fumigatus* (97,101). While it is known that amphotericin B may induce secretion of oxidative and non-oxidative metabolites and immunoenhancing cytokines, such as TNF-γ and IL-1β, and may enhance phagocytosis of fungal spores, the immunomodulatory effects of azoles and echinocandins are not well understood. Cytokines may up-regulate host antifungal mechanisms (oxidative burst or antifungal peptides), which can interact with antifungal drugs, enhance penetration of antifungals into phagocytes, where the drugs may be more effective against ingested fungi, and restore defense mechanisms, which can be depressed by an antifungal drug.

C. Cytokine Administration

Two patient populations are at high risk for IFIs: those with neutropenia and those with functional deficiencies of lymphocytes and phagocytes. The HGFs and other cytokines have a role in prophylaxis and as adjunctive treatment of IFIs in combination with antifungal drugs in both patient categories. However, due to limitations in clinical trial design and defining patient populations at risk, definitive data on the efficacy of recombinant HGFs and other cytokines have not been well-demonstrated.

1. Prevention of IFIs by Use of Cytokines in Neutropenic Patients

Malignancies and disease- or therapy-related neutropenia constitute the broadest field of acquired defects in host defenses and the greatest need for immune reconstitution. Thus, most of the studies have focused on this patient population. Although the cytokines have been extensively evaluated in preclinical studies, there is still controversy with regard to their utility in these patients. The main reason is that the number of IFIs as sequelae of immune compromise is relatively small, and no study has had the statistical power to demonstrate significant differences in the proportions of IFIs between the patients receiving or not receiving a HGF/cytokine prophylactically or empirically. Nevertheless, there are several case reports and small, uncontrolled studies that have been published suggesting the potential beneficial effects of immunotherapy. Unfortunately, the conclusions of all these studies are limited by the caveats characterizing uncontrolled studies and case reports. These include desperate use of cytokines only in the most seriously ill patients with grave prognosis, and investigators' as well as publications' bias towards improved outcome that make any definitive conclusion very difficult to be drawn. Thus, conclusive clinical data are still missing, making the issue of their use in the management of IFIs not definitive.

The clinical use of G-CSF and GM-CSF has been mainly based on the ability of either factor to abbreviate the depth and duration of neutropenia as well as to enhance the antifungal function of phagocytes (43,103,104). Both are clinically used in patients with neutropenia associated with chemotherapy and/or hematopoietic stem cell transplantation (HSCT), myelodysplastic syndromes, and aplastic anemia in order to promote bone marrow recovery (43). Both HGFs have assumed a central role in the supportive care of cancer, stem cell transplant, aplastic, and congenital neutropenic patients. Since susceptibility to IFIs is proportional to the duration and degree of neutropenia (105), the outcome of neutropenic patients with IFIs who receive a HGF is expected to be better.

The HGFs/cytokines have been administered at different settings of immunosuppression for the management of IFIs. For prophylaxis from infections they have been given at the onset of neutropenia (106–108) (Table 5). Although beneficial effects were noted in some of these studies, the number of IFIs that developed was too small to evaluate any potential effect. In a retrospective study of prophylactic administration of GM-CSF to patients with autologous bone marrow transplantation (BMT) for lymphoid cancer (105), the 28-day post-BMT incidence of infections occurring in those who had taken GM-CSF was compared with those who had not. The GM-CSF resulted in a trend towards fewer IFIs and decreased use of amphotericin B.

The GM-CSF has been used in patients with malignancies undergoing chemotherapy or HSCT, and has been found to improve survival and decrease the rate of bacterial and fungal infections (108–111). A retrospective study (109) suggested that GM-CSF has some advantages compared to G-CSF as preventive therapy of IFIs in patients receiving high-dose chemotherapy, with or without autologous stem cell transplantation.

The only prospective, randomized study in which there were enough IFIs to show significant differences has been the Eastern Co-operative Oncology Group study (108). In this placebo-controlled study, GM-CSF administration to elderly patients with myelogenous leukemia resulted in a reduction in the IFI-related mortality (2% in the GM-CSF group as compared to 19% in the placebo group), and a higher rate of complete response. Among the patients with IFIs, 11 patients had aspergillosis, seven candidiasis and two other IFIs. Only one of eight patients

Table 5 Use of Cytokines for Prophylaxis Against IFIs in Cancer Patients

Reference	Cytokine	Outcome
105	GM-CSF	Overall ↓ infections, a trend of ↓ IFIs, ↓ IV antibiotics, and ↓ days of amphotericin B usage
108	GM-CSF	More complete responses, ↑ survival, and ↓ IFI-related mortality
109	GM-CSF[a]	Overall ↓ infections, more complete responses, and prevention of IFIs in patients receiving high-dose chemotherapy
107	G-CSF	Overall ↓ incidence of fever with neutropenia and culture-confirmed infections, duration and severity of grade IV neutropenia, and in the total number of days of treatment with IV antibiotics and days of hospitalization

[a]Retrospective analysis of GM-CSF vs. non-macrophage enhancing cytokines.

who had been randomized to receive GM-CSF and developed IFI died (13%) as compared to nine among 12 patients on placebo (75%). No significant difference between aspergillosis and candidiasis was noted (111).

Furthermore, lack of consistent beneficial effects to support routine use of HGFs exists in the case of administration of G- or GM-CSF to patients at the onset of febrile neutropenia empirically or pre-emptively (112,113) (Table 6). In this setting, however, significantly less usage of antifungals was observed probably due to the effect of the cytokines on the incidence and duration of febrile neutropenia. Again, the numbers of IFIs diagnosed in the treated or the control arms were too small for any meaningful comparison to be made. The G-CSF also was studied in a randomized trial where patients with hematological malignancies and febrile neutropenia received either G-CSF with antibiotics or antibiotics alone. Although only four IFIs occurred, they were all encountered in the group receiving antibiotics alone (114).

In a double-blind controlled study, the administration of M-CSF to patients with myelogenous leukemia and febrile neutropenia decreased the incidence and duration of febrile neutropenia and significantly decreased the use of systemic antifungals (115). However, no impact on disease-free survival was found, an outcome heavily dependent on many confounding factors in these high-risk patients.

According to the American Society of Clinical Oncology (ASCO) updated recommendations regarding the use of HGFs (116), when fever persists during neutropenia

Table 6 Use of Cytokines as Adjunctive Management of Febrile Neutropenia (Early Treatment of a Possible or Probable IFI) in Cancer Patients

Reference	Cytokine	Outcome
112	G-CSF	↓ Number of days with neutropenia, ↓ time to resolution of febrile neutropenia, ↓ risk for prolonged hospitalization, and accelerated neutrophil recovery
114	G-CSF	More clinical responses, ↓ superinfections, ↓ hospitalization, ↓ antibiotic use, and ↓ mortality, IFIs only in the group treated with antibiotic alone
113	GM-CSF	No effect on clinical response and survival
115	M-CSF	↓ Incidence and duration of febrile neutropenia and ↓↓ use of systemic antifungals

and IFI is suspected, adjunctive use of a HGF with empirical antifungal therapy may be justified. The ASCO does not recommend the routine use of HGFs in afebrile neutropenia. In view of the development of new strategies for early diagnosis of IFIs such as serial high-resolution CT scans, galactomannan, and glucan assays as well as PCR, in the future one may be able to administer antifungal drugs and immunomodulators specifically to patients in whom such tests are indicative of IFI (pre-emptive therapy).

2. Adjunctive Therapy of IFIs in Neutropenic Patients

Both in vitro and experimental animal models have suggested the utility of cytokine treatment as adjunctive therapy in combination with conventional antifungal chemotherapy against refractory IFIs (7,14,117–119). There are several small studies and case reports suggesting the use of G-CSF as adjunctive therapy for certain IFIs with very poor prognosis in combination with amphotericin B or fluconazole and in some cases in addition to surgical debridement but the conclusions remain controversial (Table 7). These include reports of five children with aspergillosis (128) and patients with fungemia in the setting of hematological malignancy (132) and five patients with refractory zygomycosis (125,130). The G-CSF and GM-CSF have been also used in invasive fusariosis, another resistant IFI with mixed results (133). Similarly, some reports have suggested potential beneficial effect of the combination of GM-CSF and IFN-γ with antifungal agents (Table 7). However, statistically powered randomized clinical trials examining the utility of cytokine therapy in combination with conventional antifungal agents remain to be performed.

In a pilot study in which GM-CSF was administered to eight patients with IFIs and severe neutropenia, six had a PMN response and four of them were completely cured. However, three patients developed a capillary leak syndrome, suggesting that the dosage of GM-CSF was excessive (120). A subsequent open study of GM-CSF plus amphotericin B in 17 neutropenic cancer patients with proven IFIs did not show similar favorable results. Eight of the patients suffered from candidemia, eight from pulmonary aspergillosis and one from fusariosis (121).

The GM-CSF therapy was associated with a clinical response when administered with amphotericin B to a small number of patients with established IFIs. These patients included one with systemic infection due to *B. capitatus* (131), three with AIDS and oropharyngeal candidiasis (81), and one with refractory *Aspergillus* vertebral osteomyelitis (134). Two cases of chronic disseminated candidiasis in leukemia patients were resolved completely following six weeks of therapy with GM-CSF and IFN-γ (123). However, other clinical case reports of combination therapy with IFN-γ and conventional antifungal therapy have had mixed results. Thus, there is an urgent need of well-structured, randomized clinical trials to determine optimal dose, duration, and timing for different combinations of immunotherapy and antifungal agents in high-risk patients.

As with the other HGFs, M-CSF was used as an adjunct to antifungal therapy in patients with established IFIs. In the first clinical trial examining combination immunotherapy, M-CSF was administered to patients with proven IFIs at escalating dosages (50–2000 μg/m^2, IV) in combination with the appropriate antifungal agent (amphotericin B, fluconazole, or flucytosine) at maximally tolerated doses (135). There was a trend toward better survival in the patients receiving M-CSF (122,136). Moreover, this increase in survival was significant in patients with candidiasis and a Karnofsky score $> 20\%$ when compared with historical controls.

Table 7 Use of Cytokines for Treatment of Documented IFIs in Cancer Patients

Reference	Fungal Infections	Antifungal Therapy	Cytokine	Outcome
120	*Candida* 5 *Aspergillus* 2 *Trichosporon* 1	Amphotericin B	GM-CSF	6/8 Responses, 4/8 complete response, and 2/8 partial response
121	*Candida* 8 *Aspergillus* 8 *Fusarium* 1	Amphotericin B	GM-CSF	No effect on outcome (six deaths)
122	*Candida* 30 *Aspergillus* 15 Other 1	Amphotericin B	M-CSF	Trend of ↓ IFIs Significant improvement of survival of patients with candidiasis and Karnofsky score > 20 %
123	Chronic disseminated candidiasis	Liposomal amphotericin B	GM-CSF + IFN-γ	2/2 Responses
124	*Trichosporon beigelii* bloodstream infection	Amphotericin B	G-CSF	Response
125	Disseminated zygomycosis	Liposomal amphotericin B	G-CSF	Response
126	Disseminated *Fusarium oxysporum* infection	Amphotericin B + 5-FC	G-CSF	Response
127	Invasive thoracopulmonary mucormycosis	Amphotericin B	G-CSF	Response
128	Invasive pulmonary aspergillosis	Liposomal amphotericin B	G-CSF	3/5 Responses
129	Disseminated *Fusarium* infection	Amphotericin B	GM-CSF (WBCTx)	Response
130	Rhinocerebral mucormycosis	Liposomal amphotericin B	G-CSF	4/4 Responses
131	*Blastoschizomyces capitatus* septicemia	Amphotericin B + 5-FC	GM-CSF	Response

The issue of cost effective use of cytokines as adjunctive therapy in combination with antifungal agents has not been thoroughly studied and does not allow specific recommendations. In 29 neutropenic patients with IFIs following chemotherapy or BMT, combined therapy of conventional amphotericin B and G-CSF (3–5 µg/kg/day) was associated with an improved response rate (62% vs. 33% of control) (137). This study showed a greater cost-effectiveness of combination regimen, based on drug acquisition (all the failures were treated with liposomal amphotericin B), hospital stay, and treatment duration (138).

The only HGF that has been investigated in immunocompetent patients is G-CSF. In a multicenter clinical trial addressing the utility of G-CSF as adjunctive therapy of invasive candidiasis, 51 non-neutropenic patients were randomized to receive either fluconazole alone or fluconazole with G-CSF. While not statistically significant, there was a trend toward an earlier resolution of infection as well as reduced mortality in the patients receiving G-CSF (139). This study supports in vitro and ex vivo results that have shown that not only number, but also function of host immune cells is of importance in recovery from IFIs (56,77).

3. Phagocytic Dysfunction

Certain non-neutropenic patients are characterized by phagocytic dysfunction and are also at high risk for IFIs. Among them, patients with HSCT after recovery from neutropenia and especially during corticosteroid treatment of postengraftment graft-vs.-host disease (GVHD) are the most susceptible hosts (56). Apart from a decrease in the function of circulating phagocytes, these patients present abnormal cell-mediated immunity related to defective function of macrophages, MNCs, T, and NK cells. Indeed, IFIs, particularly aspergillosis, frequently occur in HSCT patients after the resolution of neutropenia (3,140), presumably related to an existing cytokine network dysregulation (141). These high-risk patients may benefit from cytokines administered during IFIs developed in the non-neutropenic phase after transplantation.

With the exception of a major prospective, randomized, placebo-controlled clinical trial, the clinical efficacy of IFN-γ against IFIs has not been extensively studied. As mentioned above, patients with qualitative phagocytic defects (most importantly CGD) are also at increased risk of IFIs, especially of invasive aspergillosis, an important cause of mortality in these patients (6). Long-term administration of IFN-γ has been shown to significantly reduce the incidence of serious infections in CGD patients (142). Patients in this study tended to have a reduced incidence of *Aspergillus* pneumonia compared with controls (two episodes in one patient in the IFN-γ group as compared to four episodes in four patients in the placebo group).

In addition, there is anecdotal evidence suggesting that IFN-γ can be useful adjunctive therapy for the treatment of certain unusual IFIs (143,144). Adjunctive therapy with IFN-γ has proven to be most useful in patients with defects in their immune cell function. For example, this cytokine has successfully been used for therapy of invasive aspergillosis in CGD patients in combination with antifungal agents (145,146) (Table 8).

Other non-neutropenic patients at high risk for IFIs who might benefit from immunotherapy, such as those with acquired immunodeficiency syndrome (AIDS), lymphoma, solid organ transplant recipients, and patients receiving corticosteroids or other immunosuppressants, have dysfunctional phagocytes along with cytokine dysregulation and lymphocytic defects. For example, PMNs and MNC-derived macrophages from patients with AIDS possess decreased ability to damage hyphae and to ingest conidia of *A. fumigatus*, respectively (155). In these patients, administration of recombinant IFN-γ showed a trend of decreased incidence of oral/esophageal candidiasis compared to control subjects (156).

V. RECOMMENDATIONS FOR THE USE OF HGFs AND CYTOKINES IN THE PREVENTION AND TREATMENT OF IFIs IN IMMUNOCOMPROMISED PATIENTS

As insufficient clinical data exist on the use of cytokines in the management of IFIs, definite guidelines for their routine use cannot be established. Nevertheless, reconstitution of the immune response by various actions has to be taken into serious consideration (Table 9). Reversion of immunosuppression is very important and

Table 8 Case Reports of CGD Patients with IFIs Treated with Combined Antifungal Therapy and a HGF/Cytokine

Reference	Fungal Infections	Antifungal Therapy	Cytokine	Outcome
143	*Paecilomyces varioti* soft tissue infection on the right heel	Amphotericin B followed by itraconazole	IFN-γ	Complete response
144	Disseminated infection with *Pseudallescheria boydii*	Amphotericin B followed by itraconazole	IFN-γ	Complete response
145	*P. varioti* multifocal osteomyelitis	Amphotericin B followed by itraconazole	IFN-γ	Response
146	*A. fumigatus* femoral osteomyelitis	Itraconazole	IFN-γ	Complete response
147	*Aspergillus nidulans* invasive multifocal infection	Liposomal amphotericin B	G-CSF and G-CSF-elicited PMNs	Complete response
148	*Chrysosporium zonatum* lobar pneumonia and tibia osteomyelitis	Liposomal amphotericin B	IFN-γ	Complete response
149	*A. fumigatus* brain abscesses	Various anti-fungal agents and surgery	IFN-γ	Complete response
150	*A. fumigatus* tibia osteomyelitis	Amphotericin B	IFN-γ	Response
151	*A. nidulans* femoral osteomyelitis	Liposomal amphotericin B	G-CSF	Complete response
152	*A. nidulans* multifocal osteomyelitis	Amphotericin B followed by liposomal amphotericin B plus flucytosine	IFN-γ	Complete response
153	*A. fumigatus* humeral osteomyelitis	Amphotericin B plus flucytosine followed by itraconazole	IFN-γ	Complete response
154	*A. fumigatus* thoracic vertebral osteomyelitis	Amphotericin B plus itraconazole followed by lipid complex amphotericin B plus itraconazole	IFN-γ	Complete response

when it is possible (i.e., by decreasing or discontinuing immunosuppressive therapies), it must be attempted. In particular, corticosteroids, a major risk factor of IFIs, must be decreased or discontinued. In addition, exogenous administration of HGFs and proinflammatory cytokines or inhibition of immunoregulatory cytokines appears to be a promising adjunct to our armamentarium against life-threatening IFIs. In its updated guidelines (103,116,157), ASCO recommends that high-risk patients (more than 40% risk of febrile neutropenia) receive G- or GM-CSF prophylactically. Similarly, during the onset of febrile neutropenia in patients not receiving a HGF, G-, or GM-CSF are suggested when the duration of neutropenia is predicted to be long. Although no data exist, patients who have had an episode of IFI in the past and become neutropenic again should be treated with a HGF. With regard to

Table 9 Actions That Are Indicated to Correct Antifungal Host Immune Defect When an IFI Is Diagnosed in Immunocompromised Patients

---

(1) Reversion of immunosuppression, i.e.,
    (a) Discontinuation of corticosteroids
    (b) Decrease of dose of immunosuppressive drugs
(2) Reconstitution of host defenses by
    (a) Use of G-CSF or GM-CSF (or M-CSF) in neutropenic patients with myelogenous leukemia or BMT (prevention and therapy of IFIs)
    (b) Use of IFN-γ in patients with CGD (prevention and therapy)
    (c) Infusion of G-CSF-elicited white blood cell transfusions to profoundly neutropenic patients with refractory IFIs

---

the management of documented IFIs in neutropenic patients, the 1997 Guidelines of Infectious Diseases Society of America state that these factors "may be indicated" (158) and have not been changed up to now. So far, potential direct applications of cytokines and HGFs against IFIs are limited to the following indications:

1. Use of GM-CSF or G-CSF in the prevention and treatment of IFIs in neutropenic patients, especially those with myelogenous leukemia or HSCT. The G-CSF may not be as effective as the macrophage-stimulating HGFs. In addition, patients with other types of neoplastic diseases including AIDS-related malignancies, which are associated with high probability of development of IFIs may benefit from HGF therapy. The M-CSF is used in Japan and since it has not been licensed in the United States and European Union it cannot be used clinically in these countries.
2. Prophylactic use of IFN-γ in patients with CGD.
3. Under certain conditions of defective host defenses without neutropenia (i.e., GVHD or therapy with immunosuppressive agents), IFN-γ with or without a HGF may be justified as adjunctive therapy for IFIs.

With completion of more clinical studies, indications also might include surgical and other non-neutropenic immunodeficient patients with IFIs, i.e., those with solid organ transplant or HIV-infection, neonates, and others. The role of administration of neutralizing antibodies or inhibitors of Th2 cytokines on prevention and outcome of IFIs needs further clinical study.

Two forms of G-CSF are commercially available. One is a recombinant non-glycosylated protein expressed in *Escherichia coli* (filgrastim). The other is a glycosylated form expressed in Chinese hamster ovarian cells in vitro (lenograstim). Both products have the same net effect, acceleration of myelopoiesis, and enhancement of functional responses. As an immediate effect, G-CSF causes an actual decrease of PMN count, which is followed by a sustained dose-dependent rise in PMN counts.

The G-CSF has been recommended at a dose of 5 µg/kg/day *sc* or *iv* for high-risk patients after cytotoxic cancer chemotherapy. Starting the day after the last chemotherapy dose it continues with subsequent individualized adjustment of dosage depending on the PMN count until this increases to 1000/µL for three consecutive days. A higher dosage of 10 µg/kg/day can be used in early phases of HSCT followed by a standard dose of 5 µg/kg/day or when G-CSF is administered as adjunctive therapy for a documented IFI.

The GM-CSF is a recombinant non-glycosylated protein expressed in *E. coli* (molgramostim) and glycosylated protein expressed in *Saccharomyces cerevisiae* (sargramostim) or in mammalian cells (regramostim). The GM-CSF transiently decreases leukocyte counts immediately after administration and causes sustained rises of PMN, eosinophil, and MNC counts afterwards. Various dosing regimens of GM-CSF have been used in different studies. The recommended dosage is $250 \, \mu g/m^2$ daily during the period of profound neutropenia or when a documented IFI is treated. The dosage is individualized depending on response and development of adverse effects.

The IFN-γ has been administered at a dose of $50 \, \mu g/m^2$ three times a week subcutaneously as prophylaxis in CGD patients (142). Doses up to $100 \, \mu g/m^2$ three times a week have been subsequently suggested. Similar doses have been used as adjunctive therapy.

The GM-CSF has been described in some cases as inducing pleuritic pain, pulmonary edema, and a capillary leak syndrome. Another potential complication of its use stems from its activity in stimulating recovery of leukocyte function. Massive fatal hemoptysis has been reported to follow (159). Although bone pain is described in 20% of patients receiving G-CSF, the other adverse effects associated with GM-CSF are not commonly observed in G-CSF treated patients. The toxicity of GM-CSF appears to be related to the non-glycosylated preparations expressed in *E. coli*. By comparison, the glycosylated form of GM-CSF is not associated with these adverse effects. The toxicity profile of recombinant GM-CSF is consistent with priming of macrophages for increased formation and release of inflammatory cytokines, whereas G-CSF induces production of anti-inflammatory factors, such as IL-1 receptor antagonist and soluble TNF receptor, and is protective against endotoxin- and sepsis-induced organ injury. Although administration of G-CSF to patients with acute myeloid leukemia (AML) carries the theoretical risk of accelerating the leukemic blast cells, this has not been observed. Indeed, G-CSF has been safely used in patients with AML and myelodysplasia (160). The induction of Th2 response by G-CSF may not be deleterious; indeed it may be beneficial for the mediation of excessive inflammation (161). The adverse effect of GM-CSF accelerating HIV replication in MNCs may be offset by simultaneous administration of antiretroviral agents.

With regard to IFN-γ therapy the most common adverse effects are minor and consist of "flu-like" or constitutional symptoms such as fever, headache, chills, myalgia, or fatigue. These symptoms may decrease in severity as treatment continues.

VI. WHITE BLOOD CELL TRANSFUSIONS (WBCTx)

A potential application of combined cytokine-phagocyte therapy together with antifungal chemotherapy is the transfusion of cytokine-elicited PMNs to assist recovery from antifungal chemotherapy-refractory IFIs. In a review of 32 studies, the overall efficacy of WBCTxs was 62% in 206 patients with bacterial infection (162). With regard to IFIs the data were less encouraging with a positive clinical outcome observed in only 29% of recipients. Bhatia et al. reported that there was no significant improvement in outcome of IFIs in 50 patients, despite showing the feasibility of administering WBCTx (163). However, subsequent reports have provided encouraging data with G-CSF elicited WBCTx as compared to studies that used conventional WBCTx stimulated with steroids, which necessitate follow-up studies

Table 10 Treatment of Neutropenia-Related Invasive Fungal Infections with WBCTx

Reference	Underlying Condition	No. of Pts	Fungus	Outcome
166	Aplastic anemia/BMT	1	*Aspergillus*	CR
164	Neutropenia	2	*Candida tropicalis*	2/2 CR
165	Neutropenia	15	11 molds, four yeasts	11/15 PR; (only 3/11 survived >3 months post-WBCTx)
147	CGD	1	*Aspergillus*	CR
167	Neutropenia	13	Nine *Aspergillus*	5/9 CR
			Four *Candida*	2/4 CR
168	Stem cell transplant	15	Eight molds	0/8 R
			Seven yeasts	4/7 CR
133	Hematologic cancer	7	*Fusarium*	3/7 CR
169	Neutropenia	12	Nine *Aspergillus*	4/9 CR and 1/9 PR
			Three *Candida*	2/3 CR
Total		66	46 molds	14/35 CR (40%)
			20 yeasts	10/16 CR (63%)

Abbreviations: CR, complete response; R, response; PR, partial response.
Source: Modified from Ref. 170.

(133,147,164–169) (Table 10). Indeed, in non-G-CSF strategies the number of neutrophils collected ranged between 10^9 and 10^{10}, whereas in strategies where G-CSF was combined with a corticosteroid the range was 10^{11}–10^{12} (170).

A pilot study evaluated the safety and efficacy of G-CSF-elicited WBCTxs in 15 patients with neutropenia-related IFIs that were refractory to therapy with amphotericin B alone (165). There was a favorable response reported in 11 patients at the end of therapy. Although only three of the 11 patients were alive at three months after starting WBCTx, the IFI contributed to the death in six of eight patients in the setting of persistent or progressive immunosuppression (relapsed or refractory leukemia, or allogeneic BMT). The beneficial effect of the transfusions seemed to be enhanced by their administration to patients with good performance status, as well as administration early during neutropenia and soon after onset of the IFI.

A separate prospective multicenter phase I/II clinical trial evaluated the feasibility and tolerability of WBCTxs in neutropenic patients with infection, 13 of whom had IFIs (167). A favorable outcome was observed in five of nine patients with aspergillosis, and two of four patients with yeast infections. In addition to WBCTxs, treatment consisted of amphotericin B (partly liposomal preparation) and itraconazole, as well as surgical resection of the lesions in five patients following stabilization of the septic condition. Another multicenter trial evaluated the feasibility and tolerability of PMN transfusions in neutropenic patients with refractory infections. A favorable outcome was observed in a portion of patients with yeast infections (168).

A study of WBCTx in children with cancer evaluated 15 courses of WBCTx in 13 neutropenic children with refractory bacterial and fungal infections (171) and reported a 60% response rate and without serious adverse events.

Another study evaluated WBCTx in 22 patients with hematological malignancies who developed refractory neutropenia-related bacterial and fungal infections (172). Control of infection at day 30 after the first WBCTx could be achieved in 50% of patients. In this study, the ultimate recovery of the patient's marrow was the only parameter that significantly and independently correlated with a favorable response to WBCTx.

The prophylactic use of WBCTx was described in nine allogeneic stem cell transplant recipients with either previous invasive aspergillosis or considered to be at high risk for aspergillosis during their transplant. Compared to a control, untransfused group, these nine patients had a significant reduction in the incidence and duration of fevers and maximum C-reactive protein and fewer days of neutropenia ($p < 0.05$). Radiological improvement of pulmonary infiltrates was also noted in some patients (173).

In addition, a number of successful case reports using G-CSF-mobilized WBCTxs have been reported. For example, a CGD patient with invasive aspergillosis due to *A. nidulans*, who failed five months of treatment with liposomal amphotericin B and IFN-γ, was successfully treated with BMT, G-CSF-mobilized PMNs, and liposomal amphotericin B (147). In these studies, yeast infections tended to respond to WBCTx better than mould infections (Table 10). Thus, the rapid increase in PMNs coupled with the relatively low adverse effects, suggest that WBCTx in combination with cytokines may be a useful approach and deserves further study in the setting of refractory IFIs.

The major indication for WBCTx continues to be restricted to progressive, documented infection in the profoundly and persistently neutropenic host (162). Drug-refractory IFIs in patients with underlying phagocytic defect, namely CGD, are a particularly important indication for WBCTx adjunctive therapy. Prophylactic use of WBCTx therapy has not yet been incorporated into clinical practice, primarily because of cost and toxicity. It is still unclear that WBCTx should be widely embraced until further studies are completed, which should better define its niche in supportive care. Still, this is an approach that should be investigated in multi-institutional studies so that a satisfactory enrollment can be achieved.

Patients with evidence of alloimmunization (platelet refractoriness, antileukocyte antibodies, repeated febrile transfusion reactions, or post-transfusion pulmonary infiltrates) may not benefit from WBCTx (162). This happens because they usually have a low post-transfusion increment, more pulmonary reactions and transfused PMNs unable to migrate to the sites of infection.

The higher the number of cells transfused per square meter of body surface area, the better the clinical response to WBCTx (174–177). For mobilization of PMNs in healthy donors, most experts have favored G-CSF, which is indeed, the standard method in blood processing centers (178). Both forms of G-CSF commercially available have the same net effect, acceleration of myelopoiesis, and enhancement of functional responses (including bactericidal activity, chemotaxis, phagocytosis, respiratory burst, and surface expression of low affinity Fc receptors) (179–181). The G-CSF also delays apoptosis in PMNs, which is particularly important for harvested PMNs, because it appears that G-CSF-stimulated PMNs have a longer shelf life and perhaps, once transfused, persist longer in vivo (182,183).

The G-CSF increases the yield of PMNs by roughly five fold, which is greater than the 2–3-fold increase accomplished with prednisolone (50–100 mg given intravenously or orally once 2 hr before the donation) or dexamethasone (8 mg given orally 12 hr before the donation) (167,168). Four hundred fifty micrograms of G-CSF has been recommended as optimal safe dose required for mobilization of PMNs in adults (48). Only one dose is needed 12–24 hr prior to collection. Several recent studies have evaluated the role of the combination of G-CSF and corticosteroids, suggesting that the higher dose of the former with the latter results in the highest yield (12-fold above premobilization) (184). The functional properties of G-CSF-mobilized PMNs are essentially unchanged. Specifically, the respiratory burst activity is normal or elevated, due to priming of PMNs. The half-life of transfused PMNs previously mobilized with G-CSF is at least twice as long (184). Single dose exposure to corticosteroids probably does not represent a major suppressant of PMN function in mobilized products. No G-CSF related long-term effects have been observed to the donors, even one year later, when all hematological measurements were comparable to pre-G-CSF levels (185,186). Storage at 10°C might lengthen the shelf life of mobilized PMNs and may preserve antifungal and PMN function better (187).

The leukapheresis technique used today is the continuous flow centrifugation with the addition of a rouleauxing agent such as hydroxyethyl, which produces a better quality PMN (186). This technique is very advantageous over previous techniques. It allows processing of larger volumes of blood, which has been translated into increased yields. Traditionally, related donors have been preferred to avoid toxicity related to incompatibility, but more recently, community donors have been effectively used to safely and rapidly mobilize PMNs, thus increasing the availability of WBCTxs to a larger number of individuals for whom the indication is sound (168).

The WBCTxs have been associated with a low incidence of complications. Mild reactions to the transfusion product are common, including fever and chills, which can be reduced if the infusion rate is reduced. Severe side effects, namely hypotension or respiratory distress, are estimated to occur in ~1% of recipients. In two reports, respiratory complications have been temporally linked to co-administration of deoxycholate amphotericin B (188,189). Transfusion-related acute lung injury is rare and probably not associated with G-CSF mobilization (190). The GVHD is prevented by irradiation of the product pre-infusion with 15–30 Gy, which does not appear to adversely affect the function of the transfused PMNs (191). Alloimmunization can be a formidable problem in CGD patients, but interestingly does not occur in cancer or transplant recipients, who have received immunosuppressive therapy. A recent study in HSCT reported that recipients who received G-CSF-mobilized PMNs from an incompatible donor had a delayed engraftment (192).

VII. OTHER MODES OF ADJUNCTIVE IMMUNOTHERAPY

Antibody-mediated host defense contributes to fighting against certain IFIs. Mice with experimental *Candida* infection treated with human IV immunoglobulin (IVIG) combined with amphotericin B had modest prolongation of survival, suggesting the potential efficacy of serum antibodies against fungi (193).

In humans, IVIG has been used in liver transplant recipients receiving anticytomegalovirus prophylaxis and in patients who had undergone BMT. In the first case, IVIG therapy was associated with a significant reduction in the incidence of IFIs (194), whereas in the second group, therapy was not associated with a significant reduction (195). This finding was despite a previous finding that oral administration of bovine anti-*C. albicans* antibodies to BMT recipients reduced *Candida* colonization in seven of 10 patients (196), which suggests that pathogen-specific antibodies can be effective in patients with immune defects.

For both *C. albicans* and *C. neoformans*, several protective monoclonal antibodies have been described not always with success (reviewed in Ref. 197).

Human serum antibodies and a mouse monoclonal antibody to fungal heat shock protein 90 (hsp90) were protective against candidiasis in mice as well as a human recombinant antibody to a hsp90 linear epitope mediated protection against invasive murine candidiasis (198). Mycograb, a human genetically recombinant antibody against fungal hsp90 synergized with amphotericin B for complete resolution of infection in models of murine candidiasis (199). Antibodies to *C. albicans* polysaccharides have also been shown to be protective in murine models of infection (200).

Another approach to antibody therapy has been to engineer antibodies with dual functions, or bispecific antibodies. A bispecific antibody that binds both the Fcα receptor (CD89) and *C. albicans* has been shown to enhance PMN-mediated antifungal activity in G-CSF-primed cells (201). However, although serum antibodies may promote natural resistance to infection, they may not necessarily ameliorate established or chronic infections. Hence, their efficacy against some fungi may be dependent on intact cellular immunity (202). Therefore, their clinical use has not been recommended in the management of IFIs.

The T-cell adoptive therapy and vaccination seems to be a promising strategy of prevention or even adjunctive therapy of IFIs in immunocompromised patients. Studies have begun to assess the ability of fungal antigens to induce Th1 type reactivity as potential candidates for fungal vaccines. Treatment of immunocompetent mice with *Aspergillus* crude culture filtrate antigens resulted in the development of local and peripheral protective Th1 memory responses. This finding suggests the existence of fungal antigens useful as a potential candidate vaccine against invasive pulmonary aspergillosis (203).

VIII. FUTURE DIRECTIONS

In view of the drug-resistant nature of many IFIs, the promise of certain immunotherapeutic agents underscores the need for interdisciplinary research to establish parameters for their use, and presents a major challenge to clinicians and scientists to translate preclinical data on immunotherapeutic agents into clinical benefit. In tandem with destroying fungi using potent antifungal agents, reconstitution and up-regulation of immune response by either exogenous administration of cytokines or transfusion of cytokine-elicited allogeneic phagocytes appear to be promising adjuncts to antifungal chemotherapy for these life-threatening infections. Further evaluation of the safety and efficacy of immunotherapeutic modalities is an urgent priority for research during the near future. Well-controlled studies in patients at very high risk of developing fungal infections, such as profoundly neutropenic, HSCT patients, should be the goal of future studies. The large number of immune defects that predispose to fungal infections, the biological differences among fungi, and the variable responses to immune modulators are likely to complicate the design of clinical studies, and large sample sizes will likely be required for valid conclusions. If such studies are proved to be impossible, physicians are left with great amount of positive preclinical data but with limited clinical proof of efficacy of the immunotherapy as adjunctive treatment of IFIs that are difficult to treat otherwise. Unfortunately, this is not the only management strategy in Medicine that is supported by theoretical and preclinical data but lacks statistically significant clinical proof, as we understand this proof in the beginning of the 21st century.

IX. CONCLUSIONS

The increasing incidence of IFIs and the emergence of previously rare opportunistic fungal pathogens is of major importance in the management of immunocompromised patients. The prevention and treatment of IFIs, which are still a great challenge for clinicians, may be greatly enhanced by strategies to normalize host defense mechanisms. This has been experimentally achieved by reconstitution of effector cells numerically and/or functionally with cytokines and/or WBCTx, or by manipulation of cytokine dysbalance. Undoubtedly, immunotherapy is a promising therapy and the interest in its use as adjuncts to antifungal agents has been extremely increased. Evaluation of the benefits of the HGF/cytokine prevention and adjunctive therapy with concomitant antifungal therapy are urgent priorities for clinical research. A better understanding of the synergy between cytokines and specific antifungal agents may provide additional powerful tools for managing these serious infections.

REFERENCES

1. Denning DW. Invasive aspergillosis. Clin Infect Dis 1998; 26:781–803.
2. McNeil MM, Nash SL, Hajjeh RA, Phelan MA, Conn LA, Plikaytis BD, Warnock DW. Trends in mortality due to invasive mycotic diseases in the United States, 1980–1997. Clin Infect Dis 2001; 33:641–647.
3. Marr KA, Carter RA, Crippa F, Wald A, Corey L. Epidemiology and outcome of mould infections in hematopoietic stem cell transplant recipients. Clin Infect Dis 2002; 34:909–917.
4. Grossi P, Farina C, Fiocchi R, Dalla Gasperina D. Prevalence and outcome of invasive fungal infections in 1,963 thoracic organ transplant recipients: a multicenter retrospective study. Italian Study Group of Fungal Infections in Thoracic Organ Transplant Recipients. Transplantation 2000; 70:112–116.
5. Singh N, Wagener MM, Marino IR, Gayowski T. Trends in invasive fungal infections in liver transplant recipients: correlation with evolution in transplantation practices. Transplantation 2002; 73:63–67.
6. Winkelstein JA, Marino MC, Johnston RB, Boyle J, Curnutte J, Gallin JI, Malech HL, Holland SM, Ochs H, Quie P, Buckley RH, Foster CB, Chanock SJ, Dickler H. Chronic granulomatous disease. Report on a national registry of 368 patients. Medicine (Baltimore) 2000; 79:155–169.
7. Roilides E, Dignani MC, Anaissie EJ, Rex JH. The role of immunoreconstitution in the management of refractory opportunistic fungal infections. Med Mycol 1998; 36:12–25.
8. Roilides E, Dotis J, Filioti J, Anaissie E. Adjunctive antifungal therapy. In: Dismukes E, Pappas PG, Sobel JD, eds. Clinical Mycology. New York: Oxford University Press, 2003:125–139.
9. Romani L. Innate immunity against fungal pathogens. In: Calderone R, Cihlar R, eds. Fungal Pathogenesis: Principles and Clinical Applications. New York: Marcel Dekker Inc., 2001:401–432.
10. Ibrahim-Granet O, Philippe B, Boleti H, Boisvieux-Ulrich E, Grenet D, Stern M, Latge JP. Phagocytosis and intracellular fate of *Aspergillus fumigatus* conidia in alveolar macrophages. Infect Immun 2003; 71:891–903.
11. Calera JA, Paris S, Monod M, Hamilton AJ, Debeaupuis JP, Diaquin M, Lopez-Medrano R, Leal F, Latge JP. Cloning and disruption of the antigenie catalase gene of *Aspergillus fumigatus*. Infect Immun 1997; 65:4718–4724.
12. Philippe B, Ibrahim-Granet O, Prevost MC, Gougerot-Pocidalo MA, Sanchez Perez M, Van der Meeren A, Latge JP. Killing of *Aspergillus fumigatus* by alveolar macrophages is mediated by reactive oxidant intermediates. Infect Immun 2003; 71:3034–3042.

13. Clemons KV, Stevens DA. Overview of host defense mechanisms in systemic mycoses and the basis for immunotherapy. Semin Respir Infect 2001; 16:60–66.
14. Farmaki E, Roilides E. Immunotherapy in patients with systemic mycoses: a promising adjunct. BioDrugs 2001; 15:207–214.
15. Lin SJ, Schranz J, Teutsch SM. Aspergillosis case-fatality rate: systematic review of the literature. Clin Infect Dis 2001; 32:358–366.
16. Casadevall A, Pirofski LA. Adjunctive immune therapy for fungal infections. Clin Infect Dis 2001; 33:1048–1056.
17. Roilides E, Farmaki E, Lyman CA. Immune reconstitution against human mycoses. In: Calderone R, Cihlar R, eds. Fungal Pathogenesis: Principles and Clinical Applications. New York: Marcel Dekker Inc., 2001:433–460.
18. Polak-Wyss A. Protective effect of human granulocyte colony-stimulating factor on *Cryptococcus* and *Aspergillus* infections in normal and immunosuppressed mice. Mycoses 1991; 34:205–215.
19. Polak-Wyss A. Protective effect of human granulocyte colony-stimulating factor on *Candida* infections in normal and immunosuppressed mice. Mycoses 1991; 34:109–118.
20. Graybill JR, Bocanegra R, Najvar LK, Loebenberg D, Luther MF. Granulocyte colony-stimulating factor and azole antifungal therapy in murine aspergillosis: role of immune suppression. Antimicrob Agents Chemother 1998; 42:2467–2473.
21. Clemons KV, Grunig G, Sobel RA, Mirels LF, Rennick DM, Stevens DA. Role of IL-10 in invasive aspergillosis: increased resistance of IL-10 gene knockout mice to lethal systemic aspergillosis. Clin Exp Immunol 2000; 122:186–191.
22. Mehrad B, Strieter RM, Standiford TJ. Role of TNF-alpha in pulmonary host defense in murine invasive aspergillosis. J Immunol 1999; 162:1633–1640.
23. Kullberg BJ, van der Meer JW, Meis JF, Keuter M, Curfs JH, Netea MG. Recombinant murine granulocyte colony-stimulating factor protects against acute disseminated *Candida albicans* infection in nonneutropenic mice. J Infect Dis 1998; 177:175–181.
24. Graybill JR, Bocanerga R, Luther M. Antifungal combination with G-CSF and fluconazole in experimental disseminated candidiasis. Eur J Clin Microbiol Infect Dis 1995; 14:700–703.
25. Hamood M, Bluche PF, De Vroey C, Corazza F, Buzan W, Fondu P. Effects of rhG-CSF on neutropenic mice infected with *C. albicans*: acceleration of recovery from neutropenia and potentiation of anti-*Candida* resistance. Mycoses 1994; 37:93–99.
26. Uchida K, Yamamoto Y, Klein TW, Friedman H, Yamaguchi H. Granulocyte-colony stimulating factor facilitates the restoration of resistance to opportunistic fungi in leukopenic mice. J Med Vet Mycol 1992; 30:293–300.
27. Mayer P, Schutze C, Lam C, Kricek F, Liehl E. Recombinant murine granulocyte-macrophage colony-stimulating factor augments neutrophil recovery and enhances resistance to infections in myelosuppressed mice. J Infect Dis 1991; 163:584–590.
28. Cenci E, Bartocci A, Puccetti P, Mocci S, Stanely ER, Bistoni F. Macrophage colony-stimulating factor in murine candidiasis: serum and tissue levels during infection and protective effect of exogenous administration. Infect Immun 1991; 59:868–872.
29. Vitt CR, Fidler JM, Ando D, Zimmerman RJ, Aukerman SL. Antifungal activity of rhM-CSF in models of acute and chronic candidiasis in the rat. J Infect Dis 1994; 169:369–374.
30. Kuhara T, Uchida K, Yamaguchi H. Therapeutic efficacy of human macrophage colony-stimulating factor, used alone and in combination with antifungal agents, in mice with systemic *Candida albicans* infection. Antimicrob Agents Chemother 2000; 44:19–23.
31. Gonzalez CE, Lyman CA, Lee S, Del Guercio C, Roilides E, Bacher J, Gehrt A, Feuerstein E, Tsokos M, Walsh TJ. Recombinant human macrophage colony-stimulating factor augments pulmonary host defences against *Aspergillus fumigatus*. Cytokine 2001; 15:87–95.

32. Kullberg BJ, Van't Wout JW, Hoogstraten C, Van Furth R. Recombinant interferon-γ enhances resistance to acute disseminated *Candida albicans* infection in mice. J Infect Dis 1993; 168:436–443.

33. Cano LE, Kashino SS, Arruda C, Andre D, Xidieh CF, Singer-Vermes LM, Vaz CA, Burger E, Calich VL. Protective role of gamma interferon in experimental pulmonary paracoccidioidomycosis. Infect Immun 1998; 66:800–806.

34. Nagai H, Guo J, Choi H, Kurup V. Interferon-gamma and tumor necrosis factor-alpha protect mice from invasive aspergillosis. J Infect Dis 1995; 172:1554–1560.

35. Schelenz S, Smith DA, Bancroft GJ. Cytokine and chemokine responses following pulmonary challenge with *Aspergillus fumigatus*: obligatory role of TNF-α and GM-CSF in neutrophil recruitment. Med Mycol 1999; 37:183–194.

36. van't Wout JW, van der Meer JWM, Barza M, Dinarello CA. Protection of neutropenic mice from lethal *Candida albicans* infection by recombinant interleukin 1. Eur J Immunol 1988; 18:1143–1146.

37. Kullberg BJ, van't Wout YN, Poell RJ, van Furth R. Combined effect of fluconazole and recombinant human interleukin-1 on systemic candidiasis in neutropenic mice. Antimicrob Agents Chemother 1992; 36:1225–1229.

38. Tonnetti L, Spaccapelo R, Cenci E, Mencacci A, Puccetti P, Coffman RL, Bistoni F, Romani L. Interleukin-4 and -10 exacerbate candidiasis in mice. Eur J Immunol 1995; 25:1559–1565.

39. Cenci E, Mencacci A, Del Sero G, Bacci A, Montagnoli C, Fe d'Ostiani C, Mosci P, Bachmann M, Bistoni F, Kopf M, Romani L. Interleukin-4 causes susceptibility to invasive aspergillosis through suppression of protective type 1 responses. J Infect Dis 1999; 180:1957–1968.

40. Romani L, Puccetti P, Mencacci A, Cenci E, Spaccapelo R, Tonnetti L, Grohmann U, Bistoni F. Neutralization of IL-10 upregulates nitric oxide production and protects susceptible mice from challenge with *Candida albicans*. J Immunol 1994; 152:3514–3521.

41. Del Sero G, Mencacci A, Cenci E, d'Ostiani CF, Montagnoli C, Bacci A, Mosci P, Kopf M, Romani L. Antifungal type 1 responses are upregulated in IL-10-deficient mice. Microbes Infect 1999; 1:1169–1180.

42. Arruda C, Franco MF, Kashino SS, Nascimento FR, Fazioli Rdos A, Vaz CA, Russo M, Calich VL. Interleukin-12 protects mice against disseminated infection caused by *Paracoccidioides brasiliensis* but enhances pulmonary inflammation. Clin Immunol 2002; 103:185–195.

43. Nemunaitis J. A comparative review of colony-stimulating factors. Drugs 1997; 54: 709–729.

44. Lieschke GJ, Burgess AW. Granulocyte colony-stimulating factor and granulocyte-macrophage colony-stimulating factor (1). N Engl J Med 1992; 327:28–35.

45. Yamamoto Y, Klein TW, Freidman H, Kimura S, Yamaguchi H. Granulocyte-colony stimulating factor potentiates anti-*Candida albicans* growth inhibitory activity of polymorphonuclear cells. FEMS Immunol Med Microbiol 1993; 7:15–22.

46. Roilides E, Uhlig K, Venzon D, Pizzo PA, Walsh TJ. Enhancement of oxidative response and damage caused by human neutrophils to *Aspergilhis fumigatus* hyphae by granulocyte colony-stimulating factor and gamma interferon. Infect Immun 1993; 61:1185–1193.

47. Roilides E, Holmes A, Blake C, Pizzo PA, Walsh TJ. Effects of granulocyte colony-stimulating factor and interferon-γ on antifungal activity of human polymorphonuclear neutrophils against pseudohyphae of different medically important *Candida* species. J Leukoc Biol 1995; 57:651–656.

48. Liles WC, Huang JE, van Burik JA, Bowden RA, Dale DC. Granulocyte colony-stimulating factor administered in vivo augments neutrophil-mediated activity against opportunistic fungal pathogens. J Infect Dis 1997; 175:1012–1015.

49. Roilides E, Uhlig K, Venzon D, Pizzo PA, Walsh TJ. Prevention of corticosteroid-induced suppression of human polymorphonuclear leukocyte-induced damage of

Aspergillus fumigatus hyphae by granulocyte colony-stimulating factor and interferon-γ. Infect Immun 1993; 61:4870–4877.

50. Hubel K, Dale DC, Liles WC. Therapeutic use of cytokines to modulate phagocyte function for the treatment of infectious diseases: current status of granulocyte colony-stimulating factor, granulocyte-macrophage colony-stimulating factor, macrophage colony-stimulating factor, and interferon-gamma. J Infect Dis 2002; 185:1490–1501.

51. Ono M, Matsumoto M, Matsubara S, Tomioka S, Asano S. Protective effect of human granulocyte colony-stimulating factor on bacterial and fungal infections in neutropenic mice. Behring Inst Mitt 1988:216–221.

52. Arpinati M, Green CL, Heimfeld S, Heuser JE, Anasetti C. Grsanulocyte-colony stimulating factor mobilizes T helper 2-inducing dendritic cells. Blood 2000; 95: 2484–2490.

53. Vecchiarelli A, Morani C, Baldelli F, Pietrella D, Retini C, Tascini C, Francisci D, Bistoni F. Beneficial effect of recombinant human granulocyte colony-forming factor on fungicidal activity of polymorphonuclear leukocytes from patients with AIDS. J Infect Dis 1995; 171:1448–1454.

54. Natarajan U, Brummer E, Stevens DA. Effect of granulocyte colony-stimulating factor on the candidacidal activity of polymorphonuclear neutrophils and their collaboration with fluconazole. Antimicrob Agents Chemother 1997; 41:1575–1578.

55. Vora S, Chauhan S, Brummer E, Stevens DA. Activity of voriconazole combined with neutrophils or monocytes against *Aspergillus fumigatus*: effects of granulocyte colony-stimulating factor and granulocyte-macrophage colony-stimulating factor. Antimicrob Agents Chemother 1998; 42:2299–2303.

56. Rodriguez-Adrian LJ, Grazziutti ML, Rex JH, Anaissie EJ. The potential role of cytokine therapy for fungal infections in patients with cancer: is recovery from neutropenia all that is needed? Clin Infect Dis 1998; 26:1270–1278.

57. Smith PD, Lamerson CL, Banks SM, Saini SS, Wahl LM, Calderone RA, Wahl SM. Granulocyte-macrophage colony-stimulating factor augments human monocyte fungicidal activity for *Candida albicans*. J Infect Dis 1990; 161:999–1005.

58. Roilides E, Holmes A, Blake C, Venzon D, Pizzo PA, Walsh TJ. Antifungal activity of elutriated human monocytes against *Aspergillus fumigatus* hyphae: Enhancement by granulocyte-macrophage colony-stimulating factor and interferon-γ. J Infect Dis 1994; 170:894–899.

59. Lyman CA, Garrett KF, Pizzo PA, Walsh TJ. Response of human polymorphonuclear leukocytes and monocytes to *Trichosporon beigeli*: host defense against an emerging opportunistic pathogen. J Infect Dis 1994; 170:1557–1565.

60. Roilides E, Blake C, Holmes A, Pizzo PA, Walsh TJ. Granulocyte-macrophage colony-stimulating factor and interferon-γ prevent dexamethasone-induced immunosuppression of antifungal monocyte activity against *Aspergillus fumigatus* hyphae. J Med Vet Mycol 1996; 34:63–69.

61. Muranaka H, Suga M, Nakagawa K, Sato K, Gushima Y, Ando M. Effects of granulocyte and granulocyte-macrophage colony-stimulating factors in a neutropenic murine model of trichosporonosis. Infect Immun 1997; 65:3422–3429.

62. Karbassi A, Becker JM, Foster JS, Moore RN. Enhanced killing of *Candida albicans* by murine macrophages treated with macrophage colony-stimulating factor: evidence for augmented expression of mannose receptors. J Immunol 1987; 139:417–421.

63. Roilides E, Sein T, Holmes A, Blake C, Pizzo PA, Walsh TJ. Effects of macrophage colony-stimulating factor on antifungal activity of mononuclear phagocytes against *Aspergillus fumigatus*. J Infect Dis 1995; 172:1028–1034.

64. Wing EJ, Ampel NM, Waheed A, Shadduck RK. Macrophage colony-stimulating factor (M-CSF) enhances the capacity of murine macrophages to secrete oxygen reduction products. J Immunol 1985; 135:2052–2056.

65. Murray HW. Interferon-gamma and host antimicrobial defense: current and future clinical applications. Am J Med 1994; 97:459–467.

66. Djeu JY, Blanchard DK, Halkias D, Friedman H. Growth inhibition of *Candida albicans* by human polymorphonuclear neutrophils: activation by interferon-gamma and tumor necrosis factor. J Immunol 1986; 137:2980–2984.

67. Morrison CJ, Brummer E, Isenberg RA, Stevens DA. Activation of murine polymorphonuclear neutrophils for fungicidal activity by recombinant gamma interferon. J Leukoc Biol 1987; 41:434–440.

68. Gaviria JM, van Burik JA, Dale DC, Root RK, Liles WC. Comparison of interferon-gamma, granulocyte colony-stimulating factor, and granulocyte-macrophage colony-stimulating factor for priming leukocyte-mediated hyphal damage of opportunistic fungal pathogens. J Infect Dis 1999; 179:1038–1041.

69. Lutz JE, Clemons KV, Stevens DA. Enhancement of antifungal chemotherapy by interferon-gamma in experimental systemic cryptococcosis. J Antimicrob Chemother 2000; 46:437–442.

70. Trinchieri G. Interleukin-12: a proinflammatory cytokine with immunoregulatory functions that bridge innate resistance and antigen-specific adaptive immunity. Annu Rev Immunol 1995; 13:251–276.

71. Trinchieri G. Interleukin-12: a cytokine produced by antigen-presenting cells with immunoregulatory functions in the generation of T-helper cells type 1 and cytotoxic lymphocytes. Blood 1994; 84:4008–4027.

72. Romani L, Puccetti P, Bistoni F. Interleukin-12 in infectious diseases. Clin Microbiol Rev 1997; 10:611–636.

73. Clemons KV, Brummer E, Stevens DA. Cytokine treatment of central nervous system infection: efficacy of interleukin-12 alone and synergy with conventional antifungal therapy in experimental cryptococcosis. Antimicrob Agents Chemother 1994; 38:460–464.

74. Zhou P, Sieve MC, Bennett J, Kwon-Chung KJ, Tewari RP, Gazzinelli RT, Sher A, Seder RA. IL-12 prevents mortality in mice infected with *Histoplasma capsulatum* through induction of IFN-gamma. J Immunol 1995; 155:785–795.

75. Magee DM, Cox RA. Interleukin-12 regulation of host defenses against *Coccidioides immitis*. Infect Immun 1996; 64:3609–3613.

76. Brieland JK, Jackson C, Menzel F, Loebenberg D, Cacciapuoti A, Halpern J, Hurst S, Muchamuel T, Debets R, Kastelein R, Churakova T, Abrams J, Hare R, O'Garra A. Cytokine networking in lungs of immunocompetent mice in response to inhaled *Aspergillus fumigatus*. Infect Immun 2001; 96:1554–1560.

77. Mencacci A, Cenci E, Bacci A, Bistoni F, Romani L. Host immune reactivity determines the efficacy of combination immunotherapy and antifungal chemotherapy in candidiasis. J Infect Dis 2000; 181:686–694.

78. Romani L, Mencacci A, Cenci E, Spaccapelo R, Del Sero G, Nicoletti I, Trinchieri G, Bistoni F, Puccetti P. Neutrophil production of IL-12 and IL-10 in candidiasis and efficacy of IL-12 therapy in neutropenic mice. J Immunol 1997; 158:5349–5356.

79. Fehniger TA, Caligiuri MA. Interleukin 15: biology and relevance to human disease. Blood 2001; 97:14–32.

80. Musso T, Calosso L, Zucca M, Millesimo M, Puliti M, Bulfone-Paus S, Merlino C, Savoia D, Cavallo R, Ponzi AN, Badolato R. Interleukin-15 activates proinflammatory and antimicrobial functions in polymorphonuclear cells. Infect Immun 1998; 66:2640–2647.

81. Vazquez N, Walsh TJ, Friedman D, Chanock SJ, Lyman CA. Interleukin-15 augments superoxide production and microbicidal activity of human monocytes against *Candida albicans*. Infect Immun 1998; 66:145–150.

82. Winn RM, Gil-Lamaignere C, Roilides E, Simitsopoulou M, Lyman CA, Maloukou A, Walsh TJ. Selective effects of interleukin-15 on antifungal activity and interleukin-8 release by polymorphonuclear leukocytes in response to hyphae of *Aspergillus* spp. J Infect Dis 2003; 188:585–590.

83. Roilides E, Dimitriadou-Georgiadou A, Sein T, Kadiltzoglou I, Walsh TJ. Tumor necrosis factor alpha enhances antifungal activities of polymorphonuclear and mononuclear phagocytes against *Aspergillus fumigatus*. Infect Immun 1998; 66:5999–6003.

84. Louie A, Baltch AL, Smith RP, Franke MA, Ritz WJ, Singh JK, Gordno MA. Tumor necrosis factor alpha has a protective role in a murine model of systemic candidiasis. Infect Immun 1994; 62:2761–2772.

85. Ferrante A. Tumor necrosis factor alpha potentiates neutrophil antimicrobial activity: increased fungicidal activity against *Torulopsis glabrata* and *Candida albicans* and associated increases in oxygen radical production and lysosomal enzyme release. Infect Immun 1989; 57:2115–2122.

86. Diamond RD, Lyman CA, Wysong DR. Disparate effects of interferon-gamma and tumor necrosis factor-alpha on early neutrophil respiratory burst and fungicidal responses to *Candida albicans* hyphae in vitro. J Clin Invest 1991; 87:711–720.

87. Warris A, Bjomeklett A, Gaustad P. Invasive pulmonary aspergillosis associated with infliximab therapy. N Engl J Med 2001; 344:1099–1100.

88. De Rosa FG, Shaz D, Campagna AC, Dellaripa PE, Khettry U, Craven DE. Invasive pulmonary aspergillosis soon after therapy with infliximab, a tumor necrosis factor-alpha-neutralizing antibody: a possible healthcare-associated case? Infect Control Hosp Epidemiol 2003; 24:477–482.

89. Roilides E, Kadiltsoglou I, Dimitriadou A, Hatzistilianou M, Manitsa A, Karpouzas J, Pizzo PA, Walsh TJ. Interleukin-4 suppresses antifungal activity of human mononuclear phagocytes against *Candida albicans* in association with decreased uptake of blastoconidia. FEMS Immunol Med Microbiol 1997; 19:169–180.

90. Cenci E, Romani L, Mencacci A, Spaccapelo R, Schiaffella E, Puccetti P, Bistoni F. Interleukin-4 and interleukin-10 inhibit nitric oxide-dependent macrophage killing of *Candida albicans*. Eur J Immunol 1993; 23:1034–1038.

91. Whitehead RP, Lew D, Flanigan RC, Weiss GR, Roy V, Glode ML, Dakhil SR, Crawford ED. Phase II trial of recombinant human interleukin-4 in patients with advanced renal cell carcinoma: a southwest oncology group study. J Immunother 2002; 25:352–358.

92. Roilides E, Dimitriadou A, Kadiltsoglou I, Sein T, Karpouzas J, Pizzo PA, Walsh TJ. IL-10 exerts suppressive and enhancing effects on antifungal activity of mononuclear phagocytes against *Aspergillus fumigatus*. J Immunol 1997; 158:322–329.

93. Roilides E, Katsifa H, Tsaparidou S, Stergiopoulou T, Panteliadis C, Walsh TJ. Interleukin-10 suppresses phagocytic and antihyphal activities of human neutrophils. Cytokine 2000; 12:379–387.

94. Kimball AB, Kawamura T, Tejura K, Boss C, Hancox AR, Vogel JC, Steinberg SM, Turner ML, Blauvelt A. Clinical and immunologic assessment of patients with psoriasis in a randomized, double-blind, placebo-controlled trial using recombinant human interleukin 10. Arch Dermatol 2002; 138:1341–1346.

95. Tilg H, van Montfrans C, van den Ende A, Kaser A, van Deventer SJ, Schreiber S, Gregor M, Ludwiczek O, Rutgeerts P, Gasche C, Koningsberger JC, Abreu L, Kuhn I, Cohard M, LeBeaut A, Grint P, Weiss G. Treatment of Crohn's disease with recombinant human interleukin 10 induces the proinflammatory cytokine interferon gamma. Gut 2002; 50:191–195.

96. Akpogheneta O, Roilides E, Filioti J, Gil-Lamaignere C, Panteliadis C, Petrikkou E, Rodriguez-Tudela JL, T WJ. Combined effects of amphotericin B formulations and azoles on human neutrophil (PMN)-induced damage to hyphae of *Aspergillus fumigatus* and *Aspergillus nidulans*. 40th Interscience Conference Antimicrob Agents Chemother, Toronto Canada, 2000.

97. Roilides E, Lyman CA, Filioti J, Akpogheneta O, Sein T, Gil-Lamaignere C, Petraitiene R, Walsh TJ. Amphotericin B formulations exert additive antifungal activity in combination with pulmonary alveolar macrophages and polymorphonuclear leukocytes against *Aspergillus fumigatus*. Antimicrob Agents Chemother 2002; 46:1974–1976.

98. Chiller T, Farrokhshad K, Brummer E, Stevens DA. The interaction of human monocytes, monocyte-derived macrophages, and polymorphonuclear neutrophils with caspofungin (MK-0991), an echinocandin, for antifungal activity against *Aspergillus fumigatus*. Diagn Microbiol Infect Dis 2001; 39:99–103.

99. Gil-Lamaignere C, Roilides E, Mosquera J, Maloukou A, Walsh TJ. Antifungal triazoles and polymorphonuclear leukocytes synergize to cause increased hyphal damage to *Scedosporium prolificans* and *Scedosporiun apiospermum*. Antimicrob Agents Chemother 2002; 46:2234–2237.

100. Gil-Lamaignere C, Roilides E, Maloukou A, Georgopoulou I, Petrikkos G, Walsh TJ. Amphotericin B lipid complex exerts additive antifungal activity in combination with polymorphonuclear leucocytes against *Scedosporium prolificans* and *Scedosporium apiospermum*. J Antimicrob Chemother 2002; 50:1027–1030.

101. Vora S, Chauhan S, Brummer E, Stevens DA. Activity of voriconazole combined with neutrophils or monocytes against *Aspergillus fumigatus*: effects of granulocyte colony-stimulating factor and granulocyte-macrophage colony-stimulating factor. Antimicrob Agents Chemother 1998; 42:2299–2303.

102. Winn R, Roilides E, Maloukou A, Simitsopoulou M, Gil-Lamaignere C, Walsh T. Combined effect of interferon-gamma and voriconazole on neutrophil-induced hyphal damage of *Aspergillus fumigatus*. 40th Annual Meeting of the Infectious Diseases Society of America (IDSA), Chicago, IL, 2002.

103. American Society of Clinical Oncology. Recommendations for the use of hematopoietic colony-stimulating factors: evidence-based, clinical practice guidelines. J Clin Oncol 1994; 12:2471–2508.

104. Boogaerts MA, Demuynck HM. Consensus on the clinical use of myeloid growth factors. Curr Opin Hematol 1996; 3:241–246.

105. Nemunaitis J, Buckner CD, Dorsey KS, Willis D, Meyer W, Appelbaum F. Retrospective analysis of infectious disease in patients who received recombinant human granulocyte-macrophage colony-stimulating factor versus patients not receiving a cytokine who underwent autologous bone marrow transplantation for treatment of lymphoid cancer. Am J Clin Oncol 1998; 21:341–346.

106. Seipelt G. Clinical use of hematopoietic growth factors. Antibiot Chemother 2000; 50:94–105.

107. Crawford J, Ozer H, Stoller R, Johnson D, Lyman G, Tabbara I, Kris M, Grous J, Picozzi V, Rausch G, Smith R, Gradishar W, Yahanda A, Vincent M, Stewart M, Glaspy J. Reduction by granulocyte colony-stimulating factor of fever and neutropenia induced by chemotherapy in patients with small-cell lung cancer. N Engl J Med 1991; 325:164–170.

108. Rowe JM, Anderson JW, Mazza JJ, Bennett JM, Paietta E, Hayes FA, Oette R, Cassileth PA, Stadtmauer EA, Wiernik PH. A randomized placebo-controlled phase III study of granulocyte-macrophage colony-stimulating factor in adult patients (>55 to 70 years) with acute myelogenous leukemia: a study by the Eastern Cooperative Oncology Group (E1490). Blood 1995; 86:457–462.

109. Peters BG, Adkins DR, Harrison B, Velasquez WS, Dunphy FR, Petruska PJ, Bowers CE, Niemeyer R, McIntyre W, Vrahnos D, Auberry SE, Spitzer G. Antifungal effects of yeast-derived rhu-GM-CSF in patients receiving high-dose chemotherapy given with or without autologous stem cell transplantation: a retrospective analysis. Bone Marrow Transplant 1996; 18:93–102.

110. Giles FJ. Monocyte-macrophages, granulocyte-macrophage colony-stimulatmg factor, and prolonged survival among patients with acute myeloid leukemia and stem cell transplants. Clin Infect Dis 1998; 26:1282–1289.

111. Rowe JM. Treatment of acute myeloid leukemia with cytokines: effect on duration of neutropenia and response to infections. Clin Infect Dis 1998; 26:1290–1294.

112. Maher DW, Lieschke GJ, Green M, Bishop J, Stuart-Harris R, Wolf M, Sheridan WP, Kefford RF, Cebon J, Olver I, McKendrick J, Toner G, Bradstock K, Lieschke M,

Bruickshank S, Tomita DK, Hoffman EW, Fox RM, Morstyn G. Filgrastim in patients with chemotherapy-induced febrile neutropenia. A double-blind, placebo-controlled trial. Ann Intern Med 1994; 121:492–501.

113. Anaissie EJ, Vartivarian S, Bodey GP, Legrand C, Kantarjian H, Abi-Said D, Karl C, Vadhan-Raj S. Randomized comparison between antibiotics alone and antibiotics plus granulocyte-macrophage colony-stimulating factor (*Escherichia coli*-derived in cancer patients with fever and neutropenia. Am J Med 1996; 100:17–23.

114. Aviles A, Guzman R, Garcia EL, Talavera A, Diaz-Maqueo JC. Results of a randomized trial of granulocyte colony-stimulating factor in patients with infection and severe granulocytopenia. Anti-cancer Agents 1996; 7:392–397.

115. Ohno R, Miyawaki S, Hatake K, Kuriyama K, Saito K, Kanamaru A, Kobayashi T, Kodera Y, Nishikawa K, Matsuda S, Yamada O, Omoto E, Takeyama H, Tsukuda K, Asou N, Tanimoto M, Shiozaki H, Tomonaga M, Masaoka T, Miura Y, Takaku F, Ohashi Y, Motoyoshi K. Human urinary macrophage colony-stimulating factor reduces the incidence duration of febrile neutropenia shortens the period required to finish three courses of intensive consolidation therapy in acute myeloid leukemia: a double-blind controlled study. J Clin Oncol 1997; 15:2954–2965.

116. Ozer H, Armitage JO, Bennett CL, Crawford J, Demetri GD, Pizzo PA, Schiffer CA, Smith TJ, Somlo G, Wade JC, Wade JL 3rd, Winn RJ, Wozniak AJ, Somerfield MR. 2000 update of recommendations for the use of hematopoietic colony-stimulating factors: evidence-based, clinical practice guidelines. American Society of Clinical Oncology Growth Factors Expert Panel. J Clin Oncol 2000; 18:3558–3585.

117. Kullberg BJ, Anaissie EJ. Cytokines as therapy for opportunistic fungal infections. Res Immunol 1998; 149:478–488.

118. Stevens DA. Combination immunotherapy and antifungal chemotherapy. Clin Infect Dis 1998; 26:1266–1269.

119. Stevens DA, Kullberg BJ, Brummer E, Casadevall A, Netea MG, Sugar AM. Combined treatment: antifungal drugs with antibodies, cytokines or drugs. Med Mycol 2000; 38:305–315.

120. Bodey GP, Anaissie E, Gutterman J, Vadhan Raj S. Role of granulocyte-macrophage colony-stimulating factor as adjuvant therapy for fungal infection in patients with cancer. Clin Infect Dis 1993; 17:705–707.

121. Maertens J, Demuynck H, Verhoef G, Vandenberhe P, Zachee P, Boogaerts M. GM-CSF fails to improve outcome in invasive fungal infections in neutropenic cancer patients [abstr 560]. 13th Congress of the International Society for Human and Animal Mycology, Parma, Italy, 1997.

122. Nemunaitis J, Shannon-Dorcy K, Appelbaum FR, Meyers JD, Owens A, Day R, Ando D, O'Neill C, Buckner-D, Singer JW. Long-term follow-up of patients with invasive fungal disease who received adjunctive therapy with recombinant human macrophage colony-stimulating factor. Blood 1993; 82:1422–1427.

123. Poynton CH, Barnes RA, Rees J. Interferon gamma and granulocyte-macrophage colony-stimulating factor for the treatment of hepatosplenic candidosis in patients with acute leukemia. Clin Infect Dis 1998; 26:239–240.

124. Grauer ME, Bokemeyer C, Bautsch W, Freund M, Link H. Successful treatment of a *Trichosporon beigelii* septicemia in a granulocytopenic patient with amphotericin B and granulocyte colony-stimulating factor. Infection 1994; 22:283–286.

125. Gonzalez CE, Couriel DR, Walsh TJ. Successful treatment of disseminated zygomycosis in a neutropemc patient with amphotericin B lipid complex and granulocyte colony-stimulating factor. Clin Infect Dis 1997; 24:192–196.

126. Hennequin C, Benkerrou M, Gaillard JL, Blanche S, Fraitag S. Role of granulocyte colony-stimulating factor in the management of infection with *Fusarium oxysporum* in a neutropenic child. Clin Infect Dis 1994; 18:490–491.

127. Fukushima T, Sumazaki R, Shibasaki M, Saitoh H, Fujigaki Y, Kaneko M, Akaogi E, Mitsui K, Ogata T, Takita H. Successful treatment of invasive thoracopulmonary mucormycisis in a patient with acute lymphoblastic leukemia. Cancer 1995; 76:895–899.

128. Dornbusch HJ, Urban CE, Pinter H, Ginter G, Fotter R, Becker H, Miorini T, Berghold C. Treatment of invasive pulmonary aspergillosis in severely neutropenic children with malignant disorders using liposomal amphotericin B, granulocyte colony-stimulating factor and surgery: report of 5 cases. Pediatr Hematol Oncol 1995; 12: 577–586.

129. Spielberger RT, Falleroni MJ, Coene AJ, Larson RA. Concomitant amphotericin B therapy, granulocyte transfusions, and GM-CSF administration for disseminated infection with *Fusarium* in a granulocytopenic patient. Clin Infect Dis 1993; 16:528–530.

130. Sahin B, Paydas S, Cosar E, Bicacki K, Hazar B. Role of granulocyte colony-stimulating factor in the treatment of mucormycosis. Eur J Clin Microbiol Infect Dis 1996; 15:866–869.

131. Pagano L, Morace G, Ortu-La Barbera E, Sanguinetti M, Leone G. Adjuvant therapy with rhGM-CSF for the treatment of *Blastoschizomyces capitatus* systemic infection in a patient with acute myeloid leukemia. Ann Hematol 1996; 73:33–34.

132. Niitsu N, Umeda M. Fungemia in patients with hematologic malignancies: therapeutic effects of concomitant administration of fluconazole and granulocyte-colony-stimulating factor. Chemotherapy 1996; 42:215–219.

133. Boutati EI, Anaissie EJ. *Fusarium*, a significant emerging pathogen in patients with hematologic malignancy: ten years' experience at a cancer center and implications for management. Blood 1997; 90:999–1008.

134. Abu Jawdeh L, Haidar R, Bitar F, Mroueh S, Akel S, Nuwayri-Salti N, Dbaibo GS. *Aspergillus* vertebral osteomyelitis in a child with a primary monocyte killing defect: response to GM-CSF therapy. J Infect 2000; 41:97–100.

135. Nemunaitis J, Meyers JD, Buckner D, Shannon-Dorcy K, Mori M, Shulman H, Bianco JA, Higano CS, Groves E, Storb R, Hansen J, Appelbaum FR, Singer JW. Phase I trial of recombinant human macrophage colony-stimulating factor in patients with invasive fungal] infections. Blood 1991; 78:907–913.

136. Nemunaitis J. Use of macrophage colony-stimulating factor in the treatment of fungal infections. Clin Infect Dis 1998; 26:1279–1281.

137. Hazel DL, Newland AC, Kelsey SM. Malignancy: granulocyte colony stimulating factor increases the efficacy of conventional amphotericin in the treatment of presumed deep-seated fungal infection in neutropenic patients following intensive chemotherapy or bone marrow transplantation for haematological malignancies. Hematol 1999; 4: 305–311.

138. Flynn TN, Kelsey SM, Hazel DL, Guest JF. Cost effectiveness of amphotericin B plus G-CSF compared with amphotericin B monotherapy. Treatment of presumed deep-seated fungal infection in neutropenic patients in the UK. Pharmacoeconomics 1999; 16:543–550.

139. Kullberg BJ, van de Woude K, Aoun M, Jacobs F, Herbrecht R, Kujath P, for the European filgrastim candidiasis study group. A double-blind, randomized, placebo-controlled phase II study of filgrastim (recombinant granulocyte colony-stimluating factor) in combination with fluconazole for treatment of invasive candidiasis and candidemia in nonneutropenic patients (J-100). Program and Abstracts of the 38th Interscience Conference of the Antimicrobial Agents and Chemotherapy, San Diego, CA, 1998.

140. Wald A, Leisenring W, van Burik JA, Bowden RA. Epidemiology of *Aspergillus* infections in a large cohort of patients undergoing bone marrow transplantation. J Infect Dis 1997; 175:1459–1466.

141. Roilides E, Sein T, Roden M, Schaufele RL, Walsh TJ. Elevated serum concentrations of interleukin-10 in nonneutropenic patients with invasive aspergillosis. J Infect Dis 2001; 183:518–520.

142. The International Chronic Granulomatous Disease Cooperative Study Group. A controlled trial of interferon gamma to prevent infection in chronic granulomatous disease. N Engl J Med 1991; 324:509–516.

143. Williamson PR, Kwon-Chung KJ, Gallin JI. Successful treatment oi *Paecilomyces varioti* infection in a patient with chronic granulomatous disease and a review of *Paecilomyces* species infections. Clin Infect Dis 1992; 14:1023–1026.

144. Phillips P, Forbes JC, Speert DP. Disseminated infection with *Pseudallescheria boydii* in a patient with chronic granulomatous disease: response to gamma-interferon plus antifungal chemotherapy. Pediatr Infect Dis J 1991; 10:536–539.

145. Cohen-Abbo A, Edwards KM. Multifocal osteomyelitis caused by *Paecilomyces varioti* in a patient with chronic granulomatous disease. Infection 1995; 23:55–57.

146. Pasic S, Abinun M, Pistignjat B, Vlajic B, Rakic J, Sarjanovic L, Ostojic N. *Aspergillus osteomyelitis* in chronic granulomatous disease: treatment with recombinant gamma-interferon and itraconazole. Pediatr Infect Dis J 1996; 15:833–834.

147. Ozsahin H, von Planta M, Muller I, Steinert HC, Nadal D, Lauener R, Tuchschmid P, Willi UV, Ozsahin M, Crompton NE, Seger RA. Successful treatment of invasive aspergillosis in chronic granulomatous disease by bone marrow transplantation, granulocyte colony-stimulating factor-mobilized granulocytes, and liposomal amphotericin-B. Blood 1998; 92:2719–2724.

148. Roilides E, Sigler L, Bibashi E, Katsifa H, Flaris N, Panteliadis C. Disseminated infection due to *Chrysosporium zonatum* in a patient with chronic granulomatous disease and review of non-*Aspergillus* infections in these patients. J Clin Microbiol 1999; 37:18–25.

149. Touza Rey F, Martinez Vazquez C, Alonso J, Mendez Pineiro MJ, Rubianes Gonzalez M, Crespo Casal M. The clinical response to interferon-gamma in a patient with chronic granulomatous disease and brain abcesses due to *Aspergillus fumigatus*. An Med Interna 2000; 17:86–87.

150. Tsumura N, Akasu Y, Yamane H, Ikezawa S, Hirata T, Oda K, Sakata Y, Shirahama M, Inoue A, Kato H. *Aspergillus* osteomyelitis in a child who has p67-phox-deficient chronic granulomatous disease. Kurume Med J 1999; 46:87–90.

151. Dotis J, Panagopoulou P, Filioti J, Winn R, Toptsis C, Panteliadis C, Roilides E. Femoral osteomyelitis due to *Aspergillus nidulans* in a patient with chronic granulomatous disease. Infection 2003; 31:121–124.

152. Segal B, DeCarlo E, Kwon-Chung K, Malech H, Gallin J, Holland S. *Aspergillus nidulans* infection in chronic granulomatous disease. Medicine 1998; 77:1659–1665.

153. Heinrich SD, Finney T, Craver R, Yin L, Zembo MM. *Aspergillus* osteomyelitis in patients who have chronic granulomatous disease. Case report. J Bone Joint Surg Am 1991; 73:456–460.

154. Kline MW, Bocobo FC, Paul ME, Rosenblatt HM, Shearer WT. Successful medical therapy of *Aspergillus* osteomyelitis of the spine in an 11-year-old boy with chronic granulomatous disease. Pediatrics 1994; 93:830–835.

155. Roilides E, Holmes A, Blake C, Pizzo PA, Walsh TJ. Defective antifungal activity of monocyte-derived macrophages from HIV-infected children against *Aspergillus fumigatus*. J Infect Dis 1993; 168:1562–1565.

156. Riddell LA, Pinching AJ, Hill S, Ng TT, Arbe E, Lapham GP, Ash S, Hillman R, Tchamouroff S, Denning DW, Parkin JM. A phase III study of recombinant human interferon gamma to prevent opportunistic infections in advanced HIV disease. AIDS Res Hum Retroviruses 2001; 17:789–797.

157. American Society of Clinical Oncology. Update of recommendations for the use of hematopoietic colony-stimulating factors: evidence-based clinical practice guidelines. J Clin Oncol 1996; 14:1957–1960..

158. Hughes WT, Armstrong D, Bodey GP, Brown AE, Edwards JE, Feld R, Pizzo P, Rolston KV, Shenep JL, Young LS. 1997 guidelines for the use of antimicrobial agents in neutropenic patients with unexplained fever. Infectious Diseases Society of America. Clin Infect Dis 1997; 25:551–573.

159. Groll A, Renz S, Gerein V, Schwabe D, Katschan G, Schneider M, Hubner K, Kornhuber B. Fatal haemoptysis associated with invasive pulmonary aspergillosis

treated with high-dose amphotericin B and granulocyte-macrophage colony-stimulating factor (GM-CSF). Mycoses 1992; 35:67–75.

160. Giralt S, Escudier S, Kantarjian H, Deisseroth A, Freireich EJ, Andersson BS, O'Brien S, Andreeff M, Fisher H, Cork A, Hirsch-Ginsberg C, Trujillo J, Stass S, Champin RE. Preliminary results of treatment with filgrastim for relapse of leukemia and myelodysplasia after allogeneic bone marrow transplantation. N Engl J Med 1993; 329:757–761.

161. Hartung T, Von Aulock S, Schneider C, Faist E. How to leverage an endogenous immune defense mechanism: the example of granulocyte colony-stimulating factor. Crit Care Med 2003; 31:S65–S75.

162. Strauss RG. Granulocyte transfusion therapy for hem/onc patients. Hem/Onc Ann 1994; 2:304–309.

163. Bhatia S, McCullough J, Perry EH, Clay M, Ramsay NK, Neglia JP. Granulocyte transfusions: efficacy in treating fungal infections in neutropenic patients following bone marrow transplantation. Transfusion 1994; 34:226–232.

164. Di Mario A, Sica S, Salutari P, Ortu La Barbera E, Marra R, Leone G. Granulocyte colony-stimulating factor-primed leukocyte transfusions in *Candida tropicalis* fungemia in neutropenic patients. Haematologica 1997; 82:362–363.

165. Dignani MC, Freireich EJ, Andersson BS, Lichtiger B, Jendiroba DB, Kantarjian H, Rex JH, Vartivarian SE, O'Brien S, Hester JP, Anaissie EJ. Treatment of neutropenia-related fungal infections with granulocyte colony-stimulating factor-elicited white blood cell transfusions: a pilot study. Leukemia 1997; 11:1621–1630.

166. Catalano L, Fontana R, Scarpato N, Picardi M, Rocco S, Rotoli B. Combined treatment with amphotericin-B and granulocyte transfusion from G-CSF-stimulated donors in an aplastic patient with invasive aspergillosis undergoing bone marrow transplantation. Haematologica 1997; 82:71–72.

167. Peters C, Minkov M, Matthes-Martin S, Potschger U, Witt V, Mann G, Hocker P, Worel N, Stary J, Klingebiel T, Gadner H. Leucocyte transfusions from rhG-CSF or prednisolone stimulated donors for treatment of severe infections in immunocompromised neutropenic patients. Br J Haematol 1999; 106:689–696.

168. Price TH, Bowden RA, Boeckh M, Bux J, Nelson K, Liles WC, Dale DC. Phase I/II trial of neutrophil transfusions from donors stimulated with G-CSF dexamethasone for treatment of patients with infections in hematopoietic stem cell transplantation. Blood 2000; 95:3302–3309.

169. Illerhaus G, Wirth K, Dwenger A, Waller CF, Garbe A, Brass V, Lang H, Lange W. Treatment and prophylaxis of severe infections in neutropenic patients by granulocyte transfusions. Ann Hematol 2002; 81:273–281.

170. Roilides E, Lyman CA, Panagopoulou P, Chanock S. Immunomodulation of invasive fungal infections. Infect Dis Clin North Am 2003; 17:193–219.

171. Cesaro S, Chinello P, De Silvestro G, Marson P, Picco G, Varotto S, Pittalis S, Zanesco L. Granulocyte transfusions from G-CSF-stimulated donors for the treatment of severe infections in neutropenic pediatric patients with onco-hematological diseases. Support Care Cancer 2003; 11:101–106.

172. Rutella S, Pierelli L, Sica S, Serafini R, Chiusolo P, Paladim U, Leone F, Zini G, D'Onofrio G, Leone G, Piccirillo N. Efficacy of granulocyte transfusions for neutropenia-related infections: retrospective analysis of predictive factors. Cytotherapy 2003; 5:19–30.

173. Kerr JP, Liakopolou E, Brown J, Cornish JM, Fleming D, Massey E, Oakhill A, Pamphilon DH, Robinson SP, Totem A, Valencia AM, Marks DI. The use of stimulated granulocyte transfusions to prevent recurrence of past severe infections after allogeneic stem cell transplantation. Br J Haematol 2003; 123:114–118.

174. Appelbaum F, Bowles C, Makuch R, Deisseroth A. Granulocyte transfusion therapy of experimental *Pseudomonas* septicemia: study of cell dose and collection technique. Blood 1978; 52:323–331.

175. Freireich EJ, Levin RH, Whang J, Carbone PP, Bronson W, Morse EE. The function and fate of transfused leukocytes from donors with chronic myelocytic leukemia in leukopemic recipients. Ann NY Acad Sci 1964; 113:1081–1089.

176. Higby DJ, Freeman A, Henderson ES, Sinks L, Cohen E. Granulocyte transfusions in children using filter-collected cells. Cancer 1976; 38:1407–1413.

177. Aisner J, Schiffer C, Wiernik P. Granulocyte transfusions: evaluation of factors influencing results and a comparison of filtration and intermittent centrifugation leukapheresis. Br J Haematol 1978; 38:121–129.

178. Hubel K, Dale DC, Engert A, Liles WC. Current status of granulocyte (neutrophil) transfusion therapy for infectious diseases. J Infect Dis 2001; 183:321–328.

179. Roilides E, Walsh TJ, Pizzo PA, Rubin M. Granulocyte colony-stimulating factor enhances the phagocytic and bactericidal activity of normal and defective human neutrophils. J Infect Dis 1991; 163:579–583.

180. Nathan CF. Respiratory burst in adherent human neutrophils: triggering by colony-stimulating factors CSF-GM and CSF-G. Blood 1989; 73:301–306.

181. Allen RC, Stevens PR, Price TH, Chatta GS, Dale DC. In vivo effects of recombinant human granulocyte colony-stimulating factor on neutrophil oxidative functions in normal human volunteers. J Infect Dis 1997; 175:1184–1192.

182. Kasahara Y, Iwai K, Yachie A, Ohta K, Konno A, Seki H, Miyawaki T, Taniguchi N. Involvement of reactive oxygen intermediates in spontaneous and CD95 (Fas/APO-1)-mediated apoptosis of neutrophils. Blood 1997; 89:1748–1753.

183. Colotta F, Re F, Polentarutti N, Sozzani S, Mantovani A. Modulation of granulocyte survival and programmed cell death by cytokines and bacterial products. Blood 1992; 80:2012–2020.

184. Dale DC, Liles WC, Llewellyn C, Rodger E, Price TH. Neutrophil transfusions: kinetics and functions of neutrophils mobilized with granulocyte colony-stimulating factor and dexamethasone. Transfusion 1998; 38:713–721.

185. MacHida U, Tojo A, Takahashi S, Iseki T, Ooi J, Nagayama H, Shirafuji N, Mori S, Wada Y, Ogami K, Yamada Y, Sakamaki H, Maekawa T, Tani K, Asano S. The effect of granulocyte colony-stimulating factor administration in healthy donors before bone marrow harvesting. Br J Haematol 2000; 108:747–753.

186. Bensinger WI, Price TH, Dale DC, Appelbaum FR, Clift R, Lilleby K, Williams B, Storb R, Thomas ED, Buckner CD. The effects of daily recombinant human granulocyte colony-stimulating factor adminstration on normal granulocyte donors undergoing leukapheresis. Blood 1993; 81:1883–1888.

187. Hubel K, Dale DC, Rodgers E, Gaviria JM, Price T, Liles WC. Preservation of function in granulocyte concetrates collected from donorsw stimualted with G-CSF /dexamethasone during storage at reduced temperature [abstr]. Blood 2000; 96:820a.

188. Bow EJ, Schroeder ML, Louie TJ. Pulmonary complications in patients receiving granulocyte transfusions and amphotericin B. Can Med Assoc J 1984; 130:593–597.

189. Wright DG, Robichaud KJ, Pizzo PA, Deisseroth AB. Lethal pulmonary reactions associated with the combined use of amphotericin B and leukocyte transfusions. N Engl J Med 1981; 304:1185–1189.

190. Dry SM, Bechard KM, Milford EL, Churchill WH, Benjamin RJ. The pathology of transfusion-related acute lung injury. Am J Clin Pathol 1999; 112:216–221.

191. Anderson KC, Weinstein HJ. Transfusion-associated graft-versus-host disease. N Engl J Med 1990; 323:315–321.

192. Adkins DR, Goodnough LT, Shenoy S, Brown R, Moellering J, Khoury H, Vij R, DiPersio J. Effect of leukocyte compatibility on neutrophil increment after transfusion of granulocyte colony-stimulating factor-mobilized prophylactic granulocyte transfusions and on clinical outcomes after stem cell transplantation. Blood 2000; 95: 3605–3612.

193. Neely AN, Holder IA. Effects of immunoglobulin G and low-dose amphotericin B on *Candida albicans* infections in burned mice. Antimicrob Agents Chemother 1992; 36: 643–646.

194. Stratta RJ, Shaefer MS, Cushing KA, Markin RS, Reed EC, Langnas AN, Pillen TJ, Shaw BW. A randomized prospective trial of acyclovir and immune globulin prophylaxis in liver transplant recipients receiving OKT3 therapy. Arch Surg 1992; 127:55–63.

195. Klaesson S, Ringden O, Markling L, Tammik L. Intravenous immunoglobulin: immune modulatory effects in vitro and clinical effects in allogeneic bone marrow transplant recipients. Transplant Proc 1995; 27:3536–3537.

196. Tollemar J, Gross N, Dolgiras N, Jarstrand C, Ringden O, Hammarstrom L. Fungal prophylaxis by reduction of fungal colonization by oral administration of bovine anti-*Candida* antibodies in bone marrow transplant recipients. Bone Marrow Transplant 1999; 23:283–290.

197. Casadevall A. Antibody immunity and invasive fungal infections. Infect Immun 1995; 63:4211–4218.

198. Matthews DJ, Clark PA, Herbert J, Morgan G, Armitage RJ, Kinnon C, Minty A, Grabstein KH, Caput D, Ferrara P, Callard R. Function of the interleukin-2 (IL-2) receptor gamma-chain in biologic responses of X-linked severe combined immunodeficient B cells to IL-2, IL-4, IL-13, and IL-15. Blood 1995; 85:38–42.

199. Matthews RC, Rigg G, Hodgetts S, Carter T, Chapman C, Gregory C, Illidge C, Burnie J. Preclinical assessment of the efficacy of mycograb, a human recombinant antibody against fungal HSP90. Antimicrob Agents Chemother 2003; 47:2208–2216.

200. Han Y, Cutler JE. Antibody response that protects against disseminated candidiasis. Infect Immun 1995; 63:2714–2719.

201. van Spriel AB, van den Herik-Oudijk IE, van Sorge NM, Vile HA, van Strijp JA, van de Winkel JG. Effective phagocytosis and killing of *Candida albicans* via targeting FcgammaRI (CD64) or FcalphaRI (CD89) on neutrophils. J Infect Dis 1999; 179:661–669.

202. Vecchiarelli A, Casadevall A. Antibody-mediated effects against *Cryptococcus neoformans*: evidence for interdependency collaboration between humoral cellular immunity. Res Immunol 1998; 149:321–333.

203. Cenci E, Mencacci A, Bacci A, Bistoni F, Kurup VP, Romani L. T-cell vaccination in mice with invasive pulmonary aspergillosis. J Immunol 2000; 165:381–388.

22

Antifungal Prophylaxis

John R. Wingard
Department of Medicine, University of Florida College of Medicine, Gainesville, Florida, U.S.A.

Elias J. Anaissie
The University of Arkansas for Medical Sciences, Myeloma and Transplantation Research Center, Little Rock, Arkansas, U.S.A.

I. RATIONALE

The outcomes of various invasive fungal infections have historically been suboptimal and for certain pathogens such as *Aspergillus* and *Fusarium*, frankly poor, with most infections ending in death. Although various pharmacologic agents have demonstrable in vitro antifungal activity, clinical responses have not been as good as one might anticipate. Several reasons have been posited. First, the early diagnosis of infection is often difficult to make, as noted in foregoing chapters. This means that treatment is often started late in the course of infection. Once the burden of organisms is high, with spread of the infection to multiple sites, and the physiological status of the patient is impaired, the prospect for successful resolution of the infection is compromised. Second, the host defenses of the infected patient are crucial for resolution of the infection, and patients who become infected have substantial compromise of such protective defenses, key to resolution of infection. Unless recovery of host defenses occurs concomitantly with antifungal therapy, prospects for successful treatment are limited. Third, substantial toxicities of several of the antifungal agents (e.g., amphotericin B) have limited the ability to administer the therapy at high enough doses or for long enough. An inadequate course of therapy seriously compromises the likelihood for treatment success.

To meet the challenge of poor treatment outcomes, prophylaxis is an alternative strategy to improve outcomes. There are a number of considerations one should weigh in determining if prophylaxis is appropriate for a given patient or patient population to address a specific infection (Table 1). First, the frequency of infection should be sufficient to warrant the cost, potential toxicities, and inconvenience imposed by administration of the prophylactic agent. Second, the infection of interest should be clinically important, with substantial morbidity or risk of death. Third, the option of waiting to treat the infection should be less attractive because of poor treatment results, toxicities of the therapy, or because substantial morbidity occurs even if the eventual outcome is salutary. Fourth,

Table 1 Considerations for Antifungal Prophylaxis

Benefits	Risks
Magnitude of risk in the patient population	Effects on emergence of resistance
Seriousness of infection	Effects on patterns of superinfection
Likelihood of success of treatment of established infection	Adverse events
Availability of suitable agent which is efficacious and safe	Deleterious drug interactions

suitable agents should be available for prophylaxis, with favorable antimicrobial activity and safety profiles and formulations that are convenient and inexpensive for administration of the regimen. Fifth, the strategy should be tested in controlled trials to demonstrate that it is effective in achieving the desired goal, and untoward or unanticipated adverse sequelae are not associated with it.

The earlier-mentioned considerations are important because prophylaxis can have potential undesirable consequences. The emergence of resistance is a constant threat for any antimicrobial agent. Overuse of an agent contributes to the risk for resistance. Shifts in microbial colonization may lead to changes in patterns of infections by other less-susceptible organisms. Toxicities of an agent may offset its antifungal efficacy. Unanticipated interactions with concomitant medications may occur and lead to altered effects of medications. For all of these reasons, prophylaxis should be used only when the benefits outweigh the risks.

II. TYPES OF PROPHYLAXIS

There are several types of prophylaxis strategies. Generally speaking, prophylaxis can be regarded as "primary" when prevention targets an individual or a group that has not been infected in the past, but who is vulnerable for infection. "Secondary" prophylaxis refers to the approach used in individuals who have been previously infected, but the infection has been brought under control; continued immunodeficiency or further immune-suppressing therapy places the patient at risk for loss of infection control, exacerbation, or reinfection. This is also sometimes referred to as chronic suppressive or maintenance therapy. An example of the latter would be a patient with acute leukemia who develops aspergillosis (which is then controlled with antifungal therapy), but postremission faces additional antileukemic consolidation therapy or hematopoietic cell transplantation (HCT). Another example is an HIV-infected patient who develops an acute opportunistic fungal infection, which is controlled but continues to have severely compromised cell-mediated immunity. Continued treatment would be given with the purpose to prevent a recurrence of the acute infection.

Another way to categorize prophylaxis is global vs. targeted. Global prophylaxis refers to administration to all patients deemed at risk for a given infection. This is attractive because it standardizes the approach for all patients, but is less desirable because of potential excessive exposure to patients. An alternative is to target those at greatest risk ("targeted" prophylaxis), using some parameter of host susceptibility to determine the targeted group at risk. An example is instead of offering all allogeneic HCT patients' antimold prophylaxis, reserving it only for patients with graft versus host disease, the subgroup at greatest risk; a second example is offering prophylaxis only to HIV-infected patients with a CD4 + T-lymphocyte count below a certain threshold value instead of administration to all HIV-infected patients. In each case, certain risk factors or markers of immunodeficiency are used to define those who are offered prophylaxis. Various prophylaxis strategies have been evaluated in controlled trials, and several have been adopted in clinical practice as accepted good patient-care measures. It is important to note that prophylaxis against a specific fungal pathogen may be appropriate for one patient population, while not appropriate for another. Nearly half of all serious fungal infections occur in cancer, HIV, and transplant recipients (1). Not surprisingly, most of the studies that have evaluated prophylaxis have been conducted in these patient groups. Discussed in what follows are generally accepted practices for certain fungal pathogens and the studies that have formed their basis in various patient populations.

III. *CANDIDA*

Candida organisms are commensal organisms that cause superficial mucosal or cutaneous infections and invasive, systemic infections. Polyene and azole antifungals are highly active against most *Candida* species. Although nonabsorbable topical antifungals are available and several studies have demonstrated benefit, recent prophylaxis trials have emphasized absorbable azoles, especially fluconazole (or itraconazole) because of their systemic effect and excellent tolerability. The role of prophylaxis varies by patient population.

A. Hematopoietic Cell Transplantation

Candida has historically been the most common fungal pathogen in both allogeneic and autologous HCT recipients. Although mucosal infections occur, systemic infections are more problematic. Systemic *Candida* infections are frequent in HCT patients with infection rates of 15–20% during the first month after HCT. Prospective randomized trials have demonstrated the effectiveness of fluconazole prophylaxis when given from time of transplant until engraftment to reduce systemic infection and infection-related mortality (2,3). In one trial, prolonged administration (until day 75) after allogeneic HCT had a similar antifungal benefit but in addition was associated with a survival advantage as well (4), persisting even beyond cessation of fluconazole (5). Initial studies evaluated a dose of 400 mg/day, but one study demonstrated a dose of 200 mg/day was also efficacious (6). Emergence of resistance has not been reported to date. However, isolated reports of outbreaks of fluconazole, resistant organisms, such as *C. krusei* and *C. glabrata*, have been reported in several HCT centers (7–9). Fluconazole prophylaxis has been endorsed by consensus guidelines developed by the Center for Disease Control, the American Society of Blood and Marrow Transplantation, and the Infectious Disease Society of America (Table 2) (10) for all allogeneic HCT recipients and autologous HCT recipients transplanted for hematologic malignancies. An alternative to fluconazole is low-dose amphotericin B (dosed <0.5 mg/kg/day), which is also protective but more toxic (11,12).

B. Hematologic Malignancy

Both mucosal and systemic *Candida* infections occur because of neutropenia (especially in acute leukemia patients) or diminished cell-mediated immunity (in chronic

Table 2 Prophylaxis Against *Candida*

Patient group references	Infection type	Antifungal agent	Alternative	Prophylaxis type	Concerns
Allogeneic HCT	Systemic	Fluconazole 200–400 mg/day		Global	Drug interactions (cytochrome P450)
Autologous HCT[a]	Systemic	Fluconazole 200–400 mg/day			
Acute leukemia	Systemic	Fluconazole 400 mg/day	Itraconazole, amphotericin B	Targeted	Variable infection risk
Liver transplant	Systemic	Fluconazole 400 mg/day	Amphotericin B	Global	Interaction with calcineurium inhibitors
Pancreas transplant	Systemic	Fluconazole 400 mg/day	Liposomal amphotericin B	Global	Interaction with calcineurium inhibitors
ICU (high-risk) risk	Invasive	Fluconazole 400 mg/day	Ketoconazole	Targeted	Increase in *C. glabrata*; definition of high risk
Neonatal ICU	Invasive	Fluconazole[b]		Targeted	Extremely low birth weight (<1000 g)
HIV infection	Mucosal	Fluconazole 50–200 mg/day solution	Itraconazole	Secondary	Emergence of resistance

[a]when performed for the treatment of hematologic malignancy.
[b]At a dose of 3 mg/kg every third day for the first 2 weeks, every other day during the third and fourth weeks, and every day during the fifth and sixth weeks.

leukemias, lymphomas, and those receiving corticosteroids). The rate of systemic infection is more variable in leukemic patients than with HCT and is highly dependent on the treatment regimen. Systemic infection rates of 8–16% have been reported during induction therapy for acute leukemia. Several antifungal agents have been evaluated as prophylaxis. The benefits of the nonabsorbable antifungal agents have been mixed in various trials; tolerability has limited their use. In a meta-analysis of antifungal prophylaxis and empirical therapy trials in neutropenic cancer patients using a variety of agents (mostly agents other than fluconazole), a reduction in infection and colonization was found, but no decrease in survival, except for amphotericin B (13). In contrast, a larger meta-analysis of trials testing azoles or IV amphotericin B products demonstrated reductions in rates of superficial and invasive fungal infections, decreased use of parenteral antifungal therapy, and lower fungal-related mortality, although no reduction in overall mortality (14). In a meta-analysis of fluconazole prophylaxis trials only (15), a reduction in systemic fungal infections was noted in patient populations in which the incidence of systemic fungal infection exceeded 15%. Such patient populations would typically include HCT patients and patients with hematologic malignancy receiving intensive chemotherapy regimens (3,16). Because of the heterogeneity of risk, clearly, prophylaxis must be tailored to the intensity of antileukemic treatment approach and the degree of risk posed by the particular treatment regimen. With respect to other patients with chemotherapy-induced myelosuppression, current data do not support the routine use of fluconazole prophylaxis. Of note, no increase in systemic infections by fluconazole-resistant fungi has been noted, although colonization by fluconazole-resistant organisms has been seen (15).

C. Solid Organ Transplantation

Candida infections are problematic in recipients of liver transplants. Rates of infection have been reported in the range of 5–42% (17). Risk factors include prolonged surgical time, elevated creatinine, retransplantation, reoperation, and cytomegalovirus infection (17). Randomized trials have demonstrated a reduction in *Candida* infections by the use of fluconazole (18,19). Alternatively, liposomal or lipid-complex amphotericin B is also effective (20,21). A similar benefit in pancreatic transplantation has also been suggested (22). Serious *Candida* infections are generally infrequent after renal transplantation, unless rejection episodes necessitate intensive or prolonged immunosuppression. Accordingly, routine prophylaxis is not appropriate after renal transplantation; however, recurring candiduria may signify upper urinary tract infection, should be fully investigated, and may be grounds for "preemptive" therapy to prevent obstructive uropathy from fungal balls at the ureterovesicle junction and pyelonephritis, especially in patients with impaired bladder emptying.

D. Critical Care

The risk of invasive *Candida* infection is low in unselected patients in medical or surgical intensive care units (ICUs), ~2% (23). Because of the low risk, several consensus guidelines developed by expert panels do not recommend routine prophylaxis (24–26). The risk is higher in certain subgroups, according to the complexity of critical care administered and the duration of its necessity. Risk factors identified include central venous catheters, parenteral nutrition, multiple antibiotics, extensive surgery (especially gastrointestinal surgery), burns, renal failure, hemodialysis, mechanical ventilation, chronic intestinal perforation, poor physiological status of the patient, use of gut decontamination, prolonged ICU stay, surgery for liver or pancreatic transplantation, and colonization by *Candida* (27–29). Two small trials suggested ketoconazole or fluconazole could reduce *Candida* infections in critically ill surgical patients (30,31). In a recent prospective randomized placebo-controlled trial in patients who were expected to remain in the ICU for a minimum of ≥3 days, the frequency of invasive infections was reduced by 55% in patients given fluconazole at a dose of 400 mg/day (32). Clearly, these studies suggest there is a potential role for prophylaxis in carefully selected subgroups of ICU patients, but further study is needed to determine how to optimally select such individuals in current ICU practice environments (27).

E. Neonatal ICU

The risk of invasive *Candida* infection is high in critically ill preterm infants, accounting for 9% of late-onset sepsis in infants weighing <1500 g (33). Practices associated with the care of prematurity are relatively homogeneous in contrast to practices in the adult ICU patient population. In a randomized placebo-controlled trial conducted in infants weighing <1000 g at birth, IV fluconazole was given at a dose of 3 mg/kg every third day for the first 2 weeks, every other day during the third and fourth weeks, and every day during the fifth and sixth weeks. This regimen was effective in reducing the rate of invasive infection (from 20% to 0%) (34).

F. HIV Infection

Candida infections of the oral cavity, oropharynx, vagina, and esophagus are frequent and are perhaps the most common infection seen in HIV disease. Deep-seated candidiasis has been one of the infections included in the case definition of the acquired immunodeficiency syndrome. Most patients with advanced HIV infections develop mucocutaneous candidiasis and frequent recurrences occur (35). The risk of *Candida* infection is especially high when the CD4 lymphocyte count is low (e.g., <200 cells/μL) or the HIV burden is high. The advent of highly active antiretroviral therapy (HAART) has led to a dramatic reduction in the frequency of *Candida* infections (36,37). This appears to be independent of reconstitution of anti-*Candida* cell-mediated immune responses (36). Candidemia is infrequent except in late-stage HIV infection or in those with central venous catheters. Infections may be unresponsive to antifungal therapy when the CD4 + T-lymphocyte count is very low (e.g., <50 cells/μL). Fluconazole therapy of mucocutaneous candidiasis (38) and prolonged fluconazole prophylaxis (39,40) have also been associated with the emergence of resistance.

Multiple randomized trials have demonstrated the effectiveness of fluconazole in prevention of candidiasis in HIV-infected patients (41). Notwithstanding, consensus guidelines do not recommend routine prophylaxis in HIV-infected patients (42,24). There are several reasons. Patients with the first episode of oropharyngeal candidiasis generally respond promptly to therapy. The first episode has a low risk for serious morbidity or mortality. Chronic administration of azoles has been associated with a substantive risk for resistance, particularly in patients with CD4+ T-lymphocyte counts <200 cells/μL (43). Drug interactions and cost are other considerations. Accordingly, if recurrences of oropharyngeal or vulvovaginal candidiasis are frequent or severe, an azole such as fluconazole may be given (42) at a daily dose of 100–200 mg. Similarly, multiple episodes of esophageal candidiasis are important considerations for chronic suppressive therapy or secondary prophylaxis. Fluconazole has been best studied, but other azoles have also been evaluated including itraconazole or ketoconazole as alternatives to fluconazole. Itraconazole (in solution) appears to be as effective, but there are fewer trials. Ketoconazole appears to be not as effective as fluconazole. Fluconazole is more effective than clotrimazole (44).

IV. ASPERGILLUS

A. HCT and Hematologic Malignancy

Aspergillus is a cause of life-threatening pneumonia and, less commonly, sinusitis. Prolonged neutropenia has long been known to be a major risk factor for aspergillosis (45). The intensive chemotherapy regimens typically used to treat acute leukemia are the most common scenarios in which such prolonged neutropenias are encountered. After allogeneic HCT, development of graft versus host disease and the use of corticosteroids also pose major risks with other factors such as use of T-cell depletion of the stem-cell graft, the occurrence of postengraftment neutropenia or lymphopenia, and infection by cytomegalovirus or respiratory viruses (46). With the increasing use of hematopoietic growth factors and stem-cell products containing large numbers of hematopoietic progenitors occasioned by peripheral blood stem-cell grafts, the interval to engraftment after HCT has shortened and there has been a concomitant reduction in the incidence of early aspergillosis. Most *Aspergillus* infections now occur after engraftment 2–4 months later. Because of graft versus host disease, the risk of aspergillosis after reduced intensity allogeneic HCT is similar to allogeneic HCT using standard intensity conditioning regimens (47,48). The rate of *Aspergillus* infections after HCT is 10–15% in various series and this has increased in recent years (49). The rate of *Aspergillus* infections during acute leukemia therapy is variable depending on the chemotherapy regimen and the response of the leukemia to therapy. After an initial episode of aspergillosis, the risk of later recurrence during subsequent antileukemic therapy (either additional cycles of chemotherapy or HCT) is practically 100%. Amphotericin B given at full treatment doses (1.0 mg/kg/day) (with or without flucytosine) started at the start of subsequent antileukemic treatments has found to be effective secondary prophylaxis (Table 3) (50,51). The evaluation of mold-active azoles (itraconazole and voriconazole) as secondary prophylaxis is more limited, but recent case series suggest that they are effective as well. Liposomal amphotericin B has been tested as primary prophylaxis in randomized trials after HCT, but because of small sample sizes, these trials were inconclusive (52,53). The need for prolonged prophylaxis has placed parenteral drugs at a substantial disadvantage. Oral itraconazole has anti-*Aspergillus* activity, and a number of randomized trials in patients with chemotherapy-induced neutropenia have tested its utility as prophylaxis (54–59). These studies have indicated itraconazole to be effective in reducing invasive fungal infections, but mostly the infections prevented were *Candida*, with the rate of aspergillosis in the control groups being too low to determine efficacy. A recent meta-analysis of itraconazole trials suggests that there is a reduction in *Aspergillus* infections but only if a certain threshold of bioavailable dosing is used (60). Two recent trials in allogeneic HCT patients tested prolonged courses of itraconazole (for 100 days) to cover the extended risk period for aspergillosis (61,62). In one trial (61), there was a reduction in the overall rate of invasive fungal infections, but there were too few *Aspergillus* infec-

Table 3 Prophylaxis Against Other Fungi

Pathogen	Patient group	Prophylaxis type	Antifungal agent	Alternative	Concerns
Cryptococcus	HIV infection	Secondary	Fluconazole	Itraconazole	
Histoplasma	HIV infection	Secondary	Itraconazole	Fluconazole	
Coccidioides	HIV infection	Secondary	Fluconazole or Itraconazole		
Aspergillus	Acute leukemia	Secondary	Amphotericine B		
	Acute leukemia	Primary	Itraconazole		
	Autologous or allogeneic HCT	Secondary	Amphotericin B	Itraconazole or voriconazole	
	Allogeneic HCT	Primary	Itraconazole		Trials not conclusive, small sample size, negative inotrophic effects, variable absorption
Pneumocystis	HIV infection	Secondary	TMP–SMZ	Pentamidine, dapsone, atovaquone	Pentamidine, dapsone, atovaquone
	Autologous or allogeneic HCT	Primary	TMP–SMZ	Pentamidine, dapsone, atovaquone	TMP–SMZ may be associated with toxicity
	Childhood ALL	Primary	TMP–SMZ	Pentamidine, dapsone, atovaquone	
	Solid organ transplant	Primary	TMP–SMZ	Pentamidine, dapsone, atovaquone	
	Other T-cell-deficient states	Primary targeted	TMP–SMZ	Pentamidine, dapsone, atovaquone	Approach must be individualized according to risk

tions to determine effectiveness for *Aspergillus* per se. Moreover, there were more deaths in the itraconazole arm. In the second trial (62), a higher dose regimen of itraconazole was used, and excessive toxicity in the itraconazole arm forced premature closure of the study. Although more than 200 patients were enrolled, there was no significant reduction in *Aspergillus* infections, but in a post hoc subset analysis, there was a trend toward reduction in patients who were able to remain on itraconazole. One concern that has been raised is the possibility that exposure to an azole (used in prophylaxis) may attenuate the effectiveness of a polyene given subsequently (63). Another approach is the use of nebulized amphotericin B. Uncontrolled trials suggested a benefit (64), but a randomized trial in patients with prolonged neutropenia showed no benefit (65).

B. Solid Organ Transplantation

Lung-transplant recipients are at substantial risk for invasive aspergillosis with a frequency of 8–18% (66,67) and a dissemination rate exceeding 25%. Inhaled amphotericin (either lipid-based or conventional) has been shown in preliminary studies to reduce invasive infection (68,69), but other studies have been inconclusive. Heart-transplant recipients have a risk of ~6% (67). Liver-transplant recipients have an *Aspergillus* risk that ranges between 1% and 6% (67). *Aspergillus* infections are less frequent in other transplant types: 1% kidney, 1% pancreas (67).

C. HIV Infection

Aspergillus infection is infrequent in patients with HIV infection except in the advanced stages in which CD4+ lymphocyte counts are <50 cells/μL. Clinical signs can be subtle, and aspergillosis is often discovered after death. Thus, there may be a need for targeted prophylaxis in advanced HIV infection, but this has not been tested as yet.

V. *CRYPTOCOCCUS*

A. HIV Infection

Cryptococcus can cause meningitis, fungemia, or pulmonary infection in advanced HIV disease. This is especially common in patients in developing countries. The risk increases as the CD4 count declines and in patients with high HIV burden. Other risk factors include IV drug use and tobacco use, and blacks seem to be at greater risk (70). Prospective controlled trials indicate that both fluconazole and itraconazole can reduce the occurrence of cryptococcal disease in advanced HIV infection (42). Similar to the reasoning for *Candida*, routine primary prophylaxis is not generally recommended (lack of survival benefit, possibility of drug interactions, risk for emergence of resistance, and cost). Moreover, in contrast to *Candida*, *Cryptococcus* is relatively infrequent. Doses of fluconazole at 100–200 mg/day are generally used for patients with CD4+ T-lymphocyte counts of <50 cells/μL (44). Once infection occurs and the acute infection is successfully controlled, maintenance is generally given for a prolonged course (at least 24 weeks) (Table 3). Continued secondary prophylaxis should be given indefinitely with a potential to stop it if the CD4+ count improves (to 100–200 cells/μL and this improvement is sustained) (71,72) and the HIV burden declines with effective antiretroviral therapy. Maintenance should be restarted if the CD4+ cell count declines <100 cells/μL again. Fluconazole appears to be more effective than itraconazole for secondary prophylaxis against *Cryptococcus* (73).

B. Solid Organ Transplant

Cryptococcus infection is infrequent, generally occurring after the first 6 months, especially in patients receiving systemic corticosteroids. Heart-transplant recipients are at greater risk than liver-transplant recipients. No prophylaxis strategy has been tested for this group of patients.

VI. HISTOPLASMOSIS

A. HIV Infection

Histoplasmosis is a cause of pulmonary infection in certain geographic regions, such as the Mississippi River valley. Inhalation of the organisms can occur particularly after activities that lead to organisms in soil or detritus being stirred up, including working with soil, cleaning chicken coups contaminated with droppings, cleaning or renovating old houses, or exploring caves. These activities should be avoided by individuals with CD4 + T-lymphocyte counts <200 cells/μL (42). Disseminated infection typically occurs in patients with CD4 + T-lymphocyte counts <200 cells/μL. Older age is a risk factor (74). After treatment of acute infection, maintenance therapy with itraconazole should be administered at a dose of 200 mg twice daily, using similar guidelines as for *Cryptococcus* (75) (Table 3). Fluconazole at a dose of ≥200 mg/day can be used as an alternative for secondary prophylaxis in patients who cannot tolerate itraconazole (76). Itraconazole is effective as primary prophylaxis as well in endemic areas (77). In general, it is not recommended for primary prophylaxis except in individuals with CD4 + T-lymphocyte counts <100 cells/μL, who have occupational exposure or who live in a community with a very high rate of histoplasmosis (42).

B. Other Patient Groups

Histoplasma infections are infrequent occurrences in solid organ-transplant and HCT recipients. Prophylaxis in at-risk geographic areas has not been evaluated.

VII. *COCCIDIOIDES*

A. HIV Infection

Coccidioides immitis can cause pneumonia in certain geographic areas (especially the Southwest of the United States). Activities that stir up dust and soil in endemic areas lead to exposure and inhalation of organisms and should be avoided by at-risk individuals. The major risk factor is a low CD4+ T-lymphocyte count of <100 cells/μL. Other risk factors implicated to increase risk include black race, and history of oropharyngeal or esophageal candidiasis, and protease-inhibitor therapy lessens the risk (78). After the treatment of the acute infection, maintenance with either fluconazole (400 mg/day) or itraconazole (200 mg twice daily) should be given (79), using similar guidelines for duration as for *Cryptococcus* (42) (Table 3).

B. Other Patient Groups

Coccidioides infections are infrequent occurrences in solid organ-transplant and HCT recipients. Prophylaxis in endemic geographic areas has not been evaluated.

VIII. *PNEUMOCYSTIS JIROVECI*

Pneumocystis jiroveci (formerly *P. carinii*) can cause interstitial pneumonia in patients with impaired T-cell immunity. Although pneumonia is by far the most frequent manifestation, extrapulmonary manifestations can occasionally occur as well, especially in individuals receiving aerosolized pentamidine (see in what follows); extrapulmonary organs most frequently involved include lymph nodes, spleen, liver, and bone marrow. Patient groups in which *P. jiroveci* infections have been best described include HIV-infected patients, children with acute lymphoblastic leukemia, and HCT recipients. Consensus recommendations suggest that routine primary prophylaxis should be given to all adults with HIV-infected individuals with CD4+ T-lymphocyte count of <200 cells/µL or a history of oropharyngeal candidiasis (42,80–82) (Table 3). For HIV-infected children of age <6 years, the appropriateness for prophylaxis may vary with age (82). Secondary prophylaxis should be given indefinitely to HIV-infected individuals who have experienced an earlier episode of *P. jiroveci* pneumonia. HCT patients should receive prophylaxis for at least 6 months (the greatest risk period) and longer if the immunosuppressive regimen continues for treatment of chronic GVHD (10). Children with acute lymphoblastic leukemia should be given prophylaxis (83). For other patient groups, there are no national guidelines, and the appropriateness of primary prophylaxis must be individualized by patient risk group and individual immune status because the underlying immunodeficiency and the type of immunosuppressive regimen may vary considerably and the risk for infection may be difficult to judge. Solid organ-transplant recipients generally are given prophylaxis for 6 months. Other risk groups in which prophylaxis should be considered included immune deficiency conditions, severe protein malnutrition, illnesses that result in low CD4+ lymphocyte counts (<200 cells/uL), connective tissue diseases treated by immunosuppressive regimens, and various cancers, especially lymphoreticular cancers, in which treatment regimens result in suppression of T-lymphocyte immunity (e.g., corticosteroids, purine analogs, and anti-T-cell antibodies). Infection can be prevented by trimethoprim–sulfamethoxazole (TMP-SMZ) (84). TMP–SMZ is generally given as one double-strength tablet (160 mg TMP plus 800 mg SMZ) once or twice daily, but three times weekly also is effective. Aerosolized pentamidine given once monthly at a 300- mg dose is an alternative, avoiding some of TMP–SMZ's toxicities, but is less effective (85,86). Dapsone and atovaquone are also alternatives.

IX. DURATION OF PROPHYLAXIS

For prophylaxis to be effective, the period of vulnerability must be known to determine the duration of prophylaxis. Correction of the underlying host defense that led to the susceptibility is the key determinant. For example, resolution of neutropenia for chemotherapy-induced myelosuppression and control of active HIV infection with recovery of CD4+T-lymphocyte counts to >200 cells/µL are two examples.

Notwithstanding, there is a relative paucity of data to clearly determine the optimal duration of prophylaxis. The best data are in HIV-infected patients in which improvement in the CD4+T-Iymphocyte count takes place. Several studies have clearly shown that once a threshold level of a CD4+count of at least 200 cells/μL is achieved and maintained for at least 3 months, prophylaxis against *P. jiroveci* can be stopped with a low likelihood of recurrence (42). There is a small body of data suggesting that discontinuation of secondary prophylaxis for *Candida* and *Cryptococcus* can also be done when the CD4+T-lymphocyte count rises to above 100 or 200 cells/μL and remains above this level (76,87–90). There is a paucity of published data for discontinuation strategies for other opportunistic fungal pathogens in advanced HIV disease, but expert opinion suggests that this can be considered when the CD4+T-lymphocyte count rises to >100 cells/μL with HAART therapy (42).

For patients with hematologic malignancies, few studies have evaluated the duration of prophylaxis. Generally, cessation of prophylaxis in leukemia therapy takes place at the completion of the treatment course and recovery of myelosuppression. For HCT recipients, *Candida* prophylaxis generally is discontinued at engraftment, but some continue during the peak risk period of acute graft versus host disease (4). For solid organ transplantation, various studies have evaluated antifungal prophylaxis durations between 1 and 10 weeks in duration. The general view is that prophylaxis should continue during the peak risk period, which is early after transplant.

X. INFECTION CONTROL

As important as pharmacologic agents are in a prophylaxis strategy, even more important are the measures necessary to minimize exposure of susceptible patients to potential pathogens. For pathogens infecting or colonizing patients, measures should be taken to minimize patient to patient transmission.

Candida organisms are generally endogenous, and thus no measures are ordinarily needed to prevent acquisition. However, some studies have suggested patient to patient transmission in hospital environments, presumably by healthcare workers, in transplant recipients, leukemia patients, ICU patients, and surgical patients (91–101). Thus, hand washing is an important facet of infection control. Outbreaks of infections in which nosocomial transmission is a possibility should be investigated by the hospital infection-control team. Molecular testing for DNA polymorphisms can be quite useful to determine if one or more strains are present in multiple patients (91). Other point sources of infection that have been identified (other than healthcare workers) include IV solutions, medications, and plastic tubing.

Because *Aspergillus* conidia are exogenous organisms present in the environment and are primarily air-borne, transmission of organisms can occur in the hospital environment during construction, renovation, or other activities in which organisms can be spread and inhaled by susceptible immunocompromised patients. Accordingly, high-efficiency air filtration is important in hospital rooms in which highly susceptible patients reside to prevent outbreaks (102–107). These include HCT recipients, and the routine use of HEPA filters is recommended in consensus guidelines (10,49). The use of high-efficiency masks worn during transport when leaving their rooms may also be helpful (108). The CDC has promulgated environmental guidelines to prevent inadvertent exposures to *Aspergillus* (109).

Recently, patient-shower facilities have been implicated as potential sources of noso-comial *Aspergillus* acquisition (110,111). Avoidance or cleaning procedures have been proposed to reduce the risk to susceptible patients (112).

Cryptococcus is associated with IV drug use and tobacco use. Avoidance of invasive disease from this pathogen is yet another reason that such activities should be avoided. As noted earlier, histoplasmosis can be acquired by activities that result in dispersal of organisms from soil into the atmosphere, including working with soil, cleaning chicken coups contaminated with droppings, cleaning or renovating old houses, or exploring caves. These activities should be avoided by individuals with CD4+T-lymphocyte counts <200 cells/μL in endemic areas (42). Similarly, in cocci-diomycosis endemic areas, activities that stir up dust and soil should be avoided by at-risk individuals.

XI. CONCLUSIONS

Prophylaxis can be an important strategy to improve antifungal treatment outcomes. Toxicity, emergence of drug resistance, and financial costs may offset the benefits, however. Accordingly, careful selection of at-risk patients is important. A pre-requisite for this is an understanding of the spectrum of infectious pathogens, time of vulnerability for infection, and the risk factors that identify susceptible patients. Moreover, monitoring of the strategy over time must be performed to ascertain that the strategy continues to be effective and benefits outweigh risks.

REFERENCES

1. Wilson LS, Reyes CM, Stolpman M, Speckman J, Allen K, Beney J. The direct cost and incidence of systemic fungal infections. Value Health 2002; 5(l):26–34.
2. Goodman JL, Winston DJ, Greenfield RA, Chandrasekar PH, Fox B, Kaizer H, Shadduck RK, Shea TC, Stiff P, Friedman DJ. A controlled trial of fluconazole to pre-vent fungal infections in patients undergoing bone marrow transplantation. N Engl J Med 1992; 326(13):845–851.
3. Rotstein C, Bow EJ, Laverdiere M, Ioannou S, Carr D, Moghaddam N. Randomized placebo-controlled trial of fluconazole prophylaxis for neutropenic cancer patients: ben-efit based on purpose and intensity of cytotoxic therapy. The Canadian Fluconazole Prophylaxis Study Group.. Clin Infect Dis 1999; 28(2):331–340.
4. Slavin MA, Osborne B, Adams R, Levenstein MJ, Schoch HG, Feldman AR, Meyers JD, Bowden RA. Efficacy and safety of fluconazole prophylaxis for fungal infections after marrow transplantation—a prospective, randomized, double-blind study. J Infect Dis 1995; 171(6):1545–1552.
5. Marr KA, Seidel K, Slavin MA, Bowden RA, Schoch HG, Flowers ME, Corey L, Boeckh M. Prolonged fluconazole prophylaxis is associated with persistent protection against candidiasis-related death in allogeneic marrow transplant recipients: long-term follow-up of a randomized, placebo-controlled trial. Blood 2000; 96(6):2055–2061.
6. MacMillan ML, Goodman JL, DeFor TE, Weisdorf DJ. Fluconazole to prevent yeast infections in bone marrow transplantation patients: a randomized trial of high versus reduced dose, and determination of the value of maintenance therapy. Am J Med 2002; 112(5):369–379.
7. Wingard JR, Merz WG, Rinaldi MG, Johnson TR, Karp JE, Saral R. Increase in *Candida krusei* infection among patients with bone marrow transplantation and neutropenia treated prophylactically with fluconazole. N Engl J Med 1991; 325(18):1274–1277.

8. Wingard JR, Merz WG, Rinaldi MG, Miller CB, Karp JE, Saral R. Association of *Torulopsis glabrata* infections with fluconazole prophylaxis in neutropenic bone marrow transplant patients. Antimicrob Agents Chemother 1993; 37(9):1847–1849.

9. Persons DA, Laughlin M, Tanner D, Perfect J, Gockerman JP, Hathorn JW. Fluconazole and *Candida krusei* fungemia. N Engl J Med 1991; 325(18):1315.

10. Dykewicz C, Jaffe H, Kaplan JE. In collaboration with the Guidelines Working Group members from CDC. CDC Guidelines for preventing opportunistic infections among hematopoietic stem cell transplant recipients. Biol Blood Marrow Transplant 2000; 6(6a):659–741.

11. Wolff SN, Fay J, Stevens D, Herzig RH, Pohlman B, Bolwell B, Lynch J, Ericson S, Freytes CO, LeMaistre F, Collins R, Pineiro L, Greer J, Stein R, Goodman SA, Dummer S. Fluconazole vs. low-dose amphotericin B for the prevention of fungal infections in patients undergoing bone marrow transplantation: a study of the North American Marrow Transplant Group. Bone Marrow Transplant 2000; 25(8):853–859.

12. Perfect JR, Klotman ME, Gilbert CC, Crawford DD, Rosner GL, Wright KA, Peters WP. Prophylactic intravenous amphotericin B in neutropenic autologous bone marrow transplant recipients. J Infect Dis 1992; 165(5):891–897.

13. Gotzsche PC, Johansen HK. Meta-analysis of prophylactic or empirical antifungal treatment versus placebo or no treatment in patients with cancer complicated by neutropenia. BMJ 1997; 314(7089):1238–1244.

14. Bow EJ, Laverdiere M, Lussier N, Rotstein C, Cheang MS, Ioannou S. Antifungal prophylaxis for severely neutropenic chemotherapy recipients: a meta analysis of randomized-controlled clinical trials. Cancer 2002; 94(12):3230–3246.

15. Kanda Y, Yamamoto R, Chizuka A, Hamaki T, Suguro M, Arai C, Matsuyama T, Takezako N, Miwa A, Kern W, Kami M, Akiyama H, Hirai H, Togawa A. Prophylactic action of oral fluconazole against fungal infection in neutropenic patients. A meta-analysis of 16 randomized, controlled trials. Cancer 2000; 89(7):1611–1625.

16. Rex JH, Anaissie EJ, Boutati E, Estey E, Kantarjian H. Systemic antifungal prophylaxis reduces invasive fungal in acute myelogenous leukemia: a retrospective review of 833 episodes of neutropenia in 322 adults. Leukemia 2002; 16(6):1197–1199.

17. Collins LA, Samore MH, Roberts MS, Luzzati R, Jenkins RL, Lewis WD, Karchmer AW. Risk factors for invasive fungal infections complicating orthotopic liver transplantation. J Infect Dis 1994; 170(3):644–652.

18. Kung N, Fisher N, Gunson B, Hastings M, Mutimer D. Fluconazole prophylaxis for high-risk liver transplant recipients. Lancet 1995; 345(8959):1234–1235.

19. Winston DJ, Pakrasi A, Busuttil RW. Prophylactic fluconazole in liver transplant recipients. A randomized, double-blind, placebo-controlled trial. Ann Intern Med 1999; 131(10):729–737.

20. Tollemar J, Hockerstedt K, Ericzon BG, Jalanko H, Ringden O. Liposomal amphotericin B prevents invasive fungal infections in liver transplant recipients. A randomized, placebo-controlled study. Transplantation 1995; 59(l):45–50.

21. Singhal S, Ellis RW, Jones SG, Miller SJ, Fisher NC, Hastings JG, Mutimer DJ. Targeted prophylaxis with amphotericin B lipid complex in liver transplantation. Liver Transpl 2000; 6(5):588–595.

22. Benedetti E, Gruessner AC, Troppmann C, Papalois BE, Sutherland DE, Dunn DL, Gruessner RW. Intra-abdominal fungal infections after pancreatic transplantation: incidence, treatment, and outcome. J Am Coll Surg 1996; 183(4):307–316.

23. Petri MG, Konig J, Moecke HP, Gramm HJ, Barkow H, Kujath P, Dennhart R, Schafer H, Meyer N, Kalmar P, Thulig P, Muller J, Lode H. Epidemiology of invasive mycosis in ICU patients: a prospective multicenter study in 435 non-neutropenic patients. Intensive Care Med 1997; 23(3):317–325.

24. Rex JH, Walsh TJ, Sobel JD, Filler SG, Pappas PG, Dismukes WE, Edwards JE. Practice guidelines for the treatment of candidiasis. Infectious Diseases Society of America. Clin Infect Dis 2000; 30(4):662–678.

25. British Society for Antimicrobial Chemotherapy Working Party. Management of deep *Candida* infection in surgical and intensive care unit patients. Intensive Care Med 1994; 20(7):522–528.

26. Vincent JL, Anaissie E, Bruining H, Demajo W, el Ebiary M, Haber J, Hiramatsu Y, Nitenberg G, Nystrom PO, Pittet D, Rogers T, Sandven P, Sganga G, Schaller MD, Solomkin J. Epidemiology, diagnosis and treatment of systemic *Candida* infection in surgical patients under intensive care. Intensive Care Med 1998; 24(3):206–216.

27. Rex JH, Sobel JD. Prophylactic antifungal therapy in the intensive care unit. Clin Infect Dis 2001; 32(8):1191–1200.

28. Sobel JD, Rex JH. Invasive candidiasis: turning risk into a practical prevention policy? Clin Infect Dis 2001; 33(2):187–190.

29. Blumberg HM, Jarvis WR, Soucie JM, Edwards JE, Patterson JE, Pfaller MA, Rangel-Frausto MS, Rinaldi MG, Saiman L, Wiblin RT, Wenzel RP. Risk factors for candidal blookstream infections in surgical intensive care unit patients: the NEMIS prospective multicenter study. The National Epidemiology of Mycosis Survey. Clin Infect Dis 2001; 33(2):177–186.

30. Slotman GJ, Burchard KW. Ketoconazole prevents *Candida* sepsis in critically ill surgical patients. Arch Surg 1987; 122(2):147–151.

31. Eggimann P, Francioli P, Bille J, Schneider R, Wu MM, Chapuis G, Chiolero R, Pannatier A, Schilling J, Geroulanos S, Glauser MP, Calandra T. Fluconazole prophylaxis prevents intra-abdominal candidiasis in high-risk surgical patients. Crit Care Med 1999; 27(6):1066–1072.

32. Pelz RK, Hendrix CW, Swoboda SM, Diener-West M, Merz WG, Hammond J, Lipsett PA. Double-blind placebo-controlled trial of fluconazole to prevent candidal infections in critically ill surgical patients. Ann Surg 2001; 233(4):542–548.

33. Stoll BJ, Gordon T, Korones SB, Shankaran S, Tyson JE, Bauer CR, Fanaroff AA, Lemons JA, Donovan EF, Oh W, Stevenson DK, Ehrenkranz RA, Papile LA, Verter J, Wright LL. Late-onset sepsis in very low birth weight neonates: a report from the National Institute of Child Health and Human Development Neonatal Research Network. J Pediatr 1996; 129(1):63–71.

34. Kaufman D, Boyle R, Hazen KC, Patrie JT, Robinson M, Donowitz LG. Fluconazole prophylaxis against fungal colonization and infection in preterm infants. N Engl J Med 2001; 345(23):1660–1666.

35. Fichtenbaum CJ. Candidiasis. In: Dolin R, Masur H, Saag MS, eds. AIDS Therapy. Philadelphia: Churchill-Livingstone, 2003:531–542.

36. Cauda R, Tacconelli E, Tumbarello M, Morace G, De Bernardis F, Torosantucci A, Cassone A. Role of protease inhibitors in preventing recurrent oral candidiasis in patients with HIV infection: a prospective case–control study. J Acquir Immune Defic Syndr 1999; 21(l):20–25.

37. Martins MD, Lozano-Chiu M, Rex JH. Declining rates of oropharyngeal candidiasis and carriage of *Candida albicans* associated with trends toward reduced rates of carriage of fluconazole-resistant *C. albicans* in human immunodeficiency virus-infected patients. Clin Infect Dis 1998; 27(5):1291–1294.

38. Darouiche RO. Oropharyngeal and esophageal candidiasis in immunocompromised patients: treatment issues. Clin Infect Dis 1998; 26(2):259–272.

39. Schuman P, Capps L, Peng G, Vazquez J, el Sadr W, Goldman AI, Alston B, Besch CL, Vaughn A, Thompson MA, Cobb MN, Kerkering T, Sobel JD. Weekly fluconazole for the prevention of mucosal candidiasis in women with HIV infection. A randomized, double-blind, placebo-controlled trial. Ann Intern Med 1997; 126(9):689–696.

40. Heald AE, Cox GM, Schell WA, Bartlett JA, Perfect JR. Oropharyngeal yeast flora and fluconazole resistance in HIV-infected patients receiving long-term continuous versus intermittent fluconazole therapy. AIDS 1996; 10(3):263–268.

41. Patton L, Bonito A, Shugars D. A systematic review of the effectiveness of antifungal drugs for the prevention and treatment of oropharyngeal candidiasis in HIV-positive patients. Oral Surg Oral Med Oral Pathol Oral Radiol Endod 2001; 92(2):170–179.

42. Guidelines for the Preventing Opportunistic Infections Among Hematopoietic Stem Cell Transplant Recipients. Recommendations of CDC, Infectious Diseases Society of America, and American Society of Blood & Marrow Transplantation. Biol Blood Marrow Transplant 2000; 6; 659–734.

43. Imbert-Bernard C, Valentin A, Reynes J, Mallie M, Bastide JM. Relationship between fluconazole sensitivity of *Candida albicans* isolates from HIV positive patients and serotype, adherence and CD4+ lymphocyte count. Eur J Clin Microbiol Infect Dis 1994; 13(9):711–716.

44. Powderly WG, Finkelstein D, Feinberg J, Frame P, He W, van der HC, Koletar SL, Eyster ME, Carey J, Waskin H. A randomized trial comparing fluconazole with clotrimazole troches for the prevention of fungal infections in patients with advanced human immunodeficiency virus infection. NIAID AIDS Clinical Trials Group. N Engl J Med 1995; 332(11):700–705.

45. Gerson SL, Talbot GH, Hurwitz S, Strom BL, Lusk EJ, Cassileth PA. Prolonged granulocytopenia: the major risk factor for invasive pulmonary aspergillosis in patients with acute leukemia. Ann Intern Med 1984; 100(3):345–351.

46. Marr KA, Carter RA, Boeckh M, Martin P, Corey L. Invasive aspergillosis in allogeneic stem cell transplant recipients: changes in epidemiology and risk factors. Blood 2002; 100(13):4358–4366.

47. Fukuda T, Boeckh M, Carter RA, Sandmaier BM, Maris MB, Maloney DG, Martin PJ, Storb RF, Marr KA. Risks and outcomes of invasive fungal infections in recipients of allogeneic hematopoietic stem cell transplants after nonmyeloablative conditioning. Blood 2003; 102(3):827–833.

48. Hagen EA, Stem H, Porter D, Duffy K, Foley K, Luger S, Schuster SJ, Stadtmauer EA, Schuster MG. High rate of invasive fungal infections following nonmyeloablative allogeneic transplantation. Clin Infect Dis 2003; 36(1):9–15.

49. Marr KA, Carter RA, Crippa F, Wald A, Corey L. Epidemiology and outcome of mould infections in hematopoietic stem cell transplant recipients. Clin Infect Dis 2002; 34(7):909–917.

50. Karp JE, Burch PA, Merz WG. An approach to intensive antileukemia therapy in patients with previous invasive aspergillosis. Am J Med 1988; 85(2):203–206.

51. Martino R, Lopez R, Sureda A, Brunet S, Domingo-Albos A. Risk of reactivation of a recent invasive fungal infection in patients with hematological malignancies undergoing further intensive chemo-radiotherapy. A single-center experience and review of the literature. Haematologica 1997; 82(3):297–304.

52. Tollemar J, Ringden O, Andersson S, Sundberg B, Ljungman P, Sparrelid E, Tyden G. Prophylactic use of liposomaal amphotericin B (AmBisome) against fungal infections: a randomized trial in bone marrow transplant recipients. Transplant Proc 1993; 25: 1495–1497.

53. Kelsey SM, Goldman JM, McCann S, Newland AC, Scarffe JH, Oppenheim BA, Mufti GJ. Liposomal amphotericin (AmBisome) in the prophylaxis of fungal infections in neutropenic patients: a randomised, double-blind, placebo-controlled study. Bone Marrow Transplant 1999; 23(2):163–168.

54. Morgenstern GR, Prentice AG, Prentice HG, Ropner JE, Schey SA, Warnock DW. A randomized controlled trial of itraconazole versus fluconazole for the prevention of fungal infections in patients with haematological malignancies. U.K. Multicentre Antifungal Prophylaxis Study Group. Br J Haematol 1999; 105(4):901–911.

55. Kibbler CC. Antifungal prophylaxis with itraconazole oral solution in neutropenic patients. Mycoses 1999; 42(suppl 2):121–124.

56. Kaptan K, Ural AU, Cetin T, Avcu F, Beyan C, Yalcin A. Itraconazole is not effective for the prophylaxis of fungal infections in patients with neutropenia. J Infect Chemother 2003; 9(1):40–45.

57. Menichetti F, Del Favero A, Martino P, Bucaneve G, Micozzi A, Girmenia C, Barbabietola G, Pagano L, Leoni P, Specchia G, Caiozzo A, Raimondi R, Mandelli F.

Itraconazole oral solution as prophylaxis for fungal infections in neutropenic patients with hematologic malignancies: a randomized, placebo-controlled, double-blind, multicenter trial. GIMEMA Infection Program. Gruppo Italiano Malattie Ematologiche dell' Adulto. Clin Infect Dis 1999; 28(2):250–255.

58. Bohme A, Just-Nubling G, Bergmann L, Shah PM, Stille W, Hoelzer D. Itraconazole for prophylaxis of systemic mycoses in neutropenic patients with haematological malignancies. J Antimicrob Chemother 1996; 38(6):953–961.

59. Boogaerts M, Maertens J, van Hoof A, de Bock R, Fillet G, Peetermans M, Selleslag D, Vandercam B, Vandewoude K, Zachee P, De Beule K. Itraconazole versus amphotericin B plus nystatin in the prophylaxis of fungal infections in neutropenic cancer patients. J Antimicrob Chemother 2001; 48(1):97–103.

60. Glasmacher A, Prentice A, Gorschluter M, Engelhart S, Hahn C, Djulbegovic B, Schmidt-Wolf IG. Itraconazole prevents invasive fungal infections in neutropenic patients treated for hematologic malignancies: evidence from a meta-analysis of 3,597 patients. J Clin Oncol 2003; 21:4615–4626.

61. Winston DT, Maziarz RT, Chandrasekar PH, Lazarus HM, Goldman M, Blumer JL, Leitz GJ, Territo MC. Intravenous and oral itraconazole versus intravenous and oral fluconazole for long-term antifungal prophylaxis in allogeneic hematopoietic stem-cell transplant recipients. A multicenter, randomized trial. Ann Intern Med 2003; 138(9):705–713.

62. Marr KA, Crippa F, Leisenring W, Hoyle M, Boeckh M, Balajee SA, Nichols WG, Musher B, Corey L. Itraconazole versus fluconazole for prevention of fungal infections in patients receiving allogeneic stem cell transplants. Blood 2004; 100:1527–1533.

63. Lewis RE, Prince RA, Chi J, Kontoyiannis DP. Itraconazole preexposure attenuates the efficacy of subsequent amphotericin B therapy in a murine model of acute invasive pulmonary aspergillosis. Antimicrob Agents Chemother 2002; 46(10):3208–3214.

64. Trigg ME, Morgan D, Burns TL, Kook H, Rumelhart SL, Holida MD, Giller RH. Successful program to prevent *Aspergillus* infections in children undergoing marrow transplantation: use of nasal amphotericin. Bone Marrow Transplant 1997; 19(1):43–47.

65. Schwartz S, Behre G, Heinemann V, Wandt H, Schilling E, Arning M, Trittin A, Kern WV, Boenisch O, Bosse D, Lenz K, Ludwig WD, Hiddemann W, Siegert W, Beyer J. Aerosolized amphotericin B inhalations as prophylaxis of invasive *Aspergillus* infections during prolonged neutropenia: results of a prospective randomized multicenter trial. Blood 1999; 93(11):3654–3661.

66. Gordon SM, Avery RK. Aspergillosis in lung transplantation: incidence, risk factors, and prophylactic strategies. Transpl Infect Dis 2001; 3(3):161–167.

67. Paterson DL, Singh N. Invasive aspergillosis in transplant recipients. Medicine 1999; 78(2):123–138.

68. Palmer SM, Drew RH, Whitehouse JD, Tapson VF, Davis RD, McConnell RR, Kanj SS, Perfect JR. Safety of aerosolized amphotericin B lipid complex in lung transplant recipients. Transplantation 2001; 72(3):545–548.

69. Monforte V, Roman A, Gavalda J, Bravo C, Tenorio L, Ferrer A, Maestre J, Morell F. Nebulized amphotericin B prophylaxis for *Aspergillus* infection in lung transplantation: study of risk factors. J Heart Lung Transplant 2001; 20(12):1274–1281.

70. Aberg JA, Powderly WG. Cryptococcosis. In: Dolin R, Masur H, Saag MS, eds. AIDS Therapy. 2nd ed. Philadelphia: Churchill-Livingstone, 2003:498–510.

71. Aberg JA, Price RW, Heeren DM, et al. Discontinuation of antifungal therapy for cryptococcosis after immunologic response to antiretroviral therapy [abstr 250]. Program and Abstracts of the 7th Conference on Retroviruses and Opportunistic Infections 2000, San Francisco, CA, Jan 30–Feb 2, 2000.

72. Mussini C, Cossarizza A, Pezzotti P, et al. Discontinuation or continuation of maintenance therapy for cryptococcal meningitis in patients with AIDS treated with HAART [abstr 546]. Program and Abstracts of the 8th Conference on Retroviruses and Opportunistic Infections, Chicago, IL, Feb 4–8, 2001.

73. Saag MS, Cloud GA, Graybill JR, Sobel JD, Tuazon CU, Johnson PC, Fessel WJ, Moskovitz BL, Wiesinger B, Cosmatos D, Riser L, Thomas C, Hafner R, Dismukes WE. A comparison of itraconazole versus fluconazole as maintenance therapy for AIDS-associated cryptococcal meningitis. National Institute of Allergy and Infectious Diseases Mycoses Study Group. Clin Infect Dis 1999; 28(2):291–296.

74. Cano M, Hajjeh R. The epidemiology of histoplasmosis: a review. Semin Respir Infect 2001; 16:109–118.

75. Wheat J, Hafner R, Wulfsohn M, Spencer P, Squires K, Powderly W, Wong B, Rinaldi M, Saag M, Hamill R. Prevention of relapse of histoplasmosis with itraconazole in patients with the acquired immunodeficiency syndrome. The National Institute of Allergy and Infectious Diseases Clinical Trials and Mycoses Study Group Collaborators. Ann Intern Med 1993; 118(8):610–616.

76. Norris S, Wheat J, McKinsey D, Lancaster D, Katz B, Black J, Driks M, Baker R, Israel K, Traeger D. Prevention of relapse of histoplasmosis with fluconazole in patients with the acquired immunodeficiency syndrome. Am J Med 1994; 96(6):504–508.

77. McKinsey DS, Wheat LJ, Cloud GA, Pierce M, Black JR, Bamberger DM, Goldman M, Thomas CJ, Gutsch HM, Moskovitz B, Dismukes WE, Kauffman CA. Itraconazole prophylaxis for fungal infections in patients with advanced human immunodeficiency virus infection: randomized, placebo-controlled, double-blind study. National Institute of Allergy and Infectious Diseases Mycoses Study Group. Clin Infect Dis 1999; 28(5):1049–1056.

78. Woods CW, McRill C, Plikaytis BD, Rosenstein NE, Mosley D, Boyd D, England B, Perkins BA, Ampel NM, Hajjeh RA. Coccidioidomycosis in human immunodeficiency virus-infected persons in Arizona, 1994–1997: incidence, risk factors, and prevention. J Infect Dis 2000; 181(4):1428–1434.

79. Galgiani JN, Catanzaro A, Cloud GA, Johnson RH, Williams PL, Mirels LF, Nassar F, Lutz JE, Stevens DA, Sharkey PK, Singh VR, Larsen RA, Delgado KL, Flanigan C, Rinaldi MG. Comparison of oral fluconazole and itraconazole for progressive, nonmeningeal coccidioidomycosis. A randomized, double-blind trial. Mycoses Study Group. Ann Intern Med 2000; 133(9):676–686.

80. Center for Disease Control and Prevention. Guidelines for prophylaxis against *Pneumocystis carinii* pneumonia for persons infected with human immunodeficiency virus. MMWR 1989; 38(S-5):1–9.

81. Centers for Disease Control and Prevention. Recommendations for prophylaxis against *Pneumocystis carinii* pneumonia for adults and adolescents infected with human immunodeficiency virus. MMWR 1992; 41(RR-4): 1–11.

82. Centers for Disease Control and Prevention. Guidelines for prophylaxis against *Pneumocystis carinii* pneumonia for children infected with human immunodeficiency virus. MMWR 1991; 40(RR-2):1–13.

83. Warren E, George S, You J, Kazanjian P. Advances in the treatment and prophylaxis of *Pneumocystis carinii* pneumonia. Pharmacotherapy 1997; 17(5):900–916.

84. Masur H. Prevention and treatment of *Pneumocystis* pneumonia. N Engl J Med 1992; 327(26):1853–1860.

85. Schneider MM, Hoepelman AI, Eeftinck Schattenkerk JK, Nielsen TL, van der Graaf Y, Frissen JP, van der Ende IM, Kolsters AF, Borleffs JC. A controlled trial of aerosolized pentamidine or trimethoprim–sulfamethoxazole as primary prophylaxis against *Pneumocystis carinii* pneumonia in patients with human immunodeficiency virus infection. The Dutch AIDS Treatment Group. N Engl J Med 1992; 327(26):1836–1841.

86. Hardy WD, Feinberg J, Finkelstein DM, Power ME, He W, Kaczka C, Frame PT, Holmes M, Waskin H, Fass RJ. A controlled trial of trimethoprim–sulfamethoxazole or aerosolized pentamidine for secondary prophylaxis of *Pneumocystis carinii* pneumonia in patients with the acquired immunodeficiency syndrome. AIDS Clinical Trials Group Protocol 021. N Engl J Med 1992; 327(26):1842–1848.

87. Gripshover BM, Valdez H, Salata RA, Lederman MM. Withdrawal of fluconazole suppressive therapy for thrush in patients responding to combination antiviral therapy including protease inhibitors. AIDS 1998; 12(18):2513–2514.

88. Kaplan JE, Masur H, Holmes KK. Discontinuing prophylaxis against recurrent opportunistic infections in HIV-infected persons: a victory in the era of HAART. Ann Intern Med 2002; 137(4):285–287.

89. Aberg JA, Price RW, Heeren DM, Bredt B. A pilot study of the discontinuation of antifungal therapy for disseminated cryptococcal disease in patients with acquired immunodeficiency syndrome, following immunologic response to antiretroviral therapy. J Infect Dis 2002; 185(8):1179–1182.

90. Kirk O, Reiss P, Uberti-Foppa C, Bickel M, Gerstoft J, Pradier C, Wit FW, Ledergerber B, Lundgren JD, Furrer H. Safe interruption of maintenance therapy against previous infection with four common HIV-associated opportunistic pathogens during potent antiretroviral therapy. Ann Intern Med 2002; 137(4):239–250.

91. Pfaller MA. Epidemiology of fungal infections: the promise of molecular typing. Clin Infect Dis 1995; 20(6):1535–1539.

92. Doi M, Homma M, Iwaguchi S, Horibe K, Tanaka K. Strain relatedness of *Candida albicans* strains isolated from children with leukemia and their bedside parents. J Clin Microbiol 1994; 32(9):2253–2259.

93. Sherertz RJ, Gledhill KS, Hampton KD, Pfaller MA, Givner LB, Abramson JS, Dillard RG. Outbreak of *Candida* bloodstream infections associated with retrograde medication administration in a neonatal intensive care unit. J Pediatr 1992; 120(3):455–461.

94. Burnie JP, Odds FC, Lee W, Webster C, Williams JD. Outbreak of systemic *Candida albicans* in intensive care unit caused by cross infection. Br Med J (Clin Res Ed) 1985; 290(6470):746–748.

95. Doebbeling BN, Hollis RJ, Isenberg HD, Wenzel RP, Pfaller MA. Restriction fragment analysis of a *Candida tropicalis* outbreak of sternal wound infections. J Clin Microbiol 1991; 29(6):1268–1270.

96. Schmid J, Odds FC, Wiselka MJ, Nicholson KG, Soll DR. Genetic similarity and maintenance of *Candida albicans* strains from a group of AIDS patients, demonstrated by DNA fingerprinting. J Clin Microbiol 1992; 30(4):935–941.

97. Finkelstein R, Reinhertz G, Hashman N, Merzbach D. Outbreak of *Candida tropicalis* fungemia in a neonatal intensive care unit. Infect Control Hosp Epidemiol 1993; 14(10):587–590.

98. Moro ML, Maffei C, Manso E, Morace G, Polonelli L, Biavasco F. Nosocomial outbreak of systemic candidosis associated with parenteral nutrition. Infect Control Hosp Epidemiol 1990; 11(1):27–35.

99. Sanchez V, Vazquez JA, Barth-Jones D, Dembry L, Sobel JD, Zervos MJ. Epidemiology of nosocomial acquisition of *Candida lusitaniae*. J Clin Microbiol 1992; 30(11): 3005–3008.

100. Sanchez V, Vazquez JA, Barth-Jones D, Dembry L, Sobel JD, Zervos MJ. Nosocomial acquisftion of *Candida parapsilosis*: an epidemiologic study. Am J Med 1993; 94(6): 577–582.

101. Burnie JP. *Candida* and hands. J Hosp Infect 1986; 8(1):1–4.

102. Sherertz RJ, Belani A, Kramer BS, Elfenbein GJ, Weiner RS, Sullivan ML, Thomas RG, Samsa GP. Impact of air filtration on nosocomial *Aspergillus* infections. Unique risk of bone marrow transplant recipients. Am J Med 1987; 83(4):709–718.

103. Oren I, Haddad N, Finkelstein R, Rowe JM. Invasive pulmonary aspergillosis in neutropenic patients during hospital construction: before and after chemoprophylaxis and institution of HEPA filters. Am J Hematol 2001; 66(4):257–262.

104. Patterson JE, Peters J, Calhoon JH, Levine S, Anzueto A, Al Abdely H, Sanchez R, Patterson TF, Rech M, Jorgensen JH, Rinaldi MG, Sako E, Johnson S, Speeg V,

Halff GA, Trinkle JK. Investigation and control of aspergillosis and other filamentous fungal infections in solid organ transplant recipients. Transpl Infect Dis 2000; 2(1): 22–28.

105. Cornet M, Levy V, Fleury L, Lortholary J, Barquins S, Coureul MH, Deliere E, Zittoun R, Brucker G, Bouvet A. Efficacy of prevention by high-efficiency particulate air filtration or laminar airflow against *Aspergillus* airborne contamination during hospital renovation. Infect Control Hosp Epidemiol 1999; 20(7):508–513.

106. Aisner J, Schimpff SC, Bennett JE, Young VM, Wiernik PH. *Aspergillus* infections in cancer patients. Association with fireproofing materials in a new hospital. JAMA 1976; 235(4):411–412.

107. Hahn T, Cummings KM, Michalek AM, Lipman BJ, Segal BH, McCarthy PL Jr. Efficacy of high-efficiency particulate air filtration in preventing aspergillosis in immunocompromised patients with hematologic malignancies. Infect Control Hosp Epidemiol 2002; 23(9):525–531.

108. Raad I, Hanna H, Osting C, Hachem R, Umphrey J, Tarrand J, Kantarjian H, Bodey GP. Masking of neutropenic patients on transport from hospital rooms is associated with a decrease in nosocomial aspergillosis during construction. Infect Control Hosp Epidemiol 2002; 23(l):41–43.

109. Sehulster L, Chinn RY. Guidelines for environmental infection control in health-care facilities. Recommendations of CDC and the Healthcare Infection Control Practices Advisory Committee (HICPAC). MMWR Recomm Rep 2003; 52(RR-10):1–42.

110. Anaissie EJ, Penzak SR, Dignani MC. The hospital water supply as a source of nosocomial infections: a plea for action. Arch Intern Med 2002; 162(13):1483–1492.

111. Anaissie EJ, Stratton SL, Dignani MC, Lee CK, Summerbell RC, Rex JH, Monson TP, Walsh TJ. Pathogenic molds (including *Aspergillus* species) in hospital water distribution systems: a 3-year prospective study and clinical implications for patients with hematologic malignancies. Blood 2003; 101(7):2542–2546.

112. Anaissie EJ, Stratton SL, Dignani MC, Lee CK, Mahfouz TH, Rex JH, Summerbell RC, Walsh TJ. Cleaning patient shower facilities: a novel approach to reducing patient exposure to aerosolized *Aspergillus* species and other opportunistic molds. Clin Infect Dis 2002;35(8):E86–E88.

23

Empirical Therapy of Suspected Infections

J. A. Maertens, K. Theunissen, and M. A. Boogaerts
Department of Hematology, University Hospital Gasthuisberg, Leuven, Belgium

I. INTRODUCTION

Invasive fungal infections (IFI) have become a major cause of morbidity and mortality in immunocompromised patients (1–5). The incidence and the mortality rate varies among the different underlying diseases, with relapsed acute leukemia patients and those undergoing allogeneic hematopoietic stem cell transplantation having the highest risk, followed by solid organ transplant recipients, critically ill surgical patients, and premature neonates (6,7). *Candida-* and *Aspergillus* species still account for the vast majority of documented infections, but recent epidemiological surveys have revealed the emergence of previously uncommon pathogens that are often less susceptible to conventional antifungal agents (8,9). This shift will have an impact on the choice of appropriate agents for empirical antifungal therapy.

Hospital-acquired infections caused by *Candida* species—both superficial and deep-seated forms—have increased substantially over the past two decades. Prospective surveillance studies have shown an approximately 500% increase in the rate of nosocomial primary bloodstream infections by *Candida* species in large teaching hospitals, with *Candida* now representing the fourth most commonly isolated bloodstream pathogens in the United States (10). Today, the contribution of candidemia has placed this pathogen ahead of more traditional nosocomial pathogens, including *Enterobacter* spp., *Escherichia coli*, *Pseudomonas aeruginosa*, and *Klebsiella*. At-risk patients are encountered in various settings, but most frequently in intensive care, abdominal surgery, transplantation, and oncology units (11). However, more alarming is the high overall and attributable mortality rate. In a tightly matched historical control study, Wey et al. reported an attributable mortality rate of 38% and a significantly increased duration of hospitalization for survivors (12); these data are in accordance with European studies (13,14).

Although *Candida albicans* remains the most commonly encountered pathogenic yeast in humans, recent studies have demonstrated a shift towards infection with "non-*albicans*" *Candida* species (15–18). In the SCOPE National Surveillance System, 48% of *Candida* isolates from nosocomial bloodstream infections were non-albicans species, including *C. tropicalis*, *C. glabrata*, *C. krusei*, *C. parapsilosis*, and *C. lusitaniae* (19). Although some of these species are considered less virulent than *C. albicans*, they are also inherently less susceptible to commonly used antifungals, often resulting in a higher failure rate (2). In addition, recent data have revealed important differences between patient groups at-risk (e.g., oncology vs. non-oncology), between institutions, and between countries (2,19). The causes of this changing spectrum are multifactorial and have not yet been evaluated systematically, but the selective pressure resulting from the routine prophylactic use of fluconazole in immunocompromised patients has undoubtedly played a major role in the observed shift (20). However, institution-related differences in anti-infective protocols and treatment-specific factors may have an equally important impact on fungal colonization and subsequent infection.

In prolonged neutropenic cancer patients and allogeneic hematopoietic stem cell transplant recipients, *Aspergillus* species is the most common mold causing fungal disease (4,5). Estimating the incidence of invasive aspergillosis is more problematic given the large variations between institutions and the diagnostic difficulties, especially in patients who have a suppressed inflammatory response. However, the incidence of *Aspergillus* and other filamentous mold infections has been increasing from 18% to 29% following the routine prophylactic use of fluconazole (21).

Finally, a battery of previously uncommon species—both yeasts and filamentous fungi—is increasingly recognized as opportunistic pathogens. Of particular concern is the fact that many of these emerging pathogens display decreased in vitro and in vivo susceptibilities to current antifungal agents, including amphotericin B. These infections caused by *Trichosporon* spp. (22), *Fusarium* spp. (23), *Scedosporium* spp. (24), *Aspergillus terreus*, Zygomycetes (25), and dematiaceous or darkly pigmented fungi carry a high morbidity and mortality rate. These changing epidemiological trends reinforce the requirement of broad-spectrum antifungal agents for empirical treatment in order to prevent breakthrough infections.

II. RATIONALE AND GOAL OF EMPIRICAL THERAPY

The overall case fatality rate of an established invasive opportunistic fungal infection ranges between 40% and 90% with an average of about 60% (2,26). It is evident that the outcome of these infections depends upon the early institution of appropriate therapy (27). However, the major obstacle for the prompt institution of antifungal therapy lies in the difficulty and delay in establishing a definite diagnosis. In many instances, gold standard (invasive) diagnostic tests are not feasible due to cytopenia or due to the critical condition of the patient. In addition, withholding therapy while awaiting time-consuming laboratory tests or clinical confirmation will allow dissemination to occur and will result in a high failure rate. These problems are compounded by the fact that the clinical presentations are often non-specific and suggestive signs and symptoms are frequently absent in the early stages of disease. Also, attempts to make an accurate diagnosis may be thwarted by blunted host defense mechanisms or masked by the high incidence of concomitant clinical processes, especially in transplant recipients (28). By consequence, as evidenced by autopsy surveys, a large number of these infections are never diagnosed nor treated ante mortem (1,7).

Although primary chemoprophylaxis has been effective in the prevention of invasive *Candida* infections, especially in the setting of hematopoietic stem cell transplantation (29,30), it has thus far not been demonstrated to be protective against *Aspergillus* infections (31). Given these diagnostic and preventive shortcomings, a strategy of *empirical* initiation of antifungal therapy has been advocated, especially in profound and prolonged neutropenic cancer patients. This implies the commencement of antifungal therapy at the first suspicion (though without definite proof) of a fungal infection. The aim of this approach is to ensure that all patients with a possible systemic mycotic infection receive appropriate therapy early in the course of the disease. In neutropenic patients, these infections are usually suspected solely on the basis of a continuing or recurring fever despite a predefined period of therapy (4–7 days) to cover likely bacterial pathogens. A similar approach had already been well established during the early 1970s for the early treatment of bacterial infections in neutropenia; patients experiencing a primary febrile episode received broad-spectrum antibiotics empirically because withholding therapy while awaiting culture confirmation resulted also in a too high mortality rate (32).

III. HISTORICAL PERSPECTIVE OF EMPIRICAL ANTIFUNGAL THERAPY

A. To Treat Empirically

Although this scenario has become the standard practice of care in many cancer centers worldwide, the concept has never been firmly validated. Historically, two controlled trials in support of empirical antifungal therapy in neutropenic patients were conducted in the late 1970s and the early 1980s. The first study by Pizzo et al. at the National Institute of Health compared the outcomes of three strategies in 50 neutropenic cancer patients with persistent fever despite seven or more days of broad-spectrum antibacterial therapy (cephalotin, gentamycin, and carbenicillin) in the absence of any documentation of infection: discontinuation of antibacterial agents, no change in therapy, or the addition of amphotericin B deoxycholate 0.5 mg/kg/day (33). The primary endpoint was defervescence, which indicated that amphotericin B controlled an occult fungal infection. The addition of amphotericin B decreased the incidence of breakthrough fungal infections, but there was no improved overall survival for those treated with amphotericin B. The apparent lack of any survival benefit may be explained by the small number of patients, the insufficient dose of amphotericin B, or the rather late initiation of antifungal therapy. A second, larger multicenter trial conducted by The European Organization for Research and Treatment of Cancer (EORTC) randomized 132 patients who remained febrile after 4 days of antibacterial therapy to receive empirical amphotericin B (0.6 mg/kg/day) or to continue therapy without modification (34). No statistically significant difference was seen between the two groups in terms of defervescence (the primary endpoint of efficacy) and survival, although fewer individuals died with invasive fungal disease in the amphotericin B group. Again, the number of documented fungal infections was higher in the patient not receiving amphotericin B. Interestingly, subgroup analysis revealed a better clinical response to empirical therapy in specific subgroups: those who were not receiving any antifungal prophylaxis; those who were severely granulocytopenic ($< 100/\mu L$) at randomization; those with a clinically documented site of infection; those who were more than 15-year old. These data suggested that early institution of conventional amphotericin B may reduce the number of proven fungal infections and that the benefit may depend upon patient characteristics and laboratory values.

B. Or not to Treat Empirically

However, despite these beneficial trends towards reduced fungal morbidity and mortality, it should be noted that none of these studies was blinded and that both trials suffered from inadequate statistical power, especially for subgroup analysis. Moreover, an approach that has been established at the beginning of the 1980s may currently no longer apply to standard medical practice, given drastic changes in anti-neoplastic therapy (e.g., peripheral blood stem cells have replaced bone marrow in hematopoietic transplantation), in prophylactic strategies (widespread use of triazoles), in supportive care measures (use of hematopoietic growth factors; preemptive anti-cytomegalovirus strategies), and in availability of more accurate diagnostic tools (antigen detection and advanced radiological tools). Also, not all neutropenic patients share the same risk of acquiring a pulmonary or disseminated mycotic infection. Risk-adapted strategies need to be developed and validated. Starting antifungal therapy on the grounds of persistent fever alone will inevitably result in overtreatment, since the incidence of proven invasive fungal infections appears to be less than 10% of all febrile neutropenic episodes, whereas often as much as 40% of the patients receive antifungal therapy. This approach will inevitably induce or select for resistant pathogens and may jeopardize the quality of life of patients and/or the hospital budget. Finally, much controversy still surrounds the optimal timing, dosage, and duration of therapy.

Confirmatory evidence of efficacy of a particular antifungal agent cannot be obtained from empirical studies because of the low yield of proven fungal infections; in this setting, efficacy is often primarily (or even wholly) assessed by defervescence. However, resolution of fever is a highly imprecise and non-specific end point: it may be the result of concomitant successful therapy for a non-fungal infection, may be due to resolution of a drug-induced fever, the successful management of an underlying illness (graft-vs.-host disease and malignancy-induced fever), or following neutrophil recovery. Although the rate of breakthrough infection remains the optimal endpoint when evaluating the efficacy of empirical therapy, such a trial would require an unfeasibly large sample size. Therefore, in the mid 1990s, experts have introduced a composite score, combining defervescence as well as data on survival, breakthrough infections, and safety issues, for the alternative evaluation of "success" (Table 1).

IV. THE EVOLVING EMPIRICAL ARSENAL

Despite the small number of patients enrolled in the first two trials, as well as in other non-randomized studies, empirical institution of amphotericin B deoxycholate has become standard of care for neutropenic cancer patients with persistent fever unresponsive to 4–7 days of broad-spectrum antibacterial therapy. The clinical utility, however, is hampered by the suboptimal safety profile of conventional amphotericin B with dose-limiting renal toxicity and, to a lesser extent, infusion-related side effects.

More recently, new modes of administration (e.g., continuous infusion) (35) and commercially available delivery systems with significantly reduced nephrotoxicity [liposomal amphotericin B (AmBisome®), amphotericin B lipid complex (ABLC, Abelcet®), and amphotericin B colloidal dispersion (ABCD, Amphocil®, Amphotec®)] have resulted in an overall improvement of the therapeutic index

Table 1 Composite Endpoints Used as Primary Endpoints in Recent, Large Trials on Empirical Antifungal Therapy

Success if ALL of the following occurred	Malik (1998)	White (1998)	Walsh (1999)	Winston (2000)	Boogaerts (2001)	Walsh (2002)
Resolution of fever during neutropenia			+	+	+	+
Resolution of fever at discontinuation of therapy	+	+				
Successful treatment of any baseline fungal infection		+	+	+	+	+
Survival for 7 days beyond the end of therapy		+	+	+	+	+
No death during study period (any cause)	+					
No breakthrough fungal infection during drug administration or within 7 days of study completion	+	+	+	+	+	+
No premature discontinuation of study drug due to toxicity or lack of efficacy	+	+	+	+	+	+
No withdrawal from study by patient/physician				+		

compared with conventional amphotericin B (36). However, when evaluated in documented *Candida* and *Aspergillus* infections—the two predominant fungal pathogens in neutropenic patients—none of the lipid-associated formulations proved to be more efficacious than conventional amphotericin B (37,38). Their utility in the empirical setting has been challenged in four large, randomized, multicenter trials, comparing these formulations with the parent compound or with each other (39–42). In summary, none of these four studies shows differences in the primary efficacy end point, using a composite score of success (including defervescence, survival, breakthrough fungal infection, and major toxicity). Differences in secondary end points (such as numbers of documented fungal infections and mortality) have been reported in some though not all studies and have been explained by others by imbalances in patient characteristics (43) and/or diagnostic uncertainties (44).

With respect to toxicity, these studies report clear differences between the formulations: all three lipid formulations are considerably less nephrotoxic than is conventional amphotericin B, whereas only therapy with liposomal amphotericin B results in fewer infusion-related toxicity, both in adult and pediatric patients (39,41,42). However, whereas infusional toxicity remains mostly manageable and transient, this is not the case for renal toxicity. Several analyses now underline the increased morbidity, cost, and mortality associated with (the management of) nephrotoxicity (45,46). Unfortunately, at the high current acquisition cost, the routine first-line empirical use of lipid-based formulations is not cost-effective (only demonstrated for liposomal amphotericin B) (47). However, the risk for amphotericin B-associated nephrotoxicity varies considerably among different groups of patients and depends on factors such as sex, dose, and duration of therapy, pre-existing renal disease, and the concomitant use of other nephrotoxic drugs (in particular cyclosporine or amikacine) (48). For instance, most allogeneic bone marrow transplant recipients who receive immunosuppressants will not tolerate the nephrotoxicity of conventional amphotericin B and may benefit from a first-line empirical therapy with a lipid-based formulation. Alternatively, for low-risk patients, a strategy based on careful monitoring of their renal function while receiving conventional amphotericin B followed by a timely switch to a lipid formulation may be preferred.

Thus, the lack of cost-effectiveness associated with the indiscriminate empirical use of lipid-based formulations at their current acquisition cost and the fact that breakthrough fungal infections as well as toxicity (including renal toxicity) still occur while using these less toxic alternatives, has prompted clinicians and pharmaceutical companies to look for alternatives (Table 2).

The triazole fluconazole represented an attractive alternative by virtue of its favorable pharmacokinetics and excellent safety profile. The agent had been used successfully for the treatment of oropharyngeal and esophageal candidiasis, cryptococcal meningitis and hepatosplenic candidiasis and proved to be an equally effective (but less toxic) alternative to conventional amphotericin B in non-neutropenic candidemia (49). In addition, the prophylactic use of fluconazole prevented colonization and development of superficial *Candida* infections in patients with leukemia and reduced the incidence of both superficial and systemic fungal infections in bone marrow transplant recipients (29,30,50).

Three randomized, multicenter trials have compared fluconazole to conventional amphotericin B (51–53). Not unexpectedly, all three studies found that fluconazole at a dosage of 400 mg/day (oral or IV) was associated with less infusional toxicity, less nephrotoxicity, and less hypokalemia than was amphotericin B at a dosage of 0.5 mg/kg/day. Therapeutic response, defined by defervescence or by a composite endpoint, was similar for both therapy groups in all three studies and appeared to be adversely influenced by the presence of pneumonia and the persistence of neutropenia. However, the exclusion of patients at increased risk for azole-resistant *Candida* and *Aspergillus* infections makes it difficult to assess the efficacy of fluconazole for empirical therapy. In fact, given its widespread and often indiscriminate prophylactic use and considering the emergence of causative organisms with intrinsic or acquired resistance, fluconazole may no longer be a suitable candidate for empirical therapy in many cancer centers (2). An extended-spectrum antifungal agent will likely be needed for patients known to be colonized with *Aspergillus* species, *C. glabrata*, or *C. krusei*; for patients who develop new or progressive pulmonary infiltrates; and for those at high risk for mold infections (prolonged neutropenia, refractory disease, corticosteroids, etc.).

The broad-spectrum triazole itraconazole displays good activity against *Aspergillus* and *Candida* species, including fluconazole-resistant strains, but the erratic absorption of itraconazole capsules discouraged clinicians from using it for patients who were suffering from therapy-induced mucositis. The recent development of an oral cyclodextrin solution with increased oral bioavailability in a variety of at-risk patients and the availability of an IV solution has increased the options for the use of this drug (54). The empirical use of itraconazole has been assessed in an open-label randomized trial (55). IV itraconazole (400 mg/day for 2 days followed by 200 mg/day for 5–12 days), followed by oral solution (400 mg/day for 14 days) was compared with amphotericin B (0.7–1.0 mg/kg/day for up to 28 days) in 384 neutropenic patients. Based on a composite endpoint of success,

Table 2 Controlled Randomized Studies on Empirical Antifungal Therapy in Neutropenic Fever

Author (Year)	Trial Design	Sample Size	Primary end Point	Antifungal Agents	Response Rate
Viscoli (1996)	Open-label	112	Defervescence	Amphotericin B Deoxycholate	50%
				Fluconazole	= 52%
Prentice (1997)	Open-label	338	Safety	Amphotericin B Deoxycholate	46% <
				Liposomal Amphotericin B	64%
Malik (1998)	Open-label	106	Efficacy (composite)	Amphotericin B Deoxycholate	46% =
				Fluconazole	56%
White (1998)	Open-label	213	Efficacy (composite)	Amphotericin B Deoxycholate	43% =
				Amphotericin B Colloidal dispersion	50%
Walsh (1999)	Double-blind	687	Efficacy (composite)	Amphotericin B Deoxycholate	49% =
				Liposomal Amphotericin B	50%
Winston (2000)	Open-label	317	Efficacy (composite)	Amphotericin B Deoxycholate	67% =
				Fluconazole	68%
Wingard (2000)	Double-blind	244	Safety	Liposomal Amphotericin B	40% >
				Amphotericin B lipid complex	33%
Boogaerts (2001)	Open-label	384	Efficacy (composite)	Amphotericin B Deoxycholate	38% =
				Itraconazole	47%
Walsh (2002)	Open-label	849	Efficacy (composite)	Liposomal Amphotericin B	31[a]
				Voriconazole	26[a]
Walsh (2004)	Double-blind	1095	Efficacy (composite)	Casofungin	(33.9%)
				Liposomal Amphotericin B	= (33.7%)

=: equivalence >: superior to <: inferior to.
[a]Voriconazole failed to fulfill protocol-defined criteria for non-inferiority to liposomal amphotericin B.

itraconazole was as effective as amphotericin B. However, itraconazole was associated with significantly less severe adverse events and fewer patients were withdrawn prematurely from therapy due to adverse drug reactions. In addition, itraconazole offered the flexibility to switch to oral therapy in selected patients. Unfortunately, this study did not evaluate response to treatment in patients with a documented fungal infection and excluded patients undergoing allogeneic stem cell transplantation. Also, clinical experience with this new parenteral formulation is limited and additional data on efficacy in documented *Candida* and *Aspergillus* infections is needed.

The new generation triazole voriconazole is available in oral and IV formulation, demonstrates a broad-spectrum of activity, covering both yeasts as well as classic and emerging filamentous fungi (including *Fusarium* species but not the *Mucorales*), and displays a good pharmacokinetic profile (56). The empirical use of voriconazole has been assessed in an open-label, randomized trial that compared voriconazole with liposomal amphotericin B (57). Eight hundred and thirty-seven neutropenic patients, stratified according to their risk for fungal infection and by the use or nonuse of systemic antifungal prophylaxis, were randomized to receive either voriconazole (6 mg/kg bid on the 1st day, then 3 mg/kg twice daily) or IV liposomal amphotericin B (3 mg/kg/day). In that study, voriconazole failed to meet predefined criteria for non-inferiority on the basis of the same composite end point that was previously used by the same group. Exploratory analysis of the five individual components of the composite score favored liposomal amphotericin B except for the prevention of breakthrough infections. The better activity of voriconazole in preventing breakthrough infections—the primary goal of empirical therapy—was particularly evident among high-risk patients (allogeneic transplant recipients and relapsed leukemia). Not unexpectedly, significantly more patients in the voriconazole group suffered from visual disturbances while more patients on liposomal amphotericin B had infusional toxicity and hypokalemia. There was no difference in terms of hepatotoxicity, while more patients in the liposomal group developed mild nephrotoxicity. Interestingly, the incidence of severe renal impairment was similar in both groups. The interpretation of these results is challenging, since the overall success rate according to the composite score, the response according to each of its five components, and the subgroup analyses do not point into the same direction (58,59).

V. TOWARDS PREEMPTIVE OR EARLY-THERAPY STRATEGIES

In spite of the presumed advantages of empirical therapy, this strategy can easily be challenged: since not all neutropenic patients and transplant recipients have the same risk of fungal disease, starting therapy solely directed to the management of fever will inevitably result in overtreatment, induction or selection of resistance, increased toxicity, and higher medical costs. A more targeted therapy, directed towards the high-risk patients and based upon a battery of clinical, radiological, and microbiological data that suggest the presence of an invasive mycosis—though still without histopathological proof—would be welcome. However, the feasibility of such a targeted strategy depends upon the availability of rapid and accurate diagnostic tests. Progress may come from the incorporation of new diagnostic tests, such as the sandwich-enzyme-linked immunosorbent assay (ELISA) for the detection of galactomannan (60) or mannan (61) and/or the detection of (pan)fungal DNA by a polymerase chain reaction (62), especially in combination with modern imaging techniques (63). As evidenced in a French study, a simple CT-scan-based approach can already substantially improve the early diagnosis of invasive aspergillosis in neutropenic patients and may have a favorable impact on survival (64). Single- as well as multicenter studies comparing this preemptive or early-therapy approach (e.g., PCR-based) vs. empirical therapy are currently in progress; the impact on infection-related mortality still needs to be demonstrated in prospective studies (65). If such a strategy should prove to be sufficiently robust to withhold therapy in persistently febrile neutropenic patients, then we will steer away from an empirical approach towards a pre-emptive approach.

VI. FUTURE PERSPECTIVES

While such new treatment algorithms are being properly validated, the empirical approach continues to be the standard of care. Given the non-specific nature of "persistent neutropenic fever", an empirically used antifungal drug should not only be efficacious, but above all safe (Table 3). If it were not for dose-limiting renal toxicity, amphotericin B deoxycholate would have been used at a higher dose and longer duration for empirical therapy. An excellent safety and toxicity profile is of the utmost importance since many of these patients are receiving concomitantly nephrotoxic agents or drugs that are metabolized through the cytochrome P450 enzyme system. The candins (such as caspofungin, anidulafungin, and micafungin), a class of antifungals that target the fungal cell wall instead of the plasma membrane, appear to be very attractive candidates (66). Confirmatory data of the efficacy in the treatment of *Candida* and *Aspergillus* infections is currently available for caspofungin some agents (67,68). In addition, the drugs are very well tolerated and prove to be safe in patients with a wide spectrum of diseases and many concomitant medications (69). Recently, a randomised, double-blind, multicenter trial involving more than 1100 patients compared the efficacy and safety of casofungin (loading dose of 70 mg followed by 50 mg/d) with liposomal amphotericin B (AmBisome® 3 mg/kg/d) for empirical antifungal therapy of persistently febrile neutropenic patients. Eligible patients were randomised by risk factor (allogeneic transplants and relapsed leukaemia were considered high risk) and previous antifungal therapy. The primary efficacy endpoint was percentage of treated patients (modified intent-to-treat) with a successful outcome as defined by a classical composite endpoint. In this large study, casofungin proved to be non-inferior to AmBisome. In addition, casofungin was more successful in the treatment of baseline fungal infections and proved to be significantly better tolerated (70). Empirical studies with echinocandins are currently being conducted

Concomitantly with antifungal therapy, one should also try to restore or enhance host defense mechanisms. For some patients this is easy to obtain, while it remains problematic in others. In haemato-oncological patients the depth and duration of neutropenia remain the major independent predictor of outcome.

Table 3 Profile of the Ideal Agent for Empirical Antifungal Therapy

---

Fungicidal activity against the most common fungal pathogens, including non-albicans and azole-resistant *Candida* spp. and all pathogenic *Aspergillus* spp.

&

Activity against emerging yeasts and filamentous fungal pathogens

&

No antifungal resistance/no potential for cross-resistance with agents commonly used in prophylaxis

&

Excellent safety and toxicity profile allowing prolonged therapy without dose reductions

&

No potentially hazardous drug–drug interactions

&

Linear and predictable pharmacokinetics

&

Affordable at the recommended dose

Table 4 FDA-Approved Drugs for Empirical Therapy

Drug	Dosing regimen used in controlled trials
Amphotericin B deoxycholate	0.6–1.0 mg/kg/day (IV)
Liposomal amphotericin B	3 mg/kg/day (IV)
Itraconazole	400 mg/day for 2 days followed by 200 mg/day for 5–12 days (IV), followed by oral solution 400 mg/day for 14 days
Caspofungin	70 mg loading dose, followed by 50 mg daily dose

Increasing the number and function of circulating granulocytes and monocytes by colony-stimulating factors or cytokines has shown favorable results in vitro and in animal experiments, but confirmation from clinical studies is lacking (71). The infusion of donor elicited granulocytes remains investigational, especially in the empirical setting (72). Achieving remission of the underlying disease may be the best option for survival.

VII. CONCLUSION

In conclusion, although guidelines (including the Infectious Diseases Society of America) state that conventional amphotericin B remains the drug of choice for the empirical treatment of neutropenic fever not responding to a predefined period of antibacterial therapy (73), the lipid formulations of amphotericin B, as well as voriconazole and the new formulations of itraconazole, can be used as alternatives within certain clinical boundaries. However, only amphotericin B deoxycholate, liposomal amphotericin B, the IV and oral solutions of itraconazole, and caspofungin are currently approved by the U.S. Food and Drug Administration (Table 4). Policies of the timing and specific agents are most often made on an institutional basis and are frequently influenced by cost considerations. The implementation of validated, reliable diagnostic tests and the ongoing evaluation of new antifungal compounds may significantly impact on our future thinking about empirical or pre-emptive therapy in persistently febrile neutropenic patients. New therapeutic strategies should be based on risk-assessment with consideration of both efficacy and safety issues. At this moment empirical antifungal therapy in neutropenic patients is at least sub-optimal and improvement by novel strategies, safe and potent antifungal agents, and adjunctive immunotherapy seems hardly needed.

REFERENCES

1. Groll AH, Shah PM, Mentzel C, Schneider M, Just-Nuebling G, Huebner K. Trends in the postmortem epidemiology of invasive fungal infections at a university hospital. J Infect 1996; 33:23–32.
2. Viscoli C, Girmenia C, Marinus A, Collette L, Martino P, Vandercam B, Doyen C, Lebeau B, Spence D, Krcmery V, De Pauw B, Meunier F. Candidemia in cancer patients: a prospective, multicenter surveillance study by the Invasive Fungal Infection Group (IFIG) of the European Organization for Research and Treatment of Cancer (EORTC). Clin Infect Dis 1999; 28(5):1071–1079.

3. Singh N. Fungal infections in the recipients of solid organ transplantation. Infect Dis Clin North Am 2003; 17(1):113–134.

4. Marr KA, Carter RA, Boeckh M, Martin P, Corey L. Invasive aspergillosis in allogeneic stem cell transplant recipients: changes in epidemiology and risk factors. Blood 2002; 100:4358–4366.

5. Martino R, Subira M, Rovira M, Solano C, Vazquez L, Sanz GF, Urbano-lspizua A, Brunet S, De la Camara R. alloPBSCT Infectious/Non-infectious Complications Subcommittees of the Grupo Espanol de Trasplante Hematopoyetico (GETH). Invasive fungal infections after allogeneic peripheral blood stem cell transplantation: incidence and risk factors in 395 patients. Br J Haematol 2002; 116:475–482.

6. Denning D. Invasive aspergillosis. Clin Infect Dis 1998; 26:781–805.

7. Bodey G, Bueltmann B, Duguid W, Gibbs D, Hanak H, Hotchi M, Mall G, Martino P, Meunier F, Milliken S. Fungal infections in cancer patients: an international autopsy survey. Eur J Clin Microbiol Infect Dis 1992; 11:99–109.

8. Groll AH, Walsh TJ. Uncommon opportunistic fungi: new nosocomial threats. Clin Microbiol Infect 2001; 7(suppl 2):8–24.

9. Singh N. Changing spectrum of invasive candidiasis and its therapeutic implications. Clin Microbiol Infect 2001; 7(suppl 2):1–7.

10. Banerjee SN, Emori TG, Culver DH, Gaynes RP, Jarvis WR, Horan T, Edwards JR, Tolson J, Henderson T, Martone WJ. Secular trends in nosocomial primary bloodstream infections in the United States, 1980–1989. National Nosocomial Infections Surveillance System. Am J Med 1991; 91:86S–89S.

11. Maertens J, Vrebos M, Boogaerts MA. Assessing risk factors for systemic fungal infections. Eur J Cancer Care 2001; 10:56–62.

12. Wey SB, Mori M, Pfaller MA, Woolson RF, Wenzel RP. Hospital-acquired candidemia. The attributable mortality and excess length of stay. Arch Intern Med 1988; 148: 2642–2645.

13. Vincent JL, Anaissie E, Bruining H, Demajo W, el-Ebiary M, Haber J, Hiramatsu Y, Nitenberg G, Nystrom PO, Pittet D, Rogers T, Sandven P, Sganga G, Schaller MD, Solomkin J. Epidemiology, diagnosis and treatment of systemic *Candida* infection in surgical patients under intensive care. Intensive Care Med 1998; 24:206–216.

14. Voss A, le Noble JL, Verduyn Lunel FM, Foudraine NA, Meis JF. Candidemia in intensive care unit patients: risk factors for mortality. Infection 1997; 25:8–11.

15. Pfaller MA, Jones RN, Messer SA, Edmond MB, Wenzel RP. National surveillance of nosocomial blood stream infection due to Candida albicans: frequency of occurrence and antifungal susceptibility in the SCOPE Program. Diagn Microbiol Infect Dis 1998; 31:327–332.

16. Rex JH, Pappas PG, Karchmer AW, Sobel J, Edwards JE, Hadley S, Brass C, Vazquez JA, Chapman SW, Horowitz HW, Zervos M, McKinsey D, Lee J, Babinchak T, Bradsher RW, Cleary JD, Cohen DM, Danziger L, Goldman M, Goodman J, Hilton E, Hyslop NE, Kett DH, Lutz J, Rubin RH, Scheld WM, Schuster M, Simmons B, Stein DK, Washburn RG, Mautner L, Chu TC, Panzer H, Rosenstein RB, Booth J. National Institute of Allergy and Infectious Diseases Mycoses Study Group. A randomized and blinded multicenter trial of high-dose fluconazole plus placebo versus fluconazole plus amphotericin B as therapy for candidemia and its consequences in non-neutropenic subjects. Clin Infect Dis 2003; 36:1221–1228.

17. Abi-Said D, Anaissie E, Uzun O, Raad I, Pinzcowski H, Vartivarian S. The epidemiology of hematogenous candidiasis caused by different *Candida* species. Clin Infect Dis 1997; 24:1122–1128.

18. Nguyen MH, Peacock JE Jr, Morris AJ, Tanner DC, Nguyen ML, Snydman DR, Wagener MM, Rinaldi MG, Yu VL. The changing face of candidemia: emergence of non-*Candida albicans* species and antifungal resistance. Am J Med 1996; 100:617–623.

19. Pfaller MA, Jones RN, Messer SA, Edmond MB, Wenzel RP. National surveillance of nosocomial blood stream infection due to species of Candida other than Candida albicans:

frequency of occurrence and antifungal susceptibility in the SCOPE Program. SCOPE Participant Group. Surveillance and Control of Pathogens of Epidemiologic. Diagn Microbiol Infect Dis 1998; 30:121–129.

20. Marr KA, Seidel K, White TC, Bowden RA. Candidemia in allogeneic blood and marrow transplant recipients: evolution of risk factors after the adoption of prophylactic fluconazole. J Infect Dis 2000; 181:309–316.

21. Marr KA, Carter RA, Crippa F, Wald A, Corey L. Epidemiology and outcome of mould infections in hematopoietic stem cell transplant recipients. Clin Infect Dis 2002; 34:909–917.

22. Krcmery V, Krupova I, Denning DW. Invasive yeast infections other than *Candida* spp. in acute leukaemia. J Hosp Infect 1999; 41:181–194.

23. Boutati El, Anaissie EJ. Fusarium, a significant emerging pathogen in patients with hematologic malignancy: ten years' experience at a cancer center and implications for management. Blood 1997; 90:999–1008.

24. Maertens J, Lagrou K, Deweerdt H, Surmont I, Verhoef GE, Verhaegen J, Boogaerts MA. Disseminated infection by *Scedosporium prolificans*: an emerging fatality among haematology patients. Case report and review. Ann Hematol 2000; 79:340–344.

25. Kontoyiannis D, Wessel V, Bodey G, Rolston K. Zygomycosis in the 1990s in a tertiary care center. Clin Infect Dis 2000; 30:851–856.

26. Lin S, Schranz J, Teutsch S. Aspergillosis case-fatality rate: systematic review of the literature. Clin Infect Dis 2001; 32:358–366.

27. von Eiff M, Roos N, Schulten R, Hesse M, Zuhlsdorf M, van de Loo J. Pulmonary aspergillosis: early diagnosis improves survival. Respiration 1995; 62:341–347.

28. Erjavec Z, Verweij PE. Recent progress in the diagnosis of fungal infections in the immunocompromised host. Drug Resist Updat 2002; 5:3–10.

29. Goodman JL, Winston DJ, Greenfield RA, Chandrasekar PH, Fox B, Kaizer H, Shadduck RK, Shea TC, Stiff P, Friedman DJ. A controlled trial of fluconazole to prevent fungal infections in patients undergoing bone marrow transplantation. N Engl J Med 1992; 326:845–851.

30. Slavin MA, Osborne B, Adams R, Levenstein MJ, Schoch HG, Feldman AR, Meyers JD, Bowden RA. Efficacy and safety of fiuconazole prophylaxis for fungal infections after marrow transplantation—a prospective, randomized, double-blind study. J Infect Dis 1995; 171:1545–1552.

31. Lortholary O, Dupont B. Antifungal prophylaxis during neutropenia and immunodeficiency. Clin Microbiol Rev 1997; 10:477–504.

32. Schimpff S, Satterlee W, Young VM, Serpick A. Empiric therapy with carbenicillin and gentamicin for febrile patients with cancer and granulocytopenia. N Engl J Med 1971; 284:1061–1065.

33. Pizzo PA, Robichaud KJ, Gill Fa, Witebsky FG. Empiric antibiotic and antifungal therapy for cancer patients with prolonged fever and granulocytopenia. Am J Med 1982; 72:101–111.

34. EORTC International Antimicrobial Therapy Cooperative Group. Empiric antifungal therapy in febrile granulocytopenic patients. Am J Med 1989; 86:668–672.

35. Eriksson U, Seifert B, Schaffner A. Comparison of effects of amphotericin B deoxycholate infused over 4 or 24 hours: randomised, controlled trial. BMJ 2001; 322:579–582.

36. Barrett JP, Vardulaki KA, Conlon C, Cooke J, Daza-Ramirez P, Evans EG, Hawkey PM, Herbrecht R, Marks DL, Moraleda JM, Park GR, Senn SJ, Viscoli C. A systematic review of the antifungal effectiveness and tolerability of amphotericin B formulations. Clin Ther 2003; 25:1295–320.

37. Anaissie EJ, White M, Ozun O. Amphotericin B lipid complex versus amphotericin B for treatment of invasive candidiasis: a prospective, randomised, multicenter trial [abstr LM21]. In: Programs and Abstracts of the 35th Interscience Conference on Antimicrobial Agents and Chemotherapy. Washington, DC: ASM press, 1995:330.

38. Bowden R, Chandrasekar P, White MH, Li X, Pietrelli L, Gurwith M, van Burik JA, Laverdiere M, Safrin S, Wingard JR. A double-blind randomised controlled trial of amphotericin B colloidal dispersion (ABCD) versus amphotericin B (AmB) for treatment of invasive aspergillosis in immunocompromised patients. Clin Infect Dis 2002; 35: 359–366.

39. Walsh TJ, Finberg RW, Arndt C, Hiemenz J, Schwartz C, Bodensteiner D, Pappas P, Seibel N, Greenberg RN, Dummer S, Schuster M, Holcenberg JS for the National Institute of Allergy and Infectious Diseases Mycoses Study Group. Liposomal amphotericin B for empirical therapy in patients with persistent fever and neutropenia. N Engl J Med 1999; 340:764–771.

40. White MH, Bowden RA, Sandler ES, Graham ML, Noskin GA, Wingard JR, Goldman M, van Burik JA, McCabe A, Lin JS, Gurwith M, Miller CB. Randomized, double-blind clinical trial of amphotericin B colloidal dispersion versus amphotericin B in the empirical treatment of fever and neutropenia. Clin Infect Dis 1998; 27:296–302.

41. Wingard JR, White MH, Anaissie E, Raffalli J, Goodman J, Arrieta A, L Amph/ABLC Collaborative Study Group. A randomized, double-blind comparative trial evaluating the safety of liposomal amphotericin B versus amphotericin B lipid complex in the empirical treatment of febrile neutropenia. Clin Infect Dis 2000; 31:1155–1163.

42. Prentice HG, Hann IM, Herbrecht R, Aoun M, Kvaloy S, Catovsky D, Pinkerton CR, Schey SA, Jacobs F, Oakhill A, Stevens RF, Darbyshire PJ, Gibson BE. A randomized comparison of liposomal versus conventional amphotericin B for the treatment of pyrexia of unknown origin in neutropenic patients. Br J Hematol 1997; 98:711–718.

43. Wingard JR. Lipid formulations of amphotericins: are you a lumper or a splitter? Clin Infect Dis 2002; 35:891–895.

44. Wingard JR, White MH, Anaissie E, Buell D. Mortality rates in comparative trials for formulations of amphotericin B [letter]. Clin Infect Dis 2001; 33:583–584.

45. Bates DW, Su L, Yu DT, Chertow GM, Seger DL, Gomes DR, Dasbach EJ, Platt R. Mortality and costs of acute renal failure associated with amphotericin B therapy. Clin Infect Dis 2001; 32:686–693.

46. Rex JH, Walsh TJ. Estimating the true cost of amphotericin B. Clin Infect Dis 1999; 29:1408–1410.

47. Cagnoni PJ, Walsh TJ, Prendergast MM, Bodensteiner D, Hiemenz S, Greenberg RN, Arndt CA, Schuster M, Seibel N, Yeldandi V, Tong KB. Pharmacoeconomic analysis of liposomal amphotericin B versus conventional amphotericin B in the empirical treatment of persistently neutropenic patients. J Clin Oncol 2000; 18:2476–2483.

48. Harbarth S, Pestotnik SL, Lloyd JF, Burke JP, Samore MH. The epidemiology of nephrotoxicity associated with conventional amphotericin B therapy. Am J Med 2001; 111:528–534.

49. Rex JH, Bennett JE, Sugar AM, Pappas PG, van der Horst CM, Edwards JE, Washburn RG, Scheld WM, Karchmer AW, Dine AP. A randomized trial comparing fluconazole with amphotericin B in the treatment of candidaemia in patients without neutropenia. N Engl J Med 1994; 331:1325–1330.

50. Winston DJ, Chandrasekar PH, Lazarus HM, Goodman JL, Silber JL, Horowitz H, Shadduck RK, Rosenfeld CS, Ho WG, Islam MZ, Buell DN. Fluconazole prophylaxis of fungal infections in patients with acute leukemia. Results of a randomized, placebo-controlled double-blind multicenter trial. Ann Intern Med 1993; 118:495–503.

51. Viscoli C, Castagnola E, Van Lint MT, Moroni C, Garaventa A, Rossi MR, Fanci R, Menichetti F, Caselli D, Giacchino M, Congiu M. Fluconazole versus amphotericin B as empiric antifungal therapy of unexplained fever in granulocytopenic cancer patients: a pragmatic, multicenter, prospective and randomized clinical trial. Eur J Cancer 1996; 32A:814–820.

52. Malik IA, Moid I, Aziz Z, Khan S, Suleman M. A randomized comparison of fluconazole with amphotericin B as empirical antifungal agents in cancer patients with prolonged fever and neutropenia. Am J Med 1998; 105:478–483.

53. Winston DJ, Hathorn JW, Schuster MG, Schiller GJ, Territo MC. A multicenter, randomized trial of fluconazole versus amphotericin B for empirical antifungal therapy in neutropenic patients with cancer. Am J Med 2000; 108:282–289.

54. Boogaerts M, Maertens J. Clinical experience with itraconazole in systemic fungal infections. Drugs 2001; 61(suppl 1):39–47.

55. Boogaerts M, Winston DJ, Bow EJ, Garber G, Reboli AC, Schwarer AP, Novitzky N, Boehme A, Chwetzoff E, De Beule K. Itraconazole Neutropenia Study Group. Intravenous and oral itraconazole versus intravenous amphotericin B deoxycholate as empirical antifungal therapy for persistent fever in neutropenic patients with cancer who are receiving broad-spectrum antibacterial therapy: a randomized, controlled trial. Ann Intern Med 2001; 135:412–422.

56. Johnson LB, Kauffman CA. Voriconazole: a new triazole antifungal agent. Clin Infect Dis 2003; 36:630–637.

57. Walsh TJ, Pappas P, Winston DJ, Lazarus HM, Petersen F, Raffalli J, Yanovich S, Stiff P, Greenberg R, Donowitz G, Schuster M, Reboli A, Wingard J, Arndt C, Reinhardt J, Hadley S, Finberg R, Laverdiere M, Perfect J, Garber G, Fioritoni G, Anaissie E, Lee J. National Institute of Allergy Infectious Diseases Mycoses Study Group. Voriconazole compared with liposomal amphotericin B for empirical antifungal therapy in patients with neutropenia and persistent fever. N Engl J Med 2002; 346:225–234.

58. Marr KA. Empirical antifungal therapy—new options, new tradeoffs. N Engl J Med 2002; 346:278–280.

59. Powers JH, Dixon CA, Goldberger MJ. Voriconazole versus liposomal amphotericin B in patients with neutropenia and persistent fever. N Engl J Med 2002; 346:289–290.

60. Maertens J, Verhaegen J, Lagrou K, Van Eldere J, Boogaerts M. Screening for circulating galactomannan as a noninvasive diagnostic tool for invasive aspergillosis in prolonged neutropenic patients and stem cell transplantation recipients: a prospective validation. Blood 2001; 97:1604–1610.

61. Sendid B, Poirot JL, Tabouret M, Bonnin A, Caillot D, Camus D, Poulain D. Combined detection of mannanaemia and antimannan antibodies as a strategy for the diagnosis of systemic infection caused by pathogenic *Candida* species. J Med Microbiol 2002; 51:433–442.

62. Hebart H, Loffler J, Reitze H, Engel A, Schumacher U, Klingebiel T, Bader P, Bohme A, Martin H, Bunjes D, Kern WV, Kanz L, Einsele H. Prospective screening by a panfungal polymerase chain reaction assay in patients at risk for fungal infections: implications for the management of febrile neutropenia. Br J Haematol 2000; 111:635–640.

63. Heussel CP, Kauczor HU, Heussel GE, Fischer B, Begrich M, Mildenberger P, Thelen M. Pneumonia in febrile neutropenic patients and bone marrow and blood stem-cell transplant recipients: use of high-resolution computed tomography. J Clin Oncol 1999; 17:796–805.

64. Caillot D, Casasnovas O, Bernard A, Couaillier JF, Durand C, Cuisenier B, Solary E, Piard F, Petrella T, Bonnin A, Couillault G, Dumas M, Guy H. Improved management of invasive pulmonary aspergillosis in neutropenic patients using early thoracic computed tomographic scan and surgery. J Clin Oncol 1997; 15:139–147.

65. Lin MT, Lu HC, Chen WL. Improving efficacy of antifungal therapy by poiymerase chain reaction-based strategy among febrile patients with neutropenia and cancer. Clin Infect Dis 2001; 33:1621–1627.

66. Maertens J, Boogaerts M. Fungal cell wall inhibitors : emphasis on clinical aspects. Curr Pharm Des 2000; 6:225–239.

67. Mora-Duarte J, Betts R, Rotstein C, Colombo AL, Thompson-Moya L, Smietana J, Lupinacci R, Sabie C, Kartsonis N, Perfect J. Caspofungin Invasive Candidiasis Study Group. Comparison of caspofungin and amphotericin B for invasive candidiasis. N Engl J Med 2002; 347(25):2020–2029.

68. Maertens J, Raad I, Petrikkos G, Boogaerts M, Selleslag D, Peterson FB, Sable CA, Kartsonis NA, Ngai A, Taylor A, Patterson TF, Denning DW, Walsh TJ. Caspofungin

Salvage Aspergillosis Study Group. Efficacy and safety of caspofungin for treatment of invasive aspergillosis in patients refractory to or intolerant of conventional antifungal therapy. Clin Infect Dis 2004; 39:1563–1571.

69. Sable CA, Nguyen BT, Chodakewitz JA, DiNubile MJ. Safety and tolerability of caspofungin acetate in the treatment of fungal infections. Transpl Infect Dis 2002; 4:25–30.

70. Walsh TJ, Teppler H, Donowitz GR, Maertens JA, Baden LR, Dmoszynska A, Cornely OA, Bourque MR, Lupinacci RJ, Sable CA, dePauw BE. Caspofungin versus liposomal amphotericin B for empirical antifungal therapy in patients with persistent fever and neutropenia. N Engl Med 2004; 351(14):1391–402.

71. Roilides E, Dignani MC, Anaissie EJ, Rex JH. The role of immunoreconstitution in the management of refractory opportunistic fungal infections. Med Mycol 1998; 36(suppl 1): 12–25.

72. Schiffer CA. Granulocyte transfusion therapy. Curr Opin Hematol 1999; 6:3–7.

73. Hughes WT, Armstrong D, Bodey GP, Bow EJ, Brown AE, Calandra T, Feld R, Pizzo PA, Rolston KV, Shenep JL, Young LS. Guidelines for the use of antimicrobial agents in neutropenic patients with cancer. Clin Infect Dis 2002; 34:730–751.

24
Treatment of Invasive Fungal Infections

John R. Wingard
Department of Medicine, University of Florida College of Medicine, Gainesville, Florida, U.S.A.

Elias J. Anaissie
The University of Arkansas for Medical Sciences, Myeloma and Transplantation Research Center, Little Rock, Arkansas, U.S.A.

I. INTRODUCTION

Enormous strides have been made in the management of invasive fungal infections (IFIs). New drugs, randomized trials testing comparative efficacy and safety, and development of adjunctive measures to complement pharmacologic agents have combined to improve treatment outcomes. Sufficient studies have been done to allow evidence-based consensus guidelines for *Candida*, *Aspergillus*, and *Cryptococcus* to be developed. For other pathogens, case series with different treatment modalities permit guidance of treatment preferences. In this chapter, treatment strategies of the most common IFIs will be summarized.

II. CANDIDIASIS

Amphotericin B has been the gold standard of therapy for Candidiasis for decades. Until the past decade, however, there were few randomized trials. With the advent of new antifungals, comparative trials have allowed clinicians a better understanding of the relative merits of various treatment options. There are several excellent options for antifungal therapy supported by randomized trials (Table 1).

A. Amphotericin B Deoxycholate

Despite methodologic problems in interpretation of in vitro susceptibility testing for amphotericin B, several conclusions appear warranted from the data available (reviewed in Refs. 1 and 2). Resistance is infrequent in isolates of *Candida albicans*, *Candida tropicalis*, and *Candida parapsilosis*, while resistance is not uncommon in isolates of *Candida lusitaniae*. Some isolates of *Candida glabrata* and *Candida krusei* appear to be less susceptible and may require higher doses of amphotericin B (1 mg/kg/day).

Table 1 Randomized Comparative Trials for Therapy of Systemic *Candida* Infections

Study	Percent Success					Toxicity	Comments
	Fluconazole (400 mg/day)	Amphotericin B (0.5–1.0 mg/kg/day)	Combination[a] (Amph 0.7 mg/kg/day + Flu 800 mg/day)	ABLC (5 mg/kg/day)	Caspofungin (70 mg LD, then 50 mg/day)		
Rex (13)	70	79				Favors fluconazole (less nephrotoxicity)	Gaps in fluconazole coverage
Anaissie (5)		68		63		Favors ABLC (less nephrotoxicity)	Never published; no survival difference
Phillips (12)	50	56				Favors fluconazole	Gaps in fluconazole coverage
Rex (31)	56[b]		69			Favors fluconazole (less nephrotoxicity)	Shorter time to negative blood cultures with combination
Mora-Duarte (28)		62			73	Favors capsofungin (less nephrotoxicity)	Composite success criterion contained both efficacy and toxicity parameters, most of difference in failure was due to toxicity

[a]The combination of amphotericin B with fluconazole.
[b]800 mg/day.

There is a considerable body of treatment experience of using amphotericin B for therapy of systemic Candidiasis in various patient populations, including both neutropenic and non-neutropenic patients (1–3).

B. Amphotericin B Lipid Formulations

Intolerance to amphotericin B deoxycholate due to infusional reactions or nephrotoxicity has limited its utility. It has been especially difficult to use in patients receiving calcineurin inhibitors (4). Amphotericin B lipid complex (ABLC) given at a dose of 5 mg/kg/day has been shown to be as effective as amphotericin B deoxycholate at a dose of 0.6–1.0 mg/kg/day (5) (Table 1). Response and survival rates were not different, but there was considerably less renal toxicity. There are no randomized trials for the other licensed lipid formulations for Candidiasis. However, there is sufficient experience with the other lipid formulations to permit a reasonable conclusion that all three lipid formulations are acceptable alternatives to amphotericin B deoxy cholate.

Although the lipid amphotericin B formulations are considerably less toxic they are also much more expensive and they have not been shown to improve the rates of response or survival. Accordingly, there has been considerable debate as to when and in whom the lipid formulations should be used (6–8) and when used which one (9). Certainly, the lipid formulations are excellent substitutes for patients intolerant of amphotericin B deoxycholate. Additionally, the intolerance of the deoxycholate formulation in patients receiving concomitant nephrotoxins, those with antecedent renal impairment, and in those receiving prolonged courses of doses approximating 1 mg/kg/day make such individuals good prospects for the lipid formulations in preference to amphotericin B deoxycholate upfront.

C. Fluconazole and Other Azoles

In vitro susceptibility assays have been standardized for azole testing. Most *Candida* species are highly susceptible to fluconazole (defined as MIC ≤ 8 mg/L) (1,2,10). However, several species are not reliably inhibited by fluconazole. *Candida krusei* and *Candida dubliniensis* isolates are resistant to fluconazole. Isolates of *C. glabrata* are less susceptible to fluconazole and are characterized as "susceptible-dose dependent (S-DD)," because higher concentrations are required for in vitro inhibition (MIC 16–32 mg/L). Some *C. glabrata* strains are resistant (≥ 64 mg/L). Fortunately, *C. krusei* and *C. dubliniensis* infections are infrequent. However, *C. glabrata* infections account for 10–20% of invasive *Candida* infections in various series and these appear to be increasing over time. This increase was first noted coincident with the introduction of fluconazole into clinical practice, suggesting that its widespread use has led to selection of less susceptible fungal organisms. Fortunately, bloodstream isolates of *C. albicans* have remained largely susceptible to fluconazole now a decade later after its introduction into clinical practice (11).

The standard dose of fluconazole in the treatment of *Candida* mucosal infections is generally 100–200 mg/day. For candidemia caused by susceptible *Candida* spp., doses of 400 mg are recommended. For children, dosing for serious *Candida* infections is 6 mg/kg/day. For *C. glabrata*, doses of 12 mg/kg/day are necessary.

Randomized trials and case-controlled studies have shown fluconazole (400 mg/day) to be highly effective as therapy of systemic *Candida* (12,13) (Table 1) with response and survival rates comparable to amphotericin B (0.5–0.6 mg/day). Time to clearance of *Candida* bloodstream infections is similar although slightly slower than with amphotericin B. Most treatment trials were conducted in non-neutropenic patients, and there is a paucity of data in neutropenic patients. Thus, many experts believe amphotericin B to be preferable to fluconazole for the neutropenic patient with systemic Candidiasis.

Resistance to fluconazole occurs through several mechanisms (reviewed in Refs. 14 and 15): alteration of the target enzyme (14-alpha-sterol-demethylase encoded by ERG11) by mutation or overexpression of ERG11 or up-regulation of efflux transporters (encoded by CDR1, CDR2, and MDR1 genes). Emergence of resistance *to C. albicans* has been seen largely in patients with advanced acquired immunodeficiency syndrome with low (and declining) CD4+ T lymphocyte counts, where low doses of fluconazole (50–200 mg/day) were given for many months to suppress recurrent oropharyngeal candidiasis. This experience has contrasted to the experience in leukemia and BMT patients where shorter courses of higher doses (400 mg/day) are generally given and restoration of host defenses (neutrophil recovery and/or recovery of cell-mediated immune responses) generally occurs. It seems likely that these different trajectories of host differences are important in understanding the reasons for these different experiences. Notwithstanding, several outbreaks of *Candida* bloodstream infections have been reported in BMT patients receiving fluconazole prophylaxis by fluconazole resistant organisms (16–18). Fortunately, these have been infrequent; moreover, unpublished data of investigations of these outbreaks suggest most infections were caused by only one or several strains, suggesting a common source. However, the resistance story in advanced HIV infection should serve as a cautionary note for potential similar concerns which may pertain to patients with poor T-cell immune reconstitution after transplantation or conditions associated with poor T-cell function. Several instances of fluconazole-resistant *C. albicans* fungemia in leukemia patients have also been described (19,20).

Several azoles, in addition to fluconazole, have excellent activity against *Candida* spp. These include clotrimazole, ketoconazole, itraconazole, and voriconazole. Controlled trials have shown these agents to be effective as therapy for oropharyngeal candidiasis. Because of lack of systemic effect clotrimazole is generally used only for mucosal infections. Ketoconazole has largely been replaced by fluconazole because of variable bioavailability and dependence on gastric acidity for maximal absorption. Voriconazole has been shown to be as effective as fluconazole for the treatment of *Candida* esophagitis in HIV patients (21) and is being evaluated in a randomized trial for systemic candidiasis.

D. Caspofungin

Caspofungin has excellent in vitro activity against *Candida* (including azole-resistant species) (22–26). In vitro susceptibility studies have raised a concern of lower activity against *C. parapsilosis* and *Candida guilliermondii*, but whether these in vitro findings are clinically important is at present unclear.

Two randomized trials, one in *Candida* esophagitis in HIV-infected patients (27) and the other in systemic Candidiasis in immunocompromised adults (28) have demonstrated excellent clinical activity, comparable to amphotericin B, with substantially less toxicity than amphotericin B. In both trials response and survival rates were comparable. Caspofungin was associated with a lower rate of toxicities.

Caspofungin clearly is an excellent choice for Candidiasis, but caution is necessary if the patient is on cyclosporine, due to a potential for hepatotoxicity noted in normal volunteers receiving both concomitantly. One option is to switch cyclosporine to tacrolimus if the clinician deems that acceptable. Cyclosporine appears to increase caspofungin blood levels up to 30%. Caspofungin increases tacrolimus levels by 20% (but has no effect on cyclosporine levels). Dosing in children is still being worked out, although preliminary results indicate that a dose of at least 1 mg/kg is required and computer modeling suggests dosing based on body surface area achieves more predictable blood concentrations (Walsh, unpublished observations).

Two other echinocandins are in clinical trials. Micafungin appears to have a similar antifungal spectrum of activity and toxicity profile as caspofungin (29). No hepatic transaminase elevations have been noted in patients receiving micafungin concomitant with cyclosporine, unlike caspofungin. Anidulafungin is also in clinical trials (30).

E. Combination Therapy

Rex et al. (31) evaluated combination therapy for the treatment of candidemia in non-neutropenic adults comparing amphotericin B plus fluconazole vs. high doses (800 mg/day) of fluconazole alone. There was a non-significant trend to higher success rates with the combination therapy compared to monotherapy (69% vs. 56%, $p = 0.08$) and better clearance of the bloodstream infection by the combination therapy ($p = 0.02$). Unfortunately, there was also more toxicity with the combination therapy mitigating the net benefit. An analysis examining the association of patient physiological status with response found that the extra benefit offered by dual therapy seemed to be most evident for patients in whom treatment factors may be most germaine rather than the host status to outcomes and least in patients very ill (in which no therapy has a chance to help) and in patients least ill (in which any therapy will suffice) (31).

F. Adjunctive Measures

Most experts recommend removal of central venous catheter or any other foreign body in an infected patient wherever possible (1,2). *Candida parapsilosis* is frequently associated with vascular catheters and catheter removal is especially important for this infection. Penetration by antifungal agents of biofilms on catheters may be impeded, hindering clearance of pathogenic fungi. Several studies suggest more rapid clearance of organisms from the bloodstream with catheter removal, although a recent evidence review questioned how well founded this recommendation is in empirical data (32). Clearly, there is a role for clinical judgment necessary to ascertain when and in whom catheter removal should be done (33).

G. Practical Considerations

With several excellent therapeutic options, there are practical considerations that influence treatment decisions. With its oral formulation, favorable safety profile, relative low cost, and a proven track record in clinical trials, fluconazole has considerable advantages over the other options. However, the gaps in its activity spectrum pose a dilemma for clinicians making treatment decisions before the isolate is known to be fluconazole susceptible. Several days may pass from notification of a positive culture before the isolate is speciated. Susceptibility testing is not widely available at present and testing (even if available) adds even more time. Knowledge of what species the pathogen is provides a good estimate of susceptibility, with *C. krusei*, *C. glabrata*, and *C. dubliniensis* not reliably susceptible, and all others susceptible (1,2). Accordingly, one option for serious infections is to start with caspofungin or one of the amphotericin B formulations to provide broad coverage. Once the organism is speciated and the patient stabilizes, one may either continue the initial therapy or can change to fluconazole for susceptible isolates to complete the course of therapy.

The duration of therapy is problematic with no clear guidance from published literature. Generally, one should continue treatment until resolution of signs and symptoms, clearance of cultures, improvement of radiologic manifestations, and improvement of the host defenses that contributed to the infection.

III. ASPERGILLOSIS

There are three general categories of *Aspergillus* infections: invasive, saprophytic, and allergic. This section will address treatment approaches of invasive infection only. Early detection and prompt initiation of antifungal therapy are key determinants of success. To date, there are few randomized treatment trials of aspergillosis (Table 2).

A. Amphotericin B Deoxycholate

Most *Aspergillus* isolates are susceptible to amphotericin B. However, there are notable exceptions. Most *Aspergillus terreus* isolates demonstrate in vitro resistance to amphotericin B and do not respond well to amphotericin B. Similarly, *Aspergillus ustus* and *Aspergillus versicolor* may be resistant to amphotericin B.

As with Candidiasis, amphotericin B deoxycholate has long been the gold standard for primary therapy of invasive aspergillosis and until recently was the only licensed therapy for primary therapy of invasive aspergillosis in the United States. Unfortunately, amphotericin B deoxycholate must be given in high doses and the prolonged treatment courses needed are poorly tolerated in many individuals (due to nephrotoxicity and other toxicities) and success rates are poor.

B. Lipid Formulations of Amphotericin B

The lipid amphotericin B products are also effective against *Aspergillus*, although higher doses must be administered compared to amphotericin B deoxycholate. Two lipid formulations (ABLC and ABCD) were first licensed because of their efficacy as salvage therapy in patients with progressive *Aspergillus* infection or intolerance for amphotericin B, with responses in approximately 40%. Two randomized trials have evaluated lipid amphotericin B formulations as primary therapy (Table 2). In one study (34), liposomal amphotericin B was evaluated in a randomized trial of two doses (1 and 4 mg/kg/day). Patients were required to have probable or proven invasive aspergillosis. No differences in either response rate or survival were seen, but it is important to note that the sample size was very small and the statistical power to detect a difference if present was inadequate to reject the null hypothesis; moreover, the complete response rate in the 4 mg/kg/day group was higher than in the 1 mg/kg/day group. Many experts believe this trial is inconclusive in recommending a lower dose schedule for the therapy of invasive aspergillosis.

In a second trial, ABCD at a dose of 6 mg/kg/day was compared to amphotericin B deoxycholate in a dose of 1–1.5 mg/kg/day (35). There was no difference

Table 2 Randomized Comparative Trials for Therapy of Invasive *Aspergillus* Infections

Author	Test agent	Comparator	Response rates		Survival rates		Toxicity	Comments
			Test agent	Comparator	Test agent	Comparator		
Ellis (34)	L-amph 1 mg/kg	L-amp 4 mg/kg	64%	48%	43% (at 6 mos)	37% (at 6 mos)	Favors liposomal amphotericin B	Small sample (n = 87.evaluable), not adequately powered to detect differences; response for definite infections higher in 4 mg/kg/day group 58% vs. 37%)
Bowden (35)	ABCD 6 mg/kg	Amph (1–1.5 mg/kg)	35%	35%	50%	45%	Favors ABCD (less nephrotoxicity but more infusion reactions)	Improved tolerance did not translate into response or survival advantage
Herbrecht (36)	Vori 6 mg/kg LD, then 4 mg/kg Q12H	Amph (1–1.5 kg)	53%[a]	32%[a]	71% (at 12 weeks)	58% (at 12 weeks)	Favors voriconazole	Amphotericin B was poorly tolerated and most received other lipid amphotericin B formulations or itraconazole in the comparator arm

[a] $p < 0.05$.
Abbreviations: L-amp, liposomal amphotericin B; ABCD, amphotericin B colloridal dispersion; Amph, amphotericin B deoxycholate; Vori, voriconazole.

in response or survival rates between the two arms. However, the ABCD therapy was associated with lower rates of nephrotoxicity.

C. Aerosolized Amphotericin B

Inhaled amphotericin B and lipid formulations of amphotericin B have been tested in small numbers of patients either as prophylaxis or as adjunctive drug delivery to infected tissue. This is an appealing idea which has the potential to spare the patient systemic toxicity and deliver higher drug concentrations. Because of limited data, this remains investigational at present.

D. Voriconazole

A randomized trial compared amphotericin B deoxycholate and voriconazole as first-line therapy of invasive aspergillosis in immunocompromised adults (36). Voriconazole was dosed 6 mg/kg at 12-hour intervals for the first two doses, then followed by 4 mg/kg twice daily for at least 1 week. After stabilization, the patient could be switched to the oral formulation at a dose of 200 mg/kg twice daily.

Amphotericin B was dosed at 1–1.5 mg/kg/day. Other licensed antifungal therapy was allowed in both arms for progression or intolerance. Voriconazole was found to be more effective than amphotericin B, with higher response rates (53% vs. 32% complete or partial response at 12 weeks) and better overall survival (71% vs. 58% at 12 weeks). In addition, voriconazole was associated with fewer adverse events and greater tolerance. Based on these data, voriconazole is now considered the drug of choice for first-line therapy of aspergillosis. An important consideration for practical use is knowledge of drug interactions with a multitude of concomitant medications that are metabolized by cytochrome P450, which may need to be monitored or doses adjusted.

E. Itraconazole

This azole has long been known to have anti *Aspergillus* activity. Various case series have shown it to be an effective therapy for invasive aspergillosis (37–39) for both initial and salvage therapy. Unfortunately, there are no controlled trials testing it in comparison with amphotericin B or other treatment options. Thus, today we remain uncertain as to its role relative to other drugs. Several caveats pertain. Many of the patients treated with itraconazole were relatively less immunocompromised. Use of either of the two oral formulations (capsules or solution) is plagued by erratic absorption. The oral solution is better absorbed than the capsule (especially in the fasted state) and is preferred. Several studies suggest a correlation between trough plasma levels and response. Initially, trough concentrations of ≥ 0.25 mcg/mL were targeted, but more recent data suggest that targeting of trough concentrations of ≥ 0.5 mcg/mL are better associated with response (40). With the heterogeneity of bioavailability, measurement of plasma drug levels is advisable to ensure therapeutic levels are being achieved. The IV formulation is well tolerated and gets around some of these concerns. However, its excipient is a cyclodextrin, which is renally cleared (in contrast to the hepatic clearance of itraconazole) and accumulation in renal failure occurs and this may pose a safety concern. Thus, the IV formulation should be avoided in patients with renal failure (creatinine clearance of <30 cc/min). A negative inotropic effect has been noted. This is a concern for patients with antecedent cardiac compromise and those receiving chemotherapeutic agents which are cardio-toxic in their own right. For the IV formulation, the dose is 200 mg twice daily for 2 days, then 200 mg daily (for up to 12 days). The oral dose is 2.5 mg/kg twice daily for the oral solution. In addition to the drug interaction issue noted for voriconazole, the issue of negative inotropic effects and variable bioavailability are impediments for clinical use.

There are rare reports of itraconazole resistance of *Aspergillus fumigatus* to itraconazole (41,42). An amphotericin B formulation or echinocandin should be considered for such circumstances.

F. Other Azoles

Posaconazole and ravuconazole are in clinical trials. In vitro susceptibility studies and anecdotal experience suggest roles for these agents.

G. Caspofungin

Caspofungin was first licensed for use in salvage therapy of invasive aspergillosis, refractory to amphotericin B, or in patients intolerant to licensed therapy. Response rates of 40–45% have been noted (43). To date, there are no data using caspofungin as first-line therapy. Other echinocandins are in development, including micafungin and anidulofungin.

H. Combination Therapy

A number of labs have demonstrated additive effects of a polyene plus an echinocan-din (44–46) or voriconazole plus an echinocandin (47–51). There are some limited clinical data with this approach (52,53,53A). Not all combinations are beneficial and thus caution is urged until more definitive study is undertaken (54).

I. Adjunctive Measures

The use of hematopoietic growth factors (G-CSF or GM-CSF) have been used to speed neutrophil recovery for infected neutropenic patients. Gamma interferon has also been used in patients with chronic granulomatous disease to reverse the phago-cytic defect. Although intuitively appealing, there is a paucity of data to clearly define the use of growth factors or immune modulators in these settings. Many clin-icians administer them in treatment of serious infections, especially in those poorly responsive to antifungal therapy alone.

Similarly, the use of granulocyte transfusions is also attractive. Some pilot data using transfusions of large numbers of granulocytes obtained from donors pretreated with G-CSF have shown that circulating neutrophil counts in recipients can be greatly increased for a day or two and there is some suggestion of improvement of refractory infection (55). They have also been used in patients with chronic granulomatous disease. However, to date the true benefit of this approach is not established (56).

Surgical excision should be considered in patients with pulmonary *Aspergillus* infections, where cavitary or necrotic tissues are persistent or where lesions are centrally located adjacent to great vessels or pericardium and catastrophic hemor-rhage may occur due to invasion of pulmonary vasculature, a single lesion causing hemoptysis, or lesions eroding into pleural space, ribs, or pericardium (57). If possible, reduction in the immunosuppressive treatment regimen is desirable to enhance host defenses.

J. Approaches to Aspergillosis Involving Sites Other than the Lungs

Sinusitis is an occasional manifestation and may be isolated or associated with either pulmonary or cerebral involvement. Surgical debridement is a key component of the management. For cerebral aspergillosis, case reports show some efficacy of various anti-*Aspergillus* agents, but overall mortality rates remain high (generally 80% or greater). There may be a role for surgical resection of amenable cerebral lesions, but this has not been formally studied. *Aspergillus* endocarditis should be approached with early aggressive surgical resection where feasible, along with antifungal therapy.

K. Practical Considerations

Based on clinical trial data, voriconazole is the first-line treatment of choice. There are certain patients for whom voriconazole may not be an option: these include patients with hepatic dysfunction or those with renal impairment and cannot receive an oral medication (IV voriconazole is not recommended due to the cyclodextrin accumulation during renal failure); for those an amphotericin B formulation would be indicated, with safety considerations giving considerable weight to a lipid formulation. For infections caused by *A. terreus,* an azole is preferred over a polyene due to susceptibility considerations.

For infection progression or treatment intolerance, a change to one of the lipid formulations of amphotericin B or caspofungin would be an excellent choice. When used, a lipid amphotericin B it should be given in a dose of 4–6 mg/kg/day. Some would advocate combination therapy as salvage therapy (either addition of caspofungin or change to an amphotericin B formulation plus caspofungin) based on the strength of the in vitro data and pilot clinical data.

In addition to pharmacologic therapy, resection of localized infarcted tissue should be considered as noted above and reduction of immunosuppressive therapy should also be considered. The use of myeloid growth factors or granulocyte transfusions should be strongly considered in persistently neutropenia with progressive infection.

The duration of therapy is not well worked out. As with Candidiasis, treatment until resolution of attributable clinical signs and symptoms, resolution, or maximal improvement of radiographic signs, and to the extent possible, improvement of host defenses should be done. The use of galactomannan antigen testing may be useful in monitoring clinical response along with clinical and other laboratory monitoring, but this has as yet not been well studied. At this time, much more experience is needed to clarify whether this is both practical and useful.

Important to note is the high likelihood of recurrence of infection in the event further compromise of host defenses occurs, through relapse of the underlying disease, further immunosuppressive or myelosuppressive therapy, or use of more intensive immunosuppressive therapy.

IV. *CRYPTOCOCCUS*

Treatment approaches vary according to the underlying state of the patient's immune status (normal or immunocompromised) and the form of infection (CNS or other) (58). This allows more intensive therapy (which is also more toxic) for those with serious disease and permits more convenient and less toxic oral therapy for those at lower risk for serious sequelae. Treatment is generally broken down into three phases: induction, consolidation, and secondary prophylaxis (sometimes referred to as chronic maintenance).

A. Pulmonary and Non-CNS Disease Without CNS Involvement in Non-Immunocompromised Patients

Few studies have been performed but expert opinion has been codified in IDSA treatment guidelines (58). For the immunocompetent individual who is asymptomatic, one can consider either observation or 3–6 months of fluconazole at a dose of 200–400 mg/day (58). If mild to moderate symptoms are present, then 6–12 months of fluconazole is advised. Itraconazole (200–400 mg/day) (but not ketoconazole) is an acceptable alternative. Patients with severe disease manifestations or those who are immunocompromised should be managed like those with CNS disease.

B. Meningitis or Pulmonary Infection in Immunocompromised Patients

The CNS infection in the form of meningitis is most commonly encountered in patients with advanced HIV infection; thus, the most well-developed trials have been conducted in this patient population (Table 3). For pulmonary disease associated with mild or moderate symptoms, treatment by either fluconazole or itraconazole in doses of 200–400 mg day can be given (58). For patients with more severe disease (pulmonary disease with severe symptoms or meningitis), an initial "induction" course of the combination of amphotericin B at a dose of 0.7–1.0 mg/kg/day with flucytosine 100 mg/kg/day should be used (58–62). The duration of the initial "induction" therapy has varied in different studies (generally 2–3 weeks), but amphotericin B should be continued at least until symptoms are controlled. Liposomal amphotericin B at a dose of 6 mg/kg/day for 2–3 weeks induction followed by fluconazole 400 mg day is as effective as amphotericin B in two randomized trials (63,64). Generally, after the induction course, a "consolidation" course of fluconazole given in a dose of 400–800 mg/kg/day is given for 8–10 weeks (65). The role of newer azoles has not been defined. The echinocandins are not active.

There have been few trials to determine if adjunctive measures are useful. Elevations in intracranial pressure can be harmful and should be monitored. Acetazolamide given to reduce intracranial pressure was not helpful in a small trial and was associated with considerable toxicity (66). Steroids and mannitol also do not appear to be helpful. Drainage by repeated lumbar punctures may be necessary if pressures exceed 200 mm of water). In vitro studies suggest G-CSF and GM-CSF may be helpful in enhancing azole killing (67), but this has not been tested in clinical trials. Other proinflammatory cytokines, including IL12, TNF alpha, and gamma interferon, are important in host responses (68), but these observations have not been exploited in therapeutic interventions.

Because of a high likelihood of recurrence in HIV infection, once initial induction and consolidation therapy is completed, chronic suppressive therapy should be instituted after control of the acute infection (69). Either fluconazole (200–400 mg day) or itraconazole (200 mg once or twice daily) is acceptable for chronic suppressive therapy, but fluconazole is more effective than itraconazole (70) and once weekly

Table 3 Randomized Trials for Therapy of Cryptococcosis

Author	Indication	Test agent	Comparator	Response rates		Survival rates		Time to CSF clearance (day)		Toxicities	Comments
				Test agent	Comparator	Test agent	Comparator	Test agent	Comparator		
Larsen (60)	Induction therapy	Amphotericin B plus fluconazole	Fluconazole	100%	43%	100%	33%	15.6	40.6	Favors fluconazole	Small sample (n = 20)
Bennett (61)	Induction therapy	Amphotericin B plus fluconazole	Amphotericin B	68%	47%	76%[a]	53%[a]	< 1 week[a]	1 week[a]	Similar	Low doses of amphotericin B (0.3 and 0.4 mg/kg/day in two groups)
Saag (62)	Induction therapy	Amphotericin B	Fluconazole	40%	34%	86%	82%	42	64		2 week mortality higher for fluconazole (15% vs. 8%); low doses of amphotericin B (0.4 mg/kg/day)
Leenders (63)	Induction therapy	Liposomal amphotericin B	Amphotericin B	80% (at 3 weeks)	86% (at 3 weeks)	93% (at 10 weeks)	85% (at 10 weeks)	73% at 3 weeks	38% at 3 weeks	Non-significant trend favoring liposomal amphotericin B	

Study	Therapy	Treatment							Favors	Comments
Hamil (64)	Induction therapy	Liposomal amphotericin B (dosed at 3 mg/kg/day and 6 mg/kg/day)	86%/94%	87%	86%/90% (at 10 weeks)	88% (at 10 weeks)	63%/54% at 2 weeks	54% at 2 weeks	Favors liposomal amphotericin B (fewer infusional reactions, less Nephrotoxicity at 3 mg/kg dose)	Shorter time to CSF conversion, but this did not translate into faster clinical response nor survival advantage
		Amphotericin B								
Newton (66)	Adjunct	Acetazolamide	No decrease	No decrease	84%	100%	N/A	N/A	Favors placebo	Trial terminated due to excess toxicity with autazolamide
		Placebo		84%						
van der Horst (59)	Induction therapy	Amphotericin B plus fluconazole	78% at 2 weeks	83% at 2 weeks	94% at 2 weeks	95% at 2 weeks	60% at 2 weeks	51% at 2 weeks	No difference	More rapid CSF clearance of cultures 60% vs. 51% at 2 weeks, $p = 0.06$
		Amphotericin B								
van der Horst (60)	Consolidation	Itraconazole	47%	42%	97%	99%	60%	72%		
		Fluconazole								
Saag (70)	Maintenance	Itraconazole	23%[a]	4%[a]	90%	84%	N/A	N/A	No difference Favors fluconazole	
		Fluconazole								
Powderly (71)	Maintenance	Fluconazole	2%[a]	18%[a]	N/A	N/A	N/A	N/A	Favors fluconazole	Amphotericin B given once weekly
		Amphotericin B								

(*Continued*)

Table 3 Randomized Trials for Therapy of Cryptococcosis (*Continued*)

Author	Indication	Test agent	Comparator	Response rates Test agent	Response rates Comparator	Survival rates Test agent	Survival rates Comparator	Time to CSF clearance (day) Test agent	Time to CSF clearance (day) Comparator	Toxicities	Comments
Saag (70)	Secondary prophylaxis	Itracona-zole	Fluconazole	23% relapse	4% relapse						
Vibhagool (78)	Withdrawal of secondary prophylaxis	Withdrawal of prophylaxis	Continued prophylaxis	0% relapses at 48 weeks	0% relapses at 48 weeks					N/A	This and other studies confirm that reconstitution of immunity can permit discontinuation of antifungal maintenance therapy

[a]*p* < 0.05.

amphotericin B (71). One concern is the observation of fluconazole heteroresistance in some Cryptococcal isolates (now <5%) (72). Whether this will emerge as substantial clinical issue remains to be seen. The role of maintenance therapy in cancer patients or patients on corticosteroids is less certain. Voriconazole has activity as salvage therapy (73).

Until recently, treatment was recommended lifelong, but studies have indicated that with improvement of host immunity (as can be seen with HAART), disconti- nuation can take place if there is a sustained increase in the CD4+ T lymphocyte count to above 100–200 cells/µL (74–78).

V. HISTOPLASMOSIS

Histoplasmosis is endemic in certain geographic regions. Disease is usually self- limited in non-immunocompromised individuals. In immunocompromised patients, disease can be severe, progressive, or become disseminated.

A. HIV-Infected Patients

Therapy for the acute manifestations of infection during the first 12 weeks consists of an amphotericin B formulation (79). Clearance of Histoplasma organisms from blood by culture and antigen assay occurs quicker with liposomal amphotericin B than with itraconazole in patients with moderately severe or severe disease (80) etc. Change to itraconazole can be made for patients responding well to take advan- tage of an oral regimen (81). In a randomized comparison of amphotericin B deox- ycholate at a dose of 0.7 mg/kg/day and liposomal amphotericin B at a dose of 3 mg/kg/day, there was a higher response rate, fewer deaths, and less toxicity with liposomal amphotericin B (82) (Table 4). For patients with mild to moderate man- ifestations (and without CNS involvement), itraconazole can be given at a dose of 300 mg BID for 3 days, then 200 mg BID for 12 weeks (83). Antigen monitoring can be used to monitor response to therapy (84–86).

After control of the acute infection, maintenance should be given with itraco- nazole at a dose of 200 mg once or twice daily (87). Maintenance should be con- tinued indefinitely. If a sustained increase in the CD4+ T lymphocyte count to above 100–200 cells/µL occurs discontinuation can be considered (69).

For patients with CD4+ T lymphocyte counts <200 cells/µL in endemic areas, avoidance of exposure is important. Prophylaxis with itraconazole is effec- tive (88) and can be considered in patients with CD4+ T lymphocyte counts <100 cells/µL (69) in endemic areas at high risk due to occupational exposure or high rates of infection. It should not be used routinely, however, because of an increase in resistance to both fluconazole and itraconazole in patients receiving itraconazole (88).

B. Other Immunocompromised Patients

The treatment approach is similar. For maintenance therapy, prolonged treatment in the range of 6–18 months is generally advised (69) but this has not been formally studied.

Table 4 Randomized Trials of Antifungal Therapy in Various Other Invasive Fungal Infection

Author	Pathogen	Indication	Test agent	Comparator	Success/Relapse rates		Toxicities	Comments
					Test agent	Comparator		
Johnson (82)	Histoplasmosis	Induction therapy	Liposomal amphotericin B	Amphotericin B	88%	64%	Favors liposomal amphotericin B	
Galgiani (94)	Coccidiomycosis (non-meningeal)	Induction[a]	Itraconazole	Fluconazole	63% at 8 months; 72% at 12 months	50% at 8 months; 57% at 12 months	No difference	Relapse rates after discontinuation 28% vs. 18%

[a]$p = 0.05$.

VI. COCCIDIODOMYCOSIS

As with Histoplasmosis, Coccidiodomycosis is endemic in certain geographic areas. Its clinical course can be quite variable.

There are a number of agents with activity against coccidioides, but treatment guidelines are difficult to formulate because of the lack of controlled trials (89). Generally, oral or parenteral therapy is chosen based on the degree of illness of the patient. An azole, either itraconazole or fluconazole, is effective for progressive non-meningeal infection; responses to itraconazole appear to be slightly better than fluconazole (90,91) (Table 4). If parenteral therapy is judged more appropriate, amphotericin B at a dose of 0.5–0.7 mg/kg/day or a lipid amphotericin B formulation is recommended (90). Posaconazole, voriconazole, and caspofungin have activity but a clinical role has not yet been defined.

Treatment of meningitis is quite problematic. For amphotericin B to be effective, it must be given intrathecally or by CSF shunt in a dose of 0.5–1.0 mg. Azoles are effective but relapses are frequent. In an animal model, liposomal amphotericin B was more effective than amphotericin B (92).

Surgical resection of localized pulmonary cavities can be useful in selected patients, where a cavity is persistent, progressive over time, or if subpleurally located where communication to the pleural cavity can occur. Immunomodulators offer promise as adjuncts: gamma interferon and IL12 promote protective Th1 responses and could be important adjuncts to antifungal therapy (93,94).

For patients with advanced HIV infection, maintenance with either fluconazole at 400 mg/day or itraconazole at 200 mg BID should be done indefinitely or until a sustained increase in the CD4+ T lymphocyte count above 100 cells/μL occurs (69). Relapses may occur less frequently with itraconazole than with fluconazole. Relapses appear to be infrequent in cancer patients and the role for maintenance is uncertain. One center has reported prophylaxis with fluconazole in liver transplant recipients in an endemic area is effective (95).

VII. OTHER FUNGI

A. Other Yeasts

1. Trichosporon

Amphotericin B has traditionally been used for therapy. However, persistence of fungemia during treatment coupled with in vitro observations of inhibition but not killing by amphotericin B suggest that amphotericin B is not optimal (96–98). Azoles, including fluconazole, voriconazole, and posaconazole, are active (96,99). The combination of fluconazole and amphotericin B showed greater activity in an animal model (99). GM-CSF may enhance therapeutic potential (100). There may be a role for granulocyte transfusions as well in the presence of persistent neutropenia, but this has not been studied.

2. Blastoschizomyces Captitatus (Formerly T. capitatum)

In vitro susceptibilities for this organism are similar to those of Trichosporon with the exception of fluconazole resistance noted in some isolates (101). The combination of fluconazole, amphotericin B, and GM-CSF has been used anecdotally (102).

3.   Malassezia furfur *(Pityrosporum)*

In vitro susceptibility testing suggests amphotericin B and azoles are good treatment options (103,104). Antifungal therapy alone is inadequate, however (105). Removal of catheter and lipid nutritional supplements (upon which the organism is dependent for growth) are important components of management.

4.   *Rhodotorula*

Amphotericin B is active in vitro and is generally used for treatment. The azoles have variable activity (106). Removal of central venous catheters is generally recommended, although this has not been systemically studied (107).

B. Other Molds

1.   *Zygomycetes (Mucormycosis)*

Traditional treatment is with amphotericin B given in high doses (108,109). Surgical debridement of necrotic tissue is an important adjunct to antifungal therapy. Results have been poor. Case series with amphotericin B colloidal dispersion (110) and with amphotericin B lipid complex (111) as salvage therapy may be better options than amphotericin B. Posaconazole has in vivo activity in an animal model (112). Voriconazole and caspofungin do not have activity.

3.   *Blastomycosis*

Amphotericin B in a dose of 0.7–1.0 mg/kg/day is recommended (113). In the absence of CNS disease, a change to itraconazole may be made once the patient stabilizes. Frequent relapses in HIV infection occur. Accordingly, maintenance therapy with an azole is recommended, preferably with itraconazole (113).

3.   *Scedosporium (Scedosporium apiospermum or*
       Pneumocystis boydii and Scedosporium prolificans)

Susceptibility to amphotericin B is poor in vitro and clinically there have been few successes. The lipid formulations of amphotericin B, amphotericin B deoxycholate, and voriconazole act additively with neutrophils to exert injury to *Scedosporium* hyphae (114,115). The addition of G-CSF to liposomal amphotericin B in an animal model appeared to be more effective than liposomal amphotericin B alone (116). Voriconazole and posaconazole have inhibitory activity in vitro (117–120). Voriconazole and posaconazole have been used anecdotally with some success (73,121–125). Voriconazole may be the therapy of choice at present. The echinocandins have some in vitro activity but have not been tested clinically (119,126). Itraconazole and terbinafine have demonstrated poor activity in vitro as single agents but in combination demonstrated synergy (127); the clinical significance of this observation is unknown. Where possible, surgical debridement of necrotic tissue is important.

4.   *Fusarium*

Amphotericin B in high doses has traditionally been used, although in vitro susceptibility to amphotericin B is suboptimal and some isolates demonstrate resistance in vitro (128) and treatment results have been poor. The lipid formulations of amphotericin B have been used clinically, but treatment results have remained suboptimal. Fluconazole and itraconazole have little activity. Voriconazole and posaconazole have both shown in vitro activity (118,120,129–132) and voriconazole has demonstrated clinical efficacy in the salvage setting (73,133). In vitro testing suggest synergy of caspofungin and amphotericin B (44), but this has not been evaluated clinically. Neutrophil recovery appears crucial for successful outcomes. Growth factors and granulocyte transfusions have been used anecdotally for persistently neutropenic patients with some efficacy. Removal of vascular catheters and debridement of necrotic tissue are other adjunctive measures which can be useful (65).

5. Alternaria

Antifungal agents have poor activity. Amphotericin B, itraconazole, and voriconazole have been used (134,135). Surgical debridement and efforts to effect restoration of host responses are key.

VIII. *PNEUMOCYSTIS JIROVECI* (FORMERLY *PNEUMOCYSTIS CARINII*)

Trimethoprim-sulfamethoxazole (TMP-SMX) is the preferred treatment for *Pneumocystis carinii* pneumonia (PCP), found in various randomized trials to be more effective than a variety of alternative therapies for mild, moderate, or severe PCP. The TMP-SMX is administered either orally or intravenously in a dose of 15–20 mg/kg/day of trimethoprim and 75–100 mg/kg/day sulfamethoxazole in 3–4 divided doses. Although generally well tolerated, adverse reactions may occur, especially in HIV-infected patients, with rash, fever, cytopenias, gastrointestinal intolerance being the most frequent toxicities. Alternative therapies for mild to moderate PCP include dapsone 100 mg/day with TMP 15–20 mg/kg/day (136,137). This combination is less toxic, but adverse reactions including methemoglobinemia and hemolysis in patients with glucose-6-phosphate dehydrogenase (G6PD) deficiency can occur. A third option for mild to moderate PCP is the combination of clindamycin given at a dose of 600 mg IV every 6 hr followed by 300–450 mg orally every 6 hr plus primaquine 15–30 mg base per day orally (137,138). Hemolysis from primaquine can occur in patients with G6PD deficiency. Atovaquone at a dose of 750 mg twice daily has been found to be less effective than TMP-SMX for mild to moderate PCP but it is as effective as pentamidine (139,140); it is better tolerated than either comparator. Its bioavailability has been an issue but the oral suspension is much better absorbed than the oral tablet (47% bioavailability compared with 23%).

For moderate to severe PCP, alternatives to TMP-SMX include pentamidine isethionate at a dose of 4 mg/kg/day once daily intravenously (141–144) and trimetrexate at a dose of 45 mg/m^2 once daily (145). Response rates to IV pentamidine have generally been similar to TMP-SMX. Trimethrexate is less effective than TMP-SMX but better tolerated; notwithstanding, myelosuppression, can occur, which can be lessened by administration of folinic acid.

Since the inflammatory response to PCP can lead to worsening of respiratory symptoms and greater hypoxia, corticosteroids have been used in moderate to severe PCP and found to beneficial and improve survival (146–148). Typically prednisone is given at a dose of 40 mg twice daily for 5 days and then tapered to cease by day 20.

Several agents are useful as second-line therapies for individuals progressing, or as intolerant of TMP-SMX. In a meta-analysis of salvage therapies for PCP (149), efficacy rates for salvage therapies were clindamycin-primaquine (88–92%), atovaquone (80%), eflornithine hydrochloride (57%), TMP-SMX (53%), pentamidine (39%), and trimethrexate (30%).

IX. CONCLUSION

Treatment approaches have been well studied and rigorous trials have been conducted for *Candida* and *Cryptococcus* infections forming strong bases for management strategies. Steady progress has been made and treatment outcomes have improved. Unfortunately, for other fungal infections, there have been few randomized trials, progress has been slower, and management strategies are less certain. In large part, the small numbers of cases have impeded progress. For many years the lack of antifungals to test has also contributed to slow gains; that has changed now with the introduction of several new agents which offer advantages in efficacy and safety. Another factor that has slowed progress is the heterogeneity of host factors that must also be taken into consideration in clinical trial design and evaluation of treatment outcomes. Some effort is being made to consider new trial designs (150–153) to maximize what can be learned from small numbers of patients and, in many instances, the inability to conduct a randomized trial to definitively answer which agent or strategy may be "best." Renewed commitment of clinicians to enter patients wherever possible to clinical trials is also key for progress to be made

REFERENCES

1. Rex JH, Walsh TJ, Sobel JD, Filler SG, Pappas PG, Dismukes WE, Edwards JE. Practice guidelines for the treatment of candidiasis. Infectious Diseases Society of America. Clin Infect Dis 2000; 30:662–678.
2. Pappas PG, Rex JH, Sobel JD, Filler SG, Dismukes WE, Walsh TJ, Edwards JE. Guidelines for treatment of candidiasis. Clin Infect Dis 2004; 38:161–189.
3. Gallis HA, Drew RH, Pickard WW. Amphotericin B: 30 years of clinical experience. Rev Infect Dis 1990; 12:308–329.
4. Wingard JR, Kubilis P, Lee L, Yee G, White M, Walshe L, Bowden R, Anaissie E, Hiemenz J, Lister J. Clinical significance of nephrotoxicity in patients treated with amphotericin B for suspected or proven aspergillosis. Clin Infect Dis 1999; 29:1402–1407.
5. Anaissie EJ, White M, Uzun O, Singer C, Bodey GP, Matzke D, Azarnia N, Lopez-Berestein G. Amphotericin B lipid complex versus amphotericin B for treatment of hematogenous and invasive candidiasis: a prospective, randomized, multicenter trial. (Poster Session). In: Program and abstracts of the 35th Interscience Conference on Antimicrobial Agents and Chemotherapy Washington, DC. 1995;Abstract #LM21, page 330.
6. Bennett J. Editorial response: choosing amphotericin B formulations-between a rock and a hard place. Clin Infect Dis 2000; 31:1164–1165.
7. Rex JH, Walsh TJ. Estimating the true cost of amphotericin B. Clin Infect Dis 1999; 29:1408–1410.
8. Ostrosky-Zeichner L, Marr KA, Rex JH, Cohen SH. Amphotericin B: time for a new "gold standard". Clin Infect Dis 2003; 37:415–425.
9. Wingard JR. Lipid formulations of amphotericins: are you a lumper or a splitter? Clin Infect Dis 2002; 35:891–895.
10. Rex JH, Pfaller MA, Galgiani JN, Bartlett MS, Espinel-Ingroff A, Ghannoum MA, Lancaster M, Odds FC, Rinaldi MG, Walsh TJ, Barry AL. Development of interpretive breakpoints for antifungal susceptibility testing: conceptual framework and analysis of in vitro-in vivo correlation data for fluconazole, itraconazole, and candida infections.

Subcommittee on Antifungal Susceptibility Testing of the National Committee for Clinical Laboratory Standards. Clin Infect Dis 1997; 24:235–247.

11. Pfaller MA, Diekema DJ. Twelve years of fluconazole in clinical practice: global trends in species distribution and fluconazole susceptibility of bloodstream isolates of *Candida*. Clin Microbiol Infect 2004; 10(suppl 1):11–23.

12. Phillips P, Shafran S, Garber G, Rotstein C, Smaill F, Fong I, Salit I, Miller M, Williams K, Conly JM, Singer J, Ioannou S. Multicenter randomized trial of fluconazole versus amphotericin B for treatment of candidemia in non-neutropenic patients. Canadian Candidemia Study Group. Eur J Clin Microbiol Infect Dis 1997; 16:337–345.

13. Rex JH, Bennett JE, Sugar AM, Pappas PG, van der Horst CM, Edwards JE, Washburn RG, Scheld WM, Karchmer AW, Dine AP. A randomized trial comparing fluconazole with amphotericin B for the treatment of candidemia in patients without neutropenia. Candidemia Study Group and the National Institute. N Engl J Med 1994; 331:1325–1330.

14. Kontoyiannis DP, Lewis RE. Antifungal drug resistance of pathogenic fungi. Lancet 2002; 359:1135–1144.

15. Perea S, Patterson TF. Antifungal resistance in pathogenic fungi. Clin Infect Dis 2002; 35:1073–1080.

16. Persons DA, Laughlin M, Tanner D, et al. Fluconazole and *Candida krusei* fungemia. N Engl J Med 1991; 325:1315.

17. Wingard JR, Merz WG, Rinaldi MG, et al. Association of *Torulopsis glabrata* infections with fluconazole prophylaxis in neutropenic bone marrow transplant patients. Antimicrob Agents Chemother 1993; 37:1847–1849.

18. Wingard JR, Merz WG, Rinaldi MG, et al. Increase in *Candida krusei* infection among patients with bone marrow transplantation and neutropenia treated prophylactically with fluconazole. N Engl J Med 1991; 325:1274–1277.

19. Nolte FS, Parkinson T, Falconer DJ, Dix S, Williams J, Gilmore C, Geller R, Wingard JR. Isolation and characterization of fluconazole- and amphotericin B-resistant Candida albicans from blood of two patients with leukemia. Antimicrob Agents Chemother 1997; 41:196–199.

20. Marr KA, Lyons CN, Ha K, Rustad TR, White TC. Inducible azole resistance associated with a heterogeneous phenotype in *Candida albicans*. Antimicrob Agents Chemother 2001; 45:52–59.

21. Ally R, Schurmann D, Kreisel W, Carosi G, Aguirrebengoa K, Dupont B, Hodges M, Troke P, Romero AJ. A randomized, double-blind, double-dummy, multicenter trial of voriconazole and fluconazole in the treatment of esophageal candidiasis in immunocompromised patients. Clin Infect Dis 2001; 33:1447–1454.

22. Walsh TJ. Echinocandins—an advance in the primary treatment of invasive candidiasis. N Engl J Med 2002; 347:2070–2072.

23. Cornely OA, Schmitz K, Aisenbrey S. The first echinocandin: caspofungin. Mycoses 2002; 45(suppl 3):56–60.

24. Johnson MD, Perfect JR. Caspofungin: first approved agent in a new class of antifungals. Expert Opin Pharmacother 2003; 4:807–823.

25. Ullmann AJ. Review of the safety, tolerability, and drag interactions of the new antifungal agents caspofungin and voriconazole. Curr Med Res Opin 2003; 19:263–271.

26. Serrano MC, Valverde-Conde A, Chavez MM, Bernal S, Claro RM, Peman J, Ramirez M, Martin-Mazuelos E. In vitro activity of voriconazole, itraconazole, caspofungin, anidulafungin (VER002, LY303366) and amphotericin B against aspergillus spp. Diagn Microbiol Infect Dis 2003; 45:131–135.

27. Villanueva A, Gotuzzo E, Arathoon EG, Noriega LM, Kartsonis NA, Lupinacci RJ, Smietana JM, DiNubile MJ, Sable CA. A randomized double-blind study of caspofungin versus fluconazole for the treatment of esophageal candidiasis. Am J Med 2002; 113:294–299.

28. Mora-Duarte J, Betts R, Rotstein C, Colombo AL, Thompson-Moya L, Smietana J, Lupinacci R, Sable C, Kartsonis N, Perfect J. Comparison of caspofungin and amphotericin B for invasive candidiasis. N Engl J Med 2002; 347:2020–2029.

29. Nakai T, Uno J, Ikeda F, Tawara S, Nishimura K, Miyaji M. In vitro antifungal activity of Micafungin (FK463) against dimorphic fungi: comparison of yeast-like and mycelial forms. Antimicrob Agents Chemother 2003; 47:1376–1381.

30. Krause DS, Reinhardt J, Vazquez JA, Reboli A, Goldstein BP, Wible M, Henkel T. Phase 2, randomized, dose-ranging study evaluating the safety and efficacy of anidulafungin in invasive candidiasis and candidemia. Antimicrob Agents Chemother 2004; 48:2021–2024.

31. Rex JH, Pappas PG, Karchmer AW, Sobel J, Edwards JE, Hadley S, Brass C, Vazquez JA, Chapman SW, Horowitz HW, Zervos M, McKinsey D, Lee J, Babinchak T, Bradsher RW, Cleary JD, Cohen DM, Danziger L, Goldman M, Goodman J, Hilton E, Hyslop NE, Kett DH, Lutz J, Rubin RH, Scheld WM, Schuster M, Simmons B, Stein DK, Washburn RG, Mautner L, Chu TC, Panzer H, Rosenstein RB, Booth J. A randomized and blinded multicenter trial of high-dose fluconazole plus placebo versus fluconazole plus amphotericin B as therapy for candidemia and its consequences in nonneutropenic subjects. Clin Infect Dis 2003; 36:1221–1228.

32. Nucci M, Anaissie E. Should vascular catheters be removed from all patients with candidemia? An evidence-based review. Clin Infect Dis 2002; 34:591–599.

33. Walsh TJ, Rex JH. All catheter-related candidemia is not the same: assessment of the balance between the risks and benefits of removal of vascular catheters. Clin Infect Dis 2002; 34:600–602.

34. Ellis M, Spence D, de Pauw B, Meunier F, Marinus A, Collette L, Sylvester R, Meis J, Boogaerts M, Selleslag D, Krcmery V, von Sinner W, MacDonald P, Doyen C, Vandercam B. An EORTC international multicenter randomized trial (EORTC number 19923) comparing two dosages of liposomal amphotericin B for treatment of invasive aspergillosis. Clin Infect Dis 1998; 27:1406–1412.

35. Bowden R, Chandrasekar P, White MH, Li X, Pietrelli L, Gurwith M, van Burik JA, Laverdiere M, Safrin S, Wingard JR. A double-blind, randomized, controlled trial of amphotericin B colloidal dispersion versus amphotericin B for treatment of invasive aspergillosis in immunocompromised patients. Clin Infect Dis 2002; 35:359–366.

36. Herbrecht R, Denning DW, Patterson TF, Bennett JE, Greene RE, Oestmann JW, Kern WV, Marr KA, Ribaud P, Lortholary O, Sylvester R, Rubin RH, Wingard JR, Stark P, Durand C, Caillot D, Thiel E, Chandrasekar PH, Hodges MR, Schlamm HT, Troke PF, de Pauw B. Voriconazole versus amphotericin B for primary therapy of invasive aspergillosis. N Engl J Med 2002; 347:408–415.

37. Patterson TF, Kirkpatrick WR, White M, Hiemenz JW, Wingard JR, Dupont B, Rinaldi MG, Stevens DA, Graybill JR. Invasive aspergillosis. Disease spectrum, treatment practices, and outcomes. I3 Aspergillus Study Group. Medicine (Baltimore) 2000; 79:250–260.

38. Denning DW, Stevens DA. Antifungal and surgical treatment of invasive aspergillosis: review of 2,121 published cases. Rev Infect Dis 1990; 12:1147–1201.

39. Caillot D, Bassaris H, McGeer A, Arthur C, Prentice HG, Seifert W, De Beule K. Intravenous itraconazole followed by oral itraconazole in the treatment of invasive pulmonary aspergillosis in patients with hematologic malignancies, chronic granulomatous disease, or AIDS. Clin Infect Dis 2001; 33:e83–e90.

40. Glasmacher A, Hahn C, Molitor E, Marklein G, Schmidt-Wolf I. Minimal effective trough concentrations for antifungal prophylaxis with itraconazole: a case-control study. Proc Intersc Conf Antimicrob Agents Chemother 2002; 42:M-890.

41. Slaven JW, Anderson MJ, Sanglard D, Dixon GK, Bille J, Roberts IS, Denning DW. Increased expression of a novel Aspergillus fumigatus ABC transporter gene, atrF, in the presence of itraconazole in an itraconazole resistant clinical isolate. Fungal Genet Biol 2002; 36:199–206.

42. Warn PA, Morrissey G, Morrissey J, Denning DW. Activity of micafungin (FK463) against an itraconazole-resistant strain of *Aspergillus fumigatus* and a strain of *Aspergillus terreus* demonstrating in vivo resistance to amphotericin B. J Antimicrob Chemother 2003; 51:913–919.

43. Maertens J, Raad I, Petrikkos G, et al. Update of the multicenter noncomparative study of caspofungin in adults with invasive aspergillosis refractory or intolerant to other antifungal agents: analysis of 90 patients. Proc Intersc Conf Antimicrob Agents Chemother 2002; 42:M-868.

44. Arikan S, Lozano-Chiu M, Paetznick V, Rex JH. In vitro synergy of caspofungin and amphotericin B against *Aspergillus* and *Fusarium* spp. Antimicrob Agents Chemother 2002; 46:245–247.

45. Nakajima M, Tamada S, Toshida K, Wakai Y, Nakai T, Ikeda F, Goto T, Niki Y, Matsushima T. Pathological findings in a murine pulmonary aspergillosis model: treatment with FK463, amphotericin B and a combination of FK463 and amphotericin B. Proc Intersc Conf Antimicrob Agents Chemother 2000; 40:J-1685.

46. Kohno S, Maesaki S, Iwakawa J, Miyazaki Y, Nakamura K, Kakeya H, Yanagihara K, Ohno H, Higashiyama Y, Tashiro T. Synergistic effects of combination of FK463 with amphotericin B: enhanced efficacy in murine model of invasive pulmonary aspergillosis. Proc Intersc Conf Antimicrob Agents Chemother 2000; 40:J-1686.

47. Kirkpatrick WR, Perea S, Coco BJ, Patterson TF. Efficacy of caspofungin alone and in combination with voriconazole in a guinea pig model of invasive aspergillosis. Antimicrob Agents Chemother 2002; 46:2564–2568.

48. Luque JC, Clemons KV, Stevens DA. Efficacy of micafungin alone or in combination against systemic murine aspergillosis. Antimicrob Agents Chemother 2003; 47:1452–1425.

49. Manavathu EK, Alangaden GJ, Chandrasekar PH. Differential activity of triazoles in two-drug combinations with the echinocandin caspofungin against *Aspergillus fumigatus*. J Antimicrob Chemother 2003; 51:1423–1425.

50. Perea S, Gonzalez G, Fothergill AW, Kirkpatrick WR, Rinaldi MG, Patterson TF. In vitro interaction of caspofungin acetate with voriconazole against clinical isolates of Aspergillus spp. Antimicrob Agents Chemother 2002; 46:3039–3041.

51. Petraitis V, Petraitiene R, Sarafandi AA, Kelaher AM, Lyman CA, Casler HE, Sein T, Groll AH, Bacher J, Avila NA, Walsh TJ. Combination therapy in treatment of experimental pulmonary aspergillosis: synergistic interaction between an antifungal triazole and an echinocandin. J Infect Dis 2003; 187:1834–1843.

52. Aliff TB, Maslak PG, Jurcic JG, Heaney ML, Cathcart KN, Sepkowitz KA, Weiss MA. Refractory Aspergillus pneumonia in patients with acute leukemia: successful therapy with combination caspofungin and liposomal amphotericin. Cancer 2003; 97:1025–1032.

53. Kontoyiannis DP, Hachem R, Lewis RE, Rivero GA, Torres HA, Thornby J, Champlin R, Kantarjian H, Bodey GP, Raad II. Efficacy and toxicity of caspofungin in combination with liposomal amphotericin B as primary or salvage treatment of invasive aspergillosis in patients with hematologic malignancies. Cancer 2003; 98:292–299.

54. Wheat LJ. Combination therapy for aspergillosis: is it needed, and which combination? J Infect Dis 2003; 187:1831–1833.

55. Dignani MC, Anaissie EJ, Hester JP, O'Brien S, Vartivarian SE, Rex JH, Kantarjian H, Jendiroba DB, Lichtiger B, Andersson BS, Freireich EJ. Treatment of neutropenia-related fungal infections with granulocyte colony-stimulating factor-elicited white blood cell transfusions: a pilot study. Leukemia 1997; 11:1621–1630.

56. Liles WC, Hubel K, Dale DC. Granulocyte (neutrophil) transfusion therapy. In: Wingard JR, Bowden RA, eds. Management of Infection in Oncology Patients. London and New York: Martin Dunitz, 2003:363–372.

57. Stevens DA, Kan VL, Judson MA, Morrison VA, Dummer S, Denning DW, Bennett JE, Walsh TJ, Patterson TF, Pankey GA. Practice guidelines for diseases caused by Aspergillus. Infectious Diseases Society of America. Clin Infect Dis 2000; 30:696–709.

58. Saag MS, Graybill RJ, Larsen RA, Pappas PG, Perfect JR, Powderly WG, Sobel JD, Dismukes WE. Practice guidelines for the management of cryptococcal disease. Infectious Diseases Society of America. Clin Infect Dis 2000; 30:710–718.

59. van der Horst CM, Saag MS, Cloud GA, Hamill RJ, Graybill JR, Sobel JD, Johnson PC, Tuazon CU, Kerkering T, Moskovitz BL, Powderly WG, Dismukes WE. Treatment of cryptococcal meningitis associated with the acquired immunodeficiency syndrome. National Institute of Allergy and Infectious Diseases Mycoses Study Group and AIDS Clinical Trials Group. N Engl J Med 1997; 337:15–21.

60. Larsen RA, Leal MA, Chan LS. Fluconazole compared with amphotericin B plus flucytosine for cryptococcal meningitis in AIDS. A randomized trial. Ann Intern Med 1990; 113:183–187.

61. Bennett JE, Dismukes WE, Duma RJ, Medoff G, Sande MA, Gallis H, Leonard J, Fields BT, Bradshaw M, Haywood H, McGee ZA, Cate TR, Cobbs CG, Warner JF, Alling DW. A comparison of amphotericin B alone and combined with flucytosine in the treatment of cryptoccal meningitis. N Engl J Med 1979; 301:126–131.

62. Saag MS, Powderly WG, Cloud GA, Robinson P, Grieco MH, Sharkey PK, Thompson SE, Sugar AM, Tuazon CU, Fisher JF. Comparison of amphotericin B with fluconazole in the treatment of acute AIDS-associated cryptococcal meningitis. The NIAID Mycoses Study Group and the AIDS Clinical Trials Group. N Engl J Med 1992; 326:83–89.

63. Leenders AC, Reiss P, Portegies P, Clezy K, Hop WC, Hoy J, Borleffs JC, Allworth T, Kauffmann RH, Jones P, Kroon FP, Verbrugh HA, de Marie S. Liposomal amphotericin B (AmBisome) compared with amphotericin B both followed by oral fluconazole in the treatment of AIDS-associated cryptococcal meningitis. AIDS 1997; 11:1463–1471.

64. Note: A copy of this abstract was not available to obtain names of all authors Hamill R, Sobel J, El-Sadr W, et al. Randomized double-blind trial of AmBiosome (liposomal amphotericin B) and amphotericin B in acute cryptococcal meningitis in AIDS patients. In: Programs and abstracts of the 39th Interscience Conference on Antimicrobial Agents and Chemotherapy Washington, DC: ASM Press 1999; Abstract 1161:489.

65. Chandrasekar PH. Fungi other than *Candida* and *Aspergillus*. In: Wingard JR, Bowden RA, eds. Management of Infection in Oncology Patients. London and New York: Martin Dunitz, 2003; 203–221.

66. Newton PN, Thai lH, Tip NQ, Short JM, Chierakul W, Rajanuwong A, Pitisuttithum P, Chasombat S, Phonrat B, Maek AN, Teaunadi R, Lalloo DG, White NJ. A randomized, double-blind, placebo-controlled trial of acetazolamide for the treatment of elevated intracranial pressure in cryptococcal meningitis. Clin Infect Dis 2002; 35:769–772.

67. Chiller T, Farrokhshad K, Brummer E, Stevens DA. Effect of granulocyte colony-stimulating factor and granulocyte-macrophage colony-stimulating factor on polymorphonuclear neutrophils, monocytes or monocyte-derived macrophages combined with voriconazole against *Cryptococcus neoformans*. Med Mycol 2002; 40:21–26.

68. Vecchiarelli A. Cytokines and costimulatory molecules: positive and negative regulation of the immune response to *Cryptococcus neoformans*. Arch Immunol Ther Exp (Warsz) 2000; 48:465–472.

69. 2001 USPHS/IDSA Guidelines for the Prevention of Opportunistic Infections in Persons Infected with Human Immunodeficiency Virus. Center for Disease Control 2001:1–190.

70. Saag MS, Cloud GA, Graybill JR, Sobel JD, Tuazon CU, Johnson PC, Fessel WJ, Moskovitz BL, Wiesinger B, Cosmatos D, Riser L, Thomas C, Hafner R, Dismukes WE. A comparison of itraconazole versus fluconazole as maintenance therapy for AIDS-associated cryptococcal meningitis. National Institute of Allergy and Infectious Diseases Mycoses Study Group. Clin Infect Dis 1999; 28:291–296.

71. Powderly WG, Saag MS, Cloud GA, Robinson P, Meyer RD, Jacobson JM, Graybill JR, Sugar AM, McAuliffe VJ, Follansbee SE. A controlled trial of fluconazole or amphotericin B to prevent relapse of cryptococcal meningitis in patients with the acquired immunodeficiency syndrome. The NIAID AIDS Clinical Trials Group and Mycoses Study Group. N Engl J Med 1992; 326:793–798.

72. Yamazumi T, Pfaller MA, Messer SA, Houston AK, Boyken L, Hollis RJ, Furuta I, Jones RN. Characterization of heteroresistance to fluconazole among clinical isolates of Cryptococcus neoformans. J Clin Microbiol 2003; 41:267–272.

73. Perfect JR, Marr KA, Walsh TJ, Greenberg RN, Dupont B, Torre-Cisneros J, Just-Nubling G, Schlamm HT, Lutsar I, Espinel-Ingroff A, Johnson E. Voriconazole treatment for less-common, emerging, or refractory fungal infections. Clin Infect Dis 2003; 36:1122–1131.

74. Mussini, C., Cossarizza, A., Pezzotti, P., Antinori A, DeLuca A, Ortolani P, Rizzardini G, Mongiardo N, Esposito R. Discontinuation or continuation of maintenance therapy for cryptococcal meningitis in patients with AIDS treated with HAART. 8th Conference on Retroviruses and Opportunistic Infections, February 4–8, 2001, Chicago, IL. 2001, Abstract 546.

75. Kirk O, Reiss P, Uberti-Foppa C, Bickel M, Gerstoft J, Pradier C, Wit FW, Ledergerber B, Lundgren JD, Furrer H. Safe interruption of maintenance therapy against previous infection with four common HIV-associated opportunistic pathogens during potent antiretroviral therapy. Ann Intern Med 2002; 137:239–250.

76. Aberg JA, Price RW, Heeren DM, Bredt B. A pilot study of the discontinuation of antifungal therapy for disseminated cryptococcal disease in patients with acquired immunodeficiency syndrome, following immunologic response to antiretroviral therapy. J Infect Dis 2002; 185:1179–1182.

77. Masur H, Kaplan JE, Holmes KK. Guidelines for preventing opportunistic infections among HIV-infected persons—2002. Recommendations of the U.S. Public Health Service and the Infectious Diseases Society of America. Ann Intern Med 2002; 137: 435–478.

78. Vibhagool A, Sungkanuparph S, Mootsikapun P, Chetchotisakd P, Tansuphaswaswadikul S, Bowonwatanuwong C, Ingsathit A. Discontinuation of secondary prophylaxis for cryptococcal meningitis in human immunodeficiency virus-infected patients treated with highly active antiretroviral therapy: a prospective, multicenter, randomized study. Clin Infect Dis 2003; 36:1329–1331.

79. Wheat J, Sarosi G, McKinsey D, Hamill R, Bradsher R, Johnson P, Loyd J, Kauffman C. Practice guidelines for the management of patients with histoplasmosis. Infectious Diseases Society of America. Clin Infect Dis 2000; 30:688–695.

80. Wheat LJ, Cloud G, Johnson PC, Connolly P, Goldman M, Le Monte A, Fuller DE, Davis TE, Hafter R. Clearance of fungal burden during treatment of disseminated histoplasmosis with liposomal amphotericin B versus itraconazole. Antimicrob Agents Chemother 2001; 45:2354–2357.

81. Wheat LJ, Kauffman CA. Histoplasmosis. Infect Dis Clin North Am 2003; 17:1–19, vii.

82. Johnson PC, Wheat LJ, Cloud GA, Goldman M, Lancaster D, Bamberger DM, Powderly WG, Hafner R, Kauffman CA, Dismukes WE. Safety and efficacy of liposomal amphotericin B compared with conventional amphotericin B for induction therapy of histoplasmosis in patients with AIDS. Ann Intern Med 2002; 137:105–109.

83. Wheat J, Hafner R, Korzun AH, Limjoco MT, Spencer P, Larsen RA, Hecht FM, Powderly W. Itraconazole treatment of disseminated histoplasmosis in patients with the acquired immunodeficiency syndrome. AIDS Clinical Trial Group. Am J Med 1995; 98:336–342.

84. Wheat J, Hafner R, Wulfsohn M, Spencer P, Squires K, Powderly W, Wong B, Rinaldi M, Saag M, Hamill R, Murphy R, Connolly-Stringfield P, Briggs N, Owens S. Prevention of relapse of histoplasmosis with itraconazole in patients with the acquired immunodeficiency syndrome. Ann Intern Med 1993; 118:610–616.

85. Wheat LJ, Connolly P, Haddad N, Le Monte A, Brizendine E, Hafner R. Antigen clearance during treatment of disseminated histoplasmosis with itraconazole versus fluconazole in patients with AIDS. Antimicrob Agents Chemother 2002; 46:248–250.

86. Wheat LJ, Connolly-Stringfield PA, Baker RL, Curfman MF, Eads ME, Israel KS, Norris SA, Webb DH, Zeckel ML. Disseminated histoplasmosis in the acquired immune deficiency syndrome: clinical findings, diagnosis and treatment, and review of the literature. Medicine (Baltimore) 1990; 69:361–374.

87. Hecht FM, Wheat J, Korzun AH, Hafner R, Skahan KJ, Larsen R, Limjoco MT, Simpson M, Schneider D, Keefer MC, Clark R, Lai KK, Jacobson JM, Squires K, Bartlett JA, Powderly W. Itraconazole maintenance treatment for histoplasmosis in AIDS: a prospective, multicenter trial. J Acquir Immune Defic Syndr Hum Retrovirol 1997; 16:100–107.

88. McKinsey DS, Wheat LJ, Cloud GA, Pierce M, Black JR, Bamberger DM, Goldman M, Thomas CJ, Gutsch HM, Moskovitz B, Dismukes WE, Kauffman CA. Itraconazole prophylaxis for fungal infections in patients with advanced human immunodeficiency virus infection: randomized, placebo-controlled, double-blind study. National Institute of Allergy and Infectious Diseases Mycoses Study Group. Clin Infect Dis 1999; 28:1049–1056.

89. Chiller TM, Galgiani JN, Stevens DA. Coccidioidomycosis. Infect Dis Clin North Am 2003; 17:41–57, viii.

90. Galgiani JN, Ampel NM, Catanzaro A, Johnson RH, Stevens DA, Williams PL. Practice guideline for the treatment of coccidioidomycosis. Infectious Diseases Society of America. Clin Infect Dis 2000; 30:658–661.

91. Galgiani JN, Catanzaro A, Cloud GA, Johnson RH, Williams PL, Mirels LF, Nassar F, Lutz JE, Stevens DA, Sharkey PK, Singh VR, Larsen RA, Delgado KL, Flanigan C, Rinaldi MG. Comparison of oral fluconazole and itraconazole for progressive, nonmeningeal coccidioidomycosis. A randomized, double-blind trial. Mycoses Study Group. Ann Intern Med 2000; 133:676–686.

92. Clemons KV, Sobel RA, Williams PL, Pappagianis D, Stevens DA. Efficacy of intravenous liposomal amphotericin B (AmBisome) against *Coccidioidal meningitis* in rabbits. Antimicrob Agents Chemother 2002; 46:2420–2426.

93. Jiang C, Magee DM, Cox RA. Coadministration of interleukin 12 expression vector with antigen 2 cDNA enhances induction of protective immunity against *Coccidioides immitis*. Infect Immun 1999; 67:5848–5853.

94. Magee DM, Cox RA. Roles of gamma interferon and interleukin-4 in genetically determined resistance to *Coccidioides immitis*. Infect Immun 1995; 63:3514–3519.

95. Blair JE, Douglas DD, Mulligan DC. Early results of targeted prophylaxis for coccidioidomycosis in patients undergoing orthotopic liver transplantation within an endemic area. Transpl Infect Dis 2003; 5:3–8.

96. Paphitou NI, Ostrosky-Zeichner L, Paetznick VL, Rodriguez JR, Chen E, Rex JH. In vitro antifungal susceptibilities of Trichosporon species. Antimicrob Agents Chemother 2002; 46:1144–1146.

97. Walsh TJ, Melcher GP, Rinaldi MG, Lecciones J, McGough DA, Kelly P, Lee J, Callender D, Rubin M, Pizzo PA. Trichosporon beigelii, an emerging pathogen resistant to amphotericin B. J Clin Microbiol 1990; 28:1616–1622.

98. Walsh TJ, Melcher GP, Lee JW, Pizzo PA. Infections due to *Trichosporon* species: new concepts in mycology, pathogenesis, diagnosis and treatment. Curr Top Med Mycol 1993; 5:79–113.

99. Anaissie E, Gokaslan A, Hachem R, Rubin R, Griffin G, Robinson R, Sobel J, Bodey G. Azole therapy for trichosporonosis: clinical evaluation of eight patients, experimental therapy for murine infection, and review. Clin Infect Dis 1992; 15:781–787.

100. Bodey GP, Anaissie E, Gutterman J, Vadhan-Raj S. Role of granulocyte-macrophage colony-stimulating factor as adjuvant therapy for fungal infection in patients with cancer. Clin Infect Dis 1993; 17:705–707.

101. D'Antonio D, Mazzoni A, Iacone A, Violante B, Capuani MA, Schioppa F, Romano F. Emergence of fluconazole-resistant strains of Blastoschizomyces capitatus causing nosocomial infections in cancer patients. J Clin Microbiol 1996; 34:753–755.

102. Pagano L, Morace G, Ortu-La Barbera E, Sanguinetti M, Leone G. Adjuvant therapy with rhGM-CSF for the treatment of *Blastoschizomyces capitatus* systemic infection in a patient with acute myeloid leukemia. Ann Hematol 1996; 73:33–34.

103. Marcon MJ, Durrell DE, Powell DA, Buesching WJ. In vitro activity of systemic antifungal agents against *Malassezia furfur*. Antimicrob Agents Chemother 1987; 31: 951–953.

104. Gupta AK, Kohli Y, Li A, Faergemann J, Summerbell RC. In vitro susceptibility of the seven *Malassezia* species to ketoconazole, voriconazole, itraconazole and terbinafine. Br J Dermatol 2000; 142:758–765.

105. Powell DA, Marcon MJ. Failure to eradicate *Malassezia furfur* broviac catheter infection with antifungal therapy. Pediatr Infect Dis J 1987; 6:579–580.

106. Barchiesi F, Arzeni D, Fothergill AW, Di Francesco LF, Caselli F, Rinaldi MG, Scalise G. In vitro activities of the new antifungal triazole SCH 56592 against common and emerging yeast pathogens. Antimicrob Agents Chemother 2000; 44:226–229.

107. Kiehn TE, Gorey E, Brown AE, Edwards FF, Armstrong D. Sepsis due to Rhodotorula related to use of indwelling central venous catheters. Clin Infect Dis 1992; 14:841–846.

108. Gonzalez CE, Rinaldi MG, Sugar AM. Zygomycosis. Infect Dis Clin North Am 2002; 16:895–914, vi.

109. Kontoyiannis DP, Wessel VC, Bodey GP, Rolston KV. Zygomycosis in the 1990s in a tertiary-care cancer center. Clin Infect Dis 2000; 30:851–856.

110. Herbrecht R, Letscher-Bru V, Bowden RA, Kusne S, Anaissie EJ, Graybill JR, Noskin GA, Oppenheim, Andres E, Pietrelli LA. Treatment of 21 cases of invasive mucormycosis with amphotericin B colloidal dispersion. Eur J Clin Microbiol Infect Dis 2001; 20:460–466.

111. Walsh TJ, Hiemenz JW, Seibel NL, Perfect JR, Horwith G, Lee L, Silber JL, DiNubile MJ, Reboli A, Bow E, Lister J, Anaissie EJ. Amphotericin B lipid complex for invasive fungal infections: analysis of safety and efficacy in 556 cases. Clin Infect Dis 1998; 26:1383–1396.

112. Sun QN, Najvar LK, Bocanegra R, Loebenberg D, Graybill JR. In vivo activity of posaconazole against Mucor spp. in an immunosuppressed-mouse model. Antimicrob Agents Chemother 2002; 46:2310–2312.

113. Chapman SW, Bradsher RW Jr, Campbell GD Jr, Pappas PG, Kauffman CA. Practice guidelines for the management of patients with blastomycosis. Infectious Diseases Society of America. Clin Infect Dis 2000; 30:679–683.

114. Gil-Lamaignere C, Roilides E, Mosquera J, Maloukou A, Walsh TJ. Antifungal triazoles and polymorphonuclear leukocytes synergize to cause increased hyphal damage to *Scedosporium prolificans* and *Scedosporium apiospermum*. Antimicrob Agents Chemother 2002; 46:2234–2237.

115. Gil-Lamaignere C, Roilides E, Maloukou A, Georgopoulou I, Petrikkos G, Walsh TJ. Amphotericin B lipid complex exerts additive antifungal activity in combination with polymorphonuclear leucocytes against Scedosporium prolificans and Scedosporium apiospermum. J Antimicrob Chemother 2002; 50:1027–1030.

116. Ortoneda M, Capilla J, Pujol I, Pastor FJ, Mayayo E, Fernandez-Ballart J, Guarro J. Liposomal amphotericin B and granulocyte colony-stimulating factor therapy in a murine model of invasive infection by Scedosporium prolificans. J Antimicrob Chemother 2002; 49:525–529.

117. Carrillo AJ, Guarro J. In vitro activities of four novel triazoles against Scedosporium spp. Antimicrob Agents Chemother 2001; 45:2151–2153.

118. Espinel-Ingroff A. In vitro fungicidal activities of voriconazole, itraconazole, and amphotericin B against opportunistic moniliaceous and dematiaceous fungi. J Clin Microbiol 2001; 39:954–958.

119. Espinel-Ingroff A. Comparison of In vitro activities of the new triazole SCH56592 and the echinocandins MK-0991 (L-743,872) and LY303366 against opportunistic filamentous and dimorphic fungi and yeasts. J Clin Microbiol 1998; 36:2950–2956.

120. Johnson EM, Szekely A, Warnock DW. In-vitro activity of voriconazole, itraconazole and amphotericin B against filamentous fungi. J Antimicrob Chemother 1998; 42:741–745.

121. Bosma F, Voss A, van Hamersvelt HW, de Sevaux RG, Biert J, Kullberg BJ, Melchers WG, Verweij PE. Two cases of subcutaneous Scedosporium apiospermum infection treated with voriconazole. Clin Microbiol Infect 2003; 9:750–753.

122. Mellinghoff IK, Winston DJ, Mukwaya G, Schiller GJ. Treatment of *Scedosporium apiospermum* brain abscesses with posaconazole. Clin Infect Dis 2002; 34:1648–1650.

123. Munoz P, Marin M, Tornero P, Martin RP, Rodriguez-Creixems M, Bouza E. Successful outcome of Scedosporium apiospermum disseminated infection treated with voriconazole in a patient receiving corticosteroid therapy. Clin Infect Dis 2000; 31:1499–1501.

124. Nesky MA, McDougal EC, Peacock Jr JE. *Pseudallescheria boydii* brain abscess successfully treated with voriconazole and surgical drainage: case report and literature review of central nervous system pseudallescheriasis. Clin Infect Dis 2000; 31:673–677.

125. Girmenia C, Luzi G, Monaco M, Martino P. Use of voriconazole in treatment of *Scedosporium apiospermum* infection: case report. J Clin Microbiol 1998; 36:1436–1438.

126. Pfaller MA, Marco F, Messer SA, Jones RN. In vitro activity of two echinocandin derivatives, LY303366 and MK-0991 (L-743,792), against clinical isolates of *Aspergillus, Fusarium, Rhizopus*, and other filamentous fungi. Diagn Microbiol Infect Dis 1998; 30: 251–255.

127. Meletiadis J, Mouton JW, Rodriguez-Tudela JL, Meis JF, Verweij PE. In vitro interaction of terbinafine with itraconazole against clinical isolates of *Scedosporium prolificans*. Antimicrob Agents Chemother 2000; 44:470–472.

128. Ellis D. Amphotericin B: spectrum and resistance. J Antimicrob Chemother 2002; 49(suppl 1):7–10.

129. McGinnis MR, Pasarell L, Sutton DA, Fothergill AW, Cooper CR, Jr., Rinaldi MG. In vitro activity of voriconazole against selected fungi. Med Mycol 1998; 36:239–242.

130. Marco F, Pfaller MA, Messer SA, Jones RN. Antifungal activity of a new triazole, voriconazole (UK-109,496), compared with three other antifungal agents tested against clinical isolates of filamentous fungi. Med Mycol 1998; 36:433–436.

131. Lozano-Chiu M, Arikan S, Paetznick VL, Anaissie EJ, Loebenberg D, Rex JH. Treatment of murine fusariosis with SCH 56592. Antimicrob Agents Chemother 1999; 43:589–591.

132. Paphitou NI, Ostrosky-Zeichner L, Paetznick VL, Rodriguez JR, Chen E, Rex JH. In vitro activities of investigational triazoles against Fusarium species: effects of inoculum size and incubation time on broth microdilution susceptibility test results. Antimicrob Agents Chemother 2002; 46:3298–3300.

133. Consigny S, Dhedin N, Datry A, Choquet S, Leblond V, Chosidow O. Successsful voriconazole treatment of disseminated fusarium infection in an immunocompromised patient. Clin Infect Dis 2003; 37:311–313.

134. Sharkey PK, Graybill JR, Rinaldi MG, Stevens DA, Tucker RM, Peterie JD, Hoeprich PD, Greer DL, Frenkel L, Counts GW. Itraconazole treatment of phaeohyphomycosis. J Am Acad Dermatol 1990; 23:577–586.

135. McGinnis MR, Pasarell L. In vitro testing of susceptibilities of filamentous ascomycetes to voriconazole, itraconazole, and amphotericin B, with consideration of phylogenetic implications. J Clin Microbiol 1998; 36:2353–2355.

136. Medina I, Mills J, Leoung G, Hopewell PC, Lee B, Modin G, Benowitz N, Wofsy CB. Oral therapy for *Pneumocystis carinii* pneumonia in the acquired immunodeficiency syndrome. A controlled trial of trimethoprim-sulfamethoxazole versus trimethoprim-dapsone. N Engl J Med 1990; 323(12):776–782.

137. Safrin S, Finkelstein DM, Feinberg J, Frame P, Simpson G, Wu A, Cheung T, Soeiro R, Hojczyk P, Black JR. Comparison of three regimens for treatment of mild to moderate

Pneumocystis carinii pneumonia in patients with AIDS. A double-blind, randomized, trial of oral trimethoprim-sulfamethoxazole, dapsone-trimethoprim, and clindamycin-primaquine. ACTG 108 Study Group. Ann Intern Med 1996; 124(9):792–802.

138. Toma E, Fournier S, Dumont M, Bolduc P, Deschamps H. Clindamycin/primaquine versus trimethoprim-sulfamethoxazole as primary therapy for *Pneumocystis carinii* pneumonia in AIDS: a randomized, double-blind pilot trial. Clin Infect Dis 1993; 17(2):178–184.

139. Hughes W, Leoung G, Kramer F, Bozzette SA, Safrin S, Frame P, Clumeck N, Masur H, Lancaster D, Chan C. Comparison of atovaquone (566C80) with trimethoprim-sulfamethoxazole to treat *Pneumocystis carinii* pneumonia in patients with AIDS. N Engl J Med 1993; 328(21):1521–1527.

140. Dohn MN, Weinberg WG, Torres RA, Follansbee SE, Caldwell PT, Scott JD, Gathe JC, Jr., Haghighat DP, Sampson JH, Spotkov J. Oral atovaquone compared with intravenous pentamidine for *Pneumocystis carinii* pneumonia in patients with AIDS. Atovaquone Study Group. Ann Intern Med 1994; 121(3):174–180.

141. Hughes WT, Feldman S, Chaudhary SC, Ossi MJ, Cox F, Sanyal SK. Comparison of pentamidine isethionate and trimethoprim-sulfamethoxazole in the treatment of *Pneumocystis carinii* pneumonia. J Pediatr 1978; 92(2):285–291.

142. Wharton JM, Coleman DL, Wofsy CB, Luce JM, Blumenfeld W, Hadley WK, Ingram-Drake L, Volberding PA, Hopewell PC. Trimethoprim-sulfamethoxazole or pentamidine for *Pneumocystis carinii* pneumonia in the acquired immunodeficiency syndrome. A prospective randomized trial. Ann Intern Med 1986; 105(1):37–44.

143. Sattler FR, Cowan R, Nielsen DM, Ruskin J. Trimethoprim-sulfamethoxazole compared with pentamidine for treatment of *Pneumocystis carinii* pneumonia in the acquired immunodeficiency syndrome. A prospective, noncrossover study. Ann Intern Med 1988; 109(4):280–287.

144. Klein NC, Duncanson FP, Lenox TH, Forszpaniak C, Sherer CB, Quentzel H, Nunez M, Suarez M, Kawwaff O, Pitta-Alvarez A. Trimethoprim-sulfamethoxazole versus pentamidine for *Pneumocystis carinii* pneumonia in AIDS patients: results of a large prospective randomized treatment trial. AIDS 1992;6(3):301–305.

145. Sattler FR, Frame P, Davis R, Nichols L, Shelton B, Akil B, Baughman R, Hughlett C, Weiss W, Boylen CT. Trimetrexate with leucovorin versus trimethoprim-sulfamethoxazole for moderate to severe episodes of *Pneumocystis carinii* pneumonia in patients with AIDS: a prospective, controlled multicenter investigation of the AIDS Clinical Trials Group Protocol 029/031. J Infect Dis 1994; 170(1):165–172.

146. Warren E, George S, You J, Kazanjian P. Advances in the treatment and prophylaxis of *Pneumocystis carinii* pneumonia. Pharmacotherapy 1997; 17(5):900–916.

147. Deresinski SC. Treatment of *Pneumocystis carinii* pneumonia in adults with AIDS. Semin Respir Infect 1997; 12(2):79–97.

148. Bozzette SA, Morton SC. Reconsidering the use of adjunctive corticosteroids in *Pneumocystis* pneumonia?. J Acquir Immune Defic Syndr Hum Retrovirol 1995; 8(4):345–347.

149. Smego RA, Nagar S, Maloba B, Popara M. A meta-analysis of salvage therapy for *Pneumocystis carinni* pneumonia. Arch Intern Med 2001; 161:1529–1533.

150. Rex JH, Walsh TJ, Nettleman M, Anaissie EJ, Bennett JE, Bow EJ, Carillo-Munoz AJ, Chavanet P, Cloud GA, Denning DW, de Pauw BE, Edwards Jr JE, Hiemenz JW, Kauffman CA, Lopez-Berestein G, Martino P, Sobel JD, Stevens DA, Sylvester R, Tollemar J, Viscoli C, Viviani MA, Wu T. Need for alternative trial designs and evaluation strategies for therapeutic studies of invasive mycoses. Clin Infect Dis 2001; 33:95–106.

151. Powers JH. Counterpoint: alternative trial designs for antifungal drugs—time to talk. Clin Infect Dis 2001; 33:107–109.

152. Bennett JE. Advances in the design of antifungal clinical trials. Report of the John E. Bennett Forum on Deep Mycoses Study Design 25–27 January 2002, New York City. Clin Infect Dis 2003; 36:S111–S127.

153. Estey EH, Thall PF. New designs for phase 2 clinical trials. Blood 2003; 102:442–448.

Index

About the Editors

JOHN R. WINGARD is the Price Eminent Scholar, Professor of Medicine, Professor of Pediatrics, Director of the Blood and Bone Marrow Transplantation Program, and Associate Director of Clinical and Translational Research, University of Florida College of Medicine and Shands Cancer Center, Gainesville, Florida. Dr. Wingard is the author or coauthor of more than 500 articles, books, book chapters, and abstracts. He has been an investigator on numerous infectious disease projects and has lectured nationally and internationally on viral and fungal infections. He is a member of numerous professional societies and is a Fellow of the Infectious Disease Society of America. He is a past president of the American Society for Blood and Marrow Transplantation, serves as Journal Editor for Blood and Marrow Transplant Reviews, and is a manuscript reviewer for numerous prominent journals. He received the B.A. degree from Yale University, New Haven, CT, and the M.D. degree from The Johns Hopkins University School of Medicine, Baltimore, MD.

ELIAS J. ANAISSIE is Professor of Medicine and Director of Clinical Affairs of the Myeloma and Transplantation Research Center, The University of Arkansas for Medical Sciences, Little Rock, Arkansas. Before joining the University of Arkansas, Dr. Anaissie was an Associated Internist and Associate Professor of Medicine in the Section of Infectious Diseases, Department of Medical Specialties, University of Texas System Center, M.D. Anderson Hospital and Tumor Institute, Houston TX. The author or editor of numerous professional publications, he received the M.D. degree from the University of Beirut Medical Center, Lebanon.